Sixth Edition

Manipal Manual of Surgery

As per the latest CBME Guidelines | Competency Based Undergraduate Curriculum for the Indian Medical Graduate

Volume 2

Book Shaped by the Students

Read in Over 20 Countries

The Iconic Textbook now in 2 Volumes

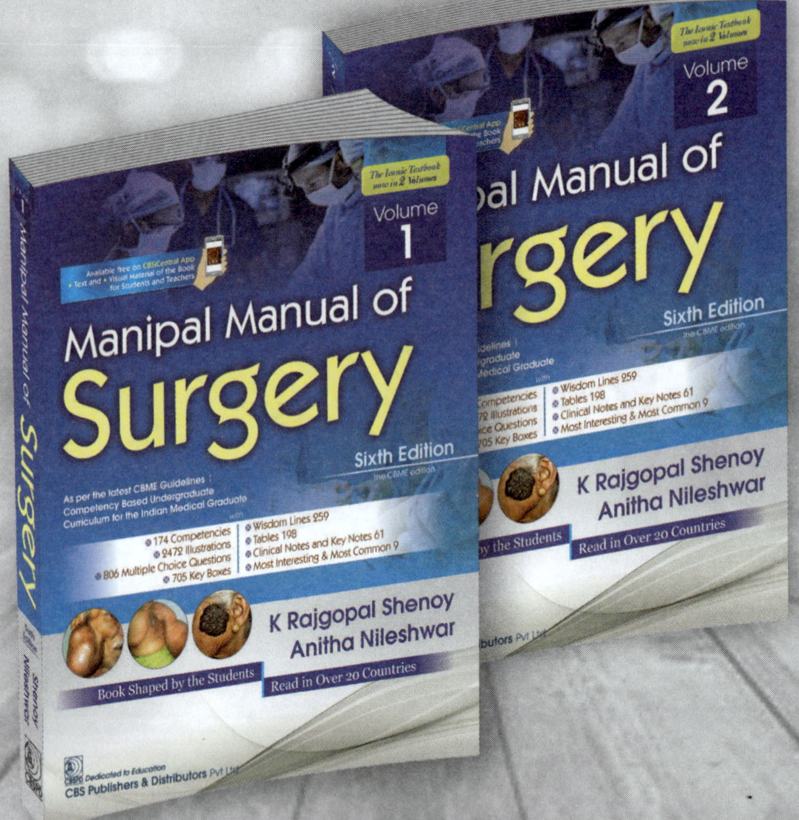

Other CBS Titles by the Same Authors

- *Manipal Manual of Clinical Methods in Surgery*
- *Manipal Manual of Instruments*, Second edition
- *Manipal Manual of Surgery with Clinical Methods for Dental Students*, Fourth edition

Sixth Edition

Manipal Manual of Surgery

As per the latest CBME Guidelines | Competency Based Undergraduate Curriculum for the Indian Medical Graduate

Volume 2

Chief Editor

K Rajgopal Shenoy MBBS, MS, FRCS (Glasgow)
Professor
Department of Surgery
Former Associate Dean-Academics and Head of the Department
Kasturba Medical College, and
Consultant Surgeon, Kasturba Hospital, Manipal 576104
Karnataka, India
Manipal Academy of Higher Education (MAHE)
email: kallyarajgopalshenoy@gmail.com

Coeditor

Anitha Shenoy (Nileshwar) MBBS, MD, FRCA
Professor and Former Head
Department of Anaesthesiology
Kasturba Medical College, and
Consultant Anaesthesiologist, Kasturba Hospital, Manipal 576104
Karnataka, India
Manipal Academy of Higher Education (MAHE)
email: anitharshenoy@gmail.com

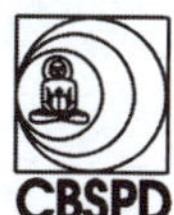

CBS Publishers & Distributors Pvt Ltd

New Delhi • Bengaluru • Chennai • Kochi • Kolkata • Lucknow • Mumbai
Hyderabad • Jharkhand • Nagpur • Patna • Pune • Uttarakhand

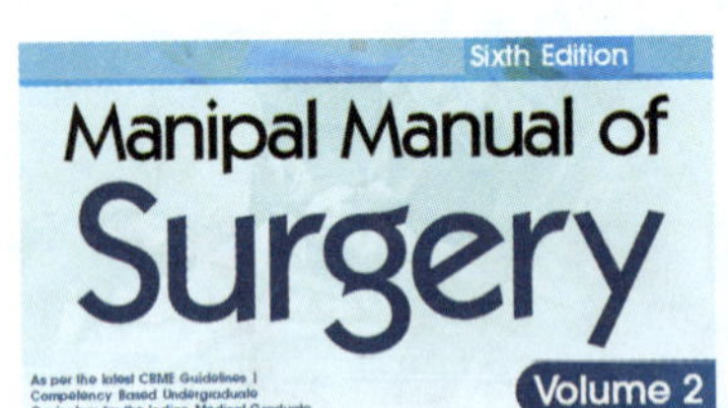

Book Shaped by the Students

Read in Over 20 Countries

ISBN: 978-93-54660-25-2

Sixth Edition: 2023
Reprint: 2024
First Edition: 2000
Reprint: 2001, 2002, 2003, 2004
Second Edition: 2005
Reprint: 2006, 2007, 2008, 2009
Third Edition: 2010
Reprint: 2011, 2012
Fourth Edition: 2014
Reprint: 2016, 2017, 2019
Fifth Edition: 2020

the CBME edition

Published by Satish Kumar Jain and produced by Varun Jain for
CBS Publishers & Distributors Pvt Ltd
4819/XI Prahlad Street, 24 Ansari Road, Daryaganj, New Delhi 110 002, India.
Ph: 011-23289259, 23266838 Website: www.cbspd.com
e-mail: delhi@cbspd.com

Corporate Office: 204 FIE, Industrial Area, Patparganj, Delhi 110 092
Ph: 011-49344934 Fax: 011-49344935 e-mail: publishing@cbspd.com; publicity@cbspd.com

Branches

- **Bengaluru:** Seema House 2975, 17th Cross, K.R. Road, Banasankari 2nd Stage, Bengaluru 560 070, Karnataka, India
  Ph: +91-80-26771678/79 Fax: +91-80-26771680 e-mail: bangalore@cbspd.com
- **Chennai:** 7, Subbaraya Street, Shenoy Nagar, Chennai 600 030, Tamil Nadu, India
  Ph: +91-44-26680620, 26681266 Fax: +91-44-42032115 e-mail: chennai@cbspd.com
- **Kochi:** 42/1325, 1326, Power House Road, Opp KSEB, Ernakulum, Kochi 682 018, Kerala, India
  Ph: +91-484-4059061-65,67 Fax: +91-484-4059065 e-mail: kochi@cbspd.com
- **Kolkata:** 147, Hind Ceramics Compound, 1st Floor, Nilgunj Road, Belghoria, Kolkata-700056, West Bengal, India
  Ph: 033-25633055/56 e-mail: kolkata@cbspd.com
- **Lucknow:** Basement, Khushnuma Complex, 7 Meerabai Marg (Behind Jawahar Bhawan), Lucknow-226001, UP, India
  Ph: +0522-4000032 e-mail: tiwari.lucknow@cbspd.com
- **Mumbai:** PWD Shed, Gala no 25/26, Ramchandra Bhatt Marg, Next to JJ Hospital Gate no. 2, Opp. Union Bank of India, Noorbaug, Mumbai-400009, Maharashtra, India
  Ph: +91-22-66661880/89 e-mail: mumbai@cbspd.com

Representatives

• **Hyderabad**	0-9885175004	• **Jharkhand**	0-9811541605	• **Nagpur**	0-8692091830
• **Patna**	0-9334159340	• **Pune**	0-9664372571	• **Uttarakhand**	0-9716462459

Printed at: Magic International Pvt. Ltd., Greater Noida, UP, India

Contents

VOLUME 2

SECTION III: GASTROINTESTINAL SURGERY

45. Peritoneum, Peritoneal Cavity, Mesentery and Retroperitoneum 719

- The peritoneum 719
- Intra-abdominal sepsis 720
- Abdominal compartment syndrome 730
- Complications of peritonitis 732
- Subphrenic abscess 733
- Special types of peritonitis 736
- Tumours of the peritoneum 741
- Mesentery 743
- Retroperitoneum 744
- Retroperitoneal abscess 745

46. Small Intestine 752

- Abdominal tuberculosis (TB) 755
- Inflammatory bowel diseases 763
- Surgical complications of enteric fever 774
- Small bowel tumours 776
- Neuroendocrine tumours (NET) 779
- Short gut syndrome 781
- Intestinal fistulae 783
- Small intestinal diverticula 786

47. Large Intestine 789

- Surgical anatomy 789
- Colonic function 792
- Tumours of the large intestine 793
- Examination of colon 796
- Carcinoma colon 796
- Surgeries in a case of carcinoma colon 809
- Colon screening 811
- Diverticular disease of colon 811
- Miscellaneous 815

48. Intestinal Obstruction 819

- Differential diagnosis of intestinal obstruction 828
- Caecal volvulus and bascule 830
- Meckel's diverticulum with a band 831
- Meckel's diverticulum 831
- Adhesions and bands 833
- Gallstone ileus—gallstone obturation 836
- Intussusception 837
- Mesenteric vascular occlusion 841
- Strictures 845
- Neonatal intestinal obstruction 846
- Anorectal anomalies 851
- Causes of intestinal obstruction as per age 852
- Paralytic ileus (neurogenic ileus) 852
- Intestinal obstruction—special causes 854
- Malrotation and midgut volvulus 858

49. Rectum and Anal Canal 861

- Surgical anatomy of the rectum 861
- Carcinoma rectum 864
- Colostomy 875
- Prolapse rectum 877
- Surgical anatomy of anal canal 882
- Anorectal physiology 883
- Haemorrhoids (piles) 884
- Stapler haemorrhoidopexy 888
- Anorectal abscess 889
- Fistula *in ano* 890
- Fissure *in ano* 893
- Pilonidal sinus (jeep-bottom) 895
- Sacrococcygeal teratoma 896
- Malignant tumours of anal canal 897
- Stricture of anal canal and rectum 897
- Anal incontinence 898
- Proctalgia fugax 899
- Pruritus ani 899
- Hidradenitis suppurativa 899

50. Lower Gastrointestinal Bleeding 902

- Causes 903
- Clinical examination 904
- Differential diagnosis of lower GI bleeding 905
- Role of colonoscopy/enteroscopy 908
- Massive lower GI bleeding 909

51. Appendix 914

- Development and anomalies 914
- Surgical anatomy of the appendix 915
- Acute appendicitis 916
- Differential diagnosis of acute appendicitis 920
- Post-appendicectomy faecal fistula 927
- Neoplasm of the appendix 928
- Mucocoele of the appendix 928
- Miscellaneous 929
- Post-appendicectomy sepsis (a case report) 929

52. Hernia 932

- Anatomy of the inguinal region 932
- Aetiology of hernia: What causes hernia? 934
- Inguinal defence mechanisms 935
- Classification of hernia 935
- Indirect hernia 935
- Direct hernia 936
- Clinical examination of a case of hernia 937
- Complications of hernia 944
- Recurrent hernia 946
- Special hernias 947
- Femoral hernia 949

- Umbilical hernia 952
- Incisional hernia 955
- Management of massive abdominal wall hernias 959
- Epigastric hernia 960
- Rare external hernias 961

53. Umbilicus and Abdominal Wall 968

- Classification of umbilical diseases 969
- Umbilical inflammation 969
- Umbilical fistulae 969
- Umbilical neoplasms 970
- Umbilical hernia 970
- Abdominal wall 970
- Burst abdomen: Abdominal dehiscence 972
- Divarication of recti 974
- Rectus sheath haematoma 975
- Meleney's progressive postoperative synergistic gangrene 975
- Fibromatoses: Desmoid tumour 975
- Endometriosis of the abdominal wall 976

54. Trauma—Initial Management, Blunt Abdominal Trauma, War and Blast Injuries and Triage 978

- Initial management of trauma victims 978
- Blast injuries 984
- Warfare injuries 984
- Missile wounds of abdomen 985
- Blunt abdominal trauma 987
- Vascular trauma 1001

55. Abdominal Mass 1004

- Clinical examination of abdominal mass (clinics) 1004
- Mass in the right iliac fossa 1012
- Firm to hard nodular mass in the umbilical region 1015
- The cystic mass in the abdomen 1016
- Mass in the epigastrium 1019
- Mass in the right hypochondrium 1020
- Mass in the right lumbar region 1022

SECTION IV: UROLOGY

56. Investigations of the Urinary Tract 1029

- Urine examination 1029
- Blood tests 1030
- X-ray KUB (kidney, ureter, bladder) 1030
- Imaging 1030
- Renal arteriography: Angiography 1033
- Micturating cystourethrography (MCU) 1033
- Computerised tomography (CT) scanning 1035
- Endoscopy 1036

57. Kidney and Ureter 1038

- Surgical anatomy of kidney 1038
- Polycystic kidneys (congenital cystic kidneys) 1039
- Horseshoe kidney 1041
- Renal stones 1042
- Ureteric stone 1046
- Hydronephrosis 1047
- Renal tuberculosis (TB) 1051
- Renal neoplasms 1054
- Wilms' tumour (nephroblastoma) 1054
- Renal cell carcinoma (RCC) 1055
- Renal mass in the surgical ward 1059
- Acute surgical infections of the kidneys 1060

58. Urinary Bladder and Urethra 1063

- Surgical anatomy of the bladder 1063
- Vesical calculus 1064
- Carcinoma of the bladder 1065
- Exstrophy of the bladder (ectopia vesicae) 1068
- Acute cystitis—urinary tract infection (UTI) 1068
- Diverticula of the bladder 1069
- Urinary fistulae 1069
- Interstitial cystitis 1070
- Schistosoma haematobium 1070
- Urinary diversion 1071
- Rupture of the urinary bladder 1071
- Surgical anatomy of the urethra 1072
- Rupture urethra 1072
- Stricture urethra 1075
- Hypospadias 1076
- Differential diagnosis of urinary retention 1077
- Posterior urethral valve (PUV) 1078
- Vesicoureteric reflux (VUR) 1078

59. Prostate and Seminal Vesicles 1081

- Surgical anatomy 1081
- Benign prostatic hyperplasia (BPH) 1082
- Carcinoma of the prostate 1084
- Prostatitis 1088

60. Penis, Testis and Scrotum 1091

- Surgical anatomy of the penis 1091
- Phimosis 1092
- Paraphimosis 1092
- Carcinoma penis 1092
- Peyronie's disease (penile fibromatosis) 1097
- Differential diagnosis of ulcer penis 1097
- Anatomy of the testis and epididymis 1098
- Hydrocoele 1099
- Cystic swellings in the scrotum 1101
- Undescended testis 1102
- Ectopic testis 1103
- Varicocele 1103
- Torsion testis (torsion of the spermatic cord) 1104
- Testicular tumours 1105
- Interstitial cell tumours 1108
- Fournier's gangrene (idiopathic gangrene of the scrotal skin) 1109
- Fracture of the penis 1110
- Male infertility 1111

61. Haematuria and Urinary Tract Infections 1114

- Causes of haematuria 1114
- History and examination 1114
- Investigations 1115
- Haematuria 1117
- Urinary tract infections 1118

SECTION V: SPECIALITIES

62. Chest Trauma, Cardiothoracic Surgery 1125

- Chest trauma 1125
- Blunt trauma to the chest 1126
- Pulmonary injuries 1127
- Injury to trachea and major bronchi 1131
- Injury to the diaphragm 1131
- Injury to the aorta (rupture of the aorta) 1132
- Myocardial contusion 1132
- Surgical emphysema 1132
- Penetrating thoracic wounds 1133
- Mediastinal emphysema 1133
- Empyema 1134
- Bronchopleural fistula 1135
- Surgical anatomy of mediastinum and mediastinal masses 1136
- Anterior mediastinal masses 1136
- Middle mediastinal masses 1138
- Posterior mediastinal masses 1139
- Pulmonary aspergilloma 1139
- Bronchogenic carcinoma 1140
- Congenital heart diseases 1143
- Coronary artery bypass surgery 1146
- Off pump coronary artery bypass surgery 1148
- Abdominal aortic aneurysms (AAA) 1148
- Ruptured abdominal aortic aneurysm 1150

63. Neurosurgery 1152

- Pathophysiology and mechanism of head injuries 1152
- Intracranial haematoma 1154
- Chronic subdural haematoma 1157
- Raised intracranial pressure 1157
- Fracture skull 1157
- CSF rhinorrhoea 1158
- Pott's puffy tumour 1158
- Hydrocephalus 1158
- Tumours 1160
- Trigeminal neuralgia 1162
- Brainstem death 1162

64. Principles of Anaesthesiology 1165

- Types of anaesthesia 1165
- Preoperative assessment and premedication 1166
- Airway management 1169
- Monitoring in anaesthesia 1173
- Local anaesthetics 1174
- Spinal and epidural anaesthesia 1176
- Other regional techniques 1180
- Complications of anaesthesia 1181
- General anaesthetic agents 1183
- Intravenous anaesthetic agents 1185
- Physiology of neuromuscular junction 1187
- Muscle relaxants 1187

65. Organ Transplantation 1191

- Principles of transplantation 1191
- Liver transplantation 1192
- Renal transplantation 1194
- Small bowel transplant 1196
- Islet cell transplantation 1198
- Medicolegal aspects of organ donation 1201

66. Principles of Clinical Radiation Oncology and Chemotherapy 1203

- Radiation 1203
- Radiotherapy—sources and methods of delivery 1204
- Source of radiation 1205
- Oncology: Concise concepts of chemotherapy 1212

SECTION VI: *VIVA VOCE* EXAMINATION

67. Principles of Radiology, Imaging, *Viva Voce* Examination 1223

- Plain X-rays 1223
- Barium studies 1226
- Angiography 1232
- Ultrasonography 1234
- Computed tomography (CT) 1235
- Virtual colonoscopy 1236
- Cholangiogram/ERCP/MRCP 1237
- Magnetic resonance imaging (MRI) 1238
- Positron emission tomography (PET scan) 1241
- Interventional radiology 1242

68. Instruments 1245

- Suture materials 1257

69. Specimens 1259

70. Operative Surgery, Laparoscopic Surgery and Accessories 1268

- History of surgery 1268
- Skin closure techniques 1269
- Excision of swellings 1270
- Surgery for hydrocoele 1272
- Incision and drainage (I and D) 1273
- Incision and drainage of breast abscess 1274
- Circumcision 1275
- Venesection or cut down 1276
- Vasectomy 1277
- Tracheostomy 1278
- Thyroidectomy 1279
- Amputations 1281
- Amputations in leg 1282
- Upper limb amputations 1285
- Abdominal incisions 1285
- Appendicectomy 1286
- Bassini's herniorrhaphy 1288
- Open cholecystectomy 1293
- Vagotomy gastrojejunostomy (GJ) 1294
- Intestinal resection and anstomosis 1295
- Colectomy 1298
- Staplers in surgery 1300
- Laparoscopic surgery 1301
- Hernia repair: TAPP (transabdominal preperitoneal mesh repair) 1305
- SILS (LESS) 1306
- Natural orifice transluminal endoscopic surgery (NOTES) 1307
- VAAFT technique 1307
- Robotic surgery 1308
- Energy sources in surgery 1309
- Harmonic scalpel 1309
- Lasers in surgery 1310
- Miscellaneous 1310

Index ***1311***

Volume 2

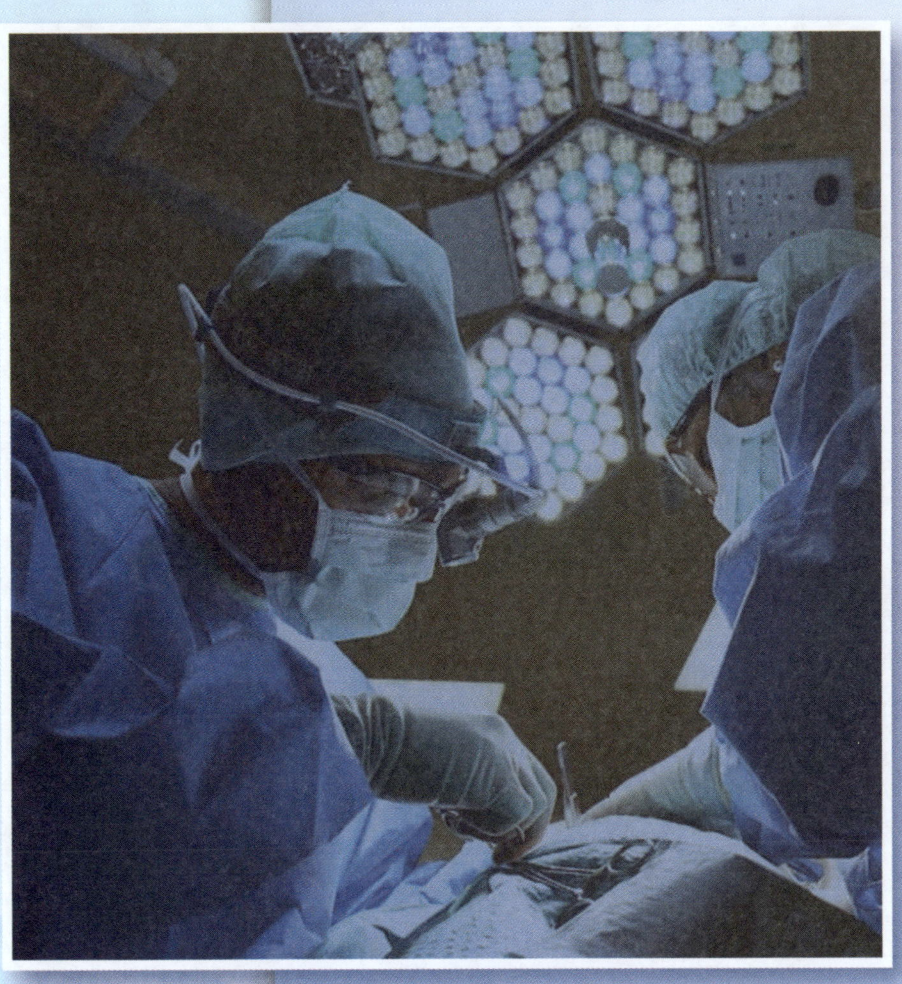

Gastrointestinal Surgery *(Continued)*

Urology

Specialities

***Viva Voce* Examination**

CHAPTER

45

Peritoneum, Peritoneal Cavity, Mesentery and Retroperitoneum

- Peritoneum
- Intra-abdominal sepsis
- Acute peritonitis–Scoring system
- Abdominal compartment syndrome
- Complications of peritonitis
  - Pelvic abscess
  - Subphrenic abscess
- Special types of peritonitis
- Tumours of the peritoneum
  - Pseudomyxoma peritonei
  - Carcinoma peritonei
- HIPEC
- Mesentery
  - Misty mesentery
  - Mesenteric cyst
- Retroperitoneum
- Retroperitoneal cyst, abscess, retroperitoneal tumour

Competency

SU28.3.1: Describe applied anatomy and physiology of peritoneum.

Introduction

Peritoneal cavity is the largest cavity in the body accommodating various viscera. It is divided into ***greater*** and ***lesser sac*** (omental bursa) which communicate through the ***foramen of Winslow*** or epiploic foramen. The peritoneum lining inner side of the parietes is called ***parietal peritoneum***. It is ***very sensitive*** and is innervated by both somatic and visceral afferent nerves. This explains the ***sharp, localised, cutting*** pain of peritonitis. Diaphragm and central part of the peritoneum is supplied by phrenic nerve (C4) and partly by intercostal nerves. Rest of the peritoneum is supplied by intercostal nerves and lumbar nerves.

Lesser omentum: It is also called hepatoduodenal ligament. It extends from the duodenum to the liver. This has two layers and within these layers are the common bile duct, hepatic artery and hepatic portal vein.

THE PERITONEUM

Lining of Peritoneum

The peritoneum is lined by simple squamous epithelium of mesodermal origin called mesothelium with surface area 1.0 to 1.7 m^2 and a thin layer of fibroelastic tissue. It is parietal peritoneum. A large peritoneal defect heals within a few hours because of these mesenchymal cells (flattened polyhedral cells—mesothelium). Applying this principle, some surgeons do not close the peritoneal layer after laparotomy. When parietal peritoneum is reflected into viscera, it is called visceral peritoneum.

It covers viscera and is supplied by autonomic nervous system. Hence, it is not sensitive. Thus, gastrojejunostomy can be done under local anaesthesia but distension and traction to the bowel causes pain. During herniorrhaphy under spinal anaesthesia, handling of bowel or traction on the bowel can produce uncomfortable upper abdominal pain.

- *In men, peritoneal cavity is completely sealed, hence cannot get infected.*
- *In women, it is communicated to exterior through fallopian tubes, hence infection can occur.*

Fluid

Peritoneal surface is a semipermeable membrane with an area comparable to that of cutaneous body surface. Nearly 1 m^2 of the total 1.7 m^2 area participates in fluid exchange with extracellular fluid space at the rate of 500 ml or more per hour.

It normally contains less than 50 ml fluid. When it is insulted by infection, a large amount of fluid can collect

Key Box 45.1

Normal Peritoneal Fluid—Transudate

- Specific gravity below 1016
- Protein concentration less than 3 g/dl
- White blood cell count less than 3000 cells/l
- Complement mediated bacterial activity
- Lack of fibrinogen related clot formation

in this space giving rise to severe fluid and electrolyte imbalance. This is described as ***III space loss***, e.g. ***peritonitis, pancreatitis***. Peritoneal fluid helps in smooth gliding of intestines. Absorption of fluid and secretion of fluid are some important functions of peritoneum (Key Box 45.1).

Absorption and Exudation

This takes place through capillaries and lymphatics present in between the two layers of peritoneum. This principle is applied in **dialysis**. The direction of circulation is towards subdiaphragmatic lymphatics.

Protective Function

It secretes prostaglandins, interferons and free radicals which help in some protection against peritonitis.

Circulation of peritoneal fluid and its surgical importance:

- Stomata are nothing but intercellular pores over the peritoneum covering inferior surface of the diaphragm. They communicate with lymphatic pools in the diaphragm.
- During expiration, diaphragm relaxes, pores open and peritioneal fluid is drawn into stomata.
- During inspiration, diaphragm contracts, the fluid particle enter into lymphatic pools in the diaphragm and through mediastinal lymphatics propelled into thoracic duct.
- Movement of the fluid is in the cephaloid direction.
- Thus in cases of severe intraperitoneal sepsis, it is no wonder that sepsis can spread so rapidly.

Fitz-Hugh-Curtis Syndrome

- It is exclusively seen in women/adolescent girls secondary to pelvic inflammatory disease.
- Caused by gonococci and chlamydial infections.
- Severe perihepatitis, irritation of diaphragm, peritonitis are features.
- Tetracycline, doxycyclines, metronidazole are a few drugs.

INTRA-ABDOMINAL SEPSIS

Introduction

Intra-abdominal sepsis is one of the most challenging situations in surgery occurs due to peritonitis. The mortality ranges from 4 to 40% in Britain. It depends upon several factors which include severity of infection, experience of the surgeon, patient's condition, comorbidity and bacterial load. They require intensive care unit with strict monitoring. An attempt has been made here to discuss common causes of sepsis and peritonitis and its management.

Types of Intra-Abdominal Sepsis

- **Complicated:** Infection process proceeds beyond the organ into peritoneum causing localised or generalised peritonitis, e.g. perforated duodenal ulcer.
- **Uncomplicated:** Infection involves only one organ and does not spread into peritoneum, e.g. appendicitis in early cases.
- **Infectious:** Primary, secondary and tertiary peritonitis.
- **Sterile.**

Competency

SU28.3.2: Describe the causes, clinical features, investigations, management and complications of localised and generalised peritonitis.

ACUTE PERITONITIS

Definition

Inflammation of the peritoneum is called peritonitis.

I. *Primary Peritonitis*

- Spontaneous peritonitis of childhood
- Spontaneous peritonitis of adults
- Tuberculous peritonitis
- Peritonitis associated with dialysis

II. *Secondary Peritonitis*

This term refers to peritonitis from an intra-abdominal source and is the most common form of peritonitis. The following are the causes for secondary peritonitis (Fig. 45.1):

1. **Perforation of a hollow viscus**
   - Perforated duodenal ulcer, gastric ulcer
   - Perforated enteric ulcer, tubercular ulcer
   - Perforated Meckel's diverticulum
   - Perforated colonic ulcer
   - Ruptured appendicitis
2. **Direct spread: Post-inflammatory**
   - Acute cholecystitis—gangrenous

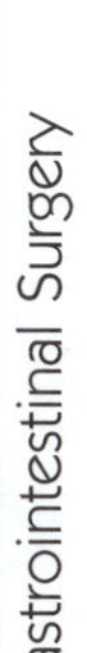

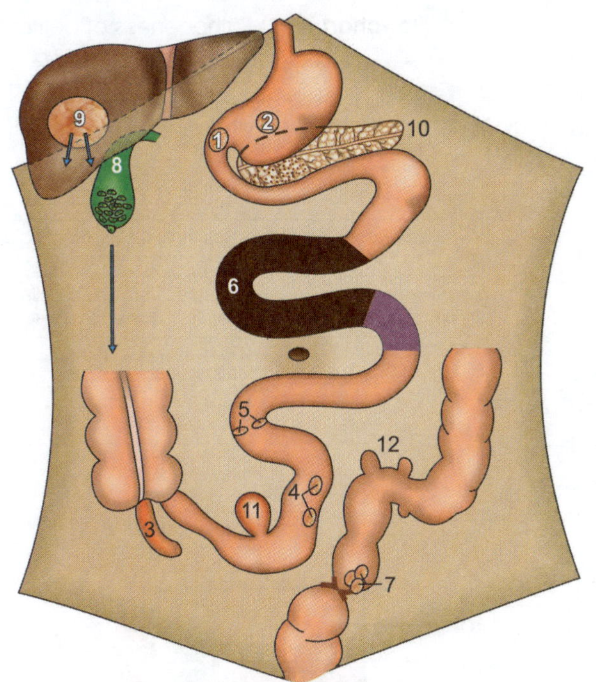

Common causes of perforation
1. Perforated duodenal ulcer
2. Perforated gastric ulcer
3. Perforated appendicitis
4. Perforated enteric ulcers
5. Perforated tubercular ulcers
6. Gangrene intestine
7. Perforated carcinoma left colon

Uncommon causes of peritonitis
8. Ruptured amoebic liver abscess
9. Perforated gall bladder
10. Necrotising pancreatitis
11. Perforated Meckel's diverticulum
12. Sigmoid diverticular perforation

Fig. 45.1: Common causes of generalised peritonitis

- Acute appendicitis
- Gangrene of the intestine
- Acute necrotising pancreatitis

3. **Penetrating injuries to the abdomen,** where the organisms gain entry from outside.
4. **Postoperative peritonitis** is due to the introduction of infection during surgery which might be due to:
   - Postoperative leaks
   - Foreign body (mop) in the abdomen
5. **Parturition peritonitis:** It refers to peritonitis after pregnancy and delivery.
6. **Blunt injuries to the abdomen:** Fluid which is spilled into the peritoneal cavity (example: Blood and bile) can travel along paracolic gutter and manifest as pain in the right iliac fossa, causing guarding and rigidity. This has been called **Valentino syndrome** (*see* later on page 723).

Classification of Peritonitis

- **Primary peritonitis:** Diffuse bacterial infection caused by single organism without loss of integrity of the GI tract.
- **Secondary peritonitis:** Loss of integrity of the GI tract, multiple organism.
- **Tertiary peritonitis:** It occurs due to recurrent infection after 48 hours—after adequate control of secondary peritonitis. A prolonged systemic inflammation is responsible leading to a higher chance of systemic inflammatory response syndrome, sepsis, severe sepsis, or septic shock. Mortality ranges between 30 and 60%.

Pathophysiology

- **Sepsis and septic shock:** Life-threatening organ dysfunction caused by dysregulated host response to infection requiring vasopressor to maintain mean arterial pressure of 65 mmHg or greater and serum lactate greater than 2 mmol/L in the absence of hypovlaemia is described as septic shock.
- Once sepsis or SIRS sets in, it results in loss of large quantity of fluids resulting in hypoperfusion. At the same time, aerobes and anaerobes act synergistically and release inflammatory mediators including toxins. Also translocation of bacteria can occur even after control of sepsis due to more oxygen delivery after control of disease. Plasma lactate or negative base excess occur resulting in acidosis. Net result is development of shock and multiorgan failure.

Scoring Systems

Many scoring systems are available. A few important ones are given below. They can predict survival or outcome. They are as follows.

A. **The Manheim Peritonitis Index (MPI) score:** It is a reliable scoring system depending upon several factors as given below.

   Presence of organ failure, time more than 24 hours, presence of malignancy, origin of sepsis, faecal peritonitis, generalised peritonitis.

B. **SOFA score:** Sequential Organ Failure Asssessment Score. The score is based on six different scores, one each for respiratory, cardiovascular, hepatic, coagulation, renal and neurological systems. Factors taken into consideration are: PaO_2/FiO_2 (mmHg), Glasgow Coma Scale, mean arterial pressure or administration of vasopressors required, bilirubin (mg/dl) [μmol/L], platelets × 10^3/μl, creatinine (mg/dl) [μmol/L] (or urine output).

C. **APACHE II score (Acute Physiology Age Chronic Health Evaluation–Knaus et al., 1985):**
- $AaDO_2$ (alveoloarterial oxygen partial pressure difference) or PaO_2 (depending on FiO_2)
- Temperature (rectal)
- Mean arterial pressure
- pH arterial
- Heart rate
- Respiratory rate
- Sodium (serum)
- Potassium (serum)
- Creatinine
- Hematocrit
- White blood cell count
- Glasgow Coma Scale

- These were measured during the first 24 hours after admission.
- The score is not recalculated during the stay; it is by definition an admission score.

Pathogenesis (Fig. 45.2 and Flowchart 45.1)

Due to any one of the reasons mentioned above, infection sets in and the causative organisms multiply in the peritoneal cavity.

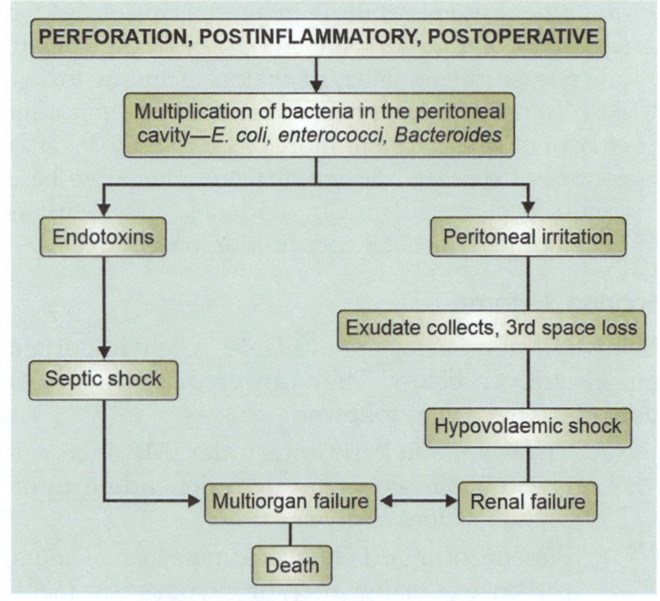

Fig. 45.2: Pathophysiology of peritonitis

Flowchart 45.1: Pathogenesis of peritonitis

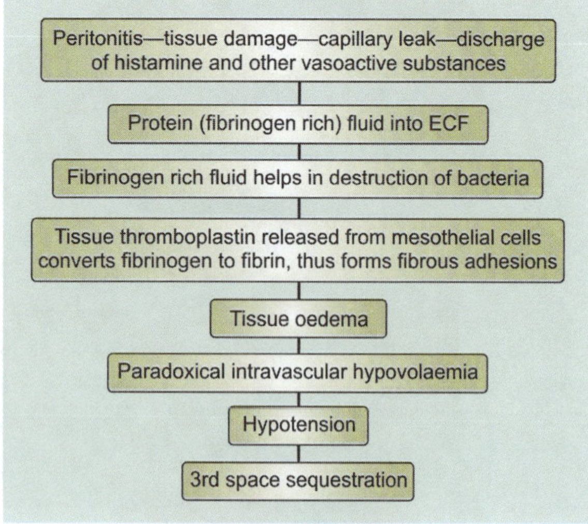

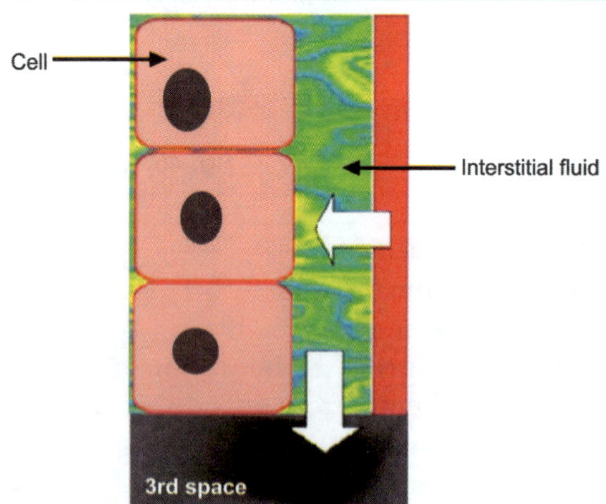

Fluid sequestration

- **Gram-negative organisms:** *Escherichia coli (E. coli), Proteus, Klebsiella*. They are present in the small and large bowel. They are the commonest organisms producing peritonitis (Key Box 45.2).
- **Enterococci:** *Streptococcus faecalis* needs bile to grow. It is present in the urinary tract, genital tract and also in the intestines. However, both aerobic and anaerobic streptococci are the second most common organisms

Key Box 45.2

Organ-specific Organisms

- **Gastric perforations:** Sterile with minimum gram-positive organisms.
- Ileal perforation, appendicitis—aerobic bacteria in 30% patients, anaerobic in 10% patients. Predominant aerobic bacteria include gram-negative *E.coli*, streptococci, *Proteus* and *Klebsiella*.
- **Colonic-rectum:** Faecal spillage produces a load of 10^{12} or more—gram-negative and anaerobic bacteria per gram of stools.

producing peritonitis. They are the chief organisms in puerperal sepsis.

- **Bacteroides:** They are anaerobic organisms, present mainly in the lower intestine.
- **Bacteria from outside alimentary canal:** Gonococci, pneumococci, tubercular organisms, etc.
- These organisms proliferate in the peritoneal cavity resulting in peritonitis. A large amount of fluid gets secreted into the peritoneal cavity resulting in 3rd space loss which leads to severe **hypovolaemic shock.** This fluid is rich in proteins, bacteria and toxins. Due to powerful endotoxins released by gram-negative bacteria, endotoxic shock or septic shock (*refer* to shock), ensues.
- The fluid is rich in fibrinogen which forms fibrin and helps in localisation of infection (Fig. 45.3).
- Peritoneum loses its shiny surface, becomes reddish and oedematous and is covered with thick fibrinous exudate.
- **Omentum:** It is a fatty apron with rich blood supply. A mobile double-layered peritoneal fold acts like a policeman to seal the area of infection or perforation. *Examples:* Perforated duodenal ulcer, acute appendicitis, acute diverticulitis, etc. Probably it also serves to supply collateral blood supply to the ischaemic viscera. In addition, it has immunological functions such as supply of phagocytes which destroy unopsonised bacteria.

Types of Peritonitis

A. **Local peritonitis:** If a perforation is small and if it is sealed off immediately by omentum, it will give rise to local peritonitis. *Examples:* Small gastric ulcer perforation, diverticular perforation, gallbladder perforation. Anatomical factors also play a role in local peritonitis. *Examples*: Retrocaecal appendicitis with perforation. It is behind the caecum and in retroperitoneum. Signs are confined to right iliac fossa only. In posterior gastric perforations or acute pancreatitis, signs are limited to upper abdomen. Pelvic peritonitis is another example—occur following septic abortions or salpingo-oophoritis.

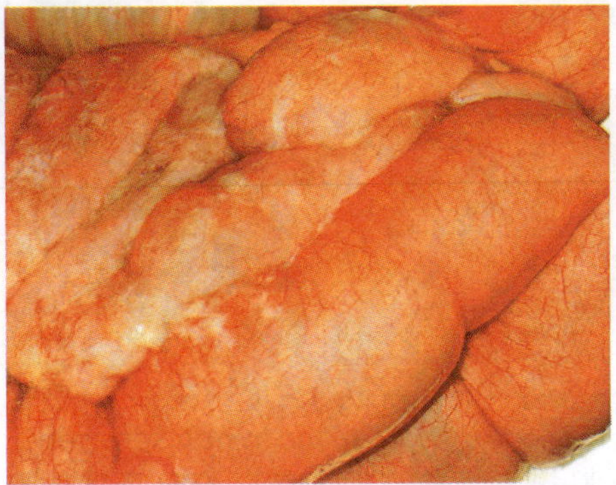

Fig. 45.3: Fibrin plaques: Early cases of peritonitis with fibrin plaques all over the peritoneal cavity

B. **Generalised peritonitis:** If the contents of the viscus leak into the peritoneal cavity with force, as it occurs in intestinal perforation or due to perforation of a free lying organ—example: Meckel's diverticular perforation. Virulence of bacteria is more as in colonic perforations with generalised peritonitis. Duodenal ulcer perforation can manifest as severe pain in the right iliac fossa mimicking appendicitis. **Many have been mistakenly operated for appendicitis because the right paracolic gutter is board and contents travel down into right iliac fossa.** This has been referred to as **Valentino syndrome** (Key Box 45.3). Before the days of ultrasound, it used to be not uncommon to do appendectomy in a patient who had acute pancreatitis. Inflammatory exudate gravitating along right paracolic gutter resulted in pain in right iliac fossa.

Factors Deciding the Severity of Peritonitis

- **Clean perforation:** Upper GI-gastric juice remains sterile for 6–8 hours. Hence, in early stages, there will be mild chemical peritonitis and early treatment gives good results.
- **Distal gut perforation and infected bile peritonitis:** Very dangerous and severe, causing sepsis and septic shock early.
- Postoperative peritonitis that usually occurs due to anastomotic leak is also dangerous.
- A perforation sealed off early by omentum causes mild peritonitis. Retrocaecal appendicitis produces minimal local peritonitis.
- On the other hand, perforated Meckel's diverticulitis produces diffuse peritonitis soon (Key Box 45.4).
- A few causes of peritonitis are shown in Figs 45.4 to 45.14.

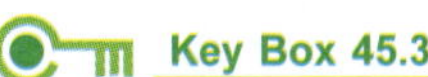

Key Box 45.3

Valentino Syndrome—Valentino Appendix

- **Rudolph Valentino** was an Italian actor who lived in early 20th century.
- On August 15, 1926, he was admitted with the diagnosis of appendicitis and gastric ulcers, with peritonitis.
- He underwent appendicectomy.
- Continued to have peritonitis.
- He developed pleural effusion and sepsis.
- Dies after a few days of surgery.
- In retrospect what he had was duodenal ulcer perforation.
- It is also called **Valentino syndrome** because in any inflammation of the upper abdominal viscera, contents can travel down the right paracolic gutter into the right iliac fossa resulting in pain and tenderness mimicking acute appendicitis.

CAUSES OF PERITONITIS

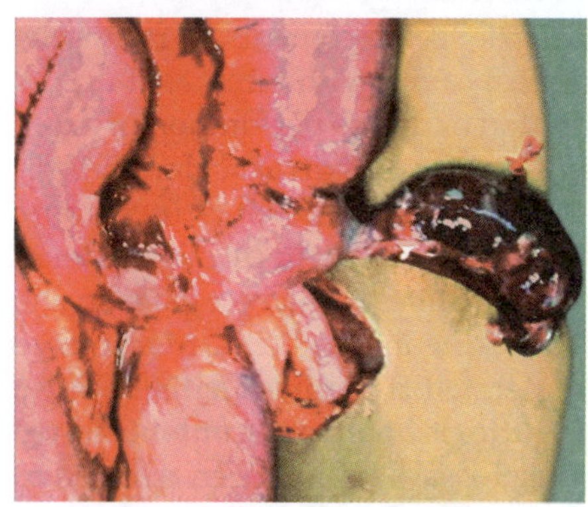

Fig. 45.4: Meckel's diverticulitis

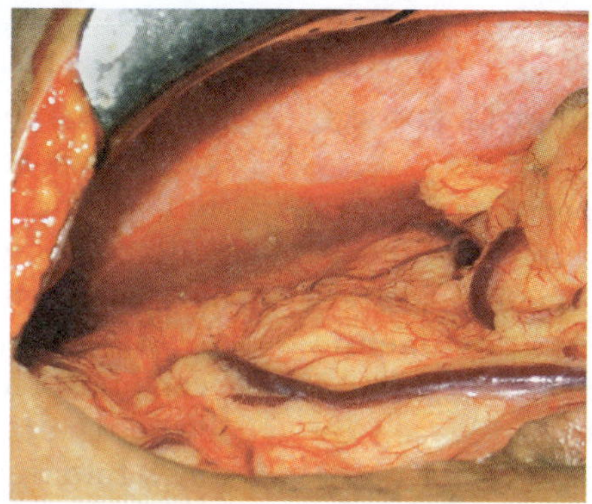

Fig. 45.5: Peritonitis due to ileal perforation consequent to tuberculosis. Usually it is an ulcerative variety

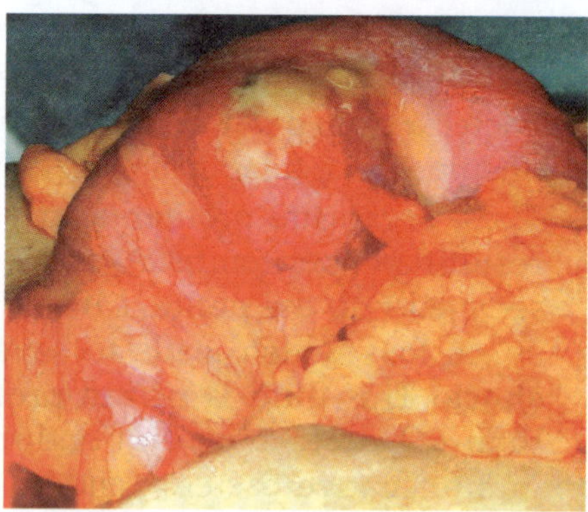

Fig. 45.6: Transverse colon injury due to steering wheel—simple closure in early cases without much peritonitis. Otherwise resection/closure with or without diversion ileostomy may be required

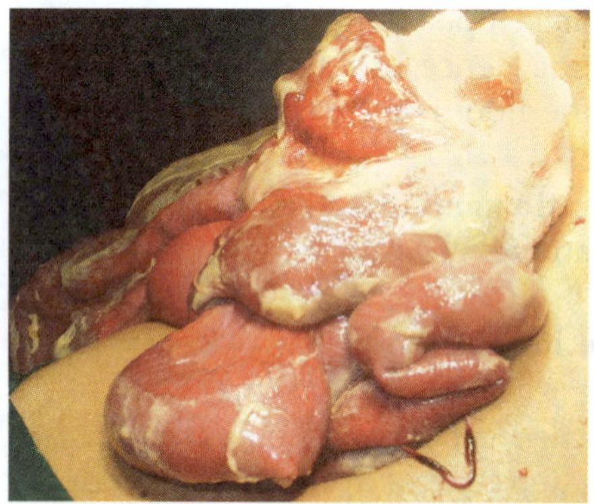

Fig. 45.7: Enteric perforation which is 4 days old—very friable edges. Re-leak after suturing is common

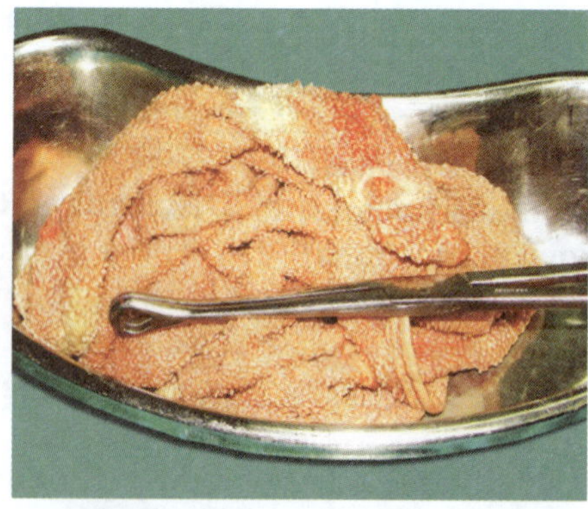

Fig. 45.8: Postoperative peritonitis due to a mop left behind following caesarean section. Always count the mops and instruments before closure of the abdomen. It is a good practice

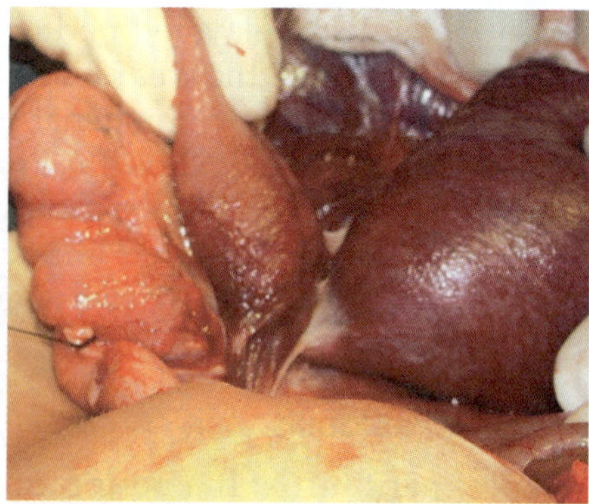

Fig. 45.9: Fibrous band causing gangrene of the terminal ileal loop resulting in peritonitis. The patient had pelvic peritonitis due to tuberculous salpingitis. That resulted in bands

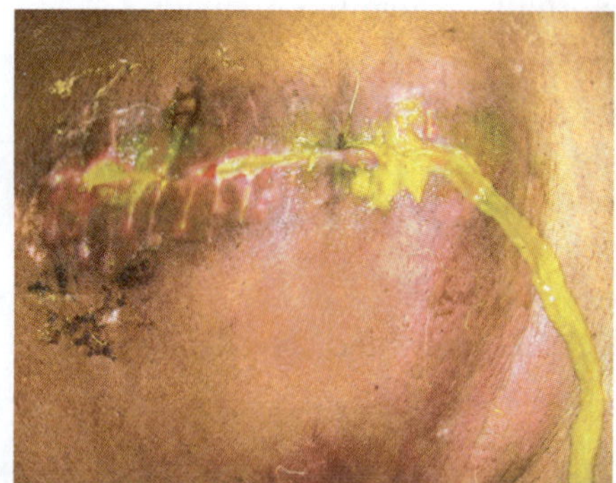

Fig. 45.10: Faecal peritonitis and faecal fistula due to anastomotic leak following right hemicolectomy. Ischaemia and tension at the suture line are the two common causes for the leak

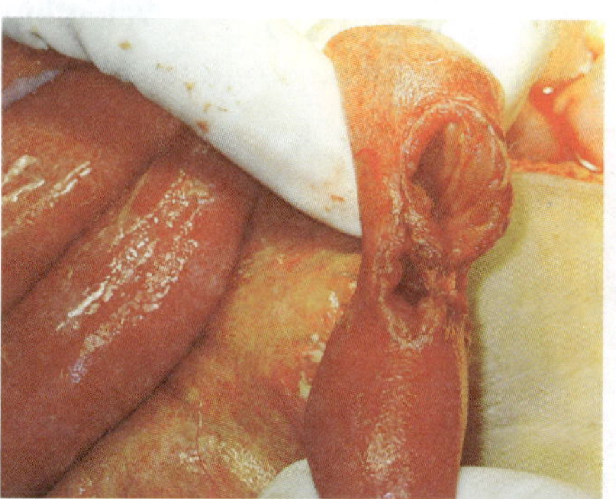

Fig. 45.11: Proximal jejunal transection following blunt abdominal trauma. It is one of the common sites affected in blunt abdominal trauma

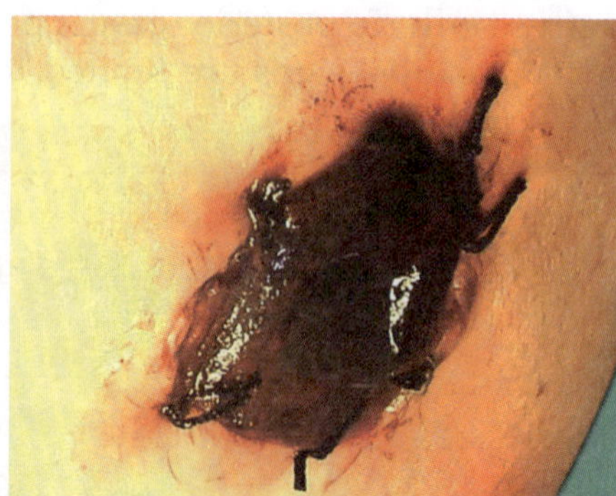

Fig. 45.12: Colostomy gangrene—the intra-abdominal segment was also gangrenous. It is important to always check for the vascularity of the colostomy site before closing abdominal incision

CAUSES OF PERITONITIS

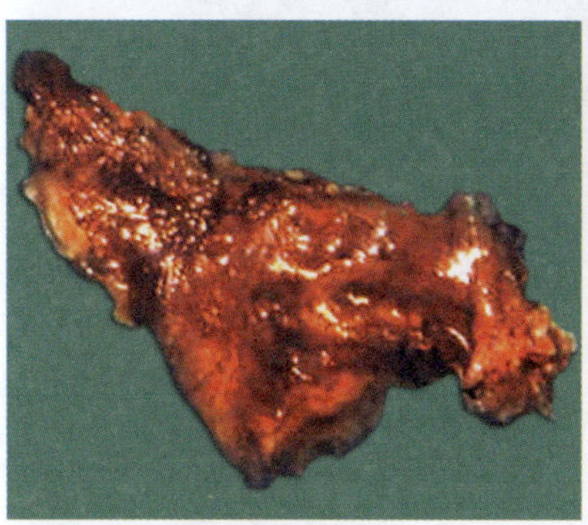

Fig. 45.13: Necrosectomy specimen—acute pancreatitis

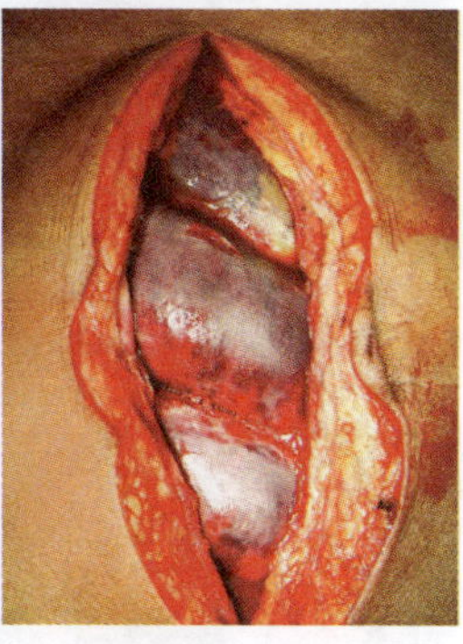

Fig. 45.14: Mesenteric ischaemia giving rise to gangrene

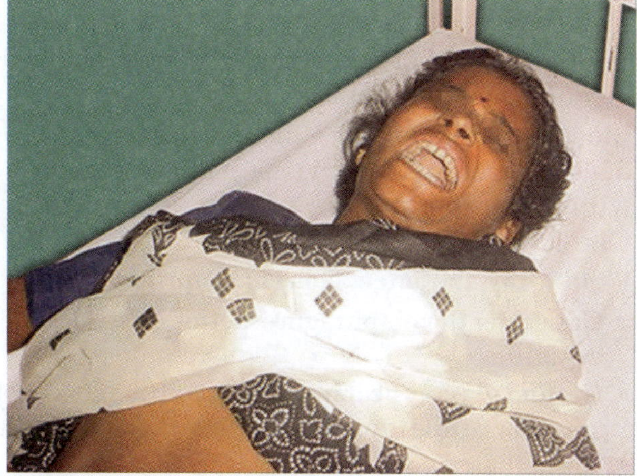

Fig. 45.15: Rebound tenderness is the diagnostic sign of peritonitis

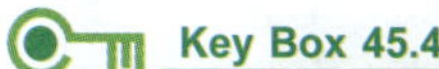

Key Box 45.4

Factors Affecting Diffuse Peritonitis

- Speed of peritoneal contamination, e.g. perforation of Meckel's diverticulum
- Stimulation by purgatives
- Virulence of organisms
- Perforation in a closed loop obstruction
- Immunocompromised status
- Young children. Omentum is thin and small

Clinical Features

It depends upon whether it is localised peritonitis or generalised. In cases of retrocaecal appendicitis, the abdominal signs may be minimal but guarding and rigidity of the back muscles is characteristic. Features of generalised peritonitis are as follows:

- **Severe abdominal pain** which is cutting in nature, becomes worse on movement of the abdominal wall. Hence, the patient lies still on the bed.
- **Persistent vomiting** is due to irritation of parietal peritoneum.
- **The pulse rate is increased.** An increase in the pulse rate may be an early indication of peritonitis, in cases of gangrene of the bowel or peritonitis following perforation of bowel.
- **High-grade fever with chills and rigors** indicates a septicaemic process.
- **Cough tenderness** indicates parietal peritoneal inflammation. Abdominal tenderness is elicited in all quadrants of the abdomen **(Dunphy's sign)**.
- **Rebound tenderness (Blumberg's sign):** Abdomen is pressed for a few seconds. The patient experiences pain. Sudden release of pressure causes severe pain. It is due to sudden movement of the sensitive parietal peritoneum (Fig. 45.15).

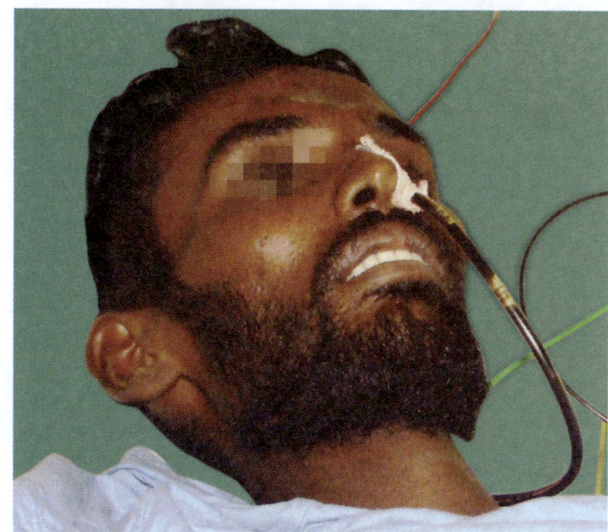

Fig. 45.16: Hippocratic facies: Sunken eyes, drawn in cheeks, dehydrated, blood in the Ryle's tube

- **Guarding** and **rigidity** of abdominal wall.
- Bowel sounds are absent. Distension of the abdomen occurs within a few hours due to accumulation of fluid and paralytic ileus.
- **End-stage disease:** Hippocratic facies (Key Box 45.5 and Fig. 45.16).

Key Box 45.5

Hippocratic Facies

- Hollow, bright eyes
- Pale and pinched face
- Cold perspiration in the head and brows
- Blue lips
- Dry, cracked tongue

Investigations

1. **Complete blood picture** shows **high total count** with predominant neutrophil count.
2. **Blood** examination for **sugar** is done to rule out diabetes mellitus. Empyema gallbladder with or without perforation can present as septic shock. Often, they are diabetic.
3. **Plain X-ray abdomen, chest and upright**
   - **Gas under the diaphragm**—perforation (Figs 45.17 to 45.19).
   - **Ground glass appearance**—a smooth homogeneous appearance due to accumulation of fluid (Fig. 45.20).
   - Air in the bowel wall—gangrene (Fig. 45.21).
   - Obliteration of psoas shadow and preperitoneal fat planes.

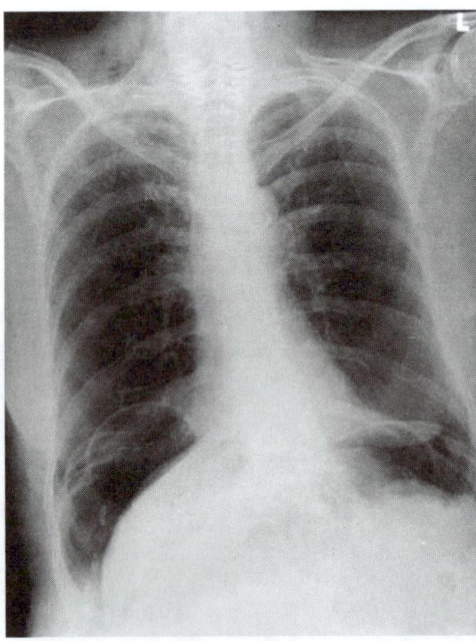

Fig. 45.17: Chest X-ray showing free gas under diaphragm

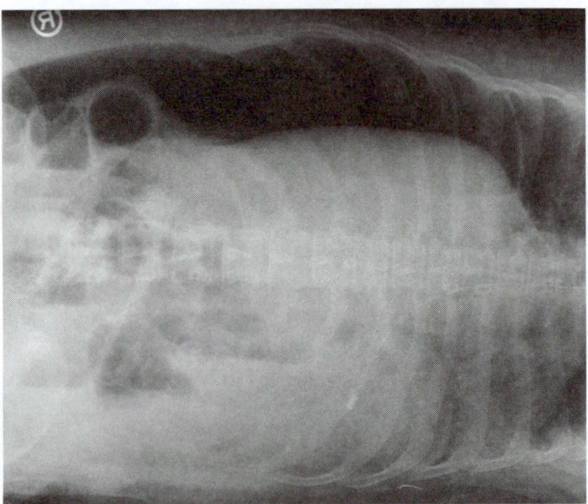

Fig. 45.18: Lateral decubitus X-ray showing free gas in the peritoneal cavity. (This position of the patient is used when patient is in shock or no able to stand)

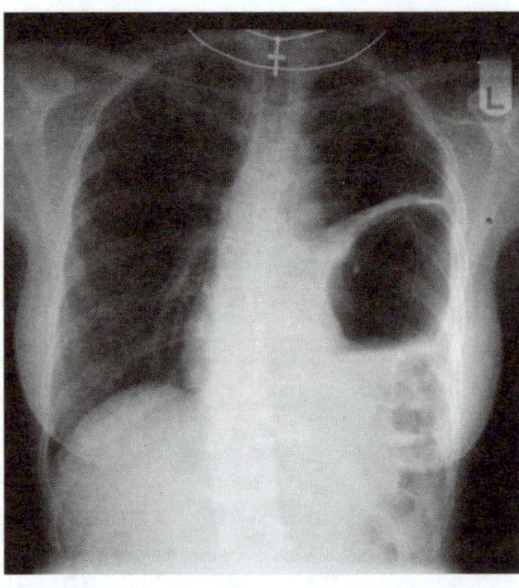

Fig. 45.19: Diaphragm is elevated—fundic air bubble is in the chest—traumatic diaphragmatic hernia

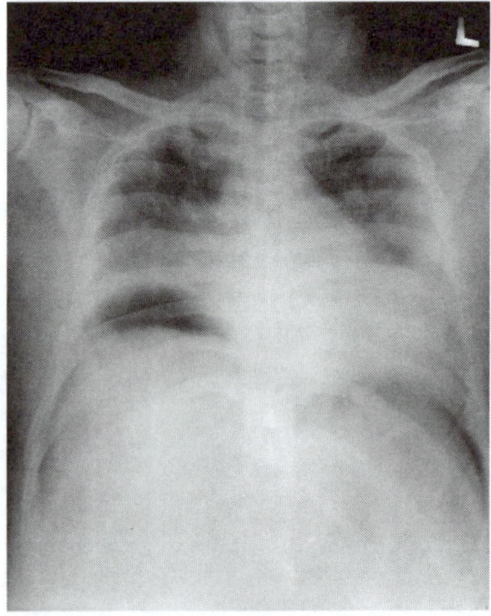

Fig. 45.20: Subphrenic abscess—mild pleural effusion on both sides

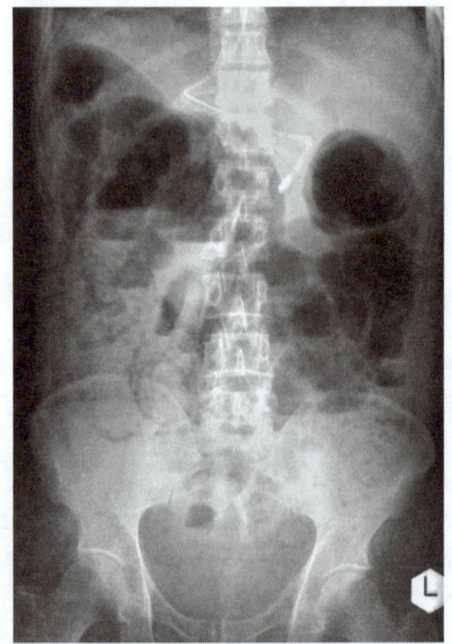

Fig. 45.21: Gas in the bowel wall (pneumatosis) indicates gangrene of the bowel

4. **Abdominal USG** to detect **fluid in the abdomen**.

   Following are different fluids which may give clue to the diagnosis:
   - Frank pus—peritonitis of more than 48 hours old
   - Bile—green coloured—duodenum, stomach, gallbladder perforation
   - Faeculent—dark green coloured thick aspirate with faecal odour—ileal perforations, postoperative anastomotic leaks
   - Serous—exudative—early acute pancreatitis, tuberculous peritonitis
   - Haemorrhagic—haemorrhagic pancreatitis
   - Food particles—hollow viscus perforation

   Thus ultrasound has so many advantages even though it may not point at the specific site. However, probe tenderness with fluid in the right iliac fossa may suggest acute appendicular perforation. It may not be possible to aspirate very thick contents such as anchovy sauce pus from ruptured amoebic liver abscess but ultrasound will provide clue about the liver abscess.

5. **Contrast-enhanced CT scan**
   - When the signs and symptoms are equivocal, CT is the ideal investigation.
   - CT can diagnose hollow viscus perforation, especially when there is no gas under the diaphragm.
   - CT can detect ischaemic changes due to gangrene of the bowel-gas in the bowel wall-pneumatosis (Figs 45.22 and 45.23).
   - CECT has higher sensitivity and specificity but it has radiation exposer of almost 200 chest X-rays.
   - CT can diagnose unsuspected and unexpected lesions in the abdomen including diverticular perforations, internal herniation and gangrene, acute pancreatitis, etc.
   - Adequate hydration and normal renal function (as indicated by normal creatinine values) are important before a contrast-enhanced CT scan.

6. **Abdominal tap**
   - Aspiration of blood indicates haemoperitoneum or gangrene of the bowel.
   - Aspiration of bile indicates biliary peritonitis due to perforation of duodenal ulcer, gallbladder or intestine.
   - **Aspiration of frank pus** indicates peritonitis due to gram-negative bacteria. Foul-smelling pus is due to anaerobic bacteria producing free fatty acids and their esters. Always send the fluid for culture sensitivity (Fig. 45.24).
   - Amylase estimation should be done to rule out pancreatitis.

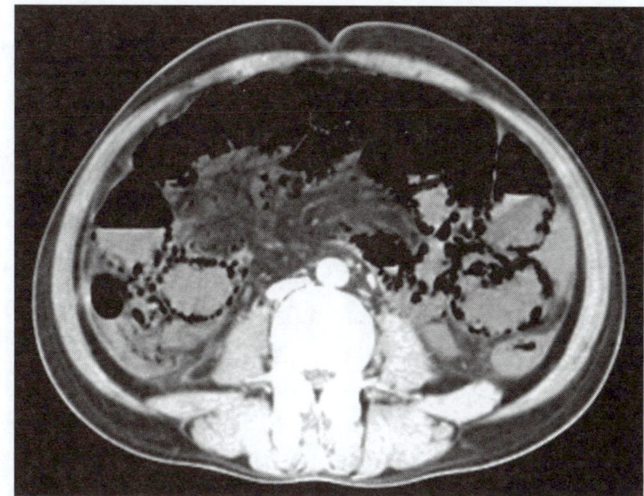

Fig. 45.22: CT showing air in the bowel wall—case of superior mesenteric ischaemia

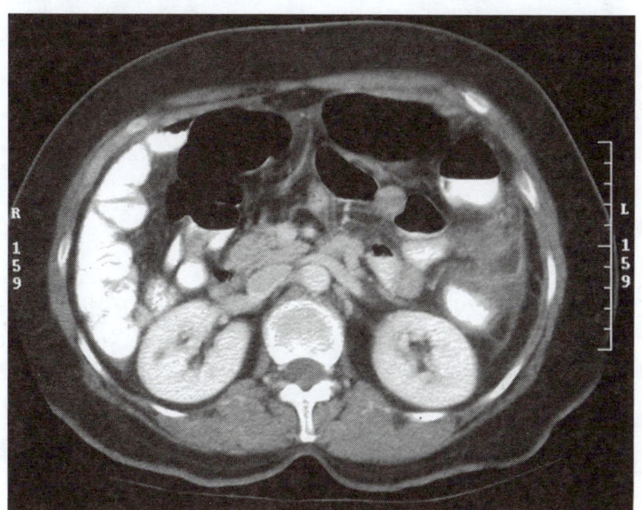

Fig. 45.23: CT showing hypodense lesion in the left iliac fossa—a case of sigmoid diverticular perforation

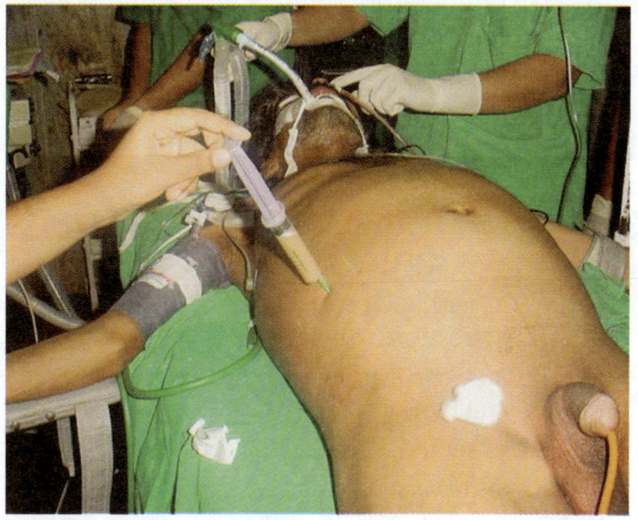

Fig. 45.24: Diagnostic tap showing pus following rupture of empyema of gallbladder

7. **MRI:** It is costly, may not be available all the time. Indicated in pregnant patients with abdominal pain and ultrasound is inconclusive.
8. **Diagnostic laparoscopy** can be used in suspected cases of peritonitis (Key Box 45.6).

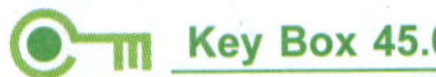 Key Box 45.6

Diagnostic Laparoscopy

- It can be used to reconfirm peritonitis.
- It can diagnose pancreatitis (laparotomy may be avoided).
- It can also treat primary cause, e.g. laparoscopic closure of duodenal ulcer perforation.
- Peritoneal toilet can be given.
- It can rule out other causes.
- In blunt injury, **it can detect diaphragmatic injury**—herniation of bowel, etc.

Pearls of Wisdom

When in doubt, do laparoscopy: It can reveal 'hidden' pathology.

Treatment

1. **Aspiration:** Nasogastric aspiration with Ryle's tube helps in decreasing gastrointestinal secretion. Thus it reduces abdominal distension. It also prevents vomiting and gives rest to the gut. Indirectly, it reduces 'bacterial load' contaminating peritoneum.
2. **Bowel care and blood:** Purgatives should not be given as it may result in perforation. Blood is arranged for surgery.
3. **Charts:** Temperature, pulse rate, respiratory rate, intake-output charts are maintained.
4. **Drugs** are given against gram-positive, gram-negative and anaerobic organisms (Key Boxes 45.7 and 45.8).

Key Box 45.7

Selection of Antibiotics

- 2nd or 3rd generation cephalosporins should be started as early as possible.
- Once culture and sensitivity reports are available (after surgery), antibiotics can be changed.
- Antibiotics should also cover aerobes and anaerobes.
- Should not have serious toxicity, especially amikacin which has nephrotoxicity. Hence, use them carefully (check creatinine).

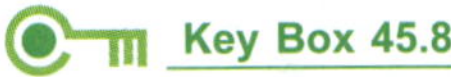 Key Box 45.8

Early Aggressive Resuscitation

- **Restore** intravascular volume. **Crystalloids:** Ringer lactate or isotonic saline stay in the intravascular space for a short period, larger volumes required.
  Colloids: Longer duration of action, smaller volumes are sufficient and can be used in cardiac patients. Not the choice.
- **Restore** oxygenation by face mask or mechanical ventilation, as necessary.
- **Restore** perfusion: Dopamine/dobutamine/noradrenaline.
- **Restore** normality by 'war' against sepsis—**ANTIBIOTICS** and surgical removal of **SEPSIS**.

5. **Exploratory laparotomy** and appropriate surgery is done followed by thorough peritoneal toilet/wash with normal saline.
6. **Fluids:** IV fluids are given before, during and after surgery. Central venous cannulation and measurement of central venous pressure (CVP) is indicated in unstable patients to guide fluid therapy. If not possible, an ***emergency cut down*** (venesection)—cephalic or basilic vein, is done followed by fluid infusion. Preoperatively, the aim is to maintain at least 30 ml/hr of urine output.
   - Ringer lactate solution is an ideal replacement.

PRINCIPLES OF SURGERY FOR PERITONITIS

Exploratory laparotomy
- Generous incision
- Extendable

Exudative secretions drained out
- Drain the fluids, send for culture and sensitivity
- Thorough peritoneal wash

Explore the diseased region
- Gently by separating loops and in between loops

Establish the diagnosis
- Identify site of perforation, gangrene, etc.

Eradicate cause of sepsis
- Resection anastomosis
- Suturing, appendicectomy, etc.

You explore the abdomen; Establish the diagnosis; Eradicate the cause and Eliminate the exudate

Principles of Surgery for Peritonitis
(Key Box 45.9, Figs 45.25 to 45.29)

1. Adequate **incision** is used—upper/mid/lower midline.

Key Box 45.9

Principles of Surgery

- Incision
- Establish the diagnosis
- Exploration
- Pus culture and sensitivity
- Treat the cause—control of sepsis
- Peritoneal toilet
- Drain
- Closure

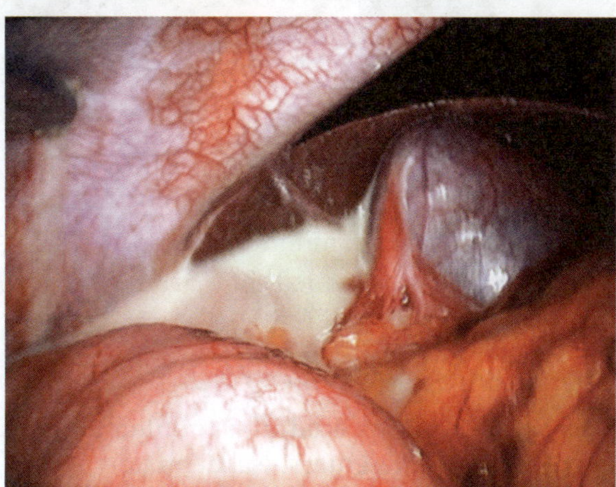

Fig. 45.25: Laparoscopy showing pus

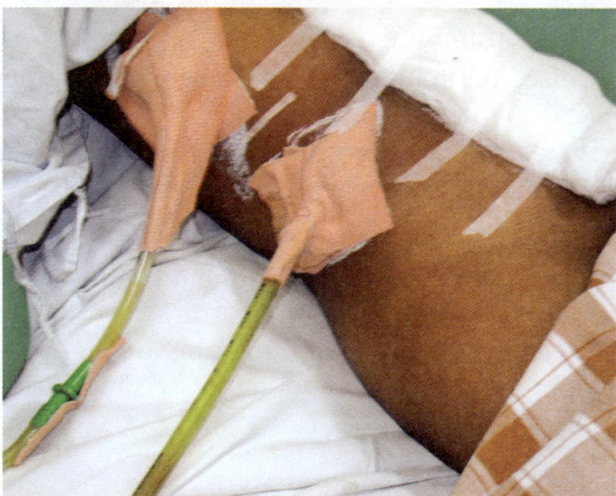

Fig. 45.26: A late case of duodenal ulcer perforation who presented with peritonitis with sympathetic pleural effusion. Laparotomy, closure of perforation and feeding jejunostomy were done. Drains in the subhepatic space and right pleural cavity were placed. Patient had stormy postoperative period with biliary fistula, which was closed after 6 weeks

2. As soon as the peritoneal cavity is opened, purulent fluid comes out. The fluid is collected and sent for **culture** and **sensitivity**. Greenish fluid indicates a hollow viscus perforation. All the fluid is drained,

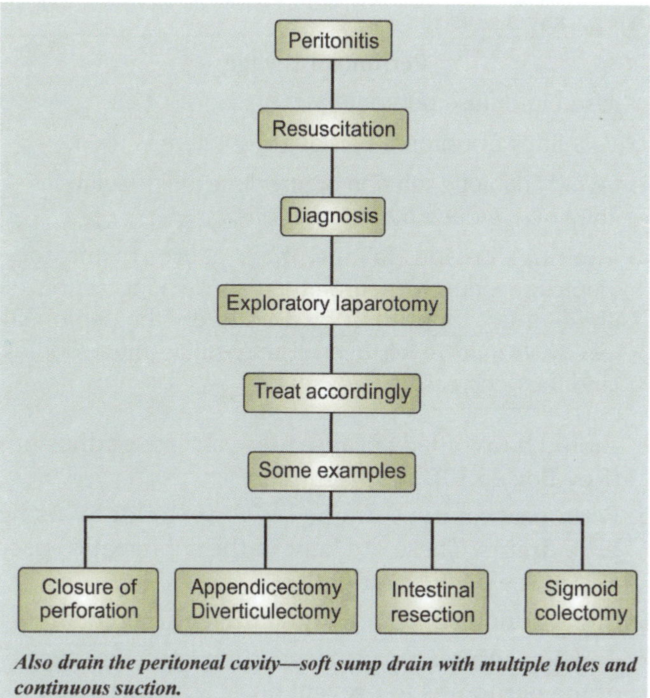

Fig. 45.27: Principles of management of peritonitis—identifying the source of sepsis and elimination is the key to success

the source of peritonitis is identified and appropriate surgical procedure is done. **Examples are:**

- Appendicectomy for appendicitis.
- Closure of perforation for perforated peptic ulcer.
- Closure or resection for ileal perforation.
- Resection of the bowel for gangrene.

Control of sepsis: This is the most important step of treatment of peritonitis. Removal of septic focus is a primary aim—examples: Appendicectomy, perforation closures (duodenal ulcer) or resection (intestinal or colonic perforation) or cholecystostomy in difficult perforated gallbladder diseases. However, all the septic foci in the abdomen have to be removed—necrotic material, pus pockets and food particles. Thorough irrigation with warm saline cleans up subhepatic spaces, pelvic spaces and interloop collections. Primary anastomosis in presence of sepsis may result in leak and postoperative peritonitis. It is better to do colostomy or ileostomy in such cases. Incision can be partially closed leaving the skin open—sutures can be tied after 2 days in the ward.

3. It is better to use **nonabsorbable suture** material such as silk for intestinal anastomosis or for closure of perforation. In the presence of infection, absorbable sutures, such as catgut, get absorbed very fast.
4. A thorough **peritoneal wash/lavage** is given by using warm saline (up to 3–5 litres) to avoid intraperitoneal abscesses. Antiseptic agent such as betadine solution

Key Box 45.10

Peritoneal Lavage

- Used in diffuse peritonitis.
- 3–5 litres of isotonic crystalloid solution is used.
- Avoid antibiotic solution or povidone iodine solutions—they may induce more adhesions.
- Aminoglycoside lavage may cause respiratory depression due to neuromuscular blocking action of these drugs. Mops must be used to dry the peritoneal cavity. If fluid is left over, it may dilute the opsonins and thus decrease phagocytosis.

should be avoided because they can cause adhesions (Key Box 45.10).

5. Peritoneal cavity is drained to the exterior by using **tube drains**. These are kept in the subhepatic space and in the pelvic cavity.
6. The wound is irrigated with **antiseptic agents**.
7. **Tension sutures** are put depending upon the severity of the peritonitis to prevent burst abdomen.
8. **Laparostomy (*vide infra*):** This method of exposing the peritoneal cavity can be done in selected cases, if abdominal compartment syndrome is suspected.

Nutrition in sepsis

- Sepsis is a catabolic event.
- Cytokines and TNF, insulin resistance play a role.
- Glucose is an essential part of nutrition and should amount to at least 500 kcal per day.
- Glucose gets converted to carbon dioxide and when in excess, can increase respiratory load.
- To reduce this, 50% daily energy requirements can be provided using lipids.
- Proteins should also be provided, bearing in mind, the increased protein catabolism in sepsis.

Laparostomy

This refers to leaving peritoneal cavity exposed to outside without approximation of the anterior abdominal wall. Some situations arise, especially in emergency cases, where this is required. Hence, it is important to know how to deal with this situation (Figs 45.28 and 45.29).

Types

1. **Open laparostomy:** Abdominal fascia and peritoneum are not sutured.

   Advantages: Abdominal compartment syndrome can be prevented. Details are given later.

   Disadvantages: Significant fluid loss and secondary infection.

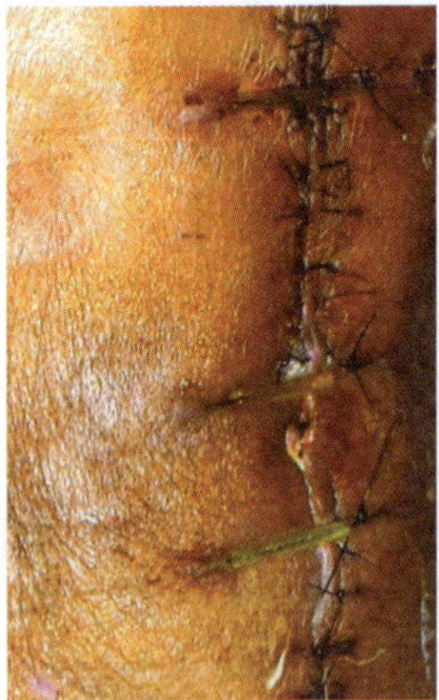

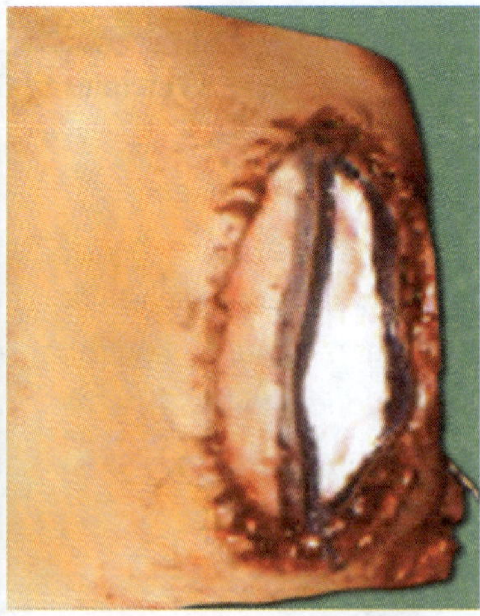

Fig. 45.28: Tension sutures **Fig. 45.29:** Zip closure of peritoneum

2. **Closed laparostomy or mesh laparostomy:** Here the fascial layer is closed by using marlex mesh or prolene mesh or even a zip to protect exposed viscera.

   Advantages: One can minimise infection.

   Disadvantages: Abdominal compartment syndrome and perforation of bowel can occur.

Indications of Laparostomy

When a second look procedure is contemplated, e.g. acute pancreatitis, mesenteric ischaemia.

Nonoperative Treatment of Peritonitis

1. Too sick a patient to tolerate the surgical procedure.
2. Sealed perforation
3. Localised peritonitis—may resolve with treatment.

ABDOMINAL COMPARTMENT SYNDROME

Introduction

The phrase "abdominal compartment syndrome" was coined in 1984 when Irving Kron, described the measurement of intra-abdominal pressure as a means of developing criteria for abdominal decompression to improve organ function.

Definition

- Abdominal compartment syndrome (ACS) is defined as a sustained increase in IAP more than 20 mmHg with or without an abdominal perfusion pressure (APP) < 60 mmHg)] that is associated with new organ dysfunction/failure (Fig. 45.30).
- Intra-abdominal pressure (IAP) is the pressure concealed within the abdominal cavity. Normal IAP is 0–5 mmHg showing phasic variation with respiration.
- Intra-abdominal pressure is measured to detect abdominal compartment syndrome and to decide on

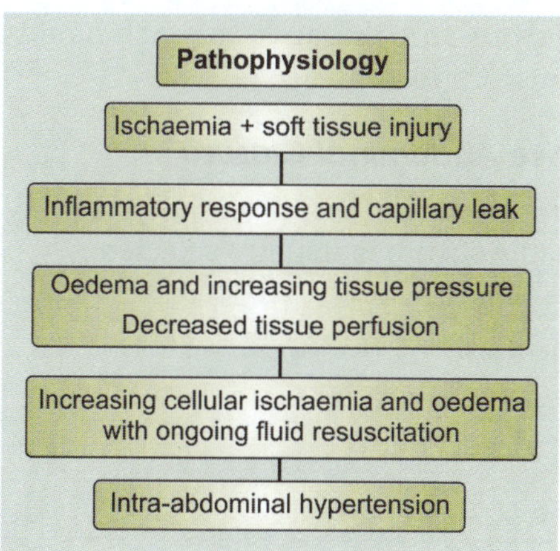

Fig. 45.30: Pathophysiology of abdominal compartment syndrome

the requirement of a decompression so as to improve organ function.

Final Effects

The adverse physiological effects of intra-abdominal hypertension (IAH) affect almost every organ system resulting in ACS. The major systems affected, in decreasing frequency of incidence and morbidity are: Pulmonary, cardiovascular, renal, splanchnic, central nervous system. Thus, the end result can be:

- Intractable hypoxia, hypercarbia, ARDS
- Cardiac insufficiency and cardiac arrest
- Oliguria, anuria, acute renal failure
- Cerebral oedema and anoxia

Grading of IAP (Burch)

Grade I	:	IAP 12–15 mmHg
Grade II	:	IAP 16–20 mmHg
Grade III	:	IAP 21–25 mmHg
Grade IV	:	IAP >25 mmHg

Risk Factors

A. Diminished abdominal wall compliance

- Acute respiratory failure with elevated intrathoracic pressure.
- Abdominal surgery with primary fascial or tight closure. Example: Reduction of massive hernia (Figs 45.31 and 45.32).
- Major trauma/burns
- Prone positioning, head of bed >30°
- High BMI, central obesity

B. Increased intraluminal contents

- Gastroparesis
- Acute gastric dilatation
- Ileus
- Colonic pseudo-obstruction

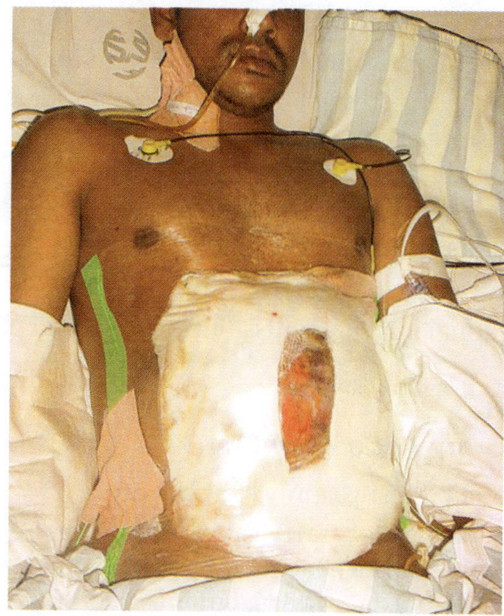

Fig. 45.31: This boy had abdominal compartment syndrome after reduction of intestinal contents from left thoracic cavity (a case of left diaphragmatic hernia) and we could not close the abdomen. It was covered with a thin plastic sheet—you can see the intestine. It took two months for granulation tissue to cover the defect. Eventually, he recovered with an incisional hernia. Bogota bag or VAC are the other alternative methods of closure

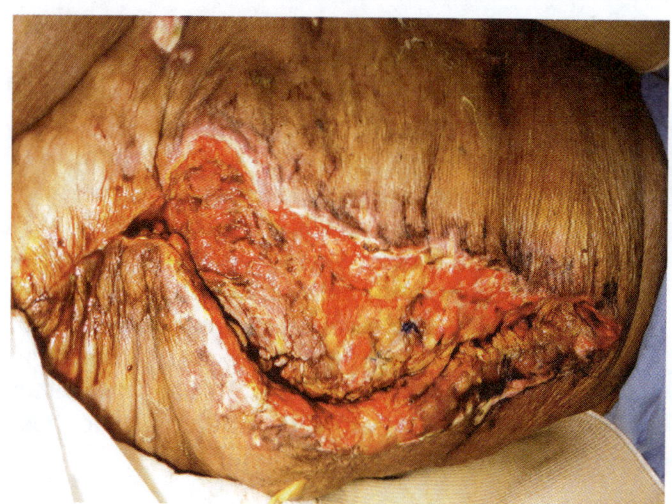

Fig. 45.32: Loss of abdominal layers following reduction of a massive ventral hernia

C. Increased abdominal contents

- Haemoperitoneum/pneumoperitoneum
- Ascites/liver dysfunction
- Laparoscopy

IAP Measurement—Principles

- Expressed in mmHg (1 mmHg = 1.36 cm H_2O).
- Measured at end expiration
- Performed in supine position
- Zeroed at mid-axillary line at the level of iliac crest.

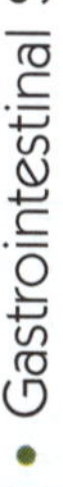

- Performed with an instillation volume of no greater than 25 ml of saline (for bladder technique).
- Measured 30–60 sec after to allow bladder detrusor muscle relaxation (for bladder technique).

Medical Treatment

- Close monitoring of patient's vitals
- Blood transfusion when required
- Nutritional supplements—intravenous/TPN

Surgery

I. *Temporary Abdominal Closure*

- Towel clip closure, only skin closure.
- Mesh—commercially available meshes with absorbable surface facing intraperitoneum and non-absorbable surface facing outer aspect of the wound are used. Example: Mesh with polygalactin (vicryl) inside and polopropylene (prolene) outside can be used.
- **PTFE mesh repair:** Expanded polytetrafluoro-ethylene (ePTFE) is another mesh which is used. It is a surgical biomaterial with two antimicrobial preservative agents—chlorhexidine diacetate and silver carbonate. It also enhances tissue ingrowth.
- **Bogota bag: A Bogota bag** is a sterile plastic bag used for closure of abdominal wounds.[1] It is generally a sterilised, 3-litre genitourinary irrigation bag that is sutured to the skin or fascia of the anterior abdominal wall. The Bogota bag acts as a hermetic barrier that avoids evisceration and loss of fluids. Another advantage to the Bogota bag is that the abdominal contents can be visually inspected which is particularly useful in cases of ischaemic bowel. Thus, it is useful in resections following mesenteric ischaemia. In our country, we can use urosac bag (which can be split open) or even a thin plastic sheet can be used like a Bogota bag (Fig. 45.31).

Clinical Notes

A young boy of 18 years, who suddenly had breathlessness was found to have diaphragmatic hernia. After reduction and closure, patient developed ACS. Reopening of abdomen was done and peritoneum was not closed but a 'cover' was given by using 'urosac' bag which was split open. Wound was allowed to heal by granulation tissue.

- **Vacuum-assisted closure (VAC):** It has been extensively used in the management of leg ulcers specially diabetic ulcers. It has been used in a few cases of severe pancreatitis. Here it is called open abdomen negative pressure therapy system. It removes debris, inflammatory exudates.

II. *Definitive Abdominal Closure*

- Primary closure. It is done layer by layer. Non-absorbable suture is usually selected.
- Synthetic mesh
- Biologic mesh
- Component separation
- Plastic surgery

Pearls of Wisdom

No doubt, drainage of the septic focus is the most important step in controlling sepsis.

COMPLICATIONS OF PERITONITIS

1. **Severe hypovolaemic shock** giving rise to renal failure. It can be prevented by adequate hydration of the patients and careful usage of antibiotics such as gentamicin.
2. **Septic shock, multiorgan failure** and death occur in late cases of peritonitis.
3. **Subacute intestinal obstruction** due to postoperative adhesions. They are easily separable adhesions.
4. **Pelvic abscess**
5. **Subphrenic abscess**

Competency

SU28.4.1: Etiopathogenesis of intraperitoneal abscess.

Pelvic abscess and subphrenic abscess are two major groups. Intraperitoneal abscesses including interloop collections can occur in acute appendicitis or following acute Meckel's diverticulitis, etc. More details are given later.

PELVIC ABSCESS

This refers to accumulation of pus in the rectovesical pouch or pouch of Douglas (rectouterine pouch).

Causes

- **Any peritonitis,** commonly following perforation due to ***acute appendicitis*** or following salpingo-oophoritis can result in pelvic abscess. The rectovesical pouch is the most dependent part in the body. Hence, the septic emboli accumulated in peritoneal space give rise to pelvic abscess.
- **Anastomotic leakage** is also an important cause.
- Perforated duodenal ulcer, perforated ileal ulcers are the other common causes.

[1]Bogota bag's use was first described by Oswaldo Borraez in Bogota, Colombia.

Clinical Features

- History of surgery/peritonitis
- Postoperative ***high-grade fever***
- History of **discharge of mucus per rectum** for the first time in a patient who is **recovering from peritonitis** suggests pelvic abscess. It occurs due to irritation of the rectum. Increased frequency of micturition occurs due to irritation of bladder.
- Deep tenderness in the suprapubic region.
- Continuing infection even after surgery—leak from an anastomotic line.
- Inadequate peritoneal toilet at the time of first surgery
- Inappropriate antibiotics.

Diagnosis

- Confirmed by **per-rectal examination**. A **tender boggy** swelling is felt in the anterior wall of rectum. **Ultrasound** can define an abscess and can detect the size of the abscess.
- **CT scan** is very useful in defining pelvic abscess, its extent and to detect presence of a foreign body (Fig. 45.33).

Treatment (Fig. 45.34)

- Under general anaesthesia, a proctoscope is introduced and a nick is made in the anterior wall of the rectum to open into the abscess cavity. Pus is drained with a sinus forceps through the rectum. There is no peritoneal contamination. The cavity collapses after a few days. Postoperatively, the patient is given broad-spectrum antibiotics.
- In females, pus can be drained through posterior fornix.

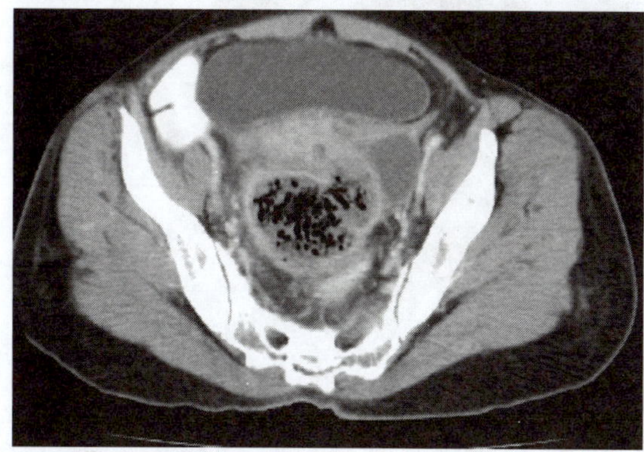

Fig. 45.33: CT scan showing gauze pieces—she had persistent foul-smelling vaginal discharge

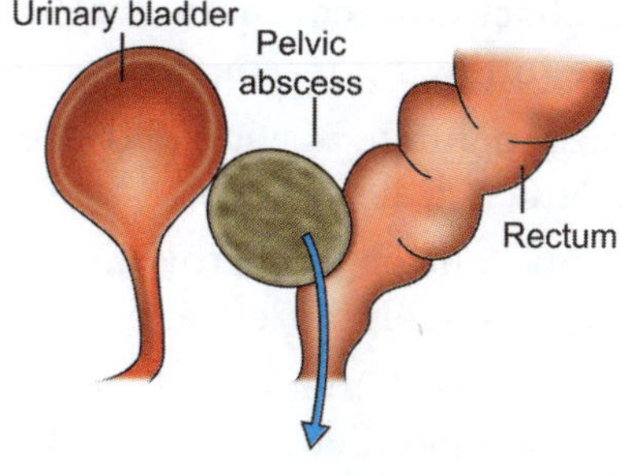

Fig. 45.34: Drainage of pelvic abscess through the rectum

Clinical Notes

A 36-year-old lady underwent vaginal hysterectomy for dysfunctional uterine bleeding. To control the bleeders, several gauze pieces were used without a proper count. After 2 weeks, purulent discharge per vagina, fever, ill health were reported. Ultrasound done showed a pelvic abscess. CT scan done in our hospital showed foreign body with air trap suggesting gauze pieces. Her abdomen was explored, abscess drained and the gauze pieces were removed.

SUBPHRENIC ABSCESS

Introduction

- As a result of peritonitis, residual abscess can collect in the intraperitoneal cavity. Pus that collects under the diaphragm is described as subphrenic abscess. Subphrenic abscess is the commonest intra-abdominal abscess.
- Gastrointestinal perforations, postoperative leaks, penetrations, trauma and puerperal sepsis are the common causes of subphrenic abscess.
- Blood clots, bacteria laden fibrin and neutrophils contribute to an abscess.

Surgical Anatomy

There are five subphrenic spaces between the diaphragm and the liver bounded by various peritoneal folds. Four are intraperitoneal and one is extraperitoneal. The spaces, boundaries and the common causes of pus in these spaces are described in Table 45.1 and Figs 45.35 to 45.37.

Aetiopathogenesis (Fig. 45.38)

- The causative organisms of peritonitis are *Escherichia coli*, enterococci, *Klebsiella, Enterobacter, Proteus, Bacteroides*, etc.
- The high incidence of subdiaphragmatic abscess is due to constant circulation of fluid from below upwards because of the following reasons:
  1. Upward movement of diaphragm during expiration.
  2. Decreased intra-abdominal pressure
  3. Capillary action

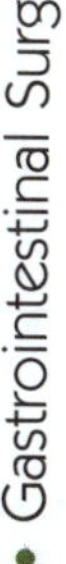

Table 45.1 Subphrenic spaces, boundaries and common causes of involvement

Spaces	Boundaries	Common causes
1. Right anterior intraperitoneal space	It lies between right lobe of the liver and diaphragm Posteriorly—anterior layer of the coronary ligament and right triangular ligament. On the left side is the falciform ligament	Perforated duodenal ulcer, gastric ulcer, cholecystitis
2. Right posterior intraperitoneal space (Rutherford Morrison's hepatorenal pouch)	It lies below the right lobe of the liver Inferiorly—hepatic flexure and transverse colon Medially—second part of the duodenum Laterally—abdominal wall. This is the biggest intraperitoneal space	Appendicitis, cholecystitis Perforated duodenal ulcer Upper abdominal surgery
3. Left anterior intraperitoneal space	Above—diaphragm. Posteriorly—left triangular ligament, left lobe of the liver, lesser omentum, anterior surface of the stomach. Right side—falciform ligament Left side—spleen	Surgery on stomach—gastrectomy. Distal pancreatectomy. Left hemicolectomy
4. Left posterior intraperitoneal space (lesser sac)	In front—by lesser omentum and posterior surface of the stomach. Behind—pancreas, suprarenal, left kidney On the right side—foramen of Winslow through which it communicates with the greater sac	Pseudopancreatic cyst Perforated gastric ulcer
5. Midline extraperitoneal space (bare area of the liver)	Above—upper layer of coronary ligament Below—lower layer of coronary ligament Left—inferior vena cava	Amoebic hepatitis Pyogenic liver abscess

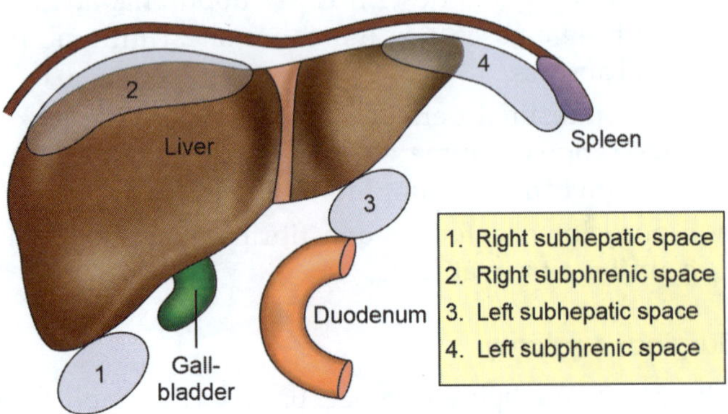

Fig. 45.35: Subphrenic spaces in sagittal section

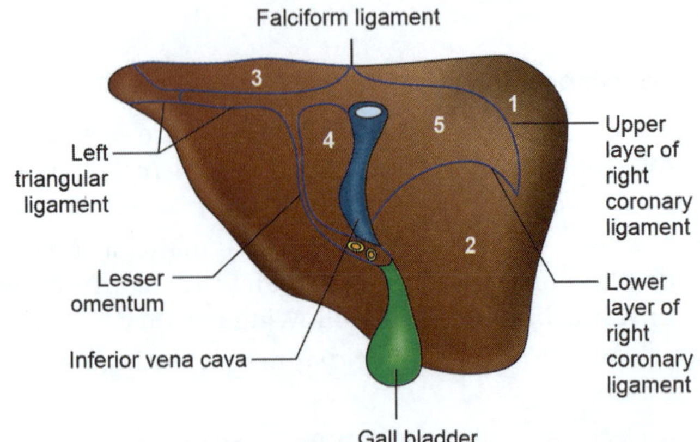

Fig. 45.36: Subphrenic spaces (Table 45.1 for numbers)

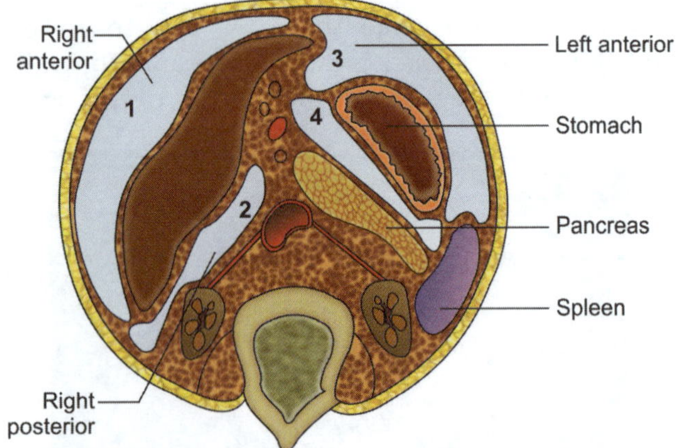

Fig. 45.37: Cross-section showing subphrenic spaces: (1) Right anterior intraperitoneal space, (2) right posterior intraperitoneal space, (3) left anterior intraperitoneal space, (4) left posterior intraperitoneal space (lesser sac)

Subphrenic abscess is common on the right side because of the following reasons:

1. Right paracolic gutter is wide and deep and colophrenic ligament is absent.
2. Left paracolic gutter is narrow and colophrenic ligament is present on the left side.
3. Majority of diseases affect right side (perforation, liver abscess, appendicitis, gallbladder disorders, etc.) (Fig. 45.38).

Section III • Gastrointestinal Surgery

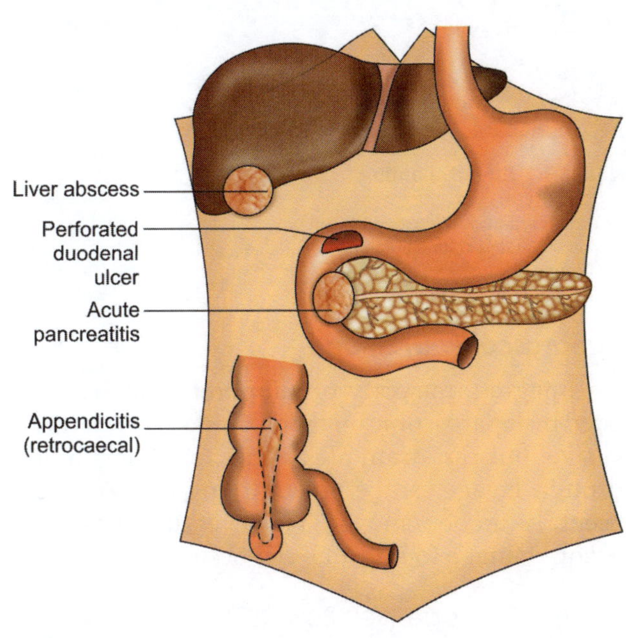

Fig. 45.38: Common causes of subphrenic abscess

Clinical Features

- A patient who is recovering from peritonitis complains of ***fever with sweating***. Initially, fever is low grade, continuous. Later, there is high-grade fever with chills and rigors.
- **Deterioration of health** occurs very fast with wasting and anorexia.
- **Shoulder pain** is due to irritation of undersurface of the diaphragm by the pus (sensory fibres of the phrenic nerve are irritated—C3, C4).
- Postoperative patient is not doing well—prolonged ileus.
- Anorexia, wasting, hiccup, dry cough.

Pearls of Wisdom

A postoperative patient who has pyrexia, prolonged ileus, poor appetite and progressive deterioration of health has subphrenic abscess.

- **Tenderness** is present in the epigastrium on deep palpation.
- Common causes of postoperative fever are absent, e.g. thrombophlebitis, urinary tract infection.

Pearls of Wisdom

Pus nowhere, pus somewhere, pus under the diaphragm—Harold Barnard.

Investigations

1. **Total count** with neutrophil count.
2. **Plain X-ray abdomen** (erect)—may show gas and fluid level under the diaphragm (Fig. 45.39).

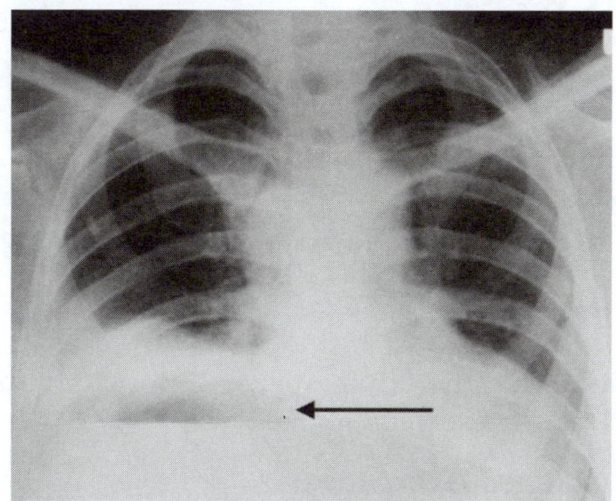

Fig. 45.39: Plain X-ray—gas and fluid level under diaphragm: PA view and lateral view

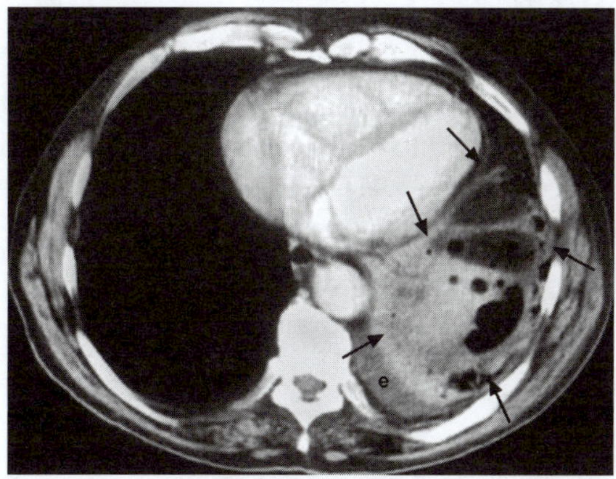

Fig. 45.40: CT scan showing left subphrenic collection following acute pancreatitis—a pigtail catheter is inserted (also see Fig. 45.41)

3. **Fluorescent radiography** may reveal absence of movement of right side of diaphragm on inspiration.
4. **Ultrasonography** confirms the site of abscess, number of abscesses, loculations, etc.
   - Abscess is characterised by hypoechogenic cavity surrounded by sharp distinct echogenic wall. It can be therapeutic to insert catheter for drainage.
5. **CT scan** demonstrates well defined, low density mass, the rim of which is enhanced after intravenous injection of contrast medium. The mass tends to be round because of centripetal expansion—high sensitivity >95% (Fig. 45.40).
6. **Isotope imaging** using Gallium 67 citrate or Iridium 111. Gallium binds to proteins—**lactoferrin and transferrin** which are present in **high concentration** in an abscess.

Treatment (Flowchart 45.2)

Today with the availability of sophisticated imaging facilities, percutaneous drainage has become the choice

Flowchart 45.2: Goals of the treatment

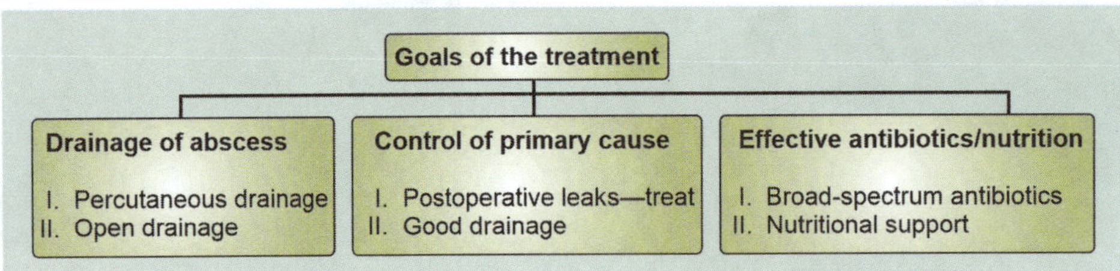

of therapy rather than surgery. Both have been described in next column.

I. *Percutaneous Drainage*

It can be done with the help of ultrasound or CT scan, provided the abscess cavity is unilocular, and the track is safe.

Types

A. ***Pigtail catheter*** (using Seldinger's technique): It is a small tube used to drain bile, urine, pancreatic fluid or abscess (Fig. 45.41).

B. ***Trocar catheter:*** 12–16 F trocar is used.

C. ***Sump catheter:*** It has a double lumen which permits irrigation as well as drainage and allows a good suction (Key Box 45.11).

Pearls of Wisdom

More than 90% of subphrenic abscesses are managed by percutaneous drainage successfully.

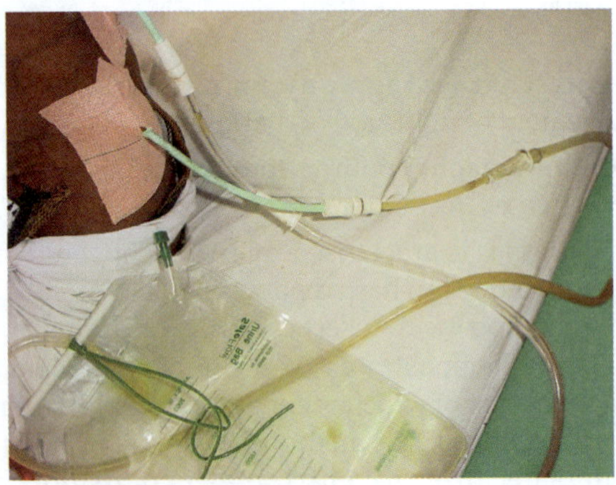

Fig. 45.41: Pigtail catheter drainage of left subphrenic abscess following gastric ulcer perforation

Key Box 45.11

Indications for Removal of Catheter

- Drainage less than 10 ml/day
- No fever, no pain
- WBC counts return to normal

II. *Laparoscopic Drainage*

With imaging, majority of subphrenic abscesses are treated by laparoscopic method. It is not only minimally invasive, but can drain all cavities, open loculi and a thorough lavage can be given. If any foreign body is present, it can be removed. However, if adhesions are present, damage to intestine can occur.

III. *Open Drainage* (Key Box 45.12)

- The anterior subcostal or posterior (bed of 12th rib) approach is used. Both are extraserous approaches.
- However, lesser sac abscess and abscesses connected with the bowel, discharging pus or bile, are drained by intraperitoneal route.
- Open drainage is ideal in cases of multiloculated abscesses.
- Surgery is always done under the cover of broad-spectrum antibiotics.

Key Box 45.12

Indications for Open Drainage

1. Multiloculated abscess
2. Persistent fistula discharging pus—communication with bowel.
3. Thick viscid content
4. Failure of percutaneous aspirations
5. Abscess very close to IVC/diaphragm

SPECIAL TYPES OF PERITONITIS

Competency

SU28.3.3: Summarize the tubercular peritonitis, spontaneous bacterial peritonitis, pneumococcal peritonitis, familial mediterranean fever (periodic peritonitis).

POSTOPERATIVE PERITONITIS

Introduction

This is not an uncommon problem encountered in the surgical wards. Often this is a patient who has undergone intestinal or biliary surgery and a few days later, develops vague symptoms and signs. It is difficult to diagnose, if one takes a casual approach. It has high mortality. Hence, it requires early detection, and demands early and effective solution.

It should be suspected following surgery on intestines or biliary tract, when a patient who is recovering from paralytic ileus starts deteriorating or when paralytic ileus does not return back to normal.

Aetiology (Figs 45.42 and 45.43)

- Leakage from anastomotic line—most common
- Iatrogenic visceral trauma
- Foreign bodies
- Others

Causes of Delay in the Diagnosis

- Presence of fever is attributed to other sources of infection such as urinary tract infection, thrombophlebitis, etc.
- Presence of pain and tenderness is attributed to recent laparotomy scar.

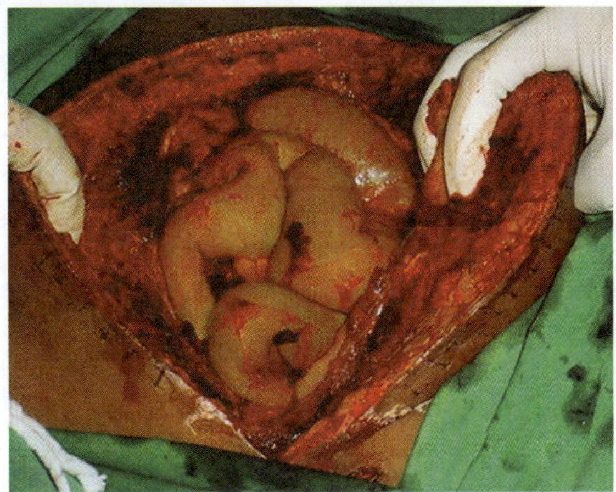

Fig. 45.42: Postoperative peritonitis due to post-cholecystectomy leak

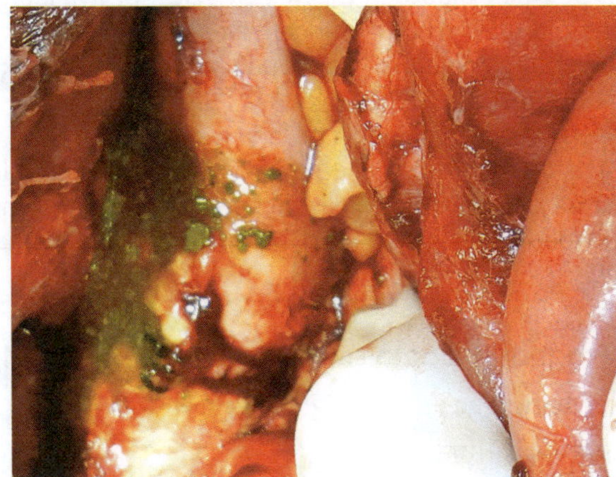

Fig. 45.43: Postoperative peritonitis due to anastomotic leak with faecal peritonitis

- Tachypnoea, and hypotension are attributed to preexisting medical conditions, such as COPD, cardiac failure.
- Steroid therapy masks the local signs and symptoms.
- Administration of antibiotics would have reduced the severity of peritonitis (masking effect) only to manifest as septicaemia some time later.

Bacteriology

1. Common organisms in postoperative peritonitis

A. Gram –ve bacilli: *E. coli*, *Klebsiella*, *Proteus*, *Pseudomonas*

B. Anaerobes: Bacteroides, *Clostridium*, Peptostreptococci, Fusobacteria

C. Gram +ve cocci: Enterococci, Staphylococci, Streptococci

2. Foreign bodies responsible for postoperative peritonitis

Macroscopic	***Microscopic***
• Gossypiboma	• Barium
• Textiloma	• Cloth piece
• Surgical drains	• Faecal matter
• Suture materials	• Necrotic tissue
• Surgical clips	• Talcum powder
• Implants	
• Instruments	

3. Presentation of foreign body

- Abdominal pain
- Mass abdomen
- Granuloma, fever
- Intestinal obstruction
- Fistula and sinus
- Extrusion—sometimes the foreign body may be visible to the exterior

How to Suspect Postoperative Peritonitis

- Patient who is recovering from initial laparotomy complains of abdominal pain and distension. He is not well. Has fever (Fig. 45.44).

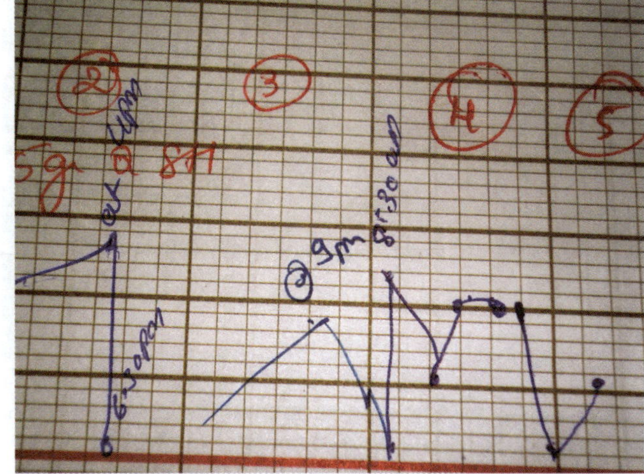

Fig. 45.44: Postoperative peritonitis due to anastomotic leak with faecal peritonitis—look at the temperature chart

- Tenderness is a feature.
- Deterioration after 3–5 days of operation (the time when anastomotic dehiscence takes place).
- Delay in recovery from paralytic ileus—abdominal distension.
- Evidence of toxaemia—tachycardia, tachypnoea.
- Free drainage of bile and faecal matter or pus from the drain site or the main wound.
- Oliguria may be an early indicator of postoperative sepsis.
- Guarding, rigidity may be present but minimal.

Treatment of Postoperative Peritonitis (Fig. 45.45)

I. Anastomotic leak: Majority of the cases are due to anastomotic leak.

- Wait and watch policy is done, if contents are coming out freely and patient is haemodynamically stable, no tachycardia, no tachypnoea, no hypotension.
- CECT of abdomen is done to rule out fistula tract/communication/foreign bodies, etc.
- However, if patient deteriorates, he is subjected to exploratory laparotomy and treated depending upon the findings at laparotomy.

  Examples: If a leak is detected from duodenal ulcer perforation closure site, re-suture it. Then add feeding jejunostomy and drain peritoneal cavity.
- If right hemicolectomy has leaked, explore, trim the edges, suture healthy tissue and do a protective proximal ileostomy.
- If a colocolic anastomosis has leaked, redo the anastomosis, with or without proximal stoma.

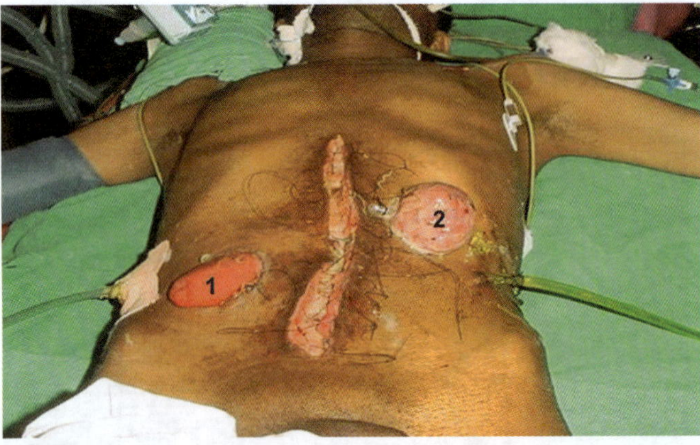

Fig. 45.45: Postoperative peritonitis due to leak following right hemicolectomy for carcinoma caecum. There were 2 sites of leak: 1. Ileocolic anastomotic site, 2. proximal jejunum. Both were exteriorized. You can see the wound left open with loose skin sutures—they will be tied after 3–4 days. This is to prevent wound infection (almost inevitable)

Pearls of Wisdom

1. While doing an ileocolic or colocolic anastomosis for 2nd time, check for adequate vascularity of both ends of the bowel. Suture, if bowel is pink and mesentery shows pulsations. The suturing must be gentile but tight. It should not be too tight.
2. A proximal diversion ileostomy or colostomy is better.
3. Improve nutrition by total parenteral nutrition.

II. Prevention of gossypiboma (MOP)

- Double counting
- Sponges with radio-opaque markers
- No hurried counting
- Additional counting—when change of OT personnel
- Avoid using packs—fascial closure
- Intraoperative radiology
- High degree of suspicion (*see* clinical notes)

III. Specific treatment (Key Box 45.13)

Key Box 45.13

Treatment

- Danger lies in delay, not in reoperation
- Leak or abscess cavity is confirmed by abdominal ultrasound/CT scan.
- Exploration (preparation similar to a routine laparotomy)
- Resection or resuturing, ileostomy, colostomy
- Drainage of abscess cavity
- Refashioning of colostomy, if it is retracted
- Appropriate antibiotics
- Delayed closure of skin
- Peritoneal lavage
- Once abscess is drained or leakage is prevented, recovery is wonderful.

Clinical Notes

In 1973, when ultrasound facilities were not available, a 35-year-old male who had undergone appendicectomy for a gangrenous appendix, was found to have high spiking fever on the 3rd postoperative day. All possible causes of postoperative fever including malaria were ruled out. On the 10th postoperative day, the patient developed a purulent discharge of 100 ml through the lower part of the main wound following which he had a spontaneous and dramatic recovery.

Poor Prognostic Factors in Postoperative Peritonitis

- Increasing age
- Organ(s) failure
- Colonic perforation
- Multiple abscess

- Lesser sac abscess
- Malnutrition
- Postoperative pneumonia
- **Anergy:** It (immunologic tolerance) refers to the failure to mount a full immune response against a target.

BILIARY PERITONITIS

- Leakage of bile into the peritoneal cavity results in biliary peritonitis.
- It will be more obvious and can be detected early, if a drainage tube has been kept.

Causes

1. **Surgery on the gallbladder**
    - Leakage from the cystic duct
    - Injury to the right hepatic duct
    - Leak from accessory cholecystohepatic duct
2. **Surgery on the CBD**
    - Retained stones in the lower CBD (postoperative)
    - Loose sutures over CBD
    - T-tube not anchored properly
3. **Surgery on the duodenum**
    - Sphincteroplasty
    - Partial gastrectomy
    - Perforation of sutured duodenal ulcer
4. **Injury to the duodenum**
    - During nephrectomy, hemicolectomy
    - Blunt injury
5. **Instrumentation:** ERCP, stenting or following duodenal polypectomy.
6. **Diseases of the gallbladder:** Perforation or gangrene of the gallbladder.

Clinical Features (Fig. 45.46)

- In majority of the cases, the local signs are confined to one quadrant of the abdomen in the form of guarding and rigidity.
- There may be excoriation of the skin due to drainage of bile to the exterior.
- However, when the anastomosis gives way, generalised peritonitis can occur.
- In untreated cases, septicaemic shock can develop.
- Final stage will be multiorgan failure and death.
- It has a very high mortality rate.

Treatment

1. Most of the biliary fistulae heal within 2–3 weeks with conservative line of treatment.
2. If it does not heal, re-exploration and resuturing or resection has to be done.

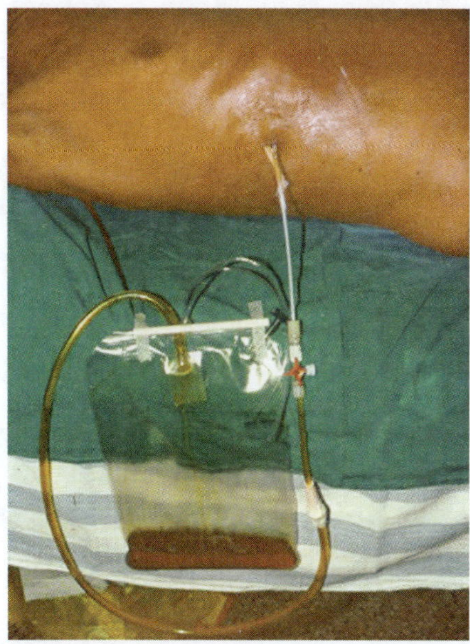

Fig. 45.46: Post-cholecystectomy bile leak due to injury to the common bile duct. Majority of such leaks can be managed conservatively. If the leak continues, get an ERCP done and treat the cause accordingly

3. Feeding jejunostomy is a very useful procedure in all cases of reperforation of sutured duodenal ulcers or difficult duodenal ulcer closures.

It should be remembered that feeding jejunostomy is temporary and is kept till it is assured that there is no leak from the operated site. If there is no peritonitis, the patient has passed flatus and stools, jejunostomy tube is removed.

Feeding jejunostomy should be done carefully with proper placement of catheter within the small bowel, fixing it firmly both inside and outside the abdominal wall and fixing to the bowel wall.

Complications of feeding jejunostomy

- Bile leak from the entry point.
- Tube blockage, if it is not flushed properly after feeding.
- Bleeding, displacement and intussusception.

PNEUMOCOCCAL PERITONITIS

- Primary variety is more common. Girls of 3–6 years of age are usually affected. Infection spreads from female genital tract through vagina.
- Malnourishment precipitates pneumococcal peritonitis.
- In boys, blood spread can occur following upper respiratory tract infection.

Clinical Features

- High grade fever with features of toxaemia.

- Bloody diarrhoea and frequency of micturition are indicative of pelvic peritoneal inflammation.
- Other features of peritonitis are present.

Diagnosis

Aspiration of peritoneal fluid demonstrates high WBC count—30,000/mm^3. More than 90% are polymorphs.

Treatment

Laparotomy and drainage of pus (odourless and sticky initially and creamy or purulent in the later stages), to be followed by appropriate antibiotics.

PRIMARY STREPTOCOCCAL PERITONITIS

- Infants and children less than 4 years are commonly affected.
- Peritoneal exudate is cloudy and contains flakes of fibrin.
- Symptoms of gastroenteritis—greenish watery stools are present.
- Source of infection is tonsillitis, pharyngitis, etc.
- Treated with injection crystalline penicillin.

PARTURITION PERITONITIS

- This occurs after delivery, if proper aseptic precautions are not taken. The incidence has come down in the recent years. Attempted abortions by using instruments which are not sterile results in peritonitis. Most of the time, peritonitis is confined to pelvis with paralytic ileus, mucous diarrhoea and offensive lochia (Key Box 45.14). Late cases develop generalised peritonitis, intra-abdominal abscess, intestinal obstruction and infertility. Table 45.2 gives summary of various types of peritonitis.
- Other name for this type of peritonitis is abortion peritonitis.

Key Box 45.14

Abortion Peritonitis

- Instrumentation
- Puerperal sepsis
- Offensive lochia
- Pelvic peritonitis
- Infertility

SPONTANEOUS BACTERIAL PERITONITIS (SBP)

As the name suggests, in this condition, there is no demonstrable intra-abdominal disease responsible for peritonitis, such as perforation, abscess, gangrene, etc.

Types

1. **In infants:** It is more common in female children. Spread is by haematogenous route. The causative organisms are *Streptococcus pneumoniae.* It may follow respiratory tract or urinary tract infection (Key Box 45.15).
2. **In adults:** Male alcoholic patients are commonly affected followed by patients with chronic liver disease. Causative organisms are *E. coli, S. faecalis,* etc.
   - **Portal hypertension** increases **permeability of gut wall**, thus increasing bacterial migration. These bacteria which colonise in the small bowel reach systemic circulation **because of shunting of blood around liver** sinusoids. **Portal lymph also gets contaminated** giving rise to increased ascitic fluid. So, this is translocation of bacteria.

Key Box 45.15

Risk Factors

CHILDREN

- Malnutrition
- Malignancy
- Chemotherapy
- Splenectomy

Low protein in the ascites prevents opsonisation of bacteria

ADULTS

- Cirrhosis ⟶ *Usually associated with SBP*
- Nephrotic syndrome
- Chronic renal failure

Table 45.2 Summary of various types of peritonitis

Type	Age	Route	Exudate
Pneumococcal	3–6 years	Vagina	Odourless, sticky, turbid pus with high-grade fever
β-haemolytic streptococci	Children	Vagina	Cloudy and fibrin flakes +
Parturition	20–40 years	Vagina	Thick pus +
Tuberculous	20–40 years	Pulmonary tuberculosis	Straw-coloured fluid + tubercles +
Perforation peritonitis	20–40 years	Hollow viscus	Foul-smelling exudate +

- It is interesting to note that it is rare for anaerobic microorganism to produce SBP. Due to high volume of oxygen in the intestinal wall, they cannot translocate.

Clinical Features

- **Dull aching** pain in the abdomen with low-grade fever.
- **Rebound tenderness** is present, bowel sounds are absent or sluggish—abdominal distension.
- Cirrhotic patients may develop ***coma*** with onset of primary bacterial peritonitis.
- **Septic shock** is a late feature with a high mortality rate.

Investigations

- Leucocytosis, ↓albumin, ↑prothrombin time suggests sepsis.
- **Peritoneal tap and Gram staining** of the fluid.
- The diagnosis of SBP is made when ascitic fluid contains more than 250 neutrophils/mm^3. Ascitic fluid also has low protein.
- Ascitic fluid culture is usually monomicrobial.
- **Laparoscopy** may help to rule out intra-abdominal emergencies, such as perforations, etc.
- **Ultrasound** can detect nature of the liver and amount of fluid in the abdomen.
- **CT scan** when in doubt about the diagnosis.

Treatment

- Conservative treatment is followed, provided secondary bacterial peritonitis is ruled out.
- Broad-spectrum antibiotics, such as aminoglycosides with 3rd generation cephalosporins are the ideal choice. Metronidazole can also be added.
- Instillation of antibiotic solution into ascitic fluid to achieve a quick and high concentration.
- If laparotomy is done, peritoneal wash or toilet is given.

PERIODIC PERITONITIS

- Also called familial Mediterranean fever.
- It is of unknown aetiology.
- It affects children, young adults and females.
- Presents as abdominal pain, tenderness, pyrexia and increased total WBC count.
- When in doubt, laparotomy should be done.

Some Salient Features (Observe 11Ps)

- **Pyrin**—a protein product from the gene—MEFVgene mutation causes this.
- **Pain** abdomen and tender abdomen
- **Pyrexia**
- **Pain** in the thorax
- **Period** of 2–3 days, it occurs and slowly remission occurs.
- **Patients** are usually ***children***
- **Principally** occurs in ***Arabs, Armenians*** and ***Jews.***
- **Primarily** runs in families
- **Peritoneal** inflammation is present
- **Polymorph** leucocyte count is increased
- **Prevent** recurrence—colchicine therapy

TUMOURS OF THE PERITONEUM

- **Primary:** Mesothelioma is the tumour to be remembered. It is more common from the pleura. In the abdomen, pelvic peritoneum is the common site.
- **Secondary** tumours are—pseudomyxoma peritonei and carcinoma peritonei.

PSEUDOMYXOMA PERITONEI

- In this condition, peritoneal cavity is filled with mucoid substance (jelly-like) brownish or yellowish.
- **Mucinous adenocarcinoma of the ovary** is the cause.
- Primary tumour is **very slow growing** and metastasis is exceptional.
- Ruptured mucinous adenocarcinoma appendix and/or ovarian adenocarcinoma are the causes.
- Once rupture takes place, peritoneal cavity is studded with jelly-like mucous-secreting tumours which appear as large loculated cystic masses.
- From the appendix (Key Box 45.16), it can be benign-mucinoma of appendix to mucinous adenocarcinomas.

Key Box 45.16

Sites

- Appendix—common site
- Ovary—common site
- Intestines—not uncommon sites
- Uterus, urachus—rare sites

Clinical Features

- Age group: 40–50 years. Equal incidence in both sexes.
- The patients can present with slow, painless and progressive abdominal distension. No shifting dullness.

- A few patients present with features of intestinal obstruction.
- Recurrence can occur because the tumour is locally malignant.

Investigations

CECT of abdomen/pelvis is done to get details about any previous pathology in the appendix or ovary.

Treatment

- Remove as much as possible **(debulking)**. This is described as cytoreduction.
- Appendicectomy, omentectomy, peritonectomy.
- Reject the involved organs (adjacent to tumours) may be colon, small bowel, etc.
- Hyperthermic intraperitoneal chemotherapy (HIPEC) (Key Boxes 45.17 and 45.18).

CARCINOMA PERITONEI

This name is applied to an advanced stage of intra-abdominal malignancy involving the entire peritoneal cavity.

Carcinomas of the stomach, colon, pancreas, breast and ovary are the common causes.

Features at Laparotomy

- Multiple firm to hard nodules on the visceral and parietal peritoneum.
- Dense adhesions between the intestinal loops and other viscera.
- Plaques on the intestinal surface
- Widespread secondaries in the liver
- Entire omentum will be studded with hard nodules. It is called omentum cake.
- Ascites: Straw-coloured or haemorrhagic
- Greater omentum being the **policeman** and a great drain pipe of the abdomen with rich lymphatics, is studded with nodules.

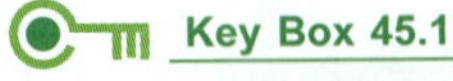

Key Box 45.17

Treatment of Pseudomyxoma Peritonei

- Remove as much as possible cytoreduction.
- Reject the adjacent involved tissues.
- Kill cancer cells by hyperthermia intraperitoneal chemotherapy.
- Doxorubicin, mitomycin, oxaliplatin are the common drugs.
- Technique of HIPEC is called coliseum technique.

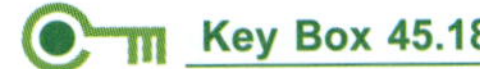

Key Box 45.18

Hyperthermic intraperitoneal chemotherapy (HIPEC)

- Advantage of HIPEC is high concentration of drugs locally and low levels in the systemic circulation.
- Also these drugs from the peritoneal cavity get into portal veins, act on metastasis, if present in the liver.
- Hyperthermia kills the malignant cells locally at the temperature around 41 to 43°C.
- Hyperthermia added by cytoxic drugs results in increased cytotoxicity.

Two methods are available for HIPEC

1. **Open method:** It is called coliseum technique by Sugarbaker.
   - A Tenchkhoff catheter with 4 closed suction drains is used. They are passed through abdominal wall.
   - 30 to 90 minutes perfusion is done.
2. **Closed technique:** Laparotomy is done and skin edges are closed. It is much more rapidly acting.

Drugs used:

- These are the primary drugs used to treat original cancer.
- Carrier solutions are 1.5% dextrose isotonic solution which is used for peritoneal dialysis, most commonly used.
- Mitomycin C 15 mg/m^2 for appendicular carcinoma, Doxorubicin 15 mg/m^2 for colonic carcinoma and ovarian carcinoma are used.

- Low protein ascites is more vulnerable for risk of developing peritonitis. **Incidence of peritonitis in malignant ascites cases is low because of increased immunoglobulin levels in malignant ascites and increased opsonic activity.**

Differential Diagnosis

- The most common differential diagnosis is tuberculosis (peritoneal). These nodules are firm and greyish.
- Acute pancreatitis with fat necrosis: This is due to calcium soap. They are yellow and soft.
- Ruptured hydatid cyst
- Lymphomatous nodules
- Ruptured GIST (not common, Fig. 45.47)

Treatment

1. Radioactive gold (^{198}Au) instillation into peritoneal cavity.
2. Tamoxifen is useful for ascites due to carcinoma of the breast.

GRANULOMATOUS PERITONITIS

- Talc, gauze, starch, etc. are causative factors.
- It occurs many weeks after surgery.

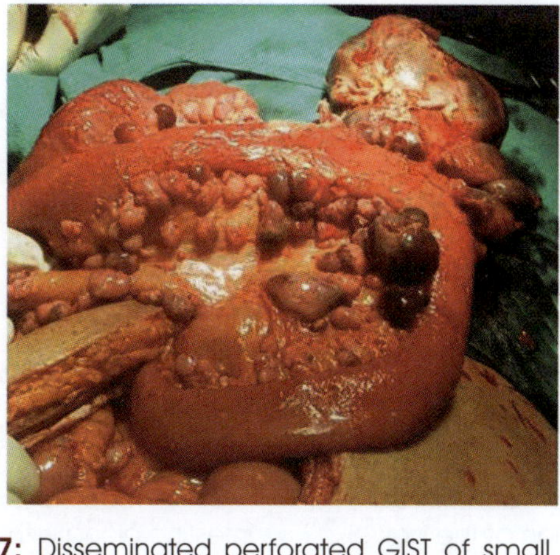

Fig. 45.47: Disseminated perforated GIST of small intestines. (*Courtesy:* Dr Jyothi, Head, Department of Surgery, GIMS Gadag, Karnataka)

- Low-grade fever, weight loss, distension, crampy abdominal pain are the features.
- Laparoscopy is the key investigation. One can visualise granuloma and biopsy can be taken. Also, fluid can be aspirated and sent for histopathology. High concentrations of lymphocytes are present in both.
- Symptomatic treatment—sinus, fistula needs to be treated.
- Intravenous prednisolone followed by oral prednisolone for 2–3 weeks is given.

Prevention

- Cleaning the gloves by wiping before handling bowel, prevents many cases of granulomatous peritonitis.
- In the initial surgery, all the foreign bodies including ova, cysts of parasites, ascariasis and ingested food particles have to be removed.

THE OMENTUM

Surgically important diseases in the omentum are:

1. **Tuberculous peritonitis:** Here omentum is involved. It becomes nodular because it is studded with tubercles. Classically seen in children who are brought with abdominal distension. On palpation, omentum is felt as granular mass in the upper abdomen which moves with respiration. Laparoscopy, biopsy and antitubercular treatment is given in Fig. 45.48.
2. **Metastasis:** Carcinoma stomach, colon, pancreas commonly result in metastasis and they give rise to omental cake (Fig. 45.49).
3. **Tumour (cyst):** Omentum is the site of omental cyst which is a lymphatic cyst (Fig. 45.50). It is a slow-growing, painless swelling in the upper abdomen. On examination, the patient is a child or an adult,

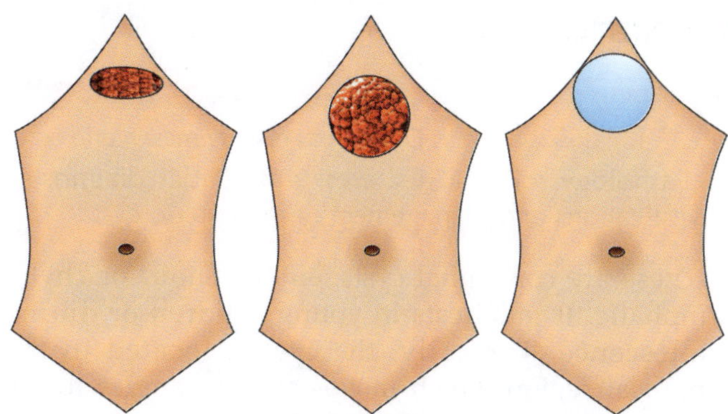

Fig. 45.48: Rolled up omentum in tuberculosis **Fig. 45.49:** Omental cake in metastasis **Fig. 45.50:** Omental cyst (lymphatic)

   with a smooth, firm mass in epigastrium which moves with respiration. Excision of the lymphatic cyst is the treatment. Massive cyst can be confused for ascites.
4. **Torsion:** It is a rare surgical emergency wherein torsion of omentum occurs due to old **adhesions** or it is primary due to lengthy mobile omentum. It produces symptoms/signs similar to that of appendicitis. Laparotomy and excision of gangrenous omentum have to be done.
5. **Non-Hodgkin's lymphoma** can affect ometum and can give rise to granularity.

   Complications: Haemorrhage into the cyst.

MESENTERY

- **Anatomy:** Given on page 752.
- Mesenteric tear has been discussed on page 753.
- Mesenteric lymphadenitis has been discussed on page 760.

MISTY MESENTERY

- It means increase in the mesenteric fat and it is a finding in the multi-detector CT scan.
- **A few pathological conditions which may give rise to this entity are:** Acute pancreatitis, retroperitoneal haemorrhage, malignancies.
- Once the source is treated, the findings may reduce or may disappear.
- Hence, follow-up CT scans are required.
- **Weber-Christian disease:** Lipodystrophy and mesenteric lipogranuloma are the features. In this condition, it should be called mesenteric panniculitis. Findings include inflammation of the mesentery, fibrosis, shortening and ischaemia. It is difficult to treat.

MESENTERIC CYST

Competency

SU28.4.3 and SU28.4.4: Define and classify mesenteric cyst.

Pathology, clinical features, differential diagnosis, investigations and management of mesenteric cyst.

These are congenital cysts, enterogenous or chylolymphatic. It manifests in young children or during adolescence. Typically, the cyst is located in the umbilical region which moves at right angles to the direction of mesentery (Fig. 45.51).

Types of Mesenteric Cysts (Figs 45.52 to 45.54, Key Box 45.19)

A. **Chylolymphatic cyst** is a lymphatic cyst arising from mesentery of ileum. It is a thin-walled cyst with clear fluid or chyle. It has a separate blood supply. Hence, enucleation is the treatment without sacrificing the bowel.

B. **Enterogenous cyst** is a duplication cyst from the intestine or due to diverticulum of the mesenteric border of the intestine. It is thick walled and contains mucus. This cyst is treated by excision of cyst with bowel segment because both share the same blood supply.

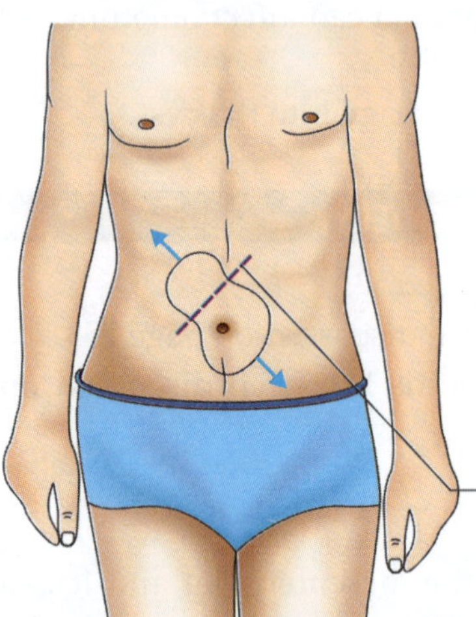

Tillaux's Triad

1. Fluctuant swelling near the umbilicus.
2. Movement perpendicular to the line of mesentery.
3. It is dull surrounded by a zone of resonance and traversed by band of resonance.

Line of attachment of mesentery

Fig. 45.51: Mesenteric cyst and its movements at right angles to the direction of mesentery (diagrammatic)

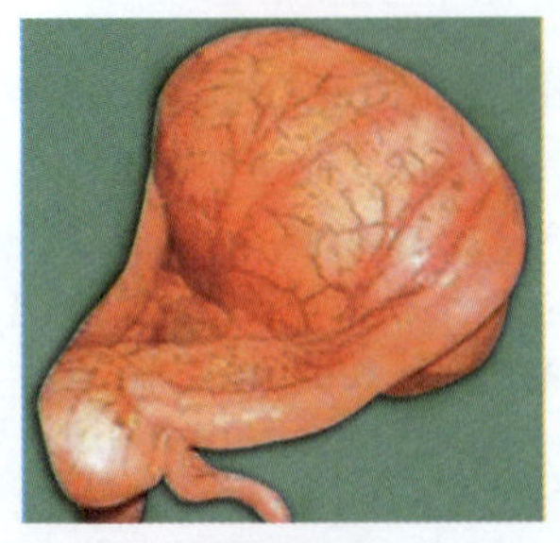

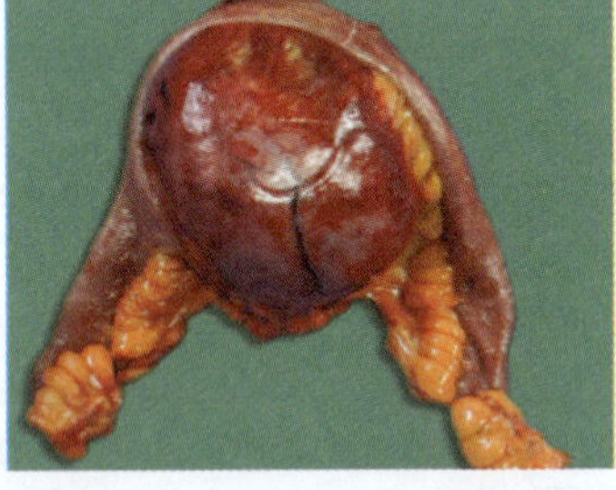

Fig. 45.52A and B: A. Mesenteric cyst excised in toto; B. Enterogenous cyst. (*Courtesy:* Dr Jayan, Professor of Surgery, Calicut)

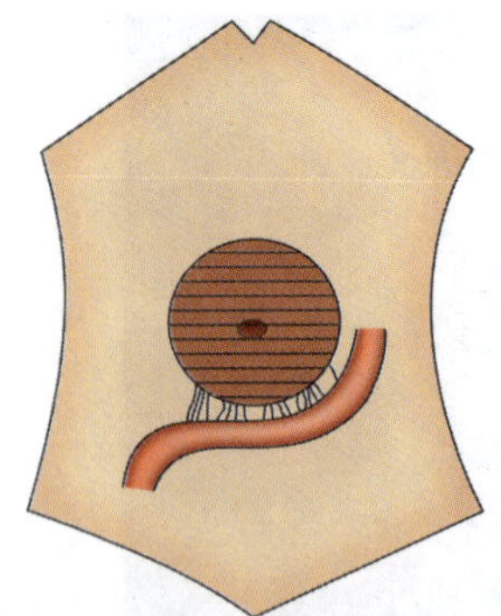

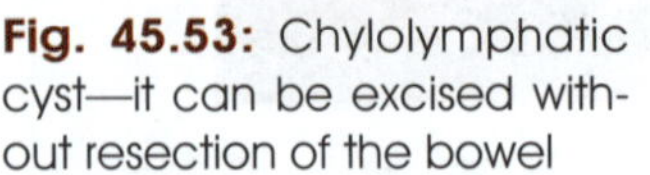

Fig. 45.53: Chylolymphatic cyst—it can be excised without resection of the bowel

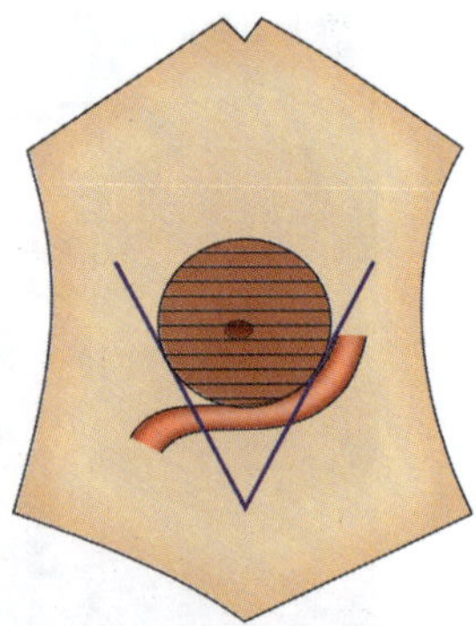

Fig. 45.54: Enterogenous cyst—it requires excision of intestine along with the cyst

Key Box 45.19

Mesenteric Cyst—Types

- Chylolymphatic cyst
- Enterogenous cyst
- Urogenital remnant
- Teratomatous dermoid cyst

Complications

- Torsion of the cyst resulting in acute abdominal pain.
- Rupture of the cyst due to trauma
- Haemorrhage into the cyst

RETROPERITONEUM

ANATOMY

Retroperitoneal space: The retroperitoneal space lies between the peritoneum and the posterior parietal wall of the abdominal cavity and extends from the diaphragm to the pelvic floor.

- **Superiorly**—12th thoracic vertebra and lateral lumbocostal arch.
- **Inferiorly**—base of the sacrum, iliac crest, and iliolumbar ligament.
- **Anteriorly**—posterior parietal peritoneum.
- **Posteriorly**—fascia overlying the quadratus lumborum and psoas major muscles.

Important Anatomical Organs (Fig. 45.55)

1. **Urinary:** Adrenal glands, kidneys, ureter, bladder
2. **Circulatory:** Aorta, inferior vena cava
3. **Digestive:** Oesophagus (thoracic part), rectum (part of middle third and lower third is extraperitoneal).
4. The head, neck, and body of the pancreas, the duodenum, except for the proximal first segment, ascending and descending portions of the colon.

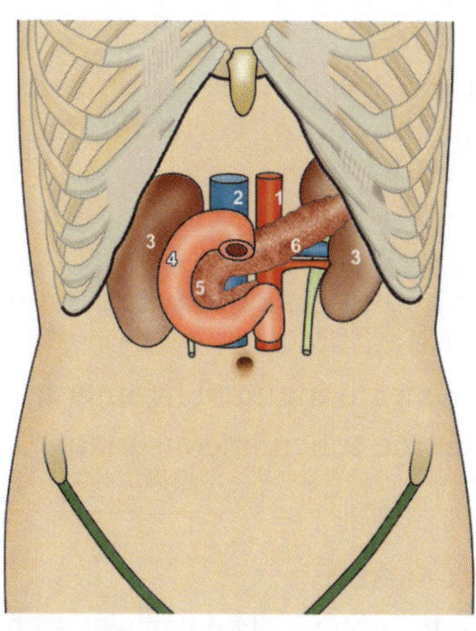

Posterior abdominal wall includes the study of the following structures

1. Abdominal aorta
2. Inferior vena cava
3. Right and left kidneys with ureters
4. Duodenum on the right side
5. Head of pancreas in the concavity of duodenum
6. Body and tail of pancreas across the posterior abdominal wall towards the left kidney

Fig. 45.55: Anatomical organs in the retroperitoneal space

IDIOPATHIC RETROPERITONEAL FIBROSIS—ORMOND'S DISEASE

Competency

SU28.4.6: Describe etiology, clinical features, differential diagnosis and management of retroperitoneal fibrosis.

- This is one of a group of fibromatosis (other being Dupuytren's contracture and Peyronie's disease).
- Other types of fibrosis such as mediastinal fibrosis, sclerosing cholangitis may also be associated features.
- Riedel's thyroiditis may be associated with this condition.
- As collagen encases ureters, they present with ureteric obstructions, requiring ureteric stenting.
- Steroid therapy is the treatment of choice.
- Tamoxifen may help.
- It can present with lower back pain, renal failure, hypertension, deep vein thrombosis and other obstructive features.

  See Key Box 45.20 and Clinical Notes.

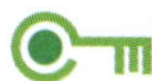 **Key Box 45.20**

Idiopathic Retroperitoneal Fibrosis—Causes

Idiopathic—Ormond's disease
Drugs—chemotherapy, methysergide, β-adrenoreceptor antagonists
Irritation—blood, urine, bowel contents
Others—autoimmune
Peritoneal disease—secondaries
Aortic aneurysm—inflammatory type
Trauma
Hereditary/familial
Inflammation—chronic
Carcinoid
Remember as **IDIOPATHIC**

Clinical Notes

- One day I was urgently called to assist the urosurgeon who had opened the abdomen for ureterolysis. Following was the clinical picture.
- A 76-year-old lady was admitted under urology for the diagnosis of renal failure. An ultrasound abdomen showed bilateral hydronephrosis. She was diagnosed to have idiopathic retroperitoneal fibrosis and posted for ureterolysis. To my surprise, when I explored, the patient had carcinoma colon in three places (synchronous), carcinoma caecum infiltrating right ureter, carcinoma sigmoid colon infiltrating left ureter and carcinoma transverse colon. She underwent total colectomy with ileorectal anastomosis. Ureteric reimplantations were done into bladder. She lived for 3 years and then succumbed due to liver metastasis.

RETROPERITONEAL CYST

- Very often, it is a painless, smooth, firm enlargement.
- May have minor degree of mobility.
- These cysts are either lymphatic cysts or derived from the remnant of Wolffian duct. A few of them are teratomatous dermoids.
- Benign retroperitoneal cysts are usually mesothelial or mesonephric in origin; rarely, rupture of the biliary tree can result in bile-filled cysts.
- **Gross:** These cysts are not connected to the kidney or adrenal; usually filled with clear or straw-coloured fluid.
- **Histology:** These cystic structures may be lined by mesothelial, enteric (glandular), or columnar epithelium.
- They can be unilocular or multilocular.
- CT scan is required to differentiate it from hydronephrosis.
- Excision is the treatment.

RETROPERITONEAL ABSCESS

Causes

1. Renal source: Pyonephric abscess
2. **Spine: Tuberculosis (details below)**
3. Haematoma: Fracture spine/pelvis
4. Acute pancreatitis (on right side)
5. Retrocaecal appendicitis (on right side)
6. Sigmoid diverticulitis

Diagnosis

- Ultrasound or CT scan-guided aspiration
- Culture of the pus and antibiotic sensitivity.

Treatment

Aspiration, appropriate antibiotics and open drainage.

PSOAS ABSCESS

Three types have been recognised

1. **Primary psoas abscess:** It is caused by haematogenous spread of *Staphylococcus aureus*. Source may be occult—tonsils, middle ear, etc. More common in children and young adults. Poor nutrition, may be a contributing factor—it is **monomicrobial**.
2. **Secondary psoas abscess:** Secondary to intestinal perforation, e.g. Crohn's disease. It is **polymicrobial.** Other causes are diverticular perforation, acute pancreatitis, etc.

   Clinical features

   Fever, flank pain, and flexion of the hip joint are triad of psoas abscess. Pain on extension confirms the diagnosis.

   Management

   - CT scan is the diagnostic test. Gas bubbles are diagnostic of an abscess.
   - Treatment include percutaneous catheter drainage, treatment of the source of infection with antibiotics.
   - If necrotic tissue does not drain well or if patient is not improving, open drainage should be done.
3. **Tuberculous spine:** Lower thoracic (T10) and upper lumbar spine are commonly affected (Fig. 45.56).

Clinical Features

- Pain in the back (localised to lesion) or referred pain, if there is a collapse.

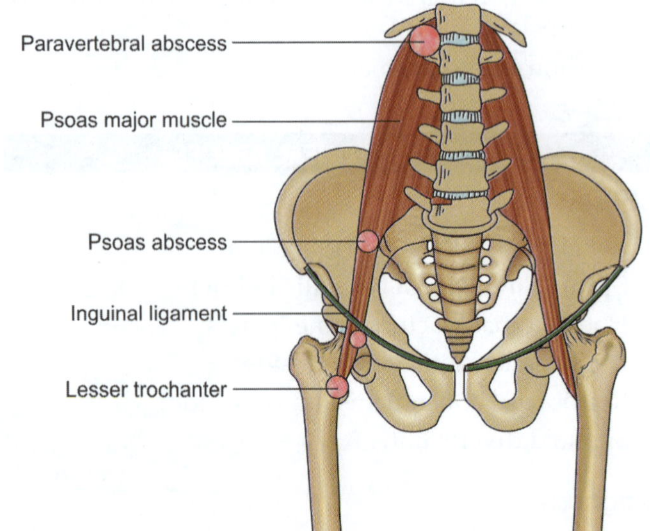

Fig. 45.56: Various sites of tubercular cold abscess arising from tuberculosis of the spine

- Evening pyrexia
- Protective muscular spasm, especially of sacrospinalis.
- Collapse of the anterior portion of vertebral body results in angular deformity—gibbus.

Route of Psoas Abscess

- Pus enters psoas sheath and tracks downwards and causes mass in the iliac fossa.
- From here, it traverses beneath inguinal ligament.
- If untreated, it collects in the subcutaneous plane.

Investigations

- **Chest X-ray, ESR, sputum AFB**
- **Spine X-ray**—AP and lateral view. The earliest sign is a decrease in the intervertebral space.
- **MRI** can detect spine lesion, cold abscess
- **CT/MR-guided aspiration of pus**/biopsy to prove histological diagnosis.

Treatment

- Cold abscess—aspiration followed by antitubercular treatment.
- Unstable/collapse spine—costotransversectomy—lateral thoracotomy.

RETROPERITONEAL TUMOUR

Competency

SU28.4.7: Describe classification, clinical features, investigation to make diagnosis and management of retroperitoneal tumours.

Definition

- The term retroperitoneal tumour (**RPT**) is usually confined to primary tumours arising in other tissues in this region, e.g. muscle, fat, lymph nodes, nerves (Tables 45.3 to 45.5). (**Jean Lobstein**, French pathologist and surgeon in 1829—coined the term **retroperitoneal tumour.**)
- Other tissues refer to—tumours of retroperitoneal organs such as kidneys, ureters, pancreas and

Table 45.3 Tumours of mesodermal origin (75%)

Fatty tissue origin	*Lipoma/liposarcoma*
Smooth muscle origin	*Leiomyoma/leiomyosarcoma*
Connective tissue origin	*Fibroma/fibrosarcoma*
Lymphatic origin	*Lymphangioma/lymphangiosarcoma*
Mesenchymal origin	*Myxoma/myxosarcoma*
Vascular origin	*Haemangioma/haemangiosarcoma/ haemangiopericytoma*
Unknown origin	*Xanthogranuloma*

Table 45.4 Tumours of notochordal or embryonic rests origin

Embryonic origin	*Benign or malignant teratomas*
Notochordal origin	*Chordomas*

Table 45.5 Tumours of neurogenic origin (25%)

Germ cell origin	*Benign or malignant teratomas*
Sympathetic origin	*Chordomas*
Adrenochromaffin origin	*Cortical carcinoma/ paraganglioma/ pheocromocytoma*

adrenals are conventionally not included in retroperitoneal tumours.

Introduction

- Uncommon (0.2–0.6% of all tumours)
- **Malignant** in 80–85% of cases (of these, 35% are sarcomas).
- **Sex:** No differences
- **Age:** Most occur between the sixth and seventh decade of life.
- Because of their location, these lesions usually demonstrate **indolent growth** and present as relatively large lesions.
- Their proximity to vital structures (especially vascular) makes **resection difficult**.

Aetiology

1. Idiopathic: The actual cause is not known.
2. History of radiation: Accidental or given for lymphoma.
3. Exposure to vinyl chloride/thorium dioxide
4. **Familial disorders:** Gardner's syndrome, familial neuroblastoma, neurofibromatosis, Li-Fraumeni syndrome.

Symptoms of RPT

- **Abdominal mass (80%):** Slow growing painless mass is the most common presentation. Typically confined to one side rather than centre.
- **Nausea, vomiting** and weight loss in about 20 to 30% of patients.
- **Compressive symptoms:** Abdominal pain, constipation, recent haemorrhoids, haematochezia can occur. Back pain and sciatica (30%) are common and are confused for spine pathology.

  Unilateral lower extremity oedema and pressure symptoms including secondary varicosities are common.

  Acute urine retention, dysuria and increased frequency can occur due to compression on urinary bladder.
- **Paraneoplastic syndrome,** such as intermittent hypoglycaemia, can occur in liposarcoma/fibrosarcoma and catecholamine excess in paragangliomas (Key Box 45.21).

Key Box 45.21

When to Suspect Retroperitoneal Sarcoma

- Recent finding of large abdominal mass
- Recent lower limb swelling
- Recent varicosities
- Recent varicocele
- Recent haemorrhoids
- Recent loss of weight

Signs of RPT (Fig. 45.57)

- Usually large abdominal mass, firm to hard, irregular.
- Nonmobile, restricted mobility
- Not moving with respiration
- Does not fall forward (knee elbow position)
- Resonant tone on percussion—due to bowel anteriorly.
- Transmitted pulsations may be felt.

Differential Diagnosis

- Lymphoma
- Germ cell tumours
- GIST
- Metastatic testicular cancers

Please note: When you suspect any of these as differential diagnosis, a CT-guided biopsy may be required to decide the management.

Investigations

Preoperative planning to assess the extent of the disease is essential because successful surgery is defined by complete excision of the mass with adequate margins of normal tissue.

1. **CBP**
2. **LFT:** Increased alkaline phosphatase may indicate secondaries.
3. **RFT:** Compressive uropathy with high urea and creatinine.
4. **Tumour markers:** AFP, beta-HCG—germ cell tumour.
5. **LDH in lymphoma/GCT:** LDH levels indicate tumour burden and growth rate.
6. **CT scan** (Key Box 45.22)
   - Delineate the anatomic limits of the lesion.
   - Vascular involvement—vena cava, aorta, renal vessels.

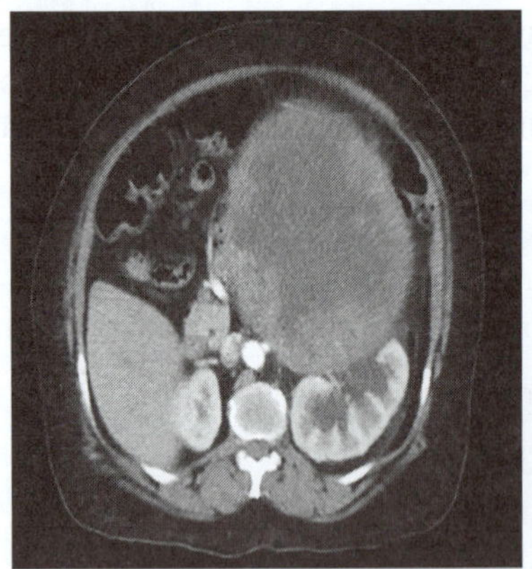
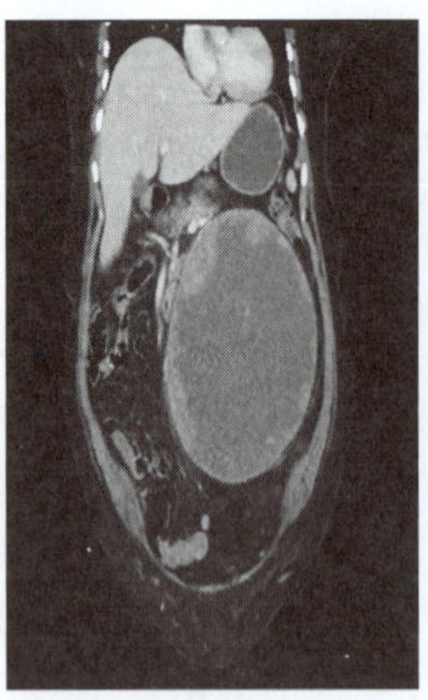
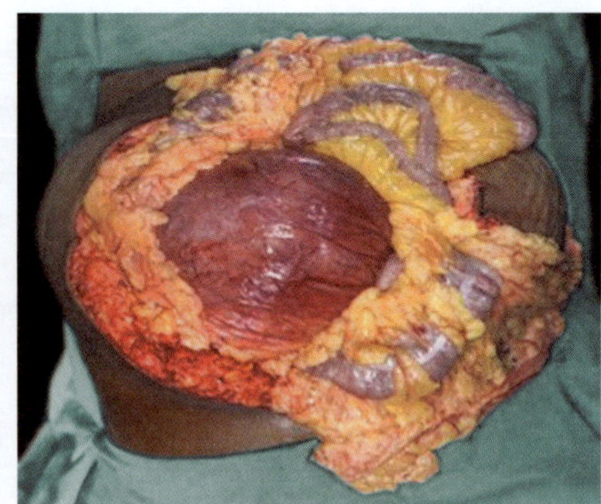

Fig. 45.57: A large well-defined peripheral nodular enhancing mass lesion with central non-enhancing areas (necrotic areas) and few peripheral chunks of calcification is noted arising from the retroperitoneum.

- Assess the integrity and function of adjacent organs—renal function is one of the important advantages of CT scan.
- Visceral metastases +/–. If present, it is inoperable but still worth trying a resection after giving neoadjuvant therapy.
- Para-aortic, iliac, mesenteric lymphadenopathy.
- Axial skeleton and renal involvement (Key Box 45.22).

7. **CT-guided core biopsy:** Reserved for cases in which a diagnosis will change therapy, such as the need for neoadjuvant chemotherapy for:
   - GIST—imatinib mesylate
   - Germ cell tumours
   - Lymphomas
8. **Laparoscopic biopsy/retroperitoneoscopy**
   - Equivocal history and diagnostic dilemma
   - Unusual appearance of the mass
   - Unresectable tumour
   - Distant metastasis

Treatment

Surgery is the main modality and the most effective modality of the treatment. It can be curative, if R-0 resection is achieved. Chemotherapy, radiotherapy are complementary to surgery. A few cases are also managed by neoadjuvant therapy.

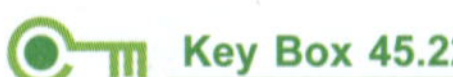

Key Box 45.22

CT Scan: Typical Findings

- **Lipoma:** Homogenous fatty density
- **Malignant fibrous histiocytoma:** Calcifications
- **Neurofibroma:** Homogenous low density
- **Teratoma:** Mixed components
- **Paraganglioma:** Para-aortic location
- **Neuroblastoma:** Calcified tumour, usually in children
- **Leiomyosarcoma:** Large areas of necrosis
- **Liposarcoma:** Heterogenous fatty density
- **Hemangiopericytoma:** Hypervascularity

I. *Surgery*

Principles: Extirpative surgery is the principal and most effective form of therapy for primary retroperitoneal tumours. **Tumour histology, tumour size, or patient age are** *not significant factors in survival* in multiple-variable analysis. Therefore, carefully planned and skillfully executed surgical therapy is critical for any chance at long-term success.

Adjuvant therapy: High local recurrence rate and eventual mortality from this disease has prompted the exploration of adjuvant therapeutic modalities. **Post-operative radiation increases toxicity to surrounding structures.**

II. *Radiotherapy*

- Radiotherapy: Two types:
  1. EBRT—external beam radiotherapy
  2. Brachytherapy for retroperitoneal leiomyosarcoma.

Advantages

- The viscera are often displaced by the tumour volume and a lack of surgical adhesions further reduces dose to the bowel.
- Effective radiation dose is lower in the preoperative setting.

III. *Chemotherapy*

- Doxorubicin is the foundation for chemotherapy in advanced sarcoma.
- **MAID regimen:** Mesna, adriamycin (doxorubicin), ifosfamide, and dacarbazine have been successful in neoadjuvant programmes for sarcomas of the extremities compared with historical controls.

TEN COMMANDMENTS

1. Complete R-0 resection should be the aim—single most important positive predictive feature.
2. Generous incision should be given to get into good access to the tumour.
3. Intra-abdominal adhesions should be released to separate the tumour. Should use of sharp, curved Mayo scissors for meticulous dissection.
4. Should never do enterotomy (accidental) because an enterotomy and subsequent fistula formation can cause major morbidity.
5. Should preserve all important vessels.
6. Should preserve important organs such as kidney, ureter, colon, etc.
7. Should resect the organs, if found infiltrated and if R-0 resection is possible.
8. Should do a centripetal dissection. It allows one to dissect those areas that are amenable to dissection.
9. Should use surgical clips, should be placed to mark the periphery of surgical field and other relevant structures to help guide potential future radiation therapy.
10. Both radiotherapy and chemotherapy are given.

DIFFERENTIAL DIAGNOSIS OF RETROPERITONEAL SARCOMA

These are pathological variants. It is difficult to consider them as a diagnosis on clinical grounds. However, more common ones have to be considered first such as liposarcoma. Patients with von Recklinghausen's disease may have neural tumours. A few differential diagnosis are given below.

Liposarcoma

Most common of primary RPT, 20% from retroperitoneum.

- **Histological types**
  1. Well-differentiated liposarcoma (low grade)
  2. Myxoid/round cell liposarcoma (50%—most common)
  3. Pleomorphic liposarcoma (10–15%—high grade)
  4. Dedifferentiated liposarcoma—the rate of metastasis depends on the degree of tumour differentiation, with nearly 90% of poorly differentiated tumours metastasizing.
- **Pathology:** The key feature of a liposarcoma is the lipoblast, which is essentially an immature fat cell. **LIPOBLASTS** have multiple fat vacuoles which compress the nucleus, creating a scalloped appearance.

Leiomyosarcoma

- 50% from retroperitoneum—Female: Male—2:1
- Site of origin (soft tissue, vascular or superficial), although many of the soft tissue lesions are believed to originate from smaller blood vessels.
- Immunohistochemistry stain for smooth muscle myosin, vimentin, and actin and less often for desmin. (*Leiomyomas stain positive for desmin, which separates them from their malignant counterpart.)*
- They stain negative for S-100.

MFH (Malignant Fibrous Histiocytoma)

- Less common in the retroperitoneum.
- Derived from fibroblast differentiation *(previously defined as a sarcoma of primary histiocytic origin)*
- Storiform-pleomorphic (40–60%) and myxoid type (25%) are subtypes. Other types being giant cell type and inflammatory.

Retroperitoneal Teratoma

- These are the tumours arising from totipotential cells. Thus, they can have ectoderm, mesoderm or endoderm elements.
- 10% of all primary RPT.
- Rare in adults because of its congenital nature.
- Solid teratoma malignant (likely).
- Malignant mature cystic teratomas (0.2 to 2% of cases) have the potential to metastasise to sites such as the retroperitoneal lymph nodes and lung parenchyma.

Rhabdomyosarcoma

- 6% in retroperitoneum
- More common in children
- Sporadic—most common
  - Genetic risk factor—10–33%: Li-Fraumeni syndrome, neurofibromatosis.

Schwannoma

- Majority has mutations in *NF2* gene.
- Majority are sporadic tumours.
- A minority (10%) are associated with syndromes, such as neurofibromatosis type 2, schwannomatosis and multiple meningiomas.
- Hallmark of schwannoma is alternating areas of cellular (Antoni A) and hypocellular (Antoni B) areas.
- Retroperitoneal tumours are larger and often show degenerative changes, such as cystic change, haemorrhage and calcifications.
- Immunohistochemistry: Diffuse S-100+ is characteristic.

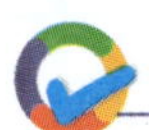

Multiple Choice Questions

1. **One need not close peritoneal layer after laparotomy because:**
   A. The peritoneum can get stuck to the bowel
   B. Flattened mesothelial cells heal within a few hours
   C. The peritoneum tears when closure is attempted
   D. It is very painful postoperatively

2. **Peritoneum can be used for dialysis because:**
   A. It is close to kidney
   B. It is faster than haemodialysis
   C. Capillaries and lymphatics between two layers of peritoneum help in absorption and exudation
   D. It covers entire abdomen

3. **Which of the following is an example of primary peritonitis?**
   A. Tuberculous peritonitis
   B. Perforation peritonitis
   C. Postoperative peritonitis
   D. Parturition peritonitis

4. **Which of the following organisms are most commonly involved in secondary peritonitis?**
   A. Enterococci
   B. Streptococci
   C. Staphylococci
   D. Pneumococci

5. **The following are the typical features of acute generalised peritonitis *except:***
   A. Abdominal pain
   B. Persistent vomiting
   C. Bradycardia
   D. High-grade fever with chills

6. **Abdominal tap is done in peritonitis for all of the following roles *except:***
   A. Aspiration of blood to indicate haemoperitoneum
   B. Aspiration of pus indicating infection with gram-negative bacteria
   C. Aspiration of bile indicating biliary peritonitis
   D. Aspiration of urine indicating ureterocele

7. **The following suture material is best suited for closure of bowel perforation:**
   A. Silk B. Catgut
   C. Nylon D. Thread

8. **History of discharge per rectum for the first time in a patient who is recovering from peritonitis suggests:**
   A. Anal prolapse B. Pelvic abscess
   C. Proctitis D. Colitis

9. **What forms the anterior relationship of Rutherford Morrison's space?**
   A. Liver B. Kidney
   C. Diaphragm D. Duodenum

10. **Subphrenic abscess is common on the right side because of the following reasons *except:***
    A. Majority of the diseases affect right side
    B. Right lung is larger
    C. Left paracolic gutter is narrow and colophrenic ligament is present on the left side
    D. Right paracolic gutter is large and colophrenic ligament is absent on the right side

11. **Indications for open drainage of subphrenic abscess include the following *except:***
    A. Persistent fistula discharging pus
    B. Thick viscid pus
    C. Abscess very close to IVC/diaphragm
    D. Single loculus

12. **Intra-abdominal pressure exceeds ________ cm H_2O in abdominal compartment syndrome.**
    A. 15 B. 25
    C. 35 D. 45

13. **Following are features of tuberculous peritonitis *except:***
    A. Tubercles over peritoneal surface
    B. Encysted form
    C. Can be a miliary form
    D. Transudate

14. **Nonoperative treatment for peritonitis may be followed in the following *except:***
    A. Moribund patients
    B. Sealed perforation
    C. Localised peritonitis
    D. Generalised peritonitis

15. **The following catheters are commonly used for percutaneous drainage of subphrenic abscess:**
    A. Pigtail catheter B. Trocar catheter
    C. Sump catheter D. Foley's catheter

16. More reliable sign of peritonitis is:

A. Cough tenderness B. Tenderness on pressure
C. Rebound tenderness D. Guarding

17. Presence of sunken eyes, pale and pinched face, dry cracked tongue, cold perspiration and cyanosis are all typical features of:

A. Hippocratic facies B. Gargoyle facies
C. Marshall hall facies D. Mask like facies

18. Following are risk factors for spontaneous bacterial peritonitis *except:*

A. Cirrhosis B. Nephrotic syndrome
C. Chronic renal failure D. Carcinoma stomach

19. Which of the following is true for pneumococcal peritonitis?

A. Common in young boys
B. Age is around 15 years
C. Peritoneal fluid is transudate
E. It is typically odourless

20. Following are about pseudomyxoma peritonei *except:*

A. Common in women
B. Ovary is the main source
C. Surgery cannot cure the disease
D. Chemotherapy is also used

Answers

1. B	**2.** C	**3.** A	**4.** A	**5.** C	**6.** D	**7.** A	**8.** B	**9.** D	**10.** B
11. D	**12.** C	**13.** D	**14.** D	**15.** A	**16.** C	**17.** A	**18.** D	**19.** D	**20.** B

CHAPTER

46

Small Intestine

- Embryology and development
- Anatomy
- Physiological functions
- Abdominal tuberculosis
- Tuberculous peritonitis
- Tuberculous mesenteric lymphadenitis
- Glandular tuberculosis
- Intestinal tuberculosis
- Inflammatory bowel diseases
- Ileostomy
- Crohn's disease
- Surgical complications of enteric fever
- Intestinal amoebiasis
- Radiation enteropathy
- Peutz-Jeghers syndrome
- Adenocarcinoma
- GIST
- Neuroendocrine tumours
- Short gut syndrome
- Intestinal fistulae
- Small intestinal diverticula

Introduction

Truly speaking small intestines extends from pylorus to ileocecal junction. However, for all practical purposes, it is discussed as starting from duodenojejunal flexure till caecum. Small intestines play an important role not only in the transfer of food contents distally but in the digestion, absorption and secretion of the contents. Being the central portion of the GI tract with long length, many diseases affect the intestine. Surgically important topics such as intestinal tuberculosis, inflammatory bowel diseases and few tumors are discussed in this chapter.

EMBRYOLOGY AND DEVELOPMENT

Competency

SU28.13: Appreciate anatomy and physiology of the small intestine.

- Small intestine develops from midgut.
- This midgut loop has cranial and caudal limbs.
- As the elongation starts from 5th week of foetal life, cranial limb develops into distal duodenum, jejunum and proximal ileum.
- Distal ileum and proximal two-thirds of transverse colon are developed from caudal limb.
- Midgut also rotates 270°. Thus, proximal jejunum will go to left side and ileum will go to right side.
- Anomalies can occur during rotation resulting in malrotation.
- Vitellointestinal (VI) duct joins the junction of cranial and caudal intestines which is about 2 feet away from ileocaecal junction.
- When VI duct is not obliterated, various anomalies occur. One of them is Meckel's diverticulum.
- Caecum which is present in the right hypochondrium descends into the right iliac fossa region.

ANATOMY

- Small intestine consists of proximal 2/5 jejunum and distal 3/5 ileum. It is about 6 metres in length.
- Small intestine starts at duodenojejunal flexure just to the **left of the inferior mesenteric vein**.

  Surgical importance: To identify the first (short) loop of jejunum for gastrojejunostomy.
- Small intestine ends at ileocaecal junction. In cases of intestinal obstruction, trace up to ileocaecal junction. If caecum is distended, it is a case of large bowel obstruction. If caecum is collapsed, it is a case of small bowel obstruction.

Key Box 46.1

Differences between Jejunum and Ileum

	Jejunum	Ileum
Length	2/5	3/5
Diameter	Wider (2–4 cm)	Less (2–3 cm)
Wall	Thick and double (mucous membrane can be felt)	Thin
Colour	Deep red	Pale pink
Peyer's patch	Very, very less	More
Blood supply	Long and a few vasa recta (1 or 2)	Short and numerous (5 or 6)
Mesentery	Transparent, less fat	More fat

- Jejunum resides in the left side of the peritoneal cavity and ileum on the right side.
- Differences between jejunum and ileum have been given in Key Box 46.1.

Blood Supply (Fig. 46.1)

- Superior mesenteric artery is the **artery of the midgut** which supplies the entire midgut (entire small intestine). Jejunal arteries are end-arteries.
- Mesenteric border of the intestine gets more blood supply when compared to anti-mesenteric border. Hence, in cases of diminished blood supply, anti-mesenteric border becomes ischaemic first.
- Venous drainage is through superior mesenteric vein.

Mesentery

- It is a fan-shaped fold of peritoneum which attaches jejunum and ileum to posterior abdominal wall.
- Blood vessels and lymphatics course in between the folds of peritoneum.
- It extends from the left of duodenojejunal flexure (left of L2) vertebra to the right sacroiliac joint, thus fixing the ileocaecal junction there.

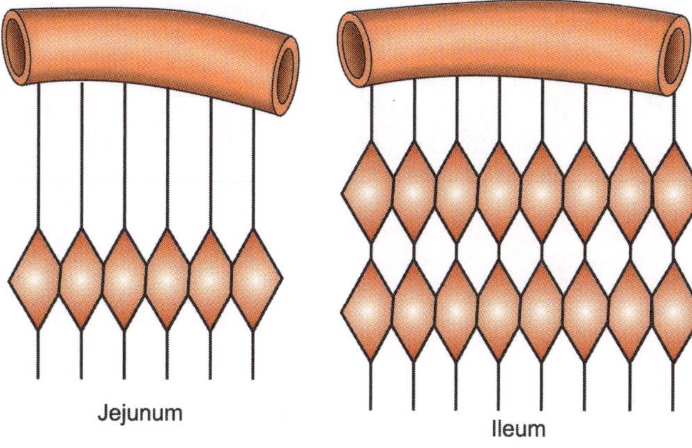

Fig. 46.1: Blood supply—jejunum and ileum

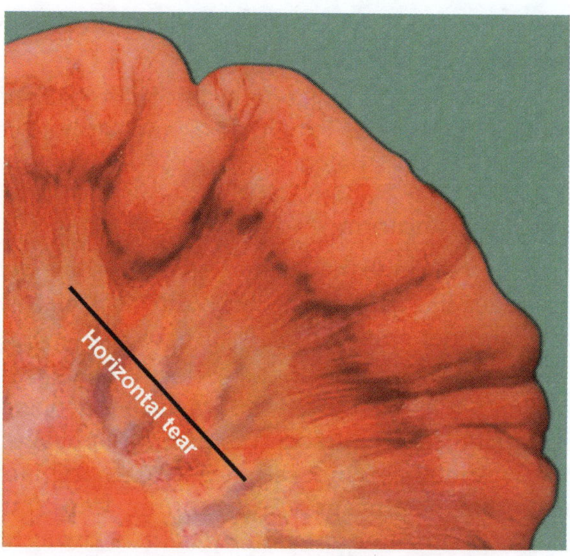

Fig. 46.2: Observe blood supply of the mesentery and it is natural that a horizontal tear causes more gangrene

- The importance of direction of the mesentery is appreciated in the following examples:
  A. **Mesenteric cyst** moves at right angles to the direction of the mesentery (*see* page 744).
  B. **Mesenteric lymph nodes** can be clinically palpable as a nodular or a smooth mass (*see* page 760).
  C. **Horizontal tear** in the mesentery causes more gangrene of the bowel than vertical tear (Fig. 46.2).
- **Structures crossed by mesentery:** Duodenum, aorta, inferior vena cava, right ureter, right psoas major and right gonadal vein.

Innervation

- **Parasympathetic:** These are derived from vagus. It is secretomotor, thus helping in secretion and motility of small intestines. Nerve fibres traverse through coeliac ganglion. Afferent fibres do not carry pain impulses.
- **Sympathetic:** These fibres arise from three sets of splanchnic nerves. Their ganglion cells are located in a plexus around base of superior mesenteric artery. Pain is mediated through sympathetic system.

Lymphatics

- From mucosa, lymphatics pass through the wall of the bowel to regional lymph nodes, then into lymph nodes at base of superior mesenteric artery.
- Then it flows into cisterna chyli and then into thoracic duct and empty into venous system at confluence of left internal jugular and subclavian veins. Extravasation of few tumour emboli outside this confluence results in enlargement of supraclavicular lymph nodes. They are about 4 to 6 in number and

are called **Virchow's nodes. This clinical sign is described as Troisier's sign**[1].

- Peyer's patches are major deposits of lymphatic tissue in the distal bowel. Tuberculosis and typhoid fever affect the Peyer's patches.

Microscopic Anatomy

- Basic unit of small bowel mucosa is the villus, which is a finger-like projection. Each villus is covered with tall columnar epithelium.
- Goblet cells, Paneth cells and endocrine cells are seen in the crypts. Goblet cells are mature mucous cells. Endocrine cells (enterochromaffin cells) have cytoplasmic granules which secrete 5-hydroxytryptamine, neurotensin, glucagon and motilin. Importantly, mucosal cell-mediated immunity is brought by mucosal T lymphocytes.

PHYSIOLOGICAL FUNCTIONS

- **Motility:** Two types of muscle contractions occur—one which does not propagate—it exposes the food contents to the absorptive surface for a longer time by causing segmentation allowing better absorption of the food. Another type is peristaltic which propagates the food contents. Control of peristalsis is done by myenteric plexus. Time taken by the solid food contents to reach from mouth to colon is about 4 hours (Key Box 46.2).
- **Absorption and digestion:** Except calcium and iron, almost everything is absorbed in the small intestines.

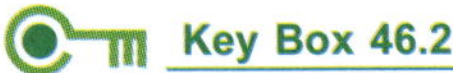
Key Box 46.2

Functions of the Small Intestine (SI)

- Digestion and absorption
- Synthesis of lipoproteins
- Secretion of regulatory peptides
  - Secretin
  - Cholecystokinin
  - Somatostatin
  - VIP
- Immune function: Production of immunoglobulins (IgA). The **B** cells and **T** cells help in phagocytosis and secretion of cytokines.

To give a few examples: Out of 6–10 litres of water, almost 80% water is absorbed in the small intestine and only 10–20% is discharged into colon. Thus in cases of terminal ileal obstruction, about 8–10 litres of fluid accumulate resulting in gross distension of the abdomen and dehydration. Carbohydrates and fat are mainly absorbed in duodenum and proximal jejunum. Proteins require pancreatic enzymes. Hence, they are broken down in the jejunum into amino acids and peptides. Conjugated bile acids are absorbed in the terminal ileum wherein enterohepatic circulation takes place and again they are secreted in the bile. Thus in ileal resections or diseases like Crohn's disease, more amount of bile acids enter colon resulting in diarrhoea due to increased secretion of water and electrolytes (Table 46.1).

Table 46.1 Absorption and digestion

	Amount (normal)	Absorption	Process	Any other
Water	8 to 10 litres/day enters into SI	Almost 90–95% only 500 ml enters the colon	Simple diffusion	Also along with water, there is active transport of sodium, glucose or amino acids
Na^+	130–140 mEq/μL	Active transport through basolateral membranes	Na^+ absorbed, H^+ secreted into lumen	H^+ combines with HCO_3^- and forms carbonic acid
Calcium	9–11 mg%	Proximal jejunum and duodenum	Enhanced by vitamin D and PTH	
Iron	Ferritin levels—12 to 300 nanogram per ml of blood for males and 12 to 150 nanogram per ml for females	Absorbed as **heme** in the duodenum	Absorbed as ferritin or transformed to plasma bound to transferrin	Helps in erythropoiesis
Vitamins	The normal range for vitamin B_{12} in the blood is between 200 and 900 nanograms per millilitre (ng/mL)	Most of vitamins are absorbed in proximal jejunum except vitamin B_{12} which is absorbed in the terminal ileum		

[1]Virchow's nodes are named after Rudolf Virchow (1821–1902), the German pathologist who first described the nodes and their association with gastric cancer in 1848.

ABDOMINAL TUBERCULOSIS (TB)

Introduction

Abdominal tuberculosis is a common extrapulmonary manifestation of tuberculosis. Disease is caused by *Mycobacterium tuberculosis*. Approximately 15–25% of cases with abdominal TB have concomitant pulmonary TB. Tuberculosis (TB) is a life-threatening disease which can virtually affect any organ system. Incidence in the West has also increased due to immigrant population and increased incidence of HIV infections. In India, extrapulmonary TB is also showing re-emergence due to incomplete treatment and occurrence of multidrug-resistant strains.

Definition

The term abdominal tuberculosis includes tuberculous infection of gastrointestinal tract, mesenteric lymph nodes, peritoneum, omentum and solid organs related to gastrointestinal tract such as liver and spleen.

Classification (Key Box 46.3)

The commonly encountered four forms of tuberculosis are given below:

1. Tuberculous peritonitis
2. Tuberculous mesenteric lymphadenitis—glandular tuberculosis
3. Intestinal tuberculosis
4. Tuberculosis of solid viscera such as liver and spleen.

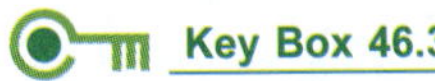 **Key Box 46.3**

Various Forms of Abdominal TB

I. Peritoneal tuberculosis: Acute, chronic

- A. Chronic forms
  1. Ascitic type (wet)
     - Generalised
     - Localised
  2. Fibrous type (dry)
     - Adhesive, plastic
     - Miliary nodule type
- B. Tuberculosis of peritoneal folds
  1. Mesenteric adenitis
  2. Mesenteric cysts/abscesses
  3. Bowel adhesion

II. Gastrointestinal

1. Ulcerative
2. Hyperplastic
3. Sclerotic/plastic

III. TB of solid viscera

1. Liver
2. Spleen

Routes of Spread of Infection and Pathogenesis

1. Intestinal tuberculosis is caused by *Mycobacterium tuberculosis* from **swallowed sputum** (pulmonary tuberculosis) or milk (milk-borne infection—*Mycobacterium bovis*). From intestinal tuberculosis, mesenteric nodes get involved and later, the peritoneum can get involved.
2. **Blood spread:** Infection from pulmonary tuberculosis can spread through blood during bacteraemic phase.
3. **Lymphatic spread** from tuberculosis of intestines.
4. **Genitourinary tuberculosis:** From here, cephalad spread occurs and thus, peritoneum gets affected.
5. **From bile:** Granuloma in liver. Bacilli are excreted in bile.

Pathology and Pathogenesis (Fig. 46.3A and B)

It is given on the next page.

Investigations

It is important to realise that there are so many investigations for abdominal tuberculosis. **Although it is essential to have a theoretical knowledge about all these investigations, all of them need not be done during clinical management**.

To give an example: If chest X-ray and sputum AFB are positive, one should start ATT (need not do costly investigations such as CT scan or even diagnostic laparoscopy, etc.). Investigations done by the clinician should be complementary to each other.

1. **Complete blood picture (CBP)** which includes Hb%, TC, DC and ESR. Haemoglobin may be low indicating anaemia. Anaemia has to be corrected before surgery.
2. **ESR** will help in equivocal cases. High values and the clinical situation may force the clinician to start antituberculous treatment in selected patients. However, with treatment, if ESR comes down and patient is symptomatically better with weight gain, settling fever, improving appetite, it suggests tubercular pathology.
3. **Sputum AFB (acid-fast bacilli):** Demonstrated by Zeihl-Neelsen method. Many patients, with abdominal tuberculosis will not have pulmonary tuberculosis. However, if sputum is present, it must be tested for AFB.
4. **Chest X-ray** may suggest tuberculosis in the form of cavity, calcification, etc. In such patients, bronchoscopy washings or biopsy may clinch the diagnosis.
5. **Mantoux test** is nonspecific but a strong ulcerated Mantoux test result suggests tuberculosis.
6. **Ultrasound,** being a noninvasive investigation, is an imaging of choice.

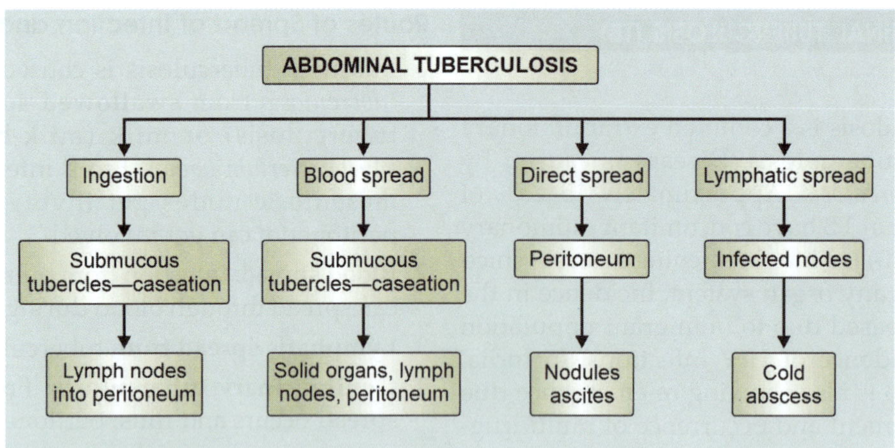

Fig. 46.3A: Abdominal tuberculosis—pathology and pathogenesis

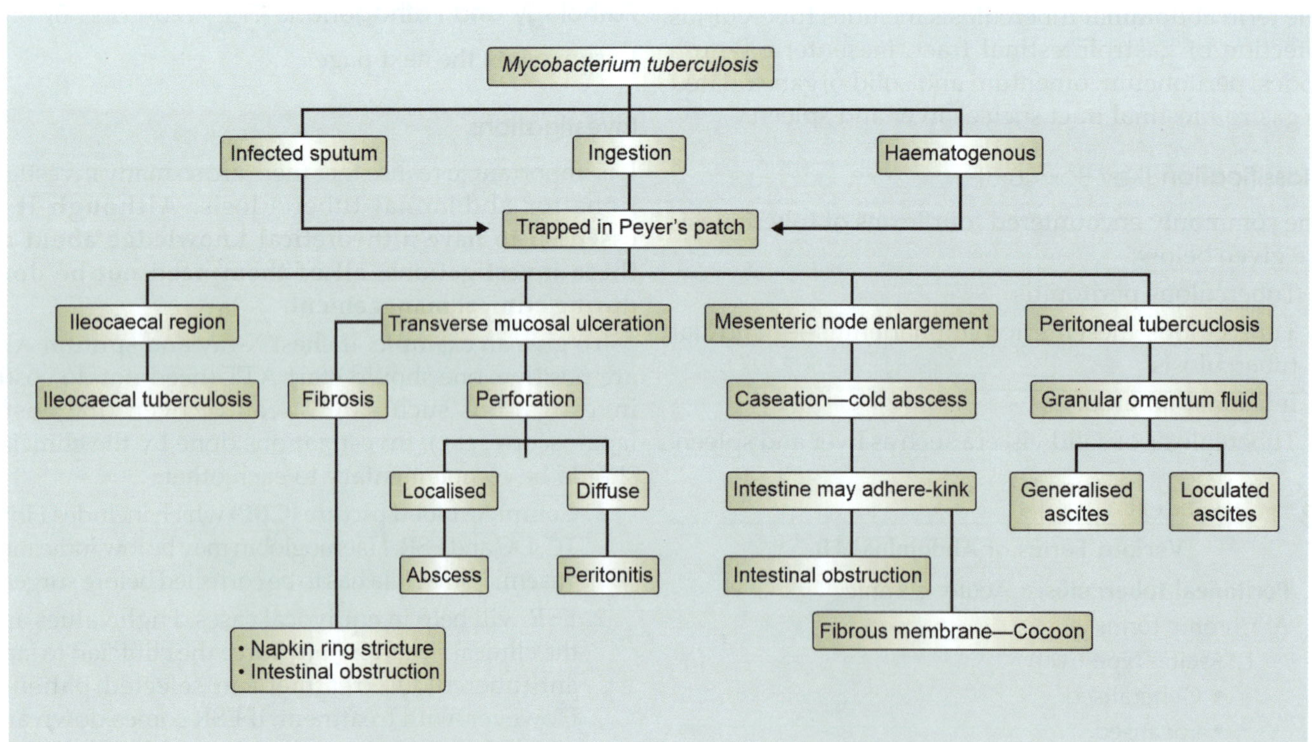

Fig. 46.3B: Abdominal tuberculosis—pathogenesis

- Ascites can be demonstrated and the aspirated fluid is sent for analysis.
- Focal ascites between loops of bowel—**Club sandwich sign** may be seen.
- Enlargement of mesenteric lymph nodes (common) and retroperitoneal nodes (uncommon) can be detected.
- Dilated loops and sometimes peritoneal tubercles are seen as echo-poor shadows.
- Thickening of omentum, mesentery, peritoneum can be found out. (However, ultrasound is not the best investigation to detect these findings.)
- **Pseudokidney sign:** Pulled caecum identified in the right hypochondrium.
- Hepatosplenomegaly may be present.

7. **Ascitic fluid analysis:** Ultrasound-guided fluid is aspirated and about 20–40 ml is sent for analysis (Key Box 46.4).
8. **CECT: Contrast enhanced CT scan of the abdomen:** CT scan is objective. All the findings which can be detected by ultrasound can be confirmed by CT scan. Addition of the contrast is definitely more superior in detecting strictures, dilatations, perforations, and more importantly loculated ascites and

Key Box 46.4

Ascitic Fluid Analysis (Straw-Coloured Fluid)

- Specific gravity is increased—2020 or more
- Glucose <30 mg%
- AFB is rarely demonstrated <3% of cases
- Increased white cell count (>500/cells/cumm), predominantly lymphocytic
- Increased total protein (>2.5 g/dl)
- Serum/ascitic fluid albumin gradient (SAAG*) <1.1 g% units
- LDH >90 units/L
- Decreased pH
- Increased adenosine deaminase
- Bacterial isolation and culture is possible in 20–45% of patients

***SAAG** = Serum albumin level—ascitic fluid albumin level

intra-abdominal collections. CT-guided biopsy can be done. If distension or matting of loops and adhesions are present, it is not safe.

9. **Barium studies:** These are not done routinely. If diagnosis is possible by the various investigations mentioned above, there is no necessity to do them. In fact, it can harm the patient by precipitating obstruction and barium peritonitis, if there is a perforation. Few finding in barium studies can be:
   - Small bowel enema—enteroclysis: Dilatation and narrowed segments in partial obstruction, narrowing of terminal ileum (**Fleischner's sign**), fibrotic terminal ileum opening into the contracted caecum (**Stierlin's sign**).
   - Barium enema: Pulled up caecum, normal acute ileocaecal angle becomes obtuse or sometimes straightening of the ileocaecal angle.
10. **Endoscopy: Upper gastroduodenoscopy** may detect tubercles in the stomach or duodenum—rare.
    - **Push enteroscopy also called small bowel enteroscopy:** Ulcers in the proximal jejunum can be detected and biopsy can be taken—chances of perforation are high.
    - **Colonoscopy** can detect nodular lesions, ulcerations in the colon—caecum and terminal ileum (last 10 cm of ileum should be entered and biopsy should be taken).
11. **Laparoscopy:** This is a diagnostic investigation as it gives the tissue diagnosis (Figs 46.4 and 46.5). One can also evaluate all possible viscera, peritoneum, omentum and pelvic organs. **Biopsy is possible under direct vision**. Findings can be: Straw-coloured peritoneal fluid, abscesses secondary to perforation, rolled up omentum, tubercles on the peritoneal surface, matting of the loops of bowel, adhesions, bands, strictures and dilatations. Other findings which can be appreciated are: Shortened mesentery, caseation of lymph nodes (pseudomesenteric cyst), pulled up caecum and hepatosplenomegaly. Laparoscopy can also be therapeutic, if a stricture is identified, the diseased loop is isolated, brought out and resection and anastomosis/stricturoplasty done (Key Box 46.5).
    - Adhesiolysis can also be done.

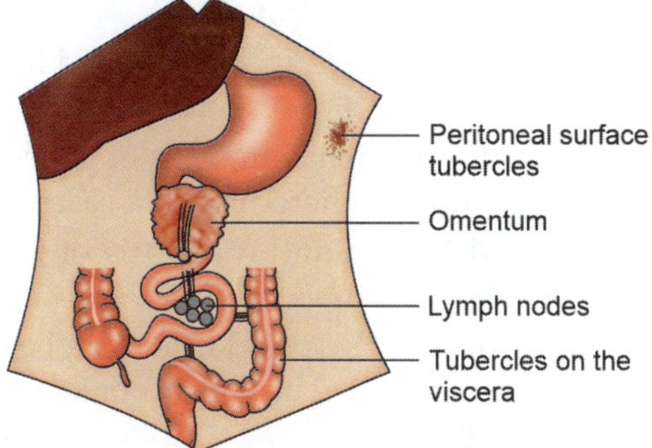

Fig. 46.4: Various sites from where laparoscopic biopsy can be taken in suspected case of abdominal tuberculosis. Biopsy from peritoneal surface and omentum is safe. Otherwise lymph node biopsy can be done

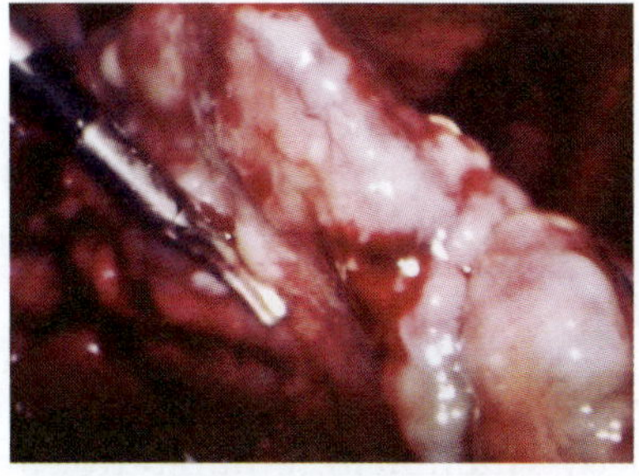

Fig. 46.5: Extensive abdominal tuberculosis. Laparoscopic biopsy being done

Nucleic acid amplification testing (NAAT)—CBNAAT (cartridge based NAAT)/Xpert MTB/RIF helps in both diagnosis of TB and about rifampicin resistance should be done in all patients (page 25).

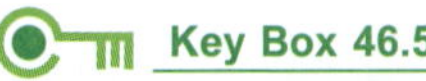

Key Box 46.5

Laparoscopy—Important Findings

- **L**ymph nodes enlargement
- **A**dhesions, matting
- **P**eritoneal nodules
- **A**scites—aspiration—AFB staining
- **R**olled up omentum
- **O**bstruction, stricture

You can remember as **LAPARO**

12. Polymerase chain reaction (PCR):
- It is a technique used in medical and biological research labs.
- One can do functional analysis of genes; useful in the diagnosis of hereditary diseases.
- Helps in detection and diagnosis of infectious diseases, such as tuberculosis.
- Laparoscopically biopsied tissue can be sent for PCR. It can detect 1–2 organisms or 8 fg of mycobacterial DNA.
- Positive PCR indicates infection but it need not be active infection. Hence, it is inferior to tissue diagnosis.
- PCR has 97% sensitivity and 99% specificity.

Antituberculous Treatment

- Details are given in medicine textbooks. However, 4-drug regimen for 2 months followed by 3-drug regimen for 4 months is recommended as a first line of treatment.
- First line of drugs include INH, rifampicin, ethambutol and pyrazinamide given for 2 months. This is followed by rifampicin, ethambutol and INH for 4 months. Refractory cases are treated by kanamycin, ofloxacin, ciprofloxacin, amikacin, etc. *see* clinical notes.

TUBERCULOUS PERITONITIS

Competency

SU28.3.3: Summarize the tubercular peritonitis.

It can be of two types: Acute and chronic. Basically, it produces the following pathological changes:
1. Intense exudation which causes ascitic form
2. Exudation with minimal fibroblastic reaction—loculated form
3. Extensive fibroblastic reaction—plastic form
4. Fibroblastic with secondary infection—purulent form
   - In most of the cases, tuberculous peritonitis results from reactivation of latent primary peritoneal focus (Key Box 46.6).

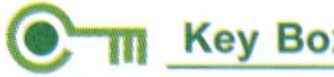 **Key Box 46.6**

Tuberculous Peritonitis

- Cirrhosis
- HIV infection
- Diabetes mellitus
- Underlying malignancy
- Dialysis
- CAPD

Types

1. Ascitic form (Fig. 46.6) (generalised variety)
- It is common in children and young adults. The child is brought to the hospital with abdominal distension.
- Omentum can be felt as a rolled up transverse mass, which is nodular due to extensive fibrosis. Abdomen has a doughy feel with fluid giving rise to shifting dullness.
- Aspiration of peritoneal fluid reveals exudate, which is rich in lymphocytes (Key Box 46.7).
- Peritoneal cavity contains pale-straw-coloured fluid and the peritoneal surface is studded with tubercles.
- Umbilical hernia or congenital hydrocele appears in children due to increased intra-abdominal pressure.

2. Loculated or encysted form (Fig. 46.7)
- In this variety, ascitic fluid is present in one quadrant of the abdomen which is sealed off by matted intestinal coils surrounded by omentum. It gives rise to localised swelling. These patients have no shifting dullness.
- It commonly presents in adults.

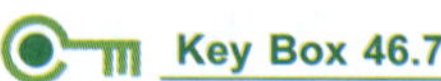 **Key Box 46.7**

Causes of Exudative Ascites—Increase in Protein

Pancreatic ascites
Rare cause: Meig's syndrome
Occlusion: Budd-Chiari syndrome
Tubercular peritonitis
Excess of chylomicrons
Infective: Peritonitis
Neoplasm of peritoneum (carcinoma peritonei)
Remember as **PROTEIN**

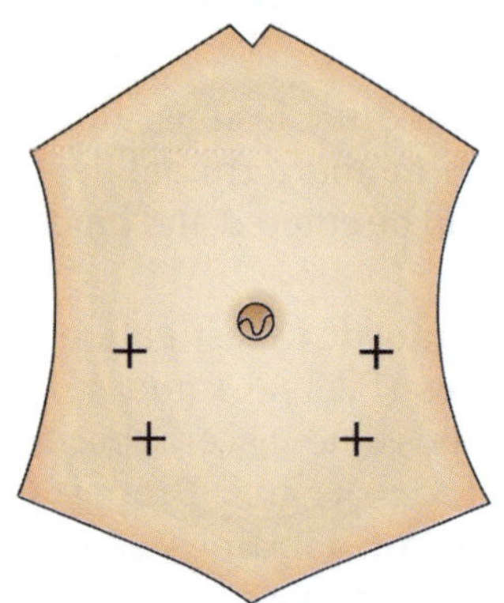

Fig. 46.6: Ascitic form

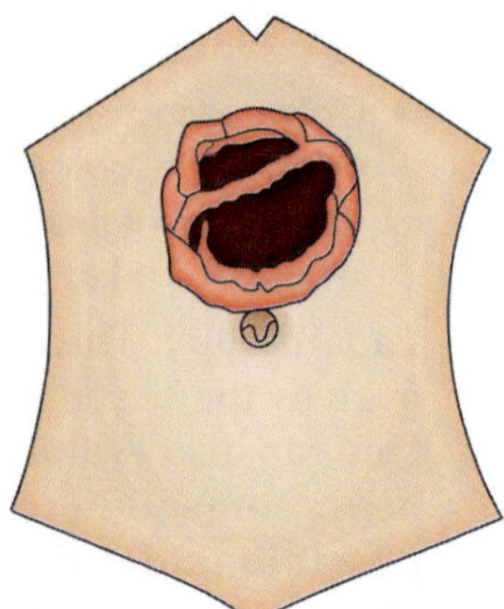

Fig. 46.7: Encysted ascites

- **Differential diagnosis:** Other cystic swellings in the abdomen such as pseudocyst of the pancreas, mesenteric cyst, retroperitoneal cyst.

3. **Fibrous peritonitis (plastic)** (Fig. 46.8)
   - In this variety, **there is no ascites** but there is extensive fibrosis which results in **dense adhesions** between the coils of intestines. Intestines are matted, distended and not able to empty properly due to adhesions and bands. It is associated with **strictures**.
   - This gives rise to blind loop with **steatorrhoea** and **emaciation**.
   - Usually, it presents with **intestinal obstruction** at a later date due to fibrous band which needs to be divided to relieve the obstruction. In some occasions, it is not possible to enter the peritoneal cavity, due to dense adhesions.
   - It is **not uncommon** to create openings in the bowel at laparotomy and end with a helpless situation wherein one will not be able to close the perforation. The net result is fistula formation.
4. **Purulent variety** (Fig. 46.9)
   - Seen in females as a complication of genitourinary tuberculosis (tuberculous salpingitis).
   - The spread occurs through the female genital tract and there is always secondary infection.
   - It presents with acute peritonitis at laparotomy, the peritoneal cavity is seen studded with tubercles, cold abscesses and pus.
   - Laparotomy, drainage of pus, followed by antituberculous treatment is the choice of therapy.
   - It carries poor prognosis because of complications such as toxaemia and faecal fistula formation.
   - Tuberculous peritonitis can be associated with infections of pleural space and pericardial space (effusion). It is called **polyserositis** syndrome.
   - *See* also Figs 46.10 to 46.13.

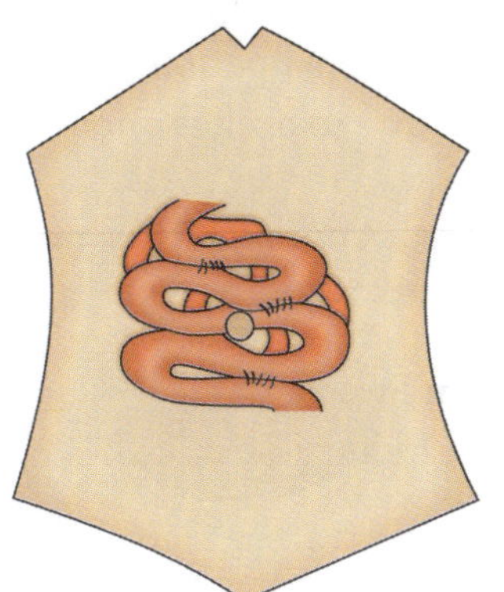

Fig. 46.8: Fibrous peritonitis

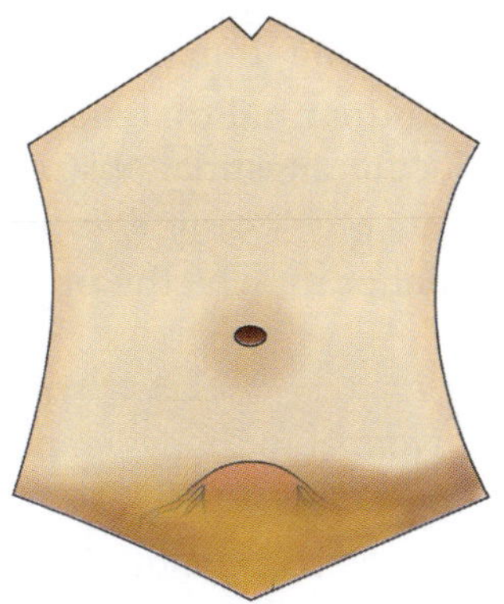

Fig. 46.9: Purulent type

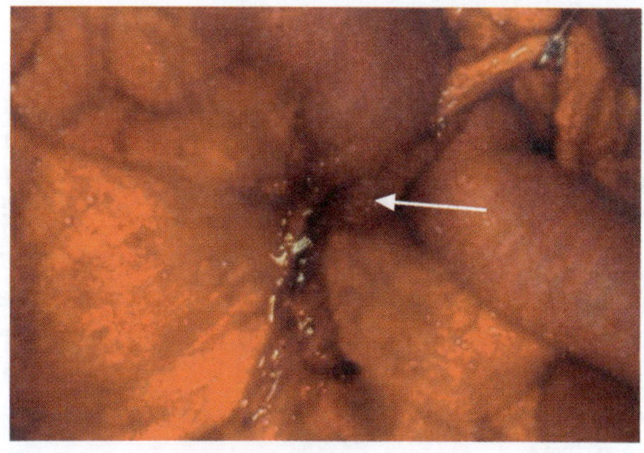

Fig. 46.10: Fibrous bands

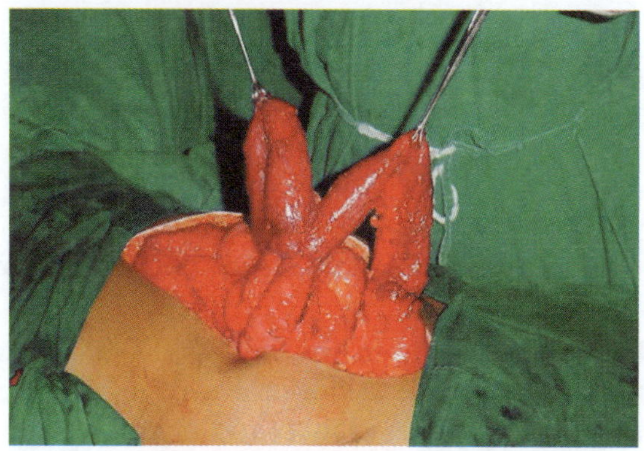

Fig. 46.11: Adhesive form

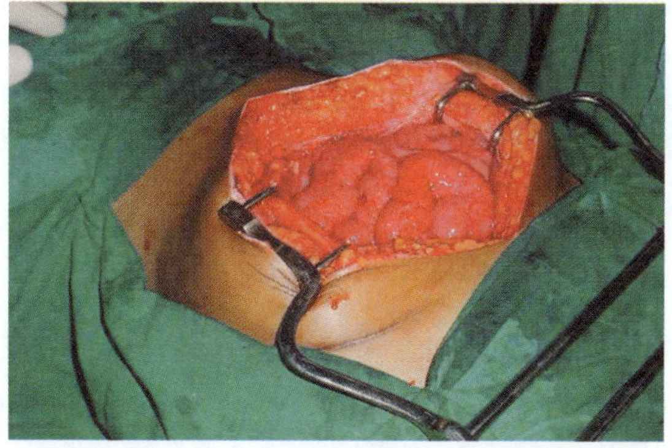

Fig. 46.12: Tubercles on the peritoneal surface

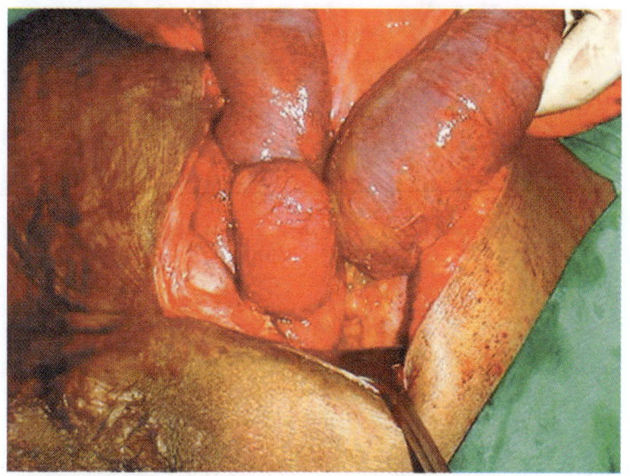

Fig. 46.13: Tuberculous peritonitis

TUBERCULOUS MESENTERIC LYMPHADENITIS

Clinical Presentation

1. **As a calcified lesion** (Fig. 46.14) along the line of mesentery, which extends from L2 vertebra, at the left of vertebral column to the right sacroiliac joint. In 50% of cases, there is no active infection but in the remaining, there is infection. If the symptoms are that of tuberculosis, antituberculous treatment should be given. The shadows caused by lymph nodes are round to oval, mottled and may be regular or irregular.
2. **Acute mesenteric lymphadenitis** (Fig. 46.15)
   - Common in children, clinically mimics acute appendicitis.
   - Pain in the right iliac fossa, vomiting, fever, rigidity can be present.
   - On palpation, tender mass of swollen lymph nodes can be felt in the right iliac fossa.
   - Laparotomy, appendicectomy and biopsy of the lymph node is the procedure of choice.
3. **Chronic lymphadenitis** (Fig. 46.16) in children presents as **failure to thrive**. Fever, loss of weight, loss of appetite, emaciation and pallor are present. Abdomen is protuberant. On deep palpation, nodes can be felt in the right iliac fossa. These nodes have to be differentiated from nodes that enlarge due to lymphoma.
4. **Pseudomesenteric cyst** (Fig. 46.17)
   - This is due to caseation of mesenteric lymph nodes confined within two leaves of mesentery.
   - Due to adhesions, intestines can get kinked or twisted causing intestinal obstruction.

Treatment

- Antituberculous treatment (details in medicine books).

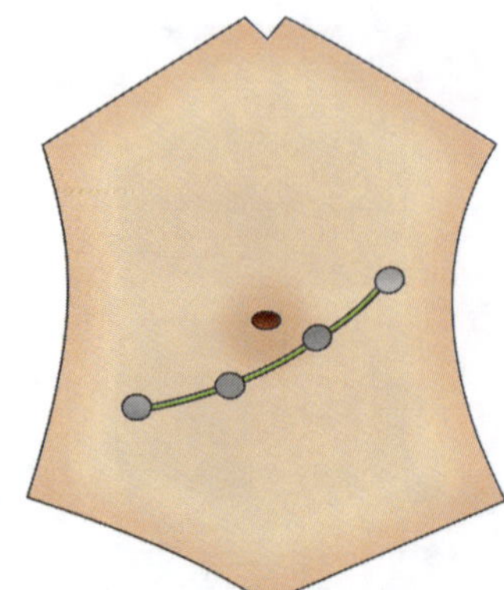

Fig. 46.14: Mesenteric lymph nodes

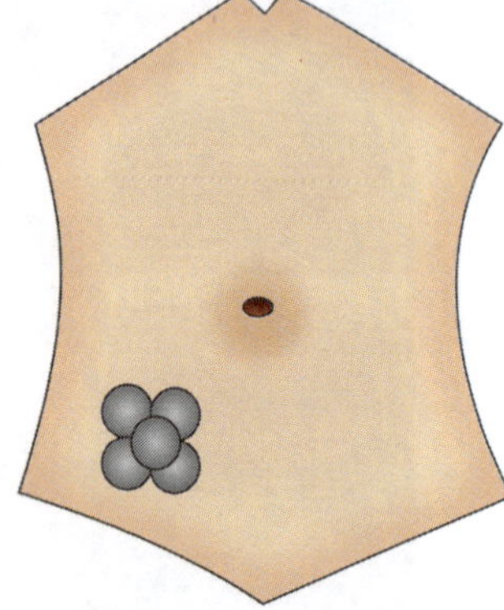
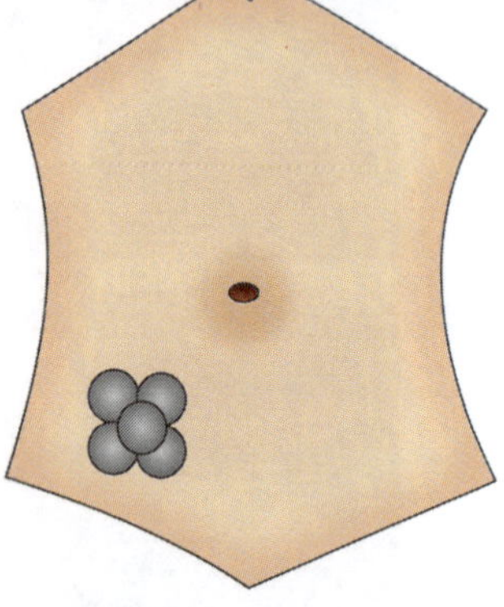

Fig. 46.15: Acute lymphadenitis

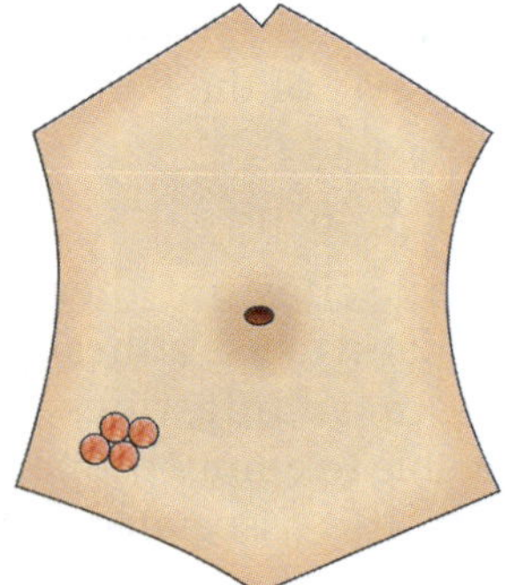

Fig. 46.16: Chronic lymphadenitis

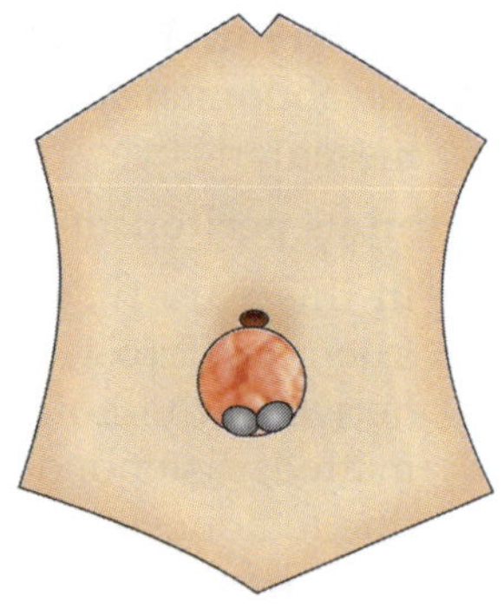

Fig. 46.17: Pseudomesenteric cyst

INTESTINAL TUBERCULOSIS

Ileocaecal region is commonly involved in tuberculosis because of the following reasons:

- Abundant Peyer's patches
- Alkaline media
- Bacterial contact time is more
- Minimal digestive activity
- Maximum absorption in the area
- Stasis due to valve—**ileocecal valve** or **Tulp's valve** or **Tulpius valve** or **Bauhin's valve**

Types (Table 46.2 for comparison)

1. Ulcerative variety
2. Hyperplastic variety
3. Mixed (sometimes)

Clinical Features (Figs 46.18 to 46.20)

- Few features of intestinal tuberculosis such as vague ill health, noisy abdomen, loose stools, evening rise in temperature, not putting on weight are common.
- **Abdominal pain:** It is the most common symptom. It can be a dull, vague pain or colicky pain (stricture) which increases after taking food or relieved by vomiting. Severe colicky abdominal pain vomiting and distension indicate intestinal obstruction.
- **Diarrhoea:** Watery, small quantity, abnormally foul smelling. It may alternate with constipation.
- **Abdominal distension:** It is due to ascites and subacute intestinal obstruction.
- Weight loss is very common. Anorexia, tiredness, pallor may be the presenting features.

Fever with Night Sweats

- Normal for body temperature to increase at night
- Activation of immune system
- Decrease in cortisol and adrenaline levels at night
- Attention of the patient

Table 46.2 Comparison of two forms of intestinal tuberculosis (TB)

	Ulcerative variety	Hyperplastic variety
1. Aetiology	Secondary to pulmonary TB. Occurs due to swallowing of TB bacilli (*Mycobacterium tuberculosis*)	It is a primary intestinal TB, due to *M. bovis*. Milk-borne infection or due to *Mycobacterium tuberculosis*—low grade infection
2. Site	Terminal ileum	Ileocaecal region
3. Virulence of the organism	More virulent	Less virulent
4. Resistance of body	**Very poor**	Good
5. Pathology	Multiple ulcerations in the terminal ileum with/without involvement of lymph nodes. **Ulcers are transverse.** Serosa is reddened and oedematous.	It is **low grade, chronic continuous inflammation** involving ileocaecal region resulting in cicatrising **granuloma** in right iliac fossa (mass in right iliac fossa).
6. Clinical features	Symptoms of **pulmonary TB,** blood and mucus in stool resulting in gross emaciation and cachexia. Diarrhoea is also a feature.	Abdominal pain and diarrhoea may be the initial symptoms for a long time and later fever, weight loss and subacute intestinal obstruction occur.
7. Complications	• **Acute** TB, ulcer perforation—ulcers are transverse because they follow the lymphatics. Treatment is laparotomy and resection of bowel. • **Chronic:** Healing of ulcer results in **stricture** of terminal ileum and **subacute intestinal obstruction.**	Nodular, mobile, **firm mass** in the right iliac fossa which later produces subacute **intestinal obstruction**. Plain X-ray abdomen shows multiple gas and fluid levels (Fig. 46.26)
8. Barium meal follow through (Figs 46.24 and 46.25)	Demonstrates a stricture, or multiple strictures. In the initial stages, ileum is not seen due to hypermotility.	**Barium enema** can demonstrate (i) contracted caecum, (ii) pulled up caecum (subhepatic), (iii) luminal obstruction, and (iv) obtuse ileocaecal angle.
9. Chest X-ray and sputum AFB	Positive	Negative
10. **Colonoscopy and biopsy** (Fig. 46.27)	To confirm the diagnosis	To confirm the diagnosis

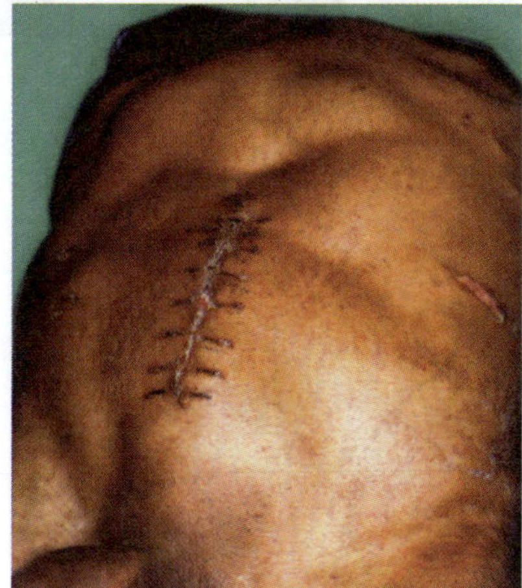

Fig. 46.18: Step ladder peristalsis is seen in a patient who underwent appendectomy for pain in the right iliac fossa. A diagnosis of appendicitis was made and appendicectomy was done. Postoperatively, he had step ladder peristalsis. The case was ileocaecal tuberculosis

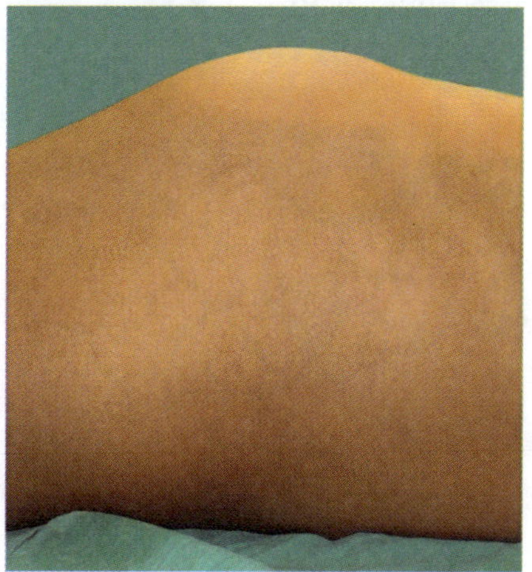

Fig. 46.19: Distension of the abdomen due to ascites—in such cases, there is uniform distension and shifting dullness is positive

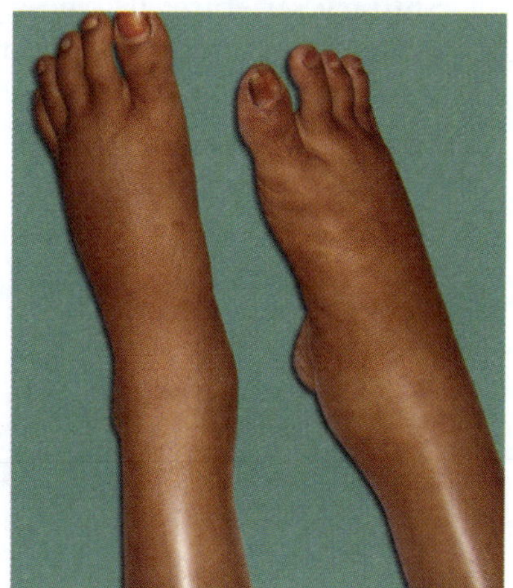

Fig. 46.20: Severe hypoproteinaemia—you can see bilateral pedal oedema. Such cases are mistaken for nephrotic syndrome and were treated also

Signs

- Typically patients are **malnourished and pale.**
- **Visible intestinal peristalsis** may be seen.
- **Distended bowel loops** can be palpated.
- **Doughy abdomen** in case of peritoneal involvement.
- **Rolled up omentum in the epigastrium,** mass in the right iliac fossa due to hyperplastic caecum or in the lumbar region due to pulled up caecum, loculated ascites as encysted mass surrounded by intestines, etc. are other features (Figs 46.21 to 46.23).

Investigations (Refer Table 46.2)

A. **The caseation necrosis** in granulomas is the histologic hallmark of TB.

   In intestinal tuberculosis, the granulomas are multiple, larger (more than 200 μm) and coalescent in mucosa and submucosa—**Langhan type of giant cells.** CB-NAAT has to be done in all cases to look for rifampicin resistance. Few investigations and pictures are given below (Figs 46.24 to 46.27).

B. **The yield of organisms on smear and culture is low. Staining for acid-fast bacilli is positive in less than 3% of cases. A positive culture is seen in only 20% of cases.**

Management of Intestinal Tuberculosis

1. **No evidence of intestinal obstruction:** Antituberculous treatment.
2. **With obstruction (stricture): More details are given in the chapter of intestinal obstruction.**
   A. **Solitary stricture:** It is best treated by stricturoplasty by incising the stricture longitudinally and suturing it transversely (Fig. 46.28).
   B. **Multiple strictures** at long intervals: Stricturoplasty is the ideal treatment.

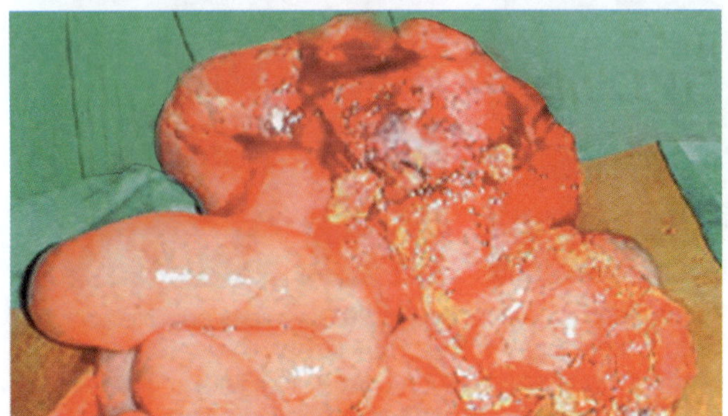

Fig. 46.21: Mass in the right iliac fossa—hyperplastic variety

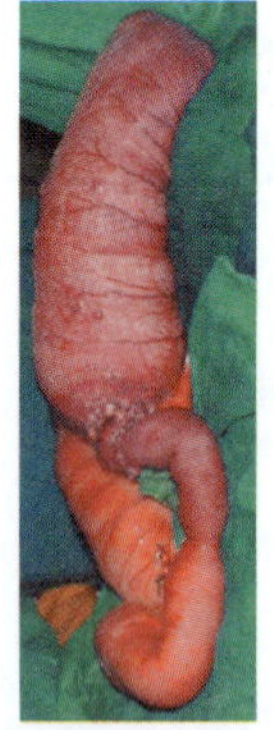
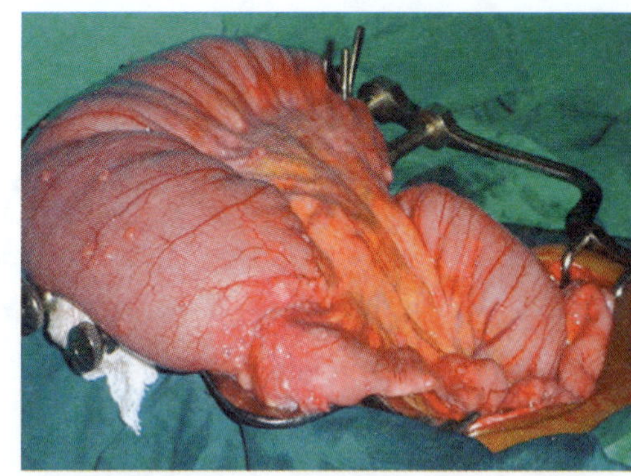

Figs 46.22 and 46.23: Tuberculous stricture with intestinal obstruction—observe the stricture, tubercles and massive proximal dilatation

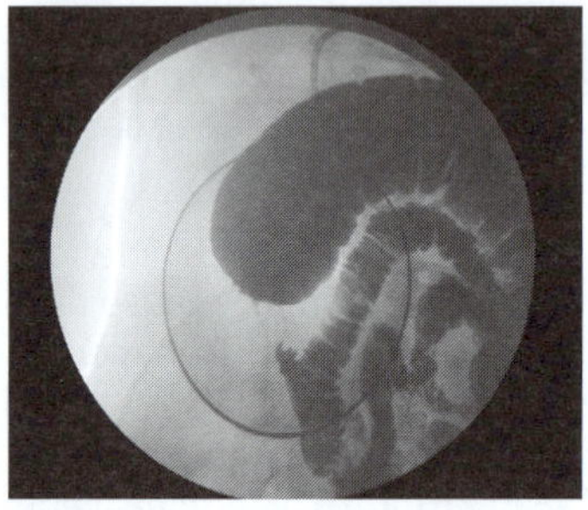
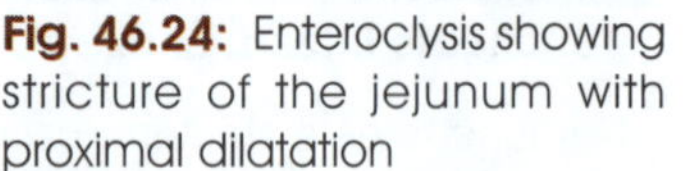

Fig. 46.24: Enteroclysis showing stricture of the jejunum with proximal dilatation

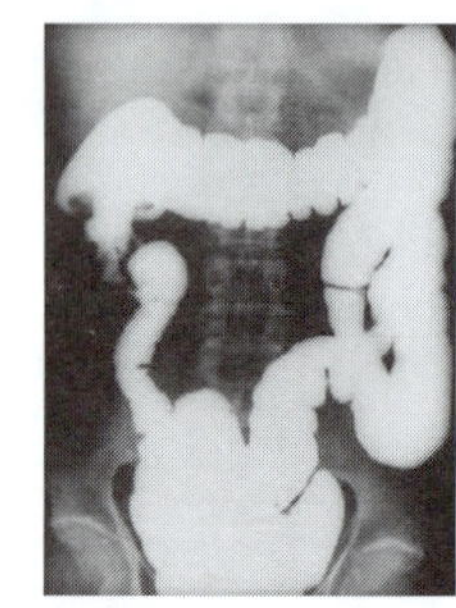

Fig. 46.25: Barium enema—'pulled up' caecum

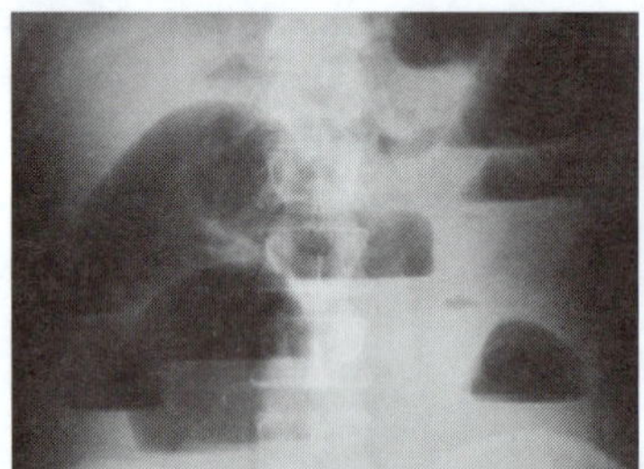

Fig. 46.26: Plain X-ray showing dilated air fluid levels

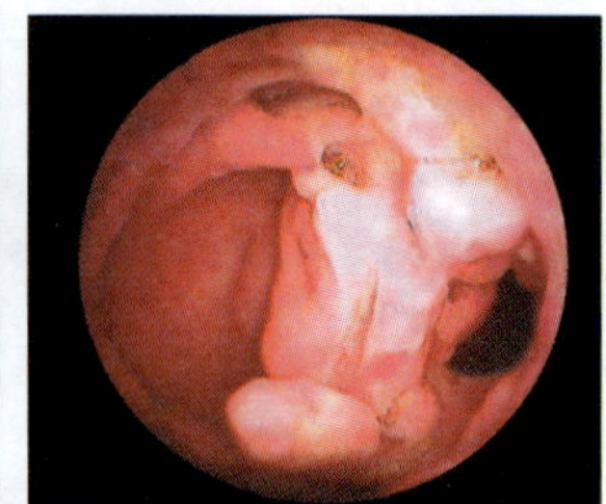

Fig. 46.27: Colonoscopy showing nodular leison in the ascending colon. Biopsy proved tuberculosis

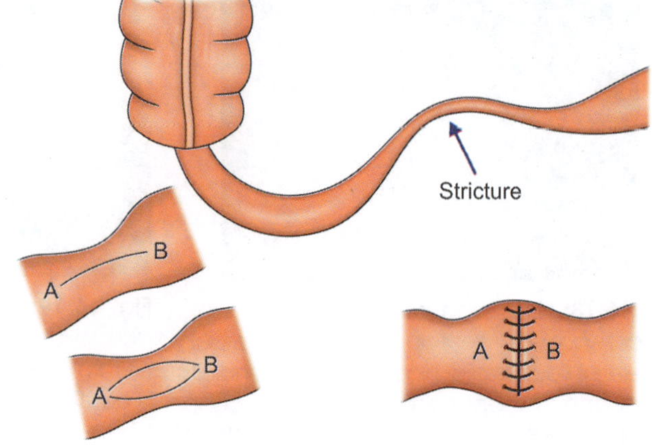

Fig. 46.28: Stricturoplasty

C. **Multiple strictures within a short segment.** Resection is the ideal treatment (Fig. 46.29).

3. **Surgical treatment of hyperplastic tuberculosis:** Limited resection is the treatment of choice. It includes removal of terminal 8–10 cm of the diseased ileum, caecum with appendix, diseased portion of the ascending colon, followed by ileocolic anastomosis. All these cases have to be given antituberculous treatment for a period of 9–12 months. Nutritional supplementation to improve albumin and haemoglobin levels and, if necessary, blood transfusion before and after surgery help in smooth recovery in the postoperative period.

Pearls of Wisdom

Stricture within 10 cm from the ileocaecal junction is best resected.

Complications of Abdominal Tuberculosis

1. **Intestinal obstruction:** Usually it is ileal or jejunal obstruction—details have already been discussed.
2. **Perforation:** It is not uncommon. Carries 6–8% mortality rate specially in late cases with peritonitis.
3. **Malnutrition:** Diarrhoea, loose stools, and blind loop syndromes contribute to malnutrition.
4. **Faecal fistula** is usually due to operated cases of intestinal tuberculosis by resection and anastomosis. In such cases, anastomotic dehiscence may result in faecal fistula. The faecal fistula is not due to direct internal involvement of viscera unlike in Crohn's disease.
5. **Disseminated tuberculosis** *per se* from abdominal tuberculosis is not common. Most of such cases have fulminant pulmonary tuberculosis. This happens in untreated cases and immunocompromised cases.

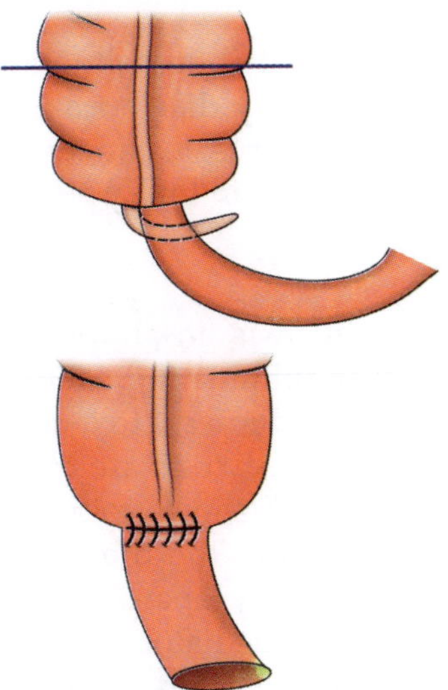

Fig. 46.29: Limited colectomy followed by ileocolic anastomosis

INFLAMMATORY BOWEL DISEASES

Competency

SU28.13.5: Understand the vascular anatomy of small and large intestines and apply the same pathologies like congenital, inflammatory, traumatic, benign and malignant, etc.

Introduction

These are the diseases involving small and large bowel, of unknown aetiology, characterised by multiple ulcerations in the bowel, clinically manifesting as blood and mucus in stools. Ulcerative colitis and Crohn's disease (regional enteritis) are included under this heading. Both diseases can present as acute abdomen with intestinal obstruction and complications such as perforation toxaemia, etc. Also both are premalignant conditions for carcinoma colon. **Ulcerative colitis is a mucosal disease and Crohn's is a transmural disease.**

ULCERATIVE COLITIS

Aetiology

1. **Autoimmune factor:** Even though exact mechanism of ulcerative colitis is not clear, there are some factors which may point out to autoimmune reaction. They are:
   - Presence of **cytotoxic T lymphocytes** against colonic epithelial cells in the lamina propria of the bowel.
   - Presence of **anticolon antibodies**.
   - Whatever be the immune mechanisms, activation of inflammatory mediators such as cytokines, growth factors and arachidonic acids takes place and they are responsible for the disease.
2. **Dysfunctional immunoregulation** in the intestinal wall results in inappropriate production of **cytokines**. This creates an imbalance between various interleukins resulting in inflammatory changes.
3. **Psychosomatic and personality factors:** Ulcerative colitis is more common in western women. Emotional stress, family stress, and stress from divorce are the contributing factors. Periods of activity and remission is common.

Pearls of Wisdom

Western, white, worrying women's disease is ulcerative colitis.

4. **Dietary factors**
   - Westernisation of the diet which is rich in red meat has been blamed. Vegetarian diet is supposed to protect the colonic mucosa.
   - **Allergy to milk protein** is responsible for ulcerative colitis in a few patients.
5. **Defective mucin production** and a defective mucosal immunological reaction is considered as a chief factor responsible for ulcerative colitis.

Pearls of Wisdom

Appendicectomy and smoking have been protective factors for development of ulcerative colitis.

6. **Genetic:** 15% of patients have first degree relatives with ulcerative colitis.

Pathology (Key Box 46.8)

- The disease always starts in the rectum and spreads in a backward manner, thus involving the entire colon in majority of cases. In 5% of cases, terminal ileum can also be involved—**back wash ileitis.**
- **Anus is not involved in ulcerative colitis.**
- The disease manifests as multiple, small superficial ulcers—**pinpoint ulcers.**
- As the disease progresses, inflammation spreads into the submucosa of the colon.
- Destruction of muscle is described as myocytolysis. Attempt at healing may produce **pseudopolyp**. There are areas of epithelial hypertrophy in between the ulcers, resembling polyp. Healing with fibrosis results in a narrow, contracted colon, called **pipe stem colon**.
- Microscopy: **Pus** (abscess) in the crypts and pus cells (inflammatory cells) in the lamina propria are typical of ulcerative colitis.
- Long-standing cases will change into dysplasia of the epithelium—dysplasia associated lesion (DAL).

Key Box 46.8

Pathology of Ulcerative Colitis

Pinpoint ulcers
Pseudopolyposis
Pipe stem colon
Pus cells
Observe **4 Ps**

Clinical Features

- More common in females. Female:male ratio is 2:1.
- Age: Common age of presentation is 3rd decade followed by 4th and 2nd decades.
- The disease is characterised by passage of 15–20 stools per day and contains blood and mucus. Sometimes, it may be watery diarrhoea (Key Box 46.9). As the rectum loses elasticity and lumen collapses, tenesmus occurs.
- Relapses and remissions are common and are related to emotional disturbances. Tenesmus, urgency with severe inflammation result in incontinence.
- Severe dehydration, malnutrition, anaemia, hypoproteinaemia are late features.

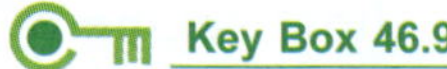

Key Box 46.9

Types—Depending Upon Severity

- **Mild colitis:** Refers to <4 stools/day without systemic signs and symptoms.
- **Moderate colitis:** Refers to <6 stools/day without systemic toxicity.
- **Severe colitis:** Refers to >6 stools/day with systemic toxicity—fever over 37.5°C, tachycardia more than 90/min, hypoalbuminaemia less than 3 g/dl, weight loss more than 3 kg

- Acute fulminating attack is associated with high grade fever, bloody dysentery, distension and tenderness all over the abdomen with profound weakness. Hypokalaemia, acidosis, anaemia and shock are the other features.

Clinical findings in severe disease

Temperature
Tachycardia
Tender colon—abdomen
Tenesmus—anaemia, hypoproteinaemia
Terrific disease—dehydration, hypokalaemia, acidosis, shock

Types of Ulcerative Colitis (depending upon the extent of the colon involved)

1. **Proctitis:** In about 20–25% of the patients, the disease involves only rectum. In such patients, stools are semisolid because of absorption of water by normal colon. Also, the intensity of the disease is not severe and risk of cancer is 2–5%.
2. **Left-sided colitis:** It is found in 15% of patients. It presents as severe recurrent attacks of diarrhea with blood in stools, without systemic toxicity (Fig. 46.30).
3. **Total proctocolitis:** It is seen in about 25% of the patients. Severe bloody diarrhoea and hypoproteinaemia are its features. Chances of cancer and complications are high in this group (Fig. 46.31).

Complications

1. **Toxic megacolon:** It is an abdominal emergency encountered with fulminating colitis. Severe abdominal pain and tenderness, toxaemia, high fever, tachycardia and leucocytosis are the features. Plain X-ray abdomen which shows colon with a diameter more than 6 cm gives the diagnosis. It requires emergency treatment by laparotomy and colectomy. Local inflammatory mediators such as interleukins and nitric oxide are released from smooth muscles. Activities of macrophages are also increased. This

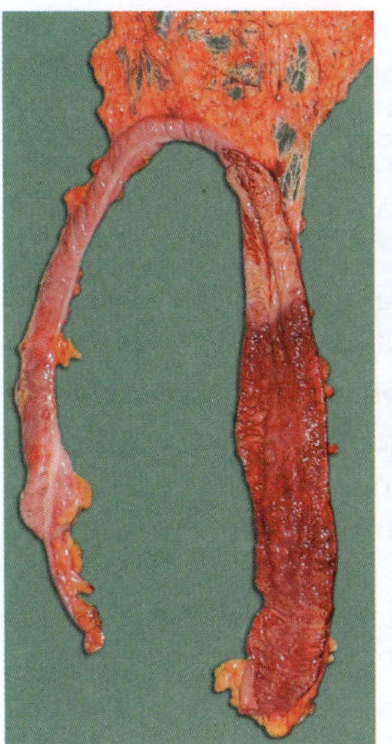

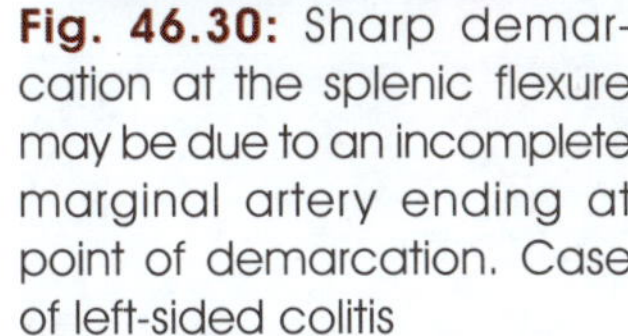

Fig. 46.30: Sharp demarcation at the splenic flexure may be due to an incomplete marginal artery ending at point of demarcation. Case of left-sided colitis

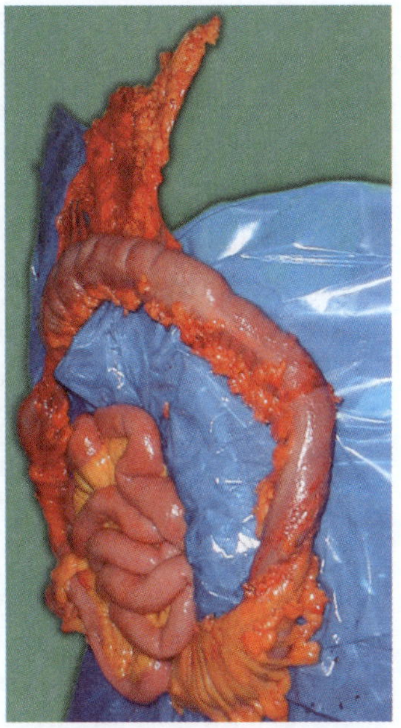

Fig. 46.31: Fully mobilised colon. Observe loss of haustrations. Total proctocolectomy with ileal pouch to anal anastomosis was done. A case of total proctocolitis

results in colonic dysmotility and toxic dilatation. As a result, mucosal sloughing, bacterial translocation, perforation/septicaemia and death can occur in untreated cases. Antidiarrhoeals, anticholinergics, narcotics, and hypokalaemia exaggerate this condition. Supportive treatment and intravenous corticosteroids are necessary (Key Box 46.10 and Figs 46.32 and 46.33).

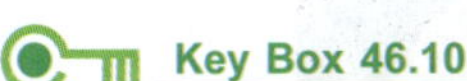

Key Box 46.10

Factors Precipitating Toxic Megacolon

- Barium enema
- Opiates, antidiarrhoeal drugs, anticholinergic agents
- Not known
- Ulcerative colitis, salmonella colitis
- Pseudomembranous colitis, amoebic colitis

2. **Massive haemorrhage** per rectum is uncommon. It is treated by blood transfusion.
3. **Perforation** is treated as peritonitis with resection of colon. Mortality rate is around 25–50%. Steroids may mask the symptoms. In an emergency situation, saving life is more important. Hence, resection followed by ileostomy should be done.
4. **Carcinoma of the colon** (Key Box 46.11)
   - Overall incidence is 3% when the disease has been present for 15 years.

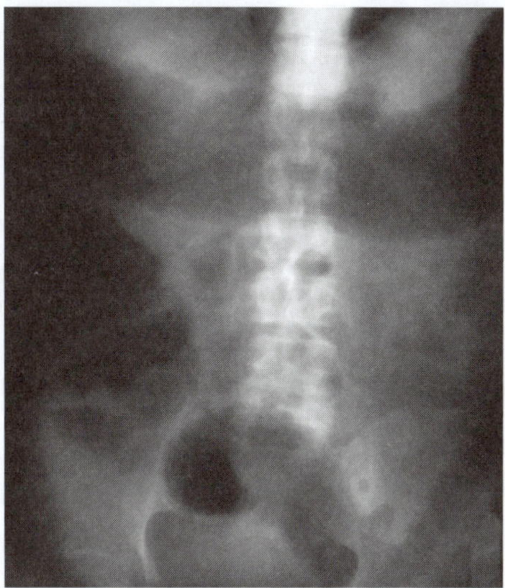

Fig. 46.32: Plain X-ray abdomen showing dilated transverse colon more than 6 cm is suggestive of toxic megacolon

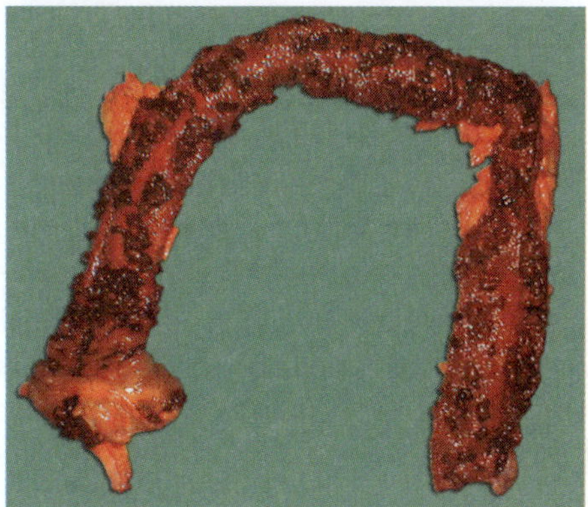

Fig. 46.33: Total colectomy for toxic megacolon specimen showing pseudopolyposis

Key Box 46.11

Ulcerative Colitis (UC) and Colorectal Cancer (CRC)

- CRC is more aggressive
- Multicentric and synchronous cancers
- UC patients with primary sclerosing cholangitis (PSC) have increased risk of CRC
- More advanced stage at the time of presentation
- Risk increases with duration of the disease
- Malignancy develops on a background of dysplasia [dysplasia associated lesion or mass **(DAL-M)**]

   - At the end of 25 years, the incidence may be around 20%.
   - Hence, routine sigmoidoscopy and biopsy have to be done when the disease is present for more than 10 years and if it shows epithelial dysplasia, it should be considered as premalignant.
   - Incidence is more in total proctocolitis and when the disease has started in the early age group.

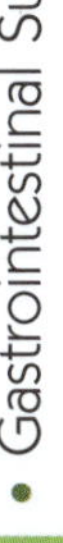

5. **Recurrent perianal abscess** resulting in perianal fistula, occurs in about 15–20% of patients.
6. **General complications (extraintestinal)**
   - **Protein malnutrition** resulting in cirrhosis. Primary sclerosing cholangitis is also found in many cases. Fatty acid infiltration is seen in 40% of cases. It is reversible after control of disease.
   - **Skin ulcerations**, pyoderma, erythema nodosum, etc. reflect protein malnutrition.
   - Conjunctivitis, iritis, arthritis involving large joints are also other features.
   - Incidence of **bile duct cancer** is high in these patients.

Pearls of Wisdom

Peripheral arthritis and ankylosing spondylitis are the two most common extraintestinal manifestations.

Differential Diagnosis

- **Crohn's disease** should be ruled out first. The differences between the two inflammatory bowel diseases have been discussed at the end of the chapter. In general, diarrhoea and bleeding are more common with ulcerative colitis than Crohn's disease.
- **Dysenteries:** Bacillary dysenteries, shigellosis, salmonellosis, amoebiasis and other dysenteries have to be kept in mind specially in developing countries including tuberculosis which has been already discussed.
- **Diverticular disease of the colon:** However, when complications including bleeding occur, diverticular disease of the colon and in cases of perforations, malignant perforation must be considered as a differential diagnosis.

Investigations

1. **Stool:** It is done mainly to rule out various causes of infective diarrhoea—amoebiasis, *Shigella, Clostridium difficile.* Most common cause of infective colitis in UK is *Campylobacterium.*
2. **Sigmoidoscopy** (Key Box 46.12): Can demonstrate inflammatory changes in the mucosa. Mucus, pus and blood are visible. Multiple ulcers are visible with bleeding.

Key Box 46.12

Sigmoidoscopy—Findings

Amoebic ulcer	Ulcerative colitis
Large	Small, pinpoint
Deep, flask shaped	Superficial
Mucosa in between ulcer is healthy	Mucosa in between ulcers unhealthy

3. **Barium enema findings in ulcerative colitis** (should not be done in acute cases) (Figs 46.34A and B)
   - Contracted colon/pipe stem colon
   - Absence of haustrations and mucosal irregularity
   - Pseudopolyposis appears as stippled appearance
   - Retrorectal space is increased.
4. **Colonoscopy** (Figs 46.35 and 46.36)
   - To confirm the diagnosis by biopsy
   - To find out the extent of involvement of colon
   - To follow up patients who are on treatment
   - To rule out carcinomatous changes
5. **Plain X-ray abdomen:** To rule out megacolon and perforation.
6. **C-reactive protein:** Its levels are very high in case of acute fulminating attack or toxic megacolon.
7. Electrolytes, albumin levels are low. They have to be corrected especially in severe cases.

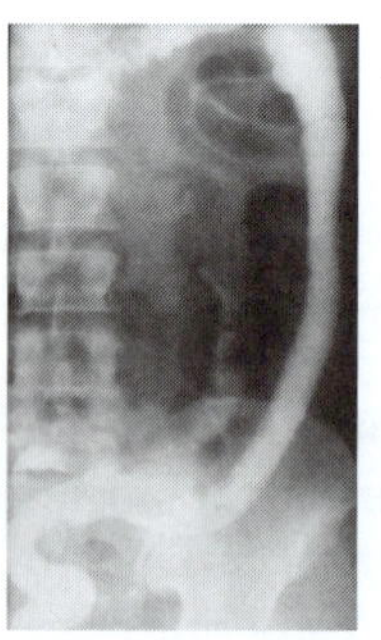

Fig. 46.34A: Barium enema showing pipe stem colon

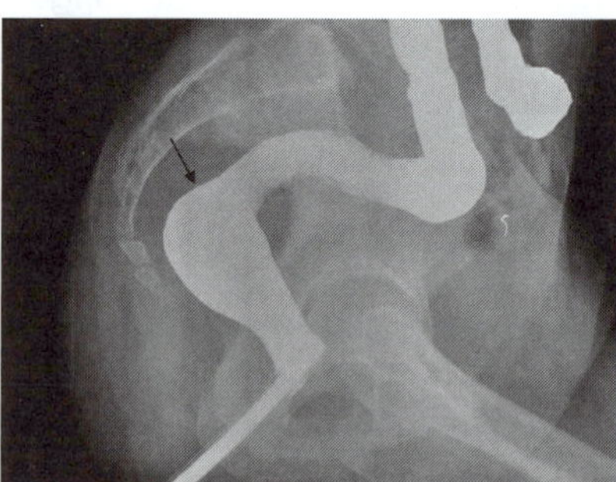

Fig. 46.34B: Barium enema demonstrating increased space between the rectum and sacrum

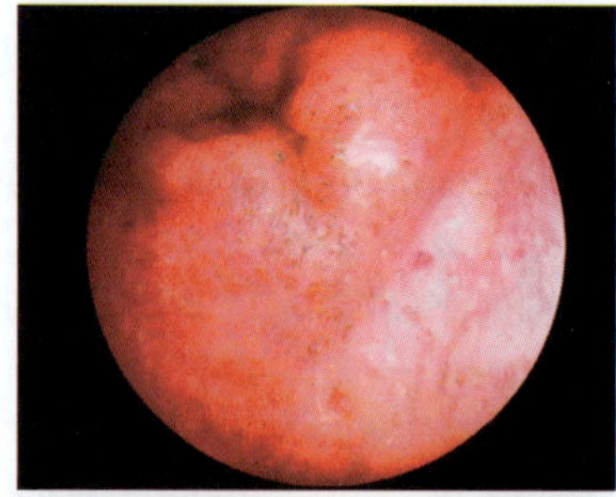

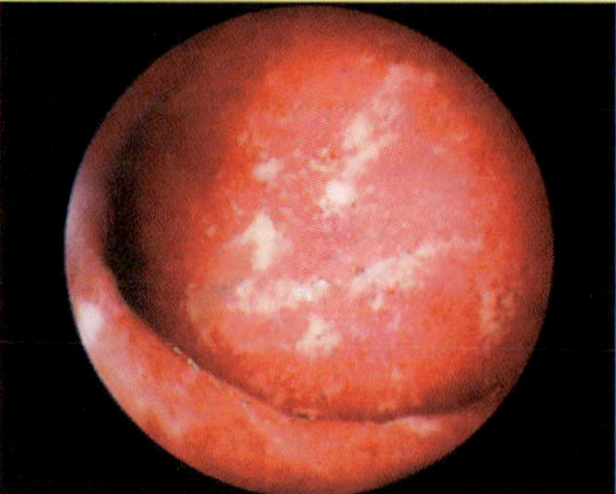

Figs 46.35 and 46.36: Colonoscopy—pinpoint ulcers with bleeding (*Courtesy:* Dr Filipe Alvares, Former Medical Gastroenterologist, KMC, Manipal)

Treatment of Ulcerative Colitis

I. Conservative Line of Management (Table 46.3)

- Hospitalisation and bed rest
- Correction of fluid and electrolyte imbalance
- Blood transfusions to correct anaemia and TPN for hypoproteinaemia (Fig. 46.37).
- **Salazopyrines** are given in the dose of 2 g/day. Mode of action: When given orally, it gets split into 5-aminosalicylic acid and sulphapyridine in the colon. This suppresses activity of prostaglandins E_1 and E_2 and thus reduces inflammation. They are used mainly to induce remission. They act as inhibitors of the cyclooxygenase enzyme system.
- **Corticosteroids:** Less severe cases not responding to salazopyrines are given a trial of oral prednisolone 60 mg/day. They decrease the frequency of stools. The dose is tapered off over 3–4 weeks.
- In acute attacks, IV hydrocortisone 100 mg is given.
- Prednisolone retention enema: 20 mg in 200 ml saline in intractable diarrhoea. It avoids systemic toxicity. Prednisolone 20–40 mg/day can also be given orally for 3–4 weeks.
- **Role of cyclosporine:** Those patients who do not respond to corticosteroids, can be given IV cyclosporine 4 mg/kg/day. It can induce remission.
- **Role of monoclonal antibodies:** These drugs act against antitumour necrosis factor alpha. They regulate inflammatory cascades. Infliximab or adalimumab are drugs. Vedolizumab is a rescue agent which blocks integrins.

II. Surgery

Indications for Surgery

- Complications—toxic megacolon, perforation.

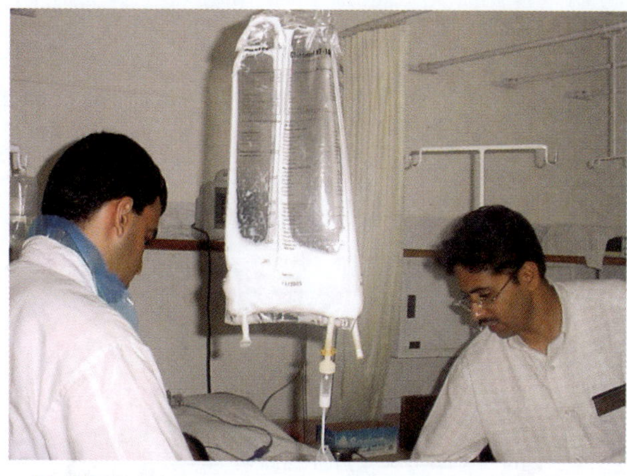

Fig. 46.37: Total parenteral nutrition (TPN) before and after surgery for ulcerative colitis plays an important role in the recovery of the patient, as these patients are grossly emaciated and hypoproteinaemic

- Active disease in spite of medical line of management
- Severe disease not responding to medical treatment
- Dysplasia on biopsy
- Steroid dependence
- Haemorrhage

Pearls of Wisdom

Failure to improve within 7 days of maximum medical treatment with steroids and cyclosporine is an indication for surgery.

1. **Restorative proctocolectomy** with ileal pouch:
   - This can be done as one- or two-stage procedure.
   - Total proctocolectomy is done first.
   - A mucosectomy of the upper anal canal is done.
   - A pouch is created by anastomosing the loops of ileum. A J-shaped pouch is the most popular followed by W pouch (Figs 46.38 to 46.41).

Table 46.3 Pharmacotherapy in ulcerative colitis

Drug	Dose	Mode of action
1. Salazopyrines—**first choice**	• 2–4 g/day • Anti-inflammatory • Immunosuppressive	• Suppresses PGE_1 and E_2
2. Steroids—refractory cases	• IV hydrocortisone 100 mg 8th hourly • Prednisolone enema • After acute illness, prednisolone 40–60 mg/day	• Anti-inflammatory
3. Immunomodulators • Cyclosporine used in refractory cases	• Azathioprine 6-mercaptopurines	• Act at DNA level and inhibit T lymphocyte functions
4. Monoclonal antibody – Antitumour necrosis factor-alpha (TNF-α) Infliximab		• Antitumour necrosis
5. Anti-inflammatory (salicylic acid)	• Olsalazine (Dipentum) • 500 mg 1–2 times/day	• Directly targeted/released into the colon

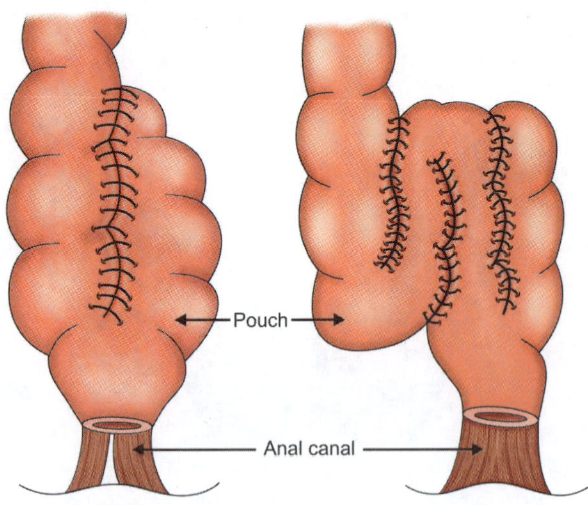

Fig. 46.38: J pouch

Fig. 46.39: W pouch

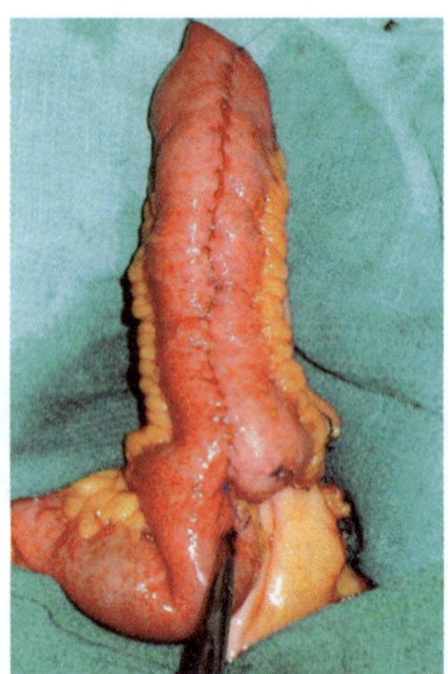

The length of the pouch is generally 15 cm and capacity around 300 ml when distended. Note that it is a two-layered anastomosis to create the pouch. The same can be achieved by linear stapling device.

Fig. 46.40: J pouch (*Courtesy:* Dr Prasad Babu TLVD Ramcharan Thyagarajan, Srikanth Gadiyaram, Prof Sadiq S Sikora, Department of Surgical Gastroenterology, Manipal Hospital, Bengaluru)

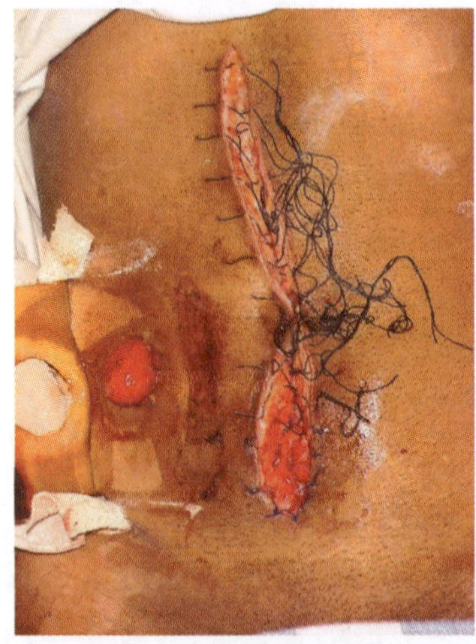

Wound was sutured after 48 hours because wound infection is a common complication after this surgery

Fig. 46.41: Total proctocolectomy with a pouch and protective ileostomy was done here

- The pouch is anastomosed to the dentate line (junction of upper and lower anal canal) by using stapler or by hand sutures.
- Protective ileostomy is done and it can be closed after two months.

2. **Total proctocolectomy** followed by permanent ileostomy (ileoanal anastomosis should not be done because of incontinence). Ileostomy is connected to ileostomy bag. Adhesive obstruction and chronic perineal sinus are late complications. This is the procedure with least complications (Figs 46.42 and 46.43).

Advantages of a pouch

- Avoids ileostomy.
- Continence is preserved and patient is able to pass the stools *via* naturalis.
- At the same time, all the diseased **mucosa** has been removed. Thus, the risk of cancer is negligible.
  - Pouchitis is a complication.
  - *See* Table 46.4 also.

Complications of pouch

- Inflammation of the pelvis due to leak.
- Adhesion causing postoperative intestinal obstruction.
- Pouch—vaginal fistula.
- Frequency of the stools around 4 to 10 times/day.
- Pouchitis: It is inflammation of the pouch. Seen in about 30% of patients. Features represent original disease such as tenesmus, frequency of stools, toxicity, etc. Metronidazole can be used to treat.

Prognosis

In general, emergency colitis is required in about 25% patients with severe attacks. Perforation has a mortality rate of up to 40% because of faecal contents and toxicity. Incidence of carcinoma colon is about 10–15%. Longer the duration of the disease, higher is the incidence.

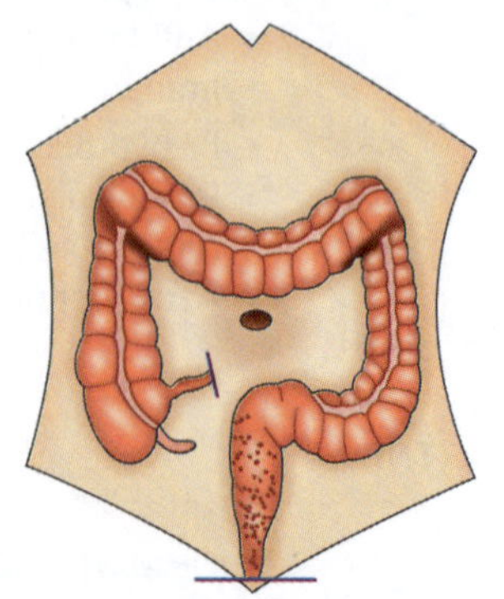

Fig. 46.42: Total colectomy

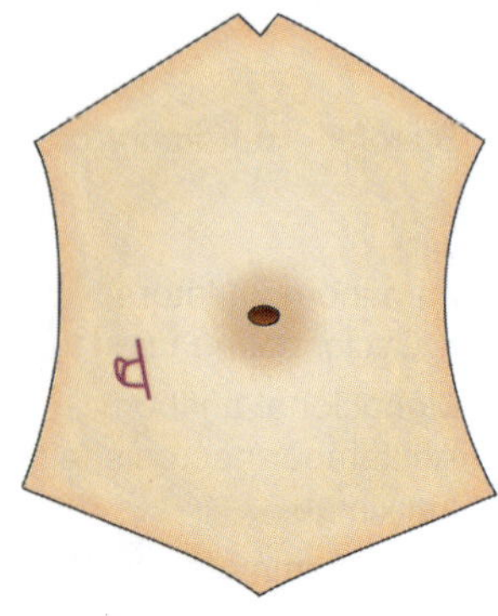

Fig. 46.43: Ileostomy

Table 46.4 Treatment of ulcerative colitis			
	Mild	**Moderate**	**Severe**
Admission	Not required	Not required	Required
Rectal steroid	Yes	Yes	No
Prednisolone	Oral 20–40 mg	Yes	IV hydrocortisone 100–200 mg/4 times/day
5-ASA	Can be given	Can be given	Not given
Nutrition	**Oral**	**Oral**	TPN/**oral/high calorie diet**
Fluid/electrolyte balance	Normal	Normal	Imbalance is very common
Blood transfusion	No	Yes	Yes
Surgery	Not done	Not done	No response for 3–5 days—**surgery**

5-ASA: Amino salicylic acid
TPN: Total parenteral nutrition

Dietary Advice

- High protein, carbohydrates, whole grains, and good fats. Meat, fish, poultry, and dairy products, breads and cereals; fruits and vegetables may be consumed.
- For vegetarians: Dairy products and plant proteins—such as soya bean products may be consumed.
- To avoid: High fibre high residue diet—thus to control diarrhoea.
- To avoid: Caffeine—coffee, dried fruits and nuts, alcohol, meat, spicy food, oily food, soda, etc.

ILEOSTOMY

- Ileostomy is a surgical procedure wherein a loop of the ileum or end of the ileum is brought to the exterior (surface of the body).
- Two types are usually done: End ileostomy and loop ileostomy.
- End ileostomy is done following total proctocolectomy. It is a permanent ileostomy. The ileum is brought out through the lateral edge of rectus abdominis. It should project at least 5 cm outside (Fig. 46.44).
- Loop ileostomy is done to divert gastrointestinal contents to protect ileo-pouch anastomosis. It is a temporary ileostomy which is closed after 6–8 weeks.
- Permanent ileostomy is also required following total colectomy for carcinoma colon. It is an end ileostomy (Figs 46.45 to 46.47).
- Ileostomy care includes maintenance of fluid and electrolyte balance, use of disposable ileostomy bag and skin protection.
- Complications of an ileostomy are similar to that of colostomy—retraction, prolapse, bleeding, stenosis.
- Precautions—living with an ileostomy.

1. Ileostomy bag has to be fitted well to the body surface. It needs to be adjusted often.
2. Ileostomy has to be emptied 4–6 times depending upon the requirement.
3. Chewed and masticated food is better.
4. Avoid gas forming diet. Patients will learn slowly what to take and what not to take.
5. Long-term complications include—gallstones, kidney stones, adhesions and intestinal obstruction.

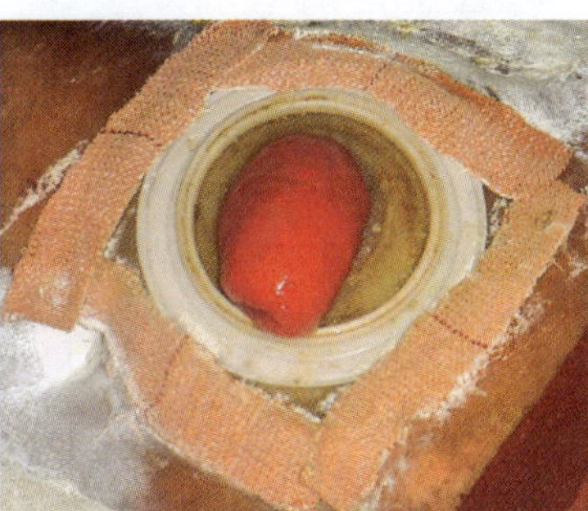

Fig. 46.44A: Ileostomy: It should project out for at least 5 cm

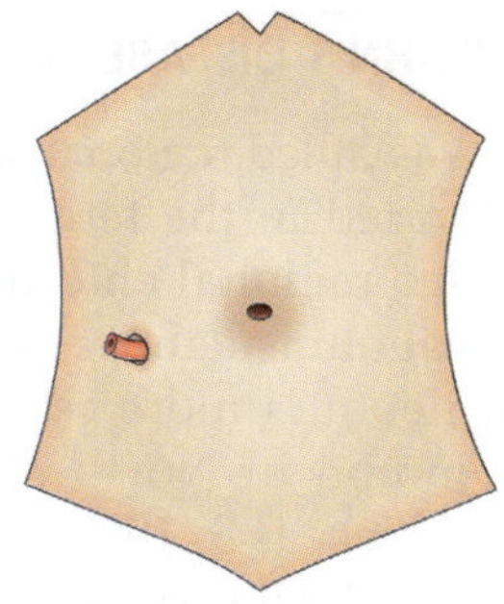

Fig. 46.44B: End ileostomy: Following total protocolectomy

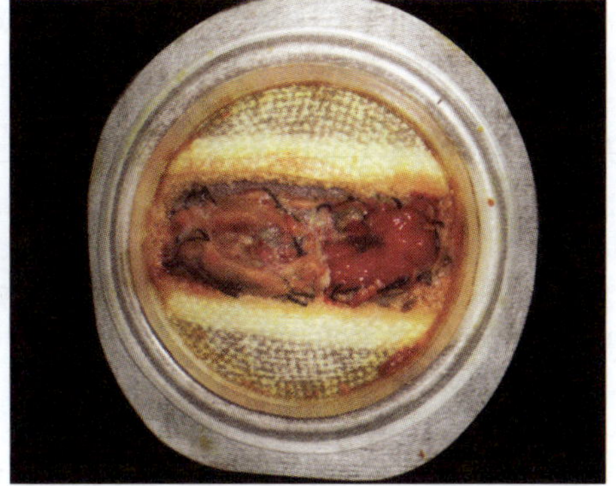

Fig. 46.45: Doubtful viability—complication of the ileostomy

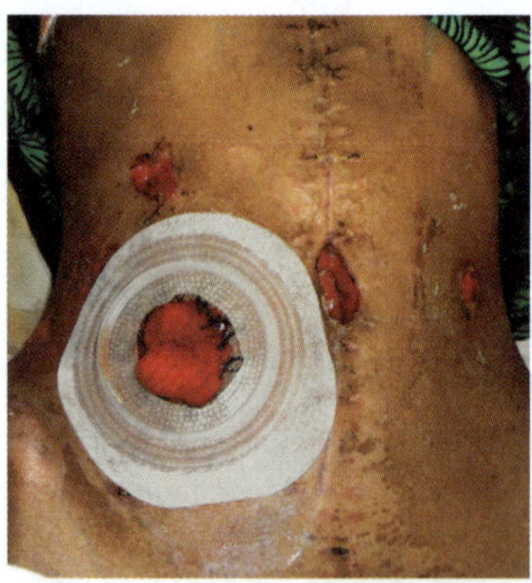

Fig. 46.46: An 18-year-old girl was diagnosed with acute appendicitis. At exploration, tuberculosis of ileum was diagnosed. Limited colectomy was done following which ileum was brought outside as temporary ileostomy

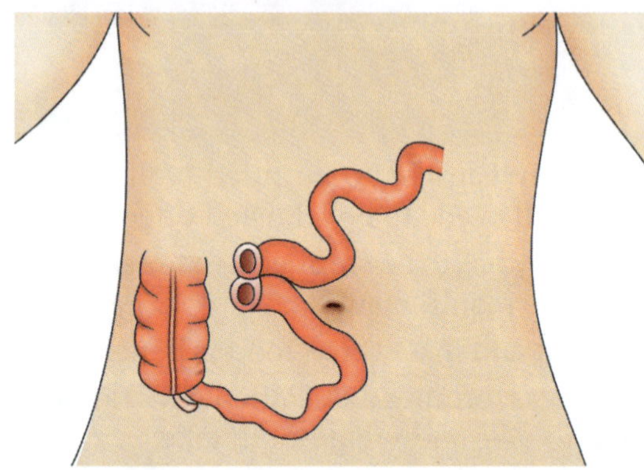

Fig. 46.47: Loop ileostomy is done following resection of perforated enteric ulcer. Distal ileum was friable and oedematous. Hence it was brought out. This is a safer option

CROHN'S DISEASE

It was called regional ileitis because the disease was first reported in the terminal ileum. However, today it is called **regional enteritis** because the disease can occur in jejunum, ileum, colon, oesophagus, etc. Involvement of ileum is more common, followed by colon. More common in North America and Northern Europe. Incidence is 8/100000 population and in UK incidence is 145/100000 population.

Definition

Crohn's disease is a chronic transmural inflammatory disease of the gastrointestinal tract of unknown aetiology. It is neither neoplastic nor tuberculous.

Aetiology

1. **Infectious agents:** *Mycobacterium paratuberculosis* and measles virus have been proposed as potential causes of Crohn's disease. However, it should be noted that antimicrobial therapy has not been effective in eradicating Crohn's disease (unlike ATT in TB). Also, no immunological reaction has been found.
2. **Immunologic factors:** Similar to UC. Focal ischaemia due to autoimmune reaction has also been considered.
3. **Genetic factors:** Single strongest risk factor for development of Crohn's is a relative with Crohn's disease.
   - Relatively high incidence is found in Ashkenazi jaws.
4. **Smoking:** It increases the risk of Crohn's disease threefold unlike its protective effect against ulcerative colitis.
5. **Diet and Crohn's disease:** Increased intake of carbohydrates and diet rich in refined food have been blamed for. Increased intake of animal protein, milk protein and increased ratio of omega-6 to omega-3 polyunsaturated fatty acids have also been blamed.

Pathogenesis of Crohn's Disease

Pathogenesis of Crohn's Disease—Early Events

Mucosa exposed to antigens
↓
Increase gut permeability
↓
Cell-mediated response
↓
Interleukin-2 and tumour necrosis factor are released
+
Defective suppressor T cells
(Normally, it prevents escalation of this response)
–
Inflammation

Pathology (Key Box 46.13)

- Disease **starts in terminal ileum** as ulcerations of intestine in about 60% of cases.
- There is extensive inflammatory oedema and mucosal ulcers are present. Fibrotic thickening of the intestine results in **hose pipe rigidity** of the intestine.

Key Box 46.13

Pathology of Crohn's Disease

Transmural inflammation
Reticulation cobblestone
Aphthoid ulcers
Noncaseating cicatrising granuloma
Skip lesions
Mesenteric lymph nodes enlarged
Ulcers are in ileum, jejunum, colon, etc.
Rigidity—Hose pipe
Adhesions occur soon
Linear ulcers
Remember as **TRANSMURAL**

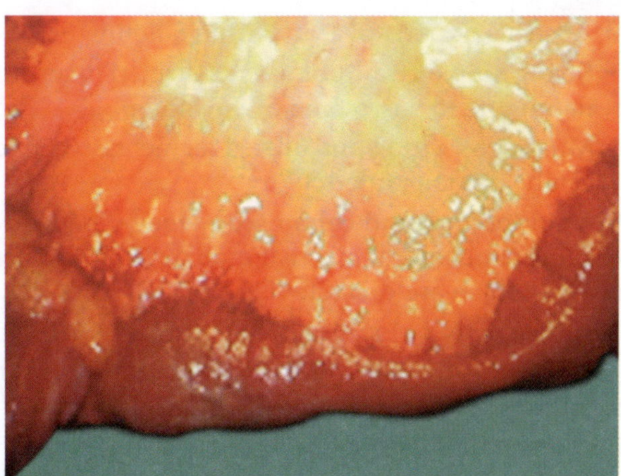

Fig. 46.48: Crohn's disease—creeping fat (*Courtesy:* Dr Ramesh Rajan, Gastrointestinal Surgeon, Trivandrum Medical College, Kerala)

- There are **skip areas** which are characteristic of Crohn's disease (segments of intestine are normal in between).
- **Mesenteric nodes are enlarged.** They can be calcified but do not show any caseation.
- **Intense infiltration of mononuclear cells** and lymphoid hyperplasia is common.
- As the disease progresses, there is cicatrizing granuloma of the bowel wall. This results in narrowing of lumen causing intestinal obstruction. **Caseation is characteristically absent.**
- Once inflammation spreads to the serosa, adhesions develop between bowel loops or other structures. Abscesses occur in the mesentery which rupture resulting in internal fistula (Fig. 46.48).

Pearls of Wisdom

Transmural inflammation is characteristic of Crohn's disease.

Clinical Features

(Key Box 46.14 and Figs 46.49 to 46.51)

The disease is often **insidious**, slowly progressive with a protracted course and commonly affects young adults in the second or third decade of life. Intermittent colicky lower abdominal pain, diarrhea and weight loss are common. Depending upon symptoms, it can be classified as follows (Table 46.5):

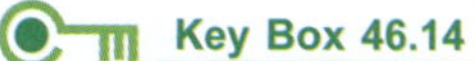

Key Box 46.14

Various Stages/Complications of Crohn's Disease

Colitis—ileocolitis
Rectal—anorectal disease
Obstruction due to stricture
Hollow viscus fistulae
Nutritional deficiencies
Remember as **CROHN**

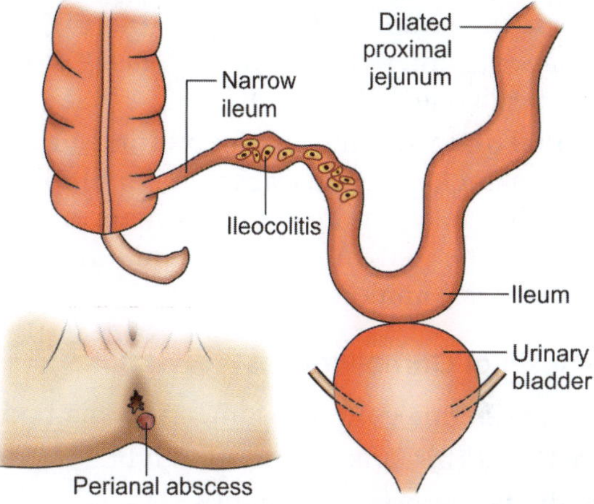

Fig. 46.49: Clinical features of Crohn's disease (*Courtesy:* Ms Vidushi, MBBS student, KMC, Manipal)

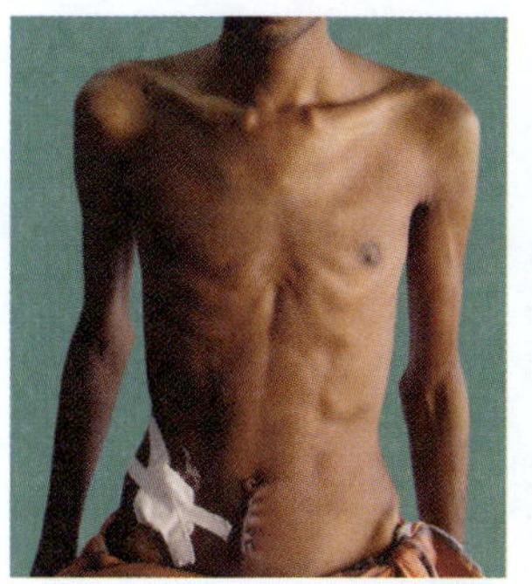

Fig. 46.50: An emaciated patient who underwent appendicectomy, only to present later with features of Crohn's disease

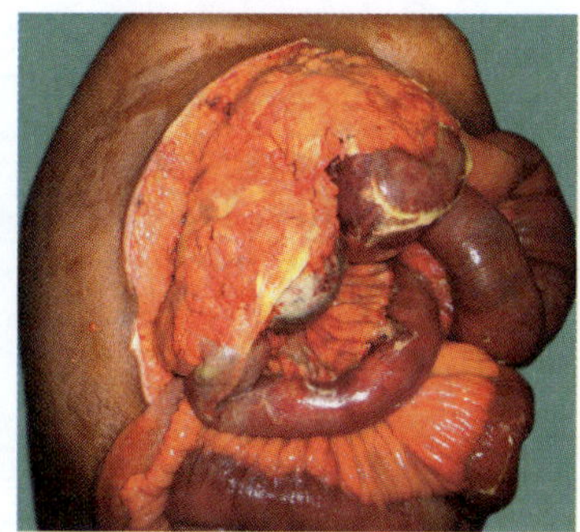

Fig. 46.51: Congested bowel loops, area of perforation, dilated loops of bowel are seen in this picture

Table 46.5 Crohn's disease

Colitis	Obstruction	Mass	Nutrition	Anorectal disease
↓	↓	↓	↓	↓
Diarrhoea	Cramps, distension	Right iliac fossa	Emaciation	Fissure, abscess
↓	↓	↓	↓	↓
Water Weight loss	Vomiting	Gurgling, tender, obstruction	Dehydration	Fistula *in ano*

1. **Stage of ileocolitis:** Clinically, it presents as pain abdomen and mucus in stools. It is seen in younger patients. It may be associated with fever. Presence of pain and tenderness in the right iliac fossa mimics appendicitis. If there is a mass, it may be confused for an appendicular mass.
2. **Stage of subacute intestinal obstruction** occurs due to stricture of the terminal ileum. Strictures can be multiple. They are not reversible.
3. **Stage of fistula formation:** It can be enteroenteric or enterocutaneous. Following are the examples of fistulae encountered in Crohn's disease—ileovesical, ileocolic, ileoileal, ileovaginal, etc.
4. **Perianal disease** in the form of multiple ulcers in the anorectal region, perianal abscesses, multiple fistulae in ano are much more common than in ulcerative colitis. Repeated infection of anal crypt due to diarrhoea is common.

Extraintestinal Complications

- Skin: Pyoderma gangrenosum, erythema nodosum
- Joints: Arthritis, ankylosing spondylitis
- Bile duct: Sclerosing cholangitis
- Eyes: Iritis, uveitis
- Nephrotic syndrome
- Pancreatitis
- Amyloidosis
- Crohn's disease that affects the ileum—increased risk of **gallstones**. This is due to a decrease in bile acid resorption in the ileum.

Pearls of Wisdom

Anal fissure is the most common anal problem in Crohn's disease. Noncaseating granuloma is most common in anorectal disease.

Differential Diagnosis

1. **Ulcerative colitis:** However, colonic symptoms are more with ulcerative colitis.
2. **Tuberculosis:** In India, tuberculosis should be considered first and ruled out.
3. **Appendicitis:** Acute pain in the right iliac fossa can be confused for acute appendicitis. For benefit of the doubt, the patient can undergo laparotomy. Laparoscopy and appendicectomy will be better.
4. **Intestinal obstruction:** Other causes of obstruction have to be kept in mind.

Investigations

1. **Small bowel enema:** Enteroclysis.
   - **Cobblestone** reticulation because of multiple ulcers with islands of normal mucosa in between.
   - Absence of peristalsis in terminal ileum.
   - **String sign of Kantor** is demonstrated in terminal ileum due to narrowing of the lumen.
   - Multiple strictures and dilated segments in between can be demonstrated.
2. **Sigmoidoscopy and colonoscopy** may demonstrate inflamed mucosa, which is granular with **aphthoid ulcers**, which are **discrete** (Fig. 46.52).
3. **Fistulography** to localise the internal fistula.
4. **CT scan:** It is done to detect thickening of bowel and extraintestinal disease (Fig. 46.53).
5. Remember to investigate upper GI tract with gastroduodenoscopy and capsule endoscopy (*see* page 907).

Treatment

I. General principles

- Complete rest, avoid stress and emotions.
- A low residue, high caloric diet such as high protein diet.
- Some patients may require total parenteral nutrition—some at home called home parenteral nutrition.

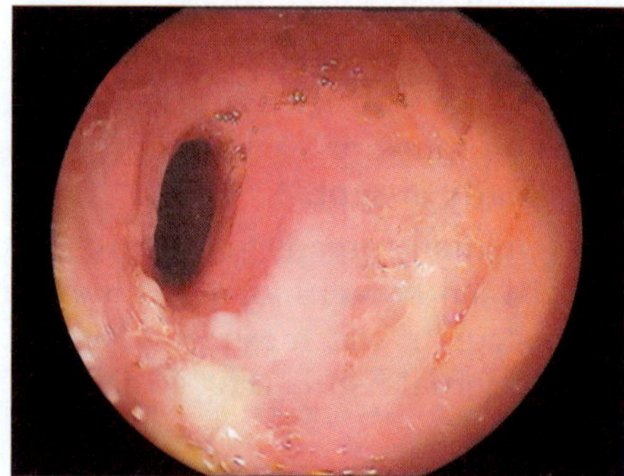

Fig. 46.52: Colonoscopic view of Crohn's disease

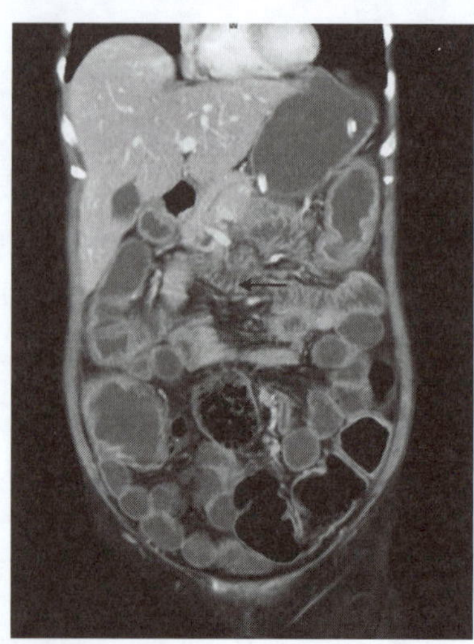

Fig. 46.53: CECT scan: Crohn's disease showing thickening of intestinal loops

II. Conservative (medical) treatment is similar to ulcerative colitis.

- Steroids are the mainstay of treatment. They are effective in inducing remission in 70 to 80% of cases.
- Steroids are most effective in treating small intestinal disease. They are anti-inflammatory. They do control diarrhoea, induce remissions. Prednisolone is used for short-term treatment. Long-term use can give rise to toxicity such as immunosuppression, bone loss, delayed wound healing, etc.
- Salazopyrines can be used especially in maintenance cases also.
- Even though salazopyrines and corticosteroids have been beneficial in Crohn's disease, salazopyrines do not induce remissions. They are used in acute ileocolitis. Steroids can be used for anorectal disease.
- Immunosuppressive therapy using azathioprine and 6-mercaptopurine are also effective.
- They are effective in treatment of colonic disease. The main concern is bone marrow toxicity. 6-mercaptopurines are known to produce pancreatitis.
- Most recent and promising drug is **infliximab**—a monoclonal antibody to tumour necrosis factor α (TNFα). It mainly helps in **closure of fistula**. It is given intravenously and is used for intestinal and perianal disease.
- Metronidazole has shown some benefit.

III. Surgical treatment: Resection is not the aim of surgery but it may have to be done in cases of obstruction, perforation, intra-abdominal abscesses, internal fistulae, bleeding and malignancies. Depending upon the involvement of the bowel, various resections are possible. Examples:

1. Stricture—stricturoplasty or resection
2. Ileocaecal resection (Figs 46.54A and B)
3. Colectomy and ileorectal anastomosis
4. If the fistulae are present, they are disconnected from the bowel and excised.

Comparison of intestinal tuberculosis, ulcerative colitis and Crohn's disease is given in Table 46.6.

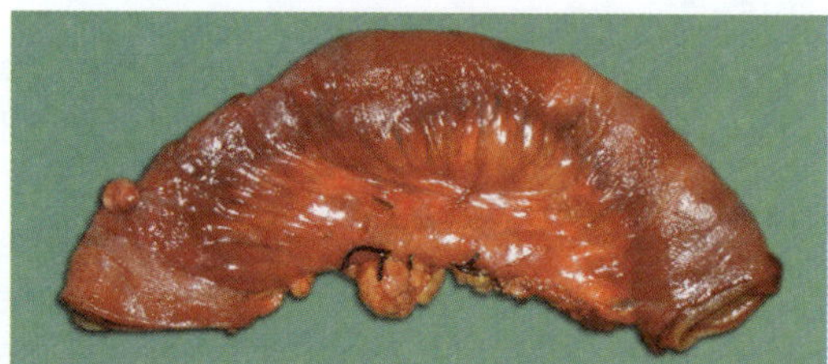

Fig. 46.54A: Resected specimen of small intestine. The patient had intestinal obstruction

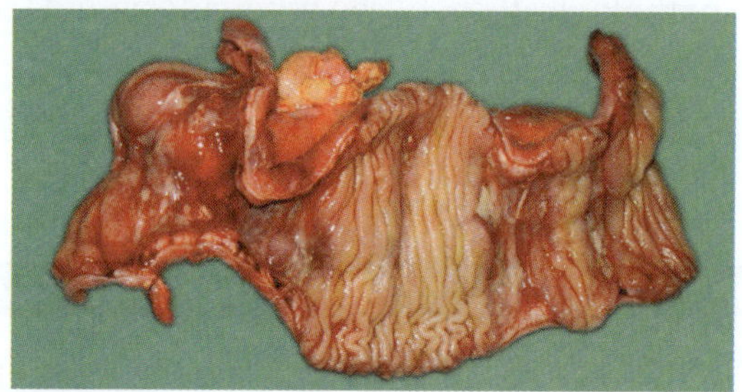

Fig. 46.54B: Opened specimen showing stricture. Biopsy proved Crohn's disease

Table 46.6 Summary of tubercular ileocolitis, ulcerative colitis and Crohn's colitis

	Tuberculosis	Crohn's	Ulcerative colitis
1. Bacteria	Mycobacterium	No	No
2. Pathology	Continuous spread. Caseating granuloma, lymph node caseation. Transmural inflammation present	Skip areas. Cobblestone granuloma present. No caseation. Deep longitudinal ulcers. Transmural inflammation	Continuous, pseudopolyposis. Pinpoint ulcers. Crypt abscesses. Superficial ulcers. Mucosa and submucosa involved
3. Site	Ileocaecal	Terminal ileum and colon	Rectum and colon
4. Bowel wall	Thick and fibrotic	Thick fibrotic	Thin
5. **Clinical**			
Bleeding	Uncommon	Uncommon	Very common
Diarrhoea	Uncommon	Very common	Very common
Fever	Common	Common	Rare
Mass	Very common	Common	Rare
Anal disease	Rare	Very common	Rare
Toxic megacolon	Never	Rare	More common
Fistulae	Uncommon	Very common	Uncommon
Stricture	Common	Common	Rare
6. Malignancy	No	Can predispose (low)	High incidence

Prognosis

- In spite of various treatment, there is no cure for the disease. About 10–20% patients come with relapses and recurrent symptoms.
- Despite for repeated treatment including surgical procedures, survival is still good as compared to general population without the disease.

A Few Observations in Crohn's Disease

- Ileum is the most common site.
- Small bowel alone is affected in 20–30% of the patients.
- Both small bowel and large bowel in 50–60% patients.
- Duodenum, stomach, oesophagus can also be involved.
- Inflammatory cells and mediators of the inflammation such as cytokines, interleukins, tumour necrosis factors produce the inflammatory changes resulting in granuloma.
- Sometimes, very difficult to differentiate clinically and pathologically between tuberculosis and Crohn's disease.
- Anus is involved in Crohn's colitis, not in ulcerative colitis.

SURGICAL COMPLICATIONS OF ENTERIC FEVER

During the third week of enteric fever, *Salmonella typhi, paratyphi* (enteric bacilli) multiply in Peyer's patches and can give rise to the following problems:

1. **Haemorrhage** is seen in about 5–10% of cases due to ulceration of Peyer's patches. It can be occult, obvious or rarely massive bleeding. It is managed conservatively in majority of cases.
2. **Perforation of terminal ileum:** An oval, vertical perforation results in peritonitis. Enteric perforation need not give rise to all signs of peritonitis. Guarding and rigidity can be minimal because of poor, immunocompromised nature of the disease and due to **Zenker's degeneration** of abdominal wall muscles. It is a single perforation in about 85% of the cases. It is situated in the antimesenteric border of the terminal ileum. Typically, it occurs in the third week of enteric fever. Bradycardia, dehydration, toxicity are the other features.
   - **Hyperplasia of reticuloendothelial system** including lymph nodes, liver and spleen is characteristic of typhoid fever (Key Box 46.15).
   - **Diagnosis of perforation** is based clinically on the acute abdominal pain, bleeding per rectum with/without guarding and rigidity. High grade fever, toxicity and bradycardia are other features that help in the diagnosis.
   - **Plain X-ray abdomen** may not reveal gas because of small sealed off performation.
   - **The most useful investigation is CT scan** which can reveal not only pneumoperitoneum but also pericolic collection, which can be missed by ultrasound (*see* the clinical notes).

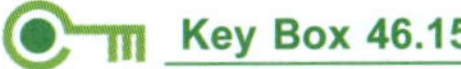

Key Box 46.15

Typhoid Fever—Salient Features

- **T**oxic—dehydrated delirious patient with diarrhoea—green pea soup stools
- **Y**oung patient
- **P**oor tone of the abdominal muscles due to Zenker's degeneration
- **H**igh grade fever
- **O**ther—hepatosplenomegaly, Rose spots
- **I**mmunocompromised status
- **D**ecreased pulse rate—**Faget sign**

You can remember as **TYPHOID**

Pearls of Wisdom

- When you suspect peritonits, no guarding and no rigidity.
- When you suspect perforation, no gas under diaphragm.
- When you suspect toxicity, no tachycardia but bradycardia, suspect enteric ulcer.

Treatment:

- Third generation cephalosporins are used.
- **Emergency laparotomy, resection of bowel** and end-to-end anastomosis or closure of the perforation by using non-absorbable sutures. Abdomen is closed with a tube drain kept in the right iliac fossa. Wound infection is common in such cases. Multiple fistulae are also common (Figs 46.55 to 46.58).

Enteric Ulcer Perforation

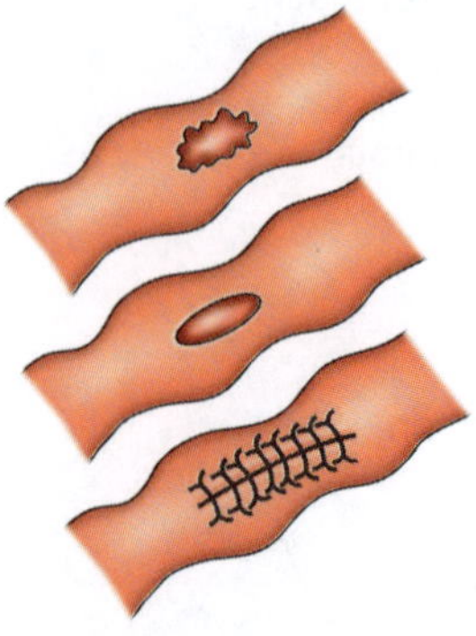

Resection

Fig. 46.55: Single ulcer, simple suturing

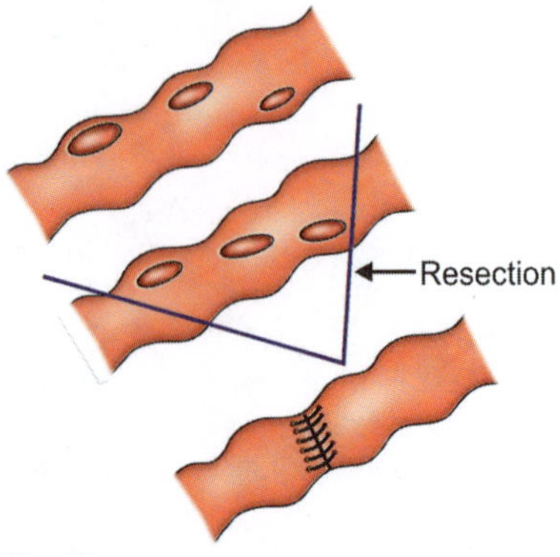

Fig. 46.56: Multiple ulcer—resection and anastomosis

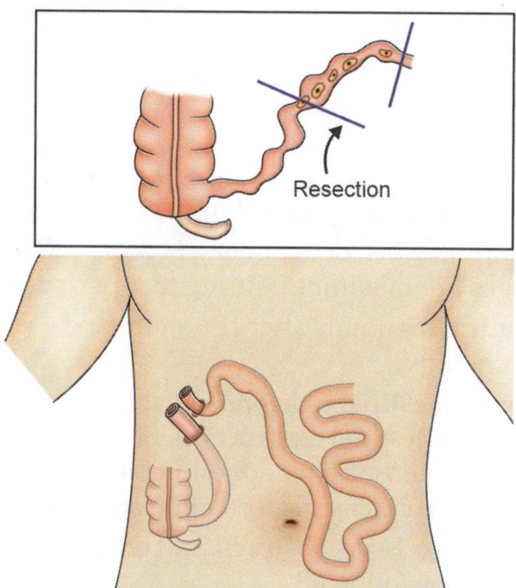

Fig. 46.57: Both ends brought outside—small bowel exteriorisation (*Courtesy:* Dr Vidushi, MBBS student, KMC, Manipal)

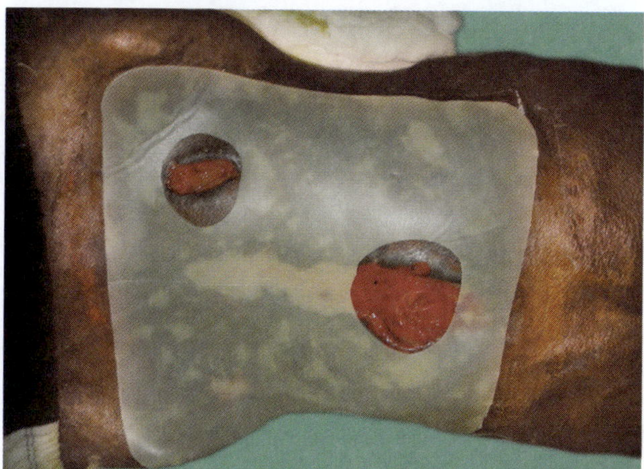

Fig. 46.58: Multiple bud fistulae developed following resection and anastomosis of typhoid ulcers treated with ostomy bags

- **Small bowel exteriorisation:** This can be considered in cases after resection when both ends of the intestine are friable. This is a very safe option. After 1–4 weeks, relaparotomy and anastomosis of resected ends is done.

3. **Paralytic ileus** due to toxic dilatation of intestine results in distension of abdomen. It is managed by drip and suction.
4. **Typhoid cholecystitis** is not uncommon. Its starts within 2 to 4 days fever. Chances of gallbladder perforation are present.
5. **Typhoid pyelonephritis,** cystitis, epididymo-orchitis.
6. **Typhoid osteomyelitis**
7. **Typhoid conjunctivitis**
8. **Thrombosis** of the common iliac vein occurs probably due to sluggish blood flow.
9. **Perforation** of large intestine can occur in paratyphoid 'B' infections.

Most of these complications occur due to bacteraemia produced in the early septicaemic phase of enteric fever. Liver, spleen, bone and bowel are commonly affected. Metastatic abscesses are common.

INTESTINAL AMOEBIASIS

- This disease is caused by *Entamoeba histolytica* and transmitted mainly by contaminated drinking water.
- After the cysts are swallowed, they are broken down in the intestine by trypsin into trophozoites which produce inflammation of the colon. **Trophozoites swallow red blood cells and multiply by mitosis. They enter into crypts of Lieberkuhn.** They produce multiple submucous loculi which later result in multiple ulcers. These ulcers are **flask-shaped (bottle neck) ulcers** with healthy intervening mucosa.
- Some trophozoites are transformed into cysts and excreted outside (Fig. 46.59).
- Lower sigmoid and upper rectum are involved in 75% of cases.

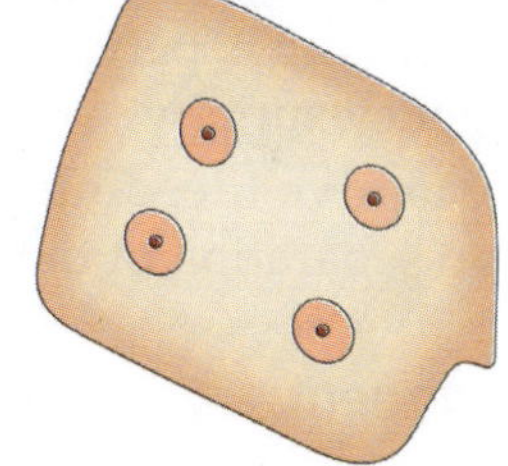

Fig. 46.59: Quadrinucleate cyst of entamoeba

Clinical Features

1. **Amoebic typhlitis:** Inflammation of the caecum by amoeba is described as amoebic typhlitis. It produces pain in the right iliac fossa and it can be confused for appendicitis. However, in this condition, there is also tenderness in the left iliac fossa. A point on the left side corresponding to McBurney point on the right side is called **Sir Philip Manson-Bahr's amoebic point of tenderness** (Fig. 46.60) and is suggestive of involvement of rectosigmoid.
2. **Amoebic dysentery:** It can be acute or chronic. An acute attack is associated with gripping pain

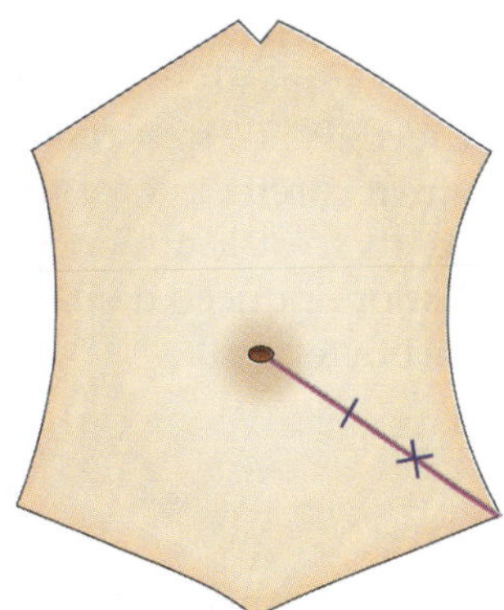

Fig. 46.60: Sir Philip Manson-Bahr's amoebic point

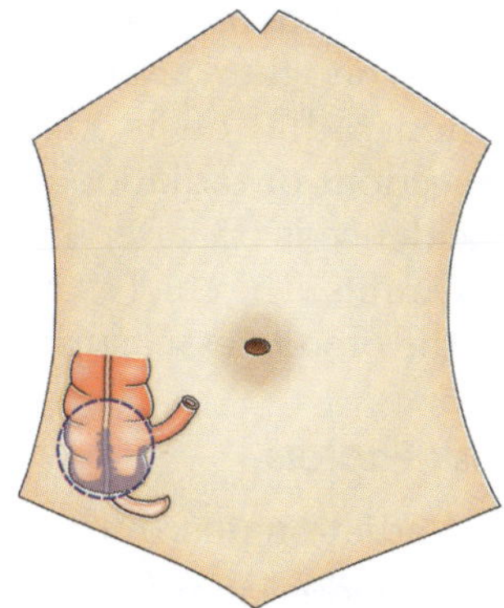

Fig. 46.61: Amoeboma is a tender thickened gurgling mass

abdomen with blood and mucus in stool, an urgency to pass stools. High grade fever and tenesmus are the other features. Chronic dysentery is more common with 2–4 foul-smelling stools per day and mild to moderate colicky abdominal pain.

3. **Amoeboma:** Chronic, low grade, persistent inflammation of the caecum produces granulomatous hyperplasia of the caecum, with thickening of the pericaecal tissue (producing mass in the right iliac fossa) (Fig. 46.61). Amoeboma can also occur in rectosigmoid junction. This is, however, uncommon nowadays because of effective treatment with metronidazole.
   - Clinically, this manifests as mass in the right iliac fossa causing dull aching pain, vague ill health, tender palpable caecum with guarding. It can be confused for ileocaecal tuberculosis or carcinoma caecum.
   - It responds very well to metronidazole.
4. **Amoebic perforation of caecum** or sigmoid can occur resulting in pericolic abscess. Peritonitis needs emergency surgery.
5. **Massive bleeding per rectum** is rare. It occurs due to separation of the slough.

Treatment

1. **Metronidazole** 400–600 mg, 3 times a day for 10 days. It acts on amoebae present in the lumen and tissue.
2. Diiodohydroxyquin 650 mg, 3 times a day for 20 days is another alternative.
3. Diloxanide furoate is ideal for chronic cases in the dose of 500 mg, 3 times a day for 10 days. It acts on luminal amoebae. It is the drug of choice in chronic cyst passers. Supportive treatment in the form of hospitalisation, correction of dehydration, antispasmodics and bedrest is also advised. Stool culture must be done before and after treatment with antiamoebic drugs.

RADIATION ENTEROPATHY

Radiation damages rapidly growing cells of intestine also when they are exposed to it. It typically happens when radiation is given to the pelvis after rectal resections or radiation given to treat carcinoma cervix. Incidence is 5% after 4500 cGy units to 30% after 6000 cGy units. The chief factor is radiation-induced damage to the blood vessel supplying the bowel wall.

Risk Factors

- Radiation dose more than 5000 cGy
- Previous laparotomy (if bowel loops are fixed due to adhesions)
- Pre-existing vascular disease
- Diabetes
- Hypertension

Clinical Types

- **Acute:** It manifests as colicky abdominal pain, bloating, loss of appetite, diarrhoea, etc. It happens during 2nd week of treatment, because inflammatory changes are maximum during that period.
- **Chronic:** This occurs after 18 months and 6 years after radiotherapy.
- **Chronic intestinal ischaemia** occurs resulting in **stricture** and intestinal obstruction. Some cases are due to fibrosis, dense pelvic adhesions, bowel entrapment into the fibrosis, fistula formation and pelvic abscess.
- When there is no obstruction, conservative line of treatment is followed.
- If there is obstruction, laparotomy with resection, bypass or any other treatment depending upon the findings.
- Surgery can be difficult because of dense adhesions.

Prevention

- Modern imaging and radiotherapy units.
- Radio-opaque markers such as titanium clips at the time of initial surgery.
- Decreasing the size of the radiation field.
- Reperitonisation of the bowel, using absorbable mesh cover over intestines, omental transposition also have been used.

Treatment

- Sucralfate, mucosal protective agent, can be used in case of bleeding due to radiation proctitis.
- Antioxidants, probiotics, statins and angiotensin converting enzyme inhibitors are used when radiotherapy treatment is on.

SMALL BOWEL TUMOURS

- Benign tumours such as lipoma, hamartoma, polyps can occur.
- Malignant tumours such as adenocarcinoma, gastrointestinal stromal tumours **(GIST)**, carcinoid and lymphoma can occur in the small intestine.

PEUTZ-JEGHERS SYNDROME (FAMILIAL HAMARTOMATOUS POLYPOSIS)

This syndrome is characterised by:

1. **Familial** tendency
2. **Melanosis** of mucosa of lip, cheek, interdigital space and even perianal skin (Fig. 46.62 and Table 46.7).

Table 46.7 Comparison of two hamartomatous polyposis syndromes

Peutz-Jeghers syndrome	Cronkhite-Canada syndrome
• Hamartomatous polyps • Polyposis of small intestine (mainly) • Melanin spots on the buccal mucosa and lips • Bleeding and intussusception are common complaints • Rarely malignancy can occur	• Hamartomatous polyps • Gastrointestinal polyposis • Cutaneous pigmentation, finger nails atrophy, alopecia • Intestinal obstruction can occur • Severe malabsorption—protein-losing enteropathy

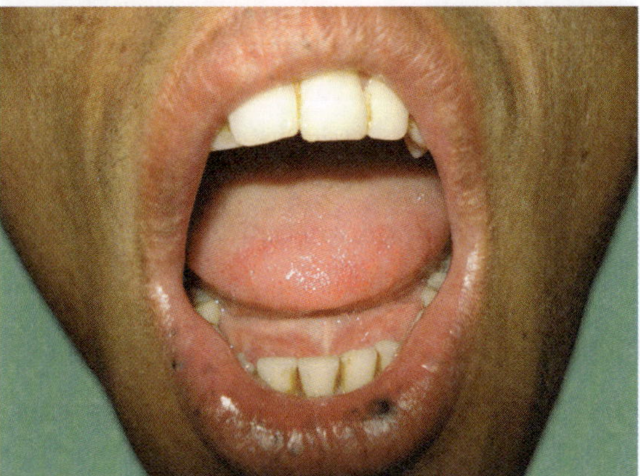

Fig. 46.62: This patient presented to hospital with abdominal pain. The registrar who examined the case reported that there was a mass abdomen. However, when he presented the case next day, there was no mass. The patient had undergone laparotomy 10 years back for similar complaints. A segment of bowel had been resected earlier. This photograph gives the clue to the diagnosis—pigmentation of lips and oral mucosa. The mass (appearing and disappearing) was due to intussusception (*Courtesy:* Prof Sreevatsa, HOD, Prof Bharathi, Prof Bagli, Dr Srikar Pai, Department of Surgery, MS Ramaiah Medical College, Bengaluru, CME 2008)

3. **Multiple polyps** in the small bowel and large bowel mainly in the jejunum. They are hamartomatous polyps.
   - It is an autosomal dominant disease.

Clinical Presentation

- Runs in families.
- As a cause of bleeding per rectum, results in chronic anaemia.
- Can cause adult intussusception.
- Rarely, it can turn into malignancy.
- Female patients have increased chances of breast and cervical cancer (*see* clinical notes).

Treatment

- Blood transfusion to correct anaemia
- Resection of that portion of bowel containing polyp, in cases of bleeding or intussusception.

Clinical Notes

We had 3 interesting cases of Peutz-Jegher syndrome.

The first case was of a boy of 14 years, who presented with acute intestinal obstruction. At laparotomy, there were 3 intussusceptions in the jejunum due to polyps. About 15 large polyps were removed after doing an enterotomy.

The second case was a 50-year-old lady, who presented with duodenal carcinoma. Endoscopy revealed polyps in the stomach and duodenum. Specimen of pancreatico-duodenectomy revealed it as a case of Peutz-Jegher syndrome. This lady did not have pigmentation of the oral mucosa.

The third case was of a 35-year-old male who has been coming to our hospital with intermittent bleeding and anaemia. Endoscopy revealed multiple polyps in the stomach and duodenum. Small bowel enema demonstrated multiple polyps in the small bowel. Even proctoscopy showed multiple polyps in the rectum. He is being managed conservatively.

ADENOCARCINOMA

- Incidence is 40% of small bowel tumours. Overall, small bowel tumours are rare. Reasons have been given in Key Box 46.16.
- Duodenum is the commonest site of adenocarcinoma. If it arises from first part and second part, it may require Whipple's pancreaticoduodenectomy. From the third part, early cases of adenocarcinoma can be resected without removal of pancreas.
- Some familial diseases predispose to adenocarcinoma. They are familial polyposis coli, adenomas, Crohn's disease, etc.

Key Box 46.16

Malignancy in Small Intestine is Rare—Why?

- No stasis, rapid transit of food
- Secretion of immunoglobulins—IgA
- Various carcinogens are diluted by secretions
- Comparatively low and inactive bacteria in the small bowel

- Clinical features include vague features like nausea, poor appetite, crampy abdominal pain, bleeding and intestinal obstruction.
- Diagnosis is by CT scan (Fig. 46.63).
- **Push enteroscopy** has the advantage of visualization of the growth and to take biopsy (Figs 46.64A and B).
- Other option is capsule endoscopy. It is time consuming and biopsy is not possible.
- Resection with at least 7 cm margin with lymphadenectomy is the treatment of choice (Figs 46.65 and 46.66).
- There is no role for radiotherapy and chemotherapy.

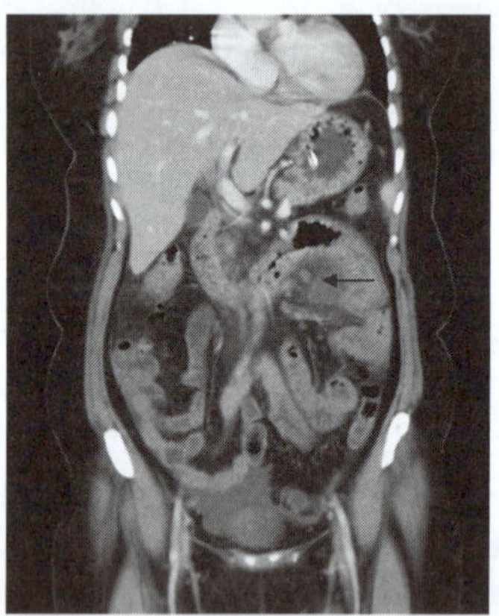

Fig. 46.63: CECT scan showing jejunal growth with narrowing of the lumen of the jejunum

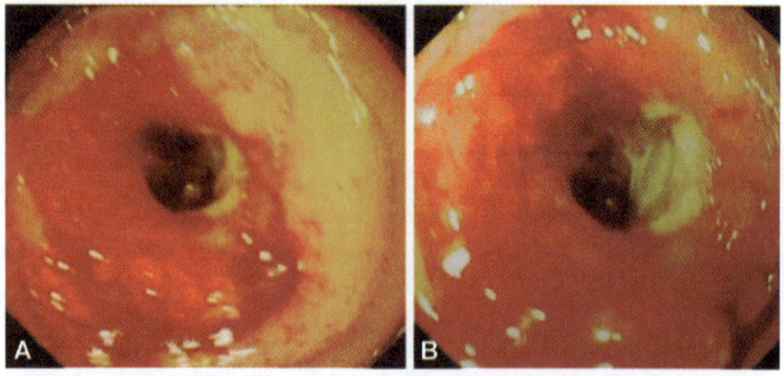

Figs 46.64A and B: Push enteroscopy showing ulcerative lesion in the proximal jejunum

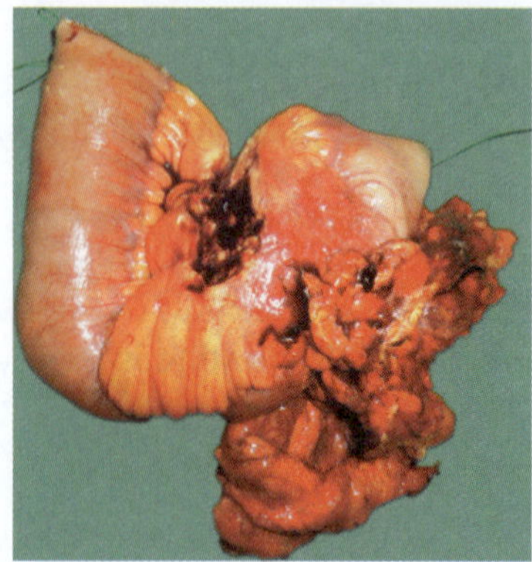

Fig. 46.65: Resection of the growth done with 6 cm margin with lymph nodes

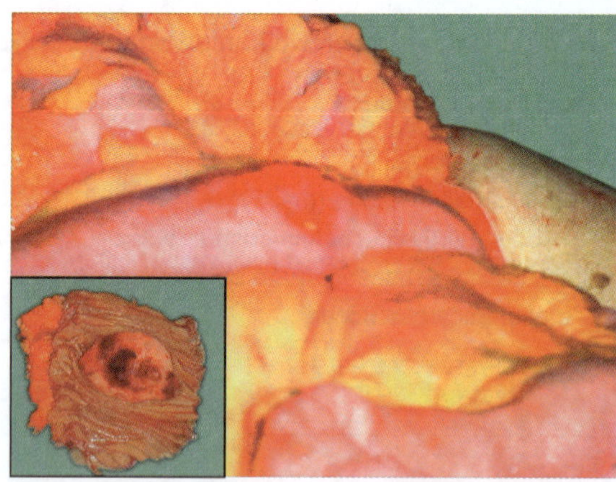

Fig. 46.66: This patient presented with abdominal pain, melaena and loss of weight. CT scan of the abdomen revealed mass in the jejunum. It was resected (inset). Mucosal surface showed ulceration. Histopathology report was adenocarcinoma

GASTROINTESTINAL STROMAL TUMOUR (GIST)

- Earlier called leiomyoma and leiomyosarcoma, they occur in jejunum or ileum. These are uncommon mesenchymal tumours (Figs 46.67 amd 46.68).

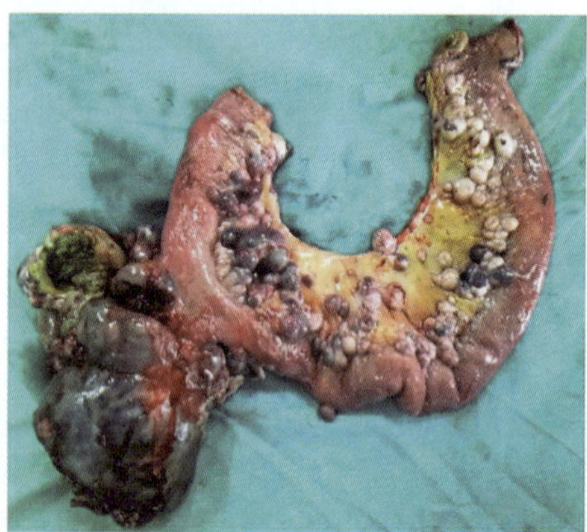

Fig. 46.67: Resected specimen of ruptured GIST of the jejunum. (*Courtesy:* Dr Jyothi, Head, Department of surgery, GIMS, GADAG, Karnataka)

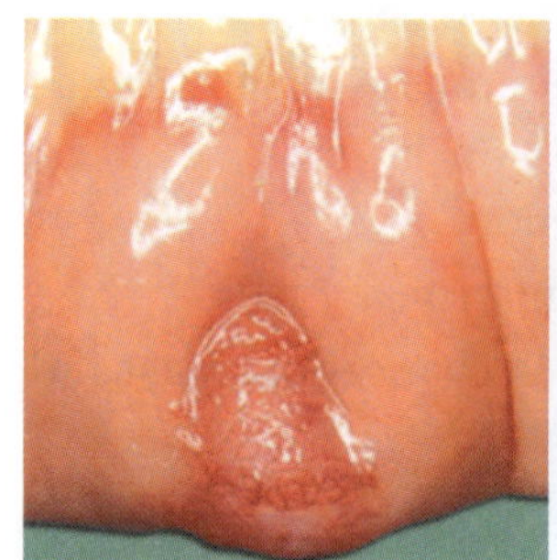

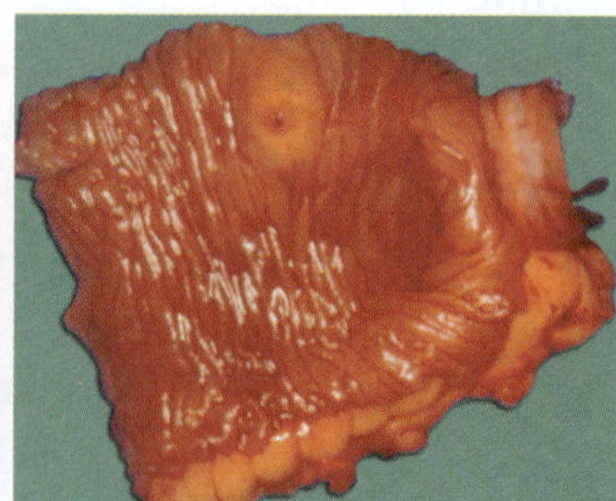

Fig. 46.68: GIST involving jejunum—resected specimen showing mucosal ulceration (*Courtesy:* Dr Padmanabha Bhat, Dept. of Surgery, KMC, Manipal and Prof HD Shenoy, Father Muller's Medical College and Hospital, Mangalore)

- **Stomach is the commonest site.** GISTs are rare in the oesophagus, whereas leiomyoma is more common.
- They constitute 20% of malignant neoplasms of the small bowel.
- More common in the 5th and 6th decades of life.
- They arise from **interstitial cells of Cajal** which are pacemaker cells that regulate motility and peristalsis.
- GISTs arise from muscularis propria. They tend to grow extramurally.

Clinical Features

- They present as bleeding/mass/perforation.
- Very often massive bleeding may be the only presentation.
- **Carney's triad:** It consists of three components:
  1. GIST
  2. Pulmonary chondromas
  3. Extra-adrenal paragangliomas
- A palpable, mobile large nodular mass suggests GIST.

Spread

- Spread is mainly locoregional. In malignant GIST of stomach, infiltration into the diaphragm is not uncommon. Haematogenous spread can occur into lungs and bone.
- Rarely lymphatic spread can occur.

Prognosis

It depends upon three factors:

- Size more than 5 cm
- High mitotic index
- Tumour invasion into lamina propria

Diagnosis

- Diagnosis is by endoscopy and biopsy. If ulcer is present, it is easy to take a biopsy. If ulcer is not present, a biopsy on a biopsy should be taken. It is difficult in cases of GIST of small intestines.
- CECT scan can define the growth and infiltration with or without lymph nodes.

Tumour Markers

They express CD117/CD34 antigen. **CD117 is known as C-kit receptor.**

Treatment

- Treatment is in the form of resection. Diagnosis of malignancy is by mitotic figures: <10 mitoses/high power field (HPF) suggests a low grade malignancy. >10 mitoses/HPF suggests high grade malignancy.
- Increased incidence of C-kit has also been found in patients with neurofibroma.
- The drug of choice for GIST is Imatinib Mesylate.

Imatinib Mesylate

- It is a tyrosinekinase inhibitor.
- It is the first drug of choice in high-risk patients.
- Given as 400 mg/day for 3 years as adjuvant treatment.
- Not given for low-risk patients of R-O resection.
- It should be given, if tumour ruptures on table.
- It is the drug of choice for unresectable and metastatic tumours. Long-term side effects include abdominal cramp, bleeding wounds, gums, swelling of face and feet, etc.
- Imatinib with doxorubicin has shown some benefit in high grade tumours.

NEUROENDOCRINE TUMOURS (NET)

- Its original name is **karzinoide**—means features resembling carcinoma.
- Today these carcinoid tumours are called **N**euro-**E**ndocrine **T**umours (NET).
- It arises from argentaffin/chromaffin cells which are present in the crypts of the villi of intestine. These cells are called **Kulchitsky cells**. These cells stain with ammonical silver salt solution to black colour. Hence, they are called argentaffinoma or chromaffinoma. They secrete 5-HT (serotonin or 5-hydroxytryptamine). They can be single or multiple and can be associated with adenocarcinoma.
- Median age of presentation is 63 years.
- NET are classified as:
  - Low grade: Grade 1, G1
  - Intermediate: Grade 2, G2
  - High grade: Grade 3, G3
- Symptoms occurring due to hormone secretion from these tumours together constitute carcinoid syndrome (Table 46.8).
- Midgut NET occurs within last 2 feet of ileum and secretes important hormones such as serotonin (5-HT) and substance-P.
- Location, pattern of growth, depth of invasion decide malignancy.
- The tumour appears as a small firm submucosal nodule with large mesenteric lymph nodal mass. Tumour produces desmoplastic reaction resulting in fibrosis, intestinal kinking and intestinal obstruction.
- Intermittent recurrent colicky abdominal pain, diarrhoea and weight loss are the features.

Table 46.8 Comparison of NET at various sites

	Foregut	Midgut	Hindgut
Site	Duodenum, stomach, bronchus, pancreas, etc.	Jejunum, ileum, right colon	Rectum
Incidence	Rare	Common	Uncommon
Hormones	Low serotonin (5-HT), 5-Hydroxytryptophan +	5-HT, prostaglandins, insulin, ACTH	Do not secrete 5-HT but somatostatin +

Bronchial carcinoid produces bronchial obstruction and produces carcinoid syndrome without secondaries in liver.

Sites

- *Appendix:* 65%. **It is the most common site.** It occurs more commonly in females. When the tumour occurs in the **appendix, it is usually benign,** hard and occurs in distal one-third of appendix (Key Box 46.17).
- **Terminal ileum:** 30%. Most of them are **malignant**. When the tumour occurs in the **ileum it is usually malignant** and produces multiple bulky secondaries in the liver, even when primary is very small. Fibrosis of the mesentery results in kinking of bowel causing periodic abdominal pain.
- The hormones produced by the tumour **5-HT** (serotonin) are not metabolised because of the secondaries. So, they are absorbed into the circulation and produce various symptoms. This is called carcinoid syndrome.

Carcinoid Syndrome

- Usually malignant NET from ileum produces classical symptoms of vasomotor, cardiac and gastrointestinal.
- Invariably it is associated with massive hepatomegaly due to metastasis.
- Hormones responsible for symptoms are serotonin, 5-HTP, histamine, dopamine, prostaglandins, etc.

Signs and Symptoms

- **Vasomotor:** These are the most common findings seen in about 80% of cases. These can be erythromatous red flushing attacks, either involving entire body or limited to areas such as face, neck and upper chest.
- **Gastrointestinal:** Episodic watery diarrhoea is seen in about 70–75% of patients. It is caused by hormone serotonin. It responds to methysergide which is a serotonin antagonist.
- **Cardiac: Pulmonary stenosis is the most common cardiac lesion** followed by tricuspid insufficiency and tricuspid stenosis.

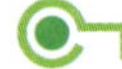 **Key Box 46.17**

'Most Common' for NET Appendix

- Most common neoplasm of the appendix
- Mostly found in distal one-third of the appendix
- Mostly tumour is yellow staining at immunohistochemistry
- Mostly benign—very rarely metastasize
- Mostly appendicectomy is sufficient. Rarely, right hemicolectomy may be required

Diagnosis

1. 5-hydroxyindole acetic acid (5-HIAA), a serotonin metabolite is elevated. It is measured in 24-hour urine sample.
2. Chromogranin-A (CgA) has a specificity around 95%. Thus a combination of 5-HIAA with CgA measurements is recommended.
3. CT scan: It can identify as NET—it appears to be solid, with spiculated borders and radiating strands. CT scan helps to locate NET and to define lymph nodal mass.
4. MRI is not used for diagnosis but can detect liver metastasis.
5. Scintigraphy is useful in detecting extra-abdominal disease. It can detect somatostatin receptor sites. Octreotide is used for scintigraphy.
6. 18FDG-PET (18F-fluorodeoxyglucose positron emission tomography) is useful only in high grade NET which has high Ki-67 expression.

Surgery

- **Excision/resection** of the NET with intestinal segment for small primary tumours less than 1 cm in size.
- **Larger tumours:** Resection of tumour, intestine and mesentery.
- **Terminal ileal NET:** Right hemicolectomy.
- **Disseminated disease:** Surgical debulking.

Pharmacotherapy

- Octreotide (somatostatin analogues) is the drug of choice in treating patients with symptoms. Mainly used in carcinoid syndrome to treat flushing and diarrhoea.

- Metastatic tumours are treated by debulking (if possible) with combination chemotherapy using Inj streptozotocin, 5-fluorouracil (5-FU) and cyclophosphamide.
- **Bromocriptine** 2.5 mg twice a day can be given to reduce the symptoms. Other agents which can be used are methysergide and diphenoxylate hydrochloride.
- Secondaries in the liver are treated by intra-arterial (hepatic artery) **streptozocin**. Localised liver metastasis can be treated with resection.
- **Therapeutic embolisation** of hepatic artery by using gel foam, etc. will reduce the size of the liver, thereby decreasing discomfort to the patient.
- Injection octreotide 100 mg IV is the drug of choice in cases of carcinoid crisis (severe bronchospasm).

Octreotide in Carcinoid Syndrome

1. It is used to suppress the tumour growth.
2. Control symptoms—flushing, wheezing, diarrhoea.
3. It controls the release of GI hormones.
4. Dose is 100 μg subcutaneously three times a day in patients with mild/moderate, non-life-threatening carcinoid syndrome.

Summary of the NET (Key Box 46.18)

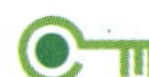

Key Box 46.18

Summary of NET

- They are APUDOMAS.
- Arise from enterochromaffin cells.
- They may be associated with multiple endocrine neoplasia (MEN) type 1 and type 2.
- About 15% of NET patients may have carcinoma elsewhere, e.g. carcinoma stomach, carcinoma lung or carcinoma colon.
- Common age is 40–50 years.
- Majority arise from midgut—almost 85% cases. They secrete 5-HT.
- Appendix is the most common site. Often appendicectomy is sufficient for malignant carcinoid tumour.
- Foregut NET do not secrete serotonin.
- Flushing and diarrhoea can be controlled by octreotide.
- Secondaries can be multiple and big, but slow growing similar to primary. Arterial embolisation has been tried in many cases.
- Since they are slow growing and prognosis is good, aggressive treatment in the form of surgery, octreotide, liver resections and rarely liver transplantation have been done.

MALIGNANT LYMPHOMA

Primary: Arising from lymphoid tissue.

Secondary: Part of systemic lymphoma. **Ileum is the most common site of lymphoma** (Key Box 46.19).

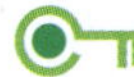

Key Box 46.19

Malignant Lymphoma

1. **Western type**
   - Non-Hodgkin's, B cell type
   - Annular ulcerating lesion
   - Bleeding, obstruction, perforation and weight loss
2. **Primary lymphoma with celiac disease**
   - Increased incidence of lymphoma
   - It is a T cell lympoma
   - Diarrhoea, pyrexia are other features
3. **Mediterranean**—associated with alpha chain disease.[1]

[1]Alpha chain disease is a disorder characterised by the secretion of a defective α-heavy chain. Patients present with steatorrhoea, often progressive and fatal.

Precipitating Factors

1. Crohn's disease
2. Celiac disease
3. Immunosuppression—AIDS—usually it is a non-Hodgkin's lymphoma of 'B' cell origin.

SHORT GUT SYNDROME

Competency

SU28.14.4: Describe the clinical features and principles of management of short gut syndrome.

Causes of Short Gut Syndrome (Key Box 46.20)

- **Short gut syndrome** occurs due to **massive resection** of the bowel resulting in loss of length of the bowel, loss of absorptive area of the bowel and loss of valves. Superior mesenteric artery being an end artery, thrombosis at its origin is invariably fatal.
- **Midgut volvulus** of neonates is congenital due to arrested rotation resulting in floating caecum and mobile intestine.

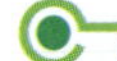

Key Box 46.20

Short Gut—Causes

- Mesenteric infarction
- Midgut volvulus
- Necrotising enteritis
- Crohn's disease[1]
- Radiation enteritis

[1]It is common cause in western countries

Clinical Notes

We had an interesting case of midgut volvulus in an 18-year-old boy consequent to a laparotomy done for perforated duodenal ulcer. While replacing the coils of bowel within the abdomen, the mesentery was probably twisted resulting in massive gangrene. This boy now has about 100 cm of the small bowel.

- **Necrotising enteritis** (enteritis necroticans) is a complication of infection of small bowel by *Clostridium perfringens*. It usually occurs after a heavy feast where pork is consumed. There is extensive suppuration of mucosal and submucosal layer of jejunum (also ileum). Serosa may show multiple dark bluish patches. Massive resection is done for a necrotic, perforated, unhealthy bowel which results in short gut syndrome.
- **Radiation enteritis** or radiation enteropathy results in patients who receive radiotherapy to the abdominal and pelvic regions, e.g. carcinoma cervix. Arrest of cell division resulting in mucosal thinning, ulceration followed by oedema and later, fibrosis are characteristics of this condition. Endarteritis and vasculitis also add to these changes resulting in stricture, perforations, abscess, malabsorption and multiple resection, etc.

Pathophysiological Effects

(Fig. 46.69 and Key Box 46.21)

It depends upon:

- Extent of resection
- Site of resection
- Presence/absence of ileocaecal valve
- Age of the patients
- Infants tolerate extensive resections better than adults. Patients with less than 100 cm of the small bowel will develop severe nutritional deficiencies and may require parenteral nutrition.

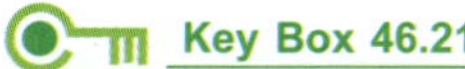

Key Box 46.21

Effects of Short Gut

- Severe malabsorption
- Gallstones
- Fatty infiltration of liver
- Urinary stones
- Gastric hyperacidity

1. **Malabsorption of fat and fat-soluble vitamins:** Can occur after ileal resections due to interruption of enterohepatic circulation of bile salts. These bile salts enter the colon and are converted into secondary bile salts. These bile salts block absorption of water and electrolytes.
2. **Gastric hypersecretion:** Due to delayed clearance of gastrin, as in proximal jejunal resections, there is increased gastric secretion of acid resulting in hyperacidity.
3. **Liver disease:** Fatty infiltration of the liver and mild hyperbilirubinaemia are seen massive resections and jejunoileal bypass. Acute fulminant hepatic failure can also occur.

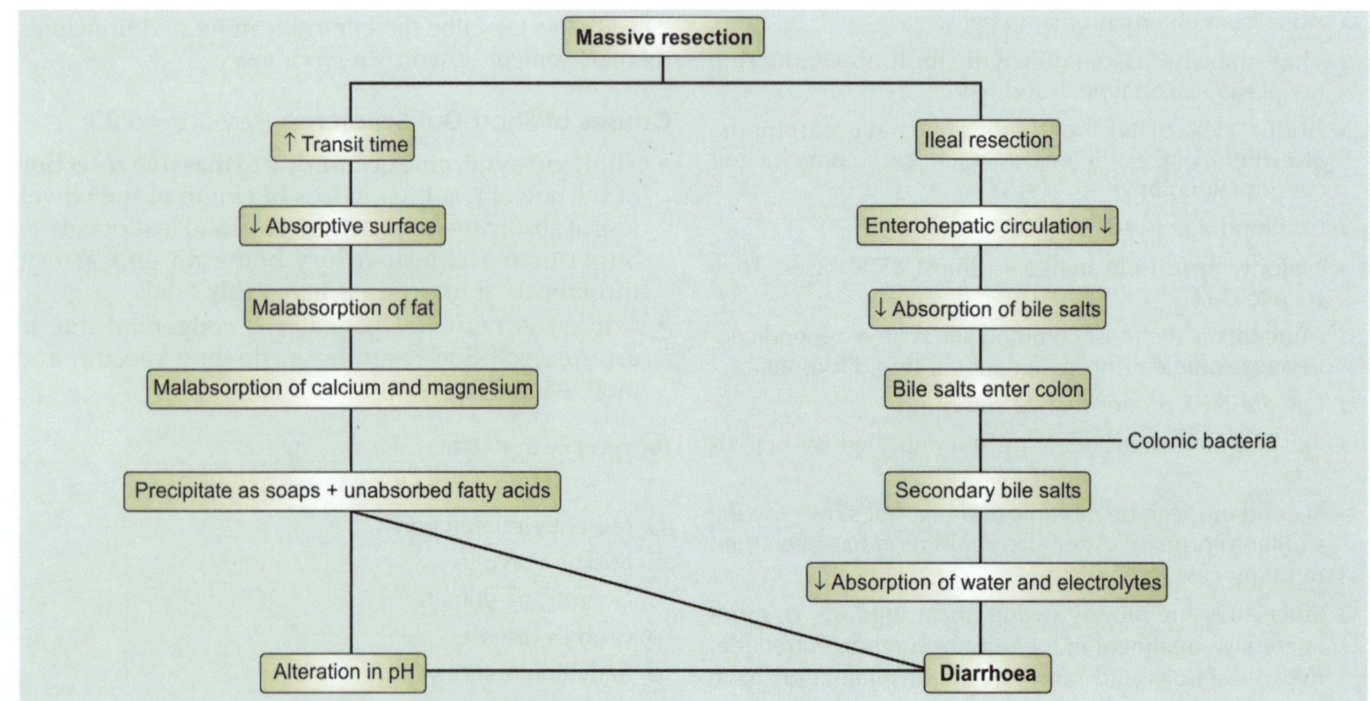

Fig. 46.69: Nutritional deficiency in short gut syndrome

4. **Gallstone formation:** There is increased incidence of cholesterol stones as a result of reduced bile salt pool, after ileal resection and jejunoileal bypass.
5. **Urinary stones**
   - All types of urinary stones are common due to low levels of calcium excretion in the urine and high levels of oxalate.
   - Water and salt depletion, and loss of K+ causes hyponatraemia and hypokalaemia.

Adaptation (Key Box 46.22)

As a result of loss of significant bowel, dilatation of the remaining intestine and villous enlargement takes place. This is brought about by a humoral agent, enteroglucagon. In children, length of the bowel is increased. Also, the number of cells in the villi is increased (work hypertrophy). There is also evidence to suggest gradual slowing of the transit time.

Treatment

- Treatment of short gut patients is difficult. It needs a special set up of dieticians who plan 'proper food' for these patients in consultation with treating surgeons. It is a gradual process of feeding the patient beginning with parenteral nutrition and progressing to normal, low fat diet after a few months.
- In the initial 2–3 months following massive resection, total parenteral nutrition including supplementation of fluid and electrolytes is the ideal treatment. Sips of plain water or oral hypotonic solutions can be allowed.
- After 2–3 months, when adaptation of bowel takes place, enteral feeding is started gradually with baby food, fat-free, fibre-free, protein-rich, liquid diet. Essential fatty acids should be supplied. Diarrhoea is a common problem and is treated with loperamide tablets.
- Enteral feeding can contain low fatty diet in addition to the other nutrients mentioned above.
- Small bowel transplantation is also being done when all measures fail specially when the bowel length is less than 50 cm. It is given in Chapter 65 on Transplantation (page 1197).

Key Box 46.22

Adaptation to Short Gut Syndrome

- Villus—size
- Length of bowel
- Transit time
- Absorption from colon

INTESTINAL FISTULAE

Introduction

- Intestinal fistulae are **abnormal communications** between two portions of the intestine, between the intestine and some other hollow viscus, or between the intestine and the skin of the abdominal wall.
- When it involves **skin and intestines, it is called enterocutaneous fistula.**
- Despite significant advances in their management, intestinal fistulae remain a major clinical problem, with an overall mortality rate of 15 to 25%.

Classification

Anatomical

- Internal: Colovesical fistula
- External: Duodenal, jejunal fistula
- Mixed: Crohn's disease

Depending on the Contents

- Low output <200 ml
- Moderate output 200–500 ml
- High output >500 ml

Aetiology

- **Iatrogenic (70%)—postoperative:** Injury to intestines unnoticed at the time of surgery or injury recognized at the time of surgery, sutured but has given way are prime causes of enterocutaneous fistula. **Anastomotic leak, partial or complete, is another important cause of enterocutaneous fistula. Meticulous surgical techniques, gentle handling of the bowel, usage of the proper suture material (Vicryl and silk), ensuring adequate blood** supply to the intestines which have to be anastomosed will largely prevent anastomotic leak (Fig. 46.70).

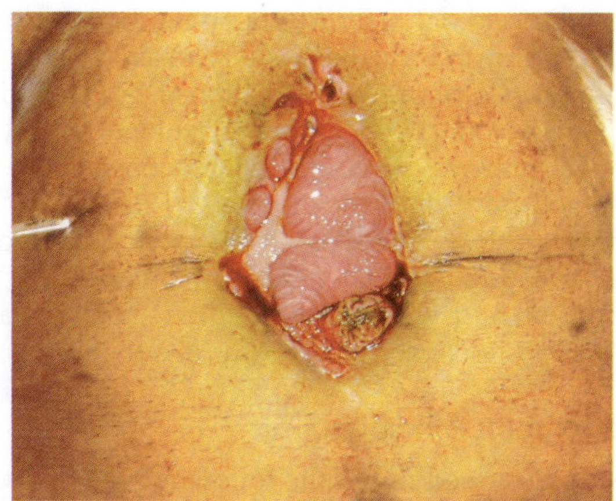

Fig. 46.70: Small intestinal fistulae due to anastomotic disruption and wound dehiscence

- **Stump blow out: Duodenal blow out: Typically happens 4–5 days following surgery** (*see* page 590).
- Inadequate resection of the **diseased segment:** In such situations, anastomosis may be in unhealthy bowel.
- **Instrumentation:** Oesophageal perforations are dangerous ones and can occur even with flexible scopies.
- **Spontaneous (30%):** Crohn's disease, diverticular disease of the colon, appendicitis are also known to give rise to fistulae.

Local Factors Precluding Spontaneous Closure

- Bleeding
- End fistula: Bowel discontinuity
- Foreign body: Swabs, tips of the suction tubes (detached), retained sponges or instruments
- Radiation
- Inflammation/infection/inflammatory bowel disease
- Epithelialisation of the tract is another important cause of the persistent fistula.
- Neoplasms
- Distal obstruction
- **Multiple fistulae** that do not heal as in Crohn's or typhoid perforations.
- **Lateral duodenal fistula** does not heal because large volume of contents are poured into the second part of duodenum and there is no rest to the part.
- When the **defect is more than 1 cm**, and the **track is more than 2 cm**, fistula does not close (*see* clinical notes).

Clinical Notes

A 60-year-old man was operated for appendicitis. On the fifth postoperative day, he developed faecal discharge from the wound. Conservative management was done for 7 days with total parenteral nutrition and other measures. Fistula persisted. CT scan was done on the 14th day. It revealed a growth in the hepatic flexure almost encircling the lumen. Colonoscopy and biopsy proved adenocarcinoma colon. He underwent re-exploration and right hemicolectomy was done. The fistula stopped and he was discharged from the hospital after 10 days. This case highlights the fact that in the presence of a distal obstruction, fistula will not close. More importantly, what the patient had was not appendicitis but subacute intestinal obstruction! The pain was due to colic.

Management: Principles

It can be discussed under the following headings.

1. Recognition and aetiology
2. Phase of stabilization
3. Nutrition—more details on page 38
4. Investigative phase
5. Phase of definitive management
   a. Surgery
   b. Skin care
   c. Abdominal wall defect

1. Recognition and Aetiology

- Delay in recovery from paralytic ileus or a common phrase used—when the ***patient is not doing well*** are early indications of a leak or a breakdown of anastomosis. Once the fistula establishes, diagnosis is easy because the drain will start draining intestinal contents including food particles (if oral intake is started). Intra-abdominal collections, abscess, fever, sepsis are other features of leak.
- Recognising the cause is important because it can dictate treatment. To give an example: **If any foreign body is left in the abdomen, exploration and removal may be urgently required.**
- If a specific disease is suspected such as tuberculosis, antituberculous treatment may cure a fistula.

2. Phase of Stabilisation

- Nil by mouth, total bowel rest, introduction of a nasogastric tube (Ryle's tube) with continuous drainage decreases fistula output.
- Proton pump inhibitors decrease gastric secretions.
- Protection of skin is by liberal zinc oxide application.
- Common fluid and electrolyte problems seen in patients with GI fistula include dehydration, hyponatraemia, hypokalaemia and metabolic acidosis. They have to be corrected.
- Drainage of collections by CT or ultrasound-guided aspiration or pig tail catheter insertions.
- Broad-spectrum antibiotics, with anaerobic coverage.

3. Nutrition (more details on page 38)

- Nutrition has been discussed in detail in the Chapter 11 on Fluid-Electrolyte Balance and Nutrition. A few points worth mentioning are that more distal the fistula, less is the requirement of **total parenteral nutrition** (TPN). TPN is safe today. One may have to wait for 4–6 weeks with TPN for the final repair of complicated fistula such as lateral duodenal fistula or ileal fistula.
- Placement of **nasogastric, nasojejunal tubes, percutaneous gastrostomy or jejunostomy** for nutrition is an important step which can be done with the help of radiology and imaging department.

4. Investigative Phase

a. Routine biochemical and haematological investigations

- Blood urea, serum creatinine, blood sugar
- Serum electrolytes
- Serum albumin, transferrin
- Blood culture helps in giving appropriate antibiotics
- Chest X-ray to rule out static pneumonia or ARDS, pleural effusions (source of sepsis also).

b. Imaging studies

- **USG:** Drainage of collections by catheters. If drainage persists, suspect fistulous communication.
- **Fistulograms** to define the exact site of fistula—proximal or distal—gastric or intestinal (Key Box 46.23).
- **Contrast CT abdomen:** To detect collections, discontinuity, diseased segments, distal obstruction and foreign body. Extremely useful investigation in intestinal fistula.
- **Colonoscopy and barium enema** are other investigations used in specific situations such as colonic fistulae.

5. Phase of Definitive Management

a. Surgical intervention

- **Drainage or aspiration of pus** urgently when there is sepsis before doing an elective repair.
- **Feeding jejunostomy** as in high fistulae, e.g. duodenal or oesophageal fistula.
- **Diversion/exclusion/colostomy/bypass** are various other treatments depending upon the location of fistula (Fig. 46.71).
- **Definitive treatment:** It includes restoration of continuity—resection and anastomosis, internal diversion or exteriorisation of bowel as in suspicious viability (mesenteric ischaemia or enteric perforations—friable bowel, known for leak and releak).

Key Box 46.23

Fistulogram/CT/Contrast GI Series

- What is the cause of the fistula?
- Is the bowel completely disrupted or is it a lateral fistula with the bowel in continuity?
- What is the length of the fistula tract?
- Is there an abscess cavity?
- What is the size of the bowel wall defect?
- Is there a distal obstruction?

b. Methods of skin care (Figs 46.72 and 46.73)

- Pouches, stoma bags of different sizes are available.
- Creams and ointments—zinc or petroleum-based
- Suction catheter placed *in situ*: Low pressure suction 60–80 mmHg.

Generally, dressings need to be changed every 4 hours. Pouch/reservoir system should be employed.

c. Abdominal wall defects: Depending upon the size of the defect, immediate or delayed closure can be achieved with tension-releasing incisions on the external oblique or laparostomy and secondary suturing, skin grafting or by using prosthetic mesh such as Marlex or Prolene.

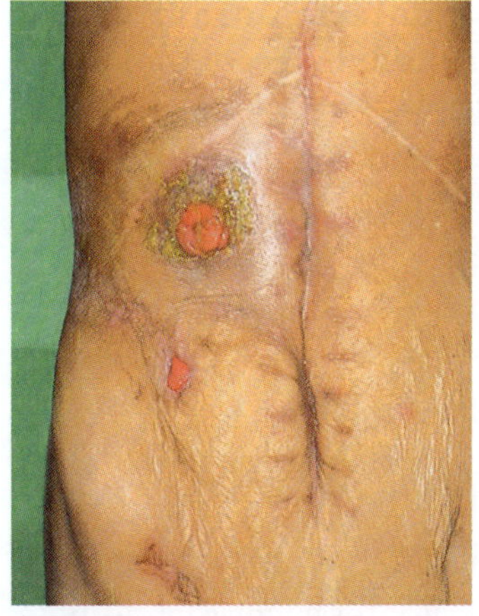

Fig. 46.71: Small bowel exteriorisation was done for enteric perforation after resection—safe option when there is gross contamination

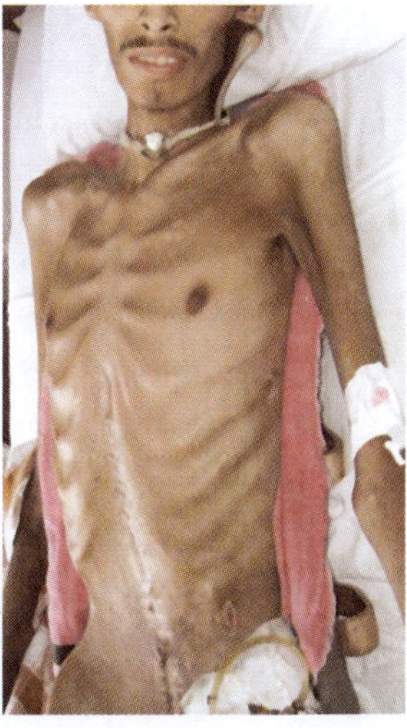

Fig. 46.72: Severe nutritional deficiency following duodenal fistula—autocannibalism

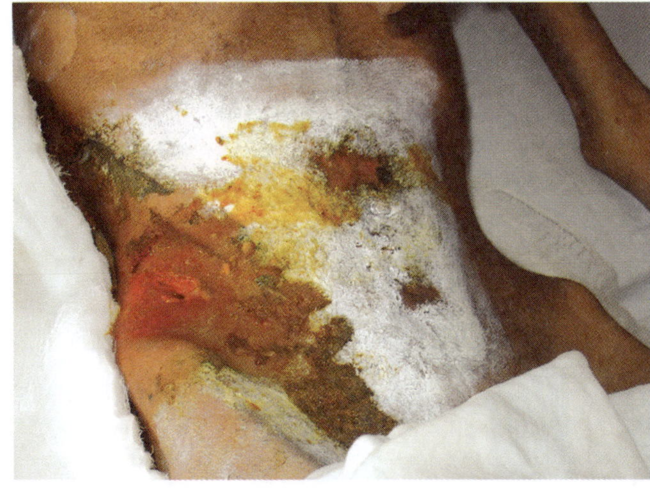

Fig. 46.73: Extensive excoriation of the skin in a faecal fistula. Zinc oxide has been applied to the abdominal wall

SMALL INTESTINAL DIVERTICULA

Introduction

Small intestinal diverticula are far less common than colonic diverticula. Multiple sac-like mucosal herniations occur through weak points in the intestinal wall where blood vessels penetrate.

Incidence

Diverticula are more common in duodenum than jejunum or ileum (Fig. 46.74).

Pathophysiology

- It is believed to develop as a result of abnormalities in peristalsis, intestinal dyskinesis and high segmental intraluminal pressures.
- **They occur in the mesenteric border unlike Meckel's which occurs in the antimesenteric border.**
- Diet low in fibre and rich in fat and some visceral myopathy have been blamed for development of diverticula.

Clinical Features

- Asymptomatic
- Occult blood in the stools—positive
- Anaemia and symptoms such as fatigue, weakness, pedal oedema
- Malabsorption—diarrhoea, flatulence, weight loss
- Pain abdomen, signs of peritonitis such as tenderness, guarding or localised abscess.

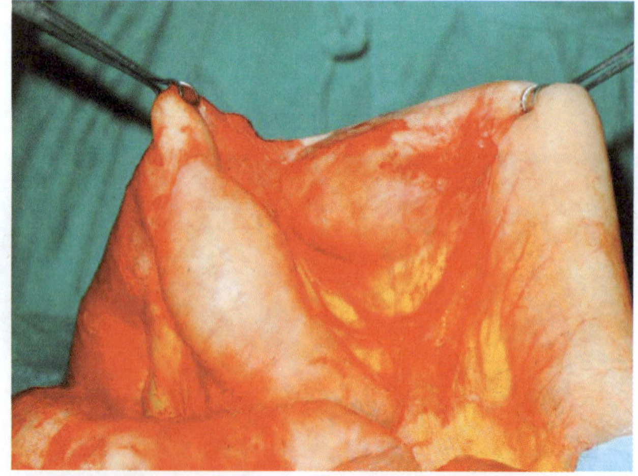

Fig. 46.74: Diverticula form mesenteric border of jejunum. It was the cause of anaemia due to occult blood loss

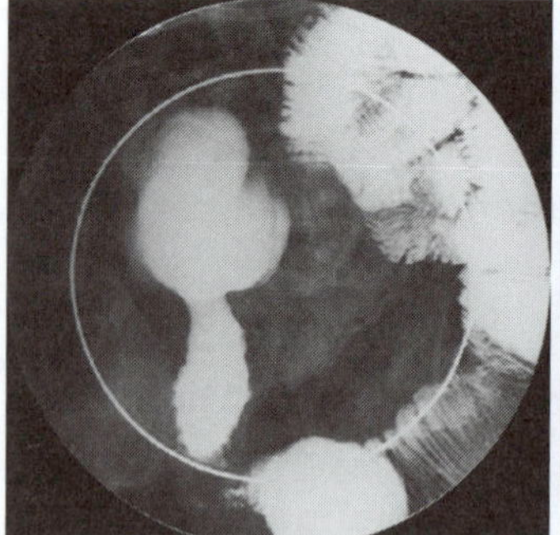

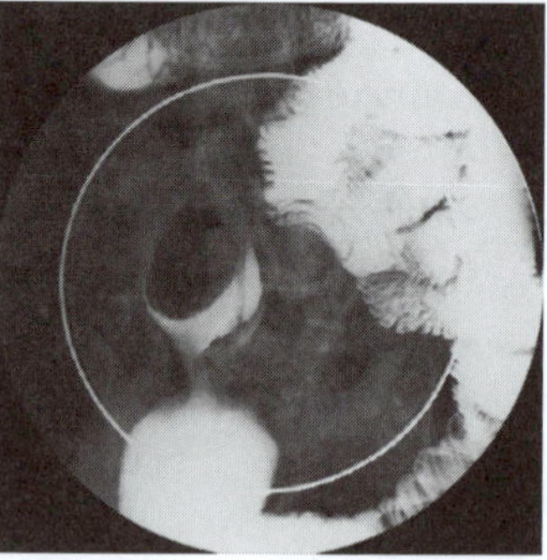

Figs 46.75 and 46.76: Enteroclysis. First picture showing filling defect and a clear view of diverticula in the second picture

Investigations

- Specific investigations are enteroclysis and enteroscopy.
- CT with contrast is the ideal investigation.
- Often diverticula are not suspected but a CT scan obtained for some pathology in the abdomen may reveal a localised abscess. Later, at laparotomy, it can turn out to be diverticula (Figs 46.75 and 46.76).

Treatment

Resection and anastomosis of the bowel containing diverticula.

INTERESTING 'MOST COMMON' FOR INTESTINES

- Most common site of gastrointestinal tuberculosis is ileocaecal region.
- Most common site of ulcerative colitis is rectum.
- Most common extraintestinal manifestations of ulcerative colitis are peripheral arthritis and ankylosing spondylitis.
- Most common site of gastrointestinal perforation in enteric fever is terminal ileum.
- Most common neoplastic lesion of small intestine is lymphoma.
- Most common anal problem in Crohn's disease is fissure in ano.
- Most common site of adenocarcinoma in intestines is duodenum.
- Most common site of malignant carcinoids is terminal ileum.
- Most common site of carcinoid in intestines is appendix.

Multiple Choice Questions

1. **Pathology of ulcerative colitis includes all of the following *except:***
   A. Punched out ulcers
   B. Pseudopolyposis
   C. Pipe stem colon
   D. Pus cells

2. **Toxic megacolon is seen in the following *except:***
   A. Intestinal tuberculosis
   B. Ulcerative colitis
   C. Amoebic colitis
   D. Salmonella colitis

3. **String sign of Kantor is seen in:**
   A. Crohn's disease B. Tubercular enteritis
   C. Typhoid enteritis D. Amoebic colitis

4. **Guarding and rigidity can be minimal in enteric perforation of terminal ileum because:**
   A. The perforation is usually small
   B. It is self-sealing and self-limiting
   C. Zenker's degeneration of abdominal muscles
   D. Occurs in the antimesenteric border of the terminal ileum

5. **Flask-shaped (bottle neck) ulcers are a feature of:**
   A. Intestinal tuberculosis
   B. Crohn's disease
   C. Intestinal amoebiasis
   D. Typhoid enteritis

6. **Malignancy in small intestine is rare because:**
   A. Bacteria in the intestine are protective
   B. Blood supply is very good
   C. No stasis, rapid transit of food
   D. Low levels of immunoglubulins

7. **Most common site of gastrointestinal perforation in enteric fever is:**
   A. Duodenum B. Jejunum
   C. Colon D. Terminal ileum

8. **Adaptation to short gut syndrome includes all of the following *except:***
   A. Decreased transit time
   B. Increased villus size
   C. Absorption from colon
   D. Increased length of bowel

9. **The symptoms of carcinoid syndrome is due to:**
   A. Histamine B. Serotonin
   C. Prostaglandins D. Epinephrine

10. **Tenderness in the Sir Philip Manson-Bahr's point is a feature of:**
    A. Rectosigmoid involvement in amoebic colitis
    B. Acute appendicitis
    C. Acute cholecystitis
    D. Crohn's disease

11. **The commonest site for gastrointestinal stromal tumour is:**
    A. Oesophagus B. Stomach
    C. Duodenum D. Jejunum

12. **Carney's triad includes all of the following *except:***
    A. Gastrointestinal stromal tumours
    B. Pulmonary chondromas
    C. Extra-adrenal chondromas
    D. Familial hamartomatous polyposis

13. **One of the drugs used in the treatment of carcinoid syndrome is:**
    A. Metronidazole B. Bromocriptine
    C. Streptomycin D. Serotonin

14. **The most common site for a carcinoid tumour is:**
    A. Stomach B. Duodenum
    C. Appendix D. Rectum

15. **Causes of short gut syndrome include all of the following *except*:**
    A. Mesenteric ischaemia
    B. Necrotising enterocolitis
    C. Crohn's disease
    D. Radiation enteritis

16. **C-kit receptor is expressed in:**
    A. Gastrointestinal stromal tumour
    B. Peutz-Jegher syndrome
    C. Carcinoid syndrome
    D. Crohn's syndrome

17. **The most recent and promising drug used in the treatment of Crohn's disease is:**
    A. Trastuzumab B. Infliximab
    C. Monteleukast D. Fab antibodies

18. Most common anal problem in Crohn's disease is:

A. Anal fistula
B. Haemorrhoids
C. Anal fissure
D. Perianal abscess

19. Transmural inflammation is characteristic of:

A. Crohn's disease
B. Tuberculous enteritis
C. Typhoid enteritis
D. Ulcerative colitis

20. 'Hose pipe rigidity' is a feature of:

A. Crohn's disease
B. Tuberculous enteritis
C. Typhoid enteritis
D. Ulcerative colitis

21. The most common symptomatic presentations of Meckel's diverticulum in children of 2 years of age is:

A. Haemorrhage
B. Perforation
C. Diverticulitis
D. Intestinal obstruction

22. The drug used to control diarrhoea in neuro-endocrine tumour is:

A. Streptozotocin
B. Sunitinib
C. Methysergide
D. Octreotide

23. Investigation of choice for gastrointestinal NET is:

A. Ultrasound B. CT scan
C. MRI scan D. FDG–PET scan

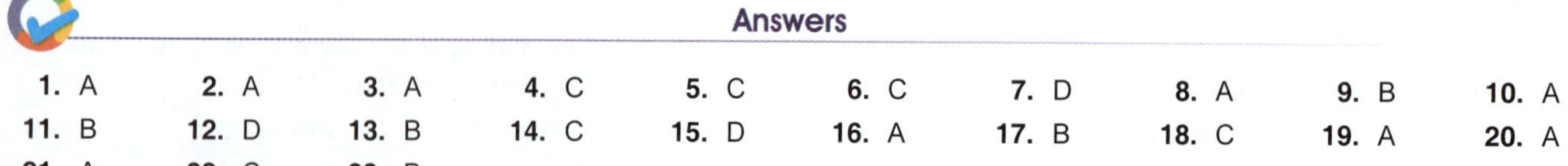

Answers

1. A	**2.** A	**3.** A	**4.** C	**5.** C	**6.** C	**7.** D	**8.** A	**9.** B	**10.** A
11. B	**12.** D	**13.** B	**14.** C	**15.** D	**16.** A	**17.** B	**18.** C	**19.** A	**20.** A
21. A	**22.** C	**23.** B							

CHAPTER

47

Large Intestine

- Surgical anatomy
- Colonic function
- Tumours of the large intestine
  - Polyps
  - Familial polyposis coli
  - Hereditary nonpolyposis colorectal cancer
- Carcinoma colon
  - ERAS
- Colon screening
- Diverticular disease of colon
- Faecal fistula
- Colonic stricture

SURGICAL ANATOMY

Competency

SU28.13.1: Appreciate anatomy and physiology of the large intestine.

Colonic blood supply is given here but resections and correlation with blood supply is given on pages 1296–1300 operative surgery section.

- Large intestine extends from ileocaecal valve to anus. It has five segments: Right colon, left colon, transverse colon, sigmoid colon, rectum and anal canal (Fig. 47.1).
- Average length is about 135–150 cm.
- Interestingly, alternating portions of the colon are mobile and fixed. Ascending colon and descending colon are fixed but caecum, transverse colon and sigmoid colon are mobile. Mobile structures can undergo twisting (volvulus).
- Layers of colon: Mucosa, submucosa, muscularis propria and serosa. Inner circular and outer longitudinal muscle layers constitute muscularis propria. In spite of 4 layers, wall of the colon is thin. Hence it distends much more in obstruction.

Caecum

- 7.5 cm in both length and breadth
- Blind pouch
- Completely covered by peritoneum except posterior surface
- Mobile

Diseases

- Carcinoma
- Tuberculosis
- Amoebic typhlitis
- Intussusception
- Volvulus—rare

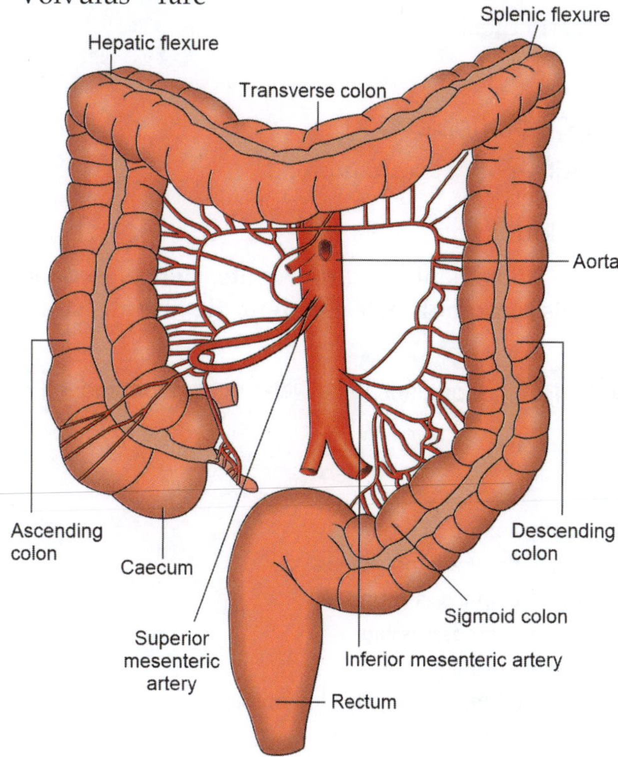

Fig. 47.1: Anatomy of the colon and parts

Ascending Colon (15 cm Long)

- Caecum continues as ascending colon.
- Covered by peritoneum in front and on both sides.
- In 25% of patients, it has a mesentery.
- Right paracolic gutter is deep on the lateral aspect of ascending colon—space for paracolic abscess in cases of perforation peritonitis.

Transverse Colon (50 cm Long)

- Most mobile part of large intestine.
- It is suspended by transverse mesocolon, loops down and is adherent to the posterior wall of omental bursa.

Diseases

- Cancer
- Ulcerative colitis

Descending Colon (25 cm Long)

- Continues as sigmoid colon
- Retroperitoneal (like ascending colon)
- Also has paracolic gutter

Sigmoid (40 cm Long)

- S-shaped
- Ends as rectosigmoid junction where taenia coli ends.

Diseases

- Volvulus
- Diverticulosis
- Cancer

Right Colon (Table 47.1)

Big and hepatic flexure is broad.

Left Colon

- Small and splenic flexure is acute. Hence, **ischaemic colitis commonly affects splenic flexure** (Table 47.1).
- Splenic flexure is deeply situated. Therefore, malignancy in this area can be easily missed.

Muscle Coat

Outer longitudinal muscle is arranged in the form of **three strips** called **taenia coli.** All three join at the rectosigmoid junction and form a complete longitudinal layer of the rectum. **These three taenia coli converge at the base of the appendix.** This is an important method to localise appendix. Inner circular muscle coalesces distally to form internal anal sphincter. **No taenia over the rectum.**

Recognise large intestine by:

1. Taenia coli
2. Omental appendices—appendicular epiploicae
3. Haustrations
4. Large diameter (calibre)

Names of three taenia coli

1. Mesocolic: Transverse colon and sigmoid colon are attached by this.
2. Omental: To which omental appendices attach.
3. Libera (free): Nothing is attached.

> *Pearls of Wisdom*
>
> Since taenia are shorter than intestine, the colon becomes sacculated between taenia forming haustra.

Arterial Supply (Fig. 47.2)

1. **Superior mesenteric artery,** a branch of abdominal aorta, arises at the level of first lumbar vertebra (L1). It supplies the entire small bowel and the right colon up to proximal 2/3rds of transverse colon. **Branches** of superior mesenteric artery (SMA) supplying colon are:
   A. **Middle colic artery** supplies ascending colon, hepatic flexure and the transverse colon mainly. It divides into right and left branches.

Table 47.1 Comparison between right colon and left colon

Right colon	Left colon
1. Big	1. Small
2. Hepatic flexure is broad	2. Splenic flexure is acute and narrow—mobilisation is difficult
3. Hepatic flexure is not deep	3. Splenic flexure is deep
4. Paracolic space is broad	4. Left paracolic space is narrow
5. Luminal diameter is big	5. Luminal diameter is narrow
6. Contents are liquid	6. Contents are solid
7. Growth pattern is usually ulceroproliferative	7. Growth is annular stricture
8. Obstruction is not common	8. Hence, obstruction is common
9. Growth is more common in women	9. Growth is more common in men

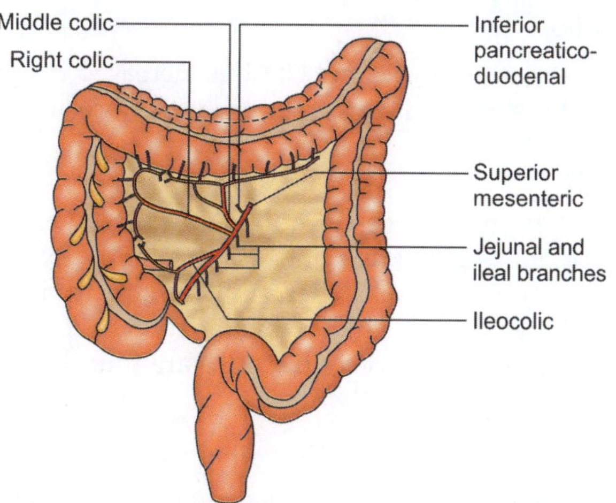

Fig. 47.2: Blood supply of the right colon

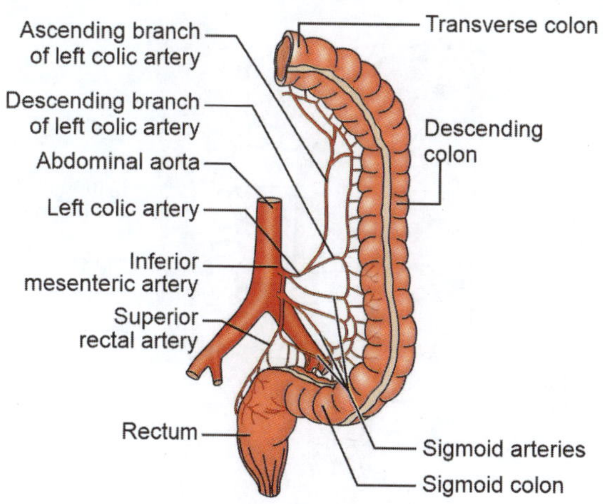

Fig. 47.3: Arterial supply of left colon

B. **Right colic artery** supplies right colon.

C. **Ileocolic artery** supplies the terminal ileum and ascending colon. It divides into anterior and posterior caecal branches and supplies caecum and appendix through appendicular artery.

2. **Inferior mesenteric artery (IMA),** a branch of abdominal aorta arising at the level of L3, supplies the left colon up to mucocutaneous junction at the lower end of anal canal (Hilton's line). Its branches are (Fig. 47.3):

A. **Left colic artery** which anastomoses with branches of middle colic artery. It divides into upper and lower branches supplying the descending colon.

B. **Three sigmoidal branches** supply sigmoid colon. Narrow point of blood supply between the first sigmoidal artery and left coelic artery is called **Sudeck's point**.

C. **Superior haemorrhoidal artery** (rectal).

- The anastomotic branches form **marginal artery of Drummond,** which is relatively narrow in the region of splenic flexure (another reason for development of ischaemia). That narrow point is called **Griffith's point**.
- **Arc of Riolan** is the anastomotic arcade formed between branches of IMA and SMA.

Venous Supply

- Follows the corresponding artery and empty into superior and inferior mesenteric veins, ultimately draining into the portal vein (Fig. 47.4).
- Thus, if the colorectal area gets infected secondary to inflammatory conditions or after surgical procedure, the infection can easily spread to the portal vein and result in portal pyaemia.

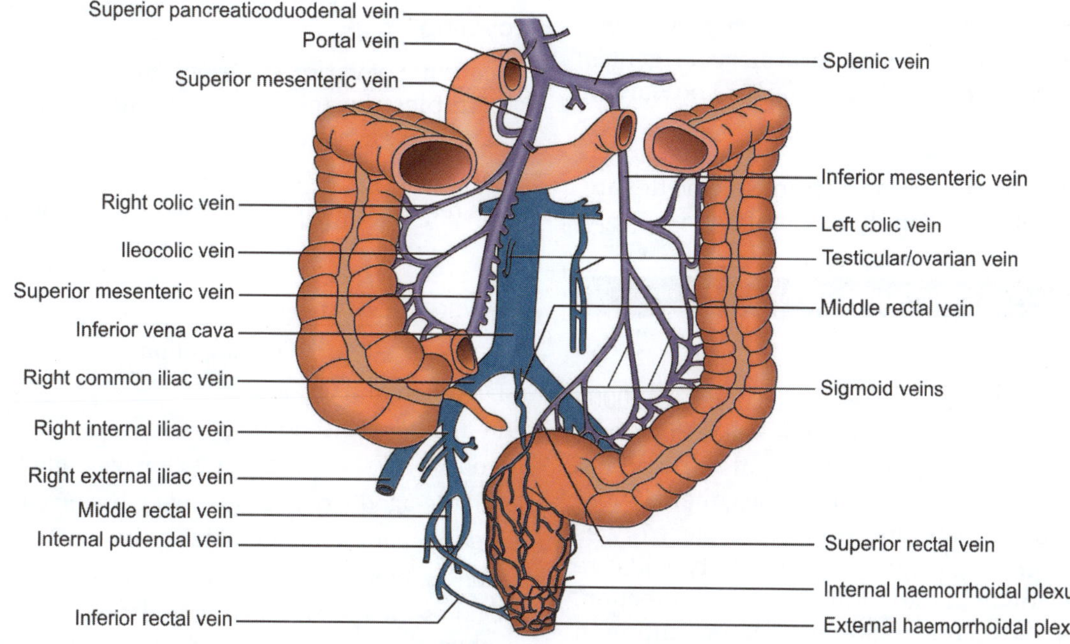

Fig. 47.4: Venous drainage

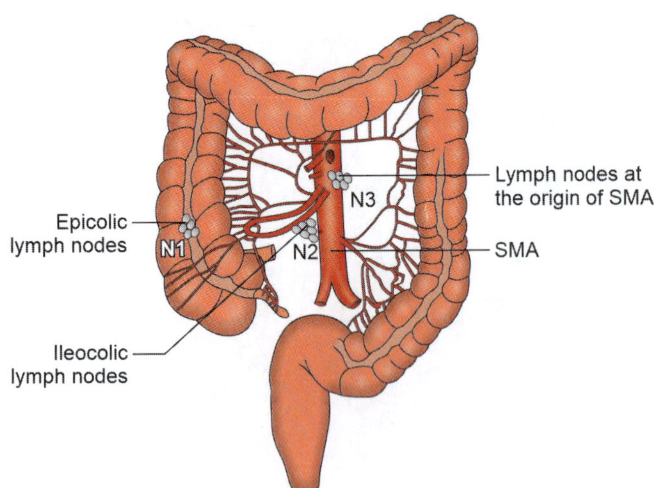

Fig. 47.5: Lymphatic drainage (see text for description of N1, N2 and N3)

Lymphatic Drainage (Fig. 47.5)

- **N1:** Epicolic, paracolic nodes are the first to get involved.
- **N2:** Nodes at the origin of ileocolic and middle colic arteries—intermediate nodes.
- **N3:** Nodes at the origin of superior and inferior mesenteric arteries. They are involved in approximately 50% of the patients with carcinoma colon at presentation to the hospital. These are called principal nodes.

Colorectal Nerve Supply

- Sympathetic (inhibitory) arise from T10–T12 and L1–L3.
- Parasympathetic (stimulation).
  A. Vagus nerve supplies right and transverse colon.
  B. Sacral nerves (S2–S4 which form nervi erigentes) supply distal colon, i.e. splenic flexure onwards.

Significance

Colonic pseudo-obstruction starts from splenic flexure. Transition zone of vagal supply to sacral nerve supply.

COLONIC FUNCTION

Absorption

Water content of faecal matter is reduced to 1000–1500 ml per day. Thus stools become solid. Similarly, sodium, potassium and bile salts are also absorbed. Significance of this is in cases of diarrhoea, there is loss of water, sodium, potassium and other electrolytes (cholerectic diarrhoea). Amino acids and fatty acids are also absorbed slowly in the colon. After ileal resection, bile salts enter the colon irritate the colon resulting in diarrhoea.

Secretion

Colon also secretes K^+ and Cl^-. It is increased in colitis. Chloride secretion is increased in cystic fibrosis.

Motility

Colon has four types of motility: Propulsive, retropulsive, mass peristalsis and gastrocolic reflux. Thus, contents travel aborally. Retropulsive activity is more in the right colon, these allowing the contents to 'churn' more and more. Mass contractions are found more in left colon—specially after meals.

Factors which stimulate the colonic motility

- Dietary fat, rich fibre diet, less water intake
- Physical activity—walking, change in posture, exercises
- Emotional activity

Constipation (Key Box 47.1)

- It depends upon several factors such as food habits, genetic, social customs.
- Generally a patient is said to have constipation, if he passes less than 2 stools per week.
- In addition to the low fibre diet, emotional feelings and many rectal diseases also cause constipation. Example—prolapsed rectum, solitary rectal ulcer syndrome. Colonic disease such as megacolon—Hirschsprung disease is an important cause of constipation in children.
- Increasing constipation in elderly patient suggest carcinoma in left colon. Needs to be evaluated by colonoscopy.

Recycling

- Recycling of various nutrients takes place in the colon. Examples: Fermentation of carbohydrates, short-chain fatty acids and urea cycling.
- Butyrate is the main product of bacterial fermentation. It is required mainly as a fuel for colonic epithelium.

Key Box 47.1

Constipation

- Digestion and absorption
- In a child—Hirschsprung's disease
- Adult women—idiopathic/following child birth
- Middle-aged women—following hysterectomy
- Elderly man—carcinoma left colon
- Constipation with severe pain—anal fissure
- Depression patient—psychotropic drugs—used to treat schizophrenia, antidepressants and antiepileptic drugs

- To accomplish this, the colon depends highly on its bacterial flora, especially for degeneration and fermentation ability.
- So broad-spectrum antibiotics inhibit production of butyrates and produce diarrhoea.

Pearls of Wisdom

More distal the colon—more is the protein metabolism and putrefaction resulting in carcinogens and greater exposure to colonic mucosa. Hence, two-thirds of colonic cancer occur in the left colon.

Colonic Bacteria

- **Anaerobic bacteria:** They constitute more than 99%. The most common pathogen is *Bacteroides fragilis* (10^{10}/g of faeces). Other organisms are clostridia, cocci, etc.
- **Aerobic bacteria:** *Escherichia coli* is the most common organism about 10^7/g of faeces. Other organisms are *Klebsiella, Proteus* and *Enterobacter*.
- **Normal function:** Bacteria degrade bile pigments, thus resulting in brown-coloured stools. They also help in colonic motility and absorption. Fatty acids produced by bacteria supply nutrition to colonic epithelium. Bacteria also supply vitamin K to the host.

Prebiotics and Probiotics

- **Prebiotics** are non-digestible food ingredients that stimulate the growth and/or activity of bacteria in the digestive system in ways claimed to be beneficial to health. Traditional dietary sources of prebiotics include soybeans, inulin sources (such as Jerusalem artichoke, jicama, soya and chicory root), raw oats, unrefined wheat, unrefined barley, and yacon.
- **Probiotic** is defined as a "live microbial feed supplement which beneficially affects the host animal by improving its **intestinal microbial balance**". They are non-degradable oligosaccharides. They stimulate the growth of beneficial intestinal bacteria.
- Probiotics are dietary supplements which contain live cultures of bacteria and yeast that are beneficial to colonic and host function. The common species used as probiotics are *Lactobacillus* and *Bifidobacterium*. Probiotics stimulate immune function, exhibit anti-inflammatory property and suppress pathogenic organism.
- **Clinical application:** When a person takes antibiotics, both the harmful bacteria and the beneficial bacteria are killed. Bacterial change in flora alters carbohydrate metabolism with decreased short-chain fatty acid absorption and results in osmotic diarrhoea. In a similar fashion, antibiotic therapy causes increase in the growth of *Clostridium difficile*. Thus, probiotics have been recommended in antibiotic-induced diarrhoea. Also, they have been used to treat diarrhoeas in ulcerative colitis, in pouchitis (inflammation of the pouch after total proctocolectomy for ulcerative colitis) and in necrotising colitis in children.

TUMOURS OF THE LARGE INTESTINE

Competency

SU28.13.5: Understand the vascular anatomy of small and large intestines and apply the same pathologies like congenital, inflammatory, traumatic, benign and malignant, etc.

Ulcerative colitis is discussed under inflammatory bowel diseases. Polyps, colonic cancer, diverticular diseases and colonic stricture are discussed here.

Benign tumours (Figs 47.6A and B) are usually referred to as polyp, which means **elevated from the surface**. Adenomatous polyps have got malignant potential. A few criteria have been incorporated into a system when malignancy develops in the polyp.

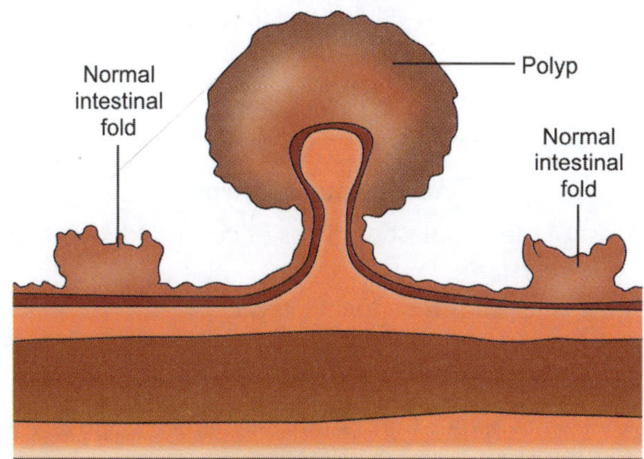

Fig. 47.6A: Polyp

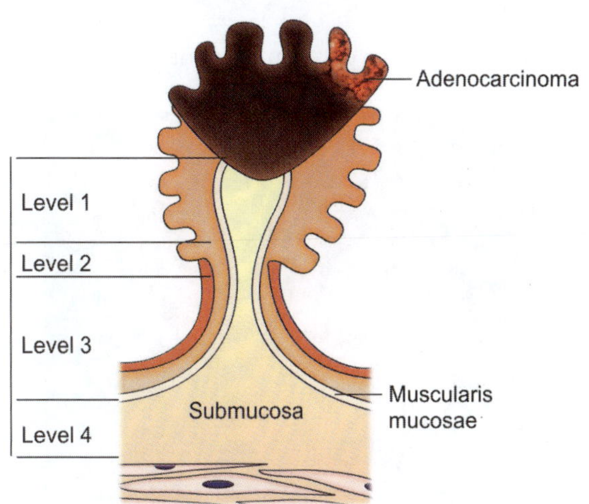

Fig. 47.6B: Pedunculated adenoma

Section III • Gastrointestinal Surgery

- It takes into consideration of level of invasion.
- Level 1: In this, carcinoma is limited to the top of the polyp. From the mucosa, it is invading through muscularis mucosa into the submucosa.
- Level 2: Carcinoma at the junction of head and stalk.
- Level 3: Carcinoma confined to anywhere in the stalk.
- Level 4: Infiltration into submucosa.

ADENOMATOUS POLYP (Key Box 47.2)

- It may be a villous adenoma which is a flat lesion or a tubular adenoma having a pedicle. Tubular is more common.
- They give rise to bleeding, mucus diarrhoea and hypokalaemia.
- They can be single or multiple.
- They are dysplastic.
- They are premalignant and the risk of malignancy is greater with increase in the size of the adenoma.
- They can be removed with the colonoscope—polypectomy.
- Malignant potential of ***villous adenoma*** is more than tubular adenoma (Fig. 47.7).
- Adenoma less than 1 cm—risk of malignancy is 1%; 1–2 cm is 10%; >2 cm is 30%.

Key Box 47.2

Adenomatous Polyps

- Most of the neoplastic polyps occur in elderly patients (>50 years).
- Most of them are pedunculated.
- Most pedunculated polyps are removed by colonoscopic snaring.
- Adenomas larger than 5 mm in diameter carry risk of malignant potential.
- More the polyps, more chances of synchronous carcinoma.
- Flat adenomas also carry malignant potential.

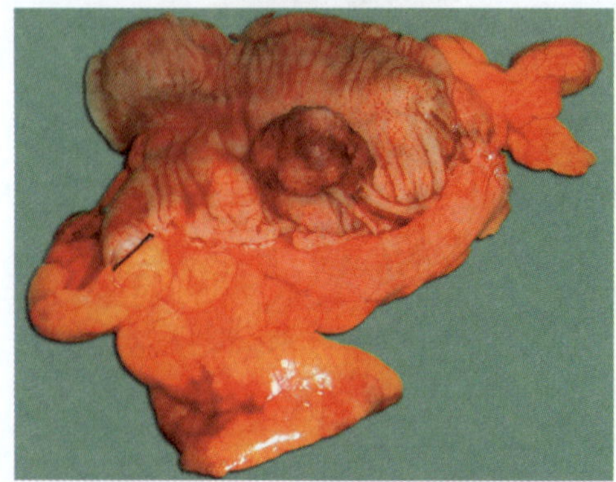

Fig. 47.7: Carcinoma in polyp

- Symptoms and signs of polyps: Bleeding per rectum is the most common symptom. Fresh bleeding is seen in rectal polyps. Typically, it is painless. It is intermittent. If it is associated with change of bowel habits means probably a malignant change. These changes include mucus discharge, tenesmus, sometimes constipation. In children, polyp may project outside the anus. In such cases, it has to be distinguished from prolapsed rectum.

Treatment

- Colonoscopy and polypectomy is the standard treatment.
- If specimen shows invasive carcinoma, radical surgery needs to be done.

Pearls of Wisdom

Although most neoplastic polyps do not evolve to cancer, most colorectal cancers originate as a polyp.

HAMARTOMATOUS POLYP (JUVENILE POLYP)

- This can occur in the colon as in Peutz-Jeghers syndrome. Risk of malignancy is very limited. Symptomatic polyps need to be treated.
- **Juvenile polyps** are usually single and occur in children. They give rise to bleeding and are easily resected. They do not have malignant potential.

FAMILIAL POLYPOSIS COLI (FPC) OR FAMILIAL ADENOMATOUS POLYPOSIS (FAP)

- FAP is a genetic disorder inherited as a Mendelian dominant. The gene APC (adenomatous polyposis coli) is located on the short arm of chromosome 5. **Prevalence:** 1 in 10,000. It is clinically defined by the presence of more than 100 colorectal adenomas (Figs 47.8 and 47.9).
- It is transmitted from both sexes. The incidence is same in either sex.

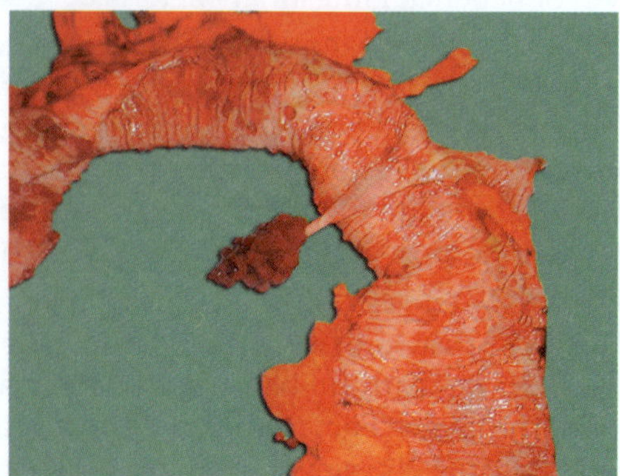

Fig. 47.8: Thousands of polyps. One of them is 2 cm and is pedunculated

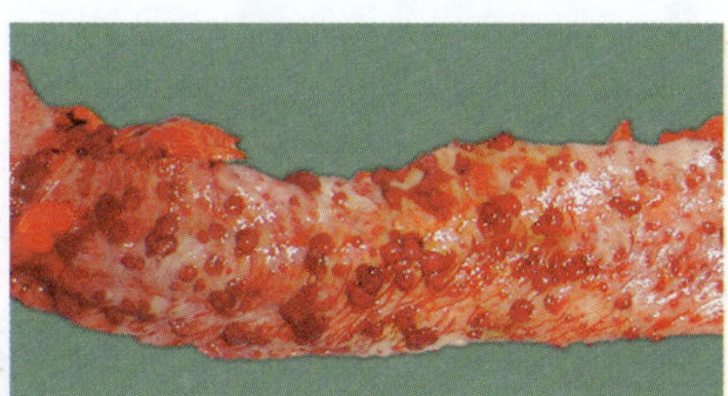

Fig. 47.9: Close-up view of the polyps

- When it is associated with desmoid tumour, craniofacial osteoma, epidermoid cysts, congenital hypertrophy of retinal pigment epithelium, it is described as **Gardner's syndrome** (Key Box 47.3).
- When familial polyposis coli is associated with central nervous system tumour and glioblastoma, it is called **Turcot's syndrome**.
- 50% of them have benign gastric polyps and 90% of them have duodenal polyps.

Clinical Features

- Runs in families; other members of the family are affected.
- Manifests at the age of 20 in the form of blood and mucus in the stool, loose stools, etc. It produces crampy lower abdominal pain.
- Anaemia, weight loss and protein malnutrition occur slowly.
- Mean age of development of carcinoma is 29 years.

Complications of FAP

Malignancy (100% risk)

Investigations

Colonoscopy—details on page 796.

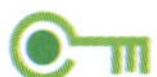 Key Box 47.3

Familial Polyposis Coli—Summary

- **P**olyps are more than 100 (colorectal adenomas).
- **O**ther mesodermal tumours—desmoid tumours, osteoma, epidermoid cysts can be present (Gardner's syndrome).
- **L**arge bowel is predominantly involved.
- **Y**ear of development of carcinoma—mean age 39 years.
- **P**olyposis gene—autosomal dominant APC gene.
- **O**ther syndrome—Turcot
- **S**igmoidoscopy from age of 15 at intervals is the investigation of choice.
- **I**leoanal anastomosis with pouch—restorative proctocolectomy—advisable above age of 30.
- **S**urgery is the only means of preventing colonic cancer.

Remember as **POLYPOSIS**

Treatment

- **NSAID: Sulindac** 300 mg, twice a day and **aspirin** 325 mg once a day have been found to decrease the size of polyps.
- Patients with FAP who are above the age of 30 have high chances of having a carcinoma in the colon. Hence, even when there is no malignancy, surgery is advisable.

Types of Surgery (Figs 47.10 and 47.11)

- Many patients do not like ileostomy. Hence, a subtotal colectomy with ileorectal anastomosis can be done. This is done provided that rectum is examined frequently and endoscopic snaring of the polyps is done regularly, especially in a young patient.
- **Restorative proctocolectomy** with ileoanal anastomosis by using a pouch is another alternative. However, it is a major surgical procedure and should be undertaken only by an experienced surgeon.

Screening

Starts from the age of 10–12 years, repeat every 1–2 years until the age 35.

Pearls of Wisdom

If there are no adenomas by the age of 30 years, FAP is unlikely.

METAPLASTIC POLYP

Also called hyperplastic nodules. They are of viral aetiology. They do not have malignant potential.

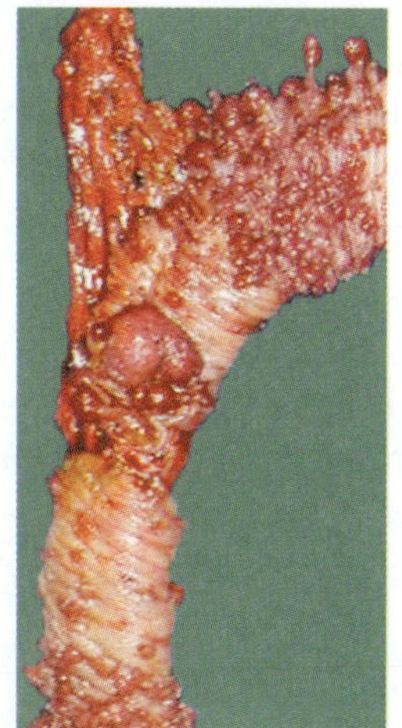

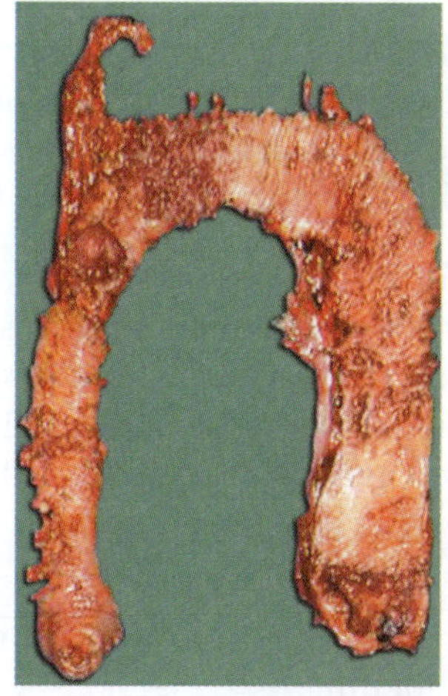

Figs 47.10 and 47.11: Familial adenomatous polyposis with two malignancies—lower rectum and hepatic flexure. This patient was being treated for chronic diarrhoea for 7–8 years with various medications. 'He underwent colonoscopy for the first time in our hospital.' Total proctocolectomy specimen (*Courtesy:* Dr Challa Srinivas Rao, Professor, Dept of Surgery, and Dr Ravi, Konaseema Institute of Medical Sciences (KIMS), Amalapuram—Andhra Pradesh)

HEREDITARY NONPOLYPOSIS COLORECTAL CANCER (HNPCC)

- Autosomal dominant, **no polyps**
- **Lynch's syndrome I:** Site-specific colorectal cancer.
- **Lynch's syndrome II:** Cancer family syndrome—they have extracolonic cancers such as endometrial cancer, ovarian cancer, transitional cell cancer, etc.
- Lifetime risk of developing colorectal cancer is 80%.
- **Synchronous carcinoma means more than one cancer at the time of diagnosis. Metachronous carcinoma which means appearance of second carcinoma after 6 months can occur here.**

Diagnostic Criteria (Amsterdam Criteria II)

1. At least 3 members in a family should have colorectal cancer—two of whom are first degree relatives.
2. At least two consecutive generations.
3. At least one relative should have had colorectal cancer by less than 50 years of age.
4. Exclusion of FAP.

Screening

Increased incidence of **proximal colonic cancer**.

EXAMINATION OF COLON

Anoproctoscopy: One can examine up to 10–12 cm of anal canal and rectum. Rubber band ligation (for piles) and polypectomy can be done with this instrument.

Flexible sigmoidoscopy: The scope measures about 60 cm in length. One can easily reach up to splenic flexure. Bowel wash or an enema is given before the procedure. No sedation is required (Figs 47.12 and 47.13).

Fibreoptic colonoscopy can assess the entire colon. It is 100–160 cm in length. Usually, there will be multiple polyps varying from a few millimetres to centimetres. Biopsy has to be taken. Polyps are visible after 15 years and certainly by the age of 30 years.

- It is the investigation of choice in most of the large intestinal lesions.
- It permits examination of entire colon and terminal ileum.
- Colon is prepared by polyethylene glycol given orally.
- Risk of perforation of colon is less than 0.1%.

Indications

Diagnostic

- Lower gastrointestinal bleeding

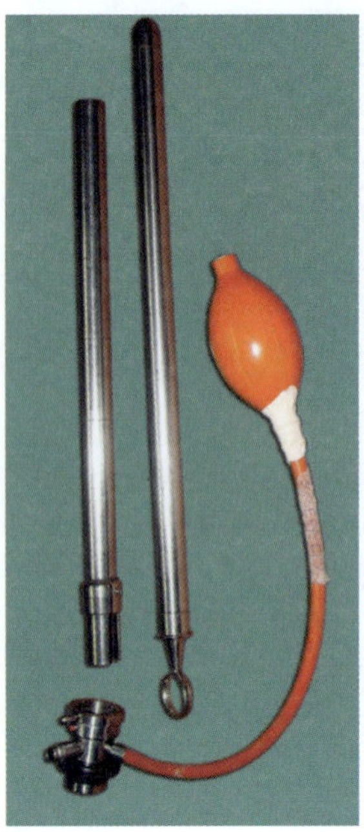

Fig. 47.12: Rigid sigmoidoscope

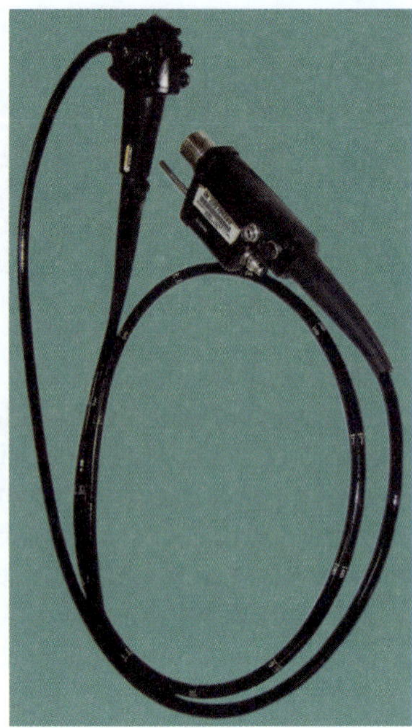

Fig. 47.13: Flexible sigmoidoscope

- Inflammatory bowel diseases
- Abnormal finding in barium enema
- Family history of colorectal cancers
- Biopsy of caecum/ileum in suspected cases of cancer
- Ileocaecal tuberculosis—to take biopsy

Therapeutic

- Control of bleeding—coagulation or injection sclerotherapy
- Snaring of polyps
- Removal of foreign body
- Detorsion of volvulus
- Decompression of pseudo-obstruction

CARCINOMA COLON

Introduction

It is the second most common cancer and cancer-related death cases in the Western world next only to lung cancer. The incidence increases with age. Multiple synchronous lesions (more than 1 malignancy at the time of diagnosis) are found in about 5% of the patients. Colon is also one of the sites of metachronous cancer (new malignancy appearing after 6 months of curative surgery). More than 95% are adenocarcinoma and surgery remains the most effective treatment. Survival has improved because of early diagnosis and multimodality of the treatment.

Over a period of years, the understanding of development of carcinoma has changed and more and more molecular biology of colonic cancer is being discussed. The **Fearon-Vogelstein adenoma–carcinoma multistep model** of colorectal neoplasia represents one of the best known models of carcinogenesis (Key Box 47.4).

- **Terminology:** Before we start the discussion on carcinoma colon, we shall study a few terminologies used in carcinoma colon. They are synchronous carcinoma, metachronous carcinoma, familial colorectal carcinoma.

SYNCHRONOUS CARCINOMA

- **Moertel's definition:** Synchronous cancers as those occurring within 6 months of the first primary cancer, or two or more histologically distinct simultaneously detected malignancies or more than one malignancy at the time of initial diagnosis. This will happen especially in cases of colon and upper aerodigestive tract wherein the stimulus or aetiological factor for malignancy affects different parts of the organ.
- Colon, head and neck, oesophagus are the sites of synchronous carcinomas.
- In cases of carcinoma colon with specific aetiological factors such as familial polyposis coli, ulcerative colitis, hereditary non-polyposis cancer, often carcinoma is synchronous.
- Thus, it is important to do a complete colonoscopy when a patient comes with colonic carcinoma because he/she may be having another synchronous carcinoma elsewhere. *See* the clinical notes.

Key Box 47.4

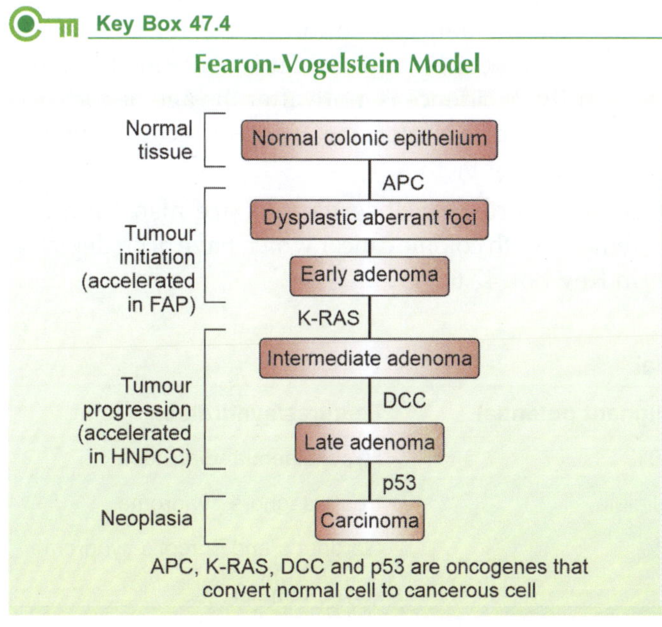

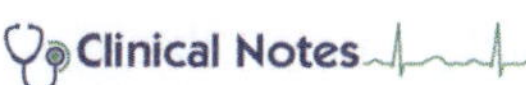
Clinical Notes

A 68-year-old lady was admitted with large bowel obstruction. Plain X-ray abdomen showed intestinal obstruction. Exploratory laparotomy was done. A 3 cm constricting growth was identified at rectosigmoid junction and high anterior resection and anastomosis was done. On the 4th postoperative day, the patient was allowed liquid diet. Distension increased. For another 3 days, distension went on increasing. Plain X-ray abdomen revealed obstruction with more gas than before. The patient was having colicky abdominal pain. Exploratory laparotomy was done. Findings at 2nd laparotomy—anastomosis was intact. Transverse colon was hugely dilated. Careful palpation of splenic flexure revealed one more growth. A resection and anastomosis was done again. Patient was discharged after 10 days. The first surgeon agreed that after finding the rectosigmoid growth, he did not look for any other lesions (mistake). This was obviously a case of synchronous carcinoma.

METACHRONOUS COLONIC CANCER

- Metachronous cancer was defined as those cancer occurring more than 6 months following resection of one malignancy.
- A few examples of metachronous site are: Colorectum, breast, kidney.
- Family history of hereditary, nonpolyposis colorectal cancer (HNPCC or Lynch syndrome), an autosomal dominant disease, also can present with both synchronous or metachronous colorectal cancers.
- It is more common in females.
- Common usually at young age.
- The associated genetic defect lies at the mismatch repair genes, responsible for the correction of DNA bases mismatch.
- The coexistence of adenomatous polyps is also considered a risk factor for the development of metachronous lesions. Thus, after treating one carcinoma, example—carcinoma sigmoid, annual colonoscopy is recommended. If polyps are detected, patients have to be informed about the polyps and their potential of malignancy.
- Survival is better.

FAMILIAL COLORECTAL CANCER

- All these have a carrier gene and thus, run in families. Malignancies occur in young age group. Often they are synchronous. Metachronous lesions are not uncommon.
- Certain criteria have been laid upon for the diagnosis of these conditions which have been discussed already.

- Genetic instability is the chief factor responsible. The instability can be at chromosomal level called chromosomal instability or **at DNA level called microsatellite instability—MSI.** As a result of this after the cell division by duplication, mismatched genes develop. These genes cannot be repaired. This predisposes to mutation, results in a cancer gene.
- **Familial polyposis coli** accounts for about 1% of colorectal cancers. However, incidence of malignancy is 100%. Gardner's and Turcot's syndromes are the variants of FPC.
- **HNPCC** accounts for about 5 to 10% of colorectal cancers. They also have extracolonic cancers such as endometrial, ovarian and urinary bladder cancers.
- Other familial syndromes are **Cronkhite-Canada syndrome.** It is more common in females. Multiple polyps develop in stomach, duodenum and in the colon. Diarrhoea is the clinical presentation. Other features include pigmentation, alopecia, loss of weight and cachexia. Chances of developing malignancy is about 15%.

PRECANCEROUS CONDITIONS (Key Box 47.5)

1. **Polyps:** Environmental and genetic factors favour the development of colonic polyps and their transformation into malignancy. The incidence of malignancy is increased when the polyp is more than 1 cm, polyps are multiple or flat (Table 47.2).

Key Box 47.5

Risk Factors Associated with Colon Cancer

Risk factor	Incidence of cancer
Familial polyposis coli	100% chances of colorectal cancer
HNPCC	80% chances
Ulcerative colitis	10–20% after 20 years
Crohn's colitis	5% after 10–20 years
Adenomatous polyps	1–20% depending upon the size

Pearls of Wisdom

Familial polyposis coli has 100% chance of carcinoma.

2. **Inflammatory bowel disease:**
   - A. **Ulcerative colitis** is a definite precancerous condition. Presence of dysplasia diagnosed by colonoscopic biopsy is an indication for colectomy.
   - B. **Crohn's** involving colon also has a mildly increased risk of developing carcinoma when compared to ulcerative colitis.
   - C. **Schistosomal colitis:** The risk of colorectal cancer is increased in patients with long-standing schistosomal colitis. Long-standing cases are associated with mild to severe grades of colonic epithelial dysplasia. Thus ulcers or pseudopolyps can occur. These dysplastic changes are considered as premalignant.
   - D. **Radiation exposure:** Usually, it is mucin-secreting adenocarcinoma with poor prognosis.
   - E. **Ureterosigmoidostomy** increases risk of colonic cancer over 100–500 times.

AETIOLOGICAL FACTORS

SAD factors: It is sad to know that **SAD** factors are responsible for carcinoma colon. They are **S**—Smoking, **A**—Alcohol, **D**—Dietary factors. Diet rich in red meat has high animal fat. This alters intestinal bacteria, which convert primary bile acids into secondary bile acids. ***This is the beginning of formation of carcinogenic polycyclic aromatic compounds.*** After cholecystectomy, there is increase in free bile acid concentration, thus increasing the risk of colonic cancer. Thus increased roughage is associated with increased transit time which in turn reduces exposure of mucosa to carcinogens.

- Increase incidence is found in western countries wherein diet rich in animal fat is consumed in large quantity. Incidence is more after the age of 50 years. Obesity, poor exercise and smoking are the contributing factors.
- Some interesting observations are also found in females with colonic cancer which have been depicted in Key Box 47.6.

Table 47.2 Summary of colonic polyps and malignant potential

Type	Cause	Malignant potential	Features/syndrome
1. Adenomatous polyp	Benign tumour	1–10%	Hypokalaemia, diarrhoea
2. Hamartomatous polyp	"Misfire"	Negligible	Peutz-Jeghers syndrome
3. Familial polyposis coli	Genetic disorder	100%	Gardner's and Turcot's syndrome
4. Metaplastic polyps	Hyperplasia	Nil	Asymptomatic

Key Box 47.6

Women and Colonic Cancer

- **Caecum** is more commonly involved than other parts.
- Women with **breast cancer** have increased incidence of colonic cancer.
- Women **smokers** have increased chances of colonic cancer.
- Women who have undergone **cholecystectomy** have increased chances of colonic cancer.
- Metastasis to ovary is mostly haematogenous (1 to 10%).

Pearls of Wisdom

Calcium salts are protective. They form insoluble bile salt complexes, thus reducing the concentration of bile acids in the colon.

PATHOLOGICAL TYPES (Fig. 47.14)

- It is an adenocarcinoma—columnar epithelium. Rectum (40%) and sigmoid (20%) take a major share in colorectal carcinoma followed by caecum (12 to 15%). Multiple synchronous cancers are also common in the colon.
  - A. **Annular stricture:** Common in left colon (splenic flexure, pelvic colon). So obstruction is common.
  - B. **Tubular stricture:** Common in left colon and at the rectosigmoid junction.
  - C. **Ulcerative lesion:** Ascending colon or caecum, they present with anemia.
  - D. **Proliferative growth:** More in right colon, the least malignant, fleshy and bulky polypoid lesion (Fig. 47.15).
- It is a columnar cell adenocarcinoma. In about 5% of cases, it undergoes mucoid degeneration. Such tumours carry poor prognosis. They spread to the liver very fast and secondaries produce mucoid material.

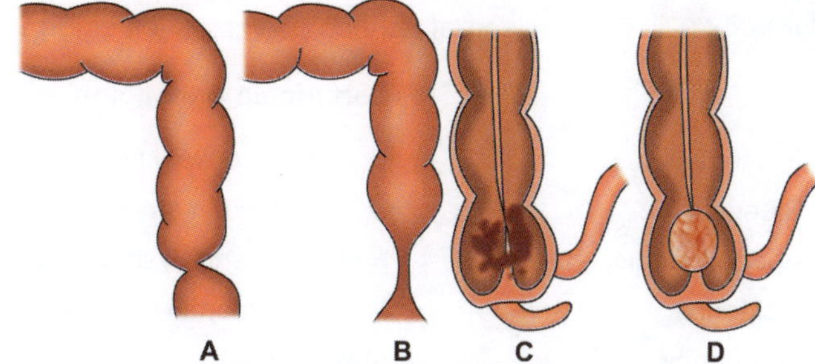

Figs 47.14A to D: Types of carcinoma colon

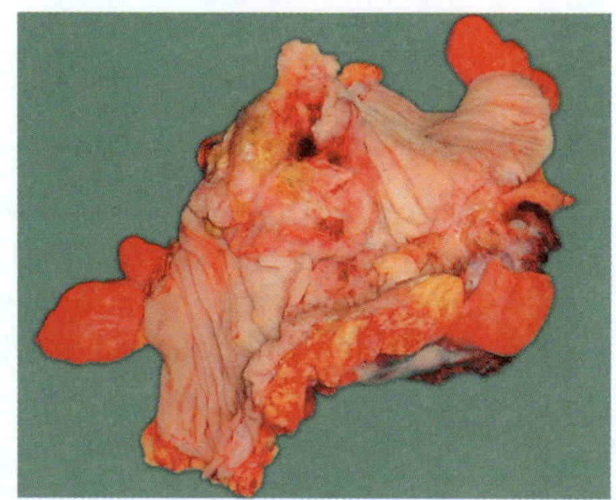
Fig. 47.15: Ulceroproliferative growth in the descending colon

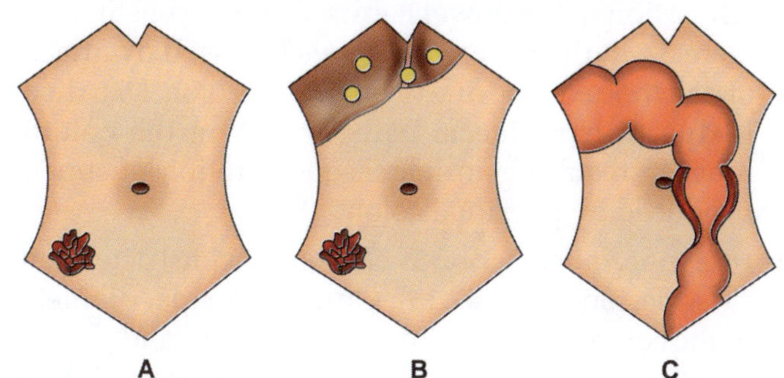

Figs 47.16A to C: (A) Carcinoma caecum, (B) Carcinoma caecum with secondaries in the liver, (C) Carcinoma left colon with intestinal obstruction

CLINICAL FEATURES OF CARCINOMA COLON

(Figs 47.16A to C and Table 47.3) (*Mnemonic:* **TMA Pai**)[1]

1. **Tumour:** The mass produced by carcinoma caecum and even hepatic flexure is palpable. It is firm to hard, irregular and with or without fixity.
   - Occasionally, growth at pelvirectal junction can be felt on rectal examination.
   - However, on left-sided constrictive lesions, growth is not often felt. It is the hard faecal matter and lymph nodes which are felt as a mass.
2. **Metastasis:** 5–10% of the patients present with metastasis to liver (mucoid adenocarcinoma), lungs ascites, etc. Distant metastasis is not common (Fig. 47.17).

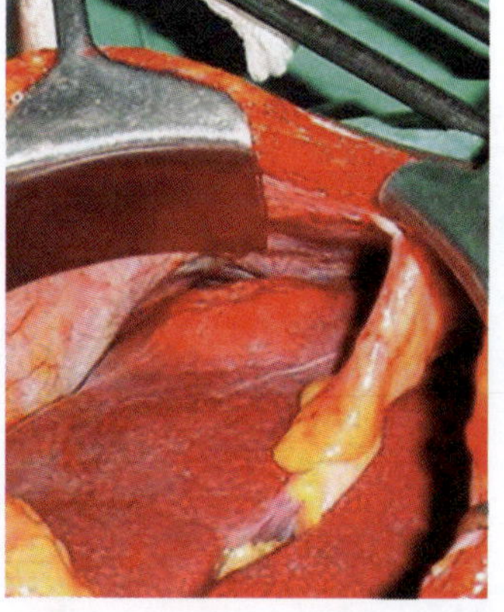
Fig. 47.17: Large secondary in the liver. Look at the umbilication resulting due to central necrosis of the secondary

[1]Late Padmashree Dr TMA Pai, was the founder of Kasturba Medical College which he started in 1953. He was also a banker and educationist. He is called 'Modern Architect of Manipal', where Manipal Academy of Higher Education (MAHE)—deemed to be the university is situated.

Table 47.3 Comparison of right colon versus left colon

	Carcinoma right colon	Carcinoma left colon
• Presentation	Unexplained weakness, anaemia	Change in bowel habits
• Bleeding	Occult blood in stools	Gross blood in stools
• Abdominal discomfort	Right side and dyspeptic symptoms also	Constipation and obstruction
• Incidence	More common in women	More common in men
• Frequency	About 10–20%	About 60–70% (including rectum)
• Pathology	Ulcerative/proliferative lesion	Strictures (rectosigmoid)
• Investigation	Colonoscopy	Flexible sigmoidoscopy
• Complication	Obstruction—less common	Obstruction, perforation, pericolic abscess—common

3. **Anaemia** is an important feature of carcinoma caecum. It may be due to blood loss or a proliferative growth secreting toxins causing suppression of bone marrow. Asthaenia and anorexia are the other features.
4. **Pain abdomen:** Dull aching pain may be present. Colicky pain is due to chronic obstruction as in left-sided growths (napkin ring stricture).
5. **Alteration in the bowel habits:** A recent constipation, increase in the dose of laxatives followed by attacks of diarrhoea can be due to carcinoma colon. Diarrhoea is due to hard faecal balls, irritating the colonic mucosa resulting in increased secretion of mucus produced by proximal colon.
6. **Intestinal obstruction** is caused by constricted left-sided lesions (Fig. 47.18). On the left side, diameter of the colon is narrow, contents are solid and growth is constrictive. Lower abdominal distension, right to left peristalsis are the late features. Carcinoma sigmoid can cause colovesical fistula.

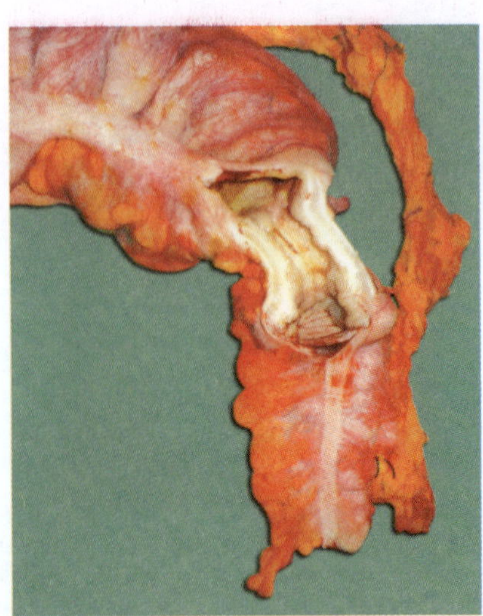

Fig. 47.18: Tubular stricture at rectosigmoid junction—cut opened specimen after resection

To Summarise

- **Early cases:** It can be easily missed—such as change in bowel habits such as diarrhoea, vague ill health, weakness (due to anaemia), intermittent bleeding per rectum, often attributed to piles or some other cause. Mass is usually not palpable.
- **Late cases:** It can present with obstruction (recto-sigmoid junction growth), perforation, intussusception (right-sided tumours), mass abdomen, secondaries in the liver, left supraclavicular nodes (Troisier's sign), etc.

See Key Boxes 47.7 to 47.9.

Key Box 47.7

Peculiarities of Carcinoma of Caecum
(Figs 47.19 to 47.25)

- Incidence is more in females.
- Presents with anaemia and a mass.
- Can present as acute appendicitis when the lumen of appendix is obstructed—called secondary appendicitis (in elderly patients).
- It is a cause of intussusception (secondary).
- Can present with flexion of hip due to infiltration of iliopsoas.

Key Box 47.8

Peculiarities of Carcinoma Splenic Flexure

- Presents as obstruction.
- It is easily missed unless carefully looked for.
- Carries poor prognosis as many cases present with obstruction.
- Often, it is inoperable.

Pearls of Wisdom

Obstructed and perforated carcinoma colon have poor prognosis.

Key Box 47.9

Peculiarities of Carcinoma Sigmoid
(Figs 47.26 and 47.27)

- Commonly presents as **obstructive lesion**—constipation and intestinal obstruction.
- **Colovesical fistula:** Carcinoma sigmoid is the 2nd commonest cause. 1st cause is diverticulosis.
- It can cause **colovaginal fistula.**
- It can also **infiltrate ureter, uterus and ovary.**
- It can present as **abscess in the lateral abdominal wall.**

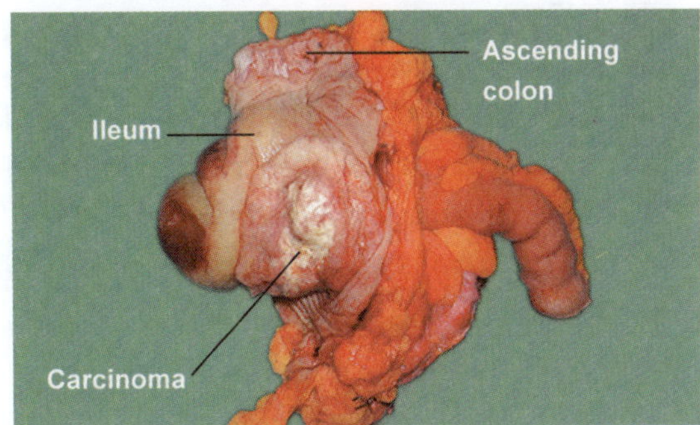

Fig. 47.19: Intussusception due to carcinoma caecum

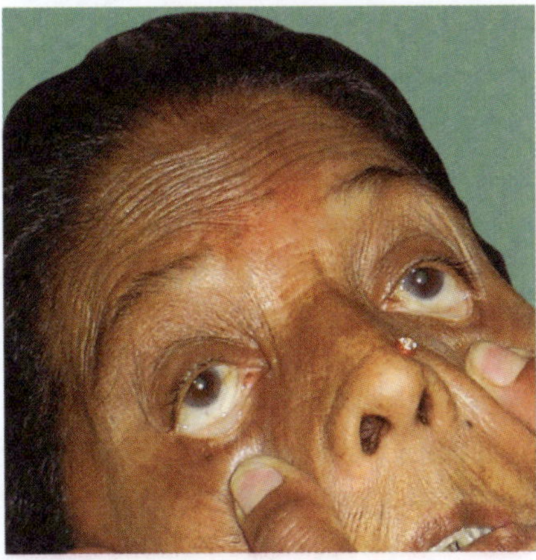

Fig. 47.20: Pallor disproportionate to the blood loss—typical of carcinoma caecum

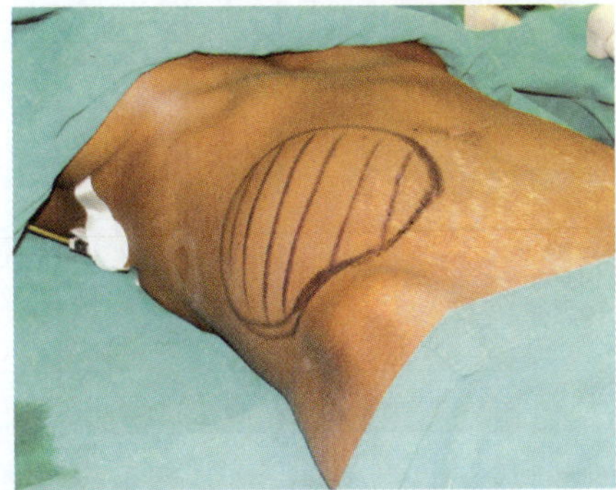

Fig. 47.21: A 34-year-old lady presented to the hospital with mass in the right iliac fossa with slight flexion of the right hip. Mass was hard and irregular. She also had anaemia

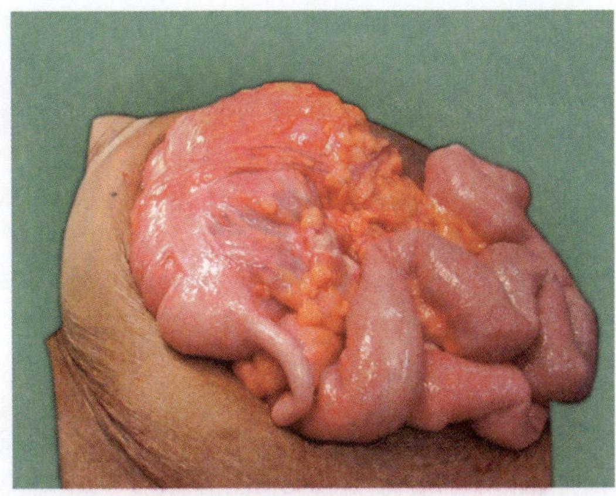

Fig. 47.22: Exploration of the mass (caecum). It was mobile. Entire right colon is mobilised by incising right paracolic gutter and dividing colo-phrenic ligament

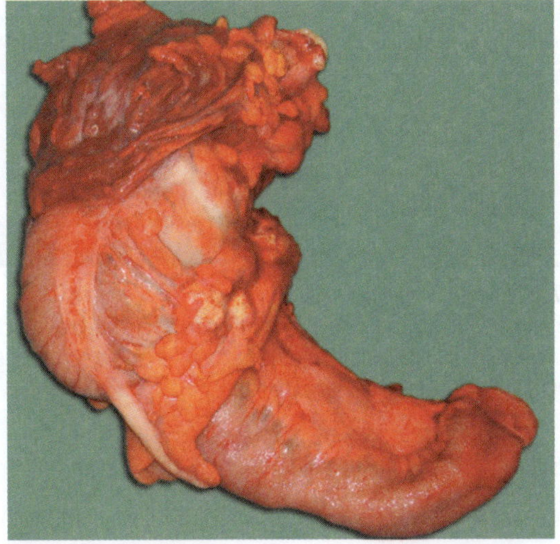

Fig. 47.23: Right hemicolectomy specimen—a case of carcinoma caecum

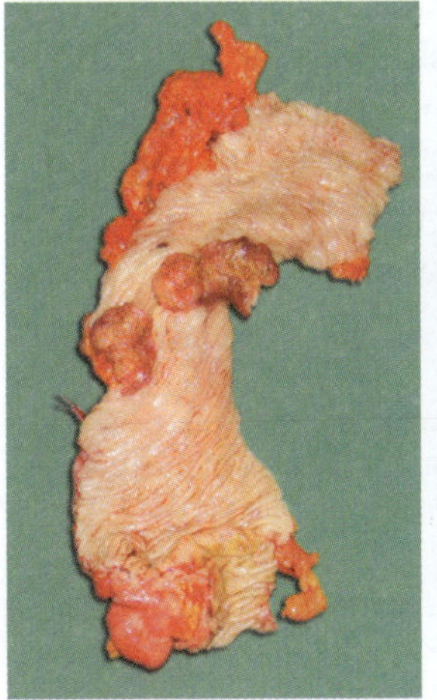

Fig. 47.24: Carcinoma hepatic flexure with partial obstruction

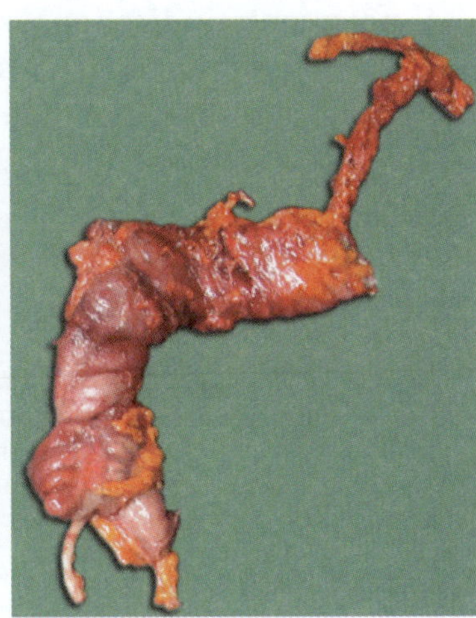

Fig. 47.25: Extended right hemicolectomy specimen

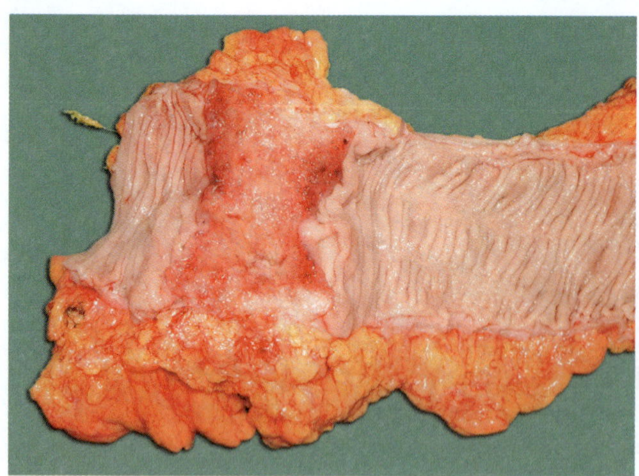

Fig. 47.26: Rectosigmoid stricture. Patient underwent high anterior resection. 5 cm proximal margin is enough for radical cure

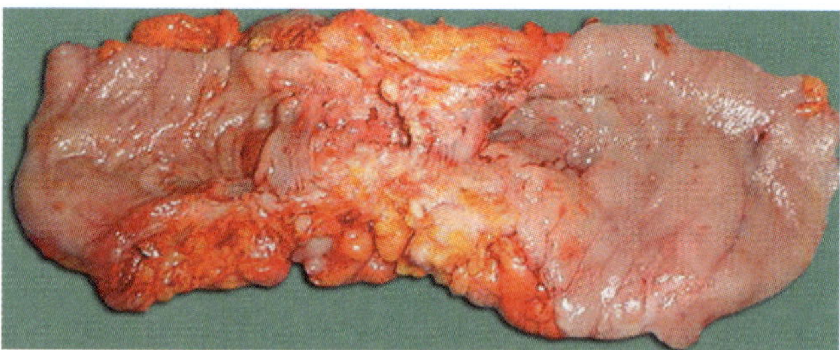

Fig. 47.27: Intestinal obstruction due to rectosigmoid stricture—a common complication. **Tumour rarely goes beyond 2 cm from the edge of the tumour** unless there is concomitant spread to lymph nodes

Spread

1. **Local:** For a long time, the lesion is confined to mucosa and submucosa. They grow in annular fashion and later longitudinally. Once serosa is involved, spread occurs rapidly into neighbouring structures such as ureter, bladder, uterus, etc. The involvement of these structures is **not a contraindication** for surgery (TNM staging).
   - Local perforation may result in pericolic abscess.
   - Hollow viscus perforation results in internal fistula.
2. **Lymphatic spread** (*see* page 792 and refer TNM staging).
3. **Blood spread:** It occurs late, resulting in secondaries in the liver, lungs, etc. Cannonball in lung, nodule in the liver.

Pearls of Wisdom

Because of the drainage into the portal system, colonic cancers spread to the liver first. On the other hand, rectal cancers spread to the lungs because of drainage into inferior vena cava.

Staging/Classifications

There are many classifications and staging for carcinoma colon/rectum. They are not important. A few important ones have been given here.

I. Dukes' Staging for Colorectal Cancer

- **Stage A:** Invasion of but not breaching the muscularis propria.
- **Stage B:** Breaching the muscularis propria but not involving the lymph nodes.
- **Stage C:** Lymph nodes are involved.

A few authors describe a stage D for metastatic disease. Since it has not been described by Duke, it is called modified Dukes' staging.

II. Astler-Coller's Modification of Dukes' Staging

Stages (Fig. 47.28)

A	Limited to mucosa—no nodes
B1	Extension into muscularis propria—no nodes
B2	Extension into entire bowel wall—no nodes
B3	Extension into adjacent organs—no nodes
C1	Extension into muscularis propria—positive nodes
C2	B2 + Lymph nodes
C3	B3 + Lymph nodes
D	Distant metastasis

III. WHO Classification

It is based on histology.

- Majority are adenocarcinoma—90%
- Mucinous adenocarcinoma—5–10%
- Signet ring cell carcinoma
- Small cell carcinoma
- Squamous cell carcinoma
- Undifferentiated carcinoma

IV. TNM Staging (see text on the next page)

A few clinical photograph, staging pictures and operative pictures have been given in the next page.

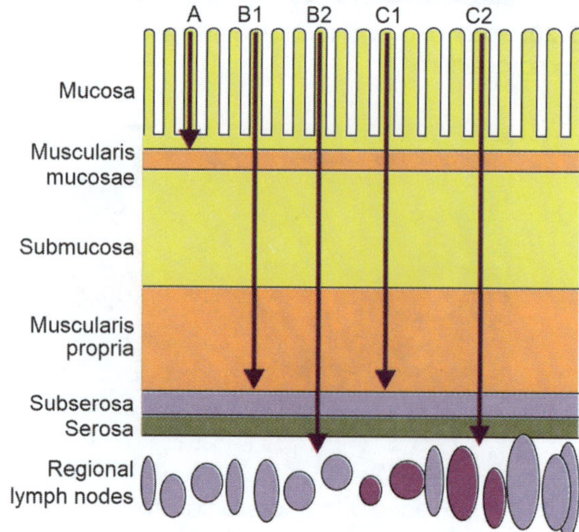

Fig. 47.28: Astler-Coller staging

TNM STAGING Colorectal cancer

Tumour—T
Tx—Primary tumour cannot be assessed
T0—No evidence of tumour
Tis—Carcioma *in situ*—intraepithelial/invasion into lamina propria
T1—Invasion into submucosa
T2—Invasion into muscularis propria
T3—Invasion into pericolorectal tissues/fat
T4a—Invasion into surface of the visceral peritoneum
T4b—Direct invasion or adherent to adjacent structures/ organs

Regional nodes—N
Nx—Nodes cannot be assessed
N0—No nodal spread
N1—Regional nodes 1–3 involved
- N1a—1 regional node
- N1b—2 to 3 regional nodes
- N1c—Tumour deposits in serosa/mesentery/non-peritonealised pericolic or perirectal tissue without regional nodes

N2a—Regional nodes 4 or more involved
- N2a—4–6 regional nodes
- N2b—7 or more regional nodes

Distant metastases M
M0 No distant spread
M1 Distant spread present
M1a Spread confined to one organ or site—liver/lung/ ovary/nonregional nodes
M1b Spread to more than one organ or site/peritoneum

Histological grade G
Gx—Grade cannot be assessed
G1—Well-differentiated
G2—Moderately differentiated
G3—Poorly differentiated
G4—Undifferentiated

Residual tumour R
R0—No residual tumour after resection
R1—Microscopic residual tumour after resection
R2—Macroscopic residual tumour after resection

Stage Group
0—Tis N0 M0
1—T1 N0 M0; T2 N0 M0
IIA—T3 N0 M0
IIB—T4a N0 M0
IIC—T4b N0 M'0
IIIA—T1-2 N1-1c M0; T1 N2a M0
IIIB—T3-4a N1-1c M0; T2-3 N2a M0; T1-2 N2b M0
IIIC—T4a N2a M0;T3-4a N2b M0;T4b N1-2 M0
IVA—Any T any N M1a
IVB—Any T any N M1b
V0—No venous invasion; V1—presence of venous invasion
L0—No lymphatic vessel invasion; L1—presence of lymphatic vessel invasion

Complications (Fig. 47.29)

1. **Intestinal obstruction**
2. **Pericolic abscess:** Pain is present in the tumour site and may radiate to back, leg or hip as in caecal perforations. It is due to irritation of the psoas muscles or due to irritation of femoral nerve.
    - Diagnosis is confirmed by ultrasound/CT scan.
    - Percutaneous aspiration, followed by elective resection is the best treatment.
3. **Faecal fistula** (Fig. 47.30)
    - Pericolic abscess when it is incised or drained to the exterior may result in faecal fistula, if there is malignancy.
    - Carcinoma caecum may result in appendicitis and appendicectomy may invariably result in faecal fistula.
4. **Internal fistula:** Colovesical (commonest), colocolic, coloenteric are not uncommon complications of malignancies. They are managed by resection. However, preoperative assessment of fistulae by investigations should be done.

Pearls of Wisdom

Involvement of local structures is not a contraindication for radical resection.

Investigations (Fig. 47.31)

1. **Complete blood picture**—demonstrates low Hb%
2. **Occult blood** in stools

Pearls of Wisdom

Occult blood in the stools may be the finding which gives a 'clue' in many cases of 'anaemia for evaluation'.

3. **Double contrast barium enema** may show irregular filling defect—intrinsic, persistent. It may also show an apple core deformity (Figs 47.32 and 47.33 and Key Box 47.10) not routinely done.

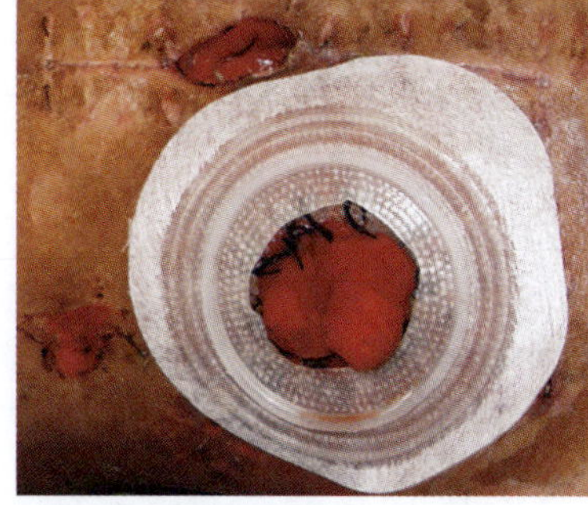

Fig. 47.29: Limited colectomy leak—managed by refashioning of the stoma followed by ileostomy

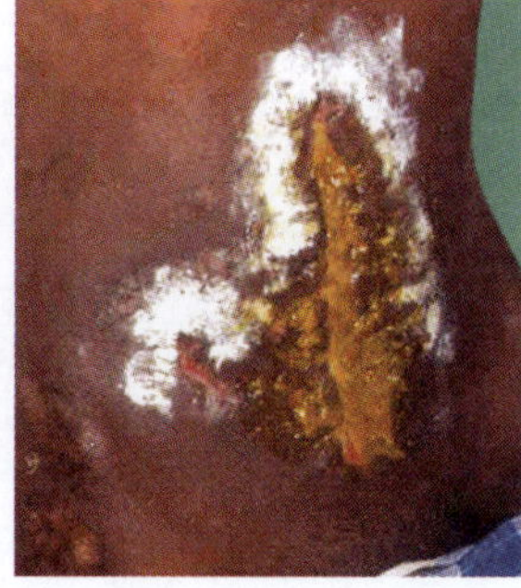

Fig. 47.30: Carcinoma colon perforated—pericolic abscess which on draining resulted in faecal fistula

Carcinoma colon—investigations

Routine tests/general fitness
1. **Complete blood count**
   - Hb%: Low indicating anaemia
   - TC, DC: If it is high, it indicates perforation, pericolic abscess
   - ESR: May be increased
2. **Stool:** Occult blood positive
3. Liver function tests, renal function tests and blood sugar estimation
4. Cardiac ECHO/ECG for fitness before surgery

ECOG performance score—page 681

Diagnostic tests
1. **Ultrasound:** Simple, baseline noninvasive investigation
   - Can pick up 'colonic mass'
   - Can detect liver metastasis
   - Can demonstrate ascites, para-aortic nodes
2. **CT scan**
   - Objective, more precise about mass, infiltration to vascular pedicles, lymph nodes, ureters
3. **Colonoscopy**
   - Invasive but diagnostic and **Gold standard investigation**
   - Biopsy should be taken for final confirmation

Metastatic workup—investigations to know spread
1. Chest X-ray to look for cannonball secondaries
2. CEA: Gross elevation may suggest advanced stage
3. CT is also done to know local and distant spread
4. PET scan: If CEA levels start increasing during follow-up of cases of carcinoma colon.

Fig. 47.31: Carcinoma colon—investigations

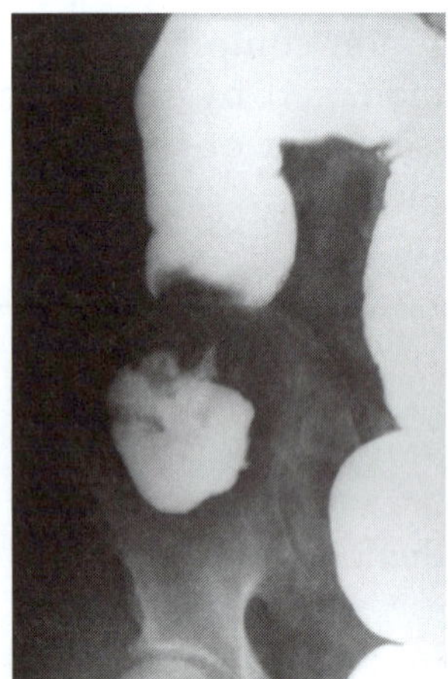

Fig. 47.32: Barium enema showing apple core deformity

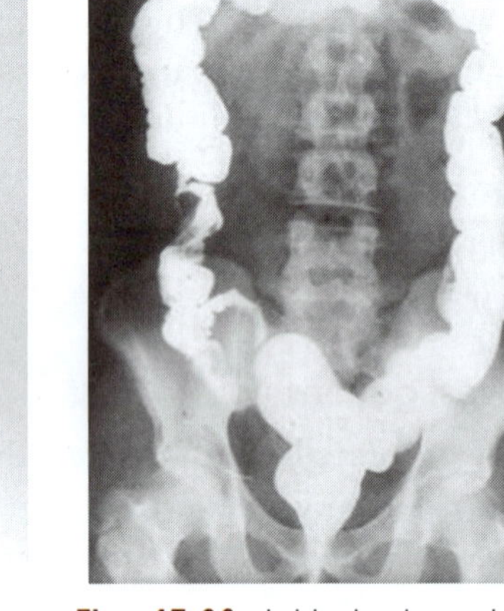

Fig. 47.33: Intrinsic, irregular, persistent filling defect

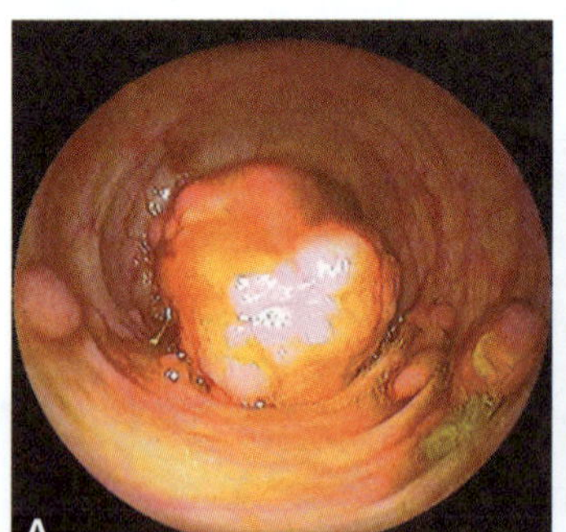

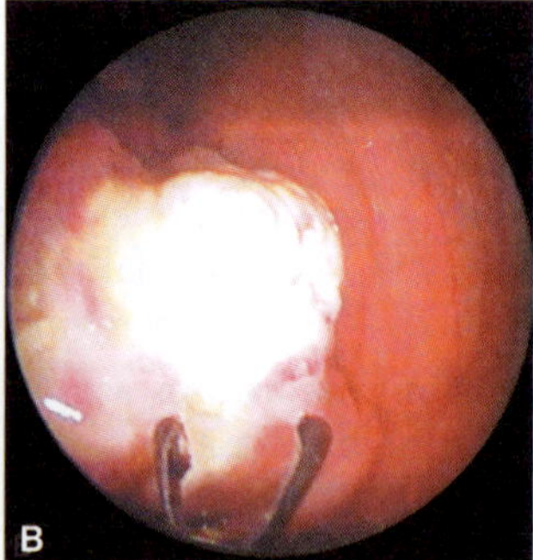

Figs 47.34A and B: Colonoscopy shows growth and biopsy is being taken (*Courtesy:* Dr Filipe Alvares, Consultant, Medical Gastroenterologist, KMC, Manipal)

Key Box 47.10

Barium Enema

- Gives good anatomic and topographic information.
- Can detect associated diverticular disease.
- Small ulcerative lesions can also be diagnosed.

4. **Flexible sigmoidoscopy:** 60 cm of colon can be visualised. It is an outpatient procedure. It is indicated in rectal bleeding. An enema is given before the procedure.
5. **Colonoscopy** is done to take a biopsy from growth and also to rule out synchronous malignancy as seen in 5% of the cases (more than one malignancy at the time of diagnosis). If biopsy cannot be taken, as in obstruction, brush cytology can be taken (Fig. 47.34).
   - Small risk of perforation is present and it is invasive procedure.
   - **Virtual colonoscopy** can pick up polyp of 6 mm size also but biopsy cannot be taken.
6. **Ultrasound:** It is the first baseline investigation to be obtained.
   - It can detect colonic mass.
   - It can detect hydronephrosis, liver metastasis, ascites, para-aortic nodes.
   - Ultrasound-guided biopsy is possible in advanced cases.
   - Definitely it cannot pick up early mucosal or lesions which have penetrated up to muscularis mucosa or serosa.
7. **CT scan in carcinoma colon**
   - Other than a biopsy, it has all the advantages and it is the investigation of choice after colonoscopy.
   - Anatomical location of the tumour, involvement of serosa.
   - Infiltration of local adjacent structures like ureter (right side)—preoperative stenting is required in such cases.

- Metastasis in the liver, ascites, para-aortic nodes.
- Other associated diseases specially in elderly such as aortic aneurysm, gallstone, hiatus hernia, etc.
- 90% and 95% sensitivity and specificity in detecting liver lesions greater than 1 cm.

8. **Carcinoembryonic antigen (CEA)** (Key Box 47.11).
   - It is a foetal glycoprotein, not present in normal human beings (minute quantities). It is present in the cell membranes of many tissues including colorectal cancer.
   - It is present in the last trimester in the foetus.
   - It has a prognostic rather than a diagnostic value. After treatment of the primary, CEA level should come back to normal. If it does not come back to normal, it indicates residual disease. If it is increased, it suggests either recurrent tumour or secondaries in the liver.
9. **Role of PET scan**
   - Routine use of PET—positron emission tomographic scanning in the primary management of colorectal cancer is not recommended.
   - It is useful in the follow-up cases wherein CEA levels are increasing and the actual cause for the rise is being evaluated.
   - **Chest X-ray:** Colonic carcinoma spreads more often to lungs than carcinoma of stomach giving rise to cannonball secondaries.

Prognostic Factors of Carcinoma Colon

- **Spread:** If it is limited to mucosa and there are no nodes, 5-year survival is 90–100%.
- **Age:** Younger patients have poor prognosis.

Key Box 47.11

Carcinoembryonic Antigen—CEA

- Discovered by Gold and Freedman.
- It is a surface glycoprotein.
- Produced by colorectal epithelium but cleared by Kupffer cells of liver. Its half-life is prolonged (normal—10 days) in cholestasis and hepatocellular dysfunction.
- Normal levels: 0–4 mg/ml.
- Significant increase in the levels is also found in pancreatic carcinoma, gastric carcinoma, lung carcinoma, breast carcinoma.
- Increased CEA in the follow-up period of colorectal cancer suggests metastasis. PET scan may help in these patients when CT/US are normal.
- It has very low sensitivity.
- If preoperative CEA is increased in node-negative colonic cancer, chemotherapy is recommended.

- **Grade:** Poorly differentiated tumours have worse prognosis.
- **Obstruction and perforation:** Poor prognosis is due to dissemination of malignant cells.
- **Blood transfusion:** Perioperative blood transfusion has poor prognosis.

Pearls of Wisdom

Blood transfusion increases number of suppressor T lymphocytes, thus causing immunosuppression. Hence, follow bloodless surgery or autologous blood transfusion.

PREOPERATIVE PREPARATION IN COLONIC SURGERY

1. **Mechanical bowel preparation (MBP):** It was believed that mechanical bowel preparation had the following benefits: It decreases intraoperative contamination, prevents disruption of anastomosis, improves the handling of the bowel, prevents postoperative infectious complications such as wound infection, intra-abdominal abscess and anastomotic leak, and reduces the bacterial count within the colon. However, studies have proved that often liquid faecal matter is present at the site of anastomosis. Liquid faeces are more difficult to handle than solid faeces and spillage of liquid faeces results in increased chance of contamination. MBP damages colocytes, causes oedema and inflammation of colon and facilitates bacterial translocation and anastomotic leak. MBP does not reduce colonic bacterial count/surgical site infection (SSI). The patient needs prior hospitalization and it delays fast-track colonic surgery. In addition to this, MBP prolongs postoperative ileus. In spite of this, many surgeons still use mechanical bowel preparation by using polyethylene glycol (PEG). It is the agent used for cleansing of the gut. PEG is an osmotic laxative and is a balanced solution that is not absorbed. Hence, it is safe for patients with electrolyte imbalances (i.e. renal failure patients) or patients who may not be able to tolerate fluid shifts (i.e. congestive heart failure patients, patients with ascites from liver disease). In addition, **PEG solution is the method of choice for bowel cleansing of infants and children.**
2. **Oral antibiotics:** Colorectal resections have a higher SSI rate than other elective abdominal operations because of the high bacterial load present within the colon lumen, estimated to be 10^{12} colony-forming units per gram of stool. Metronidazole 500 mg given may be substituted for erythromycin for better tolerability. Metronidazole has excellent anaerobic activity, enterohepatic circulation, and has been shown to be clinically effective.

3. **Parenteral antibiotics:** There is a little doubt among surgeons that administration of preoperative parenteral antibiotics prevents SSI. Second generation cephalosporins with nitroimidazole are given 0 to 2 hours before incision. The dose needs to be repeated in 2 to 6 hours depending upon the antibiotic used and the duration of surgery. **Do not continue these drugs after their use for surgical prophylaxis.**
4. **Diet:** Patients are routinely fasted before an anaesthetic but the required duration of fasting varies with substances ingested. Fasting for 2 hours is advised for clear fluids. The patients must abstain from taking solid food and milk for 6 hours before surgery. Fried/fatty food or meal needs a longer time for gastric emptying. Hence, they should fast for 8 hours after fatty food meal. Prolonged fasting is not advisable and hence, **ingestion of carbohydrate-rich clear fluids is recommended until 2 hours prior to surgery.** Advantages of carbohydrate-rich drink are that it reduces postoperative thirst, reduces postoperative hunger and decreases anxiety. It also reduces postoperative insulin resistance and postoperative weight loss. In anabolic state, postoperative nitrogen and protein losses are reduced and hence, lean body mass and muscle strength are better maintained.
5. **Thromboprophylaxis:** Patients undergoing colorectal resections are considered moderate to high-risk group for deep vein thrombosis (DVT)/pulmonary embolism (PE) and, therefore, should receive thromboprophylaxis as a rule. Chemical thromboprophylaxis is given using low molecular weight heparin—enoxaparin/dalteparin are the heparinis. Unfractionated heparinis equally effective but APTT needs to be monitored. Mechanical thromboprophylaxis can also be done in the operation theatres by using DVT stockings. **The drug used for thromoprophylaxis must be continued for minimum 4–6 weeks in the postoperative period.**
6. **Nasogastric tube:** It is not recommended routinely. Presence of a nasogastric tube will keep the oesophagogastric junction sphincter open and may cause increased chances of aspiration pneumonia. It may delay recovery from paralytic ileus. However, it is definitely indicated in cases of obstructed colon.

Preoperative Preparation of the Colon

1. Mechanical bowel preparation	Yes/No
2. Oral antibiotics	May be/yes
3. Fasting for 6 hours	Yes
4. Thromboprophylaxis	Yes
5. Intravenous antibiotics prophylaxis	Yes
6. Nasogastric tube	No

Surgery

Over a period of years, radical resections for carcinoma of colon have become less radical pertaining to the extent of bowel resection. For example: One need not remove terminal 30 cm of ileum for carcinoma caecum today. Only 6–8 cm of ileum removal is sufficient in a right hemicolectomy.

TEN COMMANDMENTS OF SURGERY FOR CARCINOMA COLON—OPEN SURGERY

1. Should mark the ostomy site preoperatively—in cases of emergency colectomy.
2. Should give an adequate incision.
3. Should explore the peritoneal cavity for metastasis.
4. Should remove the growth with at least 7 cm margin, with all groups of regional nodes, fat fascia and lymphatics called *en block* resection—R-0 resection.
5. Should do the resection without touching or handling the tumour—follow no touch technique or Turnbull.
6. Should divide the vascular pedicle first and should ligate the vessels as high at the origin—high tie.
7. Should ensure the cut ends bleed well before anastomosis.
8. Should ensure there is no tension at the suture line.
9. Should do one stage procedure in all elective cases—resection and anastomosis.
10. Should consider temporary ileostomy after resection anastomosis in obstructed colon cancer.

Different Types of Surgery

1. **Carcinoma right colon including caecum:** If it is operable, the treatment is right radical hemicolectomy. Structures removed in this operation are (Fig. 47.35 and Key Box 47.12):
   - **Terminal 6–8 cm of ileum**[1]
   - Caecum, appendix and ascending colon
   - One-third of transverse colon
   - Fat, fascia, lymphatics and lymph nodes like ileocolic nodes, pericolic nodes, nodes at the origin of SMA. At least 16 lymph nodes should be removed.

Key Box 47.12

Structures that can get Injured during Right Hemicolectomy

- Duodenum
- Ureter
- Gonadal vessels

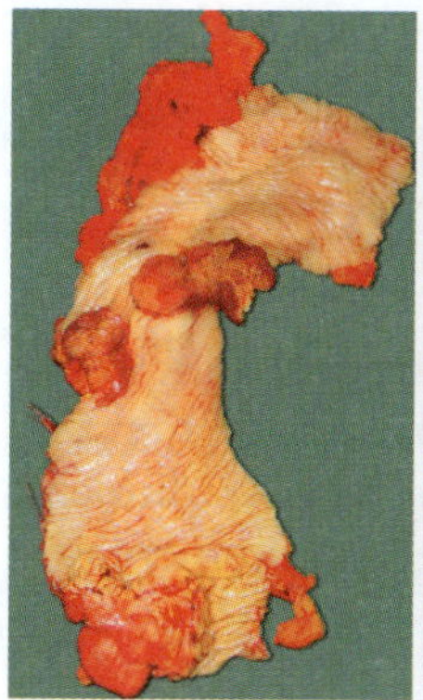
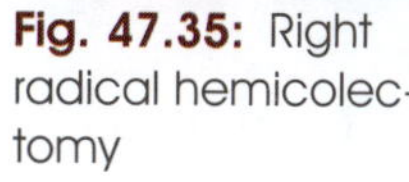

Fig. 47.35: Right radical hemicolectomy

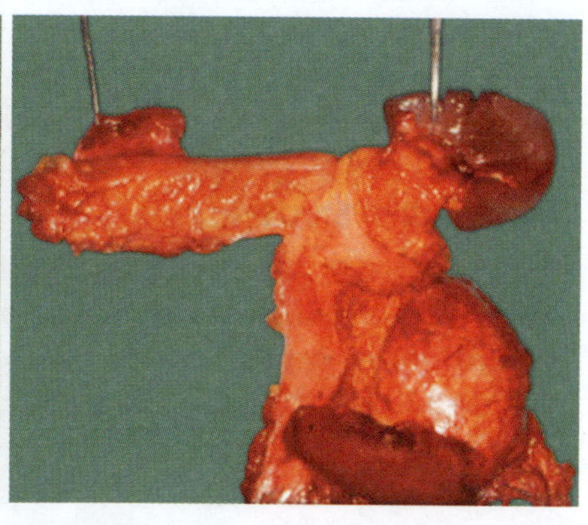

Fig. 47.36: Left radical hemicolectomy including removal of the spleen as the growth was infiltrating the spleen—routine removal of spleen should not be done

- If the growth is fixed to posterior abdominal wall and common iliac vessels, ileostomy is done first followed by neoadjuvant chemotherapy is given to downstage the tumour followed by resection. This is the only indication for neoadjuvant chemotherapy in carcinoma colon.
- However, in advanced cases and elderly patients with poor performance status, palliative ileo-transverse colostomy can be done.

2. **Carcinoma transverse colon**—'V' resection. The area supplied by middle colic artery is removed followed by end-to-end anastomosis. The patient may need removal of entire transverse colon depending upon lesion.
   - When lesion is at hepatic flexure or in the transverse colon, extended right hemicolectomy should be done.
3. **Carcinoma left colon**—left radical hemicolectomy.
   - Left half of the transverse colon and descending colon are removed followed by anastomosis of transverse colon to sigmoid colon—this is the area supplied by left colic artery (Fig. 47.36).
4. **Carcinoma sigmoid colon**—radical sigmoid colectomy followed by anastomosis of descending colon to the rectum (colorectal anastomosis). Or in a few cases, left hemicolectomy may have to be done.
5. **Left-sided colonic tumours with intestinal obstruction**—an emergency temporary transverse colostomy is done to divert the faecal matter and to relieve intestinal obstruction (for more details on colostomy, *see* page 875). Resection is not done because many patients are elderly with comorbid illness such as diabetes, hypertension, and cardiac illness.
   - General condition of the patient is poor with gross abdominal distension and dehydration.
   - Left colon is loaded with faecal matter. Hence, high chances of anastomotic leakage and faecal peritonitis are present.
   - After 2 weeks, laparotomy is done once again. The primary tumour is resected and end-to-end anastomosis done.
   - This is followed by closure of the colostomy 8 weeks later—**three-stage operation.**
   - Single-stage resection can also be done provided, thorough colonic irrigation through appendicular stump (after appendicectomy), is given and it should be successful in cleaning the entire colon. This is the concept of on-table irrigation and lavage.

On-Table Irrigation and Lavage (Fig. 47.37)

Indication

In cases of left-sided colonic obstructions—classical example being carcinoma rectosigmoid with obstruction.

Procedure

- Resection is done first. Clamps are applied to both ends.
- Appendicectomy is done and purse string suture applied but not tied.
- Through the appendicular stump lumen, a 30 Fr Foley catheter is passed into colon.
- The position of the catheter is checked to be lying safely in the caecum and its balloon is inflated. A purse-string suture, previously applied to the appendix base, is tied.

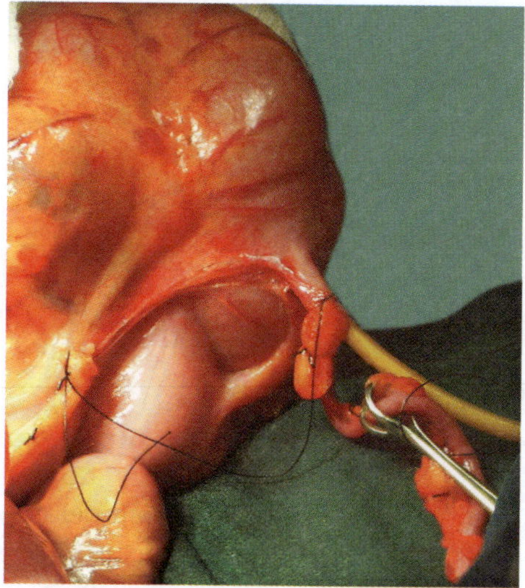

Fig. 47.37: 'On-table' irrigation through appendicular stump

[1]Removal of a foot of ileum is not necessary unless it has a doubtful vascularity after ligation of pedicles.

- Saline is irrigated at the rate of 50 to 100 ml per hour speed. Proximal clamp is opened into a container (kidney tray).
- It takes about an hour or so for the whole gut irrigation.
- This is done till the returning fluid is clear.

Advantage

It avoids a stoma, decreases stay in the hospital and thus less expensive.

Caecostomy Tube

Once anastomosis is completed, Foley catheter is brought out through an opening in the abdominal wall and connected to a bag. It is sutured to the inside of the parietes by Vicryl sutures and kept open.

Tube Removal

Tube is removed after 7–10 days provided there is no leak from the suture line.

Note: *A few diagrammatic representations of the colectomies are shown in the next page* (Figs 47.38 to 47.43).

ENHANCED RECOVERY PROGRAMME

Enhanced **Re**covery **A**fter **S**urgery (ERAS)

- It is also described as ERP (enhanced recovery programme), also called **fast track surgery.**
- Traditionally hospital stay following colorectal surgery is about 10–14 days. Now, with a few important steps taken in the pre-, peri- and postoperative periods, it is possible to decrease hospital stay to 2–5 days.

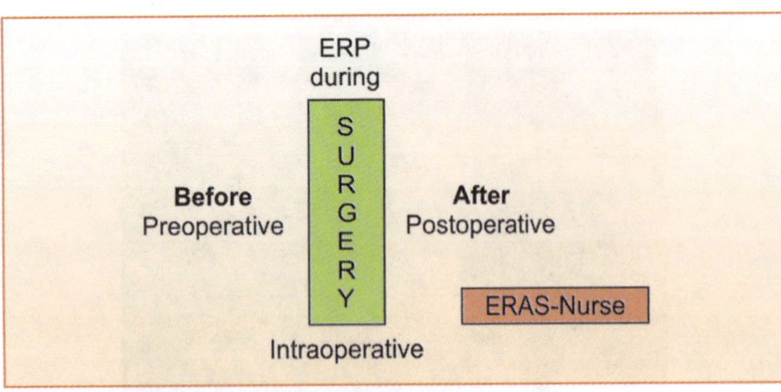

Preoperative Steps

- Metabolic response to injury/surgery produces increasing metabolic demands and nitrogen consumption. A few days in the postoperative period, there will be catabolic phase resulting in loss of muscle mass. Carbohydrate loading done a few hours before surgery decreases postoperative complication by decreasing postoperative insulin resistance and negative nitrogen balance.
- Only patients with anterior resection need to have bowel preparation. For all other colonic surgery, a single enema is more than enough.

Perioperative Steps

- Laparoscopic surgery gives the best results in the form of less pain, less wounds, less manipulation, less handling of bowel, no exposure to environment. (Thus recovery is fast.) Anaesthetic requirements are less including analgesia.
- Avoid long-acting narcotic analgesics.
- Avoid pre-medication.
- Mid-thoracic epidural block can be offered.
- Avoid tubes and catheters such as nasogastric tube (Ryle's tube) unless there is distension, postoperative drains (unless suspicious of doubtful anastomosis).
- Avoid central line and arterial lines.
- Preoperative-fluid restrictions—do not overload with water and sodium. Fluids should be less than 2 litres.
- Meticulous technique decreases the time taken for surgery, decrease in number of ports and small incisions for retrieval of specimen—all matters in ERAS.

Postoperative Steps

- Analgesics should be planned well—epidural blocks.
- Early mobilisation.
- Look for ileus/complications. If present, one should ready to manage.
- Early feeding—carbohydrate liquids.

POSTOPERATIVE CHEMOTHERAPY

1. pT1-2N0M0 do not require any adjuvant treatment, such patients can be kept on follow-up with routine 3 monthly CEA and annual CECT thorax/abdomen/pelvis.
2. pT3N0M0 or node positive disease requires adjuvant treatment in the form of concurrent chemoradiotherapy and chemotherapy. 2 cycles of FOLFOX (5-FU + Leucovorin + Oxaliplatin) → Concurrent 5-FU/Leucovorin and radiation → 2 more cycles of FOLFOX. Oral Capecitabine can be used in place of IV 5-FU.
3. It is preferable to add Oxaliplatin in the chemotherapy regimen, if nodes are positive for metastatic disease. In older population (>65–70 years), it might be of less benefit.
4. Oxaloplatins have been shown to downsize liver metastasis. Chief complication of Oxaliplatins is peripheral neuropathy.

SURGERIES IN A CASE OF CARCINOMA COLON (Figs 47.38 to 47.43 and Table 47.4)

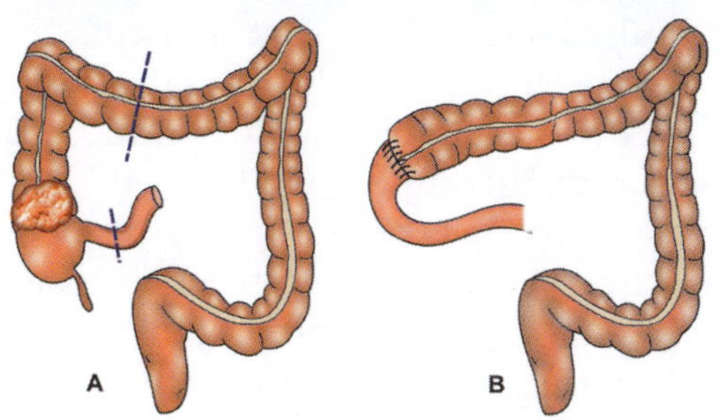

Figs 47.38A and B: Right hemicolectomy followed by end-to-end anastomosis—ileocolic

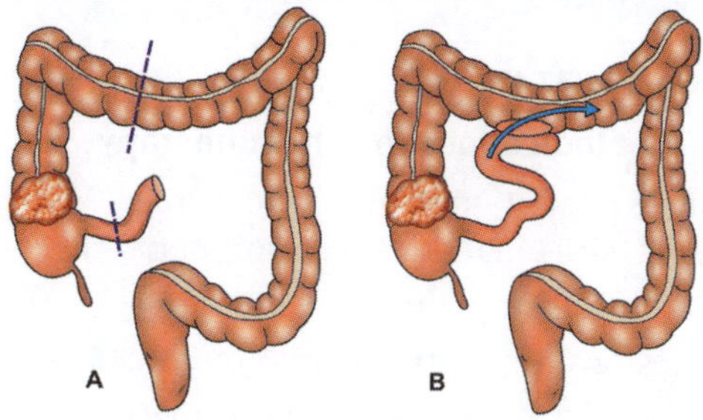

Figs 47.39A and B: Palliative ileotransverse anastomosis inoperable case

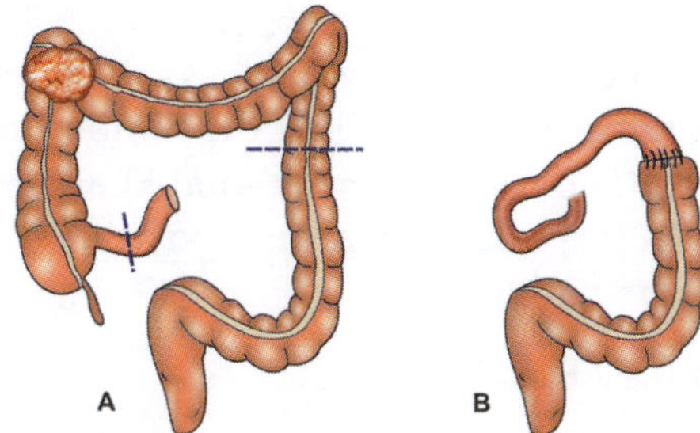

Figs 47.40A and B: Extended right hemicolectomy—growth in the hepatic flexure

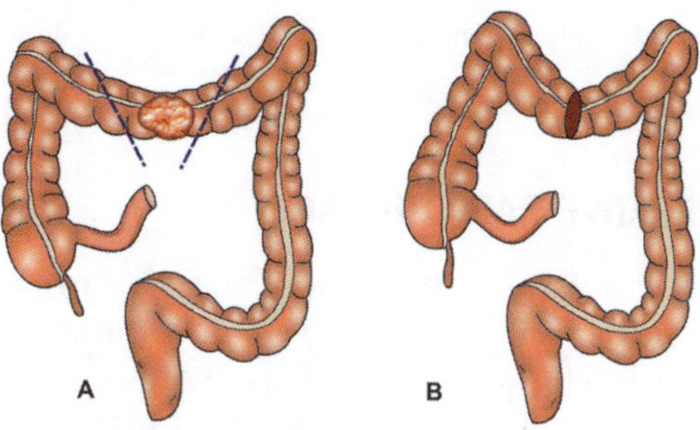

Figs 47.41A and B: Transverse colectomy followed by colocolic anastomosis

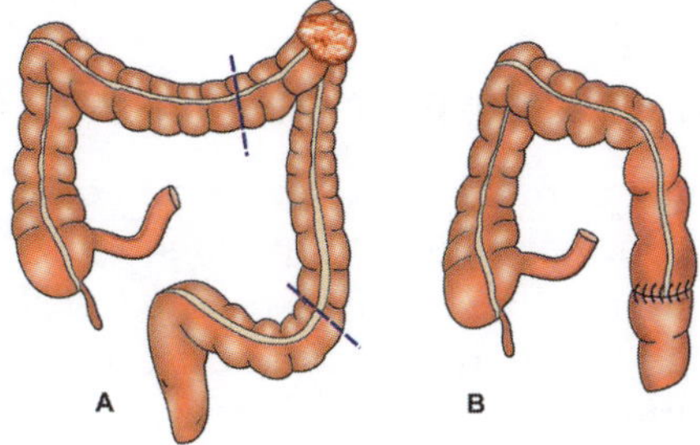

Figs 47.42A and B: Left hemicolectomy for growth in the splenic flexure

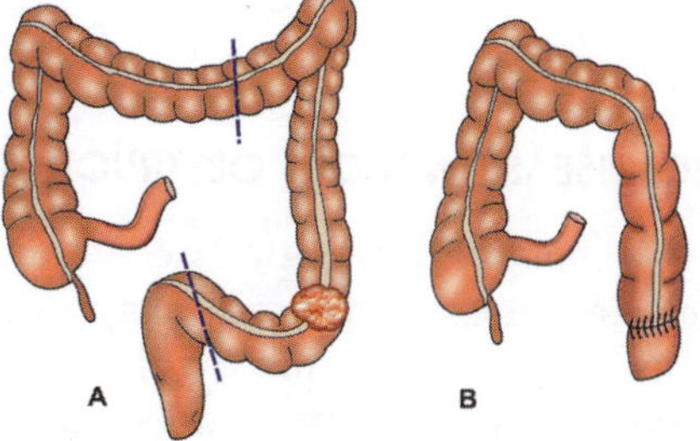

Figs 47.43A and B: Resection of rectosigmoid growth followed by colorectal anastomosis

(Figures 47.38 to 47.43 are contributed by Ms Vidushi, MBBS student, KMC, Manipal)

Table 47.4 Summary of the resections for carcinoma colon

Site of the tumour	Name of surgery	Part of the bowel resected	Artery supplying	Safe margin
Caecum	Right hemicolectomy	Terminal ileum to midtransverse colon	Ileocolic, right colic Right branch of middle colic	5 cm
Ascending colon	Right hemicolectomy	Terminal ileum to midtransverse colon	Ileocolic, right colic Right branch of middle colic	5 cm
Hepatic flexure	Extended right hemicolectomy	Terminal ileum to descending colon	Ileocolic, right colic Middle colic	5 cm
Transverse colon	Extended right hemicolectomy	Terminal ileum to descending colon	Ileocolic Right colic Middle colic	5 cm
Splenic flexure	Extended left hemicolectomy	Right flexure to rectosigmoid	Middle colic Left colic IMA	5 cm
Descending colon	Left hemicolectomy	Left flexure to sigmoid	IMA Left branch of middle colic	5 cm

- Indications for chemotherapy have been given in Key Box 47.13.

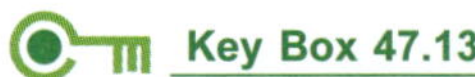 Key Box 47.13

Indications for Chemotherapy

- All node positive patients. If less than 12 nodes are harvested, it is inadequate lymph node clearance
- In node negative patients, if:
  - T4 lesions are involving free mesothelial surface
  - Major microscopic vein involvement
  - **Signet cell carcinoma**
  - High preoperative CEA
  - Aneuploidy on flow cytometry
  - Microsatellite instability

POSTOPERATIVE RADIOTHERAPY

Adenocarcinoma colon does not respond well to radiation. Routinely, it is not given. Small bowel is adjacent to the large bowel and so it cannot tolerate high dose of radiation without developing radiation enteritis. Surgery remains the gold standard for carcinoma colon. Soft tissue infiltration into psoas muscle or abdominal wall or inoperable recurrent tumours are indications for radiotherapy.

METASTATIC DISEASE WITHOUT OBSTRUCTION

Patients with isolated liver/lung secondaries should also undergo treatment with a radical approach as even in these cases with resection of the primary and adequate liver/lung resection, a good disease control can be achieved.

1. A typical course of neoadjuvant therapy comprises concurrent 5-FU/Capecitabine and radiation in cases of large lesions abutting the abdominal wall or down into the pelvis. A dose of 45–50 Gy is used to treat the pelvis including the growth and the draining lymphatic regions followed by 5 Gy boost to the tumour itself.
2. Following neoadjuvant therapy, patient should be re-evaluated using CT/MRI for possibility of resection.
3. Surgery is usually considered after 6–8 weeks following neoadjuvant therapy as the maximal response to the treatment may take up to 2 months.
4. Further adjuvant treatment is to be given following surgery depending upon the histopathological report.

MANAGEMENT OF LIVER SECONDARY

- CT scan and PET scan are done to evaluate local/systemic disease. Provided there is no systemic spread, liver secondaries have to be treated aggressively. Pattern of recurrence in colonic carcinomas is more commonly distant, i.e. they tend to recur more commonly at distant sites such as liver, and lungs. As a result, systemic treatment is essential.
- Liver-directed therapies such as hepatic arterial chemotherapy infusion/embolisation, radiofrequency-ablation, radiotherapy should be used in treatment of isolated liver metastasis.
- Isolated liver metastasis is not a contraindication for definitive resection of the primary.
- Indications for liver resection are given in Key Box 47.14.

Novel Agents in Colorectal Cancers

1. Bevacizumab—anti-VEGF (vascular endothelial growth factor) monoclonal antibody. It has anti-angiogenesis property, thereby controlling the tumour growth.
2. Cetuximab and panitumumab—anti-EGFR (epidermal growth factor) monoclonal antibody is given, only if K-RAS is negative.

Follow-up (Key Box 47.15)

Most of the colonic cases are curable, if diagnosed and treated early. Also metachronous lesion can occur in the rest of the colon. Hence, certain tests are necessary during follow-up.

TREATMENT OF RECURRENT OR METASTATIC CANCER

- Recurrence or metastasis is suspected during follow-up by abnormal values of investigation.
- Recurrent tumour should be resected *en bloc*—it may amount to a more radical procedure including resection of duodenum, liver, kidney.
- Metastasis in the liver (Key Box 47.14).

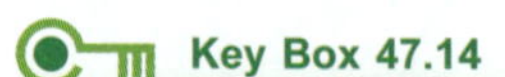 Key Box 47.14

Indication for Resection of Liver Metastasis

- Solitary metastasis or metastasis confined to one lobe
- <3 metastasis in both lobes
- Absence of extrahepatic disease

Key Box 47.15

Follow-up of Colorectal Cancer

Tests	Duration	In years
1. Haemo-occult	Once in 3–6 months	3
2. Colonoscopy	6 months after surgery, later once in a year	3
3. Alkaline phosphatase	Once in 3–6 months for 3 years	3
4. CEA	Once in 6 months	3
5. CECT chest and abdomen	Yearly	3

CHEMOPREVENTION OF COLONIC CANCER

1. **Folic acid:** It is an important vitamin with many functions. In the absence of folic acid, hypomethylation can occur. As a result of this overexpression of proto-oncogenes such as K-RAS and c-Myc can occur. Deficiency of folic acid causes imbalances in the nucleotide pool leading to DNA break and mutation. Thus folic acid supplementation should be given in adenoma specially when baseline levels of folic acid is low.
2. **Dietary fibres:** Fibres decrease the transit time, they dilute the carcinogens and are used to present development of cancer. Cellulose, hemicelluloses and pectin are a few examples. Fibres also produce short chain in fatty acids causing fermentation by faecal flora. Thus colonic pH becomes more acidic which in turn inhibits carcinogenesis.
3. **Aspirin, calcium, and sulindac** also have been used to prevent cancer developing in an adenoma.

COLON SCREENING

- Large bowel is the 4th most common site for cancer after lung, stomach and breast.
- More common in North America, North Europe and Australia. Lowest rates in Africa, India.
- 75% of CRC develop in people with no known risk factors apart from older age.

Screening Options

1. **Faecal occult blood test (FOBT)**
   - It is guaiac test which will detect elevated level of blood in stool. It requires two samples from each of three consecutive stools which are smeared onto cards.
   - **False positive:** Vegetables, fruits, red meat, aspirin or any other bleeding lesion proximal to colon screening, FOBT has shown to decrease mortality by 20 to 30%.
2. **Flexible sigmoidoscopy (FS)**
   - Reduces incidence and mortality of distal CRC by around 60%.
   - Single FS at the age of 60 is recommended in UK.
   - In US, 5-yearly screening is being done.
3. **Colonoscope screening**
   - Should be done if there is distal adenoma (chances of proximal adenoma are high).
   - 70% of all advanced colorectal neoplasia will be detected with this strategy.
   - Procedure is painful, requires sedation and analgesics.
   - Chances of perforation are 1 in 500 to 2000 cases.
   - It requires skills of an experienced endoscopist.
4. **Virtual colonoscopy**
   - It is an alternative but not yet become popular because of time, cost and preparation.
   - It is done with the help of CT scan.
   - Biopsy cannot be taken.

DIVERTICULAR DISEASE OF COLON

It is an acquired condition, in which colonic mucosa herniates through the circular muscle fibres at weak points, where blood vessels penetrate the colonic wall. Since it is acquired, it lacks the muscle coat. They are thin, more prone for infections and perforation. Hence, they are termed pseudodiverticuli.

Aetiopathogenesis

- The disease is common in western population wherein diet is very **poor in fibres** because of refining of sugar and flour. **Nonstarch polysaccharides (NSP)** or low dietary fibres are the chief factor for **diverticulosis of colon** (Key Box 47.16).
- It requires very high pressure for propulsion of faecal matter and this is believed to cause characteristic thickening of muscles and herniation of mucosa (Figs 47.44 and 47.45). Hence, it is called pulsion diverticulum.

Key Box 47.16

NSP and Diseases

- Diverticular disease
- Obesity and diabetes mellitus
- Constipation, and piles
- Breast cancer and colonic cancer

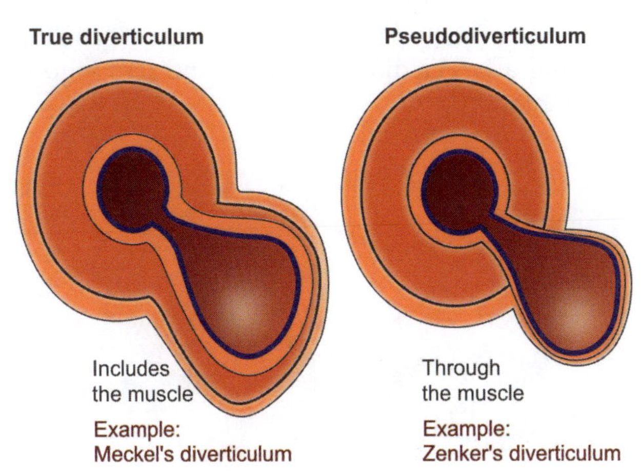

Figs 47.44 and 47.45: Diverticulum

- In Africans and Indians, the disease is rare because of high fibre content of the diet.
- The disease starts after the age of 40. Any stress or emotional disorders may add to the constipation already caused by dietary factors and result in diverticular formation.
- **90% of them affect sigmoid colon.** Rectum is spared in majority. Rarely, it affects right colon.
- Diverticulae project between antimesenteric and mesenteric borders with taenia but they never penetrate taenia (Fig. 47.46).
- There is **muscle hypertrophy,** which project into the lumen as obstructive folds. The mucosa is essentially normal. Slowly, luminal diameter is narrowed.
- **Inflammation** occurs in the pericolonic tissue with or without abscess formation.

Structural Changes in Colonic Wall of Patients with Diverticulosis

- Mycosis
- Thickening (neither hypertrophy nor hyperplasia) of the circular muscle layer.
- Shortening of the taenia coli
- Luminal narrowing
- ↑ elastin deposition in taenia coli
- ↑ type III collagen synthesis
- ↑ collagen cross-linking

Segmentation

- Law of Laplace: Pressure = K × Tension/Radius
- Sigmoid colon has small diameter resulting in highest pressure zone.
- Segmentation = motility process in which the segmental muscular contractions separate the lumen into chambers.
- Segmentation → increased intraluminal pressure → mucosal herniation → diverticulosis.
- May explain why high fibre prevents diverticuli by creating a larger diameter colon and less vigorous segmentation.

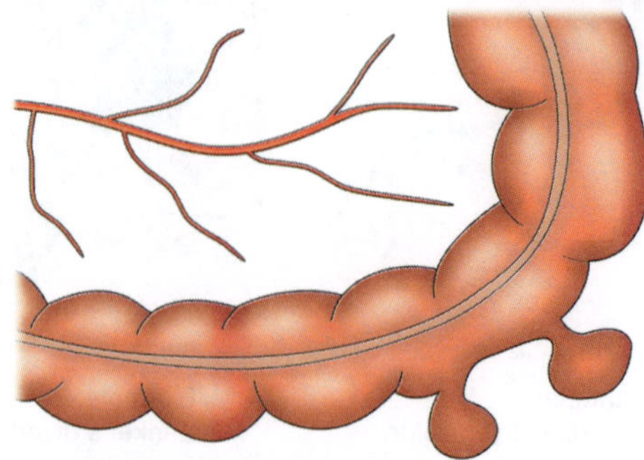

Fig. 47.46: Sigmoid diverticulae

- Collagen connective tissue diseases such as Ehlers-Danlos syndrome, Marfan's syndrome, and autosomal-dominant polycystic kidney disease result in structural changes in the bowel wall, leading to decreased resistance of the wall to intraluminal pressures and thus allowing protrusion of diverticula.

Clinical Features

1. **Diverticulosis:** It refers to presence of diverticulosis without much symptoms. But on careful questioning, patients do have lower abdominal distention, heaviness, flatulence, etc. Vague abdominal pain is also felt in the left iliac fossa.
2. **Diverticulitis:** Left-sided lower abdominal pain, moderate to severe, is associated with passage of loose stools. The pain is partially relieved on passing flatus.
   - Bleeding per rectum can be the presenting feature, sometimes it can be massive.
   - Low-grade fever, tenderness, rigidity and even mass may be present in the left iliac fossa (like left-sided appendicitis). The mass is thickened, inflamed, tender and sigmoid. Such attacks result in abscess which rupture into hollow organs and give rise to fistulae (Fig. 47.47).
3. **Internal fistulae:** Colovesical fistulae (commonest) give rise to pneumaturia (flatus in the urine) and rarely faeces in the urine (Key Box 47.17). Other fistulae are colovaginal, coloenteric, and colocutaneous.

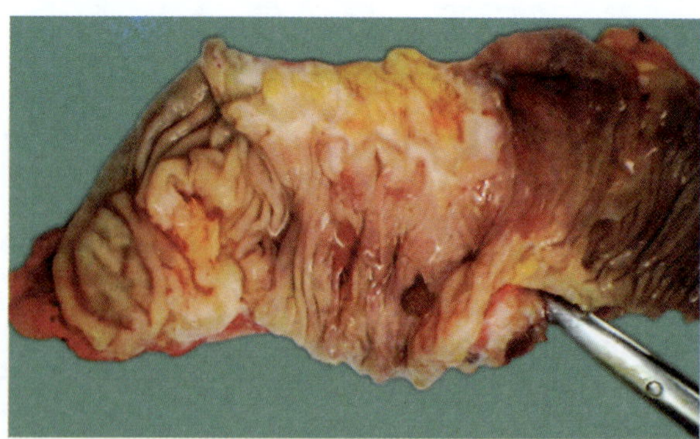

Fig. 47.47: Perforated diverticula at surgery—resected specimen (*Courtesy:* Dr Ramesh Rajan, Surgical Gastroenterologist, Trivandrum Medical College, Kerala)

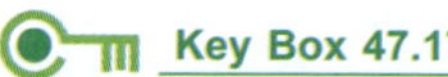

Key Box 47.17

Causes of Internal Fistulae

- Diverticular disease of colon (commonest)
- Carcinoma of colon
- Crohn's disease
- Radiation
- Tuberculosis

For summary of diverticular disease *see* Fig. 47.48

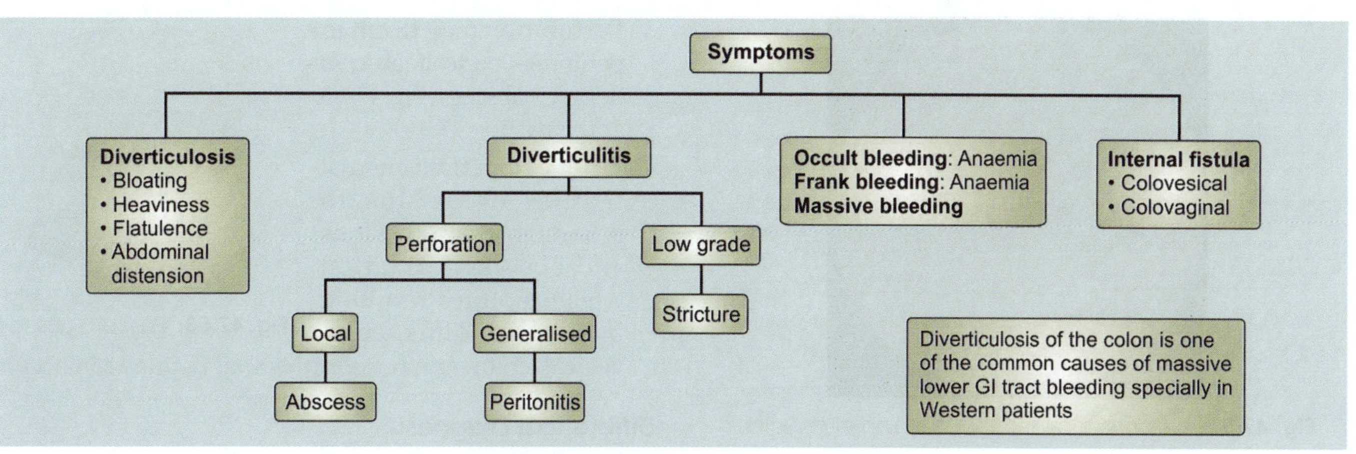

Fig. 47.48: Summary of diverticular disease

Classification/Staging System

Hinchey Classification (Fig. 47.49)

I. Pericolic abscess
II. Walled off pelvic abscess
III. Generalised purulent peritonitis
IV. Generalised faecal peritonitis

Hinchey stages I and II may be treated by sigmoid colectomy and primary anastomosis (a one-stage operation).

Hinchey stages III and IV are treated by sigmoid colectomy followed by end-colostomy and Hartmann pouch.

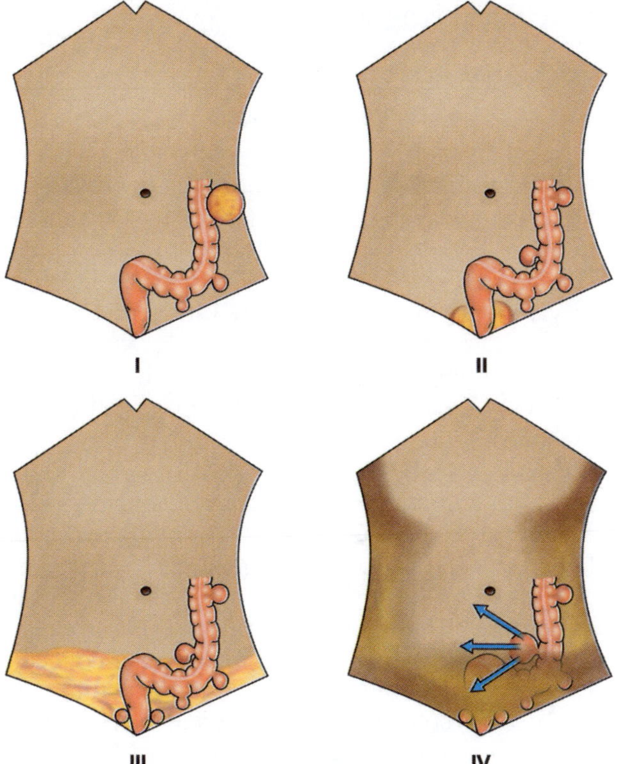

Fig. 47.49: Hinchey classification

Pearls of Wisdom

The most common fistula in acute diverticulitis is colovesical followed by colovaginal fistula.

Investigations

1. **Sigmoidoscopy:** Mucosa may be normal or may show erythematous and oedematous changes. Ulcers are absent. Opening of diverticulae can be seen.
2. **Barium enema: Contraindicated in acute cases.**
   - It may show **saw-tooth** appearance due to muscle hypertrophy.
   - It may show a long stricture.
   - **Champagne glass sign:** Partial filling of diverticula by barium with stercolith inside the diverticula.
3. **Colonoscopy** to confirm the findings and to rule out **carcinoma colon** (Figs 47.50 and 47.51). It is the investigation of choice in diverticulosis.

Pearls of Wisdom

Sigmoidoscopy, colonoscopy and barium enema are contraindicated in acute diverticulitis.

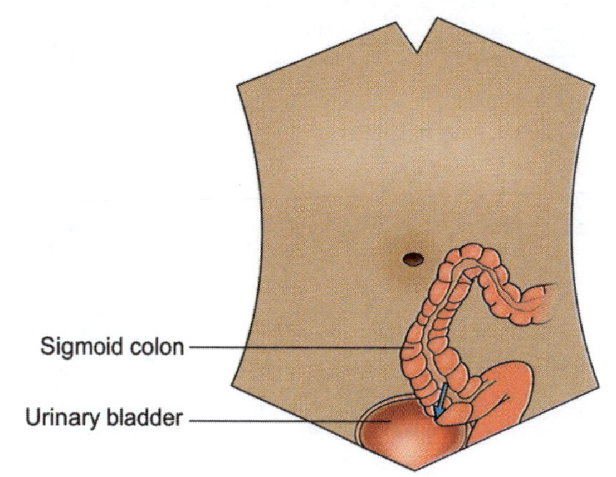

Fig. 47.50: Colovesical fistula (arrow)

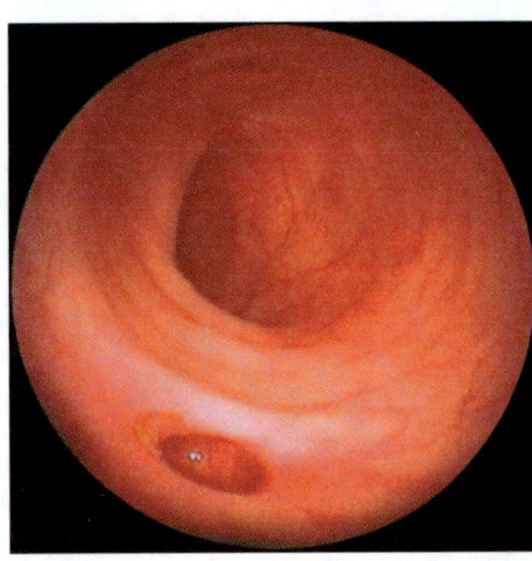

Fig. 47.51: Colonoscopy showing opening of diverticula

4. **Ultrasound and CT scan** (Key Box 47.18) are the investigations of choice in acute diverticulitis (Fig. 47.52).

Complications

1. **Massive haemorrhage** per rectum: Haemorrhage is due to vessels in the base of diverticulae, more so in atherosclerotic or hypertensive patients.
2. **Stricture** of sigmoid colon can develop due to recurrent attacks resulting in intestinal obstruction.

Key Box 47.18

CT Scan Acute Diverticulitis

- Can detect thick muscular folds—confirms the diagnosis.
- Detects an abscess and can confirm complication.
- Detects extraluminal air or contrast—confirms perforation.
- Can rule out other causes—acute pancreatitis with pericolic collection, etc.
- **It is the investigation of choice in acute diverticulitis.**
- Thickened colonic wall >4 mm.
- Pelvic abscess can be diagnosed.

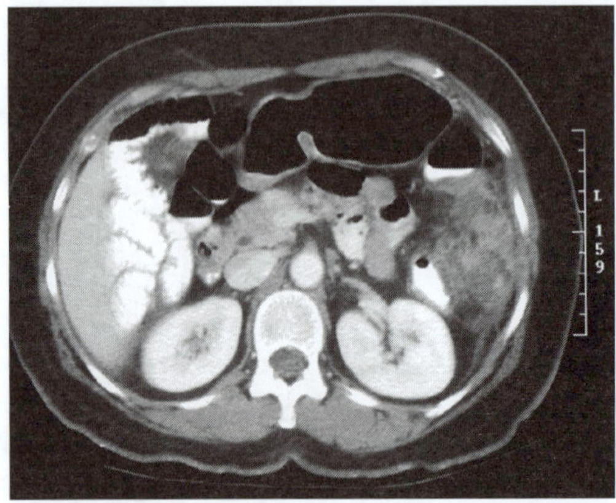

Fig. 47.52: CT scan showing pericolic abscess on the left paracolic space

3. **Perforation** may result in peritonitis, pericolic abscess or pelvic abscess (Fig. 47.53 and Key Box 47.19).
4. **Fistula formation:** Internal fistulae occur due to inflammatory adhesions and abscess formation which ruptures resulting in fistulae. Thus, colovesical, colovaginal, colointestinal fistulae can occur.

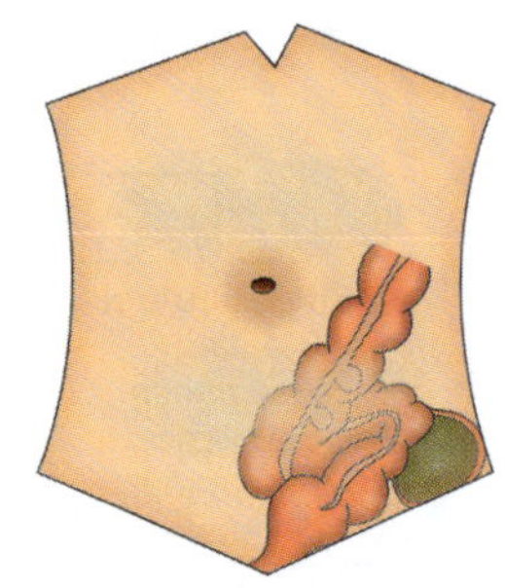

Fig. 47.53: Pericolic abscess

Differential Diagnosis

- Carcinoma of the colon
- Inflammatory bowel disease
- Ischaemic colitis
- Irritable bowel syndrome
- Pelvic inflammatory disease

Indications for Surgery

1. Failure to respond to conservative/dietary advice
2. Two attacks of diverticulitis
3. Complications

Treatment

1. **Stage of diverticulosis** or in those patients who have recovered from one attack of diverticulitis.
   - High residue diet
   - Fruits and vegetables

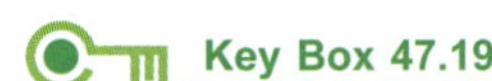

Key Box 47.19

Pericolic Abscess

- Abscess depends on the ability of the pericolic tissues to localise the spread of the inflammatory process.
- Intra-abdominal abscesses are formed by—anastomotic leakage: 35%—diverticular disease: 23%.
- Limited spread of the perforation forms an inflammatory phlegmon, while further (but still localised) progression creates an abscess.
- Signs and symptoms: High grade fever with or without leukocytosis despite adequate antibiotics, tender mass.
- Treatment:
  A. **Small pericolic abscess:** 90% will respond to antibiotics and conservative management alone. Often it is retrocolic. May present as swelling in the loin.
  B. **Percutaneous abscess drainage** (PAD) is the treatment of choice for small, simple (>4 cm), well-defined collections. 100% success in simple unilocular abscesses.
  C. **Open drainage:** In cases of multilocular collection, abscesses associated with enteric fistulas, and abscesses containing solid material, drainage of pus, resection and Hartmann's operation is the ideal choice. Closure of colostomy is done after 6–8 weeks.

- Whole meal bread and flour
- Bulk purgative
- To avoid constipation

Diet

- High fibre diet, optimal amount of daily fibre is unknown.
- 20 to 30 g per day is widely recommended.
- Recommendation to avoid seeds, nuts and popcorn.

2. **Acute diverticulitis with pericolic abscess**
   - Rest, hospitalisation, correct hydration
   - IV antibiotics: Bactericidal against gram –ve and anaerobes.
   - Abscess is aspirated under ultrasound guidance.
   - After 4–6 weeks, elective sigmoid colectomy and anastomosis is done.
3. **Diverticulitis with peritonitis**
   A. **Hartmann's procedure** is the choice: Sigmoid colon is resected, end-colostomy is done by using descending colon followed by closure of rectal stump (Figs 47.54A and B).
   - After 4–6 weeks, colorectal anastomosis is done.
   B. However, if a **perforation is small** and the general condition is good after the resection, the colon is irrigated with 8–10 litres of saline till the contents are clear. This is followed by colorectal anastomosis in the same sitting.
4. **Treatment of fistulae:** As an elective procedure, with good preparation, after confirming the site of fistula, resection of the sigmoid colon with closure of fistula can be done.

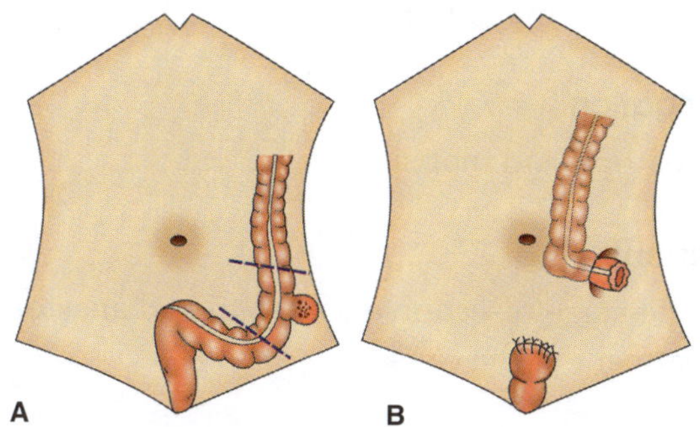

Figs 47.54A and B: Hartmann's procedure

MISCELLANEOUS

FAECAL FISTULA

Classification

Depending upon the Nature of the Disease or a Surgical Procedure

I. **Primary or type I fistula:** It develops as a result of an underlying disease affecting gut. Example: Carcinoma colon infiltrating urinary bladder resulting in colovesical fistula or rupture through the skin resulting in pericolic abscess, fistula.

II. **Secondary or type II fistula:** It occurs after injury to otherwise normal gut. Examples: Left colonic/right colonic injury in percutaneous nephrolithotomy (PCNL) for renal stones or following anastomotic leak.

Depending upon the Site of the Fistula

A. **Lateral fistula:** It occurs after a colocolic or ileocolic anastomosis wherein a few sutures would have given way in the immediate postoperative period.

B. **End fistula:** This means both ends of the intestines are open following resection and anastomosis giving rise to postoperative peritonitis.

- A few fistulae in diverticular disease of the colon are given in Key Box 47.20.

Bacterial Flora

- More than 99% of faecal bacterial flora are **anaerobic**.
- Most common anaerobe is ***Bacteroides fragilis***, with a count of 10^{10}/g of wet faeces. Clostridia, Lactobacillus are other organisms.
- ***E. coli*** is the predominant **aerobic organism**. Count is 10^7/g of faeces. Klebsiella, Proteus, and Enterobacter are other **aerobes**. ***Streptococcus faecalis*** is the principal enterococcus.

Clinical Manifestations

- Postoperative patient 'not doing well'—prolonged paralytic ileus, faeculent discharge from wound or drainage site, etc. is an indication of faecal fistula.
- Features of septic shock: Often patient may not complain of abdominal pain but manifestations can be of renal failure, tachycardia, tachypnoea and hypotension.

Diagnosis

- Total counts are elevated—it indicates infection.
- Creatinine and urea values are high indicating renal failure.
- Ultrasound to detect any collection.
- CECT can detect intraperitoneal collection, pneumoperitoneum, anastomotic leak. However, creatinine should be normal before doing CT scan. Often patients are in sepsis with renal failure.

Key Box 47.20

Types of Fistula Related to Diverticular Disease

- Colovesical: 65%
- Colovaginal: 25%
- Colocutaneous
- Coloenteral

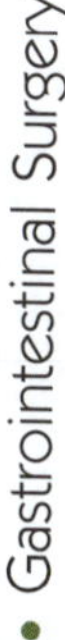

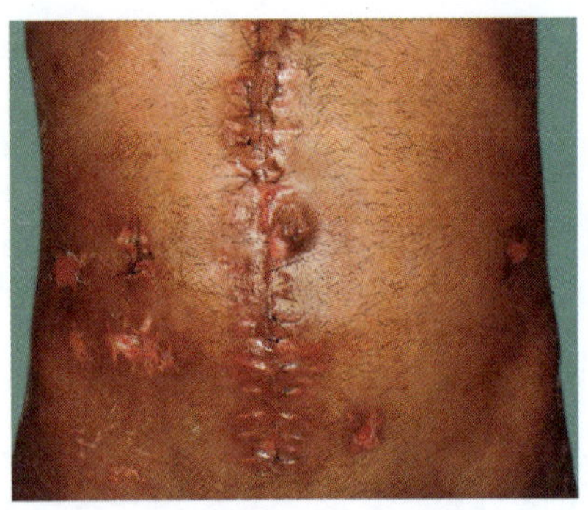

Fig. 47.55: This patient underwent three surgical procedures for treatment of fistula. Initial surgery was right hemicolectomy for ileocaecal tuberculosis. Second surgery (Fig.47.58) was resection and a proximal diversion ileostomy because of the leak and finally after two months, closure of ileostomy was done followed by ileotransverse anastomosis

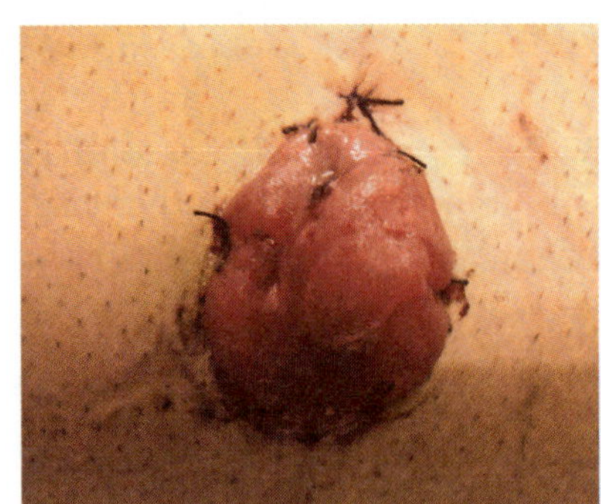

Fig. 47.56: Ileostomy was done to divert the proximal intestinal contents. To have the maximum benefit it should be an end ileostomy and the distal end can be brought out as mucus fistula. However, often during exploration of this type of cases, it is not possible

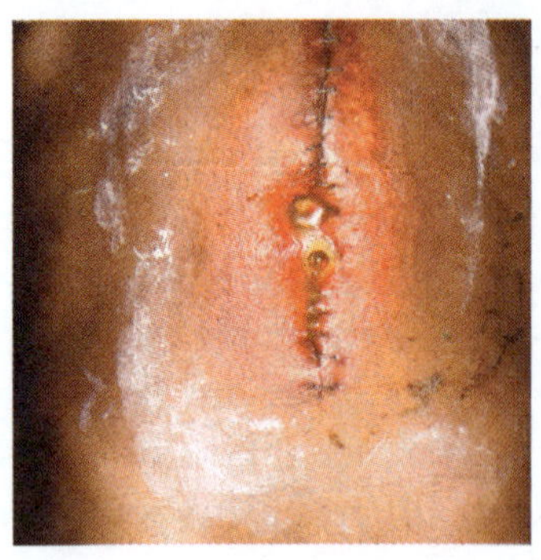

Fig. 47.57: A case of faecal fistula following ileal resection for obstruction caused by a band. Following resection anastomosis on the fifth postoperative day, air-mixed faecal matter started coming out from the wound. CT scan revealed small lateral fistula. The patient responded to conservative treatment with TPN given for 14 days. Fistula subsided

Treatment (Figs 47.55 to 47.57)

- Control of infection
- Drainage of sepsis—laparotomy, resection and anastomosis, ileostomy or colostomy may be necessary.
- Lateral fistula may heal with total parenteral nutrition provided there is no distal obstruction (TPN).
- End fistula may require resuturing with or without proximal diversion colostomy/ileostomy.

COLONIC STRICTURE

Causes

1. Malignant: Adenocarcinoma colon is the commonest cause of stricture colon (rarely lymphomas, carcinoid).
2. Tuberculosis: Uncommon cause of stricture in the ascending colon.
3. Ischaemic: Uncommon/rare cause—left colon may be affected.
4. Inflammatory bowel disease: Any ulcers, including amoebic, may heal with fibrosis resulting in stricture.
5. Diverticular stricture
6. Radiation stricture
7. Endometriomas: Ectopic endometriosis tissue responds to cyclic hormonal stimulation causing inflammation and fibrosis.

Clinical Features

- Progressive constipation
- Change in bowel habits
- Bleeding per rectum
- Features of large bowel obstruction
- Mass may/may not be felt

Investigation

Colonoscopy and biopsy

Treatment

- Single-stage resection and end-to-end anastomosis.
- Treatment of the cause.

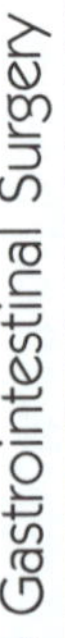

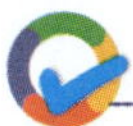

Multiple Choice Questions

1. The following feature is true of adenomatous polyps of the large intestine:

A. Most are sessile
B. Most can be removed by colonoscopic snaring
C. Adenoma smaller than 15 mm in diameter do not carry the risk of malignant potential
D. Young people are more likely to have these polyps

2. Common premalignant conditions for colonic cancer include the following *except*:

A. Familial polyposis coli
B. Ulcerative colitis
C. Adenomatous polyp
D. Peutz-Jeghers syndrome

3. Flexion of the hip can be present in:

A. Carcinoma splenic flexure
B. Carcinoma caecum
C. Carcinoma sigmoid colon
D. Carcinoma hepatic flexure

4. Abscess in the lateral abdominal wall can be a feature of:

A. Acute pancreatitis
B. Perforated carcinoma caecum
C. Diverticular perforation
D. Meckel's diverticular perforation

5. Mechanical bowel preparation is best given using:

A. Plenty of saline
B. Oral mannitol
C. Glycerine enema
D. Whole gut irrigation using oral polyethylene glycol

6. Which one of this is true in colonic surgery?

A. No touch technique of Turnbull
B. Right-sided lesions are treated by colostomy
C. Left-sided lesions are treated by resection
D. Removal of 30 cm of ileum along with colon

7. Following is true about prognostic factors of carcinoma colon *except:*

A. Elderly patients have poorer prognosis
B. Perioperative blood transfusion has poor prognosis
C. Survival is good if it is limited to mucosa and there are no nodes
D. Obstruction and perforation is associated with poor prognosis

8. Regarding colonoscopic screening, which one of the following is true?

A. It is done if there is distal adenoma
B. It is painless and easy to perform
C. It is not useful for screening of colonic cancer
D. Detection of all advanced colorectal neoplasia is only up to 20%

9. Proliferative growth is more common in the ________ colon:

A. Right B. Left
C. Rectosigmoid D. Splenic flexure

10. The 'Gold standard' investigation for detection of colonic cancer is:

A. Ultrasound abdomen
B. CT scan
C. Barium enema
D. Colonoscopy and biopsy

11. Following are the features of intestinal tuberculosis *except:*

A. It can be secondary to pulmonary tuberculosis
B. Terminal ileum and caecum are commonly involved
C. Ulcers are transverse
D. Ulcers do not result in stricture

12. In which of the following malignancies anaemia is an important method of presentation?

A. Malignant melanoma B. Carcinoma breast
C. Carcinoma caecum D. Carcinoma pancreas

13. The most common fistula in diverticulitis is:

A. Colovesical B. Colovaginal
C. Colorectal D. Colocolic

14. Which of the following is a true diverticulum?

A. Sigmoid diverticulum
B. Meckel's diverticulum
C. Parabronchial diverticulum
D. Laryngeal diverticulam

15. In hereditary nonpolyposis colorectal cancer, which carcinoma is more often seen?

A. Rectum
B. Rectosigmoid
C. Transverse colon
D. Caecum and ascending colon

16. Incidence of malignancy in familial polyposis coli is:

A. 10% B. 30%
C. 50% D. 100%

17. Following are true for carcinoembryonic antigen *except*:

A. It is a glycoprotein
B. It is tumour marker for carcinoma colon
C. It should be done in all cases of carcinoma colon before surgery
D. Produced by colorectal epithelium and cleared by kidney

18. Following are true for right hemicolectomy for carcinoma caecum *except:*

A. Right one-third of transverse colon is also removed
B. Greater omentum should be removed
C. Terminal 30 cm of the ileum should be removed
D. Duodenum can get injured during surgery

19. Indications for postoperative chemotherapy following colectomy for carcinoma include following *except*:

A. Signet ring carcinoma
B. Lymph nodes are positive
C. Lymphovenous involvement
D. Involvement of muscularis propria

20. The most common aerobic organism present in a sigmoid colonic faecal fistula is:

A. Clostridia
B. Lactobacillus
C. *Bacteroides fragilis*
D. *E. coli*

Answers

1. B	**2.** D	**3.** B	**4.** D	**5.** D	**6.** A	**7.** A	**8.** A	**9.** A	**10.** D
11. D	**12.** D	**13.** A	**14.** B	**15.** D	**16.** D	**17.** D	**18.** C	**19.** D	**20.** D

CHAPTER

48

Intestinal Obstruction

- Pathophysiology, basic principles in management
- Sigmoid volvulus
- Meckel's diverticulum
- Adhesions and bands
- Gallstone ileus
- Intussusception
- Mesenteric vascular occlusion
- Hirschsprung's disease
- Atresia and stenosis
- Arrested rotation with bands
- Volvulus neonatorum
- Meconium ileus
- Imperforate anus
- Paralytic ileus
- Food bolus obstruction
- Abdominal coccoon
- Malrotation and midgut volvulus

INTRODUCTION

- Intestinal obstruction is a challenging surgical emergency encountered by general surgeons. This can affect any age group starting from neonate to an old man. It can affect a school going boy, working woman or a man during their peak of life. Sometimes it can be fatal either due to delay in the diagnosis, delay in the treatment or complications related to surgery. Abdomen is a Pandora's box. Sometimes, it is difficult to pinpoint the cause of obstruction.
- Adhesions and hernia are the two most common causes of intestinal obstruction. Adhesions are more common than hernias nowadays. Laparoscopic surgery has definitely decreased incidence of adhesions. In Western countries more than 50% cases of intestinal obstruction are due to adhesions and only 10–15% are due to obstructed hernia (Fig. 48.1). However, students should be able to diagnose intestinal obstruction, resuscitate the patients and refer the patient for further surgical treatment. With the availability of sophisticated investigations such as CT scan, diagnosis can be established in majority of cases before surgery. However, in other cases, **'exploratory laparotomy'** will give the diagnosis.

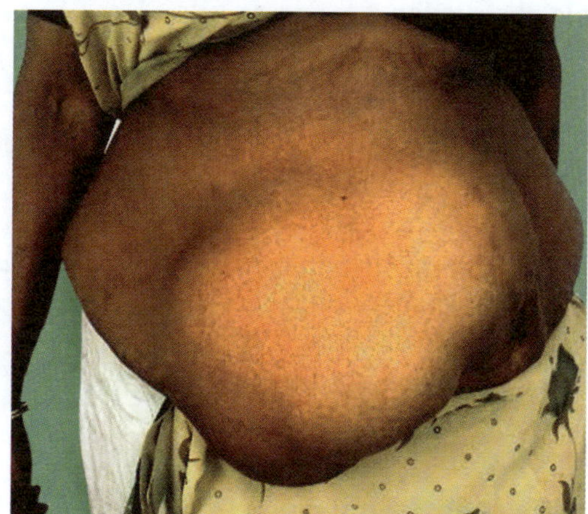

Fig. 48.1: Obstructed incisional hernia (*Courtesy:* Prof. (Late) Manjunath Shenoy, JSS Medical College and Hospital, Mysore)

Pearls of Wisdom

Fatty female with fatty fold of abdomen concealing a small femoral hernia. In all cases of intestinal obstruction, examine hernia orifices.

DEFINITION

When the intestinal contents fail to move distally, it is called intestinal obstruction. It is the most common surgical disorder (emergency) of the intestines.

A few important facts about intestinal obstruction:

- 80% occur in small bowel
- 20% occur in large bowel
- Majority (more than 80%) of small bowel obstructions are benign in nature.
- In the large bowel, more than 70% of colonic obstruction is due to malignancy—others being inflammatory bowel diseases, ileocaecal tuberculosis, volvulus, etc.

Classification

I. Depending upon the Nature of Obstruction

(Key Box 48.1)

A. Dynamic obstruction/mechanical obstruction.

B. Adynamic obstruction—paralytic ileus or neurogenic ileus.

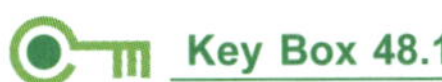

Key Box 48.1

Commonly used Terminology

- **Mechanical obstruction**
  There is a physical barrier which prevents the normal progress of intestinal contents.
- **Paralytic ileus**
  There is no physical barrier but failure of peristalsis to propel intestinal contents due to neurogenic causes.
- **Simple obstruction**
  It refers to obstruction to lumen only (early cases)
- **Strangulated obstruction**
  It refers to obstruction with impairment of blood supply to the gut.
- **Closed loop obstruction**
  In this condition, the intestine is occluded in two places. More chances of gangrene and perforation are present, e.g. volvulus.
- **Pseudo-obstruction:** No mechanical cause.

II. Depending on the Blood Supply

A. **Simple obstruction:** Blood supply is not seriously impaired.

B. **Strangulated obstruction:** Blood supply is seriously impaired, resulting in gangrene of the bowel and gram-negative shock.

C. **Closed loop obstruction:** It means both proximal and distal ends are blocked. This occurs in carcinoma of hepatic flexure—the right colon with constrictive lesions. If the ileocaecal valve is competent and the obstruction is total, the intraluminal pressure within the colon increases. As a result of this, the caecum may perforate. Thus, closed loop obstruction can be dangerous (Fig. 48.2). Another example is sigmoid volvulus.

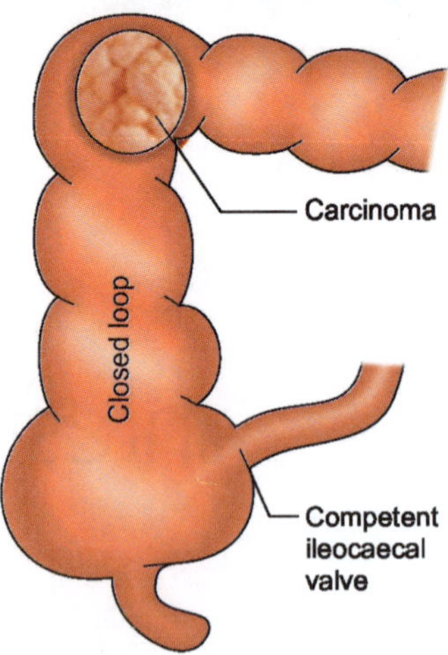

Fig. 48.2: Closed loop obstruction: In 40% of patients, ileocaecal valve is competent

III. Depending upon the Cause of Obstruction

Competency

SU28.14.6: List the causes of small bowel and large bowel obstruction.

A. **In the lumen of the gut**
- Gallstone ileus
- Food bolus obstruction
- Roundworm mass
- Foreign body (rare)
- Meconium ileus

B. **In the wall of the gut**
- Stricture, e.g. tuberculosis
- Crohn's disease
- Carcinoma
- Atresia
- Adhesions

C. **Outside the wall of the gut**
- Volvulus, intussusception
- Congenital bands
- Meckel's diverticulum with band
- Obstructed hernia

IV. Depending upon Severity of Obstruction

A. **Acute obstruction:** Signs and symptoms appear very early. Usually, it affects small bowel, obstructed hernia, bands.

B. **Chronic obstruction** (e.g. carcinoma colon) affects large bowel (colic comes first, distension later). Diverticular disease also produces chronic obstructions (Fig. 48.3).

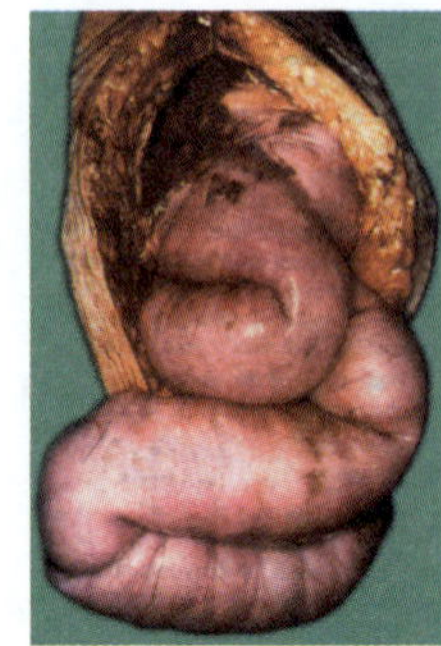

Fig. 48.3: Dilated small intestinal loops in a case of ileal obstruction

C. **Acute on chronic obstruction** develops in carcinoma colon, wherein an acute obstruction suddenly results due to the accumulation of faecal matter in the proximal bowel (Fig. 48.4 depicts various causes of intestinal obstruction).

Pathophysiology (Fig. 48.5)

> Competency
>
> **SU28.14.5:** Differentiate pathophysiology of dynamic and adynamic intestinal obstruction.

A. Pathophysiology of Dynamic Obstruction

- As a result of obstruction, the proximal bowel undergoes hyperperistalsis which is responsible for colicky pain abdomen. The peristalsis may continue for a few days and later the intestine may be paralysed and flaccid. After 3–4 hours, distal to the obstruction, all physiological activities of the bowel are stopped. Intestine becomes contracted, pale and does not exhibit peristalsis. After a few hours, the proximal bowel gets dilated secondary to obstruction.

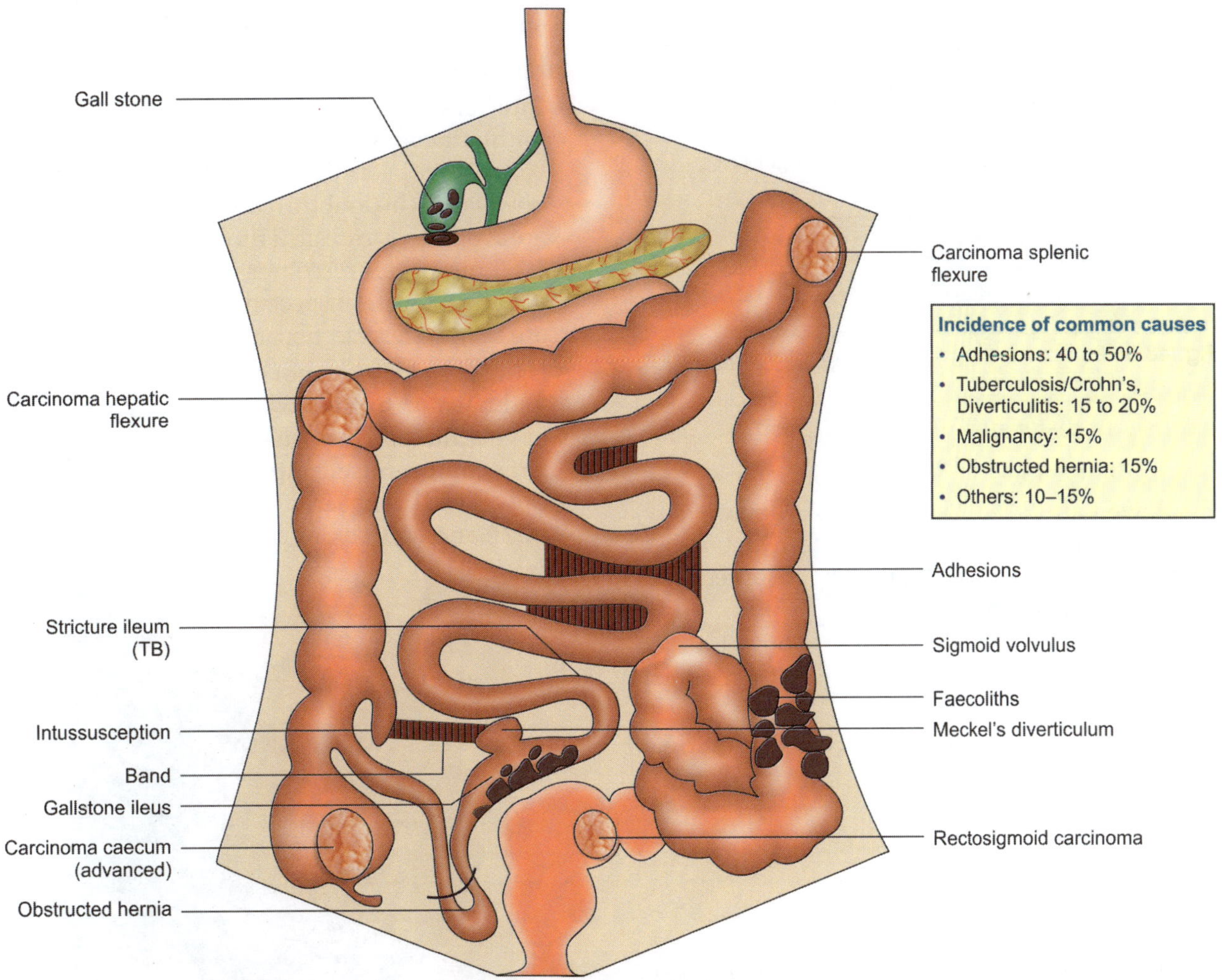

COMMON CAUSES OF ILEAL OBSTRUCTION

- Adhesions
- Obstructed hernia
- Stricture
- Intussusception
- Ileocaecal tuberculosis
- Bands
- Worm ball—in children
- Ileal atresia—in children

COMMON CAUSES OF COLONIC OBSTRUCTION

- Carcinoma colon
- Sigmoid volvulus
- Faecal impaction
- Mesenteric ischaemia
- Hirschsprung's disease
- Anorectal malformations
- Stricture colon—rare

COMMON CAUSES OF GANGRENE

- Volvulus
- Intussusception
- Obstructed hernia
- Mesenteric vascular occlusion
- Twisting around a band
- Necrotising enterocolitis

Fig. 48.4: Differential diagnosis of intestinal obstruction—diagrammatic representation

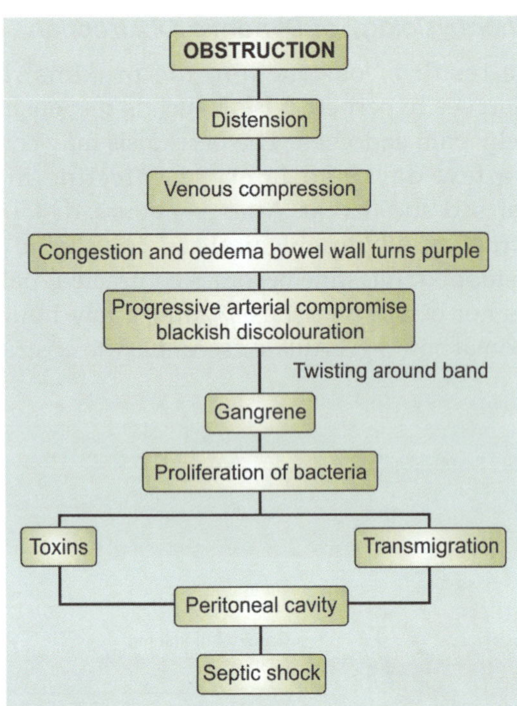

Fig. 48.5: Pathophysiology of intestinal obstruction

- The causes of distension of intestinal loop are:

A. Gaseous distension

- Swallowed air (70%). Because of olic and anxiety, the swallowed air is increased. Oxygen is absorbed and nitrogen remains as it cannot be absorbed. This results in distension.
- Diffusion of air from the blood into bowel lumen increases carbon dioxide which diffuses very rapidly.
- Gas due to bacterial activity releases H_2S, NH_3, etc.

B. Distension due to fluids

- 1500 ml of saliva
- 2 litres of gastric juice
- 3 litres of intestinal secretions
- 1 litre of bile and pancreatic juice

Normally, all this fluid is absorbed in the bowel. In cases of intestinal obstruction, this fluid absorption is delayed. It accumulates in the intestinal loop. Excretion of water and electrolytes into the lumen is also increased.

C. Role of nitric oxide: Activated neutrophils and macrophages accumulate within the muscular layer of the bowel wall due to dilatation and inflammation of the bowel wall Z. This damages the secretory and motor processes by release of reactive proteolytic enzymes and cytokines. Net result is increase in **the local release of nitric oxide**, itself a potent inhibitor of smooth muscle tone. It further aggravates the intestinal dilatation.

D. Role of bacteria

- Bacterial colony count increases following obstruction resulting in stasis. From less than 106 in jejunum and from 108 in ileum, counts increase.
- **Bacterial translocation** can occur even in simple obstruction without strangulation. Thus, bacteria can enter into lymph nodes and into systemic circulation. Abdominal distension, hypovolaemia, renal failure and sepsis set in. In addition to these changes, diaphragm gets elevated, respiration is impaired which result in respiratory complications such as atelectasis and basal pneumonia.

E. Strangulation (Fig. 48.6 and Key Box 48.2)

- Interference with blood supply: As the tension within the loops becomes more and more, venous congestion takes place resulting in oedema of the bowel wall. In doubtful cases of viability, if facilities are available, a test called **fluorescein** test can be done. 1000 mg of fluorescein is injected into peripheral vein and bowel is inspected under wood light. If loops are nonviable, resection and anastomosis is done.
- If the obstruction is not relieved, capillary rupture and haemorrhage into bowel may ensue. **In cases of volvulus and intussusception,** the **arterial supply gets compromised rapidly causing gangrene of bowel wall** very early. Bacterial proliferation takes place and endotoxins are released.

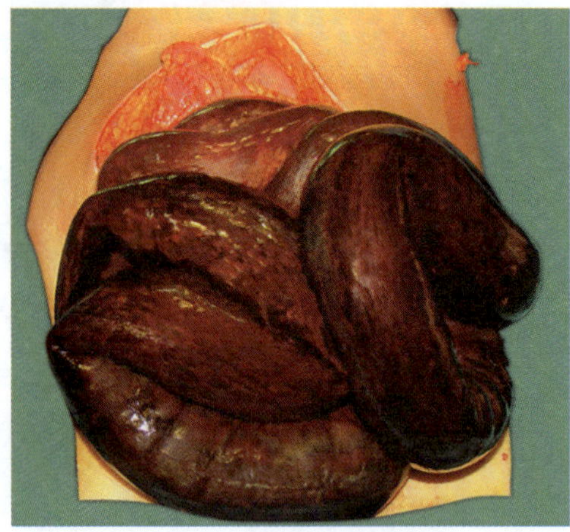

Fig. 48.6: Gangrene of the intestine due to bands

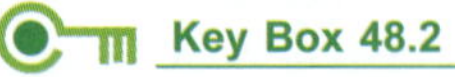 **Key Box 48.2**

Factors Predisposing Ischaemia

- Volvulus
- Mesenteric ischaemia
- Necrotising enterocolitis
- Intussusception
- Progressive distension—long standing
- Extrinsic compression by adhesions, bands, etc.

- **Transmigration** (translocation) of gram-negative organisms, anaerobes and gram-positive organisms through the gangrenous bowel results in peritonitis.
- The organisms release **powerful endotoxins** which are absorbed from the peritoneal surface and cause high mortality rate (30%).
- Early gangrene without obstruction is a feature of mesenteric thrombosis or embolism.
- Loss of blood volume is an important feature of massive gangrene.

B. Pathophysiology of Paralytic Ileus

- As a result of adynamic obstruction (no peristaltic activity), contents within the lumen do not get absorbed. Saliva, gastric and intestinal contents secreted in the lumen further add to the volume resulting in volume of fluid loss, distension and difficulty in breathing. Hypovolemia worsens and also hypokalemia resulting in further distension.
- If not treated, distension results in stretching of intestinal wall, ischemia and even perforation and septic shock.
- Difficulty in breathing results in basal atelectasis/ pneumonia.
- Fluid and electrolyte imbalance.
- Nutritional deficiencies.

Competency

SU28.14: Describe the clinical features, investigations and principles of management of small bowel and large bowel obstruction.

Clinical Features (Key Box 48.3)

1. **Pain abdomen:** Central abdominal pain is a feature of small intestinal obstruction and peripheral pain is a feature of large intestinal obstruction. The pain is colicky in nature, lasts for 5–10 minutes and is intermittent. On pressure, it decreases.

Key Box 48.3

Cardinal Features of Intestinal Obstruction

- Colicky abdominal pain
- Abdominal distension
- Vomiting
- Absolute constipation

2. **Vomiting** is due to reverse peristalsis. Vomitus consists of stomach contents initially, then bile, followed by faeculent matter. **Faeculent is not faecal matter** but **terminal ileal contents which undergo bacterial degradation** and **fermentation** resulting in the smell of faecal matter. Vomiting of altered blood indicates haemorrhage and gangrene. Frequent vomiting reflects jejunal obstruction (Fig. 48.7 and Table 48.1).

Pearls of Wisdom

Vomiting of faeculent contents indicates terminal ileal obstruction.

3. **Distension of the abdomen:** It may be central abdominal distension as seen in ileal obstruction, peripheral abdominal as in large bowel obstruction, or localised to one or two quadrants as in sigmoid volvulus.
4. **Constipation** occurs because the distal bowel does not move. Constipation to faeces and flatus is called obstipation. Exceptions are given in Key Box 48.4.
5. **Late (advanced cases):** Oliguria indicates renal failure, tachypnoea indicates acidosis due to sepsis, altered sensorium indicates sepsis, hypoxia, electrolyte imbalances suggest impending gangrene (Fig. 48.8).

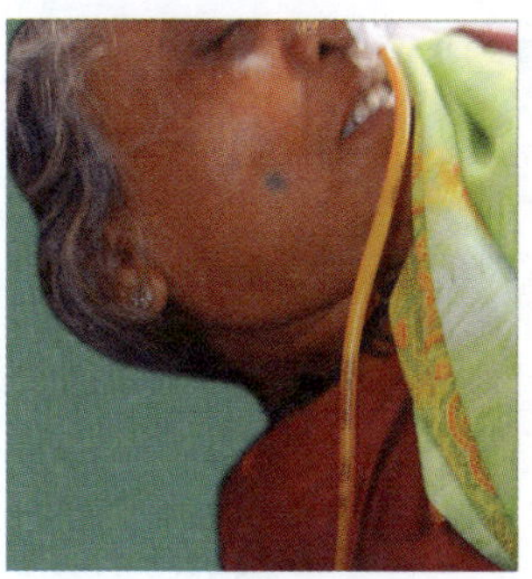

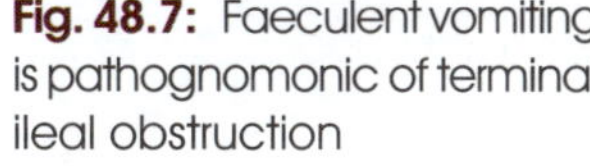

Fig. 48.7: Faeculent vomiting is pathognomonic of terminal ileal obstruction

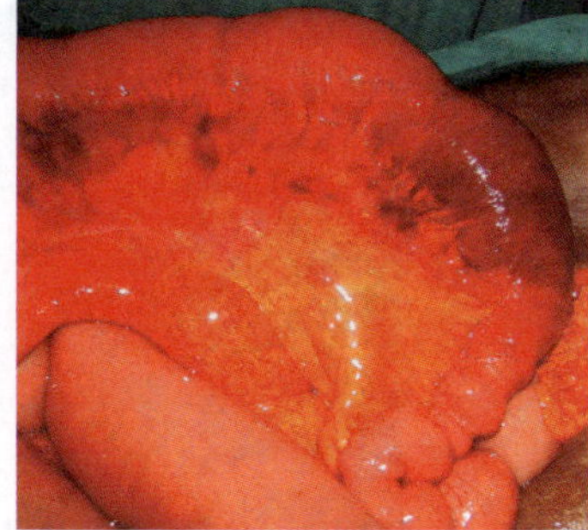

Fig. 48.8: Ischaemic area may develop stricture (intestinal stenosis of Garré) or may progress to gangrene

Table 48.1 Comparison of clinical features at different levels of intestinal obstruction

	High (jejunum)	Distal (ileum)	Low (colon)
• Vomiting	Frequent, bilious	Moderate bilious, faeculent	Late vomiting, faeculent
• Distension	No	Moderate distension	Marked distension
• Pain	Intermittent, not crescendo type	Intermittent, crescendo type, colicky	Variable pain, not classical crescendo
• Constipation	Not initially	Not initially	Initially present
• Peristalsis	Not seen	Step ladder peristalsis	Right to left peristalsis may be seen

Key Box 48.4

Intestinal Obstruction with Diarrhoea

- Faecal impaction : Page 821 (Fig. 48.4)
- Richter's hernia : Page 948
- Gallstone ileus : Page 836
- Mesenteric vascular occlusion : Page 841

Signs

1. **General signs of dehydration** such as dry skin, dry tongue, sunken eyes, feeble pulse, low urinary output are seen. Dehydration occurs due to persistent vomiting and sequestration of fluid and electrolytes. Hypokalaemia is an important finding.
2. **Abdominal findings**

- Distension, tympanitic note on percussion
- Step ladder peristalsis (Figs 48.9 and 48.10) is seen in terminal ileal obstruction. Right to left colonic peristalsis is seen in left-sided colonic obstruction, large bowel obstruction.
- On auscultation—loud, noisy intestinal sounds are heard. They are called **borborygmi**.
- Hernial orifices have to be examined, especially for a femoral hernia in females.

Signs of Strangulation

- It should be suspected when features of obstruction are present along with features of shock.

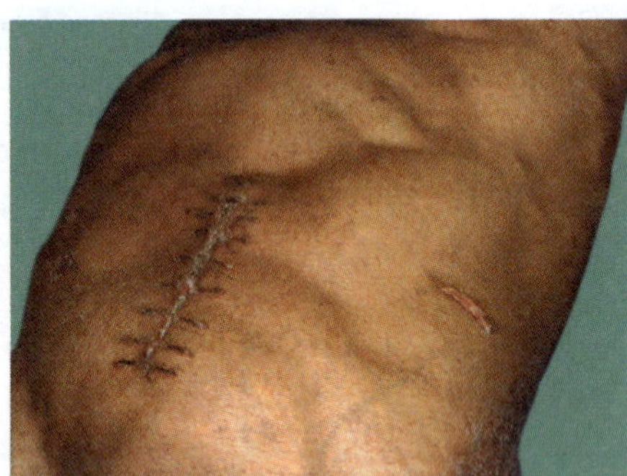

Fig. 48.9: Step ladder peristalsis

- Features of **septic shock**—fever, hypothermia, renal failure, respiratory failure (Key Box 48.5).
- **Rebound tenderness:** It is called **Blumberg's sign**. It is a classical sign of peritonitis.
- Guarding and rigidity of the abdominal wall.
- **Absent bowel sounds** because rest of the bowel loops undergo paralytic ileus.
- **Sudden symptoms**—spasmodic pain (due to peristalsis) and continuous pain suggest strangulation (Fig. 48.11).
- Features of strangulation and perforation occur quickly in cases of closed loop obstruction (Figs 48.11, 48.12 and Key Box 48.6).

Rectal Examination

- In small bowel obstruction, **rectum is empty** and is often ballooned out.

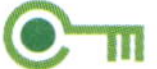

Key Box 48.5

Features of Strangulation

- Tachycardia
- Tenderness
- Temperature—fever
- Acidosis
- Drowsiness
- Altered sensorium
- Tense abdomen
- Rebound tenderness

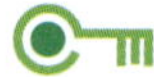

Key Box 48.6

Closed Loop Obstruction

- This occurs when the bowel is obstructed at both proximal and distal points.
- Proximal bowel is not distended as much in this condition.
- Gangrene and perforation can occur fast.
- Retrograde thrombosis of mesenteric vein, can result in distension of the bowel.
- A few examples of closed loop obstruction include sigmoid volvulus, strangulated hernia, carcinoma right colon.

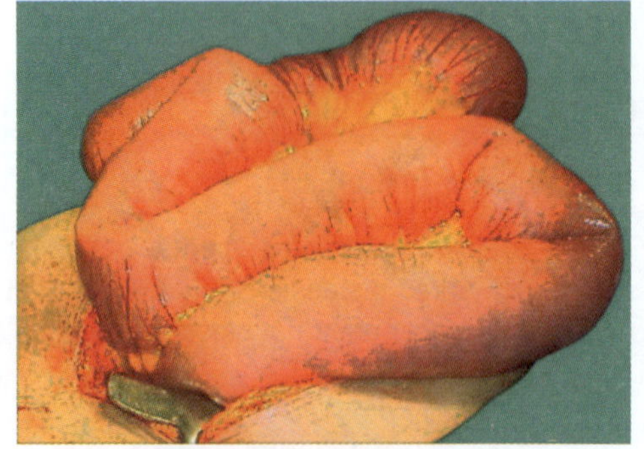

Fig. 48.10: Dilated intestinal loops

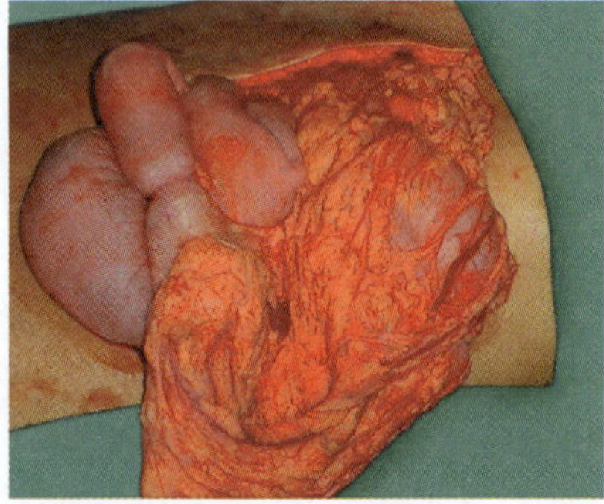

Fig. 48.11: Perforation due to obstruction

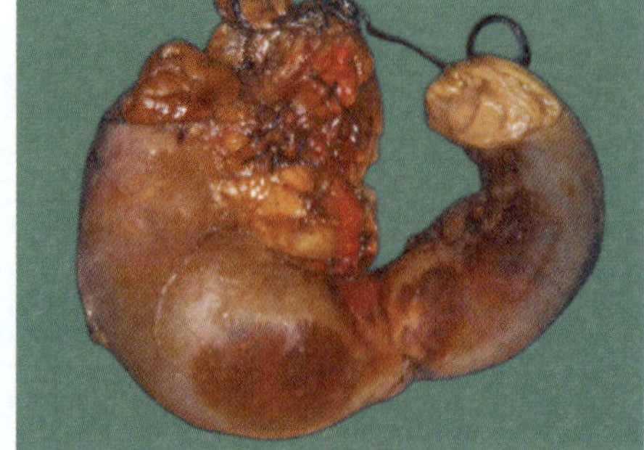

Fig. 48.12: Gangrene due to intussusception

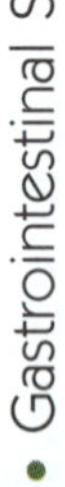

- Carcinomatous growth with or without stools can be felt.
- The finger may be stained with blood.
- Altered foul blood indicates gangrene of the bowel.
- Located colon/hard masses indicate pseudo-obstruction.

INVESTIGATIONS

- **Complete blood picture:** Low Hb% indicates underlying malignancy. Increased total WBC count indicates infection and sepsis (perforation and gangrene).
- Electrolytes: Most of the electrolytes are low in cases of intestinal obstruction and require correction preoperatively. Strangulation may be associated with deranged potassium, amylase or lactic dehydrogenase.
- Plain X-ray abdomen in the erect position may show multiple gas fluid levels. Gas levels appear earlier than fluid level. Normally, two insignificant fluid levels can be present, one in the terminal ileum and another in the first part of the duodenum (Key Box 48.7). Supine films indicate the distal limit of obstruction (Figs 48.13 to 48.17).
- The small intestine is considered dilated if loops of bowel measure more than 3 cm in diameter. Measurements for the large bowel vary among different anatomic segments, with a relative threshold of 9 cm in diameter for the proximal colon and 5 cm for the sigmoid colon.
- **Enteroclysis (Barium meal follow through):** Should not be done in total obstruction but can be done in partial obstruction by using thin barium sulfate.

Key Box 48.7

Plain X-ray Findings Upright and Supine

- First get supine films. They indicate distal limit of obstruction. Erect films are asked if any doubt exists about obstruction.
- Jejunum is characterised by regularly placed mucosal folds called **valvulae conniventes** (Fig. 48.15) placed opposite to each other **(Herringbone pattern)**. They are produced by **valves of Kerckring.**
- Large bowel is characterised by **haustrations** (Fig. 48.16): Incomplete, large mucosal folds, not placed opposite to each other.
- **Caecum has no haustrations.** It appears as a round gas shadow in the right iliac fossa.
- Ileum has no characters—**characterless loop of Wangensteen.**
- Plain X-ray may demonstrate gallstone ileus or foreign body.
- Gas is absent in the small bowel as in mesenteric vascular ischaemia.
- Sigmoid volvulus appears as a large dilated loop—inverted 'U' shape.

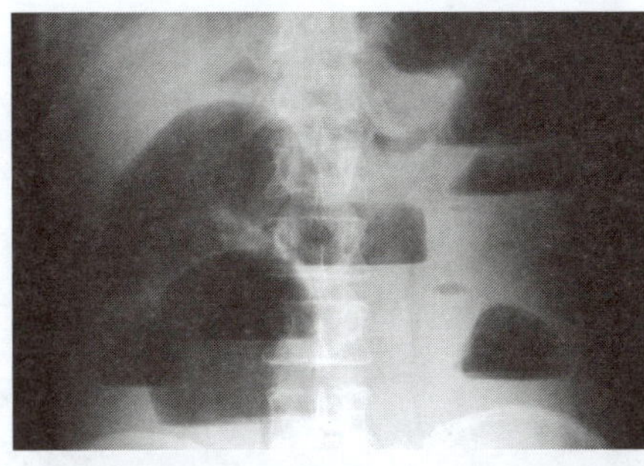

Fig. 48.13: Multiple gas fluid levels—plain X-ray erect abdomen

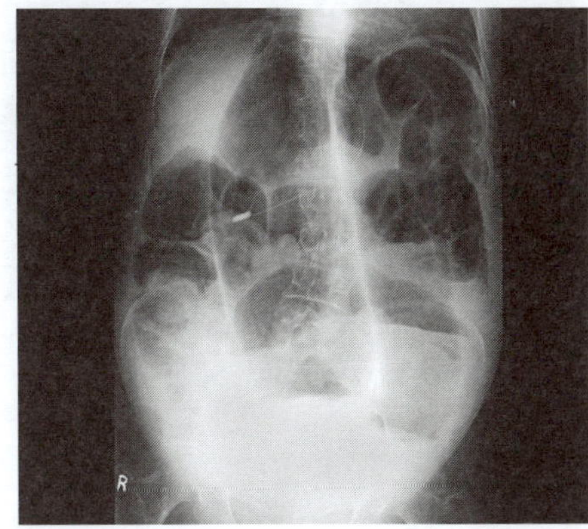

Fig. 48.14: Multiple gas fluid levels seen with a large dilated loop in the centre

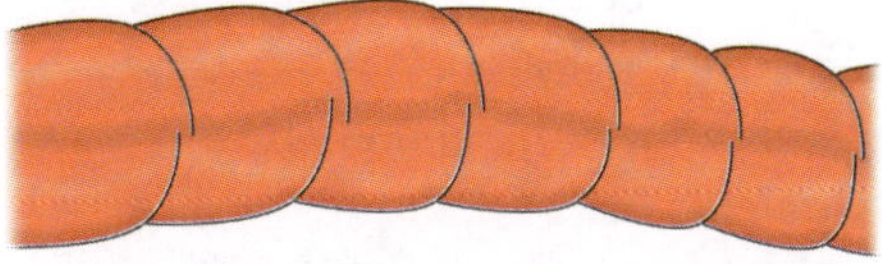

Fig. 48.15: Valvulae conniventes—typical of jejunum

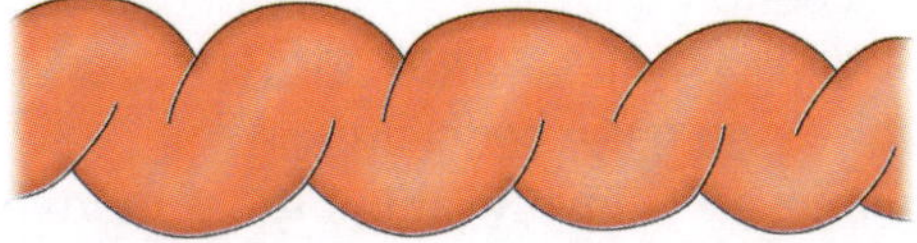

Fig. 48.16: Haustrations—typical of colon

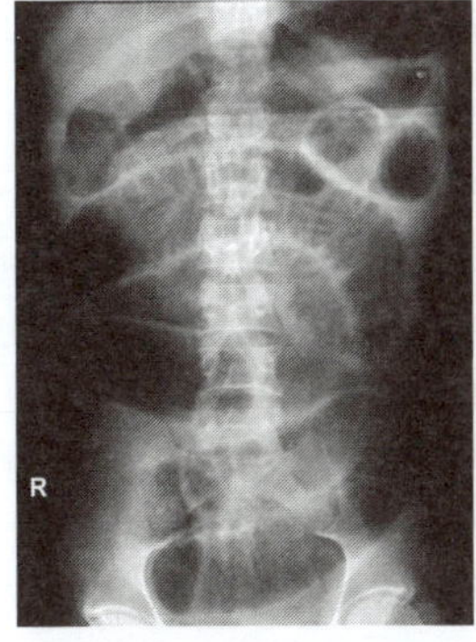

Fig. 48.17: Plain X-ray abdomen supine—distended intestines. Supine X-ray will indicate distal limit of obstruction

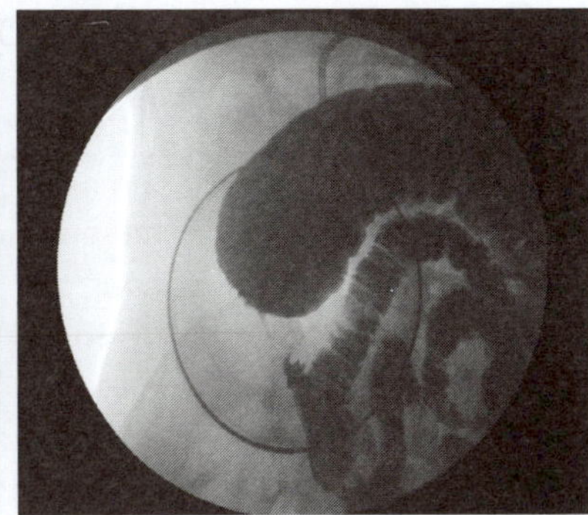

Fig. 48.18: Jejunal stricture due to tuberculosis—enteroclysis picture. You can see grossly dilated jejunal loops proximally. You can see grossly dilated jejunal loops proximally

Pearls of Wisdom

Enteroclysis is rarely performed in acute intestinal obstruction but it has greater sensitivity in the detection of partial small bowel obstruction (Fig. 48.18).

- **Ultrasound/CT scan**—Fig. 48.19, Key Boxes 48.8 and 48.9.

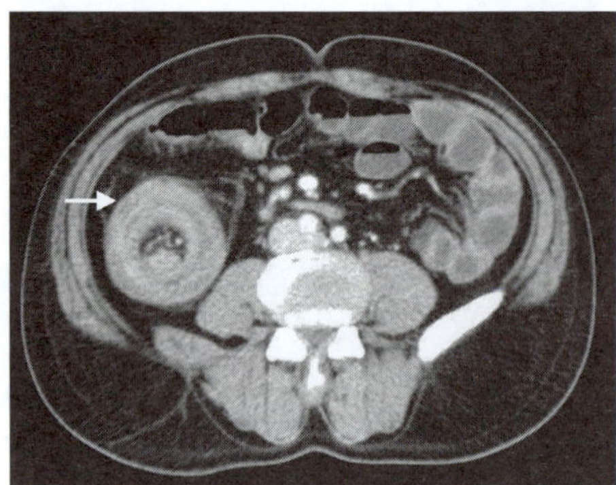

Fig. 48.19: Ileocolic intussusception—observe 'target sign' on the right side

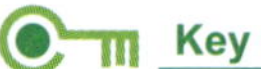 **Key Box 48.8**

Ultrasound

- It is not the investigation of choice or it may not be required

However, a good sonologist can diagnose:

a. Dilated loops of intestine
b. Presence of fluid in the abdomen
c. Gallstone ileus
d. Infarcted/ischaemic bowel/gas in the portal vein or intrahepatic gas.
e. Intussusception and can assess vascularity with the help of duplex scan.
f. It can also rule out other causes.

Being a noninvasive investigation, it has more benefits.

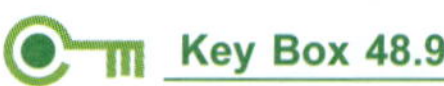 **Key Box 48.9**

CT Scan in Intestinal Obstruction

- Can detect dilated intestines proximally and collapsed bowel distally.
- If bowel wall is thick and air is present (**pneumatosis**), strangulation is likely mesenteric ischaemia
- It can detect portal venous gas (suggesting gangrene)
- CT can detect **mass lesions**—carcinoma sigmoid, caecum or ileocaecal mass (TB).
- CT has low sensitivity in detecting low grade or partial small bowel obstruction. Sensitivity increases in total obstruction.

MANAGEMENT PRINCIPLES

Preoperative preparation includes correction of dehydration, electrolytes and broad spectrum antibiotics.

Principles in the management of intestinal obstruction are as follows: **Mnemonic: A, B, C, D, E, F.**

A. **Aspiration with Ryle's tube:** This is the most important step in the management of intestinal obstruction. It helps in decreasing the distension and also prevents vomiting. This will help in preventing respiratory complications due to aspiration following general anaesthesia.
B. **Bowel care:** No purgatives because purgation can cause perforation. Do not stimulate bowel by drugs or food.
C. **Charts:** Temperature, pulse, respiration and intake output chart. In cases of conservative management such as obstruction due to adhesions, change in temperature and increasing pulse rate suggests perforation or gangrene. These cases have to be explored immediately.
D. **Drugs** to cover gram-positive, gram-negative and anaerobic organisms.
E. **Exploratory laparotomy** is done and depending upon the findings, obstruction is treated. A few examples are given in Key Box 48.10 and Fig. 48.20.
F. **Electrolytes** should be given before, during and after surgery. It forms the most important treatment of intestinal obstruction.

Key Box 48.10

Principles of Exploratory Laparotomy

- Ideally done within 6–8 hours
- Long midline incision
- Resection of gangrene and anastomosis
- Adhesions—release
- Bands—divide
- Gallstone ileus—remove the stone/stones
- Volvulus—untwist or resection
- Obstructed hernia—reduce/resect if gangrene
- Gangrene—resect
- Stricture—resection or stricturoplasty
- Advanced malignancy—bypass

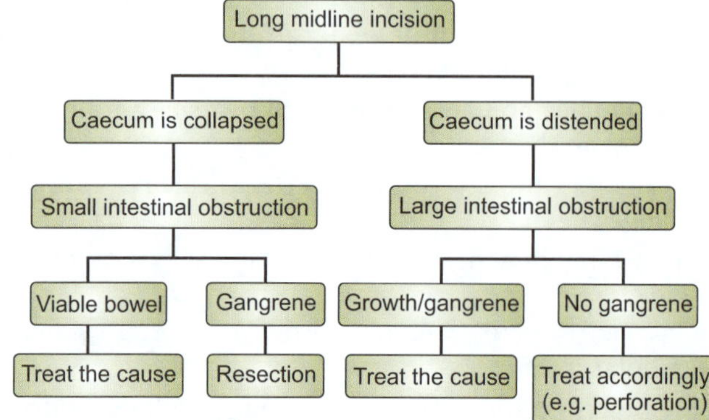

Fig. 48.20: Principles of management of intestinal obstruction

APPROACH TO THE MANAGEMENT OF INTESTINAL OBSTRUCTION—MORE DETAILS

Ask the following questions to yourself and proceed.

1. What is the probable cause of obstruction?
2. Is it small bowel obstruction at laparotomy?
3. Is it large bowel obstruction at laparotomy?
4. Is it simple obstruction?
5. Is it strangulation?
6. Is it some kind of a surprise or a difficult case?
7. Can I manage conservatively?

1. Probable Cause of Obstruction

- A previous **laparotomy scar** may indicate that it could be an adhesive obstruction (most common).
- An obvious obstructed hernia (inguinal/umbilical/incisional or femoral) can be managed with inguinal approach (Figs 48.21 to 48.23). It is treated by reducing contents, repair: Suture/mesh and resect, if gangrene is present.
- An elderly man, hypertensive and atherosclerotic, with features of blood in the stools and acute abdominal pain may be having superior mesenteric ischaemia.
- A constipated, elderly man in poor health, with acute or chronic obstruction may be having carcinoma of the colon.

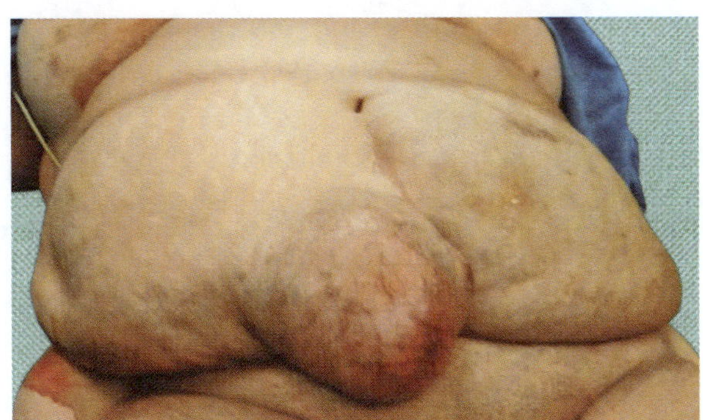

Fig. 48.21: Obstructed incisional hernia

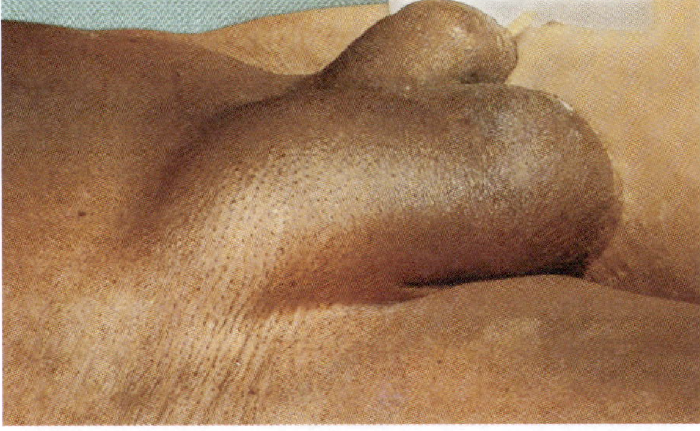

Fig. 48.22: Obstructed inguinal hernia

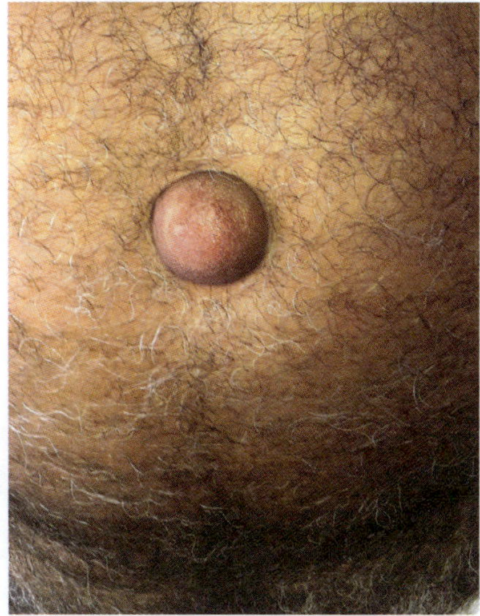

Fig. 48.23: Obstructed umbilical hernia

2. Diagnosis of Small Bowel Obstruction at Laparotomy

- Caecum is collapsed
- Dilated loops of small intestine are present.
- A stricture or a mass lesion may be obvious at laparotomy.

3. Diagnosis of Large Bowel Obstruction at Laparotomy

- Caecum is distended.
- A growth may be palpable and obvious in the transverse colon or in the hidden colon, i.e. splenic flexure.
- It is very important to examine the entire colon (synchronous carcinoma is more common).

4. Diagnosis of Simple Obstruction

- It is done when bowel is not gangrenous.
- In doubtful cases, because of long-standing ischaemia, wrapping the bowel with warm and moist pack and administration of pure oxygen may help the bowel to recover from ischaemia.
- Pink bowel, peristalsis is seen, peritoneal sheen and pulsations indicate healthy bowel.

5. Diagnosis of Strangulation

(Fig. 48.24 and Key Box 48.11)

- Black, dark, foul-smelling bowel is seen as soon as laparotomy is done.
- Peritoneal fluid contains blood-stained fluid.
- Precautions must be taken not to contaminate peritoneal cavity when gangrenous segment is removed.

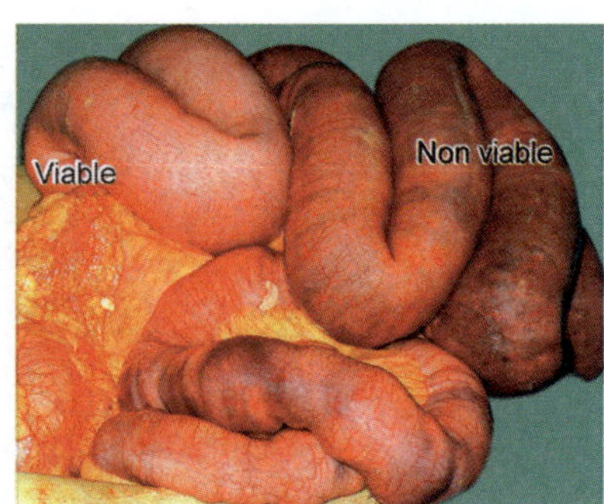

Fig. 48.24: Viable and nonviable bowel

Key Box 48.11

Viable Bowel—Features

- Normal peristalsis
- Normal peritoneal sheen is present
- Normal pulsations are visible or felt at the mesentery
- Normal pink colour is present

Do not hesitate to take the help of senior experienced surgeons in treating an uncommon situation such as massive ischaemia and gangrene of small bowel and colon (due to mesenteric vascular occlusion), synchronous carcinoma and ileosigmoid knotting, etc.

6. It is a Surprise

- Surprises are well known in intestinal obstruction. Congenital bands, foreign bodies, internal herniation, strictures are a few examples.
- The detailed management of individual cases is discussed below.

7. Can I Manage Conservatively?

- In these cases, a long intestinal tube called Miller-Abbott tube can be passed to decompress intestines (Key Box 48.12).

Key Box 48.12

Intestinal Obstruction Conservative Treatment

1. **Partial small bowel obstruction** mostly due to adhesion: Wait for 48 to 72 hours. They may show improvement. If not, surgery is required.
2. **Early postoperative obstruction:** It rarely progresses to strangulation. Hence, nonoperative management can be extended to many days (3–7) provided there is no evidence of peritonitis.
3. **Intestinal obstruction in Crohn's disease:** Aim in Crohn's disease is to 'preserve' bowel as it may respond to medications.
4. **Carcinomatosis:** Disseminated malignancy with obstruction. The aim is nonoperative treatment as nothing much can be achieved with laparotomy.

DIFFERENTIAL DIAGNOSIS OF INTESTINAL OBSTRUCTION

VOLVULUS OF THE SIGMOID COLON

- Common in North India (Punjab), Eastern Europe, Uganda.
- In certain parts of India as mentioned above, it is one of the common surgical emergencies in elderly population (Key Box 48.13).

Precipitating Factors (Fig. 48.25)

1. Long mesentery of the pelvic colon
2. Narrow attachment at the base
3. Long, redundant, pendulous sigmoid
4. Loaded colon due to high residue diet
5. Diverticulitis with a band, or adhesions

Sigmoid volvulus is a definite occurrence in mentally disturbed patients, hypothyroidism, Parkinson's disease, multiple sclerosis, etc. probably due to severe constipation due to medications.

Key Box 48.13

Certain Facts about Sigmoid Volvulus

- More common in males
- 2/3rd of the cases are sigmoid volvulus and 1/3rd are caecal volvulus.
- Common in middle age and >60 years
- It accounts for about 10 to 15% of cases of intestinal obstruction in India.
- More common in rural population
- It is not an uncommon event during pregnancy

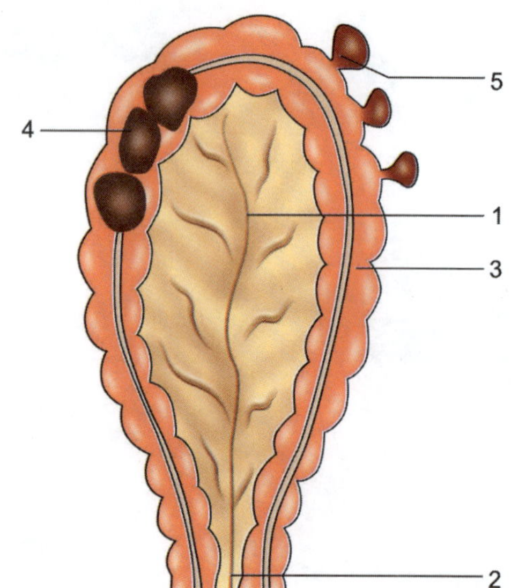

Fig. 48.25: Causes of sigmoid volvulus (see text for numbers)

Pearls of Wisdom

Ogilvie's syndrome precipitates volvulus.

Clinical Features

1. **Acute sigmoid volvulus (fulminant)** presents as intestinal obstruction. It starts usually after straining at stools. Volvulus is usually in anticlockwise direction and after one and a half turns, the entire loop becomes gangrenous.

   Enormous distension of the abdomen takes place, which gives a tympanitic note all over the abdomen. It is due to **diffusion of CO_2** (Fig. 48.26). Due to gross distension, severe hypovolaemic shock develops within 6–8 hours of volvulus. Gangrene sets in, which gives rise to features of strangulation. A dilated loop can be seen and felt. Features of peritonitis are seen within 1–2 days. Per rectal examination shows rectum to be empty.

Pearls of Wisdom

Distended tympanitic drum-like abdomen—sigmoid volvulus.

2. **Chronic (indolent) recurrent sigmoid volvulus:** It occurs due to partial twisting and untwisting of the bowel. Elderly patients present with recurrent lower abdominal pain on the left side and distension of the abdomen which is relieved on passing large amount of flatus.

Diagnosis

- **Plain X-ray abdomen erect** shows a hugely dilated sigmoid loop which is described as **'bent inner tube sign'**. The dilated loop may be visible on the right side, centre and to the left of abdomen, having two fluid levels, one on right side and one on left side. This is also described as **'omega sign'** (Figs 48.27 and 48.28).
- **Contrast enema:** As the barium enters the rectum, it tapers into the sigmoid colon—**Bird's beak sign** (not to be done in acute cases).

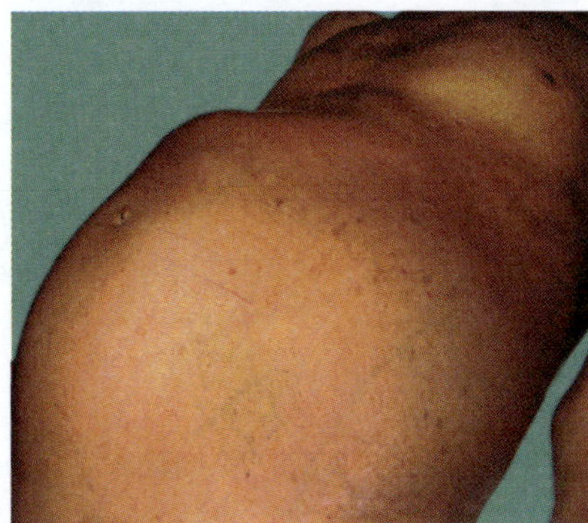

Fig. 48.26: Uneven distension due to sigmoid volvulus

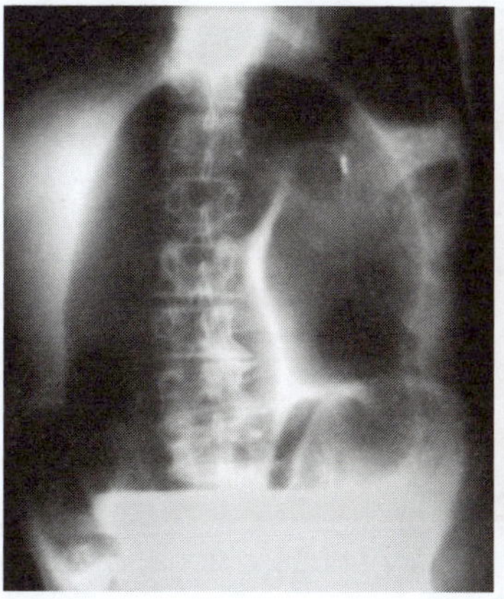

Fig. 48.27: Plain X-ray abdomen showing distended sigmoid loop

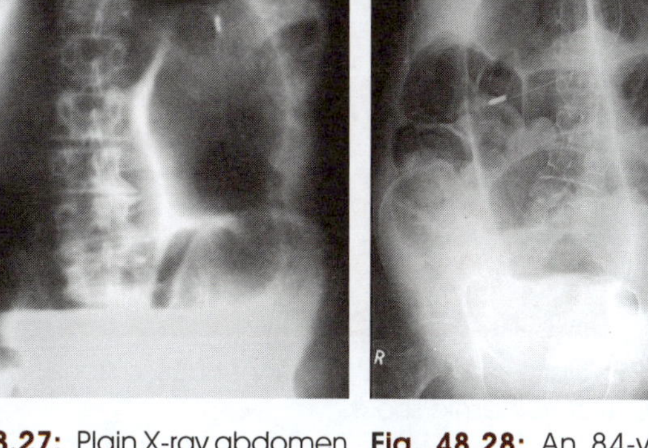

Fig. 48.28: An 84-year-old patient with sigmoid volvulus, managed by sigmoidoscopic decompression

TREATMENT

I. Nonoperative

A successful passage of flatus tube or sigmoidoscope up to 25–30 cm results in release of a large amount of flatus and fluid, and obstruction is relieved. If obstruction is completely relieved or if there is no gangrene and the general condition of the patient improves, an elective resection is done after 7 days. If resistance is found while passing flatus tube, instill barium for guidance.

II. Operative Treatment

1. **Single-stage resection:** This can be done, provided general condition of the patient is good. If the loop is gangrenous, resection followed by end to end anastomosis is done, after giving 'on table' lavage using saline washes till the contents of the colon are clear. Sigmoid colon is hugely dilated (Fig. 48.29).
2. **Hartmann's procedure:** If the loop is gangrenous and proximal bowel is loaded with faecal matter, resection of the sigmoid colon is done. Proximal descending colon is brought out as an end colostomy and rectum is closed (Hartmann's procedure). After 6 weeks, colorectal anastomosis is done.
3. **Sigmoidopexy:** If the loop is not gangrenous, untwist the sigmoid loop and fix the sigmoid to the posterior abdominal wall (sigmoidopexy). If the mesentery is long, it can be made short by plication.
4. **Exteriorisation:** Paul-Mickulicz procedure is done when general condition of the patient is poor as in elderly patients, in severely dehydrated patient with impending septicaemia. In such cases, the gangrenous loop is brought outside and resected, with a proximal colostomy and a distal mucous fistula (Fig. 48.30).

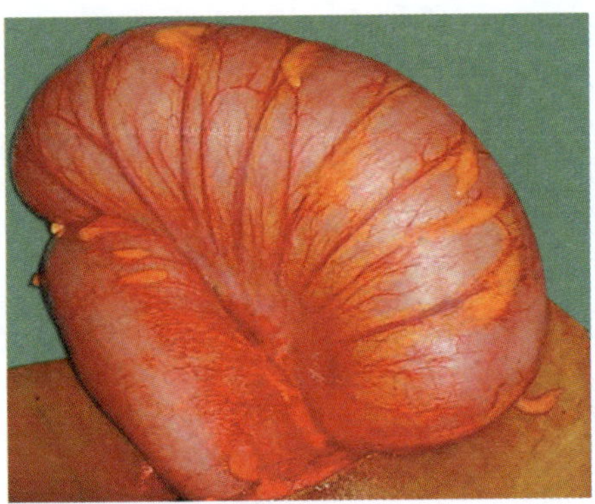

Fig. 48.29: Sigmoid colon at surgery—huge distension results in severe hypovolaemic shock

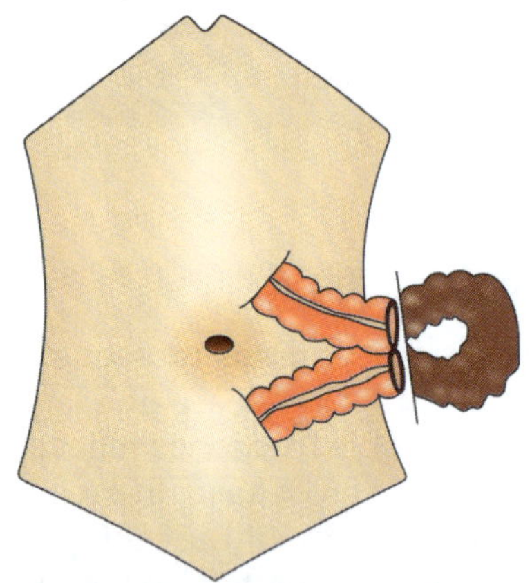

Fig. 48.30: Paul-Mickulicz procedure

CAECAL VOLVULUS AND BASCULE

- It is a rare cause of intestinal obstruction (Figs 48.31 to 48.34 and Key Boxes 48.14 and 48.15).
- Presumably, it is more likely to occur following any surgical procedure which might require some degree of medial visceral rotation or disruption of the fusion plane between the caecum or ascending colon with the lateral peritoneum, providing sufficient mobility allowing caecal volvulisation to occur.
- A constant feature of **caecal bascule** is the presence of a constricting band across the ascending colon. This may be found at laparotomy.
- In a plain X-ray abdomen, caecum produces round shadow in the centre of the abdomen.
- Resection is the ideal treatment.

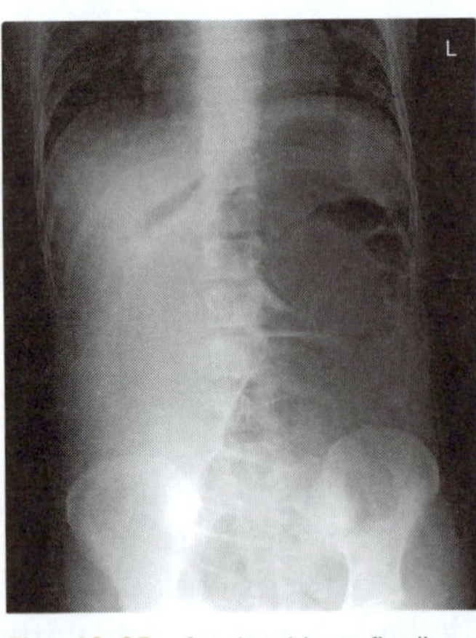

Fig. 48.31: Supine X-ray findings in caecal volvulus

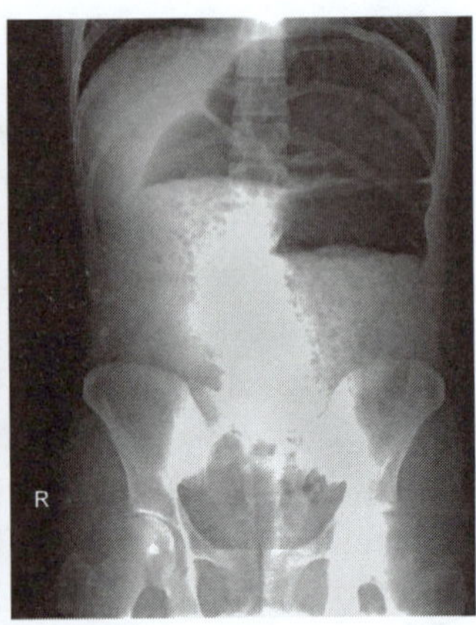

Fig. 48.32: Erect X-ray showing distended loop. Caecum was palpable in the left hypochondrium

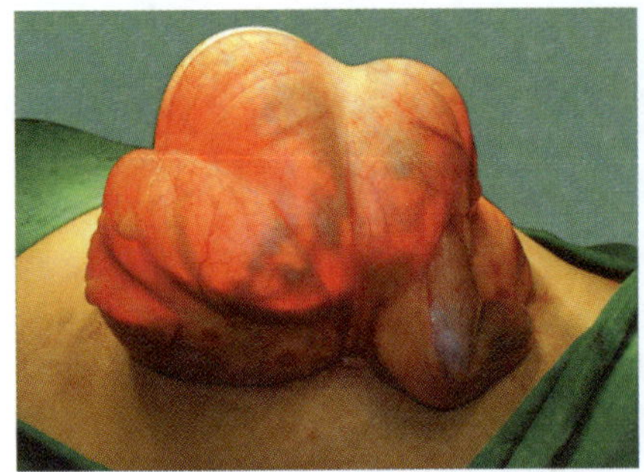

Fig. 48.33: Distended caecum at surgery. (*Courtesy:* Dr Basavaraj Patil, Dr Hartimath, Dr Rasheed, Dr Nikil, Department of Surgery, KMC, Manipal)

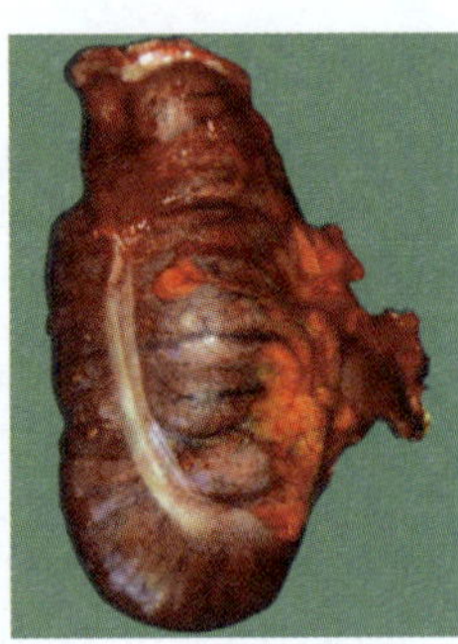

Fig. 48.34: Caecal volvulus with gangrene

Key Box 48.14

Caecal Bascule

- Caecum folds anteromedial to the ascending colon, with production of a flap-valve occlusion at the site of flexion.
- Caecum will be markedly distended and will be found in the centre of the abdomen.
- Occasionally, it is associated with malrotation of the gut.
- There will be a constricting band across the ascending colon.
- It is also argued that caecal bascule can also be due to lack of fixation of large bowel. Resection is ideal even though fixation (caecopexy) is also another alternative.
- Bascule is a French term for seesaw and balance

Key Box 48.15

Comparison of Caecal Volvulus and Sigmoid Volvulus

Caecal volvulus	Sigmoid volvulus
Rare	Common
Clockwise twist	Anticlockwise
Mobile caecum	Long mesentery is the cause
Middle-aged	Elderly, debilitated
Kidney-shaped gas shadow with single fluid level on the leftside	Omega sign or coffee shaped. Two fluid levels can be found.
Treated only by surgery	Nonoperative treatment should be attempted in all cases, provided there is no ischaemia.

Pearls of Wisdom

If loop is gangrenous, do not derotate—clamp the mesentery first, then detorsion can be done to avoid reperfusion injury.

MECKEL'S DIVERTICULUM WITH A BAND

It is a congenital diverticulum which occurs due to persistent intestinal end of vitellointestinal duct. **Being congenital, it has all the layers of the bowel**. Hence, it is a true diverticulum.

Anomalies of Vitellointestinal Duct (Figs 48.35A to F)

A. **Fibrous band** results when entire duct is obliterated and bowel can twist around the band, resulting in volvulus.

B. **Persistent intestinal end:** Meckel's diverticulum.

C. **Meckel's diverticulum with the band** attached to the umbilicus can give rise to intestinal obstruction.

D. **Umbilical fistula** results when entire duct is patent. Even though it is connected to the terminal ileum, the opening is very small. The discharge is rarely faecal. Often, it is the mucus secreted from the lining of the duct **(omphaloenteric fistula)**.

E. **Umbilical sinus** results due to persistent umbilical end discharging mucus. Slowly umbilical adenoma occurs and epithelial lining of the sinus gets everted.

F. **Intra-abdominal cyst** results when both ends are obliterated. The central portion of the duct persists and secretes mucus. This is very, very rare.

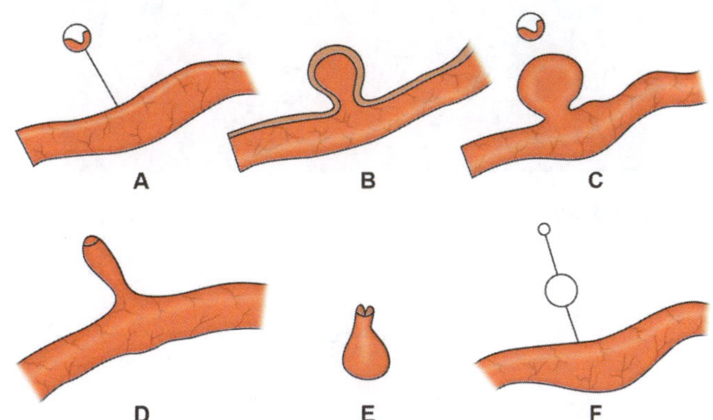

Figs 48.35A to F: Anomalies of vitellointestinal duct (A to F *see* text for details)

MECKEL'S DIVERTICULUM

- It is present in 2% of the cases, 2 inches long, 2 feet away from ileocaecal region in the antimesenteric border (ileal duplication can occur in the mesenteric border). It is two times more common in females.
- Symptomatic cases are below 2 years of age.
- In 12% of the patients, heterotopic gastric tissue is found which can produce peptic ulceration. In a few other patients, it can contain pancreatic and colonic tissue. Other anomalies (Key Box 48.16).

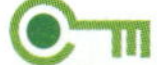

Key Box 48.16

Meckel's[1] Diverticulum and other Associated Anomalies

- Angiodysplasia of the caecum
- Anorectal atresia, atresia of the oesophagus

[1]The most common congenital anomaly of small intestine

RULE OF 2 FOR MECKEL'S DIVERTICULUM

- Incidence: 2%
- Location: 2 feet proximal to ileocaecal junction
- Length: 2 inches long
- Ectopic tissue: 2 types—gastric and pancreatic
- Presentation: 2 years or below 2 years is the most common age
- Male: female ratio—1:2

Clinical Presentation

- **Massive bleeding per rectum:** In the form of melaena, it is not uncommon. In many other patients, mild chronic bleeding can result in anaemia. Blood is maroon coloured.
- **Acute Meckel's diverticulitis:** Factors which precipitate diverticulitis are:
  - Peptic ulceration due to ectopic gastric mucosa of the diverticulum
  - Ingested foreign material, e.g. stalk of vegetable, seeds, fish or chicken bones
  - Faecolith (not common in ileum), tumours, worms causing stasis and bacterial infection
  - Inflammation and ischaemia caused by torsion due to an associated band is called mesodiverticular band
  - Association with acute appendicitis
- **Perforation:** It is impossible to differentiate it from ruptured appendix. This is treated by laparotomy and resection of diverticulum along with adjacent intestine. In majority of appendicular perforations, local abscess will occur because of retrocaecal position of the appendix (70%). However, perforation of Meckel's diverticulum, even though a rare cause of peritonitis, has a high mortality rate. This is because infection spreads very fast as **diverticulum is intraperitoneal and contents are faeculent**.
- As a cause of **intestinal obstruction**, when it is associated with a band or due to volvulus. It is the most common presentation in adults (Key Box 48.17).

Key Box 48.17

Meckel's Diverticulum and Intestinal Obstruction

- Intussusception
- Band
- Volvulus due to band
- Internal herniation beneath mesodiverticular band
- Diverticulitis with band
- Littre's hernia

Pearls of Wisdom

Older child, deformed umbilicus, scarless abdomen with intestinal obstruction—cause may be Meckel's diverticulum.

- **As a cause of intussusception:** Here also, inflamed heterotopic tissue can be found in the diverticulum (2% cases).
- **Pain** can occur due to chronic peptic ulceration.
- **Neoplasm:** Carcinoids and GIST are more common in Meckel's diverticulum than elsewhere in the small intestine although presence of Meckel's diverticulum itself is rare.

Pearls of Wisdom

Hernia of Littre is a hernial sac containing Meckel's diverticulum (Key Box 48.17).

Investigations

1. No investigation can prove diagnosis of Meckel's diverticulum. Small bowel enema may demonstrate the diverticulum if opening is wide (fluoroscopy is more ideal).
2. **^{99m}Tc-labelled pertechnetate** when given IV, may localise the heterotopic gastric mucosa in the Meckel's diverticulum, in about 90% of patients.
   - This radionuclide is taken up by **mucin-secreting cells** and **parietal cells** and it is secreted immediately. Thus, if ^{99m}Tc appears in the stomach as well as in other part of bowel, it indicates functioning heterotopic tissue.
   - Even when bleeding is at a rate of 0.1 ml/minute, it can detect Meckel's diverticulum. Hence, it is superior to angiography.
   - Very useful in children with bleeding.

Pearls of Wisdom

The pertechnetate anion ^{99m}Tc is selectively taken up by gastric mucosal cells, thyroid, salivary glands and choroid plexus.

Treatment (Fig. 48.36)

1. Incidentally found Meckel's during laparotomy for some other causes can be left alone, provided it has a wide mouth. However, a note of it must be made in the operation register (Key Box 48.18).
2. Meckel's diverticulum with bleeding, band, perforation and narrow mouth is treated by removal of diverticulum with adjacent intestine because the gastric tissue may often line the intestine also (Figs 48.37 and 48.38).

Key Box 48.18

Indications for Removal of Incidentally found Meckel's Diverticulum

- Children under 2 years of age
- Meckel's with a band
- Meckel's with adhesions
- Meckel's with narrow base
- Long Meckel's diverticulum

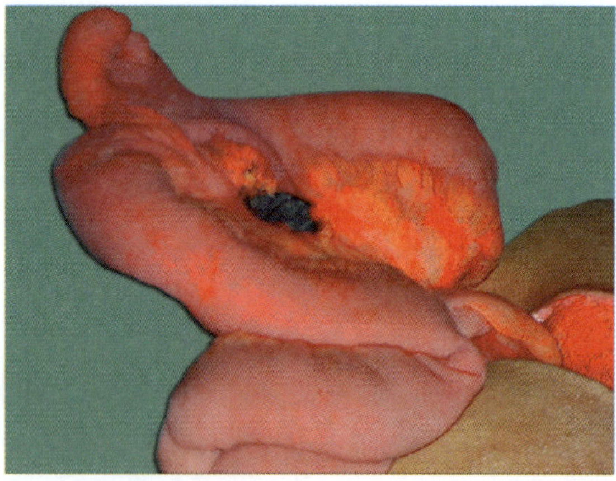

Fig. 48.36: Inflamed Meckel's diverticulum of surgery

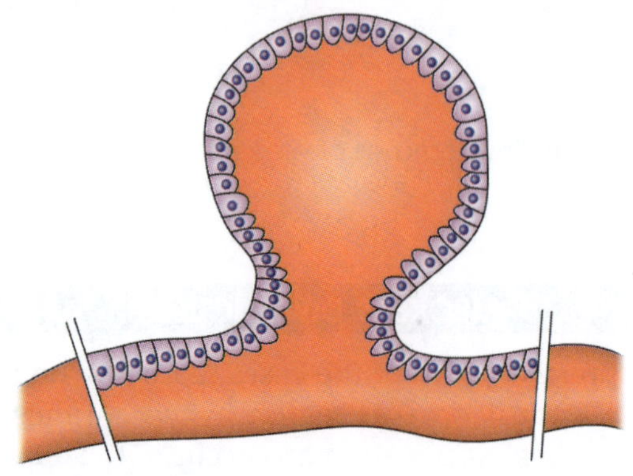

Fig. 48.37: Meckel's diverticulectomy should include normal intestine also

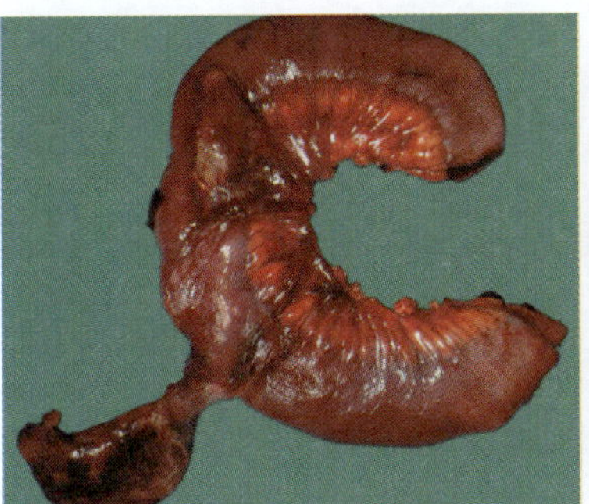

Fig. 48.38A: Resected Meckel's diverticulum with normal intestine (*Courtesy:* Dr Pramod K, Dr Deviprasad, Shetty, Kasturba Hospital, Manipal)

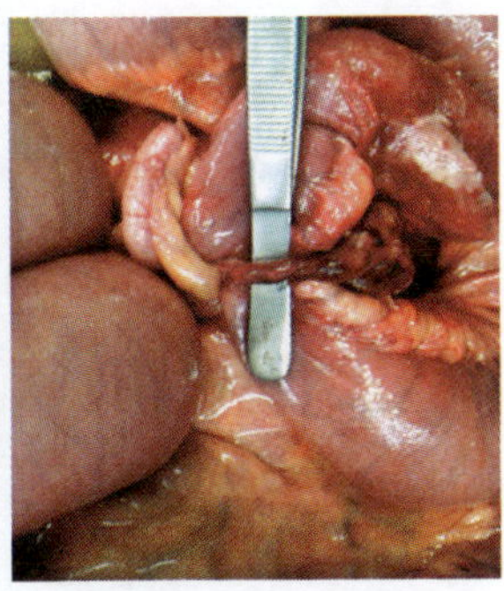

Fig. 48.38B: Meckel's diverticulum with band and obstruction

ADHESIONS AND BANDS

ADHESIONS

Introduction: Intra-abdominal adhesions develop after abdominal surgery as part of the normal healing processes that occur after damage to the peritoneum. The early balance between fibrin deposition and degradation seems to be the critical factor in adhesion formation. They also cause significant morbidity, including adhesive small bowel obstruction, infertility and increased difficulty with reoperative surgery. Thus, high chances of causing intestinal fistula after reexploration.

Definition: Peritoneal adhesions can be defined as abnormal fibrous bands between organs or tissues or both in the abdominal cavity that are normally separated. They are common causes of intestinal obstruction in the western world, Chinese population of Malaysia, etc. In India, adhesions and obstructed hernia are the two common causes in adults.

Pearls of Wisdom

It is important to realise that secondary infertility in women and ectopic gestation can occur due to adhesions.

Causes: Remember the Important 5 Is

1. **Infection:** Laparotomy done for acute appendicitis with or without perforation, perforation peritonitis, intra-abdominal abscess have higher incidence of adhesions. Surgery is the commonest cause of peritoneal adhesions.
2. **Ischaemia:** Lack of blood supply, particularly venous occlusion can cause adhesions, e.g. mesenteric vascular occlusion.
3. **Iatrogenic:** It refers to talc, silk thread, foreign body (mop), etc. used for surgery which can induce extensive adhesions due to foreign body reaction (spilled gallstone also).
4. **Injury** to the bowel can result in adhesions.
5. **Irradiation** enteritis is becoming common due to irradiation for carcinoma of the cervix.

Pathogenesis

Ischaemia and irritation of the intestines are the chief factors responsible for adhesions (Key Box 48.19).

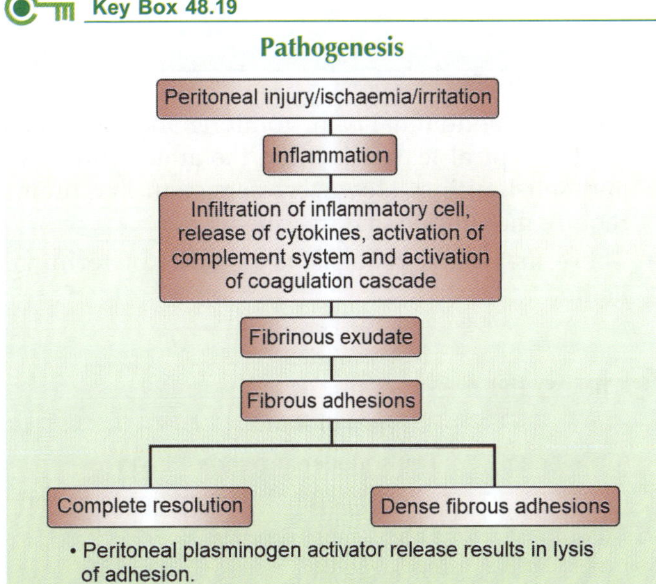

Types (Fig. 48.39)

1. **Fibrinous adhesions** (bread and butter adhesions): They are the causes of early postoperative obstruction, which settles down within 3–5 days. Majority of them disappear in due course of time.
2. **Fibrous adhesions:** If the infection is continuing or if foreign body is present, the fibrinous material is converted to fibrous band. They also occur at the site of ischaemia. They will cause late intestinal obstruction (Fig. 48.40).

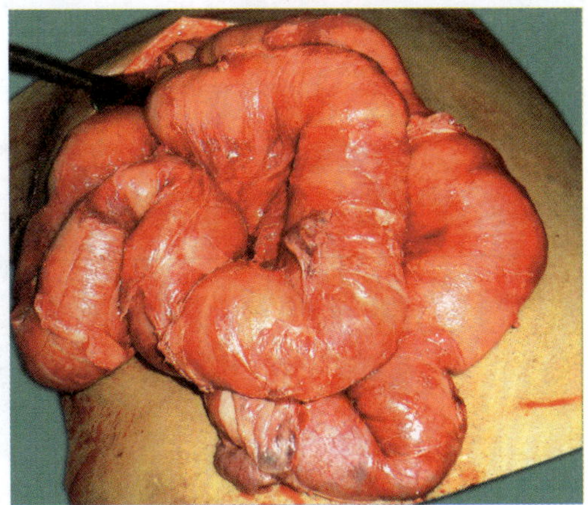

Fig. 48.39: Bread and butter adhesions—case of perforation peritonitis

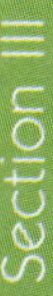

3. **Tuberculous adhesions** are dense adhesions that result in matting of intestinal coils. Separating them at laparotomy is extremely difficult (Fig. 48.41).
   - Congenital band is the 4th type of band (not due to adhesion).

Pearls of Wisdom

A congenital band, omental band, a string band of bacterial peritonitis or a fibrous band of tuberculosis is responsible for obstruction (Fig. 48.42, and Key Box 48.20).

Clinical Features

- Recurrent abdominal pain, vomiting and distension are the typical features. Often the attacks are mild and self-limiting. However, persistent symptoms require monitoring and treatment.
- There may be peristalsis as in cases of terminal ileum.

Key Box 48.20

Types of Band

❍ Congenital	:	Transduodenal band of Ladd
	:	Vitellointestinal duct associated band
❍ Acquired	:	Following peritonitis
	:	Diverticulum
	:	Greater omentum as a band

- Gangrene is not common in cases of adhesive obstruction (Fig. 48.42). However, these cases have to be closely monitored for any changes in the type of pain or new abdominal signs. Severe pain, tachycardia, temperature, tachypnoea and tenderness in the abdomen indicate gangrene or perforation (Figs 48.43 and 48.44).

- Gilroy Benan triad of adhesive pain:
  - Pain gets aggravated or relieved on change of posture.
  - Pain in the region of old abdominal scar.
  - Tenderness elicited by pressure over the scar.

Investigations

- **Plain X-ray abdomen and small bowel enema** are very useful investigations to prove the obstruction.
- **Computed tomography (CT)** enhanced with oral contrast:
  - Detects air-fluid level: Complete obstruction
  - The absence of mass lesion
  - Dilated and collapsed loop junction
  - Thickening and oedema of the bowel wall suggest intestinal ischaemia. Presence of **intramural air** is a late sign (gangrene)
  - CT has a sensitivity of 90% and specificity of 88%
  - Thus, CT and MRI are very helpful in patients with small bowel obstruction.

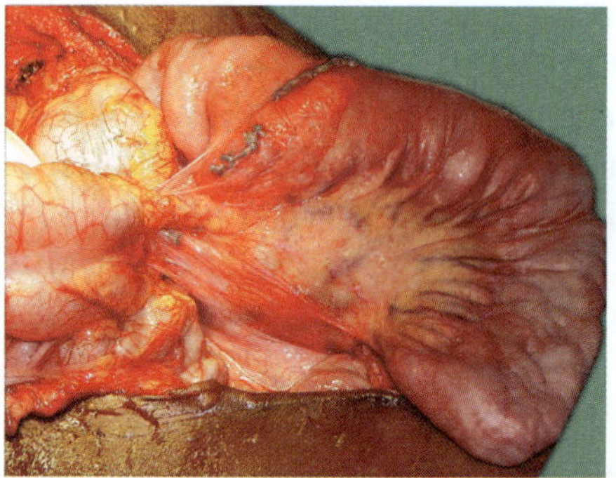

Fig. 48.40: Postappendicectomy band causing obstruction

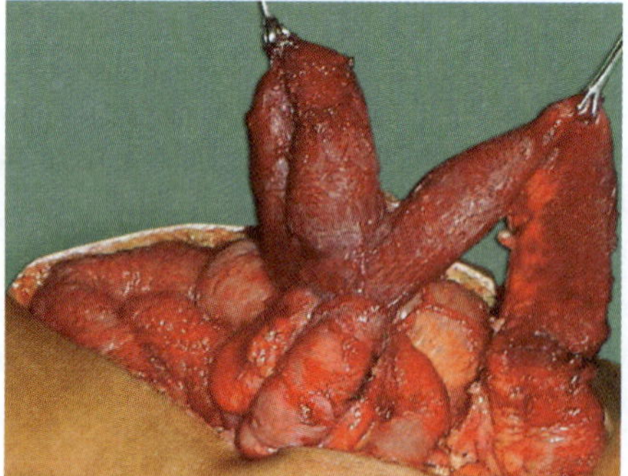

Fig. 48.41: Tuberculous adhesions and bands causing intestinal obstruction

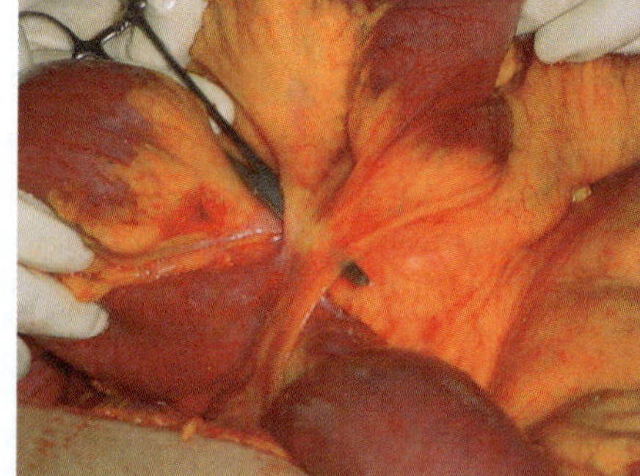

Fig. 48.42: Congenital band causing obstruction

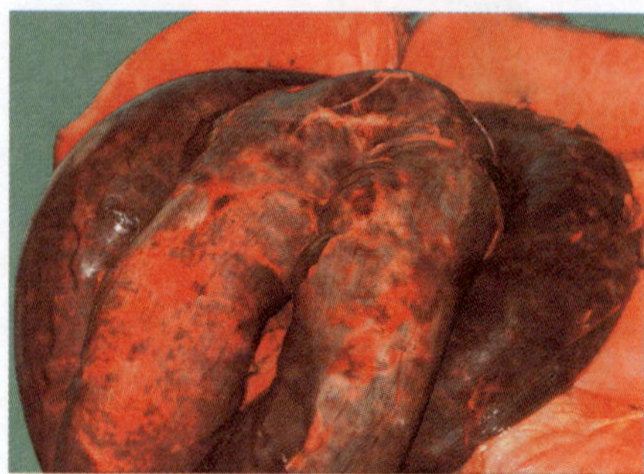

Fig. 48.43: Close up view of gangrene

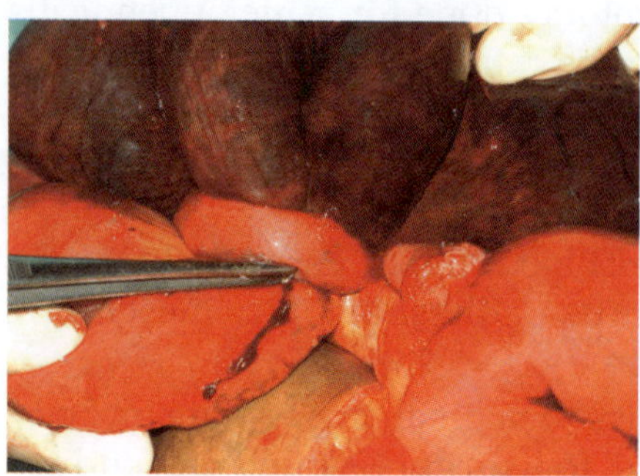

Fig. 48.44: Band secondary to peritonitis causing gangrene

Treatment

I. Conservative Treatment

- In the form of nasogastric aspiration, IV replacement of fluids and electrolytes to correct dehydration may be successful in early postoperative obstruction. If it is not successful, reoperation is required. Generally 48–72 hours is the waiting period in patients who present to the hospital as late adhesive obstruction.

  Further delay may result in perforation or gangrene of the bowel.
- Record pulse rate, blood pressure, abdominal girth and intake output. Increasing pulse rate, hypotension, increasing abdominal girth and oliguria in spite of adequate IV fluids will suggest gangrene. Such cases need to be explored immediately.

II. Surgical Methods (Key Box 48.21)

- Where fibrous bands are the cause, they need to be divided to relieve obstruction.
- Laparoscopic adhesiolysis is more often being used and it is indicated in pelvic adhesion, selected cases of abdominal adhesion, single band adhesion and obstruction with mild distension.

Key Box 48.21

How to Decrease Adhesions?

- Handle the bowel carefully. Good suturing without tension. Avoid anastomotic leak.
- Raw peritoneal areas should not be sutured
- Thorough peritoneal toilet in cases of peritonitis with saline or dextran to drain pus, bile, blood clots.
- Avoid spillage of contents—bile, faecal matter.
- Prefer a Pfannenstiel incision to midline incision.
- Noble's plication (Fig. 48.45)
- Laparoscopic method produces decreased adhesions than laparotomy.
- Membrane barriers

III. Prevention of Adhesion (Key Box 48.22)

A. Recently **absorbable and nonabsorbable membrane barriers** such as expanded polytetrafluoroethylene **(PTFE)** and membrane composed of hyaluronic acid and carboxy-methyl cellulose have been used.

B. **Noble's plication:** By suturing loops together so that they are fixed in a suitable relation to one another (not very successful) (Fig. 48.45).

Key Box 48.23 describes summary of adhesive obstruction.

Key Box 48.22

Membrane Barriers

- The bioresorbable membrane called seprafilm is currently the most effective membrane barrier.
- It consists of hyaluronic acid and carboxymethyl-cellulose.
- At the completion of surgery, these films are placed at the potential sites of adhesion formation—such as pelvis, between the intestinal loops.
- Mechanism of action: Within the next 24 to 48 hours, the seprafilm membrane hydrates to form a gel-like barrier. It slowly resorbs within 7 days.
- These barriers should not be used to cover the anastomosis—chances of leak rates are high.

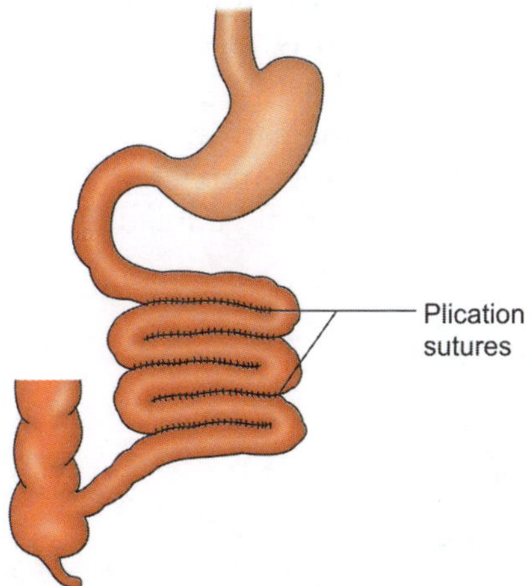

Fig. 48.45: Surgery for adhesions

Key Box 48.23

Adhesive Intestinal Obstruction

- It is the most common cause of intestinal obstruction (in the West).
- The most common cause of adhesion is inflammatory peritonitis.
- It is the cause of recurrent intestinal obstruction—often partial.
- Conservative treatment is successful in majority of cases.
- One can wait for 3–4 days with careful monitoring before a decision of laparotomy is undertaken (worsening situation).
- Repeated X-ray abdomen and CT scan will show changes and progression of the obstruction.
- Most valuable clinical signs of ischaemia/gangrene are tachycardia and tenderness.
- Adhesiolysis/resection is the treatment.

GALLSTONE ILEUS—GALLSTONE OBTURATION

Introduction: Gallstone ileus is more common in women and accounts for 1–4% of all presentations to hospital with small bowel obstruction. The term gallstone ileus is a misnomer, as the condition is a mechanical obstruction of the gut and not a true ileus.

- It should be suspected in a patient who has gallstones and present with intestinal obstruction.
- Elderly females above the age of 60 are usually affected.
- Gallstone reaches the terminal ileum by forming 'cholecystoduodenal fistula' due to recurrent attacks of cholecystitis (Figs 48.46 to 48.49).
- Due to recurrent inflammation, adhesions develop between gallbladder and duodenum (common) or gallbladder and colon or stomach (rare). Large stones cause pressure necrosis, resulting in formation of a cholecystoduodenal fistula.
- Terminal ileum is the narrowest portion of the gut wherein gallstone gets impacted. Sometimes, the stone may ulcerate from gallbladder into jejunum, colon, etc.

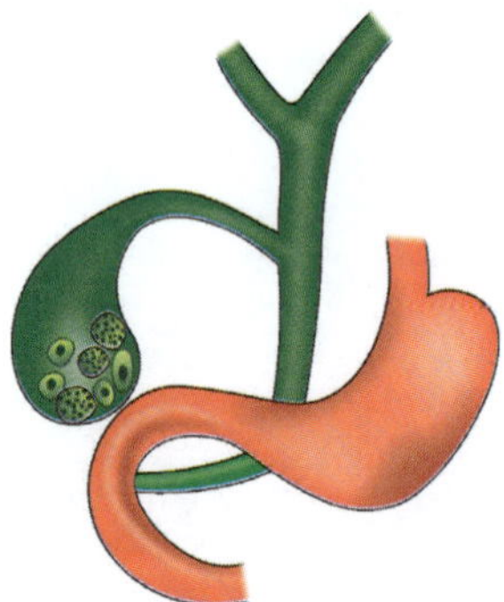

Fig. 48.46: Cholecystoduodenal fistula caused by gallstones

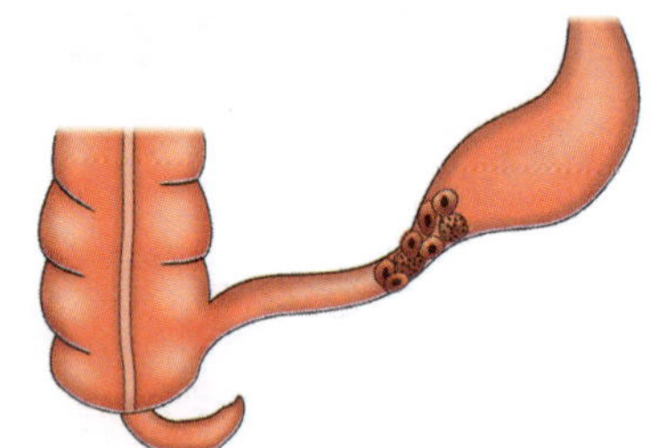

Fig. 48.47: Gallstones ileus (*Courtsey*: Both these figures are contributed by Ms Vidhushi, Kasturba Medical College, Manipal)

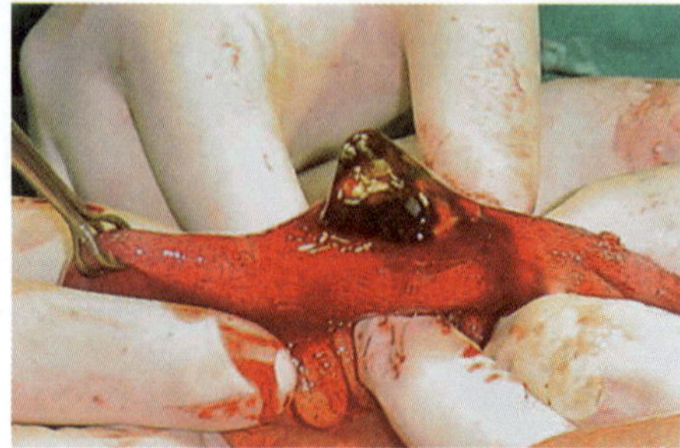

Fig. 48.48: Gallstone ileus (*Courtesy:* Prof MG Shenoy and Dr GN Prasad, KMC, Manipal)

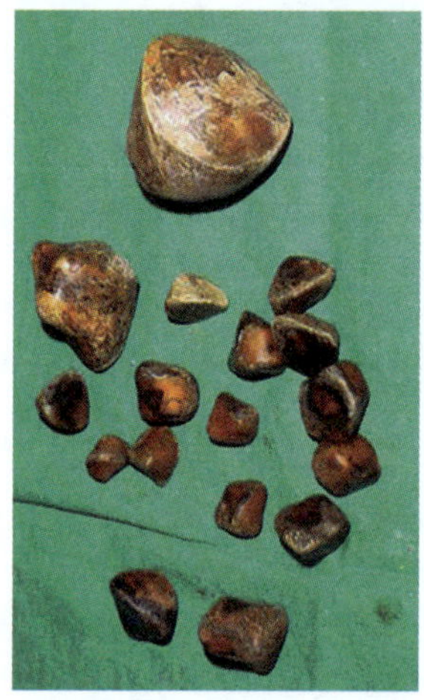

Fig. 48.49: 17 Gallstones were removed in this case

- ***Clinical features:*** They are suggestive of small intestinal obstruction—abdominal pain is severe, vomiting and distension. Step ladder peristalsis may be seen. History suggestive of recurrent cholecystitis may be present.

Rigler's triad: **Pneumobilia**, the **presence of an aberrant gallstone** and **enteric obstruction** (Fig. 48.50). *Bouveret syndrome: It is a gastric outlet syndrome secondary to stone lodged in proximal duodenum due to cholecystoduodenal fistula. Proximal migration of the stone will precipitate obstruction.

Investigations

1. **Plain X-ray abdomen** (erect position) may demonstrate multiple gas and fluid levels and stone in the gallbladder and also in the lower abdomen suggesting gallstone ileus.
   - **Air may be found**[1] in the biliary system.
2. **Small bowel enema** may demonstrate partial obstruction.

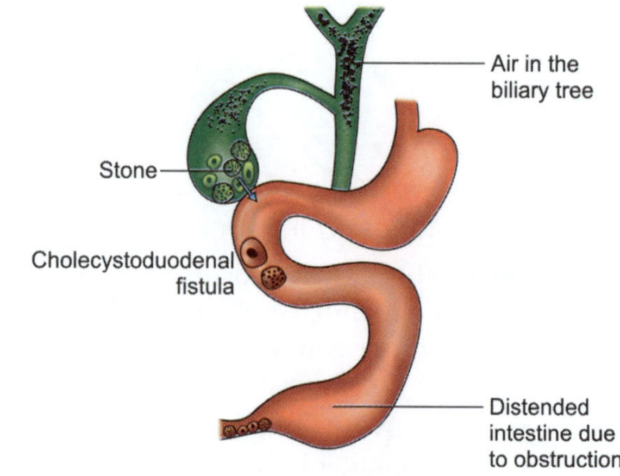

Fig. 48.50: Rigler's triad

*Cholecystoduodenal fistula, choledochoduodenostomy, sphincteroplasty, emphysematous cholecystitis are a few other conditions wherein air is found within biliary tree.

3. **Computed tomography (CT)** scanning is the investigation of choice. It has preoperative diagnosis of gallstone ileus with a sensitivity of 93%. It will also indicate any inflammation of the gallbladder, fistula—air pockets in the gallbladder, distal stone and proximal dilatation.

Treatment

There is difference of opinion regarding what is the ideal surgery to be done in case of gallstone obstruction. It is because many patients are elderly, with co-morbidity and they have intestinal obstruction (dehydration, bowel oedema, bacterial proliferation, etc). Whatever it is, the first step is always to do enterolithotomy by incising the ileum and deliver the stone/stones. It may be possible to crush the stone and pass it onto caecum, avoiding enterolithotomy. Search the proximal intestine for any other stones. What must be done next? Two types are described.

1. **Single stage procedure:** If general condition of the patient is good, and gallbladder is gangrenous or inflamed (more chances of perforation), enterolithotomy, cholecystectomy followed by closure of the duodenal fistula is done.
2. **Two-stage procedure:** If general condition is not good or with no active inflammation of the gallbladder, enterolithotomy is the procedure of choice, followed 6 weeks later by cholecystectomy with closure of the duodenal fistula (Fig. 48.51).

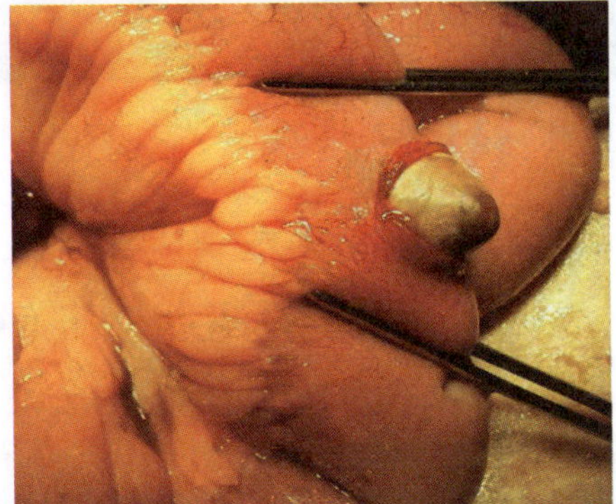

Fig. 48.51: Enterolithotomy and removal of stone

INTUSSUSCEPTION

DEFINITION

Invagination of one segment of intestine into another (usually the proximal into distal) is called intussusception.

Pearls of Wisdom

It is the most common cause of intestinal obstruction in infants aged 6 to 18 months.

Incidence: 2–4/1000 live births.

Types

1. **Simple ileocolic** is the most common type, followed by ileoileal or colocolic.
2. **Compound**—ileo-ileocolic
3. **Retrograde jejunogastric intussusception**, a complication of gastrojejunostomy (GJ) is a rare but interesting type of intussusception (*see* page 587).

Parts (Fig. 48.52)

1. **Intussuscipiens:** It is the outer tube (distal bowel which receives the intestine).
2. **Intussusceptum:** Proximal bowel (inner tube) which enters the distal segment.
3. **Apex** is the part which advances further into the distal bowel.
4. **Neck**, the narrowest portion of intussusception, is the junction of entering layer with the mass.
   - The whole mass that develops is called intussusception.

Aetiopathogenesis

1. **Idiopathic intussusception:** Actual cause is not known. It is seen in infants. Possible factors (Key Box 48.24).
   - **Dietary factor:** Around the age of 6–9 months, weaning of breast milk is done. Weaning causes alteration in the bacterial flora in the GIT, causing enlargement of the Peyer's patches. These protrude into the terminal ileum and may precipitate intussusception.

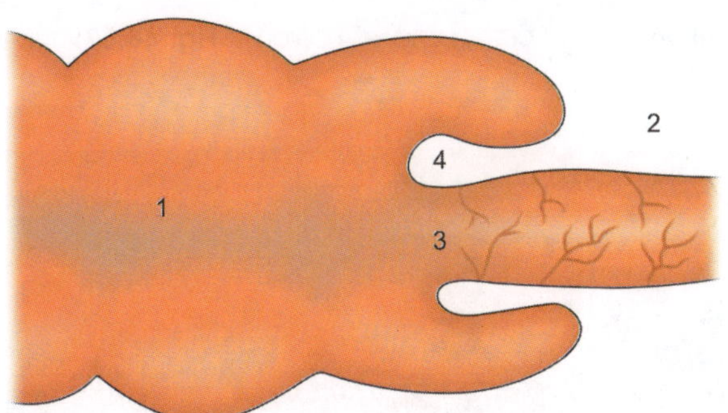

Fig. 48.52: Parts of intussusception (see the text for numbers)

Key Box 48.24

Predisposing Factors

- Recent viral infection (upper respiratory)
- Recent operation
- Henoch-Schönlein purpura
- Cystic fibrosis
- Coeliac disease
- Haemophilia

- **Infective factor:** It usually follows upper respiratory tract infection with virus (adeno rotaviruses) which produce inflammation of Peyer's patches.

2. **Adult intussusception (secondary):** In adults, there is always a cause for intussusception (Key Box 48.25 and Figs 48.53 to 48.60A, B).

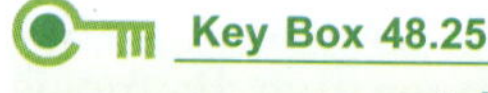

Adult Intussusception

- Meckel's diverticulum
- Polyps, tumours, submucous lipoma
- Carcinoma colon (caecum, transverse colon)

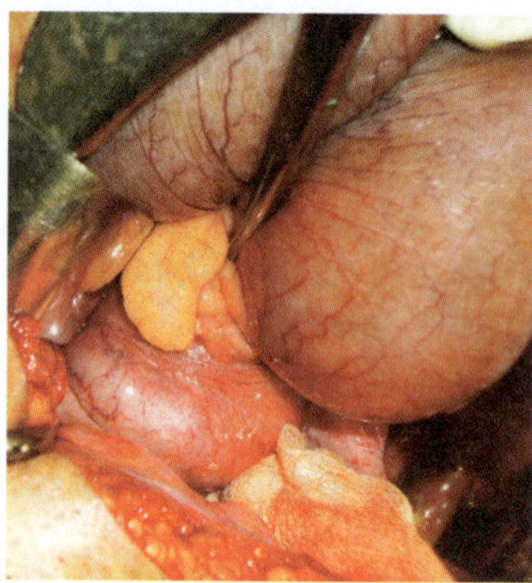

Fig. 48.53: Carcinoid of the ileum with intussusception

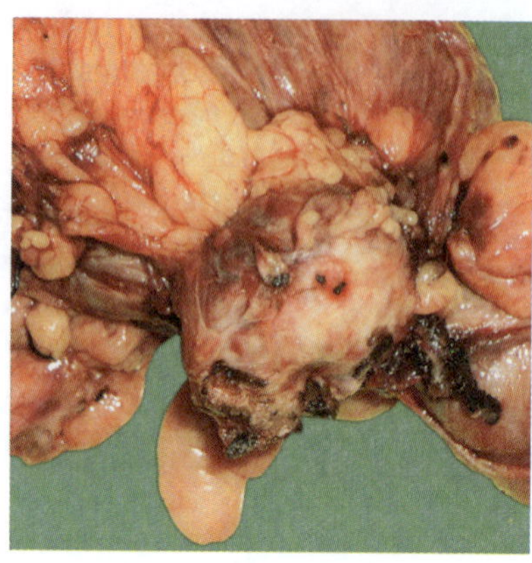

Fig. 48.54: Carcinoid of the ileum causing intussusception—resected specimen

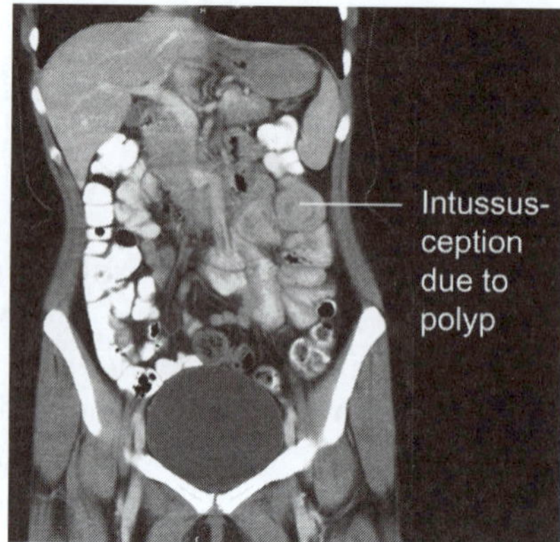

Fig. 48.55: Intussusception due to polyp

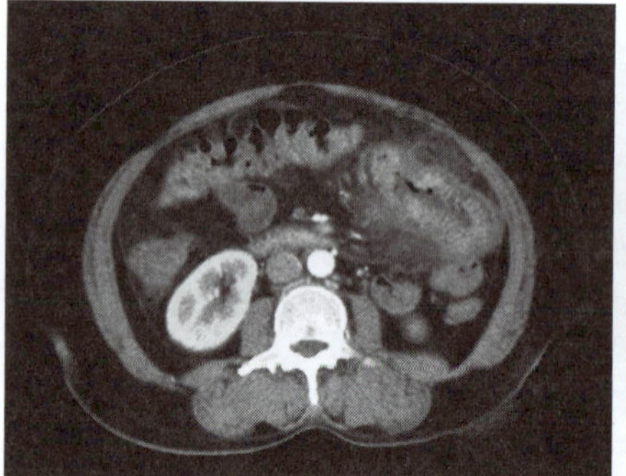

Fig. 48.56: Jejunal carcinoma—CT coronal section

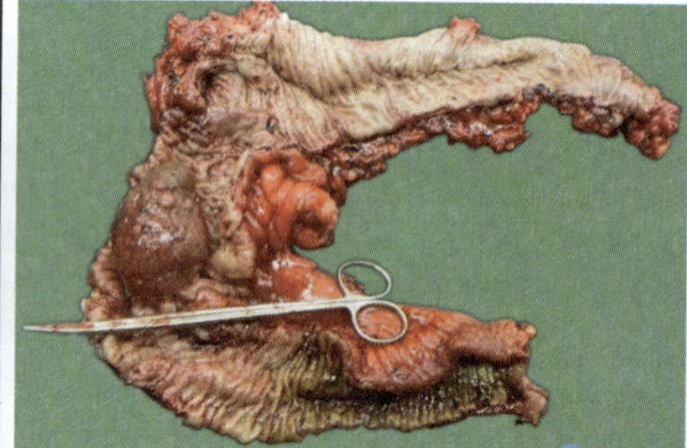

Fig. 48.57: Opened specimen showing polyp

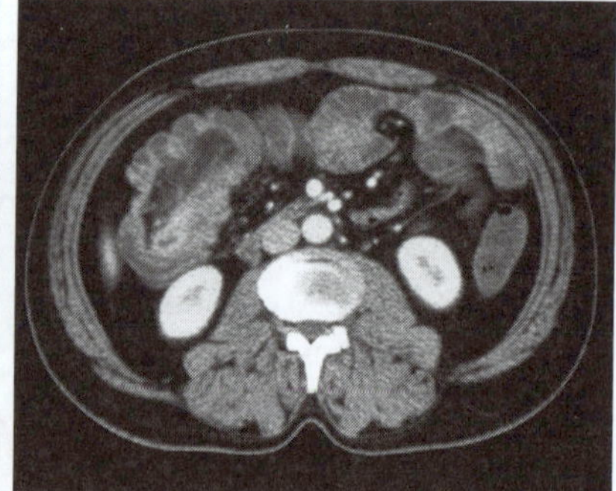

Fig. 48.58: Ileocolic intussusception CT

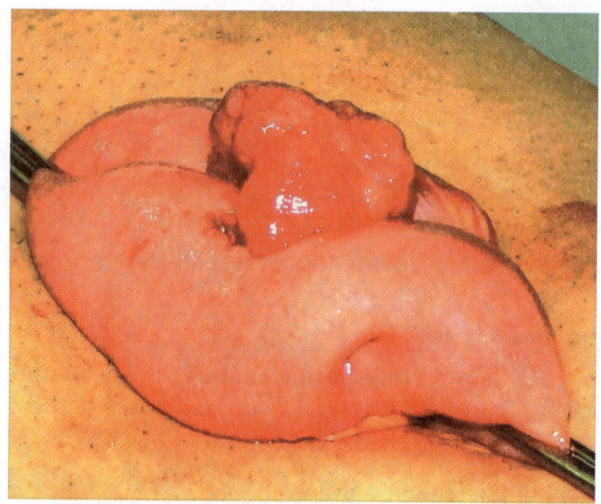

Fig. 48.59: Intussusception due to polyp. (*Courtesy:* Dr Kshama Hegde, Dr Sunilkrishna, Dept of Surgery, KMC Manipal)

[1]Hindi speaking mother says, *'Baccha sota hai aur rota hai'*

Pathophysiology

- As the apex advances, it drags the mesentery containing blood vessels which get obstructed at the neck resulting in mucosal ulcers and haemorrhages. Marked lymphadenopathy and hypertrophy of Peyer's patch is found at operation.
- If the neck is too tight, gangrene sets in very early, as in ileocolic intussusception.
- All other features of strangulation, dehydration, distension and septicaemic shock develop later.

Clinical Features

- First born male infants between 6 and 9 months are commonly affected. Boys : Girls—3 : 2.
- **Child screams** with abdominal pain[1] (intestinal colic) which is associated with facial pallor.

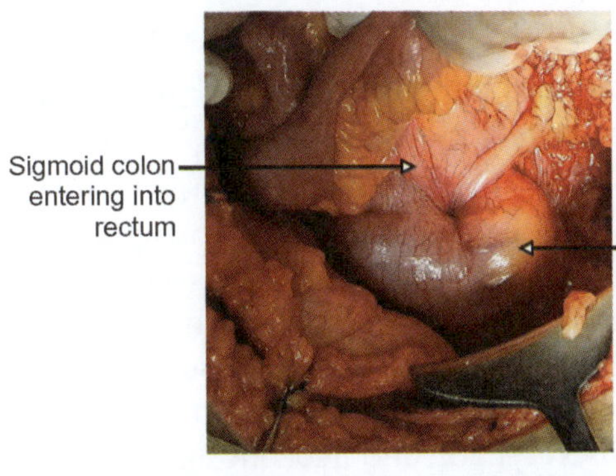

Fig. 48.60A: Sigmoido-rectal intussusception due to polypoidal lesion (opened specimen below—same patient)

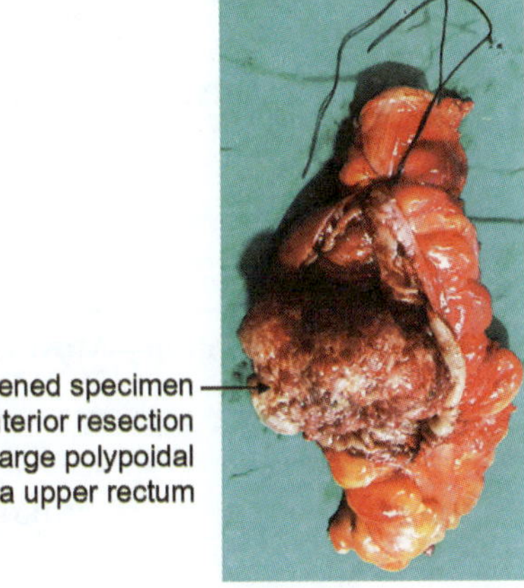

Fig. 48.60B: Low anterior resection (LAR) specimen

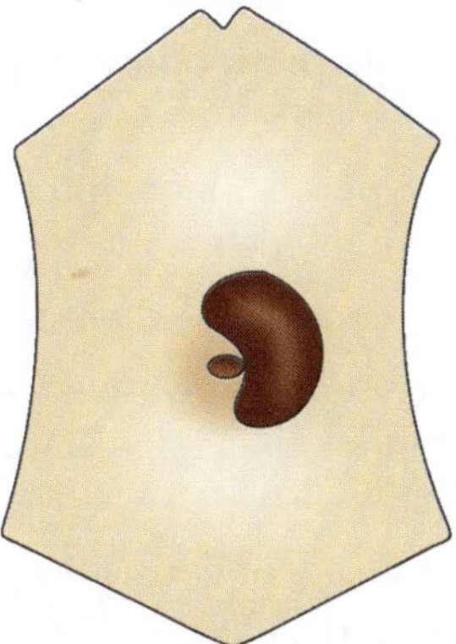

Fig. 48.60C: Sausage-shaped mass—resonant, mobile

- One attack of **red currant jelly stools** is characteristic. Bleeding is due to mucosal ulcer (venous infarction). Mucus secretion is due to irritation of intestines. This is followed by absolute constipation. **Red currant jelly stools are not found in adult intussusception.**
- Vomiting 3–4 times, initially due to pylorospasm. Later, due to obstruction.
- In between the spasms, the child sleeps but gets up suddenly with pain.

Signs

- The mother is asked to feed the baby in sitting position and examination of the baby's abdomen is done with the left hand, standing in front of the mother.
- A contracting, hardening mass in and around the umbilical region can be felt (**sausage-shaped,** Fig. 48.60C).
- **Emptiness in the right iliac fossa** (Dance's sign—*signe de dance*).
- There may be a **visible step ladder peristalsis**.
- Rarely, intussusception can be seen **outside the anus** due to long mesentery.
- Rectal examination reveals **blood-stained mucus** on the examining finger.
- Features of peritonitis occur in untreated cases.

Investigations

- **Ultrasound** (Figs 48.61 and 48.62) is the investigation of choice. It can detect target sign and detect mass **(Doughnut sign)**. With Doppler, it can be used to assess vascularity of the bowel also. Thus, barium enema has become obsolete.
- **CT scan:** It is the most sensitive imaging modality in the diagnosis of intussusception. Sausage-shaped mass, with blood vessels within bowel lumen are typical findings (*see* Fig. 48.58). Gangrene can be detected.
- **Barium enema:** 'Claw (pincer) ending' (Fig. 48.63) is diagnostic of intussusception. This is also called '**meniscus sign**'. If there is any suspicion of gangrene, this test should not be done. In many cases, the diagnosis is established on clinical grounds.

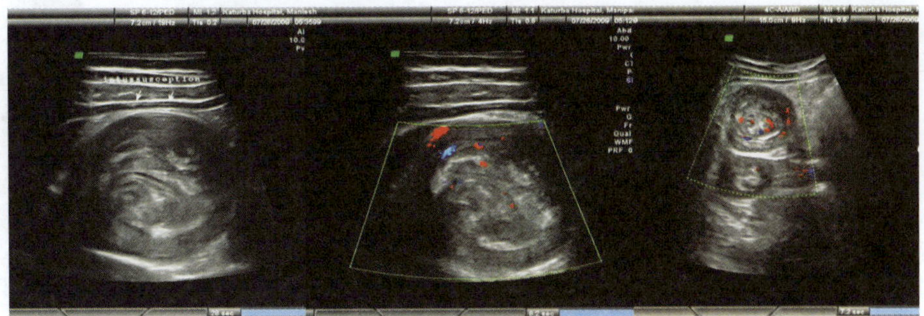

Figs 48.61 and 48.62: Ultrasound—pseudokidney sign, target sign, Duplex—assesses vascularity also

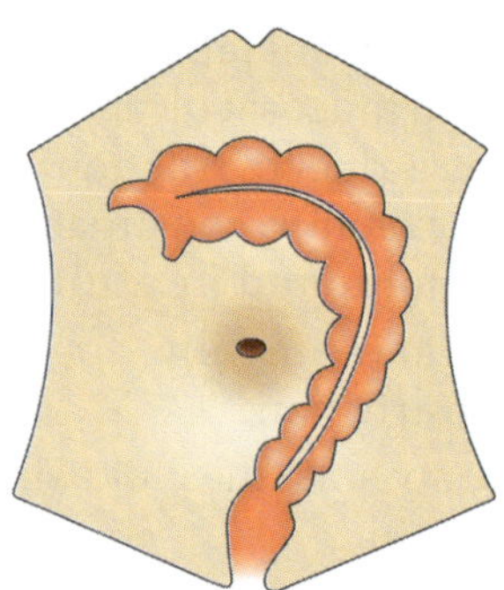

Fig. 48.63: Claw ending

Treatment

I. Conservative Treatment (Key Box 48.26)

- Hydrostatic reduction can be attempted when the gangrene is ruled out as in early intussusception. A lubricated catheter is introduced into the rectum and 1–2 litres of saline from a height of 1–2 metres is allowed to run. Catheter is removed and buttocks are pressed together. 50–70% of cases are reduced by this method, 1:3 barium sulphate in warm isotonic saline can also be used.
- Air contrast enema will not reduce gangrenous bowel. Air is pumped into the colon at a pressure of 60–80 mmHg.

  Contraindications
  - Peritonitis with shock
  - Total intestinal obstruction

Key Box 48.26

Hydrostatic Reduction is Successful when

1. Flatus and faeces are passed with barium
2. Child is symptom-free and comfortable
3. Small bowel loops are filled with contrast

Advantage

- Easy, nonoperative method

Complication

- Rarely, colonic perforation

II. Surgical Treatment (Figs 48.64 to 48.66)

Laparotomy and reduction of intussusception

- Intussusception is reduced by milking (squeezing) the colon in opposite direction, which is facilitated by breaking the adhesions at the neck using the little finger. Appendicectomy is also done, as it avoids any future confusion as to the reason for the abdominal scar. Fixing the caecum is not necessary because idiopathic intussusception rarely recurs. If the loop is gangrenous, resection and ileocolic anastomosis is done.
- **Recurrent intussusception is rare:** If it occurs, terminal ileum is sutured to the side of the ascending colon.

Key Box 48.27 for some interesting "more common" about intussusception.

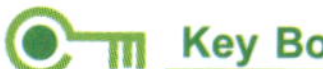

Key Box 48.27

Acute Intussusception—Most Common

- Most common in children between 5 and 10 months of age
- Most common cause of intestinal obstruction in children
- Most common cause is idiopathic (90%)
- Most common variety is ileocolic variety
- Most commonly hypertrophied Peyer's patches are reported
- Most common type of nonoperative reduction is by using air and barium enema
- Most commonly done surgical procedure is reduction
- Most commonly used noninvasive test for diagnosis is ultrasound—pseudokidney sign, target sign, Duplex-assesses vascularity also
- Most incidence of adenovirus infection, common in midsummer and midwinter

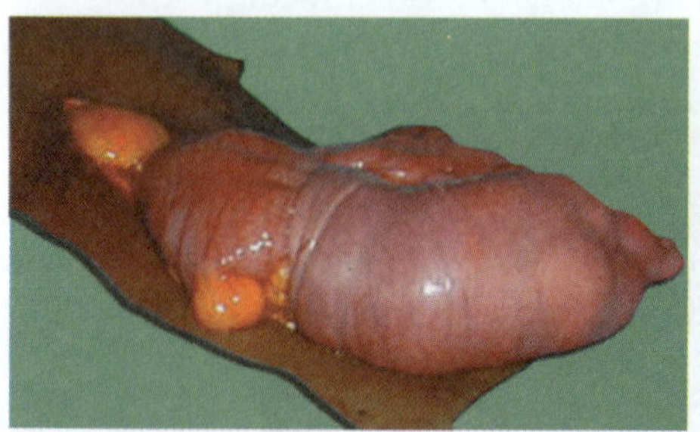

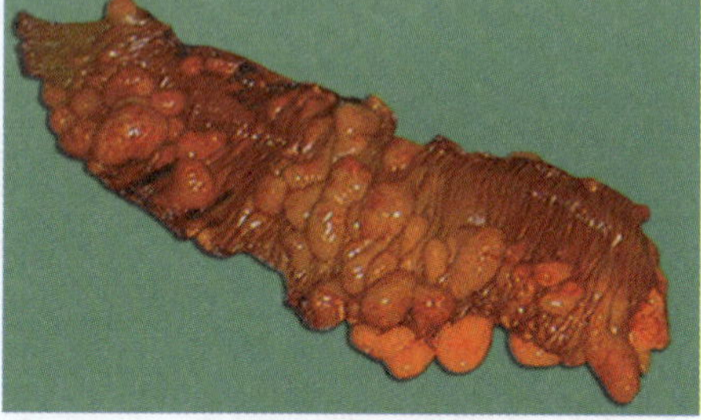

Figs 48.64 and 48.65: Adult intussusception due to jejunal lipomatosis. This patient was 24-year-old male who presented with intestinal obstruction. A mass was palpable in the umbilical region at laparotomy. This mass was resected. Opened specimen showed extensive segmental lipomatosis (*Courtesy:* Dr Gabriel Rodrigues, Dr Mahesh Gopa Setty, Dr Lavanya K, KMC, Manipal)

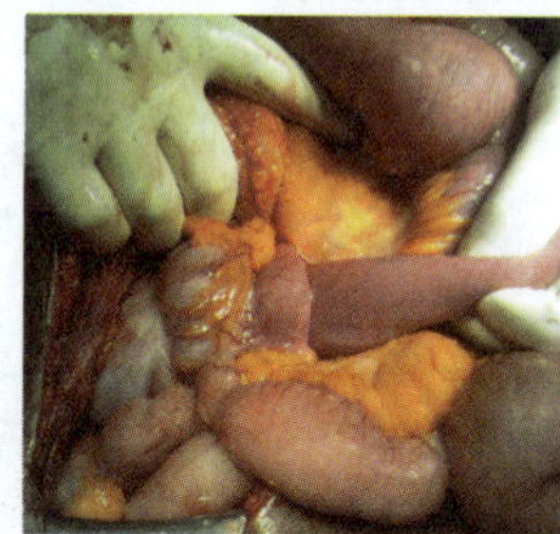

Fig. 48.66: Intussusception is reduced at surgery

MESENTERIC VASCULAR OCCLUSION

DEFINITION

Acute mesenteric ischaemia is an abrupt reduction in blood flow to the intestinal circulation of sufficient magnitude to compromise the metabolic requirements and potentially threaten the viability of the affected organs (Key Box 48.28).

Key Box 48.28

Types

1. Acute mesenteric ischaemia (AMI): It is a sudden occlusion of artery or vein resulting in gangrene. It has a mortality rate of 60 to 90%.
2. Chronic mesenteric ischaemia (CMI): It is associated with stenosis of coeliac artery, superior mesenteric artery or inferior mesenteric artery.

Competency

SU28.13.2: Understand and differentiate different parts of small and large intestines depending on length, size, vascular anatomy, mesentery and their attachment.

Anatomy of Mesenteric Vasculature

The mesenteric arterial and venous circulation of the abdominal viscera form an extensive vascular network. There are a large number of collateral pathways that protect against ischaemic changes. The three major branches of aorta responsible for the arterial supply of the intestine are: Coeliac artery supplies **foregut**, superior mesenteric artery (SMA) supplies **midgut** and inferior mesenteric artery supplies **hindgut**. The venous drainage includes the superior and inferior mesenteric vein.

Normal Anatomy and Variations

- **Coeliac axis:** Normal coeliac axis anatomy is seen in only 55% of patients. An anomalous right or left hepatic artery has been reported in about 50% of patients.
- **Superior mesenteric artery:** It supplies the entire small intestines and right one-third of transverse colon (Fig. 48.67).
- **Inferior mesenteric artery (IMA):** It supplies left colon including rectum and surgical anal canal. The IMA arises at the level of the third lumbar vertebra supplies the large bowel from mid-transverse colon to upper rectum. Several collateral networks exist in the branches of IMA. These collaterals are important when rectosigmoid or splenic flexure resection is performed (Fig. 48.68).
- **Collaterals:** Like collaterals in the leg, many collaterals exist between 3 major branches—coeliac artery, SMA and IMA. Because of this extensive collaterals,

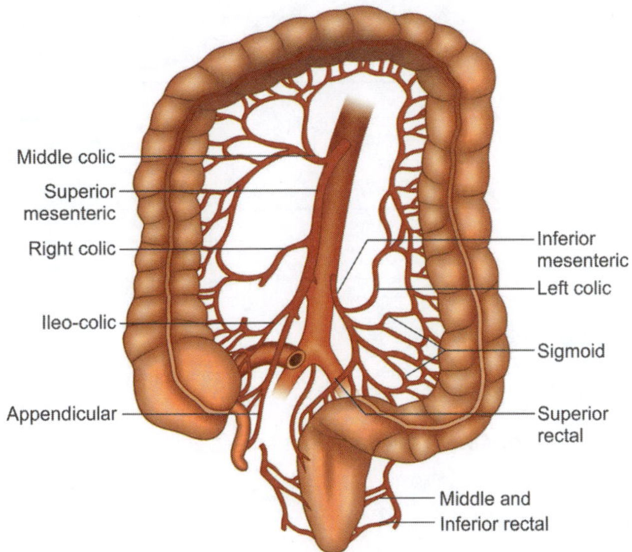

Fig. 48.67: Superior mesenteric artery and its branches

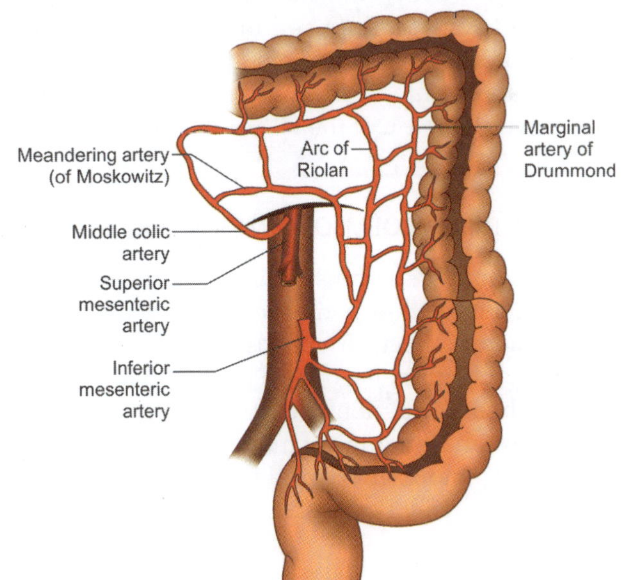

Fig. 48.68: Inferior mesenteric artery and its branches

patients remain asymptomatic with normal bowel function may have chronic occlusion of one or two mesenteric vessels.

Griffiths' point: Between branches of left colic and SMA.
Sudeck point: Sigmoidal arteries and superior rectal vessels.

Types (Fig. 48.69)

1. **Acute mesenteric ischaemia (AMI):** It is a sudden occlusion of artery or vein resulting in gangrene. It has a mortality rate of 60 to 90%.
2. **Chronic mesenteric ischaemia (CMI):** It is associated with stenosis of coeliac artery, superior mesenteric artery or inferior mesenteric artery.
3. **NOMI:** Non-occlusive mesenteric ischaemia.

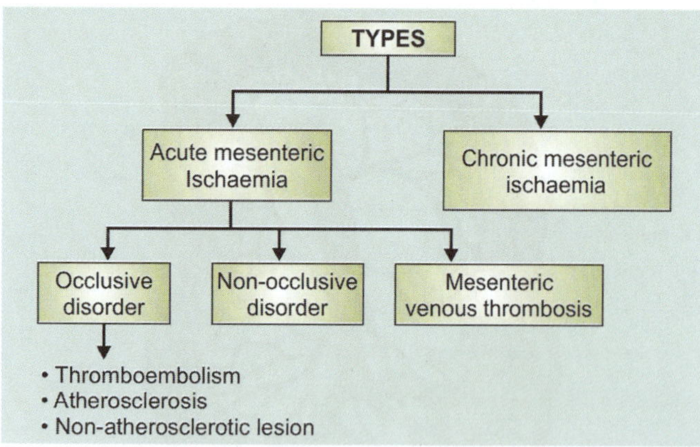

Fig. 48.69: Types of mesenteric ischaemia

Pathogenesis

Ischaemic damage to the intestine occurs with decreased blood supply to a level at which delivery of oxygen and various nutrients cannot maintain oxidative metabolism. Cell integrity is lost resulting in cell death. In low-flow states, blood is shunted from arterioles to venules near the base of the villus resulting in necrosis of the intestinal villi.

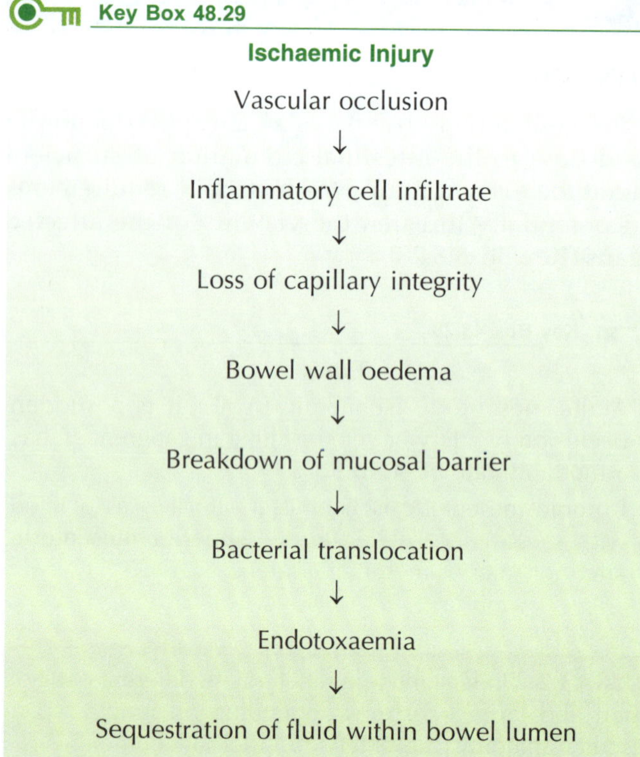

Key Box 48.29

Ischaemic Injury

Vascular occlusion
↓
Inflammatory cell infiltrate
↓
Loss of capillary integrity
↓
Bowel wall oedema
↓
Breakdown of mucosal barrier
↓
Bacterial translocation
↓
Endotoxaemia
↓
Sequestration of fluid within bowel lumen

ACUTE SMA THROMBOEMBOLIC MESENTERIC ISCHAEMIA

SMA takes off at less obtuse angle than the celiac axis. Hence thromboembolism most commonly involves the SMA. Ischaemia affects the mucosa first—most sensitive to hypoxia. Subepithelial oedema occurs within 30 min, loss of epithelial cells along the villus in 1 hour and total loss of villi with sloughing of mucosa in 2 hours. Within 4 hours gangrenous changes start. Thus the condition is rapidly fatal (Key Box 48.29).

Etiopathogenesis

- It is common in elderly patients who are hypertensive and usually obese.
- It is due to atherosclerosis causing thrombosis of the superior mesenteric artery or due to emboli which originate from atheromatous plaques or from the infarcted heart.
- Smokers are more often affected by this condition.
- **Superior mesenteric vein** can also get thrombosed due to injury during pancreatectomy or thrombosis as a result of oral contraceptive pills.

Effects

The pathological effects of arterial occlusion and venous occlusion are the same. Superior mesenteric artery supplies the entire midgut starting from the duodenojejunal flexure to right one-third of the transverse colon. It is an end-artery. As a result of thrombosis, the entire small bowel and portion of the large bowel becomes gangrenous (if there is a thrombus at the origin of superior mesenteric artery).

Splanchnic Circulation

- It is better to have some idea about the splanchnic circulation to understand the effects of ischaemia to the gut.
- The splanchnic circulation receives approximately 25% of the resting and 35% of the postprandial cardiac output.
- 70% of the mesenteric blood flow is directed to the mucosal and submucosal layers of the bowel. Hence early cases present with bleeding due to mucosal ulcerations.
- 30% supplies the muscularis and serosal layers.
- Blood flow is regulated by intrinsic (metabolic and myogenic) and the extrinsic (neural and humoral) factors.
- Reactive hyperaemia and hypoxic vasodilation are considered intrinsic controls and are responsible for instantaneous fluctuations in splanchnic blood flow.
- An imbalance between tissue oxygen supply and demand will raise the concentration of local metabolites (e.g. hydrogen, potassium, carbon dioxide, and adenosine), resulting in vasodilation and hyperaemia.

Causes of Acute Mesenteric Ischaemia

1. **Arterial emboli** are the most frequent cause of AMI and are responsible for approximately 40 to 50% of cases. Most mesenteric emboli originate from a cardiac source. They lodge in the superior mesenteric artery (SMA) because it emerges from the aorta at an oblique angle. A few emboli lodge in the origin of middle colic artery.

Embolic: Majority of emboli originate in the heart
- Valvular heart disease
- Dilated left atrium
- Recent myocardial infarction
- Atrial arrhythmias
- Ventricular dilatation with mural thrombus
- Atheroemboli
- Aneurysm

2. **Acute mesenteric thrombosis** accounts for 25 to 30% of all ischaemic cases. Atherosclerotic disease is the cause of thrombosis. It typically occurs at the origin of the superior mesenteric artery. Gangrene is more extensive in cases of thrombosis than embolism.
3. **Nonocclusive mesenteric ischaemia (NOMI):** Typically happens in cases of hypotensive patients. Low cardiac output, ICU patients on vasoconstrictors and inotropes precipitate the problem. Splanchnic vasoconstriction occurs in response to hypovolemia. Vasoactive drugs, particularly digoxin, have been implicated in the pathogenesis of NOMI.
4. **Mesenteric venous thrombosis (MVT)** is the least common cause of mesenteric ischaemia, representing up to 10% of all patients with mesenteric ischaemia related to primary clotting disorders. Thrombi usually originate in the venous arcades and propagate (Key Box 48.30).

Key Box 48.30

Aetiology of Mesenteric Venous Thrombosis

- Hypercoagulable states (e.g. polycythaemia vera, protein C and S deficiencies)
- Visceral infection
- Portal hypertension
- Blunt abdominal trauma
- Pancreatic malignancy
- Pancreatitis
- Women taking oral contraceptives
- Post-splenectomy
- Smokers

Clinical Features

Symptoms

1. **Abdominal pain:** Severe, poorly localised, unresponsive to narcotics, out of proportion to the physical findings (Fig. 48.70).
2. Onset may be abrupt (embolism) or insidious (thrombosis).
3. **Gastrointestinal emptying:** Vomiting, diarrhoea, with occult or frank bleeding once infarction sets in.

Condition presents as severe abdominal pain which is sudden onset, constant and more in the periumbilical region. It is often preceded by palpitations, arrhythmia, catheterization or myocardial infarction. There is urge to defecate. Loose stools develop within 2–3 hours of onset of symptoms. Attack of melaena indicates gangrene. Patients often present in an agitated or anxious state.

Signs

- Abdomen is flat or scaphoid with a little to no pain on palpation. Abdomen is often soft and "Pain out of proportion to the signs" is often typical of AMI. Peripheral pulses may be feeble as it is common to have multiple emboli.
- Peritoneal signs with guarding and rigidity is a late sign and implies bowel gangrene and perforation.
- Very soon septic shock develops with dehydration, cold clammy extremities, hypotension, desaturation, acidosis, oliguria.

Pearls of Wisdom

Sudden event, sudden bleeding, sudden collapse, severe pain, silent abdomen, shock progressing to sepsis is mesenteric ischaemia.

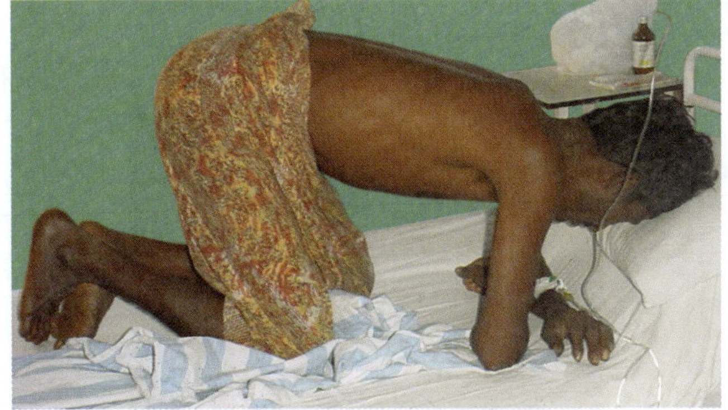

Fig. 48.70: Attitude of a patient with severe ischaemia due to superior mesenteric vascular occlusion. In these cases, the pain is disproportionate to the abdominal signs

Investigations

1. **Total counts** are raised, in about 75% of cases >15,000 cells/mm^3.
2. **Plain X-ray abdomen** (erect) reveals absence of gas within the bowel loops and intramural gas. Blunt plicae are seen. This is called **thumb printing** (Figs 48.71 and 48.72).
3. **Metabolic acidosis** in > 50% of cases.
4. **Serum phosphate** levels are raised within 3–4 hours following ischaemia as smooth muscle layer of small bowel is rich in phosphates.
5. **D-dimer** is elevated in all cases.
6. **CT angiogram** is the investigation of choice. It can detect **intramural air pockets** in the bowel wall, air within biliary radicle, perforation, etc. It can also detect thrombus or narrowing of superior mesenteric artery or superior mesenteric vein (Figs 48.73 and 48.74).
7. **Emergency angiography** is the test of choice and can be done within 6 hours of ischaemia. (It can also be therapeutic.)
8. **Hypercoagulability disorders**—protein C and protein S antithrombin III, factor V, anticardiolipin antibody (MVT).

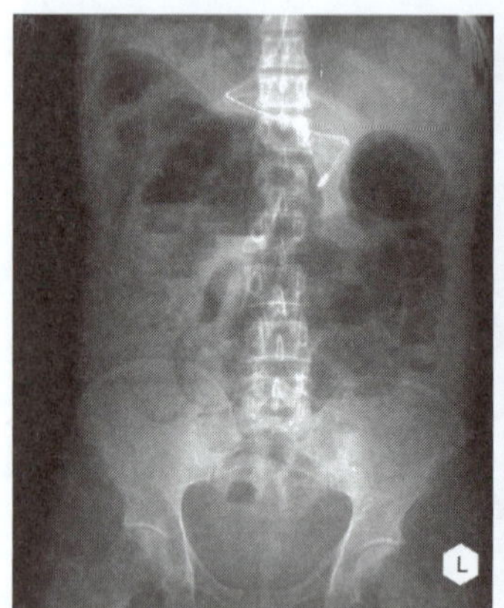
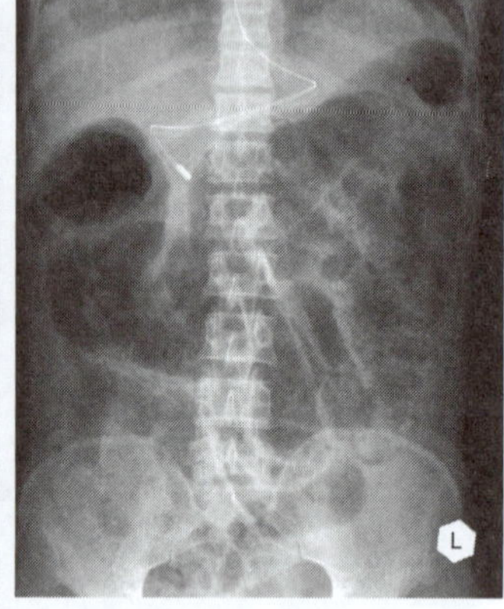

Figs 48.71 and 48.72: Plain X-ray showing presence of air in the bowel wall

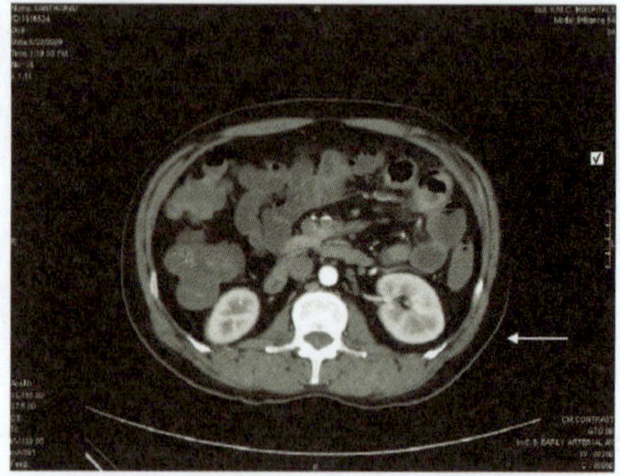

Fig. 48.73: CT showing SMA thrombosis

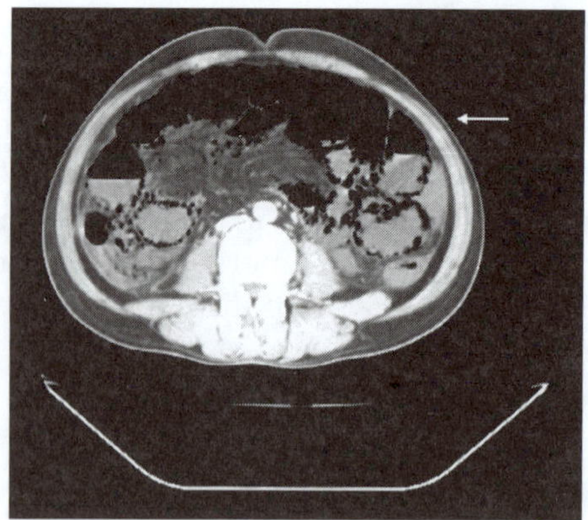

Fig. 48.74: CT confirming the same. A case of superior mesenteric arterial thrombosis with massive gangrene (see Fig. 48.75) with pneumotosis intestinalis

Treatment

- Patient is admitted in intensive care unit.
- Resuscitation is done. Nasogastric tube is inserted. Antibiotics started, heparinisation heparin given.
- Once CT confirms the diagnosis, exploratory laparotomy is done.
  1. Majority of the patients present late with massive gangrene. Massive resection of the gangrenous bowel followed by end to end anastomosis is done. These patients suffer from short bowel syndrome (*vide infra*), if they survive.
  2. If patients come within 4–6 hours of ischaemia, emergency angiography followed by papaverine infusion (30 to 60 mg/h) into the superior mesenteric artery can be tried. Otherwise, emergency laparotomy is done and the superior mesenteric artery is explored. A Fogarty catheter is introduced and embolectomy is done. These patients may require a **second look operation within 24–48 hours** to rule out gangrene developing later due to rethrombosis of the artery (Fig. 48.75). Before resection check for bowel viability.

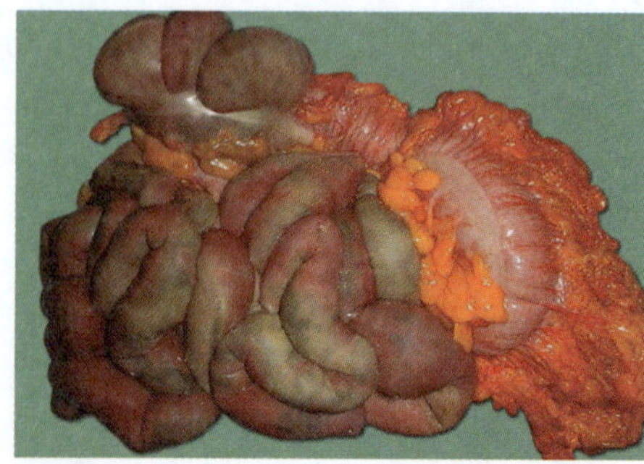

Fig. 48.75: Massive gangrene of small intestines and right side of the colon due to thrombosis at the origin of superior mesenteric artery

Assessing bowel viability
- Doppler (84%)
- Absent arterial flow on antimesenteric border of bowel.
- Absent mesenteric arterial flow
- Fluorescein test (100%)
  - Sodium fluorescein 1 g administered IV over 30 to 60 seconds and the bowel examined using a hand-held long wave UV Wood's lamp (yellow).

3. Other vasodilator agents used are: Tolazoline, glucagon, nitroglycerine, nitroprusside, prostaglandin E, phenoxybenzamine, isoproterenol.
4. Sympathetic epidural block

Recent advances in cases of mesenteric ischaemia
- Catheter directed thrombolysis
- Percutaneous transluminal angioplasty
- Endovascular fenestration of aortic dissection:
  - Techniques to assess bowel viability
  - Pulse oximetry
  - Infrared photoplethysmography
  - Bowel surface oximetry
  - Quantitative fluorescence using perfusion fluorometer.

Prognosis

Majority of the cases present with massive gangrene. Even after massive resection, they succumb to the sepsis and multiorgan failure (Fig. 48.75).

NON-OCCLUSIVE MESENTERIC ISCHAEMIA (NOMI)

It is a discrete clinical entity where mesenteric flow is impeded due to arterial spasm.
- Causes of NOMI are given below in Key Box 48.31.
- Typically these patients are critically ill in intensive care units (ICU), intubated. The pathology resides in the mesenteric arcades where severe spasm has limited flow. Like AMI, they can have loose and bloody stools, abdominal pain out of proportion to signs. Tenderness is present.

  Diagnostic arteriography is the only way to demonstrate the small vessel mesenteric arterial spasm that leads to NOMI.
- **Treatment:** Direct catheter delivery of papaverine (30–60 mg/hour) may have to be given for a few days. Systemic anticoagulants are given. Vessel spasm can be overcome by maximizing cardiac output. Peritonitis or clinical evidence of bowel perforation mandates exploration and resection of ischaemic segment. Also, primary cause of acute illness is treated.

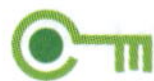 **Key Box 48.31**

Etiology

- **Pharmacotherapy**
  - Digoxin
  - Digitalis
  - Cocaine
  - Alpha agonists
  - Vasopressin
- **Sympathetically mediated stress response**
  - Hypovolaemia or haemorrhagic shock
  - Haemodialysis
  - Cardiopulmonary bypass
  - CCF
  - Arrhythmias
  - Pancreatitis
  - Septic shock
  - End stage renal disease

CHRONIC MESENTERIC ISCHAEMIA (CMI)

It is a form of severe atherosclerotic disease affecting multiple mesenteric arteries. Most of patients are asymptomatic due to rich collateral network. Most common cause—atherosclerosis. Other causes are vasculitides—Takayasu disease, coarctation of aorta. Women are more commonly affected than men. When patient is not eating, the circulatory demands of the resting bowel are easily met and there is no pain.
- After eating, in times of high demand, pain occurs. Hence called **postprandial pain**. Pain typically begins 15 to 45 minutes after eating and is described as crampy, affecting the upper and periumbilical abdomen. It is due to a phenomenon called **"Gastric steal"** phenomenon. Metabolically active stomach "steals" from the splanchnic circulation. Fixed proximal arterial obstruction does not allow for blood volume to compensate. Small bowel ischaemia and pain follow.
- Patients develop an aversion to eating or "food fear" as the disease progresses.
- Over a period of time, significant weight loss occurs.
- **Triad of CMI: Postprandial pain, food fear and weight loss.**
- CT angiography is the investigation of choice.
- Endovascular therapy and stenting and bypass grafts can be used. Endarterectomy can also be done if significant thrombus is present in the SMA.

STRICTURES

- Common causes are tubercular stricture of the ileum or jejunum in India and Crohn's disease in the Western world.
- Radiation stricture, ischaemic strictures and nonspecific strictures are the other causes.

- Malignant strictures. Carcinoma rectosigmoid junction tumours
- Small bowel enema or enteroscopy are very useful investigations (Figs 48.76 to 48.84).

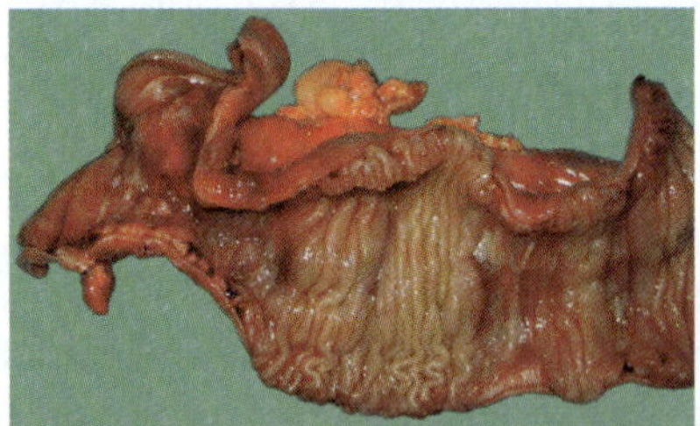

Fig. 48.76: Tubercular stricture—annular stricture

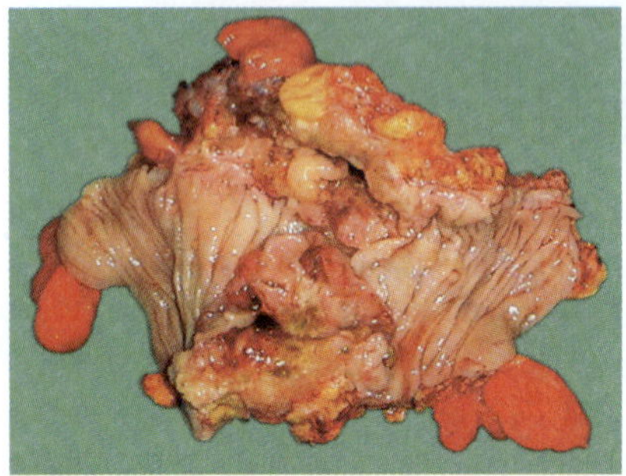

Fig. 48.77: Sigmoid stricture due to carcinoma

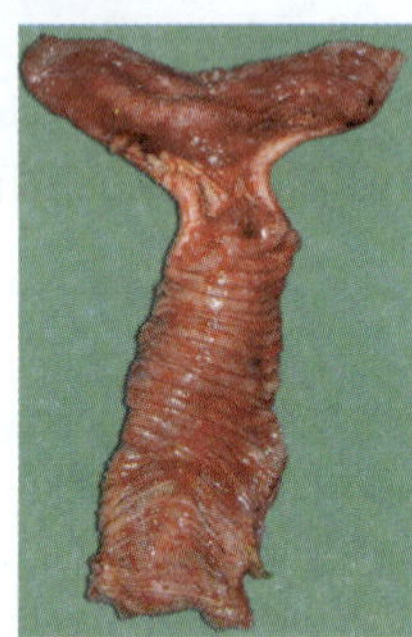

Fig. 48.78: Non-specific stricture

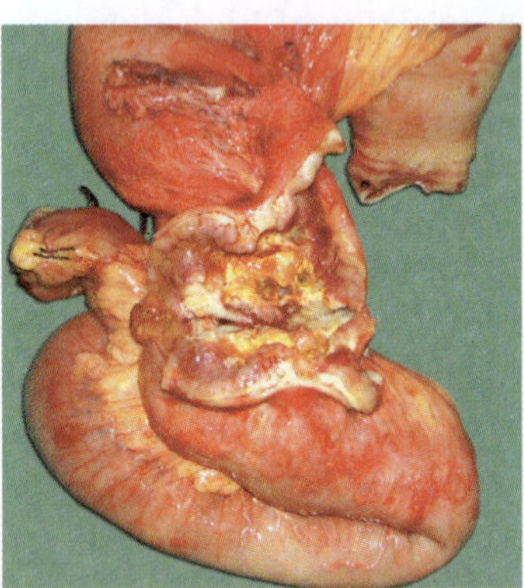

Fig. 48.79: Peritoneal metastasis causing narrowing of lumen resulting in obstruction.

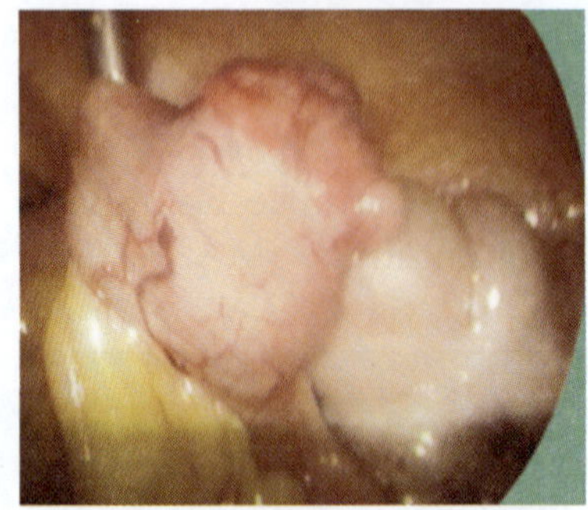

Fig. 48.80: Laparoscopy detected a lesion in the small intestine. On opening the abdomen turned out to be a jejunal GIST with obstruction

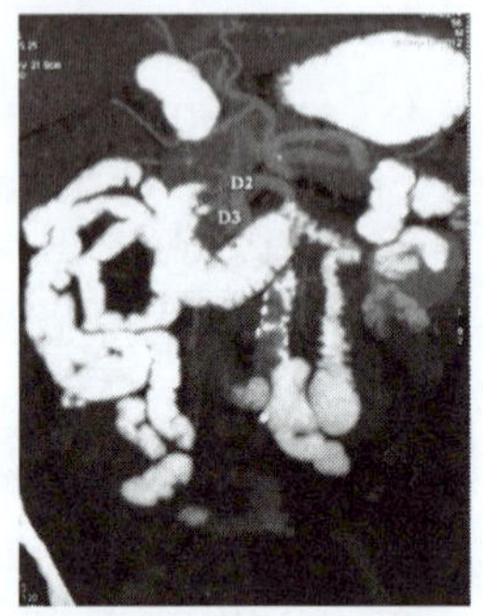

Fig. 48.81: Enteroclysis showing jejunal narrowing and aortic calcification

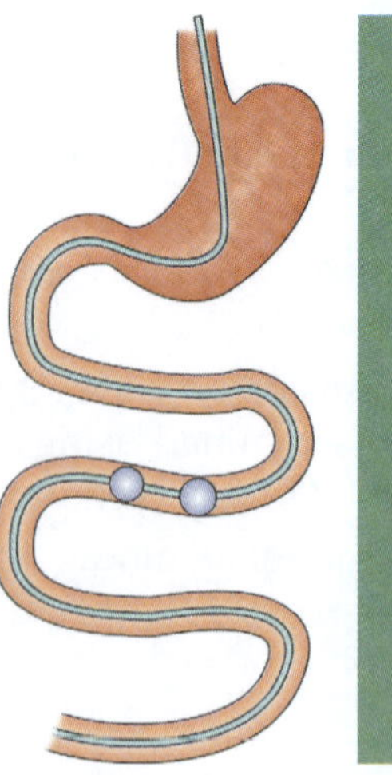

Fig. 48.82: Double enteroscopy representation

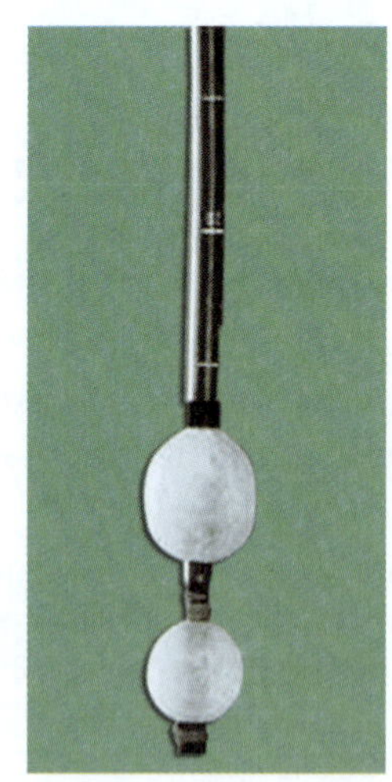

Fig. 48.83: Double balloon enteroscopy

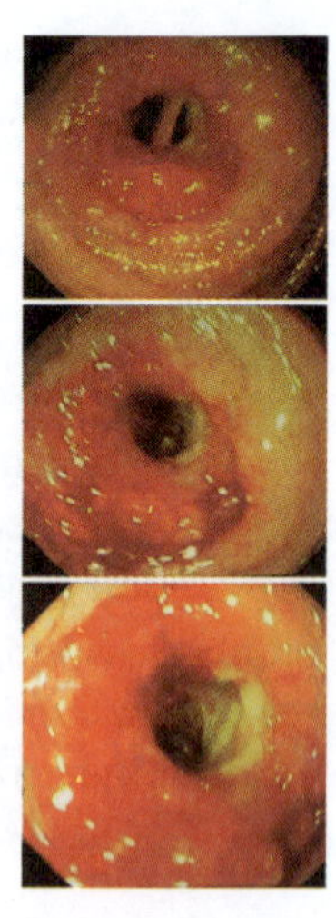

Fig. 48.84: Balloon enteroscopy showing jejunal ulcers

NEONATAL INTESTINAL OBSTRUCTION

Competency

SU28.14.3: Describe the clinical features, investigations and principles of management of neonatal obstruction.

Causes

1. **Hirschsprung's disease**—congenital megacolon
2. Atresia and stenosis
3. Arrested rotation with bands
4. Volvulus neonatorum
5. Meconium ileus
6. Imperforate anus

HIRSCHSPRUNG'S DISEASE: CONGENITAL MEGACOLON

Hirschsprung's disease is also called congenital megacolon, aganglionic megacolon or primary megacolon. It is one of the common causes of neonatal intestinal obstruction.

Pathophysiology (Fig. 48.85)

- The disease always involves the anus and rectum wherein parasympathetic ganglion cells are absent in the neural plexus of the intestinal wall. The defect involves internal sphincter.
- As a result of this, there is a terminally constricted, non-relaxing segment, in the rectum and sigmoid (lower part), above which the pelvic colon (sigmoid) is enormously dilated. Rectosigmoid area is involved in 80% of cases.
- Circular muscle hypertrophy, mucosal hyperaemia and ulcers are present in the dilated segments.

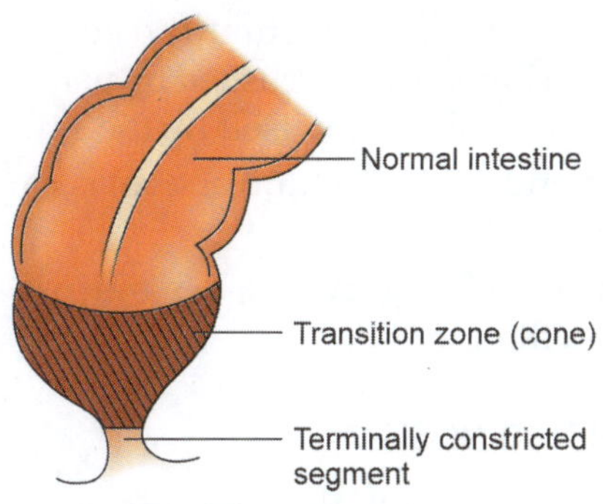

Fig. 48.85: Pathophysiology

- In between, there may be a transition zone (cone), which contains a few parasympathetic ganglion cells.
- Rarely, Hirschsprung's can also involve the entire sigmoid colon or even the entire colon.
- Hirschsprung's rarely occurs in adults also.

Types of Hirschsprung's Disease (Fig. 48.86)

1. **Ultrashort segment:** Anal canal and terminal rectum are aganglionic.
2. **Short segment:** Anal canal and entire rectum is completely involved.
3. **Long segment:** Anal canal, rectum and part of colon involved.
4. **Total colonic:** Anal canal, rectum and whole length of colon is involved.

Clinical Features

- Male children are commonly affected, when compared to females.
- **Incidence:** 1 in 4000 to 5000 live births.

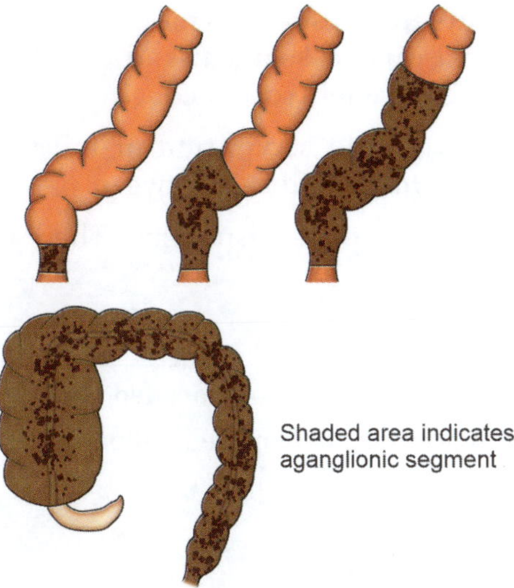

Fig. 48.86: Types of Hirschsprung's disease

Pearls of Wisdom

The most common associated anomaly with Hirschsprung's disease is Down's syndrome (5 to 10%).

- The child presents with acute neonatal intestinal obstruction as manifested by failure to pass meconium or delay in passing meconium with abdominal distension.
- Within 12–24 hours, all features of intestinal obstruction can be found. If it is complicated by enterocolitis, it may result in perforation and septicaemia. A severe diarrhoea with blood and mucus, abdominal distension and vomiting can occur within a few hours, followed by hypovolaemic shock.
- Rectal examination reveals that the rectum is empty, finger is gripped by anal sphincter and there is no perianal soiling (Fig. 48.87). On the other hand, in acquired megacolon, rectum is loaded with faecal matter, perianal soiling is present and there is no sphincter activity (Fig. 48.88).
- **Chronic variety:** Chronic constipation manifesting in the first few weeks of life. The child may be brought with abdominal distension. Stools are goat pellet-like.

Differential Diagnosis (Key Box 48.32)

Acquired megacolon: Usually manifests by one to two years of age. Rectum is loaded with faecal matter.

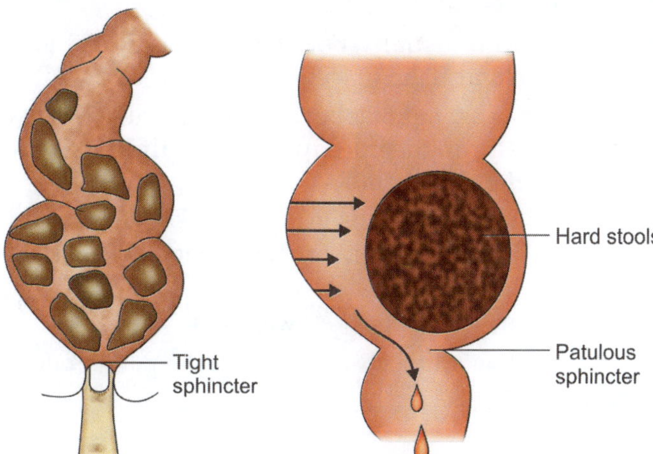

Fig. 48.87: Rectal examination in congenital megacolon

Fig. 48.88: Rectal examination in acquired megacolon

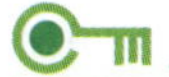
Key Box 48.32

Differential Diagnosis

- Hypothyroidism
- Meconium plug syndrome
- Intestinal pseudo-obstruction
- Colonic neuronal dysplasia

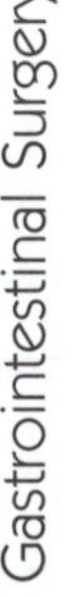

Complications

- Intestinal obstruction, perforation, peritonitis
- Enterocolitis
- Growth retardation

Investigations

1. **Full thickness rectal wall biopsy** under GA demonstrates absence of parasympathetic ganglion cells and hypertrophic nerve fibres in the nerve plexus. It should be taken above the anorectal junction. Today submucosal suction biopsy is more popular than biopsy since it avoids haemorrhage, infection and scarring.
2. **Barium enema:** 3.6% solution of barium is used, the intermediate zone appears as a cone with proximal dilatation and a distal narrow zone which is characteristic of Hirschsprung's disease.

Treatment

I. Emergency Cases

- Right transverse loop colostomy: In most of the cases, aganglionic segment is limited to rectosigmoid region.
- A full thickness biopsy of the colostomy is sent for histopathological examination.

II. Definitive Surgery

- Can be done usually between the age of 3 and 6 months (8 to 10 kg of weight).
- Resection of aganglionic bowel (anorectum) followed by a pull-through procedure. **Maintaining continence is the main aim.**
- A few points of comparison between 'Duhamel's and Swenson's pull-through' are mentioned below.

Duhamel's	Swenson's
• Retrorectal pull-through	• Endorectal pull-through
• Technically easy	• Difficult

Steps of Duhamel's Pull-through Surgery

1. The rectum is transected above the peritoneal fold and is closed.
2. The proximal ganglionic segment is pulled down behind the rectum (retrorectal space created by using blunt dissector).
3. An incision is made in the posterior wall of the anorectum above the dentate line and is deepened through the entire bowel wall.
4. The end of the proximal colon is sutured to the opening in the posterior anal canal all around.
5. The adjacent walls of rectum (posterior wall) and colon (anterior wall) are crushed by using a Kocher's forcep which falls off by itself by the 14th day.
6. The open end of the rectum (above) is closed end to side to the colon.

Other types of surgery: Soave's mucosectomy and pull-through operation.

ATRESIA AND STENOSIS

- Commonly, it affects the duodenum, followed by ileum and jejunum (Fig. 48.89).
- There may be single/multiple atresia.
- Incidence: 1 in 10,000 live births.

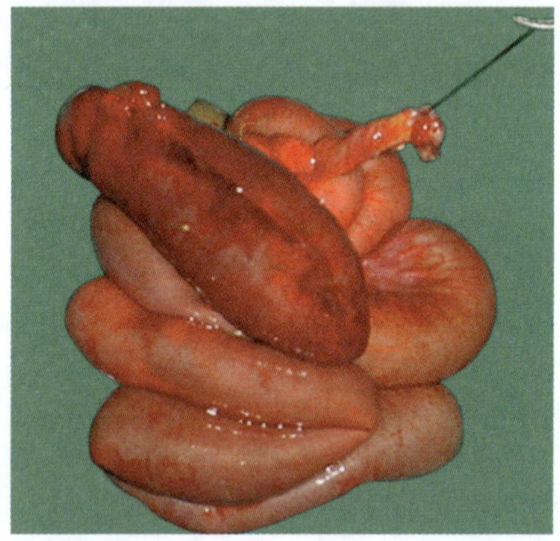

Fig. 48.89: Ileal atresia at surgery

Pearls of Wisdom

Duodenal atresia is the most common cause of intestinal obstruction in neonates.

DUODENAL ATRESIA (Key Box 48.33)

Types

Type I: Complete atresia—it is the commonest atresia. The proximal dilated segment and distal collapsed segment are completely separated.

Type 2: There is no separation of the two parts. However, a **fibrous band** is in between.

Type 3: It is incomplete obstruction: There may be a web or stenosis.

Key Box 48.33

Duodenal Atresia—Associated Lesions

- Annular pancreas, incomplete rotation of the gut
- Down's syndrome (trisomy 21)
- Maternal hydramnios
- Congenital heart disease
- Anorectal malformations

Windsock deformity: An incomplete diaphragm, with central aperture (hole) with proximal dilatation

- *Anastomosis:* A special anastomosis named after Kimura is being described. It is a diamond-shaped anastomosis between upper pouch (duodenum) which is opened transversely and lower pouch (distal duodenum) which is opened longitudinally.
- Needless to mention here that general condition has to be taken care of with supportive therapy including fluid and electrolytes, total parenteral nutrition, nasogastric decompression and adequate urinary output.
- Clinical features of obstruction manifest within 48–72 hours in the form of obstruction.
- Atresia means imperforation; stenosis means narrowing.
- Duodenal atresia presents as vomiting with or without bile, minimal distension and visible gastric peristalsis.
- Jaundice
- **X-ray abdomen erect: Double-bubble** in duodenal atresia.

Treatment

Duodenal atresia: Duodenojejunostomy by anastomosing dilated duodenum above the atresia to the jejunal loop.

SMALL INTESTINAL ATRESIA

Salient Features

- It can affect jejunum (common) or ileum.
- Like duodenal atresia, it can be associated with maternal hydramnios or malrotation of the gut.
- Exact reasons for atresia are not known. However, vascular variations in the mesentery such as V-shaped mesentery or due to occlusion of vessels in the intrauterine life are the possible factors.
- Like any obstruction, proximal bowel is dilated and distal bowel is collapsed. The colon is very small—microcolon.

GRIES FIELD MODIFICATION OF MARTIN'S CLASSIFICATION

- **Type I:** Simple stenosis. Mesentery is normal. It is mucosal atresia (Fig. 48.90).
- **Type II:** Proximal and distal bowels are connected by a fibrous band which has no lumen—atretic segment. Here again, mesentery is normal (Fig. 48.91).

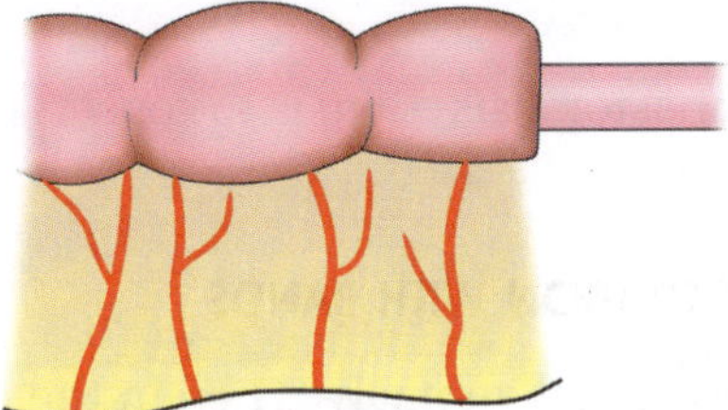

Fig. 48.90: Type I

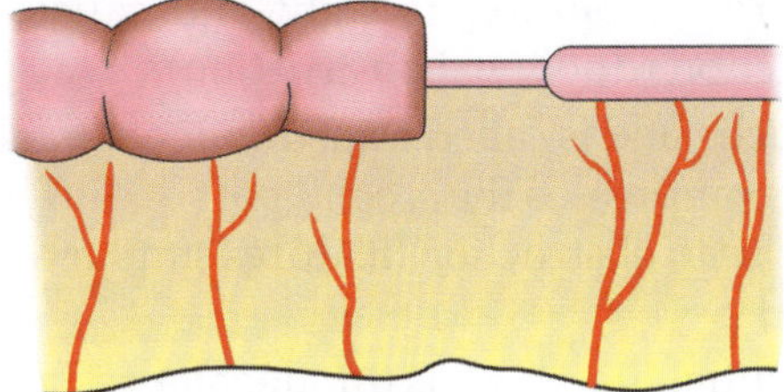

Fig. 48.91: Type II

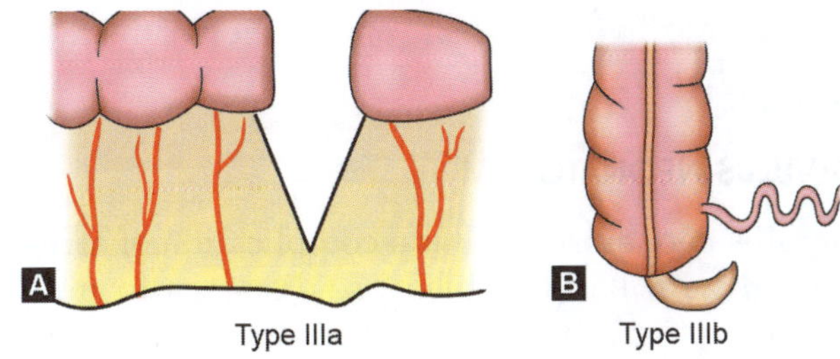

Figs 48.92A and B: Type III

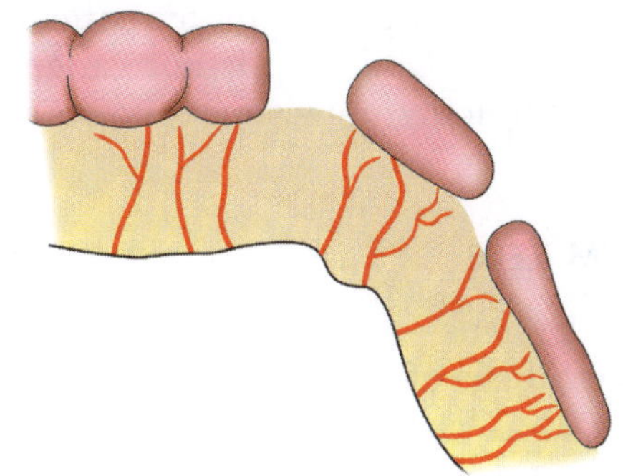

Fig. 48.93: Type IV

- **Type III:** Further divided into 2 types. IIIa refers to atresia with V-shaped loss of mesentery in between, IIIb refers to complete jejunal atresia with coiled ileum. It has been called Christmas tree deformity (Figs 48.92A and B).
- **Type IV:** Multiple atretic segments including mesentery (Fig. 48.93).

> ***Please note:*** Apple-peel or Christmas tree deformity. Here, obstruction is usually in the proximal jejunum, which is supplied by the entire superior mesenteric artery (SMA). This results in a gap in the mesentery. So, rest of the small intestine is coiled around the ileocolic branch of the SMA.

Treatment

Resection, anastomosis—aim is to conserve as much as possible.

ARRESTED ROTATION WITH BANDS

- It is a congenital anomaly wherein the caecum and right colon are found on the left side (Fig. 48.94).
- As a result of this, there are peritoneal bands which run across from left to right and cause intestinal obstruction (duodenal obstruction).
- One such band is called **transduodenal band of Ladd** which compresses the second part of duodenum and gives rise to obstruction (features similar to duodenal atresia).
- Differential diagnosis is duodenal atresia.

Treatment

Laparotomy, division of band and fixation of the caecum in the right iliac fossa.

VOLVULUS NEONATORUM

Volvulus neonatorum—it is a complication of arrested rotation with bands which pre-disposes to midgut volvulus (small bowel). These unfortunate infants undergo massive resection of the bowel if it is gangrenous (Fig. 48.95). Such massive resections give rise to short gut syndrome. Thus, the patient becomes a digestive cripple. If the loop is not gangrenous, it is treated by laparotomy, untwisting of bowel and division of bands.

MECONIUM ILEUS

- Meconium ileus—it is a neonatal manifestation of **mucoviscidosis** of the pancreas wherein the mucus is thick and viscid. This, along with meconium, produces obstruction. **There may be ileal atresia**, which might have precipitated meconium ileus (Fig. 48.96). Majority of meconium ileus is coupled by complications such as **gangrene, perforation** and **peritonitis**. As a sequel to peritonitis, calcification and adhesive meconium obstruction develop.
- Infants present with abdominal distension, bilious vomiting and failure to pass meconium.
- Plain X-ray shows distended bowel and **mottling** due to calcification.
- **Soap bubble sign** or **Neuhauser's sign:** Ground glass appearance in the right lower quadrant due to viscid meconium mixed with air.
- **Ultrasonography:** Dilated loops of bowel filled with echogenic material are highly suggestive of meconium ileus rather than ileal atresia.
- If perforation is ruled out, barium enema can be done which shows microcolon.

Treatment

I. Conservative Treatment

It is indicated if there is no peritonitis, general condition of the child is reasonably good or if there is partial obstruction. Dilute gastrograffin is introduced into the colon as enema. It fills up terminal ileum. It absorbs fluid from the interstitial space into the lumen because it is hyperosmolar. Consequently, the meconium becomes soft and it is rejected naturally. Hypervolaemia is to be corrected during this.

II. Nonresectional Procedures

A. Bishop-Koop operation (Fig. 48.97)

- Ileum is divided in the proximal healthy part. This proximal ileum is anastomosed to the ascending colon to relieve obstruction—end-to-side anastomosis.
- Distal ileum containing thick meconium pellets is brought outside as a fistula and regular saline washes are given to dilute the meconium. Mucous fistula needs to be closed after a few weeks.

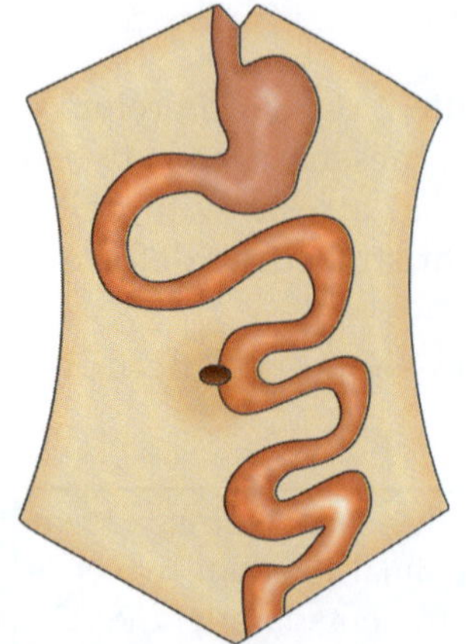

Fig. 48.94: Arrested rotation—malrotation

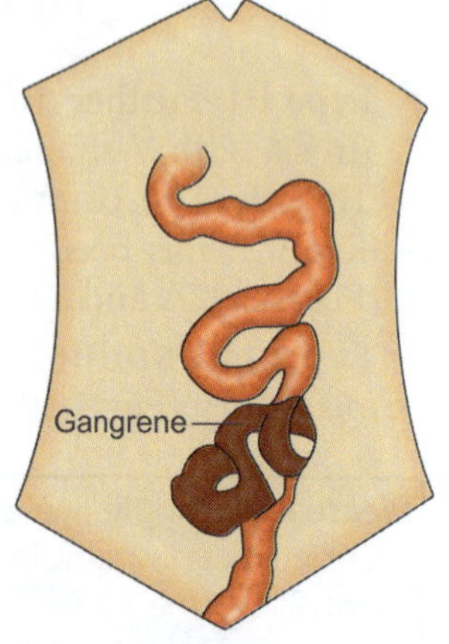

Fig. 48.95: Volvulus neonatorum

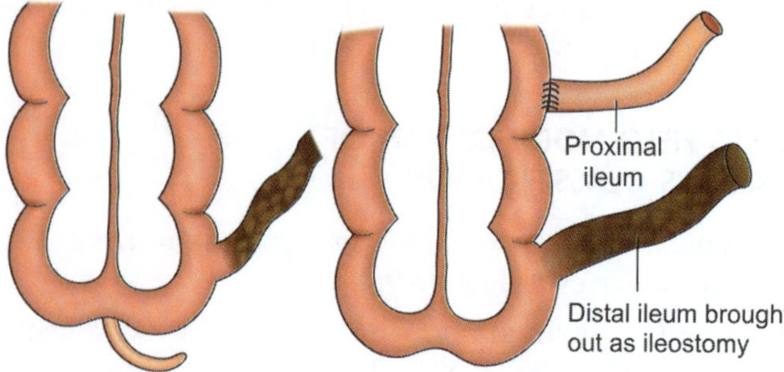

Fig. 48.96: Meconium ileus

Fig. 48.97: Bishop-Koop operation

B. Santulli operation (Fig. 48.98): In this operation, proximal ileum is brought out as ileostomy. Distal ileum is anastomosed to proximal ileum as end-to-side anastomosis.

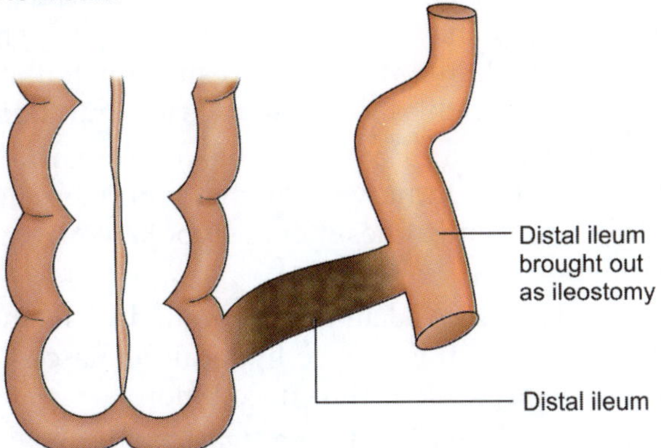

Fig. 48.98: Santulli operation

III. Resection

Resection is the surgery of choice today as more cases present with short segment obstruction. Long-term results and complications are much less than non-resectional procedures.

ANORECTAL ANOMALIES

Competency

SU28.16.2: Describe clinical presentation, diagnosis and management of imperforate anus and other congenital anorectal malformations.

Developmental Anatomy

- To start with, there is a common chamber called cloaca, which is later divided into 2 chambers, anteriorly allantois gives rise to urinary bladder and posteriorly, postallantoic gut gives rise to rectum and upper 2 cm of anal canal.
- Postallantoic gut fuses with proctodeum, thus giving rise to anal canal. If there is a defective fusion of this, it results in imperforate anus.

IMPERFORATE ANUS

Incidence

1:4500 live births. Common in female children.

Types of Imperforate Anus

I. **Low anomalies:** It refers to termination of the bowel below the anorectal bundle.
   1. **Covered anus** (Fig. 48.99A): The anal orifice is covered by a tag of skin.
   2. **Membranous anus** (Fig. 48.99B): Covered with a thin membrane.

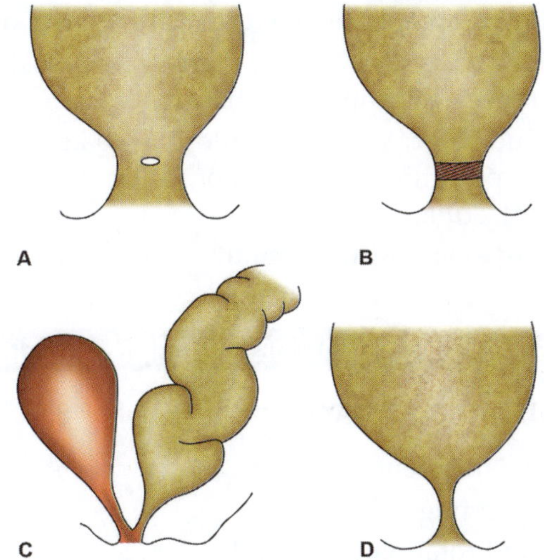

Figs 48.99A to D: Low anorectal anomalies

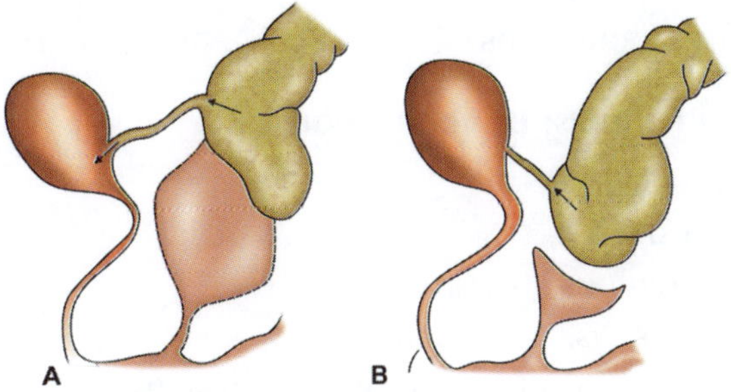

Figs 48.100A and B: High anorectal anomalies

   3. **Anterior ectopic anus** (Fig. 48.99C): Anus is situated anteriorly.
   4. **Stenosed anus** (Fig. 48.99D): Anal orifice is microscopic.

II. **High anomalies:** They are supralevator—the bowel terminates above the anorectal bundle.
   1. Anorectal and agenesis, with fistula: Rectovesical, rectovaginal, rectourethral fistulae (Fig. 48.100).

Diagnosis

12 hours after birth, the child is put in the prone position (Fig. 48.102B) (12 hours is the time for the gas shadow to reach the distal portion of the gut). A metal coin is strapped to the site of anus and X-ray is taken. If the gas shadow is above the pubococcygeal line, it is a high anomaly. If the distance between the coin and gas shadow is more than 2.5 cm, it is a high anomaly. If the gas shadow is below the pubococcygeal line, it is a low anomaly. Pubococcygeal line is called Stephen's line.

Treatment

I. **Low anomaly:** Easy to treat, division of membrane or skin followed by dilatation is all that is required with some amount of plastic reconstruction (anoplasty is necessary).

II. High anomaly: Repaired by 3-stage procedure:
- 1st stage: Preliminary transverse colostomy to relieve intestinal obstruction.
- 2nd stage: When the child is 8–10 kg of weight, a "pull-through" operation is done with division of fistula.
- 3rd stage: After 2 months, colostomy is closed.

CAUSES OF INTESTINAL OBSTRUCTION AS PER AGE

NEONATES: 0 TO 7 DAYS (Figs 48.101 to 48.108)

1. Atresia and stenosis
2. Hirschsprung's disease
3. Arrested rotation with bands
4. Volvulus neonatorum
5. Meconium ileus
6. Imperforate anus

Young Patients: Up to 30 Years

1. Obstructed hernia
2. Adhesions
3. Tuberculous stricture ileum
4. Crohn's disease of ileum
5. Tuberculous peritonitis with adhesions
6. Meckel's diverticulum with band
7. Adult intussusception

Middle-aged Patients: 30–60 Years

1. Adhesions
2. Obstructed hernia
3. Carcinoma left colon
4. Diverticulosis with stricture left colon
5. Gallstone ileus
6. Sigmoid volvulus
7. Mesenteric vascular occlusion
8. Adult intussusception

PARALYTIC ILEUS (NEUROGENIC ILEUS)

In this condition, there is a failure of transmission of parasympathetic impulses from one segment to the other. That means, there is a failure of parasympathetic mechanism, which results in paralysis of bowel. It gives rise to a large collection of fluid and gas within the bowel resulting in distension.

Causes/Etiology

- During surgery, stimulation of sympathetic nerves that inhibits gastrointestinal movement results in autonomic nervous system dysfunction(s) causing ileus.
- In sepsis, a few inflammatory mediators like *nitric oxide, prostaglandins, vasoactive intestinal peptide-VIP* are released. They cause some motility problems to the gut. Inflammation also results in leukocyte infiltration and this factor also adds to paralytic ileus.
- Hypokalaemia: Potassium is responsible for depolarization in nerve cells that innervate muscle of the small intestines, hence hypokalemia causes paralytic ileus.
- Hypocalcaemia: Calcium is associated with smooth muscle contraction, hence hypocalcaemia can give rise to paralytic ileus (it is uncommon).
- Metabolic: Uraemia, diabetes (gastropathy).
- Drugs: Central-acting drugs—loperamide, phenothiazine, tricyclic antidepressants, and anti-Parkinson's drugs. Peripherally acting drugs—anticholinergic group, calcium-channel blocker group (e.g. verapamil), alpha-2 adrenergic agonist group (e.g. clonidine), etc.

Clinical Features

1. **Abdominal distension** is gross. Tympanitic note all over is a feature. Respiratory and cardiac functions are impaired.
2. **No colicky pain abdomen** (in dynamic obstruction, colicky pain is a feature). Dull pain occurs due to distension of the abdomen.
3. **Failure to pass flatus,** effortless vomiting is also characteristic of paralytic ileus.
4. On auscultation, **tinkling sounds** are heard due to shift of fluid from one coil of bowel to the other (Key Box 48.34).
5. Severe fluid, electrolyte and protein depletion occur.

Investigations

1. Plain X-ray abdomen erect demonstrates distended loops of bowel (Fig. 48.109).
2. Electrolyte study and correction of any abnormality.

Treatment

- Basic principle of treating paralytic ileus is **drip and suction**.

Key Box 48.34

Three Types of Bowel Sounds

- Normal: Once in 20 seconds, low pitch.
- Borborygmi: Loud, noisy, which occurs once in 5–10 seconds.
- Tinkling sounds: Mild metallic sounds as in paralytic ileus.

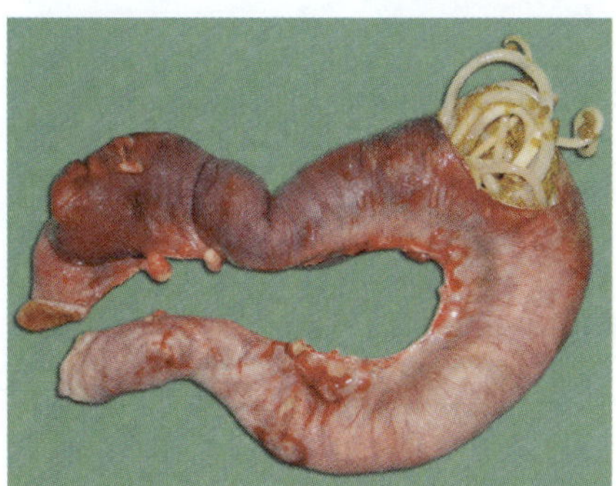

Fig. 48.101: Worm ball obstruction

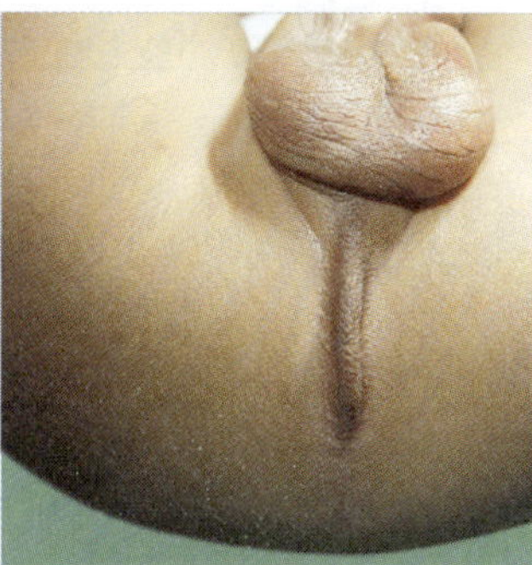

Fig. 48.102A: Anorectal malformation

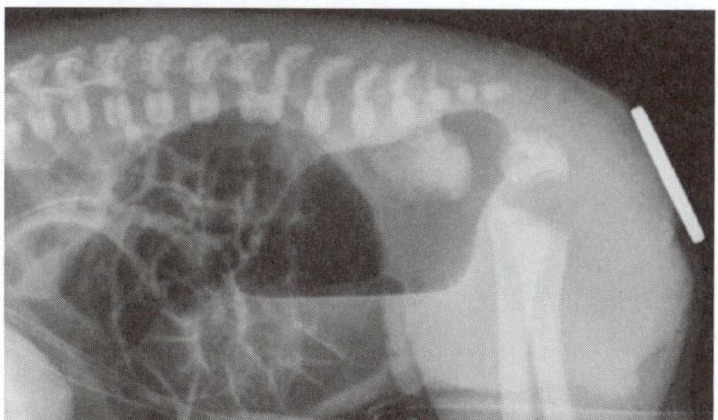

Fig. 48.102B: Prone position showing high anomaly

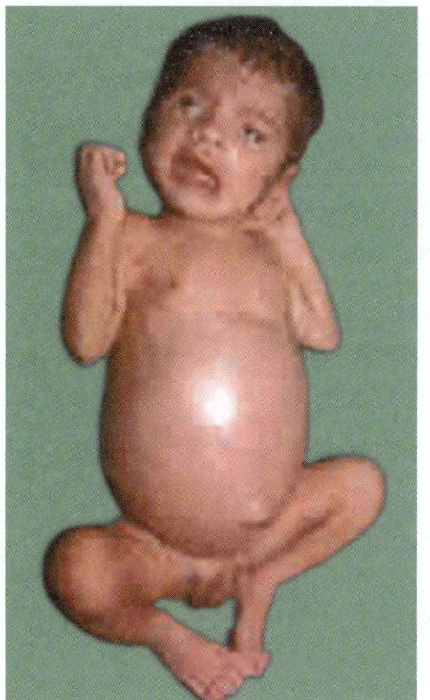

Fig. 48.103: Ileal obstruction

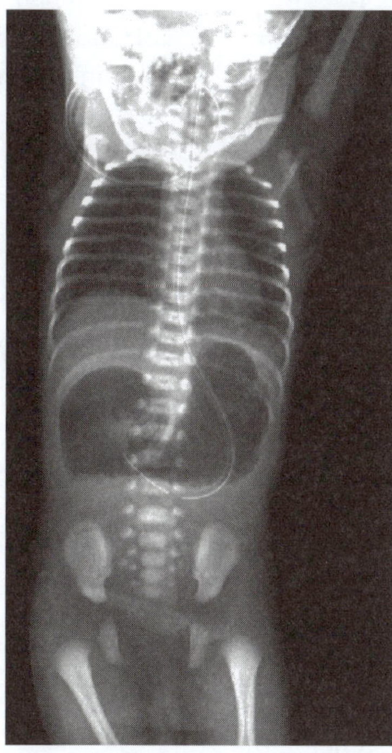

Fig. 48.104: Double-bubble appearance

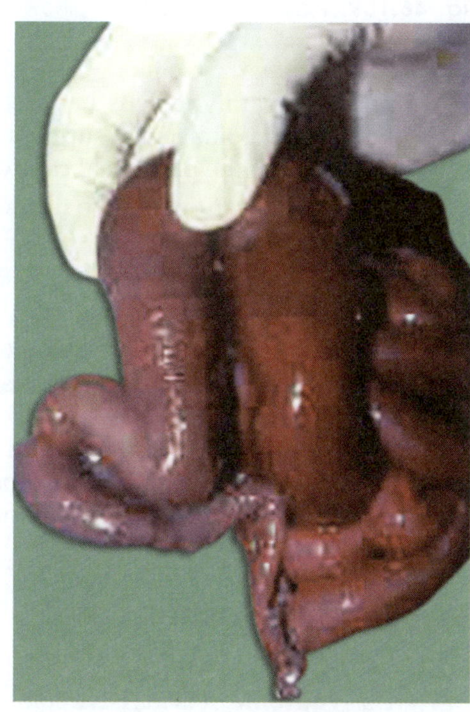

Fig. 48.105: Hirschsprung's disease

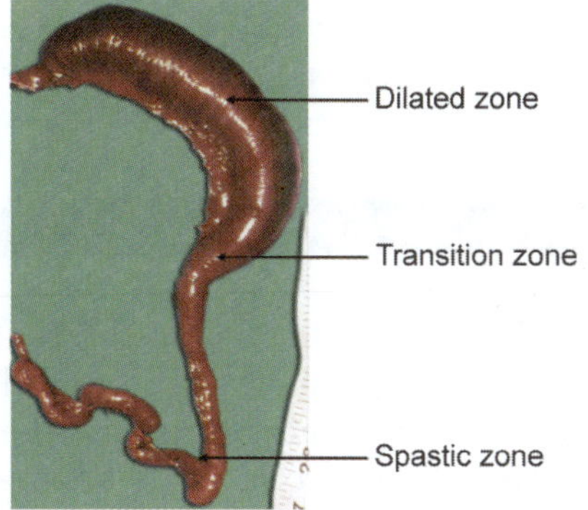

Fig. 48.106: Various segments of the large intestine in Hirschsprung's disease

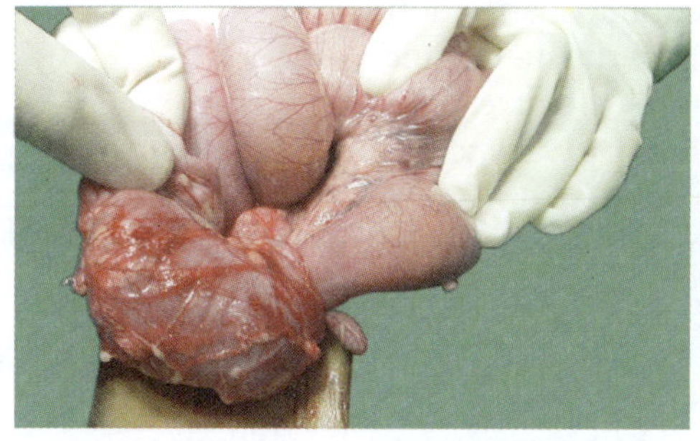

Fig. 48.107: Ileocaecal intussusception

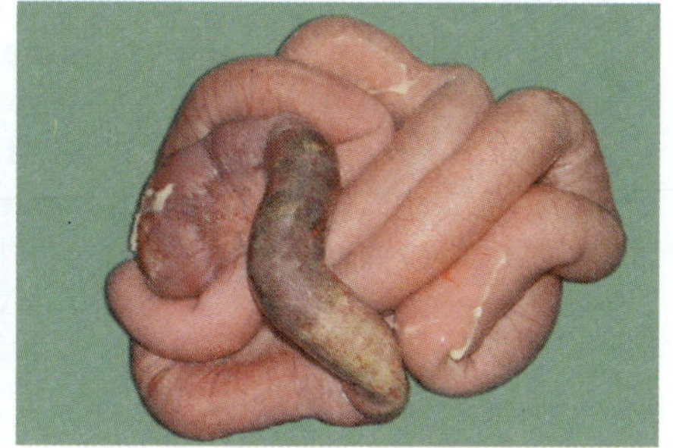

Fig. 48.108: Necrotising enterocolitis with patchy gangrene

(*Courtesy:* Professor Vijaykumar, Department of Paediatric Surgery, KMC, Manipal)

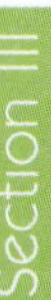

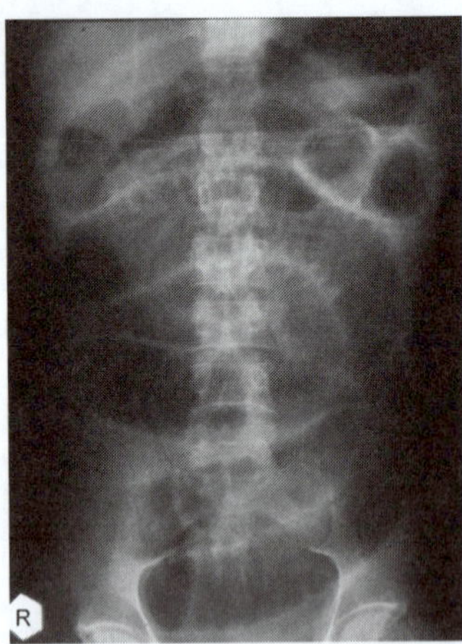

Fig. 48.109: Plain X-ray abdomen showing dilated bowel loops

- The cause of paralytic ileus has to be treated first, e.g. if there is **hypokalaemia, supplement potassium**. If there is pus in the peritoneal cavity, **drain** it.
- **Ryle's tube aspiration,** to give rest to the gut.
- Intravenous fluids, supplementation of ions, correction of dehydration, oliguria, etc. Such treatment is continued for 3–4 days.
- Ryle's tube is removed when abdomen is soft, bowel sounds are heard and patient has passed flatus. Clear oral fluids are started for 2–3 days followed by soft diet. Small bowel activity returns within 12–18 hours, followed by colon which starts functioning within 36–48 hours. However, gastric functions may return ranging from 18 hours to 4 days.

PSEUDOINTESTINAL OBSTRUCTION

Acute colonic pseudo-obstruction (ACPO) is also called **Ogilvie's syndrome**. It is massive colonic distension in the absence of a mechanically obstructing lesion.

Pathogenesis

It occurs mainly due to **malfunctioning of sacral parasympathetic nerves (S2–S4)**. It results in atony of the descending colon resulting in functional obstruction. It is interesting to note that the **junction of the dilated and collapsed bowel is near the splenic flexure. This is the place wherein parasympathetic supply by vagus ends and sacral autonomic nervous system starts**. An increased sympathetic tone results in colonic dilatation due to inhibition of contraction (Key Box 48.35).

Clinical Features

- Elderly bedridden patient with cardiac/lower respiratory illness are the victims. Aerophagia and drugs which decrease colonic mobility are precipitating factors.

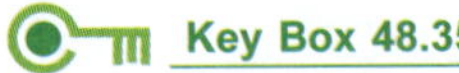

Key Box 48.35

Causes of Colonic Pseudo-obstruction

1. Retroperitoneal irritation
   - Blood
   - Urine
   - Fracture spine and pelvis
2. Drugs
   - Levodopa
   - Tricyclic antidepressants
3. Metabolic
   - Uraemia
   - Diabetes
   - Myxoedema
   - Hypokalaemia
4. Viral infections

- Failure to pass faeces and flatus for several days.
- Tachypnoea due to elevation of the diaphragm due to distended colon is common.
- Rectal examination reveals some faeces (in cases of mechanical obstruction, rectum is empty).
- Plain X-ray abdomen erect may or may not show one or two air fluid levels. Distension is mainly colonic.
- Carcinoma colon is to be differentiated by barium enema.
- Caecal perforation is a dangerous complication. Hence, look for right iliac fossa tenderness.

Treatment

- It is conservative, provided acute abdomen is ruled out.
- Colonoscopic decompression is the method of choice.
- Prokinetic drugs such as cisapride or mosapride have been tried in selected cases.
- Rarely, even after colonoscopic decompression, caecal tenderness continues. If distension persists, laparotomy followed by tube caecostomy may have to be done.

INTESTINAL OBSTRUCTION—SPECIAL CAUSES

1. ADHESIVE OBSTRUCTION

- Firstly, strangulation should be ruled out by clinical and radiological tests. **Extended nonoperative therapy** may be advised, e.g. if one can wait for 48 hours in a case of intestinal obstruction. In these cases, 4–6 days of waiting is sometimes worth, especially in a patient who has been operated many times earlier.

- During this extended period, careful monitoring is important to look for any new symptoms/signs of strangulation.
- **Early postoperative adhesions** (bread and butter adhesions) can also be given an extended nonoperative therapy because mostly it is **partial obstruction.**

2. INTESTINAL OBSTRUCTION IN CROHN'S DISEASE

- As far as possible, **resection should be avoided** in Crohn's disease because the aim is to save as much as possible.
- 30% of patients eventually develop obstruction which requires resection.
- Again, if possible do **strictureplasty**
- Strictureplasty should not be done in patients with intra-abdominal abscesses or intestinal fistulae.
- Some cases of Crohn's obstruction also **respond well to medications—one more reason for nonoperative treatment.**

3. INTESTINAL OBSTRUCTION IN PREGNANCY

- The commonest cause of intestinal obstruction in pregnancy and puerperium is **adhesive bands**.
- **Volvulus** is the second commonest cause of intestinal obstruction—intestine volvulates around an adhesive band and that is why the primary cause is adhesive bands (Fig. 48.110).
- **Inguinal hernia** and **intussusception** are the other causes.
- The consequences of intestinal obstruction in pregnancy **do not differ** from those found in nonpregnant women except that in the pregnant patient, a second entity, the foetus, is also threatened.
- Most of the intestinal obstructions tend to occur in the **third trimester**.
- Maternal **mortality** for intestinal obstruction in pregnancy (10–33%) is **higher** than in nonpregnant patients.

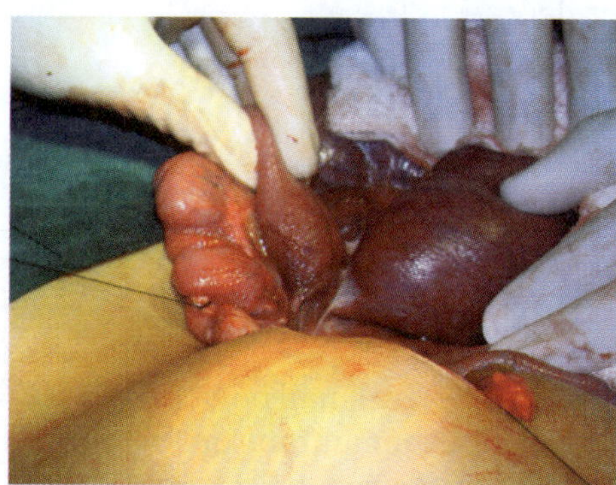

Fig. 48.110: Pregnant lady with adhesions causing intestinal obstruction

- In the first half of the pregnancy, nausea, vomiting and episodes of constipation are quite common. Hence, they are confused for hyperemesis gravidarum, acute duodenal ulcer and gastritis.
- **In the second half of the pregnancy,** symptoms can be confused for toxaemia, constipation, Braxton Hicks contractions, etc.
- **Ultrasound** can help in the diagnosis by detecting dilated intestinal loops, fluid in the peritoneal cavity and intussusception. It also helps to rule out ovarian torsion, gallstone disease, etc.
- **Premature labour can be prevented with tocolysis (abolition of uterine contraction).**
- **Abdominal surgery in the third trimester does not induce labour.**
- Negative laparotomy carries a small risk of disturbing the pregnancy.
- **Volvulus and intussusception** are the two major causes of small intestinal obstruction in pregnancy. Both can give rise to gangrene. Hence an intervention is required before gangrene sets in.
- ***The diagnosis and treatment of a pregnant patient suspected of having a bowel obstruction should be no different from those given to a nonpregnant one.***

4. ILEOSIGMOID KNOTTING

It is rare type of knotting between sigmoid and ileum carrying significant mortality if not treated timely (Key Box 48.36).

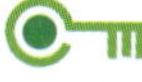

Key Box 48.36

Ileosigmoid Knotting

- It is also called compound volvulus.
- Predisposing factor is long pelvic mesocolon.
- The ileum twists around the sigmoid colon resulting in gangrene of ileum or sigmoid colon or both.
- Even though sigmoid is also twisted, features are similar to small intestinal obstruction—not massive distension as seen in sigmoid volvulus.
- Resection anastomosis of gangrenous segment followed by anastomosis of the bowel (ileoileal/colic and colocolic).

5. ILIAC CREST GRAFT HERNIA WITH OBSTRUCTION

- This is also a rare hernia following bone graft removal from the iliac crest for treatment of fractures.
- Iliac crest is the common donor site of bone graft. If the bone graft removed is large, the intestines can herniate resulting in intestinal obstruction.
- Tenderness in the surgical site scar can cause diagnostic difficulty.

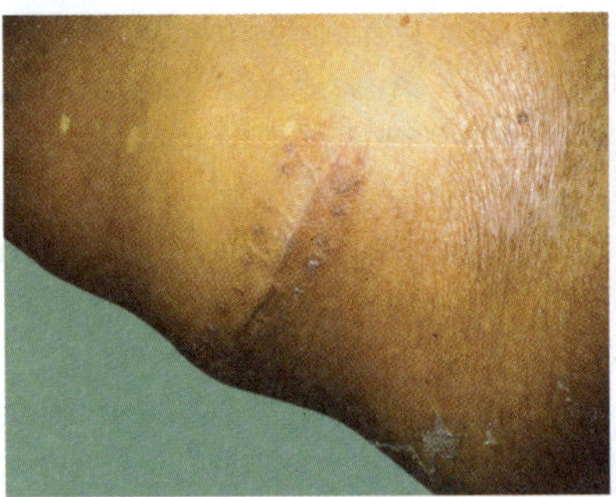

Fig. 48.111: Iliac bone graft site hernia

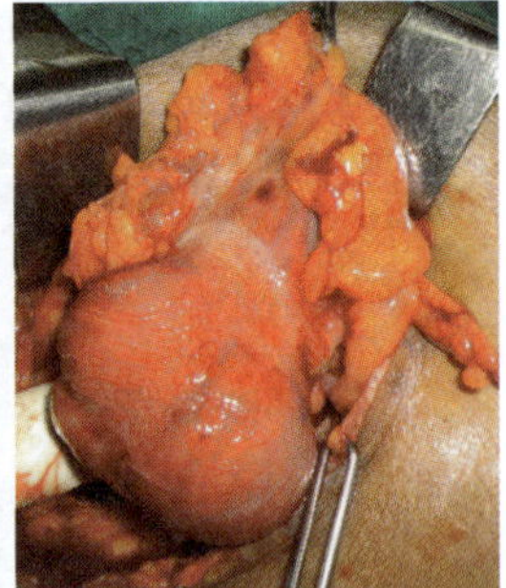

Fig. 48.112: Caecal herniation

- It is confused for haematoma.
- CT scan gives the diagnosis.

Following is the case report of a patient who had undergone iliac crest bone graft and developed hernia (Figs 48.111 and 48.112).

Clinical Notes

A 50-year-old man presented to the casualty with abdominal pain, vomiting and distension. Features were suggestive of intestinal obstruction. On examination, there was a bulge in the region of right iliac fossa—more lateral. There was a scar of bone graft incision. On questioning the patient, he says that he had fracture humerus. Two months back, nailing and bone grafting had been done. Ultrasound revealed bowel loops. CT scan showed a large bone graft defect with herniation of intestines resulting in intestinal obstruction. Emergency surgery, reduction of hernia contents and mesh repair was done. Recovery was uneventful.

6. FOOD BOLUS OBSTRUCTION

This complication can occur, particularly when a GJ or partial gastrectomy is done.

Factors Precipitating this Condition

- Unmasticated, undigested particles
- Coconut pieces, jackfruit seeds and gulped coins, etc.
- They get impacted in the terminal ileum which is the narrowest portion of the gut.

Treatment

Squeeze the bolus into the caecum. Otherwise, enterotomy and removal may be necessary.

7. OBSTRUCTION DUE TO INTERNAL HERNIA

Syn: Stammer's Hernia

1. These are rare causes of intestinal obstruction. Due to some congenital defect in the mesentery, the floating, mobile intestines can herniate (Key Box 48.37). The defect may be in:

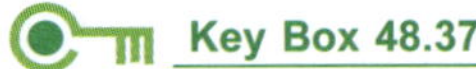

Key Box 48.37

Internal Hernia

- Wherever a defect is present which is an anatomically present recesses or congenital or following surgery, loop of small intestine can herniate resulting in hernias.
- They are difficult to diagnose. The diagnosis is by exclusion.
- Triggering factors: Inflammation in the vicinity with or without an adhesion and band trigger herniation and complications.
- Most of these cases present as acute abdomen with features of intestinal obstruction.
- CT scan is the best investigation in such cases.
- It should be remembered that an important vessel runs in the close vicinity of these sites in most of the cases.
- Treatment is reduction, suturing the defect or resection anastomosis if the intestine is gangrenous taking care not to damage the vessel. Decompression without dividing the constricting ring may be required.

   - Mesentery
   - Transverse mesocolon or
   - Broad ligament
   - Foramen of Winslow

   Hence, whenever a surgical procedure is done for resection of the bowel or GJ, etc. Once the anastomosis is completed, the rent in the mesocolon as in GJ or rent in the small bowel mesentery should be closed.
2. Herniation can also occur through one of the potential spaces (fossae) in and around a viscus.

Duodenal Fossa

- Left paraduodenal fossa: Inferior mesenteric vein lies very close to the free border here.
- Right duodenojejunal fossa: Superior mesenteric artery runs in its free border.

Colonic Fossa

- Superior ileocaecal fossa
- Inferior ileocaecal fossa
- Sigmoid fossa

Pearls of Wisdom

These are the rare causes of intestinal obstruction to be kept in mind.

8. ABDOMINAL COCOON SYNDROME

- It is characterized by small bowel encapsulation by a fibro-collagenous membrane or "cocoon". It is a rare cause of intestinal obstruction secondary to kinking and/or compression of the intestines within the constricting cocoon.

- **Three types have been recognized.**
  A. **Primary form** is probably caused by a subclinical peritonitis leading to the formation of a chemical peritonitis was caused by retrograde menstruation, leading to the formation of a cocoon. This was first reported by Foo[1] KT, *et al.* and he coined the term "abdominal cocoon" in 1978.
  B. **Secondary** causes include the placement of Le Veen shunts for refractory ascites, continuous ambulatory peritoneal dialysis, systemic lupus erythematosus, use of povidone iodine for abdominal wash-out, an adrenergic blocker practolol, etc.
  C. **Tuberculosis** also has been found to be a factor in a few cases.
- Diagnosis is established by CECT scan and treatment is separation of bowel loops and removal of the membrane in toto or in pieces.

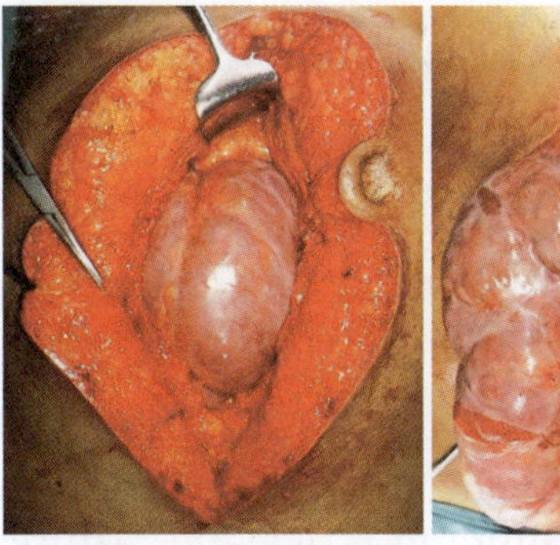
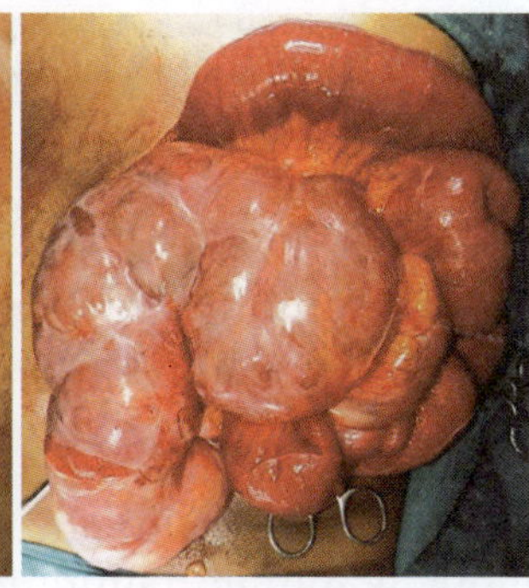

Fig. 48.113: Abdominal cocoon (*Courtesy*: Dr Sunil Krishna, Dr Keertan Upadhya, Dr Ameena, Department of Surgery, KMC, Manipal)

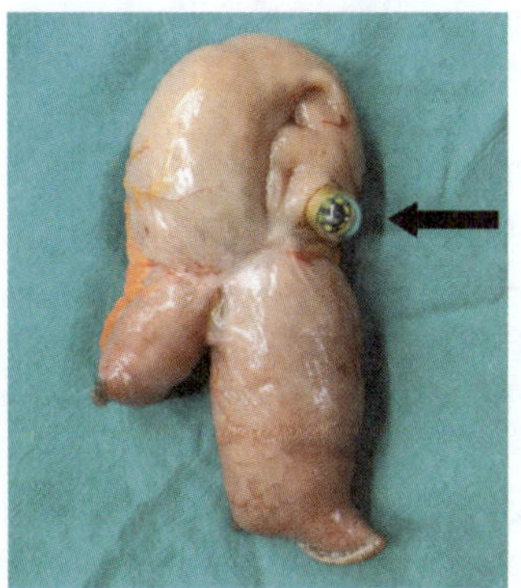

Fig. 48.114: Capsule obstruction (*Courtesy:* Dr Bharath Bhat, Dr Jegan, Dr Sridevi, Department of Surgery, KMC, Manipal)

Clinical Notes

We had a 30-year-old man with nil previous history of abdominal pain or any illness, presented to the hospital with colicky abdominal pain, 2 times bilious vomiting and distension. On examination tympanitic vague mass was palpable in the right iliac fossa. X-ray was suggestive of intestinal obstruction. Abdominal ultrasonography revealed clustering of the small bowel loops in the right iliac fossa. CECT was reported as intestinal obstruction secondary to internal herniation. Emergency exploratory laparotomy was done. A cocoon with matted loops were found in the right iliac fossa (Fig. 48.113). An attempt to separate the cocoon resulted in multiple tears, it was not possible, hence resection and anastomosis of about 20 cm of the ileum followed by ileocolic anastomosis was done. Patient recovered completely from obstruction and was discharged.

9. CAPSULE OBSTRUCTION

Capsule endoscopy (page 907) is done for evaluation of small intestines, major indication being occult bleeding or diarrhoea—causes can be tumours or tuberculosis or Crohn's disease, etc. Capsule can get stuck at the site of ulcer or stricture or a bent intestinal loop due to adhesions (Fig. 48.114). In such patients, it needs to be removed along with intestine.

10. ACUTE LARGE BOWEL OBSTRUCTION

Details about the causes of large bowel obstruction, pathophysiology and the treatment are given in Chapter 48. However, a few important points have been given in ten commandments.

TEN COMMANDMENTS WHILE TREATING INTESTINAL OBSTRUCTION

1. Should rule out pseudo-obstruction before exploring the abdomen.
2. Should do limited contrast study or CT scan
3. Should resuscitate the patient before surgery
4. Should take into account, the general condition of the patient before resection anastomosis.
5. Should consider right hemicolectomy or extended hemicolectomy for right-sided growth which is operable.
6. Should consider single stage resection anastomosis also for left-sided growth provided general condition of the patient is good and on table lavage is given before the anastomosis.
7. Should consider exteriorisation of gangrenous bowel in a very sick patient.
8. Should consider a simple diversion colostomy in moribund patients in rectosigmoid obstructions (it is a common problem).
9. Should not do anastomosis in cases with faecal contamination, peritonitis, haemodynamic instability or possible ischaemia of the remaining colonic segments.
10. Should mark the probable stoma site.

[1]Foo KT, Ng KC, Rauff A, Foong WC, Sinniah R. Unusual small intestinal obstruction in girls: The abdominal cocoon. Br J Surg 1978;65:427–30.

MALROTATION AND MIDGUT VOLVULUS

Introduction

- The incidence of malrotation is 1 in 500 infants.
- The male to female ratio is 2 : 1.
- Malrotation with midgut volvulus may become rapidly life-threatening. The previously healthy infant with bilious vomiting is a characteristic presentation of malrotation. Usually it presents with bilious vomiting, failure to thrive and features of intestinal obstruction (Fig. 48.115).
- In approximately 60% of patients, malrotation presents by one month of age. Another 20–30% of patients present at age 1–12 months. Thereafter, it can present at any age, and is seen in adults and even the elderly.

Basic Pathophysiology

- A volvulus is a complete **twisting of a loop of intestine around its mesenteric attachment site.** This can occur at various locations of the GI tract, including stomach, small intestine, caecum, transverse colon, and sigmoid colon. Midgut malrotation refers to twisting of the entire midgut about the axis of the superior mesenteric artery (SMA).
- **Malrotation is any deviation from the normal 270° counterclockwise rotation** of the bowel that occurs during embryogenesis (Figs 48.115 and 48.116).
- At the fourth week of gestation, the gastrointestinal system is a straight tube centrally located in the abdomen. During the ensuing 8 weeks, the midgut rotates and becomes fixed to the posterior abdominal wall. **Arrest of development at any stage narrows the mesenteric base and impairs fixation, leaving the bowel at high risk for volvulus.**

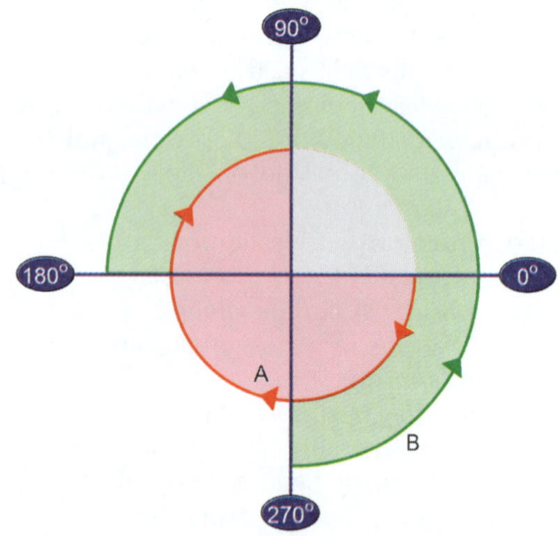

Fig. 48.115: Midgut volvulus: (A) Clockwise rotation resulting in superior mesenteric ischaemia shown in red line, (B) Anticlockwise untwisting to be done at surgery is shown as green line

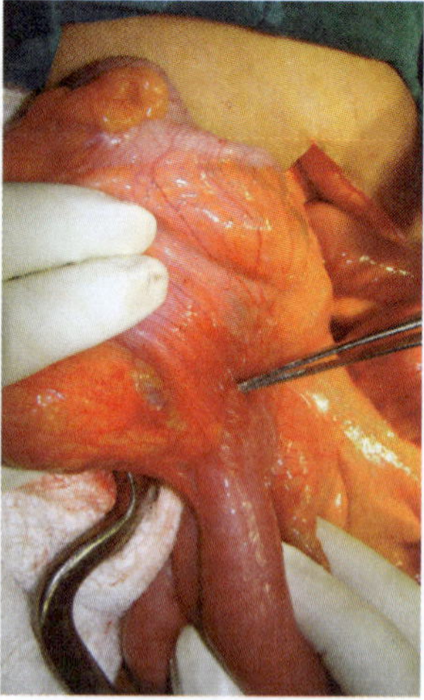

Fig. 48.116: Malrotation with band

- The resultant shortened mesenteric pedicle predisposes to midgut volvulus, a clockwise rotation around the superior mesenteric artery axis that can lead to bowel ischaemia.

Investigations

- Conventional radiographs are neither sensitive nor specific for malrotation.
- On the upper GI series, it is crucial to locate the position of the duodenojejunal junction (DJJ). The DJJ must be at least over (but more reassuringly lateral to) the left vertebral pedicle and at the same height as the duodenal bulb on a well-centred view. If the DJJ does not meet these two criteria, malrotation is diagnosed.
- **Signs of midgut volvulus include an abrupt termination, or break of the contrast column and the corkscrew (apple peel, or barber pole) sign.**
- On ultrasound (US) and computed tomography (CT), the superior mesenteric artery (SMA) and superior mesenteric vein (SMV) relationship may be reversed.
- Normally, the SMV is to the right of the SMA; with malrotation, the SMV may occupy a position directly anterior or to the left of the SMA.

Treatment

- **The Ladd procedure** remains the cornerstone of surgical treatment for malrotation today.
- ***A classic Ladd procedure*** is described as reduction of volvulus (if present), division of mesenteric bands, **placement of small bowel on the right and large bowel on the left of the abdomen, and appendicectomy.**
- A laparoscopic variation of the Ladd procedure has been used in some centres, with the general advantage of decreased adhesions and scarring, but good visualisation of the entire bowel is necessary.

Key Box 48.38

Intestinal Obstruction
'Clues' to the Causes of Obstruction

- Operative scar – Adhesions
- Groin swelling – Obstructed hernia
- Gross distended intestinal loop – Sigmoid volvulus
- Stepladder peristalsis – Small intestinal obstruction
- Red currant jelly stools – Intussusception
- Deformed umbilicus in adult child – Meckel's diverticulum with band
- Melanosis of lips, mucosa – Intussusception in adults (PJ syndrome)
- H/o constipation/ bleeding per rectum – Colonic obstruction (cancer)
- Emaciated, young patient with loose stools/weight loss/fever – Ileocaecal tuberculosis (TB) stricture
- Elderly, hypertensive severe abdominal pain, tachycardia, tachypnoea, acidotic – Mesenteric vascular occlusion

Laparoscopy is a particularly suitable investigative procedure for children presenting with acute abdomen. 'Clues' to the causes of intestinal obstruction are mentioned in Key Box 48.38.

INTERESTING 'MOST COMMON' IN INTESTINAL OBSTRUCTION

- Most commonly encountered disorder of intestines is intestinal obstruction.
- Most common cause of small intestinal obstruction is intra-abdominal adhesion.
- Most commonly performed, simple diagnostic investigation in case of obstruction is plain X-ray abdomen in erect position.
- Most common abdominal symptom of intestinal obstruction is colicky abdominal pain.
- Most common congenital anomaly of small intestine is Meckel's diverticulum.
- Most common presentation of Meckel's diverticulum in children is bleeding.
- Most common cause of intestinal obstruction in infants between 6 and 18 months is intussusception.

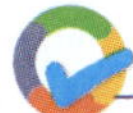

Multiple Choice Questions

1. Which of the following is true for closed loop obstruction?
   A. Can occur with constrictive growth in the hepatic flexure
   B. Ileocaecal valve is incompetent
   C. Perforation of the sigmoid colon is common
   D. Occurs with partial obstruction

2. Which of the following is not the cause of gangrene in intestinal obstruction?
   A. Ileocaecal tuberculosis
   B. Mesenteric vascular occlusion
   C. Necrotising enterocolitis
   D. Volvulus

3. Faeculent vomiting is pathognomonic of:
   A. Jejunal obstruction B. Terminal ileal obstruction
   C. Duodenal obstruction D. Colonic obstruction

4. Cardinal features of intestinal obstruction include all of the following *except*:
   A. Colicky abdominal pain
   B. Vomiting
   C. Diarrhoea
   D. Abdominal distension

5. The following is true in a plain X-ray of abdomen in intestinal obstruction:
   A. Caecum can appear as round shadow
   B. Ileum has valvulae conniventes
   C. Colon has haustrations
   D. Sigmoid appears shapeless

6. Features of strangulation includes all of the following *except*:
   A. Tachycardia
   B. Disappearance of pain abdomen
   C. Fever
   D. Acidosis

7. The features of viable bowel includes all of the following *except*:
   A. Normal peristalsis
   B. Normal pulsations are visible
   C. Normal pink colour is present
   D. Peritoneal sheen is absent

8. Conservative treatment is advocated in intestinal obstruction when there is:
A. Disseminated malignancy with obstruction
B. Complete obstruction with adhesions
C. Postoperative obstruction with peritonitis
D. Crohn's disease unresponsive to medications

9. 'Bent inner tube design', 'Omega sign', 'Bird's beak design' are all seen in:
A. Sigmoid volvulus
B. Caecal volvulus
C. Meckel's diverticulum
D. Bascule

10. The most common cause of intestinal obstruction in infants aged 6–18 months is:
A. Worms B. Bands
C. Intussusception D. Adhesions

11. Red currant jelly stools are characteristic of:
A. Worms B. Bands
C. Intussusception D. Adhesions

12. Dance's sign (signe de dance) is a feature of:
A. Worms B. Bands
C. Intussusception D. Adhesions

13. The investigation of choice in mesenteric vascular occlusion is:
A. Ultrasound abdomen
B. Plain X-ray abdomen
C. CT with or without angiogram
D. MRI

14. The most common cause of intestinal obstruction in neonates is:
A. Bands B. Duodenal atresia
C. Imperforate anus D. Meconium ileus

15. The most common congenital anomaly of small intestine is:
A. Bands B. Duodenal atresia
C. Stenosis D. Meckel's diverticulum

16. Features of paralytic ileus include the following *except*:
A. Gross abdominal distension
B. Pain abdomen
C. Failure to pass flatus
D. Tinkling sounds

17. Melanosis of lips and mucosa with intestinal obstruction should arouse the suspicion of:
A. Gardner's syndrome
B. Turcot's syndrome
C. Peutz-Jeghers syndrome
D. Down's syndrome

18. Which is the factor precipitate sigmoid volvulus?
A. Short colon
B. Broad attachment at the base
C. Empty colon
D. Long mesentery of the colon

19. Common factor precipitating sigmoid volvulus in patients with parkinsonism, multiple sclerosis, hypothyroidism is:
A. Diarrhoea
B. Constipation
C. Drugs
D. Long mesentery of the colon

20. Investigation of choice for detecting bleeding Meckel's diverticulum is:
A. CT scan B. Pet scan
C. MRI scan D. Technetium scan

21. Presence of intramural air is diagnostic of:
A. Gallstone ileus B. Sigmoid perforation
C. Duodenal atresia D. Intestinal gangrene

22. Following complications can occur after gastrojejunostomy *except*:
A. Dumping syndrome B. Intussusception
C. Volvulus D. Stomal ulcer

23. Following are the causes of adult intussusception *except*:
A. Meckel's diverticulum
B. Submucous lipoma
C. Carcinoma caecum
D. Hypertrophy of Peyer's patches

24. The most common anomaly associated with Hirschsprung's disease is:
A. Down's syndrome B. Hypothyroidism
C. Meckel's diverticulum D. Anorectal atresia

25. Following are causes of paralytic ileus *except*:
A. Anastomotic leak B. Retroperitoneal irritation
C. Hyperkalaemia D. Fracture spine

Answers

1. A	**2.** A	**3.** B	**4.** C	**5.** A	**6.** B	**7.** D	**8.** A	**9.** A	**10.** C
11. C	**12.** C	**13.** C	**14.** B	**15.** D	**16.** B	**17.** C	**18.** A	**19.** B	**20.** D
21. D	**22.** B	**23.** D	**24.** A	**25.** C					

CHAPTER

49

Rectum and Anal Canal

- Surgical anatomy
- Carcinoma rectum
- Prolapse rectum
- Surgical anatomy of anal canal
- Anorectal physiology
- Haemorrhoids
- Anorectal abscess
- Fistula *in ano*
- Fissure *in ano*
- VAAFT
- Pilonidal sinus
- Sacrococcygeal teratoma
- Malignant tumours of anal canal
- Stricture of anal canal and rectum
- Anal incontinence

Competency

SU28.16.1: Describe applied anatomy including congenital anomalies of the rectum and anal canal.

SURGICAL ANATOMY OF THE RECTUM

The rectum starts at the rectosigmoid junction, opposite the **third piece of sacrum**. It descends in the sacral hollow, passes through the pelvic floor, and ends in the anorectal junction, which is about 4 cm away from the anal verge. Anorectal junction is encircled by puborectalis muscle posteriorly and in the lateral aspects. **The rectum is 12–15 cm in length** (Key Box 49.1).

Key Box 49.1

Some Interesting Features of Rectum

1. Rectum means straight, but it is not
2. Coverings of the peritoneum are different at different levels.
3. Even though it is a part of the large intestine, taenia, appendices epiploicae and sacculations are absent.
4. Middle curve marks the anterior peritoneal reflection. It is about 12–15 cm above anus.
5. Rectal carcinoma has high recurrence rates because of lack of serosal layer and close relation to other pelvic viscera.
6. Principal route of lymphatic drainage is upwards towards para-aortic nodes.

Peritoneal Covering

- Upper one-third is **completely covered** by peritoneum (>11 cm from anal verge) (Figs 49.1 and 49.2).
- Middle one-third is **covered in front and lateral aspects** (6–11 cm).
- Lower one-third (0–6 cm) has **no extraperitoneal covering** but has two fascial condensation layers.

  Posteriorly, the strong **Waldeyer's** layer separates the rectum from lower sacral pieces and coccyx. At surgery, **stripping of this fascia results in uncontrollable bleeding from sacral plexus of veins,** which is underneath the Waldeyer's fascia.

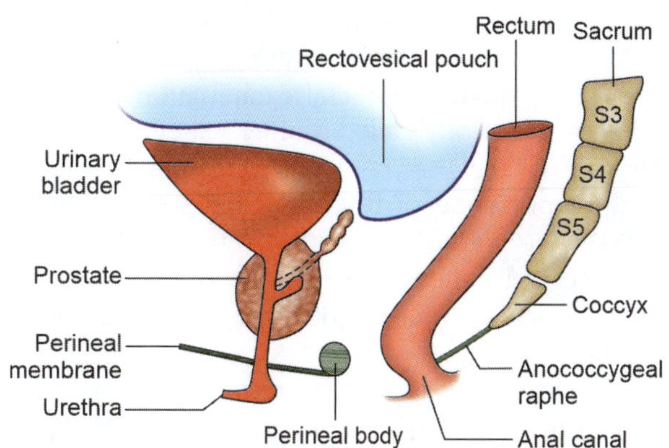

Fig. 49.1: Sagittal section through the male pelvis showing the location of the rectum and some of its anterior and posterior relations

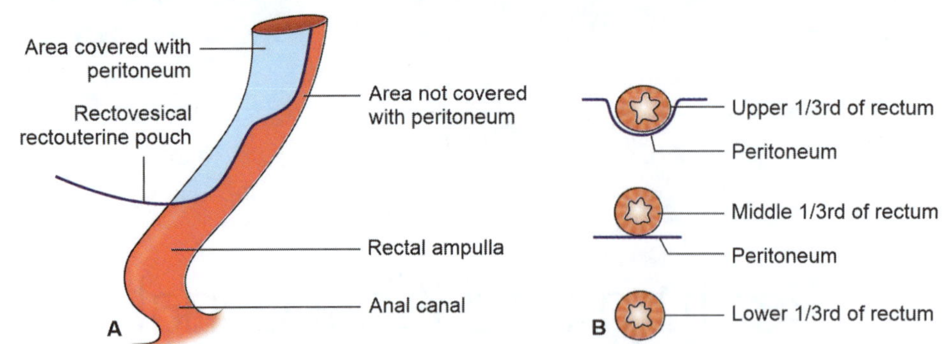

Figs 49.2A and B: Peritoneal relations of the rectum

- Anteriorly, the weak **Denonvilliers'** fascia separates the rectum from prostate and bladder. **Stripping of this fascia results in troublesome bleeding from prostatic venous plexus.**
- Rectum is attached to side wall of pelvis by **lateral ligaments**, which contain middle haemorrhoidal vessels. These need ligation or coagulation during mobilisation of lower rectum.
- **Valves of Houston:** Despite the name rectum means straight, it is **never straight in adults.** It has one convexity on the left and two convexities on the right side. There are 3 **valves of Houston** (prominent mucosal folds), two on the left and one on the right.
- That portion of the rectum resting on the pelvic floor is called **ampulla**—dilated portion of the mid-rectum.

Rectovesical pouch (Key Box 49.2)

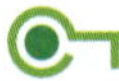 **Key Box 49.2**

Rectovesical Pouch—Rectouterine Pouch

- After investing the upper rectum, pelvic peritoneum is reflected anteriorly in males onto the urinary bladder, thus forming into rectovesical pouch. In females, it reflects onto uterus to form rectouterine pouch.
- It is one of the sites of transcoelomic spread of malignant cells.
- Malignant cells settle down in this most dependent part of the abdominal cavity and grow.
- They are palpable by rectal examination, a shelf-like finding—popularly called Blumer's shelf.
- Thus, if per rectal or per vaginal examination findings suggest presence of Blumer's shelf—it means hard deposits are felt and the case is inoperable.
- Rectovesical pouch is also the site of pelvic abscess.
- Pelvic abscess is diagnosed by per rectal or per vaginal examination.
- Pus can be drained through the rectum or posterior fornix.
- Aspiration of blood from rectovesical pouch through posterior fornix indicates intraperitoneal bleeding—may be ruptured ectopic.

Arterial Supply

1. **Superior haemorrhoidal artery** is a branch of the superior rectal artery which is the continuation of the inferior mesenteric artery. It divides into right and left branches. The right branch divides into anterior and posterior branches which supply the rectum (Fig. 49.3).
2. **Middle haemorrhoidal artery,** a branch of internal iliac artery, runs in the lateral ligament of the rectum.
3. **Inferior haemorrhoidal artery,** a branch of internal pudendal artery, supplies the lower rectum.

Venous Return (Fig. 49.4)

The rich submucous plexus of veins surrounding the ampulla forms external rectal plexus. The venous drainage from here flows in two directions.

1. **Upwards** to drain into **superior rectal veins.** These join inferior mesenteric veins, which in turn drain into the portal system.
2. **Across** to drain into middle rectal veins, which run in the lateral ligament of the rectum along with middle rectal artery. Hence, the lateral ligaments have to be ligated and divided during resection of rectum. These veins drain into internal iliac veins (systemic circulation). Hence, rectum is a site of portosystemic anastomosis.

Lymphatic Drainage of Rectum (Fig. 49.5)

- **Upper one-third of rectum** is completely enclosed by peritoneum and the **middle one-third of rectum** is covered in front and on the sides by peritoneum. From these areas, lymphatic drainage always occurs in the **upward direction,** first to **(A)** pararectal nodes of Gerota followed by superior haemorrhoidal nodes, middle haemorrhoidal nodes and nodes at the origin of inferior mesenteric artery.
- From **lower one-third of rectum**, lymphatics spread in the **lateral direction** and can involve **(B)** internal iliac nodes.

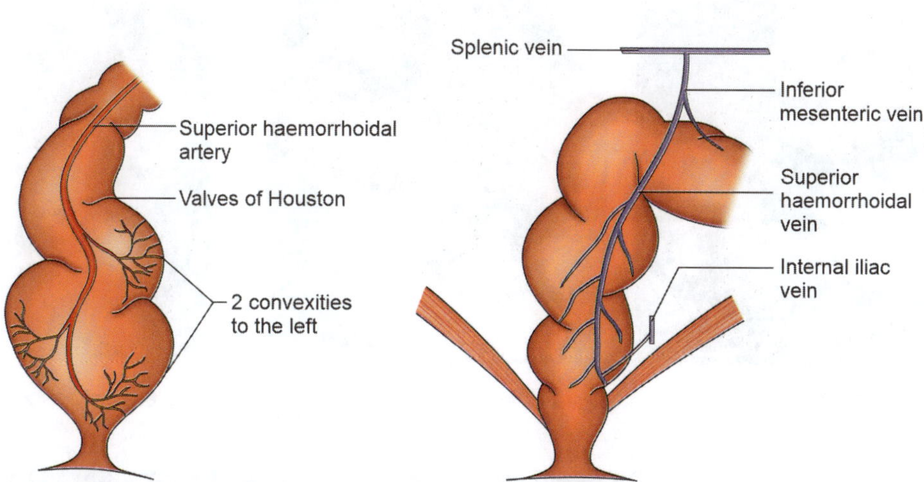

Fig. 49.3: Arterial supply of rectum

Fig. 49.4: Venous return

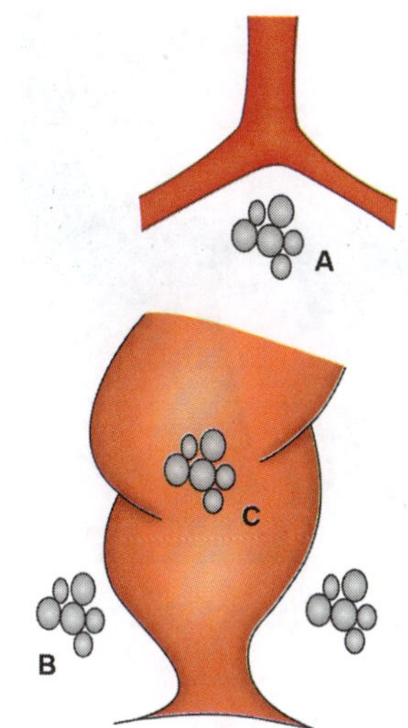

Fig. 49.5: Lymphatic drainage

- Lymph nodes are also present in the hollow of sacrum along median sacral artery **(C)**.

  Lymphatics are present in the muscularis mucosa.

Nerve Supply

- **Sympathetic:** The fibres come from hypogastric plexus, which is located at the aortic bifurcation at the level of L5. Injury to this can cause absence of erection or dry orgasm. Fibres also come along with inferior mesenteric artery and superior rectal artery.
- **Parasympathetic:** (S2, S3, S4) by means of nervi erigentes from the hypogastric plexus and supply motor fibres to detrusor. Pain and ability to distinguish flatus and faeces is because of these fibres. Loss of the rectal mucosa results in the loss of these sensations. During division of lateral ligaments or during anterior dissection of the bladder base, injury to nervi erigentes can occur.
- External anal sphincter and puborectalis are innervated by inferior rectal branches of internal pudendal nerve (somatic).

Please note: Congenital anomalies of rectum and anal canal are given on page 846.

Examination of Rectum and Anal Canal (Table 49.1)

Table 49.1 Examination of rectum and anal canal

Digital rectal examination (Fig. 49.6)	**Proctoscopy (Kelly's)** (Fig. 49.7)	**Flexible sigmoidoscopy** (Fig. 49.8)
• Lubricate the finger with lignocaine jelly • **Sim's position: Left lateral** is ideal position • Explain to the patient what you plan to do • Gently apply pressure on the external sphincter (anal opening) and slowly introduce the finger • Polyps, carcinomatous growths, strictures, thrombosed piles can be felt • Sphincter tone is poor in prolapse rectum and lumbosacral myelopathy.	• Do a per rectal examination and rule out painful condition (Fissure *in ano*) • Proctoscope with obturator is introduced to full length • Piles are seen bulging into lumen as **obturator is withdrawn** • Biopsy from growth can be taken • Piles can be injected with sclerosants • Pelvic abscess can also be drained	• Flexible sigmoidoscope is 60 cm long • An enema is given before the procedure • Growth, ulcers, bleeding diverticulae, polyps, colitis can be diagnosed and biopsy can be taken • Do not force instrument—it may perforate colon • It may deflate and derotate sigmoid volvulus—therapeutic use of sigmoidoscopy.

These are the common anal/perianal conditions which can be diagnosed by inspection (only), or palpation or per rectal examination/proctoscopic examination (Fig. 49.9).

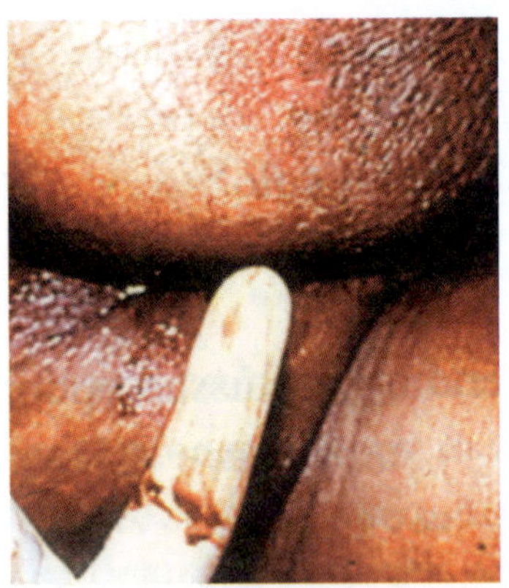

Fig. 49.6: Digital rectal examination

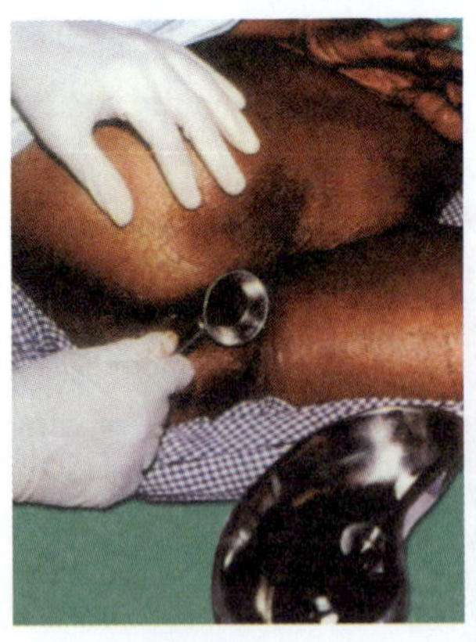

Fig. 49.7A: Proctoscopy

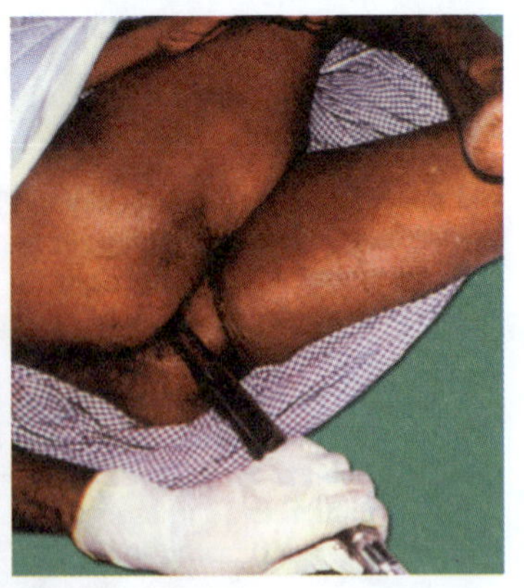

Fig. 49.7B: Rigid sigmoidoscopy

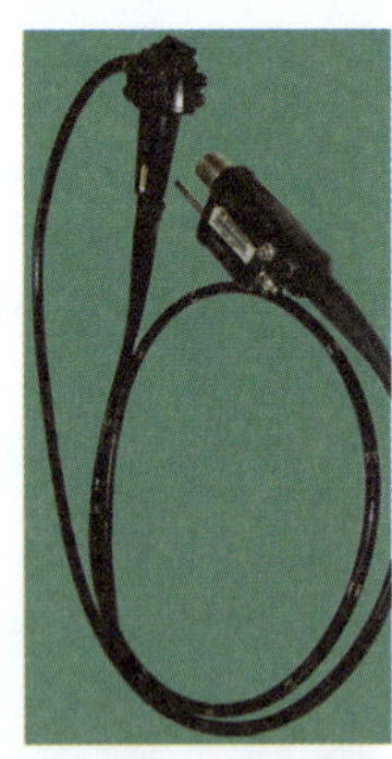

Fig. 49.8: Colonoscopy

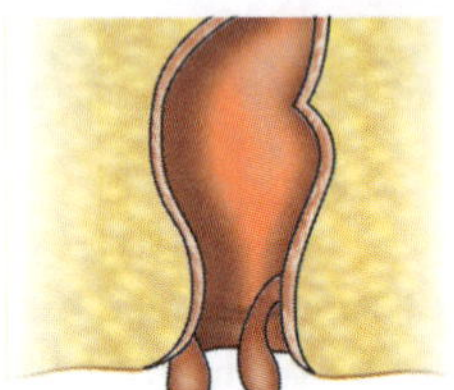

Haemorrhoids—painless

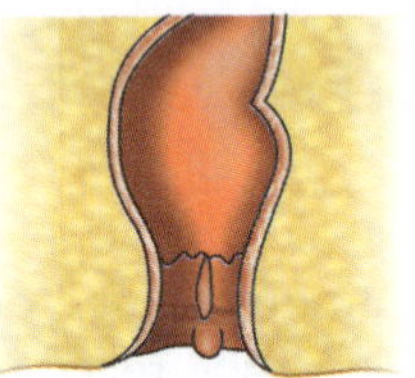

Anal fissure—painful

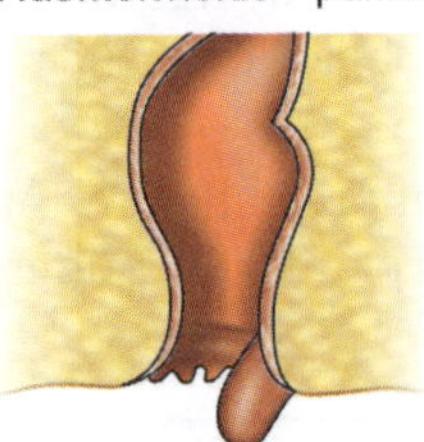

Thrombosed external haemorrhoids—painful

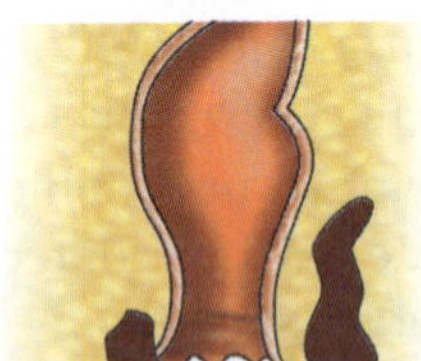

Perianal abscess—painful

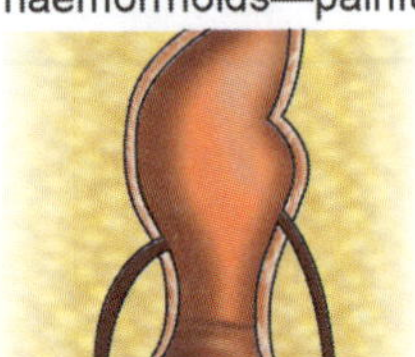

Fistula *in ano*—painless/painful

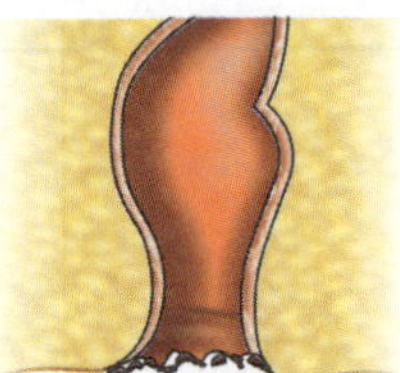

Perianal warts—painless

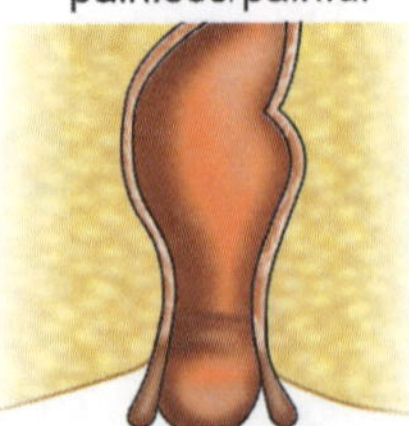

Rectal prolapse—painful/painless

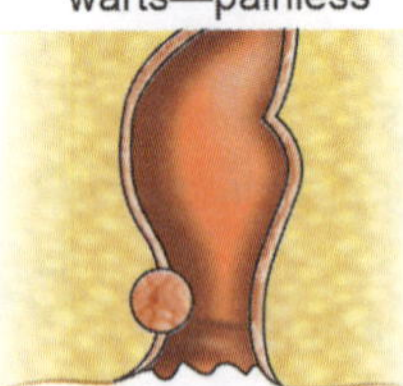

Carcinoma anal canal—painless

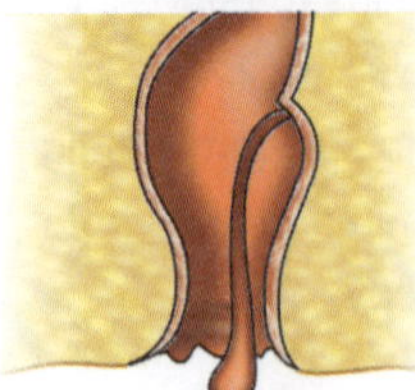

Pedunculated polyp—painless

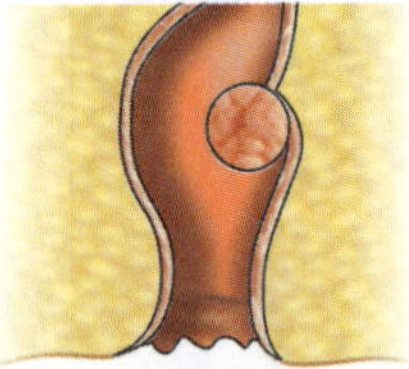

Carcinoma rectum—painless

Fig. 49.9: Common diseases of anorectum

CARCINOMA RECTUM

Competency

SU28.17.5: Describe pathology, clinical features, diagnosis and principles of treatment of carcinoma rectum.

Aetiopathogenesis: Similar to carcinoma colon events such as adenoma—dysplasia and carcinoma. However, a few precancerous conditions and risk factors are given as follows.

Precancerous Conditions

- Polyps in FAP, villous adenoma (*see* page 794)
- Ulcerative colitis (*see* page 763)
- Crohn's disease (*see* page 770)

Risk Factors

- Smoking: Smokers have 30 to 40% more likely to die of colorectal cancer.
- Obesity: Obesity and lack of exercises are associated with rectal cancers.
- Alcohol: Definite increase has been found in breast and colon cancers. Alcohol damages the cells and prevents repair of cells, thereby increases the risk of malignancy.
- Genetic: Familial adenomatous polyposis gene: In hereditary forms of colorectal cancers such as Lynch syndrome (page 796) **mutation** in one of the DNA mismatch repair genes is responsible.

Pathological Types

1. **Annular** variety is common at the **rectosigmoid** junction. It presents with constipation and intestinal obstruction. It takes about a year for the growth to completely encircle the lumen of the gut (napkin ring deformity) (Fig. 49.10).
2. **Polypoidal** lesions are common in the **ampulla** of the rectum (Fig. 49.11).

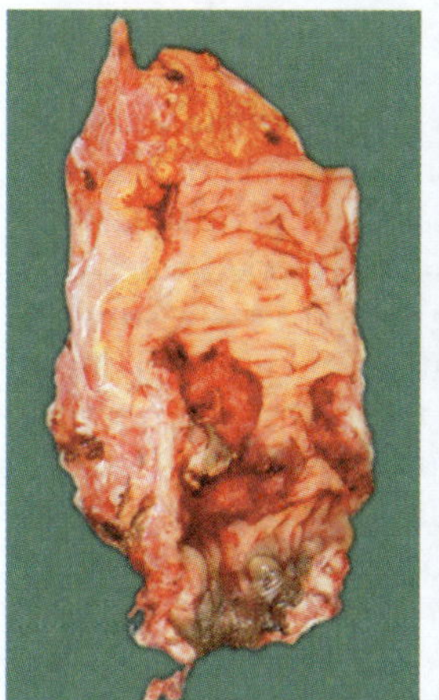
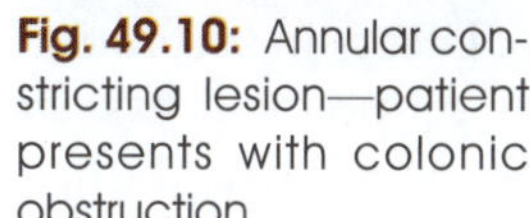

Fig. 49.10: Annular constricting lesion—patient presents with colonic obstruction

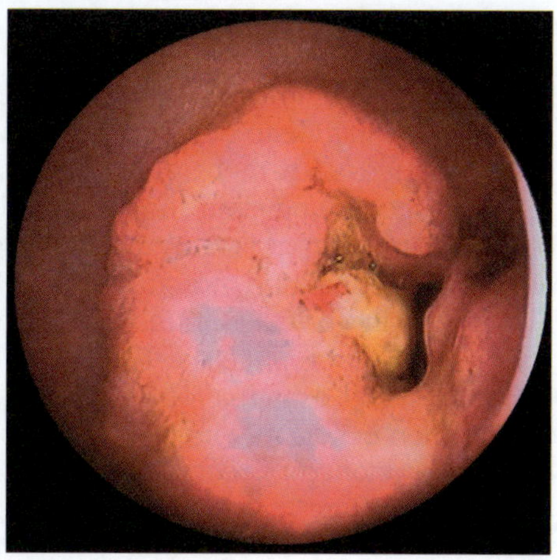

Fig. 49.11: Fibreoptic sigmoidoscopy showing growth in the upper rectum—biopsy proved signet ring carcinoma

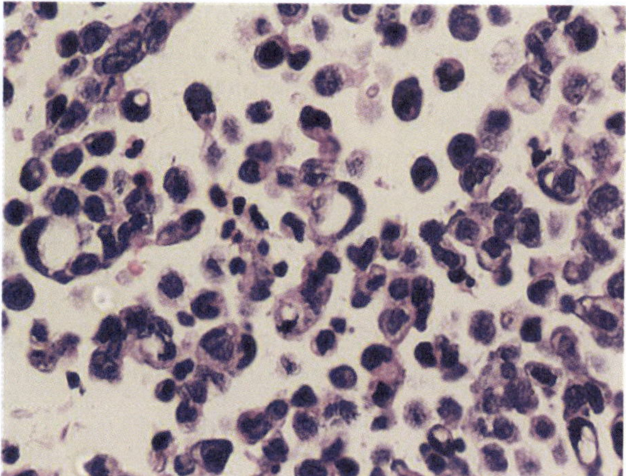

Fig. 49.12: Signet ring carcinoma colon—relatively poor prognosis (*Courtesy:* Dr Laxmi Rao, Head, Department of Pathology, KMC, Manipal)

3. **Ulcerative** lesions can occur anywhere in the rectum with **raised edges** and growth occurs in the transverse direction.
4. **Diffuse** variety is similar to linitis plastica. It develops from ulcerative colitis. It has a poor prognosis.
5. **Colloid** variety is rare. The tumour contents are **gelatinous** due to increased mucus production. This variety is seen in young patients. The cell is filled with mucus and nucleus is displaced. It is called **'signet ring' carcinoma**. It is associated with poor prognosis (Fig. 49.12).

Clinical Features of Carcinoma Rectum

- **Constipation** requiring increasing doses of purgatives due to annular growth at rectosigmoid junction. Always a sense of incomplete evacuation and altered bowel habits.
- **Bleeding per rectum,** frank blood or mixed with stools is common. It is painless, never massive and is the earliest symptom of carcinoma rectum. Very often, it is confused for haemorrhoids.
- **Early morning spurious diarrhoea** is due to accumulation of mucus overnight in the ampulla of rectum (dilated middle portion of rectum), which causes an urgency to pass stools but results in passage of only mucus with minimal stools. It is associated with a sense of incomplete defaecation.
- **Tenesmus**
  - **Painful, incomplete defaecation** associated with **bleeding** is called tenesmus.
  - This symptom is common with stricturous growths.
- **Bloody slime** (Key Box 49.3): An attempt at defaecation results in mucus mixed with blood.
- **Loss of appetite,** loss of weight due to **liver secondaries** (cancer cachexia) and abdominal distension due to obstruction are late features.

Key Box 49.3

Correlation of Symptoms to Carcinoma Rectum

Symptom	Probable site of lesion/explanation
Constipation	Rectosigmoid
Bleeding	Cauliflower-like growth
Tenesmus	Rectosigmoid stricture
Early morning spurious diarrhoea	Growth in the ampulla of rectum
Bloody slime	Blood and mucus
Sciatica-like pain	Sacral plexus infiltration
Abdominal distension	Large bowel obstruction
Loss of weight/ abdominal distension	Liver metastasis, ascites, etc.
Strangury	Infiltration of the bladder base anteriorly

ABCDEF of Rectal Carcinoma—Symptoms

1. **A**ltered bowel habits
2. **B**leeding per rectum and bloody slime—upper rectum.
3. **C**onstipation increasing—annular carcinoma at rectosigmoid junction.
4. Incomplete **d**efaecation
5. **E**arly morning spurious diarrhoea—midrectum
6. **F**atigue, weight loss

Clinical Examination

1. **Rectal examination:** In every patient with bleeding per rectum, rectal examination has to be done. More than 90% of cases of carcinoma rectum can be diagnosed by rectal examination. Always feel for the ulcer

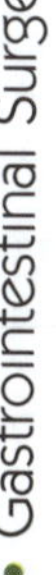

or growth, nodularity, induration, fixity to posterior sacrum, anterior bladder base and laterally to lateral ligaments. Look for the blood stains specially in ulcerative cases. It is also possible to feel the lymph nodes in the mesorectum in cases of lower third carcinomas.

2. **Vaginal examination:** When the growth is situated in the anterior wall of the rectum, accurate assessment of the growth can be done with one finger in the rectum and the other in the vagina. Large Krukenberg tumours, if present, can also be felt by vaginal and rectal examinations.
3. **Evidence of metastasis:** Palpable nodular liver, paraaortic lymph nodes, ascites and enlarged left supraclavicular nodes **(Troisier's sign).**

Pearls of Wisdom

Rectal cancer presenting as fistula *in ano* is the equivalent to a perforated colonic cancer. It is a bad prognostic sign.

Histology: They are adenocarcinomas—well differentiated, moderately differentiated and poorly differentiated. However, a few special types of adenocarcinomas are colloid carcinoma rectum and signet ring carcinoma. In colloid carcinoma, colloid-like substance is produced which can be detected macroscopically. Signet cell cancer is **a rare (less than 1%) type of cancer that starts in glandular cells.**

Signet ring carcinoma and colloid carcinoma carry poor prognosis.

Differential Diagnosis (Key Box 49.4)

1. **Villous adenomas (benign)** present as bleeding per rectum with occasionally mass per rectum. They have a frond-like appearance. They are very friable, bulky and easily bleed on touch. Biopsy is a must. If it is benign, it can be removed through the rectum—submucosally.
2. **Proctitis due to inflammatory bowel diseases:** Both ulcerative colitis and Crohn's disease produce diarrhoea, blood in the stools and multiple non-indurated ulcers. Regardless biopsy is a must before doing a major surgical resection. Ulcers in ulcerative colitis are typically described as pinpoint ulcers. In Crohn's, they are fissure type or patchy with a cobblestone appearance.
3. **Amoebic granuloma:** It is not common nowadays. It presents with a soft mass at rectosigmoid junction with or without obstruction. An ulcer over the surface will mimic carcinoma. Biopsy is mandatory because amoebomas are completely curable with antiamoebic treatment.
4. **Tuberculous proctitis:** Usually patients have pulmonary tuberculosis. Submucosal abscess ruptures and results in ulcers with undermined edges. Hypertrophic tuberculosis with stricture can also occur. Biopsy is mandatory before resection.
5. **Endometrioma:** It presents as constipation, bleeding per rectum especially during menstruation. Typically young females between the age of 20 and 40 years are affected. It produces a constricting lesion in the rectosigmoid junction. Mucosa is intact as seen by sigmoidoscopy. Treatment is biopsy followed by treatment of endometriosis.
6. **Solitary rectal ulcer syndrome (SRUS)**
   - **Site:** Commonly occurs in the anterior wall of lower rectum, an area of mucosal change.
   - **Mucosa:** It is erythematous, heaped up and bleeds on touch.
   - It is a single, depressed ulcer.
   - The cause, even though not clear, is probably due to trauma by anal digitation. Today, it is believed that it is due to **internal intussusception** or **anterior wall prolapse.**
   - **Clinical features are** passage of blood and mucus in stools. Mucosal prolapse may also be a feature.
   - A biopsy must be done to rule out carcinoma rectum.
   - **Treatment is conservative:** Avoidance of constipation and straining may treat the prolapse.

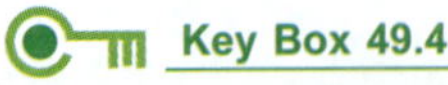
Key Box 49.4

Rectal Ulcers

1. Carcinoma rectum
2. Amoebic ulcers
3. Ulcerative colitis
4. HIV infection
5. Solitary rectal ulcers
6. Radiation proctitis

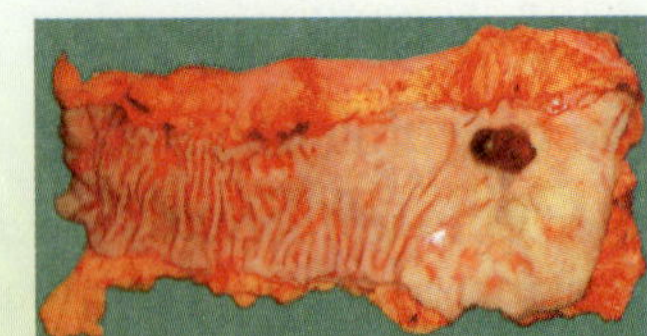
Fig. 49.13: Solitary rectal ulcers

Clinical Notes

A 22-year-old girl was treated with iron tablets for anaemia due to occasional bleeding per rectum. She was treated with metronidazole because she was passing mucus along with the stools. She developed intestinal obstruction after 6 months during which time a surgeon was consulted. Rectal examination revealed a large growth, fixed all around. She died 6 months later because of advanced disease. The case illustrates the importance of rectal examination and that carcinoma of the rectum often occurs in young patients also. Again to highlight the importance of rectal examination in a case of bleeding per rectum.

Spread of Carcinoma Rectum

1. **Local spread**
   - **It takes 18 months** for a growth to encircle the rectal lumen as in annular strictures at the recto-sigmoid junction.
   - Then, it involves muscle coat and spreads into extrarectal tissues.
   - **Anteriorly,** it involves **prostate, seminal vesicles and bladder** base in males, vagina and uterus in females.
   - **Posteriorly, sacral plexus** gets involved in late cases and causes sciatica-like pain. Posterior sacral infiltration and anterior bladder base infiltration—surgery can be very difficult and dangerous (uncontrollable bleeding from sacral plexus of veins and prostatic plexus of veins in males. Hence, preoperative chemoradiotherapy followed by surgery is done.
   - Involvement of mesorectum carries poor prognosis. Hence, the **circumferential resected margin** is important.
2. **Lymphatic spread**—chief nodes are para-aortic nodes.
3. **Haematogenous spread:** It results in secondaries in the liver, lungs, etc. It is common in young patients with anaplastic variety and in colloid carcinoma.
4. **Peritoneal spread:** It results in ascites, carcinomatous nodules over the peritoneum, etc.

STAGING

Competency

SU28.17.2: Describe investigations for diseases of the rectum including those used for staging of carcinoma rectum.

I. Modified Dukes' Staging of Carcinoma of Rectum (Fig. 49.14)

Stages

A. Growth confined to the rectal wall
B. Growth involving perirectal pad of fat and tissues. No nodes are involved.
   B1: Invading muscularis mucosa
   B2: Invading to or through serosa

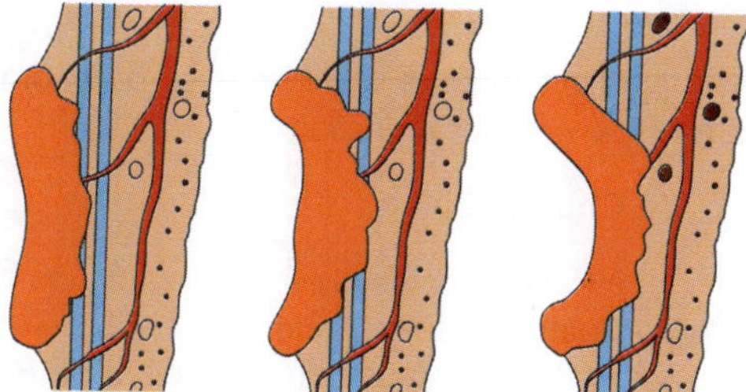

Fig. 49.14: The three cardinal stages of progression of the neoplasm

C. Nodes are involved
   C1: Local lymph nodes—pararectal
   C2: Distal lymph nodes—along the course of blood vessels
D. Distant spread—liver, lungs, etc.

II. Astler-Coller Modification of Dukes' System

Stages

A Limited to mucosa—no nodes
B1 Extension into muscularis propria—no nodes
B2 Extension into entire bowel wall—no nodes
B3 Extension into adjacent organs—no nodes
C1 Extension into muscularis propria—positive nodes
C2 B2 + Lymph nodes
C3 B3 + Lymph nodes
D Distant metastasis

Prognosis as per Dukes' Staging

- Dukes' A: 5-year survival is 90 to 100%.
- Dukes' B: 5-year survival is 50 to 80%.
- Dukes' C: 5-year survival is less than 50%.

III. TNM Staging

TNM STAGING

T	**Primary Tumour**
TX	Primary tumour cannot be assessed
T0	No evidence of primary tumour
Tis	Carcinoma *in situ*: Intramucosal carcinoma (involvement of lamina propria with no extension through muscularis mucosae)
T1	Tumour invades the submucosa (through the muscularis mucosa but not into the muscularis propria)
T2	Tumour invades the muscularis propria
T3	Tumour invades through the muscularis propria into pericolorectal tissues
T4	Tumour invades the visceral peritoneum or invades or adheres to adjacent organ or structure.
T4a	Tumour invades through the visceral peritoneum (including gross perforation of the bowel through tumour and continuous invasion of tumour through areas of inflammation to the surface of the visceral peritoneum)
T4b	Tumour directly invades or adheres to adjacent organs or structures
N	**Regional Lymph Nodes**
NX	Regional lymph nodes cannot be assessed
N0	No regional lymph node metastasis
N1	One to three regional lymph nodes are positive (tumour in lymph nodes measuring ≥0.2 mm), or any number of tumour deposits are present and all identifiable lymph nodes are negative
N1a	One regional lymph node is positive
N1b	Two or three regional lymph nodes are positive

(Contd...)

N1c No regional lymph nodes are positive, but there are tumour deposits in the subserosa, mesentery or non-peritonealized pericolic, or perirectal/mesorectal tissues
N2 Four or more regional lymph nodes are positive
N2a Four to six regional lymph nodes are positive
N2b Seven or more regional lymph nodes are positive

M Distant Metastasis
M0 No distant metastasis by imaging, etc.; no evidence of tumour in distant sites or organs
M1 Metastasis to one or more distant sites or organs or peritoneal metastasis is identified
M1a Metastasis to one site or organ is identified without peritoneal metastasis
M1b Metastasis to two or more sites or organs is identified without peritoneal metastasis
M1c Metastasis to the peritoneal surface is identified alone or with other site or organ metastases

- T1s: Does not penetrate muscularis mucosa
- T1s: Intraepithelial carcinoma—but this term is not used.
- pT4a: It should not be used for non-peritonised portion of large bowel such as ascending and descending colon, lower rectum.
- Minimum of 12 nodes should be removed. If less number of lymph nodes are removed, even if they are negative, these patients should receive chemotherapy.
- M1a: Multiple metastasis in an organ, even paired organs (ovaries lungs) M1a disease
- Stage grouping: **Stage I:** T1 or T2 N0 M0, **Stage IIA:** T3 N0 M0, **Stage IIB:** T4 N0 M0, **Stage IIIA:** T1 N2a M0, T3 or T4a N1/N1c M0, **Stage IIIB:** T2 or T3 N2a M0, T1 or T2 N2b M0, **Stage IIIC:** T3 or T4a N2b M0, T4b N1 or N2 M0, **Stage IV:** Any metastasis.

Investigations (Table 49.2)

1. **Proctoscopy:** It should be done in all cases of bleeding per rectum. It is done as an outpatient procedure. The left lateral position with buttocks elevated on a small pillow is the ideal position for proctoscopy. However, knee-elbow position can also be used. The growth appears as an ulcer with everted edges. A biopsy is taken to confirm the diagnosis. The histological grading of the tumour is as follows:
   A. ***Well-differentiated carcinoma:*** Low-grade variety (10–15%).
   B. ***Moderately differentiated carcinoma:*** The most common variety (65%).
   C. ***Undifferentiated carcinoma:*** The most aggressive variety (20–25%).
2. **Sigmoidoscopy:** To take a biopsy from rectosigmoid growths, sigmoidoscopy is essential.
3. **Colonoscopy:** **To detect any** synchronous carcinoma. It can be present in about 8 to 10% of patients. It can also detect adenomas, polyps. Biopsy should be taken in all suspicious lesions.
4. **CEA:** Increased levels of carcinoembryonic antigen indicates metastasis.
5. **Ultrasound of the abdomen:** **It is done to know the** metastasis such as secondaries in the liver, ascites with para-aortic nodes, etc. Colloid carcinoma rectum is one of the types which can present as metastasis.
6. **Endorectal ultrasonography (EUS)** (Key Box 49.5)
   Endoscopic ultrasound staging of rectal tumours
   UT1 Invasion confined to the mucosa and submucosa
   UT2 Penetration of the muscularis propria but not through the mesorectal fat
   UT3 Invasion into the perirectal fat
   UT4 Invasion into the adjacent organ
   UN0 No enlargement of lymph nodes
   UN1 Perirectal lymph nodes enlarged

Key Box 49.5

EUS

- It is also called **T**rans **R**ectal **U**ltra **S**onography (**TRUS**)
- To know the level of penetration
- Detect perirectal lymph node enlargement
- Invasion of adjacent structures—levator ani, bony pelvis, etc.
- It is superior in T-staging of rectal cancers.

7. **CECT scan: Contrast enhanced computed tomography**
   - It helps to detect the lesion, to know the extension of the tumour thus able to detect T staging.
   - To know the fixation to adjacent structures (ureter, uterus, bladder base, etc. hydronephrosis).
   - Importantly, to know nodal status
   - Detect metastasis in liver.
8. **MRI:** Both MRI and EUS are good for assessment of T-staging. MRI has the following advantages
   - It is better for T3 and T4 stages.

Table 49.2 Importance of each investigation and how it alters the treatment plan in a case of biopsy-proven carcinoma rectum. APR—abdominoperineal resection, HAR, LAR—high and low anterior resection

	Plan	Investigation finding	Changed plan
1. Carcinoma lower rectum	APR	CT—metastasis in liver	Palliative colostomy/chemoradiation
2. Carcinoma upper rectum	HAR	Colonoscopy growth in transverse colon	Subtotal/total colectomy
3. Carcinoma lower rectum	APR	MRI/endosono-extensive T4 lesion	First chemoradiation followed by APR or LAR
4. Carcinoma rectum	LAR	CT scan—hydronephrosis	Cystoscopy—ureteric stenting—LAR
5. Carcinoma lower rectum	APR	PET scan—bone metastasis present	No APR, colostomy

- High resolution MRI is better for assessment of circumferential resected margin (CRM).
- It is also good for lymph nodal staging and phased array MRI can pick up small nodes.

TREATMENT PRINCIPLES

1. Aim is to have a **curative resection.**
2. **Palliative resection** is worth doing even in the presence of metastasis, when there is obstruction.
3. Even though surgical treatment is the main modality, **radiotherapy and chemotherapy** are beneficial.
4. **At surgery, ligation of vascular pedicle is done first to prevent tumour embolisation.**
5. **Ligation of bowel,** proximal and distal to the tumour helps to prevent transluminal dissemination.
6. **Distal surgical margin should be about 2 cm.** Proximal margin—minimum 5 cm.
7. Radical surgery is described as **total mesorectal excision (TME)**—which improves quality of life (*see* Ten commandments and Key Box 49.6).
8. A double-stapled anastomosis as described or a hand-sewn anastomosis is then performed. A diverting loop ileostomy is used routinely for these ultra low anastomoses.

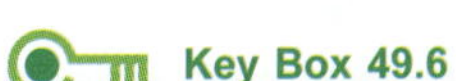

Key Box 49.6

Total Mesorectal Excision—Advantages

1. Mesorectum is the perirectal fat surrounding the rectum.
2. It preserves autonomic nerves
3. Impotence, urinary incontinence and retrograde ejaculation are lesser after TME.

TEN COMMANDMENTS OF TOTAL MESORECTAL EXCISION

1. Should perform TME in all cases of mid and lower carcinoma rectum
2. Should excise the entire mesorectum (contains fat, lymph nodes and superior rectal blood vessels)
3. Should perform the dissection with electrocautery or scissors
4. Should open the posterior plane between visceral and parietal layers of endopelvic fascia—**holy plane of Heald or avascular plane** (refer to Figs 49.15A to D)
5. Should exert good traction and countertraction to develop the planes
6. Should excise the entire mesorectum circumferentially—minimum of 5 cm of the CRM
7. Should be inside the pelvic plexus laterally
8. Should excise Denonvilliers' fascia anteriorly
9. Should excise rectosacral ligament so as to reach the pelvic floor
10. Should perform proximal diversion ileostomy.

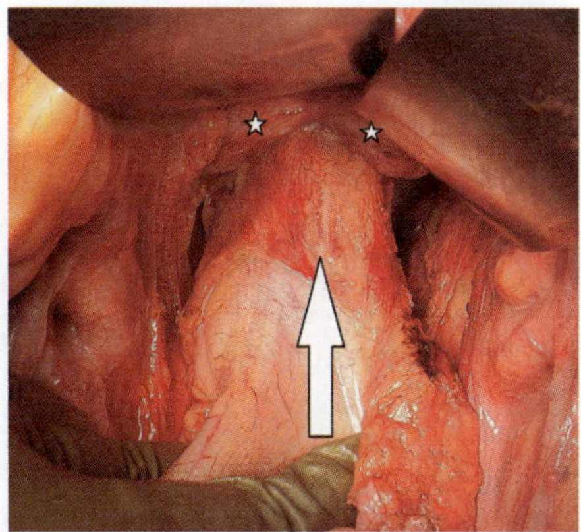

Fig. 49.15A: Anterior TME (holy plane) plane in male patient. Star (☆) indicates right and left seminal vesicles. Arrow points mesorectum covered by Denonvilliers' fascia

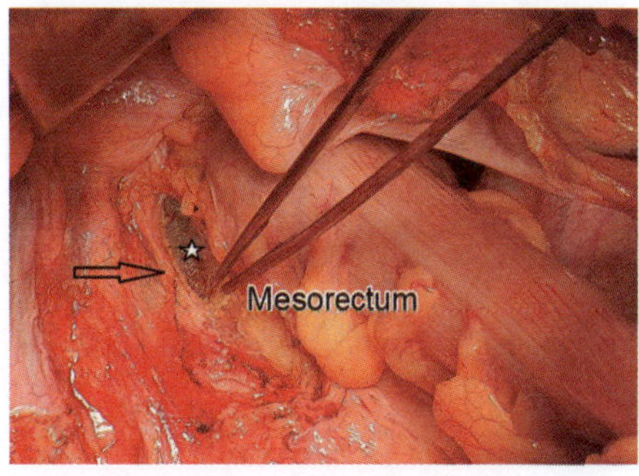

Fig. 49.15B: Left lateral dissection between lateral aspect of pelvic fascia and mesorectum. Arrow points to pelvic nerves. Forceps show plane of dissection. Star (☆) indicates exact holy (TME) plane where dissection is to be done

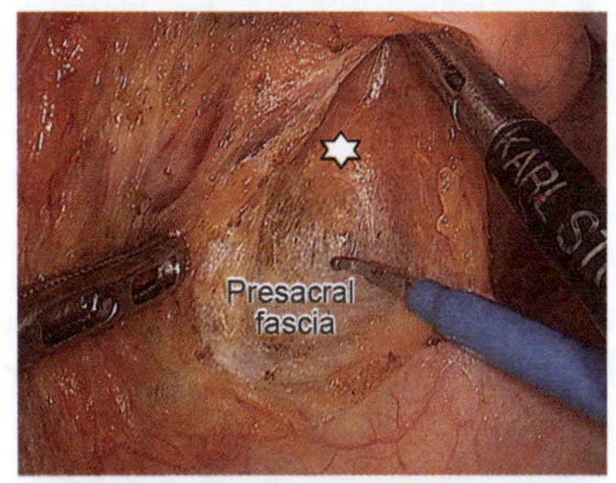

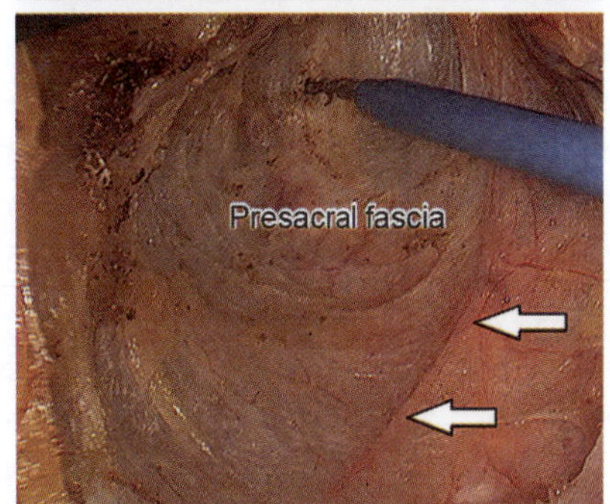

Fig. 49.15C: Posterior TME (holy) plane between presacral (Waldeyer's) fascia and mesorectum.
Arrows point pelvic nerves covered by pelvic fascia. Star (☆) indicates mesorectum with all lymph nodes

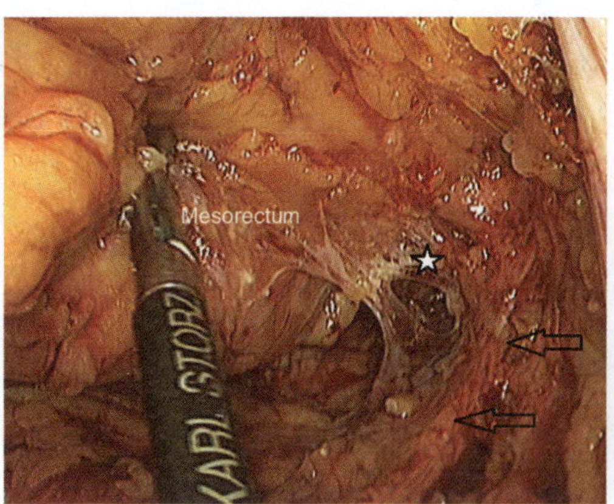

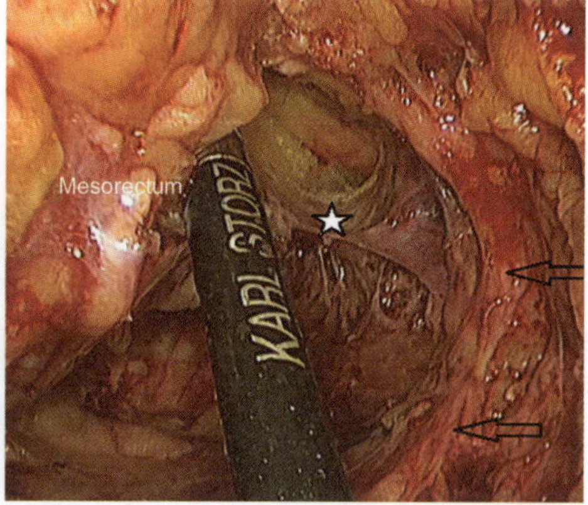

Fig. 49.15D: Right lateral dissection between mesorectum and pelvic fascia covering pelvic nerves. Arrow points to fascia covering pelvic nerves. Star (☆) indicates exact plane of dissection (*Courtesy:* Figs 49.15A to D, Dr Vipin Goel, Basavatarakam Indo-American Cancer Hospital and Research Institute, Hyderabad)

9. **Colonic pouch:** The splenic flexure is mobilised first. A 6 cm limb of sigmoid or descending colon is folded and a pouch is created. A colotomy is made at the apex of the pouch. Linear cutter is used to staple the pouch on itself to create a common lumen. A second fire of the stapler may be necessary. This pouch now acts like a neo-rectum.

LAPAROSCOPIC MESORECTAL EXCISION

Introduction

Laparoscopic anterior resection and total mesorectal excision are well-established procedures now. It is possible because of advances in the laparoscopic instruments, high definition cameras and improved technology.

Advantages

- A 30° camera allows a beautiful magnified view of the entire dissecting field specially low down in the pelvis. Thus, no part of the laparoscopic procedure is blind.
- Laparoscopic surgery allows the surgeon to adopt the principle of no touch technique. At the same time with better visualisation of the rectum and meso-rectum all around, it permits a good dissection.
- It is not uncommon in the open method that the specimen gets torn due to traction. It has been proved that this tearing is much less in laparoscopy.
- Recovery is very fast after laparoscopy.
- Better preservation of the pelvic autonomic nerves, low anastomotic leak and low mortality rates.
- For laparoscopic low resections, one needs not mobilise splenic flexure but sigmoid can be used for anastomosis.
- Wound infection, paralytic ileus are much less after laparoscopic surgery than open surgery.

Disadvantages

- **Very low resection**—because of the limited space and the lack of proper curved instruments—open method has a slight advantage.
- **Port site recurrence:** Local tissue trauma due to trocars, tumour manipulation, tumour behaviour are the factors responsible for port site recurrence. Tumour spillage, tumour cell aerosolisation due to sudden loss of pneumoperitoneum, tumour spillage during extraction and immunosuppression during pneumoperitoneum are a few factors responsible for port site recurrence. This can be minimised by using bag for extraction, minimal handling of the tumour and avoiding tearing of the specimen.

DIFFERENT TYPES OF SURGERIES FOR CARCINOMA RECTUM

Carcinoma Upper One-third of Rectum (Fig. 49.16)

High anterior resection, which includes removal of growth along with the nodes, followed by colorectal anastomosis is the treatment of choice. This is the operation of choice when the growth is situated between **11 and 15 cm** from the anal verge. The lymphatic spread from upper one-third is always in the upward direction. Hence, the sphincter is saved. If the bowel is well prepared, protective colostomy is not necessary (sphincter-saving surgery). Stapler anastomosis is popular as there is a lesser incidence of leak.

Carcinoma Lower One-third of Rectum (Figs 49.17 to 49.19)

This refers to growth within 4 cm from the anal verge. Two types of surgery can be done depending upon the

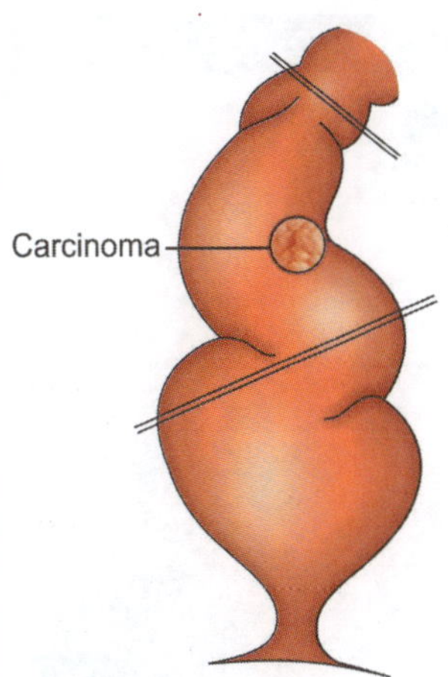

Fig. 49.16: Carcinoma upper rectum

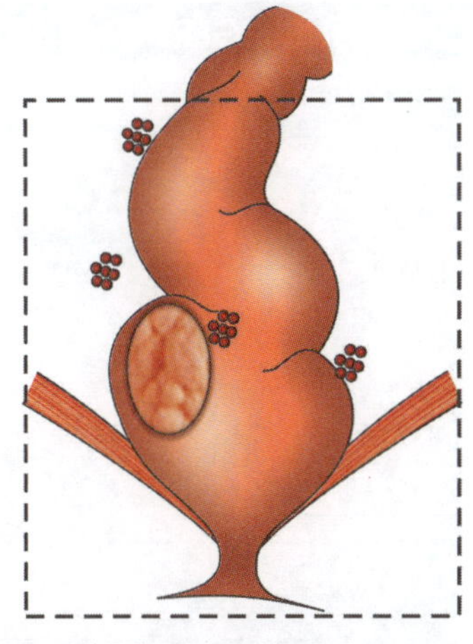

Fig. 49.17: The field of clearance in APR

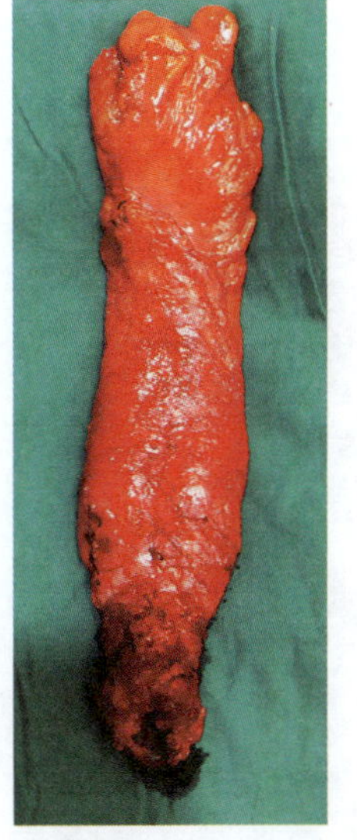

Fig. 49.18A: APR specimen showing appearance of baby bottom (*Courtesy*: Dr SS Parsad, Dr Rajendra, Dr Vijendra, Department of Surgery, KMC, Manipal)

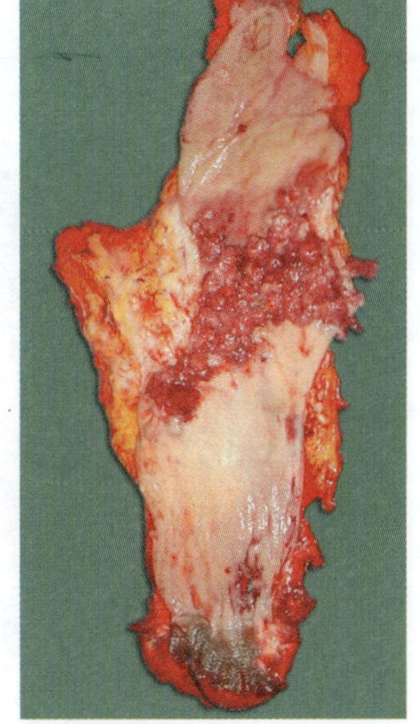

Fig. 49.18B: Nodular lesion 3 cm away from the anal verge buttock. (*Courtesy*: Dr Dinesh B, Dr Sunilkrishna, Department of Surgery, KMC, Manipal)

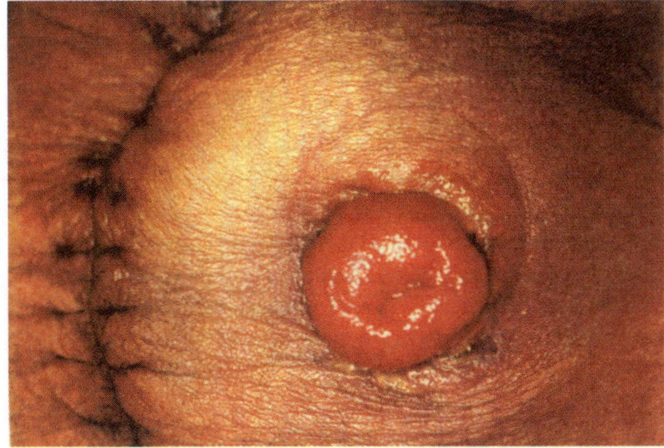

Fig. 49.19: Permanent end-colostomy following APR

degree of involvement of the growth with adjacent and surrounding tissues. When the sphincter is involved, **abdominoperineal resection** (APR) is done. In early cases, local excision can be done. In patients with low rectal cancers—T3 and T4 lesions, chemoradiation is given before surgery. This method is also followed when sphincter is involved. This is called preoperative chemotherapy. Inoperable lesions may become operable, and, in a few patients, it is possible to save the sphincter. Details are given later.

A. **Radical surgery** is called **abdominoperineal resection** (APR) or Miles-Walker operation (Key Box 49.7). The patient is put in Lloyd-Davies position (supine with lithotomy). Two surgeons operate simultaneously, one from the abdomen and one from the perineum. Abdomen is opened first and the growth is mobilised from the sacrum and urinary bladder. At this stage, anus is closed by a perineal surgeon. Rectum and anal canal are mobilised. The entire specimen of rectum, anal canal and lymph nodes are removed followed by ***permanent endcolostomy*** by bringing the sigmoid colon outside in the left iliac fossa (sphincter sacrificing surgery).

Key Box 49.7

Structures Removed in APR

- Growth with entire rectum and anal canal.
- Fascia propria with pararectal nodes.
- Two-thirds of the sigmoid colon and mesocolon with lymphatics and lymph nodes.
- Muscles and peritoneum of pelvic floor.
- Wide area of perianal skin, with part of ischiorectal fossa.

B. **Local excision:** In our country, 95% of low rectal cancers are offered and treated with abdominoperineal resection. Very small percentage of patients may be considered for local treatment—**local excision** (Key Box 49.8). This can be done only in selected group of patients.

Key Box 49.8

Local Excision of Carcinoma Rectum

- Mobile tumours less than 4 cm in diameter
- Less than 40% of rectal wall involvement
- Located within 6 cm of anal verge
- Lesion should be T1 or T2 with node negative status
- No vascular or lymphatic invasion
- No nodal involvement—preoperative MRI or EUS.
- Well/moderately differentiated

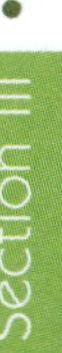

VARIOUS PHOTOGRAPHS OF CARCINOMA RECTUM AT SURGERY (Figs 49.20 to 49.24C)

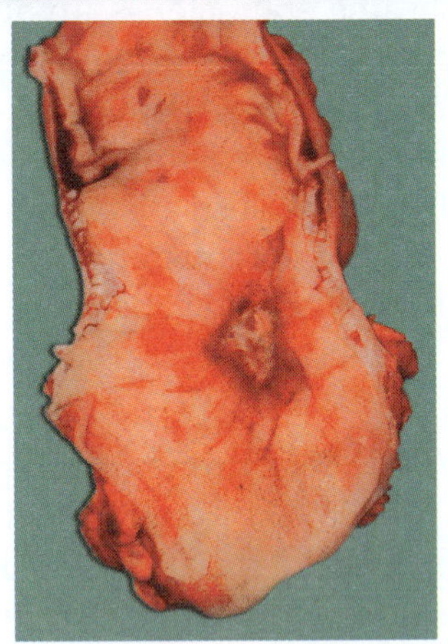

Fig. 49.20: This patient with carcinoma midrectum presented with bleeding per rectum. Low anterior resection was done. At least 3 cm margin could be achieved distally

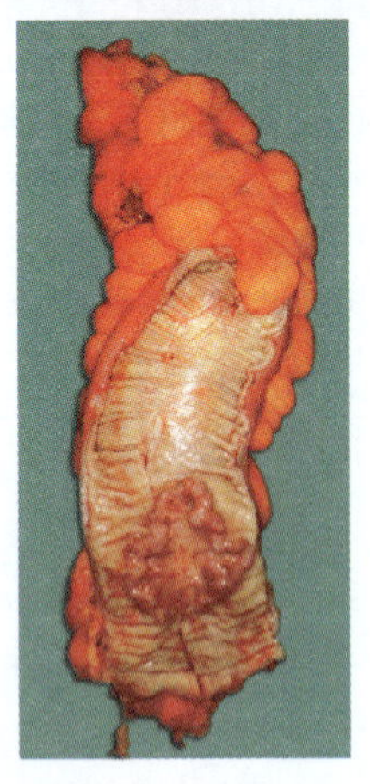

Fig. 49.21: Low anterior resection—see the lower margin

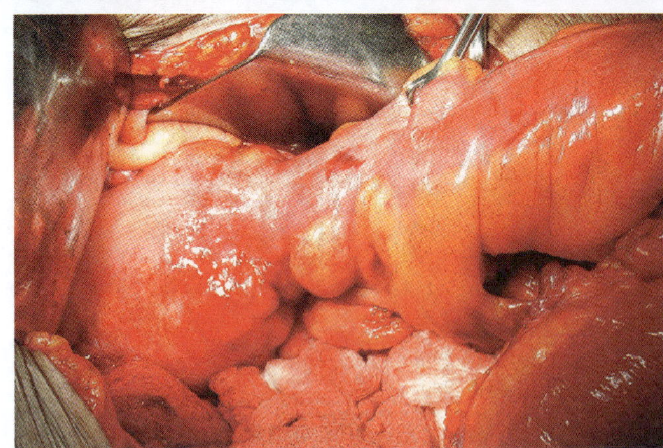

Fig. 49.22A: Low anterior resection is in progress. The rectum has been mobilised from urinary bladder anteriorly and sacrum posteriorly—carcinoma midrectum

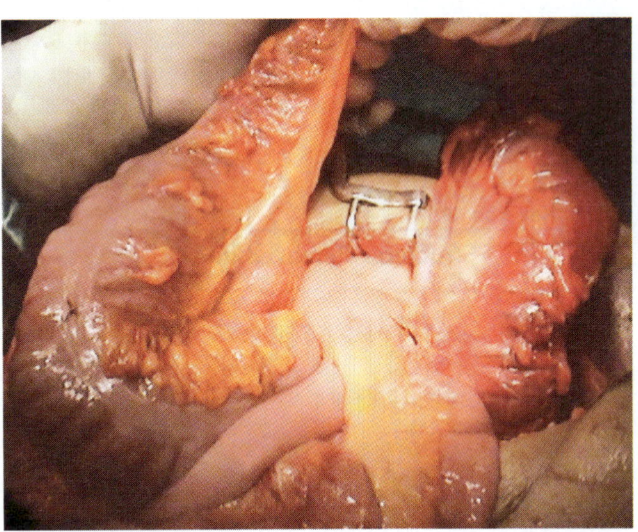

Fig. 49.22B: Proximal colon is mobilised up to the transverse colon so that it can be easily brought down without tension

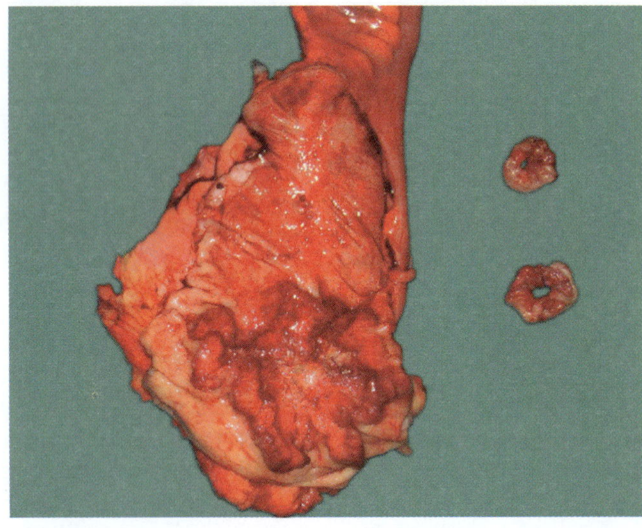

Fig. 49.23: Low anterior resection specimen—Stapler anastomosis has been done—you can see the complete doughnuts

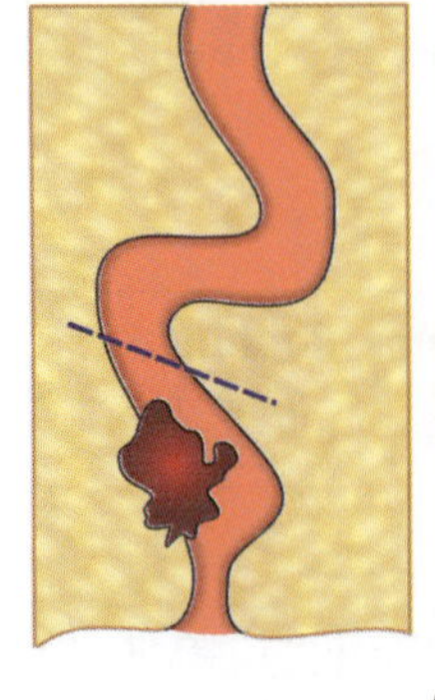

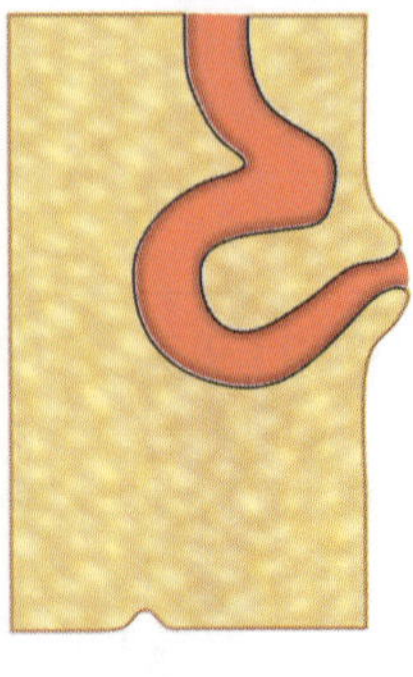

A

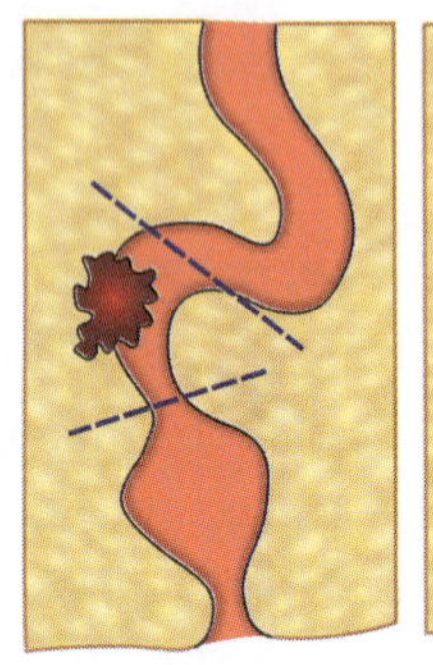

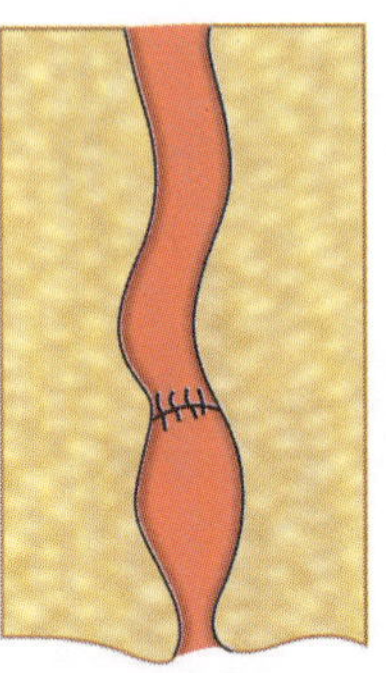

B

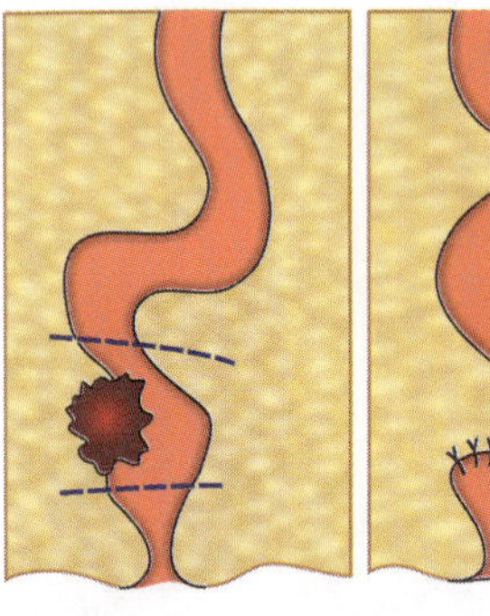

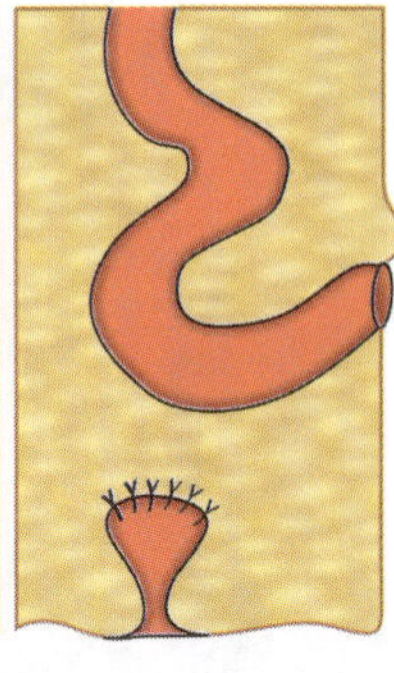

C

Figs 49.24A to C: Schematic representations of resection of the rectum. (A) AP resection followed by colostomy, (B) High anterior resection followed by anastomosis, (C) Low anterior resection with colostomy and closure of rectal stump—Hartmann's procedure—in large bowel obstruction. The colostomy is closed and colorectal anastomosis is done after 4 weeks

C. Ultra-low resection: *Low anterior resection and ultra-low resection*

- In female pelvis, broad pelvis, and even in thin males, a tumour measured at 5 cm by rigid proctoscopy, at surgery often may be moved to 8 cm from the dentate line, thus growth can be resected with a good margin and low resection can be done.
- Now with availability of the staplers, if one can give a 2 cm distal margin, ultra-low resection can be done followed by stapler anastomosis.
- Stapler anastomosis is the choice for low and ultra-low resections. A 30-, 45-, or 60-mm linear stapler is used. The bowel is clamped and transected just proximal to this point (Figs 49.25 to 49.27D).

  A diverting loop ileostomy is done in any low anastomoses (<5 cm) from the dentate line, which are associated with anastomotic leak rates of up to 17%. Other risk factors for anastomotic leak include a history of radiation, malnutrition, elderly patients undergoing preoperative combined-modality therapy with planned postoperative chemotherapy.

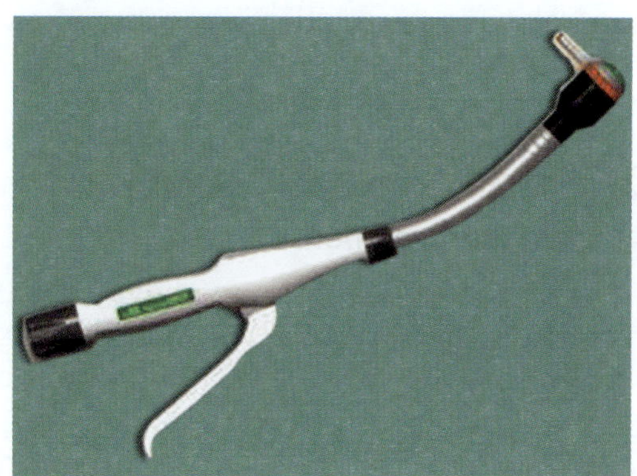

Fig. 49.25: Circular stapler used for anterior resection

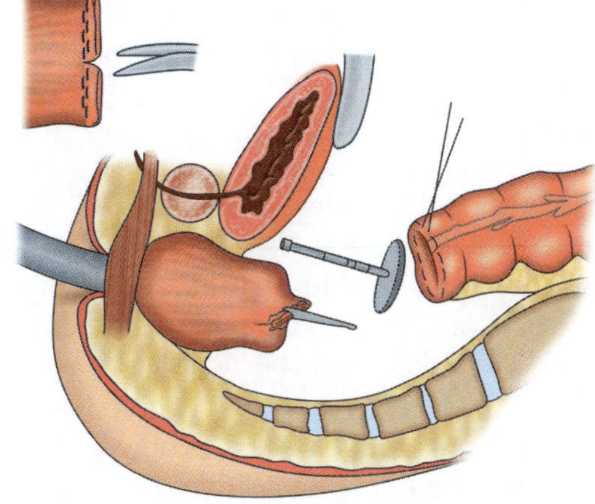

Fig. 49.26: Diagrammatic representation of anterior resection and use of staplers.

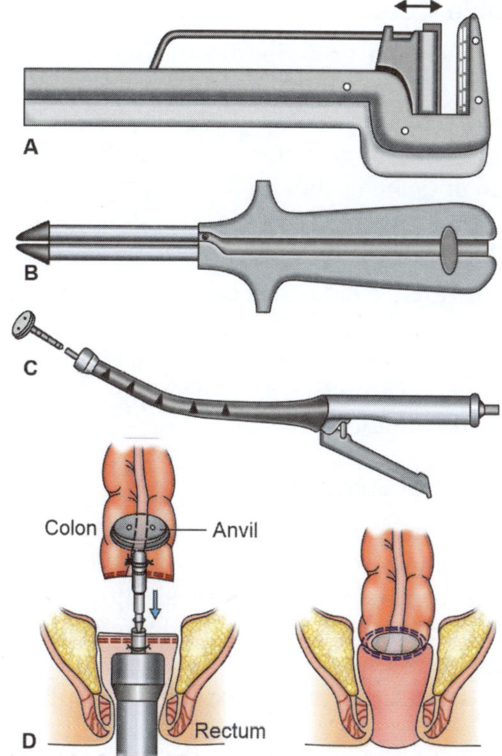

Figs 49.27A to D: (A to C) Parts of the stapler, (D) shows as the stapler is tightened, upper and lower rectum come together and the anvil fits in very well in the circular stapler

- Coloanal anastomosis is done just above the anorectal ring. It usually causes increased frequency of stool, incontinence or soilage, and impaired quality of life owing to an insufficient reservoir. Diet restrictions and time after surgery usually will improve these symptoms.These complications can be minimised by creating a colonic pouch.

Recent change in APR: In the conventional APR, dissection is within the levator ani and levator ani is preserved. The change is APR with removal of levator ani—it is called Extra Levator Abdominoperineal Excision (ELAPE). The resected specimen has a waist—it is called cylindrical APR. Aim is to get adequate CRM.

Carcinoma Middle One-third of Rectum

This refers to growth between **7 and 11 cm** from the anal verge. The decision to save the sphincter can be taken at laparotomy. In cases of well-differentiated carcinoma, 2 cm margin is adequate. **In anaplastic carcinoma, 5 cm clearance is necessary**. In female patients with broad pelvis after mobilisation of the rectum, the 7 cm growth may appear around 10 cm from the anal verge. Thus, sphincter can be saved. If the sphincter can be preserved, low anterior resection (LAR) should be done. (APR is also done, if the tumour is bulky and high-grade.)

Inoperable Cases

Locally advanced growths present with severe pain, bleeding and with subacute intestinal obstruction. Temporary loop colostomy is done in the left iliac fossa by bringing the sigmoid colon outside. Postoperatively, radiation and chemotherapy are given.

Hartmann's Operation (Fig. 49.28)

This is indicated in old and debilitated patients who may not withstand APR. The rectum is excised, the lower end of the rectum is closed and a colostomy is performed. When the growth is slow-growing, this operation gives good palliation.

Other Types of Surgeries

TEM (transanal endoscopic microsurgery): It involves wide anorectal retraction, followed by good visualisation of lesion using operating sigmoidoscope and distension of rectum by CO_2 followed by complete thickness excision and direct suturing. It can also be done by trans-sacral or trans-sphincteric approach.

ENDOSCOPIC TREATMENT OF COLORECTAL LESIONS

- **Colonoscopic polypectomy:** All adenomas and potential adenomas should be removed. Pedunculated polyps are removed by snare. Small polyps can be removed by cold or hot forceps and hot or cold snare. Bleeding can be controlled by injection of epinephrine, electrocautery, clips or endoloops.
- **Endoscopic mucosal resection:** It is indicated for flat, sessile lesions, not more than 2.5 cm in diameter. First the lesion is elevated by injecting saline or hypertonic dextrose with epinephrine. The lesion is elevated, cut and removed or sucked and cut.
- **Endoscopic submucosal dissection:** Technically more difficult. Principle of the procedure is same. More chances of perforation.

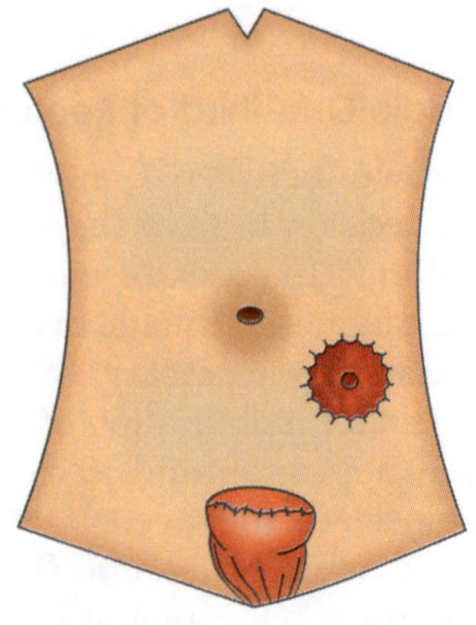

Fig. 49.28: Hartmann's operation

- **Endoscopic stents for decompression for malignant obstruction:** Large bore colorectal decompression tubes are available. They can be passed with or without endoscope with a guidewire. They are used to relieve obstruction so that bowel preparation can be done and one stage treatment—resection and anastomosis can be done. Self-expandable metal stents—SEMS have been used as palliation in cases of large gut obstruction. Quality of life is slightly better but no increase in survival rate of patients. Stent migration, tumour ingrowth, overgrowth, perforation and bleeding are the other complications.
- **Bridge to surgery: In left colonic obstruction, this is used in operable and advanced lesions.** Self-expandable metal stents—SEMS is used to relieve obstruction or an emergency ostomy without resection. Advantages of this method is: Get time for correction of fluid/electrolyte imbalance, normalization of bowel caliber, mechanical bowel preparation, provides time for the multidisciplinary team to complete staging workup. We can also screen for synchronous lesions, and initiate neoadjuvant therapy for the primary tumour, if needed. Advantage of diverting ostomy being, it offers a high success rate for relieving obstruction compared to stenting, no need for tumor manipulation, no potential risk of stent-related perforation or tumor spillage.

ROLE OF RADIOTHERAPY AND CHEMOTHERAPY

Postoperative Management

1. pT1-2N0M0 do not require any adjuvant treatment, such patients can be kept on follow-up with routine 3 monthly CEA and annual CECT thorax/abdomen/pelvis.
2. pT3N0M0 or node positive disease requires adjuvant treatment in the form of concurrent chemoradiotherapy and chemotherapy. Example: 2 cycles of FOLFOX (5-FU + Leucovorin + Oxaliplatin) → concurrent 5-FU/Leucovorin and radiation → 2 more cycles of FOLFOX. Oral Capecitabine can be used in place of IV 5-FU.
3. It is preferable to add Oxaliplatin in the chemotherapy regimen, if nodes were positive for metastatic disease. Although in older population (>65–70 years), it might be of less benefit.
4. Radiation portals should include the postoperative tumour bed, presacral nodes and internal iliac nodes. External iliac nodes should be included in T4 tumours.

   Radiation dose is usually 45–50 Gy given over 5 days a week for 5 consecutive weeks. Another 5–9 Gy boost to the tumour bed can be considered especially when there are adverse features such as lymphatic emboli, close margins, etc.

Preoperative—Neoadjuvant Chemoradiation

(Key Box 49.9)

Rationale: In locally advanced cases where the surgeon feels that complete resection may not be feasible or sphincter saving will not be possible, neoadjuvant chemoradiation can be attempted thus saving the patient from having a permanent colostomy bag and also better curative outcomes.

Key Box 49.9

Advantages of Preoperative Radiotherapy

- Decreased tumour seeding at surgery
- Increased radiosensitivity due to more oxygenated cells
- Conversion of APR to LAR

Generally, clinically T3–T4 tumors which may or may not be node positive are eligible candidates for neoadjuvant (NACT) chemotherapy.

1. A typical course of NACT comprises concurrent 5-FU/Capecitabine and radiation. A dose of 45–50 Gy is used to treat the pelvis including the growth and the draining lymphatic regions followed by 5 Gy boost to the tumors itself.
2. Following NACT, patient should be re-evaluated using CT/MRI for possibility of resection.
3. Surgery is usually considered after 6–8 weeks of NACT as the maximal response to the treatment may take up to 2 months.
4. Further adjuvant treatment is to be given following surgery depending upon the histopathological report.

Pearls of Wisdom

Rectal cancers are more radiosensitive and colonic cancers are more chemosensitive.

LOCALLY RECURRENT RECTAL CANCER

- Major cause is a positive margin on the pelvic side wall. This is the reason why preoperative chemoradiotherapy should precede excision of T3 and T4 lesions with TME.
- Usually develops within 18 months.
- Presents as pelvic pain, mass and rectal bleeding.
- Pelvic CT, MRI, CEA levels are the required investigations.
- Chemoradiation, surgery, local palliative treatment, pelvic exenteration (resection of rectum and bladder—Brunschwig's operation) are alternative treatments available.

COLOSTOMY

Opening of the colon to the exterior, either temporary or permanent, for the drainage of faecal matter is called colostomy.

TYPES

1. Temporary Colostomy

A. In cases of acute left-sided colonic obstruction, proximal half of right transverse colon is brought out through the upper part of the right rectus abdominis muscle. Later, radical resection of the left colon is done followed by closure of the colostomy.

B. In cases of traumatic or congenital fistula affecting the left colon, temporary colostomy is indicated (Fig. 49.36). The loop of the colon which is brought outside is held in place by a glass rod. This is passed through the transverse mesocolon and held by rubber tubing. This rod is removed after 10 days.

C. Colostomy/ileostomy is done, if a distal colorectal anastomosis gives way (Figs 49.29 and 49.30).

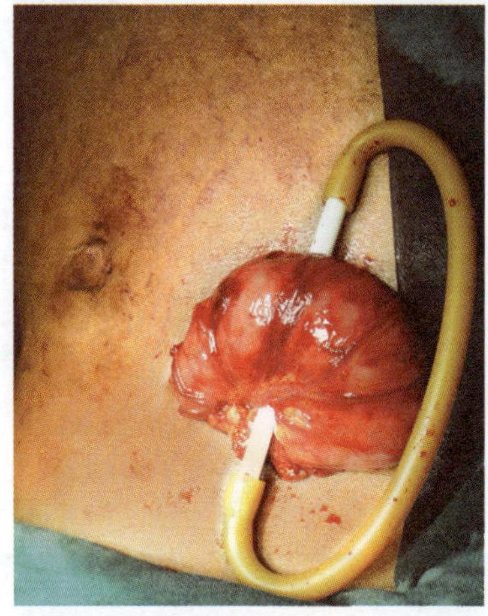

Fig. 49.29: Sigmoid colon is brought out and a glass rod connected to rubber tube is used to hold it out

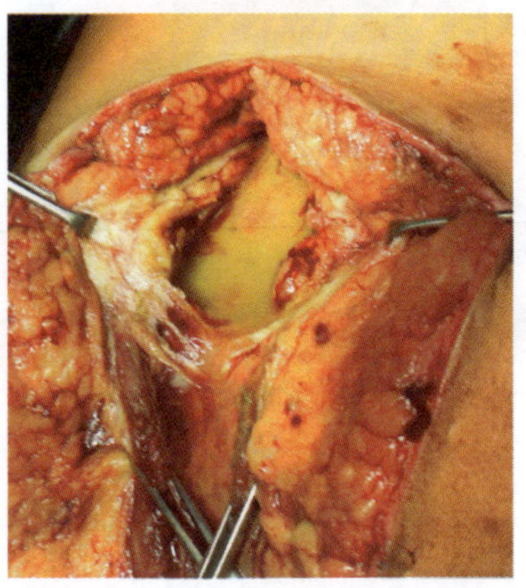

Fig. 49.30: Faeculent leak from failed anterior resection

TEN COMMANDMENTS

1. Should mark the colostomy site in the standing and sitting positions.
2. Should be at least 3 cm away from the bony landmark (anterior superior iliac spine).
3. Should be at least 3 cm away from the midline incision. Otherwise, colostomy will contaminate the incision site (Fig. 49.31).
4. Should close the paracolostomy space within the abdomen to prevent herniation of the small intestines.
5. Colostomy should be opened after 2 or 3 days and midline incision should be protected from getting infected due to bowel contents
6. Should be in flush with skin surface in the left iliac fossa.
7. Should excise a disc of skin for permanent colostomy
8. The stoma should be brought out through the rectus muscle.
9. Should avoid bringing stoma outside through scar tissue.
10. Should examine the end of the colostomy for vascularity (Fig. 49.32).

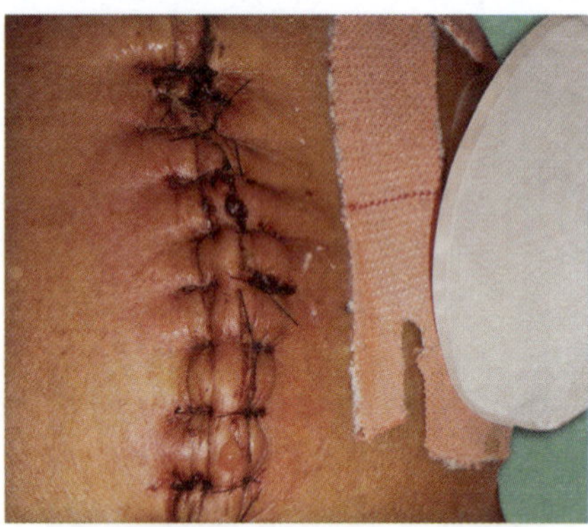

Fig. 49.31: End colostomy away from the main incision

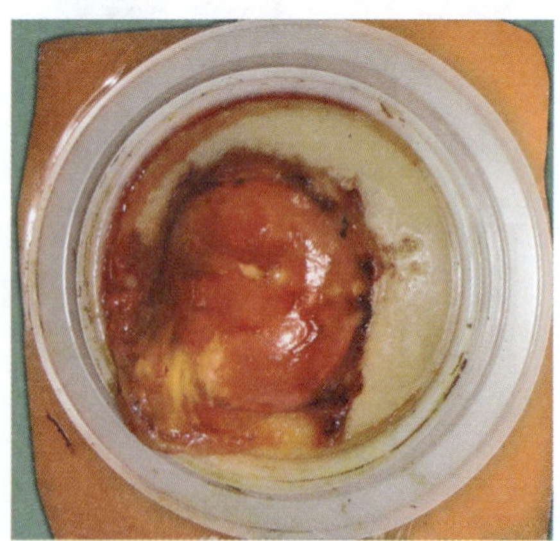

Fig. 49.32: Inspect for vascularity of colostomy following APR

Pearls of Wisdom

Transverse colostomy is bulky, contents are semiliquid and difficult to manage—try to avoid it.

2. Permanent Colostomy

It is indicated after abdominoperineal resection where the end of sigmoid colon is brought outside in the left iliac fossa as permanent colostomy (Figs 49.31 and 49.32, Key Box 49.10). The colostomy site should be 3 cm away from anterior superior iliac spine so that colostomy bag can be fitted properly (Figs 49.33 and 49.34).

Key Box 49.10

Permanent Colostomy—Left Iliac Fossa

- Avoid bony prominences
- Avoid belt lines
- Avoid marking in lying down position
- Avoid scars
- Avoid bringing out stoma lateral to rectus

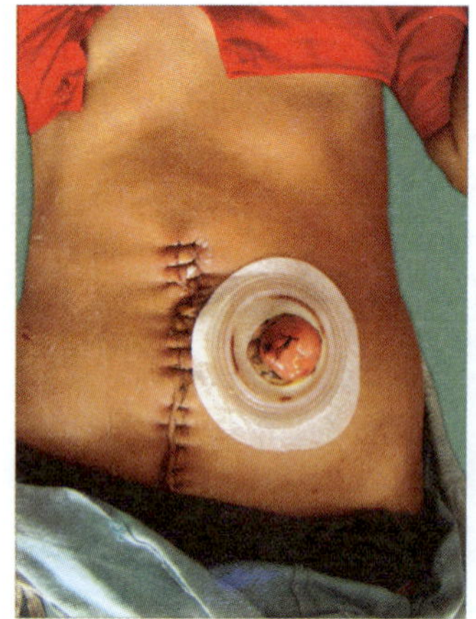

Fig. 49.33: Disposable colostomy bags are available with or without flange. Depending upon the size of the stoma, it can be cut open so as to fit into the colostomy.

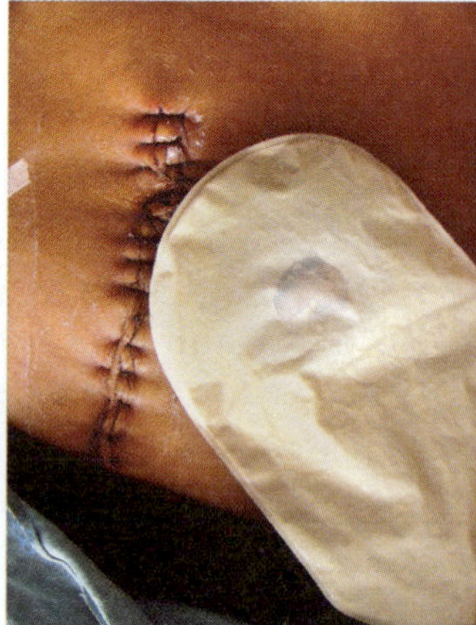

Fig. 49.34: A colostomy bag has been applied. It can be reused

3. Double-barreled Colostomy

In this, the adjoining walls of the intestine are crushed. Both ends of the loop are defunctioned. This type of colostomy is not frequently done now. It was done earlier for sigmoid volvulus, resection of colonic stricture, etc.

Indications for Colostomy

- **Congenital:** In Hirschsprung's disease and anorectal anomalies, temporary colostomy is done first.
- **Carcinoma:** Following APR, permanent end-sigmoid colostomy is done.
- **Colonic fistulae:** Fistulae due to diverticulitis, Crohn's disease or tuberculosis.
- **Colonic injuries:** Trauma due to stab injuries or operative injuries following nephrectomy, pelvic operations, PCNL (percutaneous nephrolithotomy).

Advantages of Colostomy

Distal bowel takes complete rest, regains normal size and bacterial colonisation is reduced. It becomes empty and sterile so that chances of leakage at a later operation is reduced.

Complications of Colostomy (Figs 49.35 to 49.38)

- Bleeding, necrosis, retraction, prolapse, parastomal hernia and colostomy diarrhoea are some complications.
- Colostomy obstruction, gangrene.

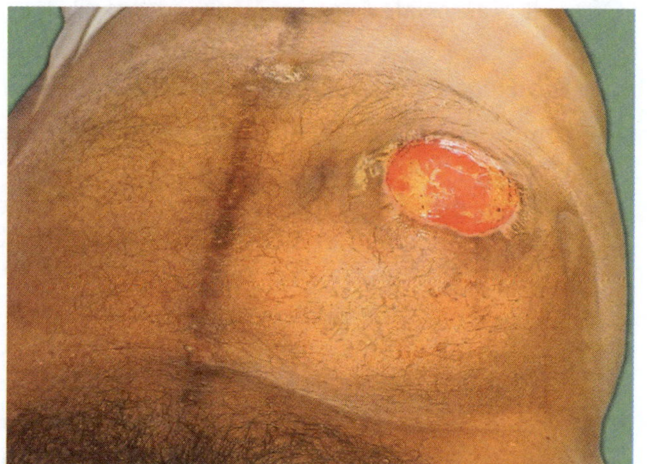

Fig. 49.35: Paracolostomy hernia: Herniation of bowel from the side of colostomy. It can give rise to intestinal obstruction. This needs to be repaired by reduction of contents, closure of defect and sometimes mesh repair

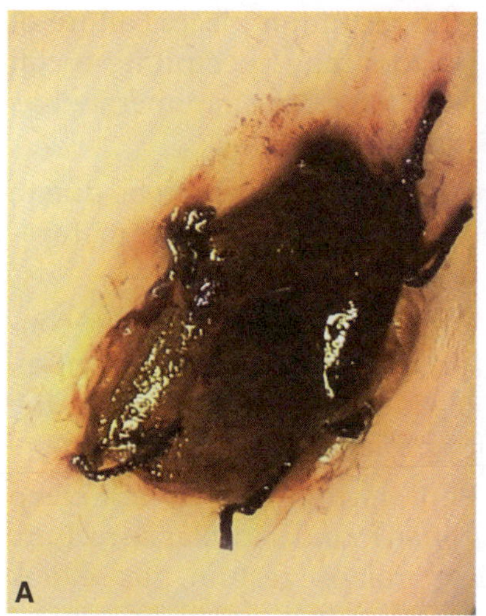

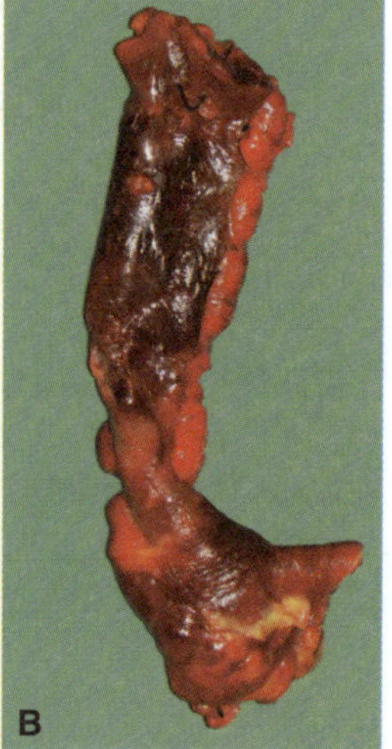

Figs 49.36A and B: Colostomy gangrene. It is mandatory to inspect the end of the colostomy everyday in the postoperative period to check for vascularity. If it is gangrenous and if it is retracted, it is better to open the abdomen again and refashion colostomy

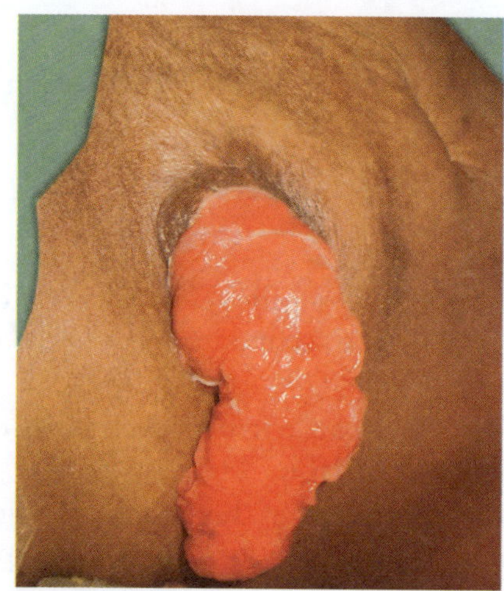

Fig. 49.37: Colostomy prolapse due to give way of sutures anchored to the aponeurotic layer. The patient also had violent cough in the post-operative period

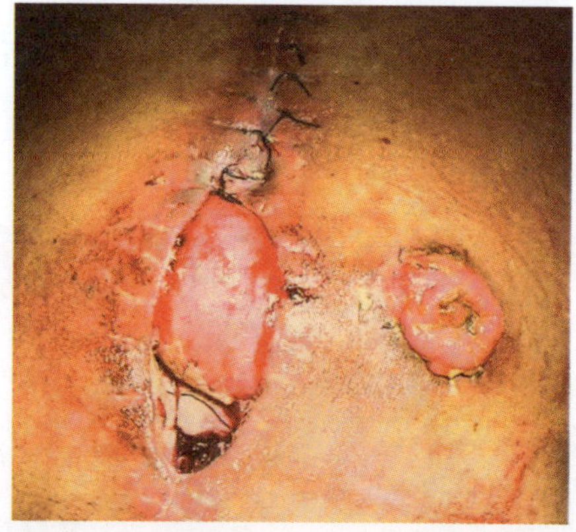

Fig. 49.38: Burst abdomen due to contamination of the wound from colostomy—proper care should be taken to isolate laparotomy site and colostomy till complete healing of laparotomy wound takes place

Pearls of Wisdom

Colostomy should be done by an experienced surgeon as patient has to live with the colostomy life long.

PROLAPSE RECTUM

Competency

SU28.17.3: Describe etiology, clinical features and management of rectal prolapse.

Protrusion of the mucous membrane or the entire rectum outside the anal verge. This condition is common in children and elderly patients.

Types

Prolapse can be of two types: Partial prolapse and complete prolapse.

Partial Prolapse

- In this variety, the protrusion is between 1.25 and 3.75 cm outside the anal verge (Fig. 49.39).
- It is usually a mucosal prolapse.

Causes

1. In infants, it is due to **undeveloped sacral curve** and in children it can be secondary to **habitual constipation.**
2. It can follow an attack of **whooping cough or excessive straining** (Fig. 49.40).
3. It can follow an attack of diarrhoea resulting in **loss of fat** in the ischiorectal fossae, which supports the rectum.
4. In adults, it is common in females mostly due to **torn perineum** caused by obstetric trauma.

Treatment

1. **Digital reposition:** In infants, partial prolapse is temporary. The mother is advised to push the prolapse inside after lubricating with lignocaine jelly.

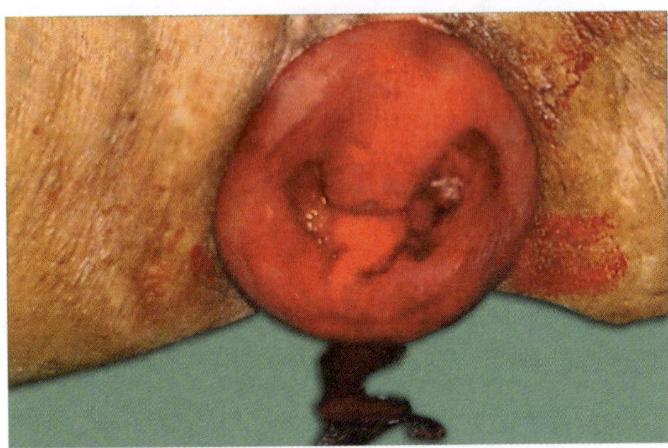

Fig. 49.39: Partial prolapse

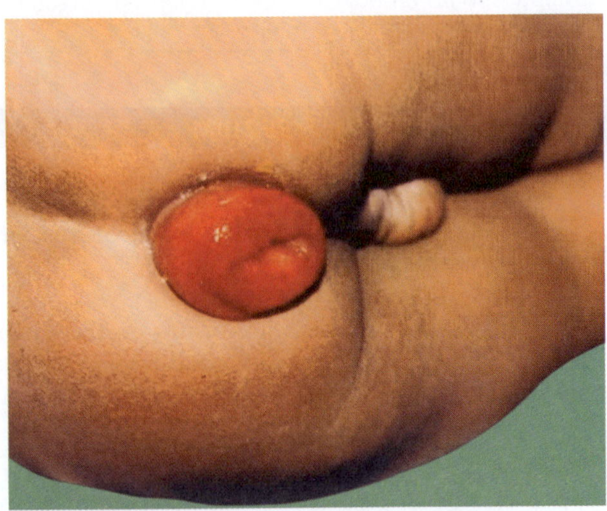

Fig. 49.40: Rectal prolapse in a child

2. **Injection of ethanolamine oleate** into the submucosa of the rectum. It causes aseptic fibrosis. Thus, mucosa gets tethered to the other layers.
3. Partial prolapse can be **excised**, after applying **Goodsall's ligature.**

COMPLETE/TOTAL PROLAPSE

- Full thickness prolapse is also called procidentia.
- It is defined as protrusion of the rectum for more than 3.75 cm outside the anal verge. Very often, it is the entire rectum which protrudes out on straining, sometimes along with the peritoneal sac.
- Often, it is associated with prolapse uterus.

The Pelvic Floor—Surgical Anatomy (Fig. 49.41)

- It is composed of **two levator ani** and a **puborectalis** muscle.
- Levator ani originates from pelvic side walls and sacrospinous ligament. It **suspends** the rectum in a muscular sling till the level of puborectalis.
- Puborectalis muscle takes origin from posterior aspect of pubis, forms a sling around rectum and returns to posterior pubis.
- **Contracted puborectalis is responsible for normal acute anorectal angle and it is critical for maintaining continence.** Thus during coughing and sneezing, anorectal angle becomes more acute, increasing continence.

Supports of the Rectum and Surgical Importance

Various supports keep the rectum in place. Failure of one or more of these factors may precipitate rectal prolapse (Fig. 49.42). They have been enumerated as follows.

1. **Pelvic floor:** Weakness of pelvic floor can be due to birth injuries or due to defective collagen maturation.
2. **Lateral ligaments:** These ligaments are either condensation of pelvic fascia on either side of the rectum. Excessive mobility of these ligaments may be the contributing factor for prolapse rectum.
3. **Fascia of Denonvilliers** (rectovesical fascia): **Deep rectovesical pouch** is often found in prolapse rectum. In all cases of complete prolapse rectum, please look for the deep rectovesical pouch and if present, it should be obliterated.
4. **Fat in the ischiorectal fossae** supports the rectum. Hence, any chronic illness and loss of fat may contribute to prolapse rectum.

PHOTOGRAPHS OF PROLAPSE RECTUM

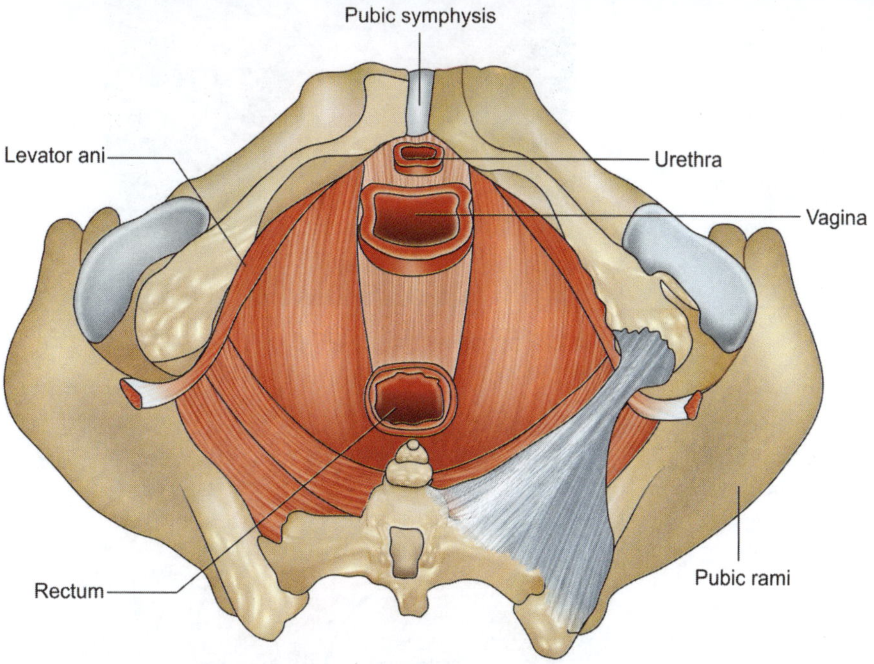

Fig. 49.41: Pelvic floor anatomy—weakness of the pelvic floor is an important cause of prolapse rectum

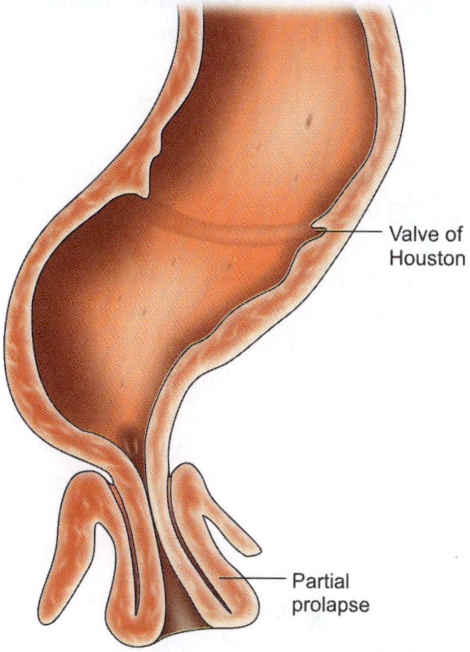

Fig. 49.42: Prolapsed rectum—diagrammatic representation, sometimes confused for prolapsed haemorrhoids

Anorectal Physiology and Investigation

These are useful in patients who have complaints of prolapse rectum, constipation, incontinence.

1. **Anorectal manometry**
   - Normal resting pressure in the anal canal—40–80 mmHg. (It is the function of internal anal sphincter.)
   - **Squeeze pressure:** It is maximum voluntary contraction pressure minus resting pressure. It is 40–80 mmHg above resting pressure. It reflects the function of external anal sphincter.
2. **Function of pudendal nerve and perineal nerve:** Injuries to the nerve are diagnosed by nerve conduction studies.

Causes or Pathogenesis (Fig. 49.43)

1. **Common in elderly women who are multipara.** It is probably due to repeated **birth injuries** to the perineum causing damage to the nerve fibres. As age advances, muscles become weak (Key Box 49.11). This, together with fatty degeneration of the muscle, results in prolapse rectum.
2. **Excessive straining** causes weakness of the supports of the rectum.
3. **Defective collagen maturation** results in failure of rectal support by levators and pelvic fascia.

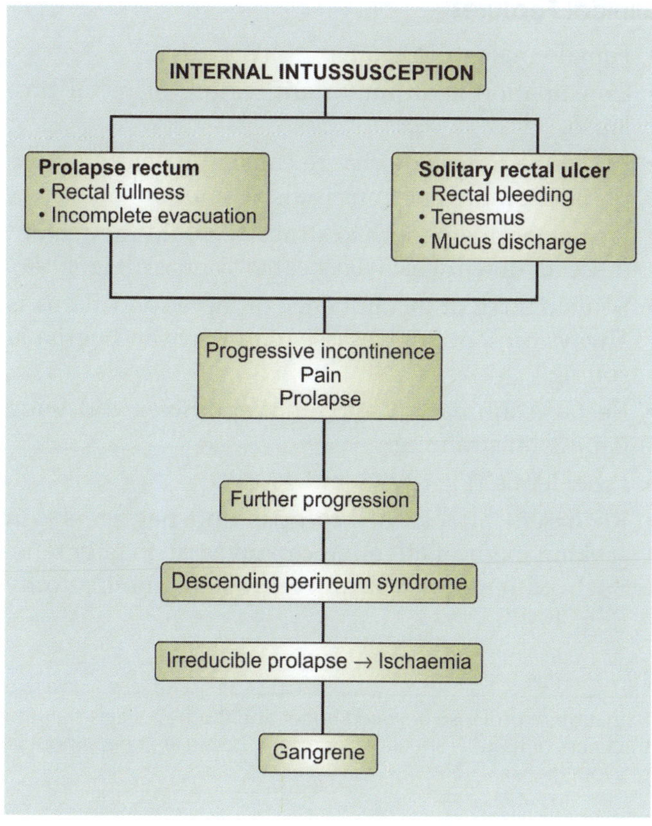

Fig. 49.43: Pathogenesis of prolapse rectum

Key Box 49.11

Obstetric Trauma

- Multiple vaginal deliveries—cause pudendal nerve stretch.
- Prolonged labour—disrupts sphincter and stretching of pudendal nerve.
- 3rd degree perineal tears—weaken the internal sphincter and pelvic floor.

4. Presence of **deep rectovesical pouch** and excessive mobility of the rectum (mesorectum) predisposes to prolapse of the rectum.
5. Many people believe that prolapse of the rectum starts as an **intussusception** in the first stage, initiated by certain factors such as diarrhoea, constipation and disorder of the pelvic floor. The process starts with anterior wall of rectum, where supporting tissues are weakest (Broden–Snellman theory).

Beahrs Classification

A. Incomplete—mucosal prolapse
B. Complete—full thickness rectal prolapse
   1st degree—concealed
   2nd degree—externally visible on straining
   3rd degree—visible without straining

Clinical Features

- Female-male ratio is 6:1.
- Constipation is an important feature of rectal prolapse.
- Excessive mucus discharge causing irritation to the perianal skin. Tenesmus is also common.
- On asking the patient to strain at stool,[1] the rectum descends down, which clinches the diagnosis (Fig. 49.44).
- Some degree of incontinence of faeces and flatus is always present. It gives rise to urgency and perianal soiling.
- Rectal examination—lax anal sphincter and wide gaping on straining.
- Procidentia (Figs 49.45 and 49.46).
- Recurrent attacks of prolapse and negligence in seeking medical attention can give rise to gangrene. Such patients may require proctosigmoidectomy (Fig. 49.47).

Pearls of Wisdom

Palpation of prolapse between finger and thumb reveals double thickness of tissue, especially anteriorly because of deep pouch of Douglas.

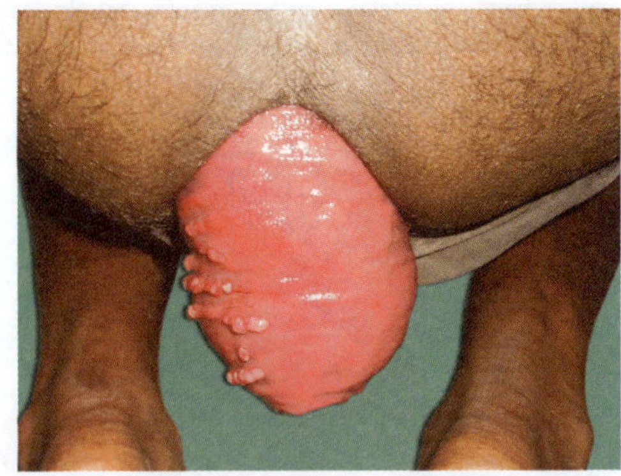

Fig. 49.44: Complete prolapse—should be tested by asking the patient to squat and strain

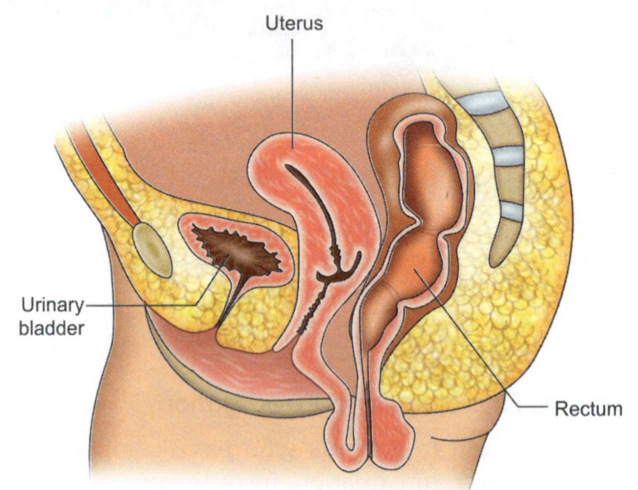

Fig. 49.45: Prolapse of the rectum with uterus: Procidentia—not an uncommon presentation specially in multipara women

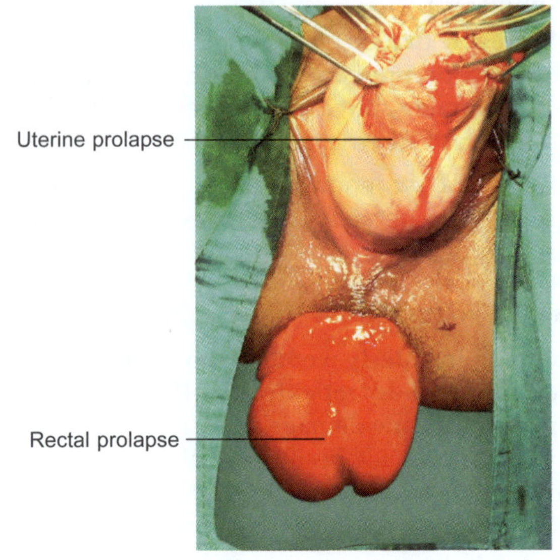

Fig. 49.46: Complete prolapse of the rectum with prolapse of uterus—procidentia

[1]In fact, the surgeon should see the prolapse of the rectum outside when patient strains to make a clinical diagnosis.

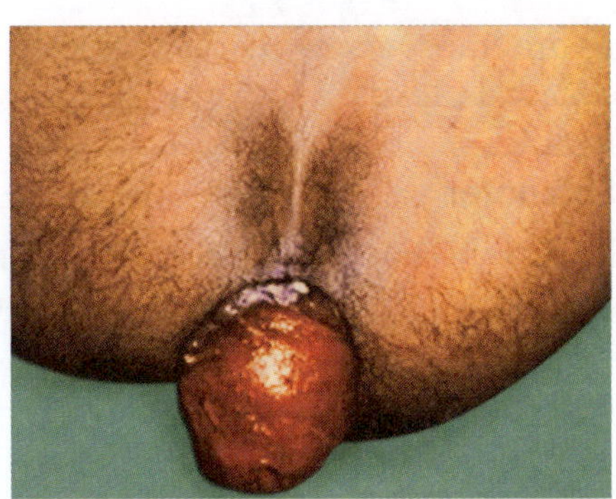

Fig. 49.47: Prolapsed rectum—slowly change in colour—would have become gangrene

Differential Diagnosis

- Large third degree haemorrhoids—not circumferential and are blue in colour.
- Large polypoid tumour
- Prolapse of sigmoid colon

Complications

- Proctitis, ulceration and rarely bleeding
- Gangrene of the rectum

Treatment

Medical management—prior to surgery, patients not fit for surgery or patients who refuse surgery

- Adequate fluid and fibre intake
- Enemas and suppositories for severe constipation

Surgical Procedures—Aim

1. Safe procedure to correct with minimal morbidity and without mortality. They are classified as **perineal procedures and abdominal procedures**.
2. To cure or to improve **incontinence**.

I. PERINEAL PROCEDURES

(Preferred for High-Risk Patients)

1. **Delorme's procedure** (reefing the rectal mucosa): In this, the prolapse is completely everted, mucosa is stripped and muscle coat is plicated. Mucosal continuity is maintained by suturing anal canal mucosa below to the rectal mucosa above. This is an easy operation to do in elderly patients. However, relapse rates are high and it does not correct the defect.
2. **Altemeier's procedure:** In this operation, full thickness of the prolapsed rectum with part of sigmoid is ***excised*** followed by ***anastomosis of part of the sigmoid*** to the ***anal canal*** from below. To improve continence, plication of levator ani and puborectalis muscle is done. ***Urgency and incontinence*** are the features because of removal of rectum.
3. **Thiersch wiring:** In this operation, a steel wire or a thick silk suture is applied all around the anus after reducing the prolapse. The knot is tightened around a finger. Patients with poor surgical compliance benefit from this operation. However, breakdown of the wire, perianal sepsis and anal stenosis are the complications.

II. ABDOMINAL PROCEDURE—MESH RECTOPEXY—LAPAROSCOPIC OR OPEN METHOD

A marlex mesh or prolene mesh can be kept behind the rectum. This is sutured behind, to the sacrum and then to the posterior and lateral surfaces of rectum. **Laparoscopic method of fixing the mesh has become popular. This is the procedure of choice today.** Constipation is one of the complications of mesh rectopexy (Figs 49.48 and 49.49).

For summary refer Key Box 49.12.

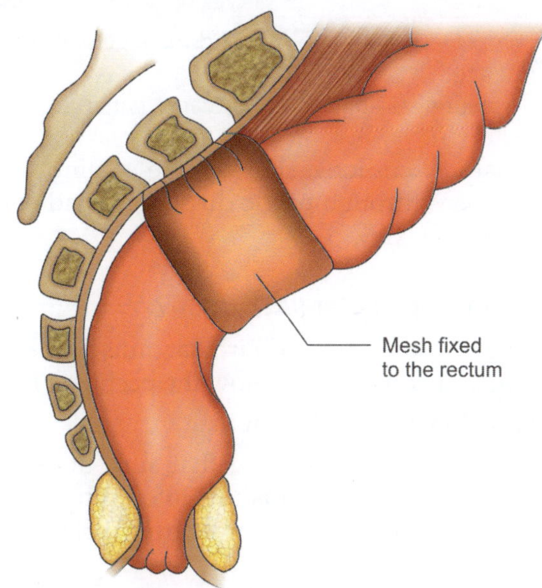

Fig. 49.48: Fixing the mesh to the rectum—mesh is sutured to the sacrum posteriorly and sutured to the sides of the rectum

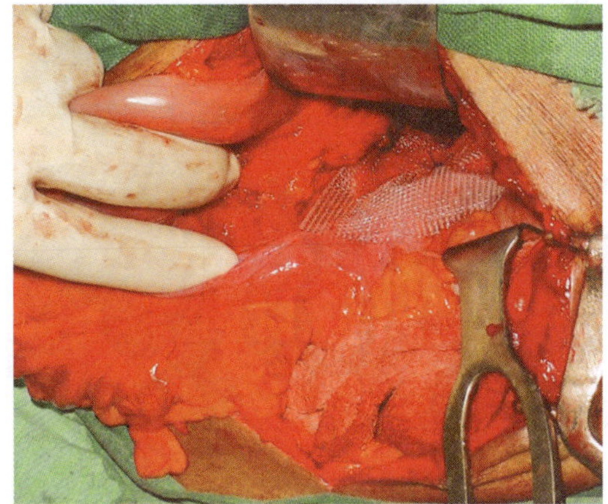

Fig. 49.49: Mesh fixation for total prolapse of the rectum—most common surgery—open or laparoscopic method

Key Box 49.12

Summary of Surgeries for Prolapse Rectum

- Mesh rectopexy corrects/prevents prolapse but does not correct chronic constipation.
- Laparoscopic mesh rectopexy has become gold standard—fast recovery, less pain, short hospital stay.
- Mesh rectopexy with resection is ideal for patients with constipation or patients with a redundant sigmoid colon.
- High operative risk patients—Thiersch wiring—anal encirclement.
- Altemeier procedure done for perineum is an alternative in patients with incontinence. Here, perineal proctectomy and posterior sphincter enhancement is done.

SURGICAL ANATOMY OF ANAL CANAL

Competency

SU28.17.7: Describe aetiology and management of anal incontinence.
First learn surgical anatomy of the anal canal.

Anal canal is 3 cm long, starts as the continuation of rectum, passes through pelvic diaphragm and ends at the anal verge (skin).

Internal Anal Sphincter (IAS) (Fig. 49.50)

- It is the continuation of circular muscle fibres of rectum and ends 0.5 cm below the pectinate line.
- It is involuntary and 2.5 cm long.
- The IAS is a muscular ring that surrounds about 2.5–4.0 cm of the anal canal. Its inferior border is in contact with, but quite separate from, sphincter ani externus muscle.
- Internal sphincter with fibres of external sphincter and puborectalis which maintains the anorectal angle, form the **anorectal bundle, and maintains continence.**

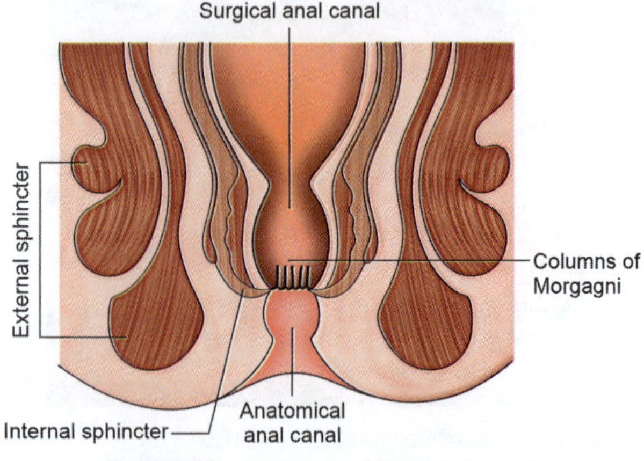

Fig. 49.50: Anatomy of the anal canal

- Its fibres are transversely placed. Motor fibres come from presacral plexus.

External Sphincter

- It is formed by **striated muscle fibres** intermingled with longitudinal muscle fibres of the rectum which are attached to the skin of perianal region.
- It has superficial, deep and subcutaneous portions.
- The funnel-shaped configuration of the paired levator ani muscles form the major part of the pelvic floor, and their fibers decussate medially with the contralateral side to fuse with the perineal body around the prostate or vagina.
- Nerve supply (motor) comes from inferior haemorrhoidal branch of internal pudendal nerve and perianal branch of the 4th sacral nerve (motor to levator ani also).
- It is voluntary and gives temporary continence.

Development

- Anal canal is developed from fusion of **post-allantoic gut** with **proctodeum**.
- The junction of these is the dentate line or pectinate line. **Anal valves of Ball** are remnants of proctodeal membrane.
- At the level of dentate line, the mucosa is folded in the form of longitudinal columns—***columns of Morgagni.***
- In between the columns of Morgagni, 4–8 anal glands open into small anal sinuses.

Lining Epithelium

- The mucosa of the upper anal canal, like that of the rectum, is pinkish and is lined by columnar epithelium, whereas the mucosa distal to the dentate line is paler and lined by squamous epithelium devoid of hair and glands.
- The change between the two types of epithelium is called transitional zone. It lies immediately proximal to the dentate line and consists of layers of cuboidal cells with a few columnar cells.
- Thus diseases affecting the rectal mucosa, such as ulcerative colitis, can extend to the transitional zone but not distal to the dentate line. *Cancers proximal to the dentate are typically adenocarcinomas, and those distal are squamous cell carcinoma.*
- Thus even after total proctocolectomy and pouch procedures for ulcerative colitis, carcinoma can occur in the transitional zone.
- At the anal verge, characteristics of normal skin with its apocrine glands are present. This is where infectious complications of the apocrine glands—hidradenitis

suppurativa can occur. This differentiation helps in sensory perception, which influences the surgical approaches to anorectal conditions. *To give an example, internal hemorrhoids can be treated with rubber band ligation without the need for local anaesthesia. On the other hand, excision of external hemorrhoids requires the application of local anaesthesia.*

Blood Supply, Lymphatic Drainage and Nerve Supply

- The superior portion of the anal canal (i.e. superior to the dentate line) is supplied by the superior haemorrhoidal artery. Below the dentate line, the inferior haemorrhoidal arteries supply the inferior most part of the anal canal. Between the two, the middle haemorrhoidal arteries form anastomoses.
- Above the dentate line, internal haemorrhoidal venous plexus drains into the superior haemorrhoidal vein. Below, veins drain into the inferior haemorrhoidal vein. Also, middle haemorrhoidal veins drain the muscularis externa and anastomose with the superior and inferior haemorrhoidal veins.
- **The lymphatic drainage:** Above the dentate line, the lymphatics drain into the internal iliac lymph nodes and below the dentate line, lymphatics drain into the superficial inguinal lymph nodes.
- **Nerve supply:** The anal canal has differing nervous innervations above and below the dentate line. Above the dentate line, the nerve supply comes from the inferior hypogastric plexus (visceral). This part of the anal canal is sensitive to stretch. Below the dentate line, the nerve supply is somatic, receiving its supply from the inferior haemorrhoidal nerves (branches of the pudendal nerve). It is sensitive to pain, temperature, and touch (refer to Table 49.3).

ANORECTAL PHYSIOLOGY

- The anal canal which has length of 4 cm, lengthens with squeezing of the external sphincter and shortens with straining during defaecation. Resting pressure, which depends largely on the internal sphincter, averages 90 cm H_2O. It is lower in women and older patients than in men and younger patients.
- This high-pressure zone increases resistance to the passage of stool. The external anal sphincter and puborectalis muscle generate pressure, by contraction which is more than double the intra-anal canal resting pressure.
- The principal mechanism that provides continence is the pressure differential between the rectum (6 cm H_2O) and the anal canal (90 cm H_2O). The anorectal angle is produced by the anterior pull of the puborectalis muscle as it encircles the rectum at the anorectal ring. This angle may act as a flap valve or have a sphincter-like function.
- Anorectal sensation allows discrimination of the enteric contents (gas, liquids, or solids). It also detects the need to pass stools or flatus. The internal sphincter will relax when enteric contents reach the anal canal, while the rectum distends and contracts. It is called rectal anal inhibitory reflex. Transient relaxation of the internal anal sphincter brings the rectal content into contact with the sensory mucosa of the proximal anal so that it can be recognized.

Mechanism of Anal Continence

- Distension of the rectum causes **tonic contraction of external sphincter**, which is controlled by the cerebrum. The centre is in the **lumbosacral region of the spinal cord.**
- Faeces in the anal canal stimulates the nerve endings. Nerve endings are also present in the puborectalis. **High pressure** in the anal canal (25–120 mmHg) and angle between rectum and anal canal (80°) are the important factors which maintain anal continence. *More details are given on page 898.*

Table 49.3 Comparison of anal canal above and below the dentate line

	Above the dentate line	Below the dentate line
1. Nomenclature	Surgical anal canal	Anatomical anal canal
2. Epithelium	Cuboidal epithelium	Skin—squamous epithelium, without hair and sweat glands
3. Nerve supply	Parasympathetic. Hence, painless	Spinal nerves, inferior haemorrhoidal nerve, very painful
4. Venous drainage	Portal system	Systemic veins (external iliac vein)
5. Colour	Pink	Skin colour
6. Development	Post-allantoic gut	Proctodeum
7 Lymphatic drainage	Para-aortic nodes	Superficial and deep inguinal nodes

HAEMORRHOIDS (PILES)

Competency

SU28.17.9: Describe aetiology, clinical features, non-surgical management and surgeries for hemorrhoidal disease.

Definition

Dilated plexus of superior haemorrhoidal veins, in relation to anal canal.

Classification—Aetiological

I. Primary/Idiopathic Haemorrhoids

1. **Standing posture:** A famous saying goes-varicosity is the penalty for verticality against gravity. This holds true for haemorrhoids. It is true that animals do not develop haemorrhoids as well. Man's upright posture and absence of valves in the portal system with other factors precipitate development of haemorrhoids.
2. **Haemorrhoidal veins** and their branches are thin veins which pass through submucosa of the rectum. They get compressed due to contractions caused by rectal musculature (the sphincters) during the act of defaecation.
3. **Genetic/familial factors:** Absence of valves, or congenital weakness of the vessel wall are few other factors contributing for the haemorrhoids.
4. **Diet:** A diet deficient in fibres which prolongs the gut transit results in constipation and the hard pellet like stools. The hard stools compress veins and result in haemorrhoids.

II. Secondary Haemorrhoids

Causes

1. **Carcinoma of rectum**, by blocking the veins, can produce back pressure and can manifest as piles.
2. **Portal hypertension**—uncommon cause of rectal varices.
3. **Pregnancy**, due to compression of superior rectal veins or due to progesterone which relaxes smooth muscle in the wall of the veins, can cause haemorrhoids.

Current view: Normally the anal cushions retract after defaecation. Latest theory is that haemorrhoids occur due to caudal displacement of anal cushions. It is due to recurrent trauma, shearing forces, loss of elasticity.

Location

Classically situated in the 3, 7 and 11 o'clock positions (Fig. 49.51) (left lateral, right posterior and right anterior, respectively).

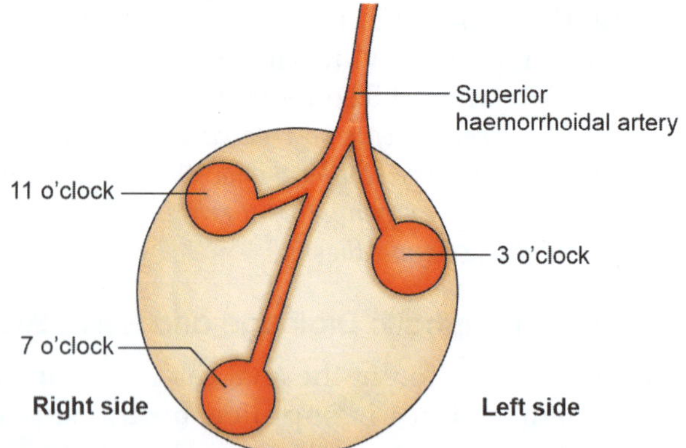

Fig. 49.51: Classic location of pile masses

- Superior haemorrhoidal artery gives 2 branches on right side and 1 branch on left side. Hence, piles are two on right side and one on left side.

Clinical Features (Table 49.4)

- Painless bleeding—fresh bleeding occurs after defaecation—**splash in the pan.** This causes chronic anaemia. Haemorrhoids which bleed are called Grade I haemorrhoids.
- The capillaries of the lamina propria are protected by only a single layer of epithelial cells. Hence, minor trauma precipitates bleeding.
- As the straining increases, the haemorrhoids partly prolapse outside. After defaecation, it returns back (Grade II) or can be digitally replaced (Grade III haemorrhoids).
- Permanently prolapsed pile outside (Grade IV haemorrhoids). The patient complains of pain or discomfort.
- Most of the patients complain of constipation.
- Discharge of mucus and soiling of perianal skin—pruritus by prolapse of haemorrhoidal cushions and mucosa (Figs 49.52 to 49.54).

Table 49.4 Grades of haemorrhoids

Grades features	Symptoms
I. Never prolapse	Bleeding per rectum
II. Prolapse on defaecation with spontaneous reduction	Mass per rectum descending down
III. Prolapse on defaecation requires manual reduction	Mass per rectum bleeding, mucus discharge, pruritus
IV. Permanent prolapse	Acute pain, throbbing discomfort

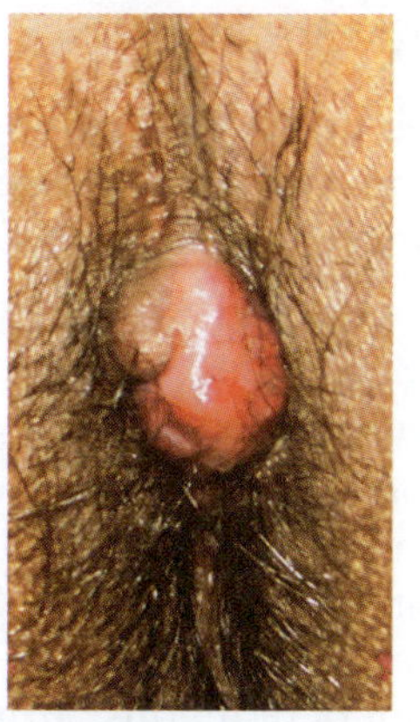

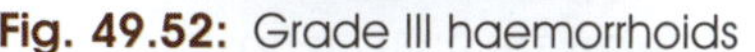

Fig. 49.52: Grade III haemorrhoids

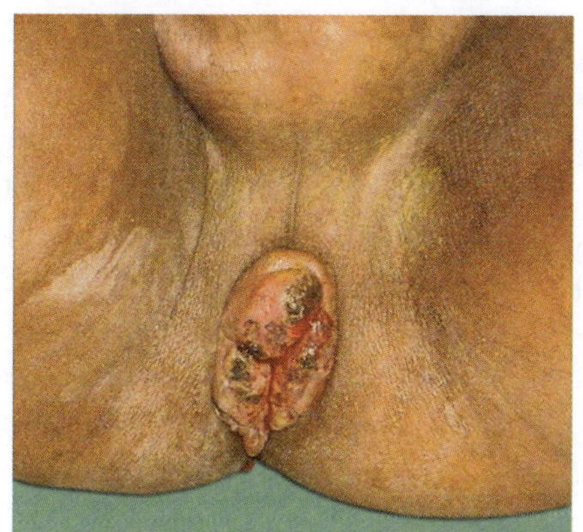

Fig. 49.53: Grade IV haemorrhoids

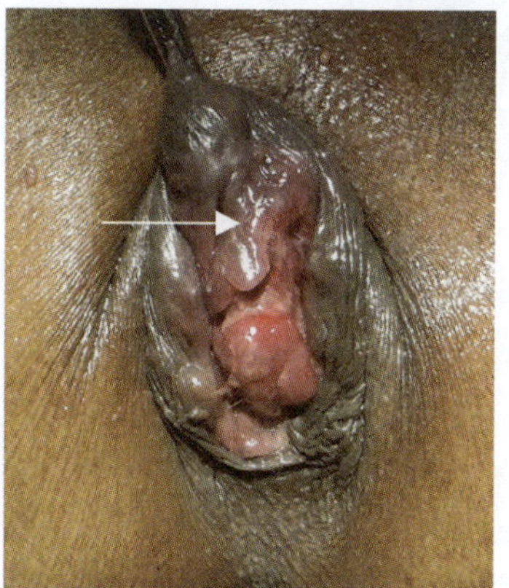

Fig. 49.54: External pile

III. *Depending upon the Location of Haemorrhoids*

1. **Internal haemorrhoids**—above the dentate line, covered with mucous membrane.
2. **External haemorrhoids**—at anal verge, covered with skin (Fig. 49.54).
3. **Interno-external**—both varieties together.

Investigations

- Per rectal examination is done mainly to rule out carcinoma rectum or other causes of bleeding per rectum. Haemorrhoids cannot be felt by rectal examination unless they are thrombosed or fibrosed.
- **Proctoscopy:** As the obturator is removed, piles prolapse into the lumen of proctoscope as cherry red masses.
- **Sigmoidoscopy and proctoscopy are done to rule out proximal cancer.**

Complications of Haemorrhoids

(Figs 49.55 to 49.57)

1. It can cause **chronic anaemia**. Rarely, massive bleeding can occur because of portal hypertension.
2. A **prolapse** outside presents with severe pain in the perianal region—piles gripped by internal sphincter results in venous congestion and oedema followed by strangulation. Such patients are treated by:

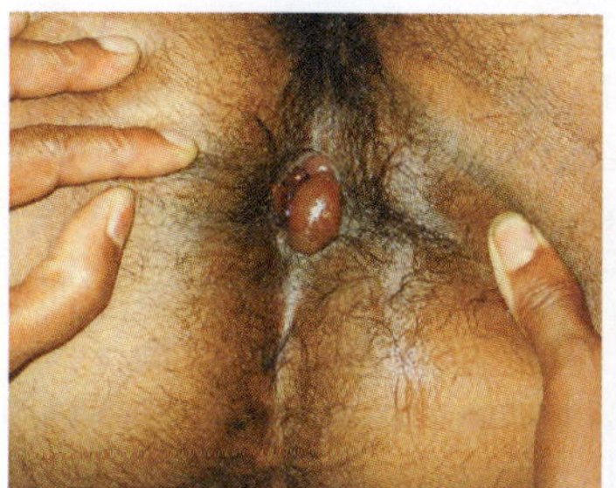

Fig. 49.55: Prolapsed piles—painful condition

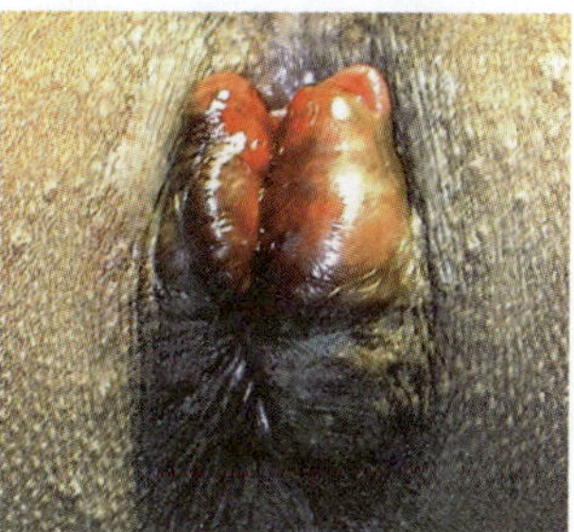

Fig. 49.56: Thrombosed pile mass

   - Elevation of foot end of bed
   - Metronidazole 400 mg, 3 times a day for 5 days.
   - Saline dressings to reduce oedema—glycerine $MgSO_4$
   - Local lignocaine jelly application
3. **Ulceration** and secondary infection
4. **Thrombosis** and fibrosis

TREATMENT OF HAEMORRHOIDS

A. Nonoperative treatment: It is indicated in Grade I and Grade II piles which are not causing significant bleeding or discomfort (Key Box 49.13).

B. Injection of sclerosant: 5% phenol in almond oil is injected into **submucosa** above the dentate line. Hence, it is painless. It produces **aseptic thrombosis**

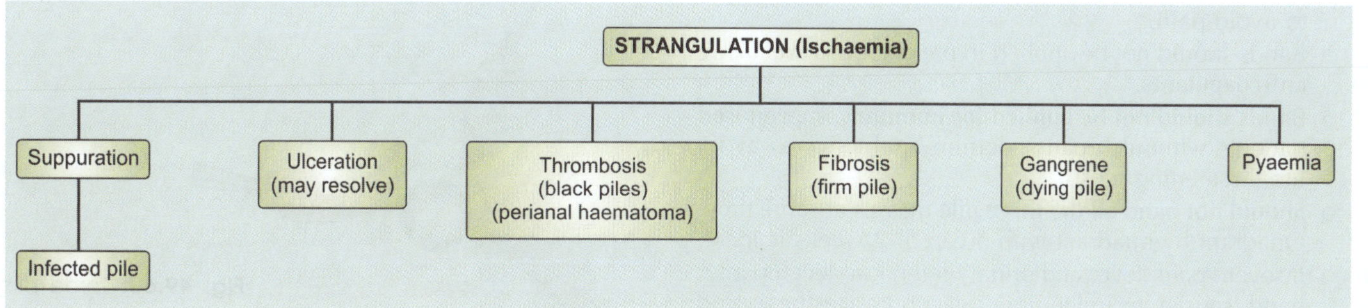

Fig. 49.57: Complications of piles

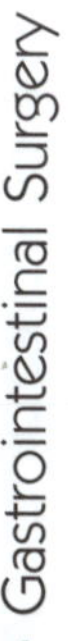

Key Box 49.13

Nonoperative Treatment

- Fibre supplementation
- Increased fluid intake
- Bulk purgative—laxatives—isabgol husk, etc.
- Reading in toilet to be discouraged (respond to call and do not strain)
- Encourage to lose weight
- Sitz-bath

Remember as **FIBRES**

of pile mass and is indicated in Grade I. The injection is **perivascular**.

C. **Barron's band application** (Figs 49.58 and 49.59): It is indicated for Grade II and Grade III haemorrhoids, wherein bands are applied at the neck of the haemorrhoids. It causes necrosis and thus, piles get fibrosed. One or two can be banded at a time (Key Box 49.14).

D. **Operative treatment:** Haemorrhoidectomy. Open method, closed method, stapler haemorrhoidopexy.

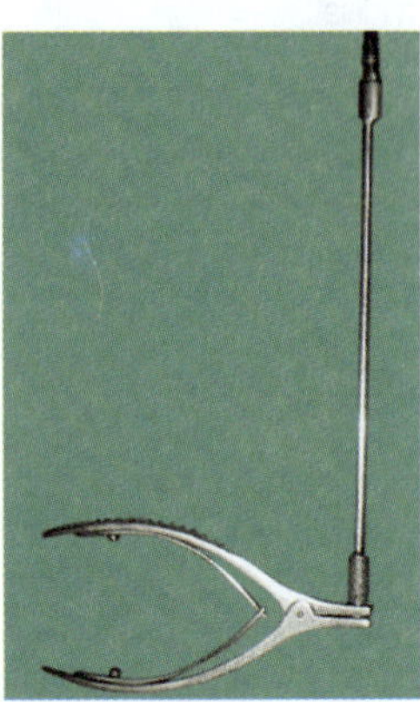

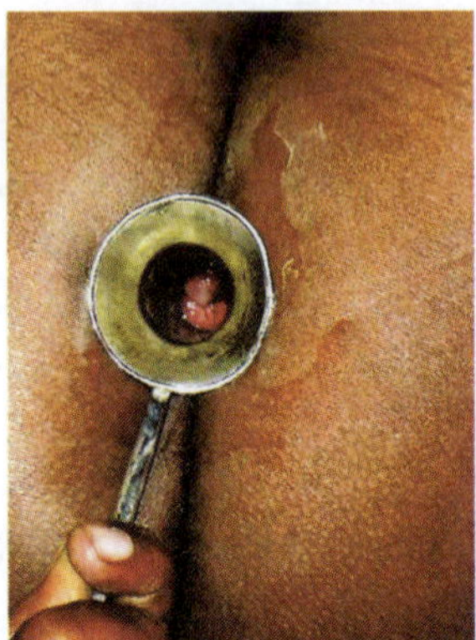

Figs 49.58 and 49.59: Barron's band ligator and band has been applied to one of the pile masses

Key Box 49.14

Band Ligation: Wisdom Lines

- Bands should be applied **1–2 cm above dentate** line to avoid pain.
- Bands should not be applied in patients who are taking **anticoagulants**.
- Bands **should not be applied for immunocompromised** patients without broad spectrum antibiotics to avoid life-threatening sepsis.
- **Should not band all the three pile** masses at same time. Quadrant by quadrant with a gap of 2 weeks is ideal.
- If severe pain, fever and urinary retention develop after band (sepsis), examine under general anaesthesia and remove band.

HAEMORRHOIDECTOMY (Key Box 49.15)

Excision of the pile masses up to base is indicated in Grade II and Grade III haemorrhoids. It can be done by 3 methods: Open, closed and with stapler (*vide infra*).

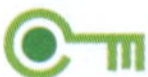

Key Box 49.15

Interesting Wisdom in Haemorrhoids

- Haemorrhoids occur due to downward prolapse of vascular cushions into and beyond anal canal.
- Minimum ideal investigation for haemorrhoids should be flexible sigmoidoscopy.
- Preserve adequate mucocutaneous bridges in excisional procedures to prevent anal stenosis.
- Urgency and tenesmus following stapled haemorrhoidoscopy responds well to oral nifedipine.
- Metronidazole is the most important agent in reducing pain after haemorrhoid surgery.
- Grades I and II can be injected: Injections should be perivascular, submucosal and above the level of dentate line.
- Grade III requires haemorrhoidectomy or haemorrhoidopexy.
- Grade IV requires initial conservative treatment followed by surgical procedure.

Pearls of Wisdom

Excisional haemorrhoidectomy produces more discomfort (pain) than stapler haemorrhoidopexy but lesser recurrences).

Types

I. Open Method: Milligan-Morgan Ligature and Excision (Figs 49.60 to 49.62)

- Stretch the sphincter
- Identify the positions of pile masses
- Dissection up to the base (pedicle)
- Transfixation ligature with **nonabsorbable silk**
- Excision of the piles with skin
- Trimming the wound
- Haemostasis obtained
- Wound packed with roller gauze

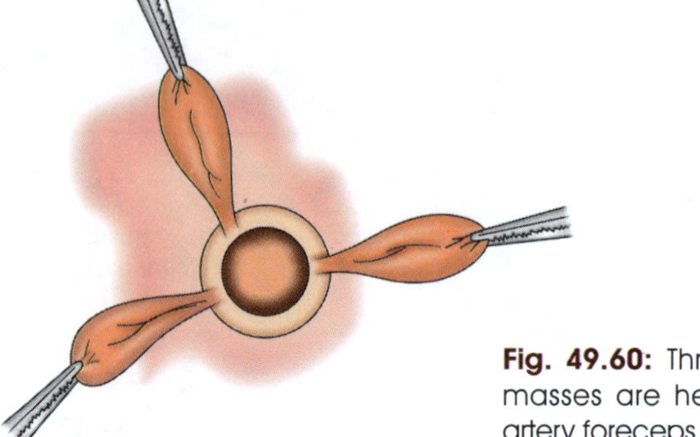

Fig. 49.60: Three pile masses are held with artery forceps

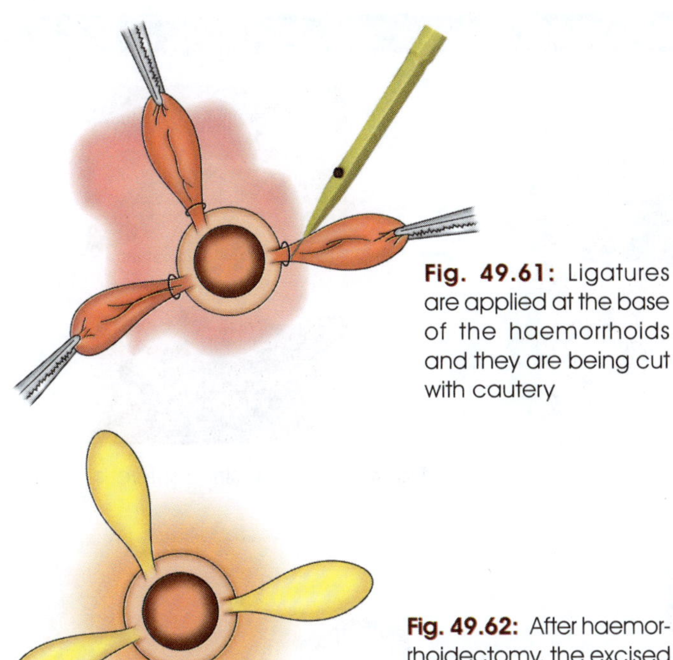

Fig. 49.61: Ligatures are applied at the base of the haemorrhoids and they are being cut with cautery

Fig. 49.62: After haemorrhoidectomy, the excised portion should look like a clover

- A tube drainage is provided so that the blood (oozing) can escape outside.

Pearls of Wisdom

Always leave a bridge of skin in between the excised pile masses to prevent anal stenosis.

II. Closed Method (Hill-Ferguson)

- Basic steps are the same as above.
- Cut mucosa and skin edges are sutured with absorbable catgut sutures.

Postoperative Management

1. Strong analgesics, in the form of injection pethidine or morphine, are given to reduce the pain.
2. Antibiotics along with metronidazole are given to prevent secondary infection.
3. Bulk purgatives are given to avoid constipation.
4. **Sitz bath** twice a day is given by using warm saline or $KMnO_4$ solution.

Postoperative Complications

They can be classified into early and late complications.

Acute retention of urine and haemorrhage are early complications. Anal stricture, anal stenosis, anal fissure and incontinence are the late complications. A few complications are described below.

1. **Retention of urine** is common in men due to severe pain. It can be managed by treating the pain and hot water fomentation in the suprapubic region. Catheterisation is done as a last resort.
2. **Reactionary haemorrhage** is more common. It is due to a loose ligature or some opened up bleedings. Generally stops by pressure packing. Otherwise, under anaesthesia, ligate or cauterise bleeding point.
3. **Secondary haemorrhage** can occur due to infection. It manifests 6 to 8 days later. If the bleeding is significant, exploration in the operation theatre may be necessary. It should be done under anaesthesia. With good illumination, it is possible to identify the bleeding points and ligate them.
4. **Anal stenosis** can occur, if too **much skin** is excised during haemorrhoidectomy. It needs regular dilatation.
5. **Anal fissure, submucous abscess, and incontinence** can occur after haemorrhoidectomy.
6. **Wound infection:** Minor degree of wound infection does occur and can be treated with sitz-bath, antibiotics and regular dressings.

Newer Techniques

- **Cryotherapy**—liquid nitrogen or nitrous oxide is used with cryoprobe infrared coagulation—used for Grades I, II and III.
- **Laser therapy**—Nd:YAG or CO_2 laser used to cause non-contact coagulation.

STAPLER HAEMORRHOIDOPEXY: NON-EXCISIONAL PROCEDURE (Figs 49.63 to 49.68)

- A novel method for 3rd and 4th degree haemorrhoids was introduced by Dr Antonio Longo in 1997.
- It is also called Procedure for Prolapse and Haemorrhoids (**PPH**).
- After reduction of prolapsed piles, a prolene purse string suture is applied circumferentially, taking good mucosal bites 3 cm above dentate line.
- This is possible by using Circular Anal Dilator (**CAD**).
- By maintaining traction in the tails of suture, the stapler is fully closed and fired.
- Slowly stapler is opened and withdrawn.
- **Look at 'doughnut'. If it is complete, nothing to worry.**
- Thus a circular ring of mucosal tissue above the level of dentate line is removed. Internal haemorrhoids are not removed, external haemorrhoids are also not removed (eventually they regress).
- Thus, **2 rows of staples** and **28 staples** are present.

Advantages

- Lesser operative time
- Less bleeding

STAPLER HAEMORRHOIDOPEXY

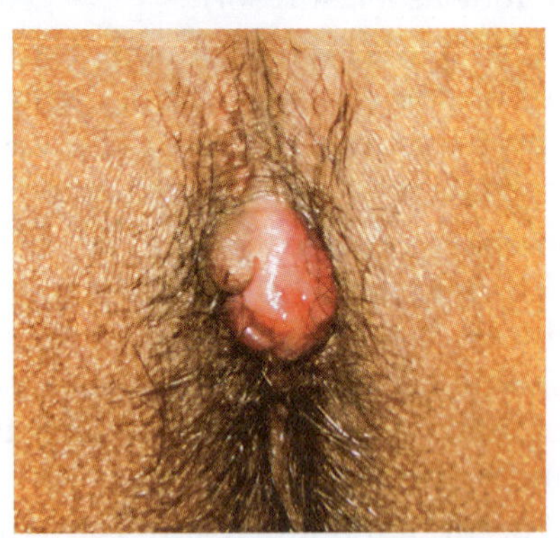

Fig. 49.63: Grade III haemorrhoids before surgery

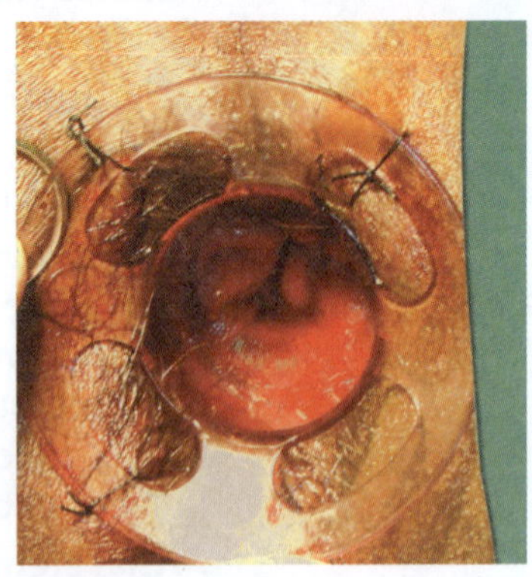

Fig. 49.64: Circular anal dilator is in place

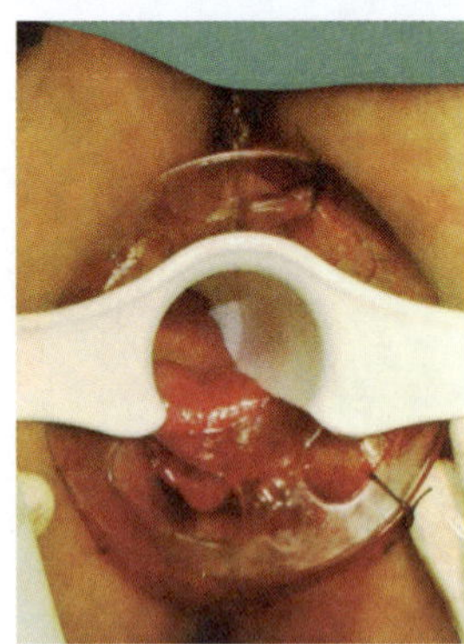

Fig. 49.65: Purse string suture is applied

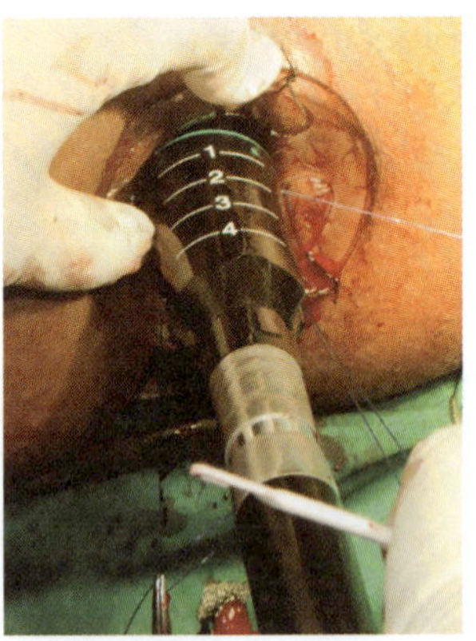

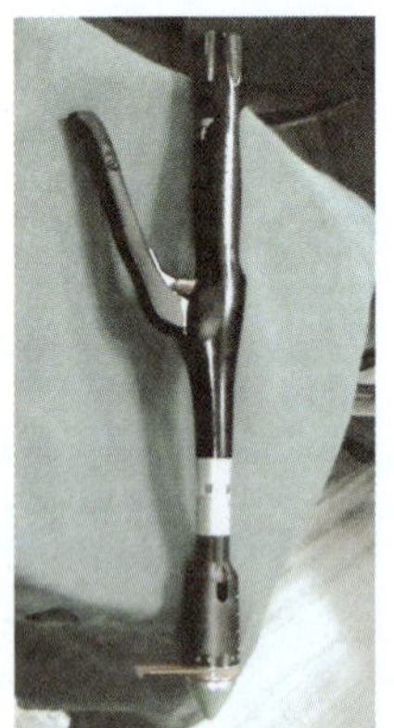

Figs 49.66 and 49.67: Maintain traction in the tails of purse string suture and stapler is closed and fired

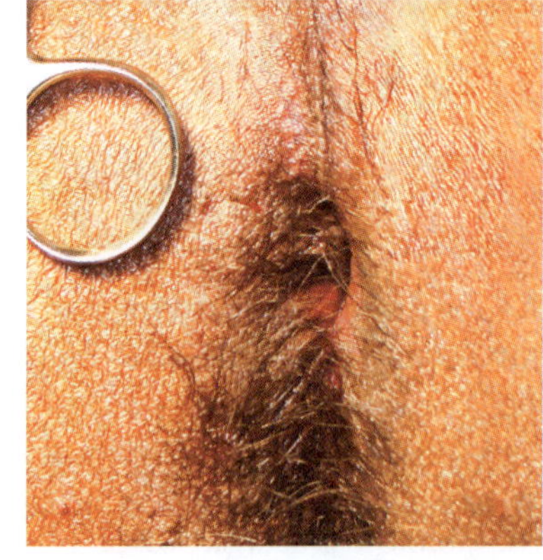

Fig. 49.68: After surgery

Courtesy: Dr BH Anand Rao, Dr Vinayak Shenoy K, Dr Ramachandra L, Dr Hartimath B, Dr Prashanth Shetty, Dr Saritha Kanth (Consultants), and Dr Akshay Nadakarni (Registrar), Department of Surgery, KMC, Manipal. Details of the study are given below.
- Study period: July 2007–2009
- Total number of patients: 186
  93 open, 93 stapled
- Follow-up: 2 years

Result of stapled group
- **Advantages:** Lesser postoperative pain, earlier return to normal activities, better satisfaction.
- **Side effects:** Mucoid discharge with tenesmus (5 patients), recurrences in 3 patients.

- Lesser postoperative pain and need for analgesia
- Lesser postoperative stay at hospital, part of day care procedures
- Earlier return to normal activities
- No major postoperative short-term and long-term complications
- No long-term side effects such as anal stenosis or chronic pain as may happen with open haemorrhoidectomy.

Disadvantages

- High cost of instrumentation.
- Difficult technically and needs special training (learning curve).
- Rare complications such as intra- and postoperative bleeding. Occasional cases of postoperative fissures, mucosal discharge, persistent tenesmus, infection and long-term complications such as rectovaginal fistulae, polyps at stapler line and recurrence.

Pearls of Wisdom

In open haemorrhoidectomy: If wound is like clover, it is over. In stapler haemorrhoidectomy: If doughnut is complete, it is time to celebrate.

DOPPLER-GUIDED HAEMORRHOIDAL ARTERY LIGATION

- Doppler principle is used to identify the feeding artery to the haemorrhoid mass and it is ligated.
- Doppler incorporated proctoscope is introduced and the artery is recognised by audible signal.
- After this, the needle is inserted into the lumen of the proctoscope.
- The artery is ligated by **figure of eight** suture. Thus, main artery supplying the haemorrhoid is blocked.
- The procedure is a simple outpatient procedure. There is no pain or blood loss. Anaesthesia is not required and recovery is early.
- Safe in all types of patients including patients with serious morbidity.

External haemorrhoids

- Described by Milligan as **5-day painful self-curing lesion.**
- Constipation and sudden straining at stools or lifting weights will result in a tender subcutaneous swelling at the anal margin.
- It is bluish in colour because it is a thrombosed vein or venule (external haemorrhoid).
- If tenderness is extreme, under local anaesthesia, incision can be given over the swelling and clot can be evacuated.
- In other cases, it will resolve within 5 days after fibrosis/ suppuration.

ANORECTAL ABSCESS

Competency

SU28.17.10: Describe aetiology, types, clinical features, complications of anorectal suppurative diseases.

Acute Anorectal Suppuration—Anorectal Abscess

- More common in men especially diabetic. Bloodborne infection is common in diabetic patients.
- Mostly originate from the anal gland opening at the base of the anal crypts. This is **cryptoglandular theory of intersphincteric anal gland infection** described by Sir Allan Parks. From here, pus spreads along path of least resistance—thus form perianal abscess or ischiorectal abscess (Key Box 49.16).
- Other source of anorectal sepsis is foreign body, trauma, sexually transmitted diseases for lower level abscesses. Crohn's disease and carcinoma rectum with perforation may form pelvirectal abscess (supralevator).

Key Box 49.16

Causes of Anorectal Abscess

- Infection
- Irritation (Crohn's disease, ulcerative colitis)
- Immunity low (diabetes, AIDS)

- Typically patients present with high grade fever with chills and rigors. On examination, a tender indurated swelling is found in the perianal region or in the ischiorectal fossa.
- Culture usually shows *E. coli* in about 70–80% of cases.
- *Staphylococcus aureus, Streptococcus, Bacteroides* are the other organisms.

Types (Fig. 49.69)

1. *Perianal Abscess*

- It occurs due to infection of anal glands in the perianal region.
- It may be due to a boil, anal gland infection or thrombosed external pile.
- It produces severe pain, throbbing in nature and on examination a soft, tender, warm swelling is found.
- Rectal examination reveals a tender, boggy, swelling under the anal mucosa.

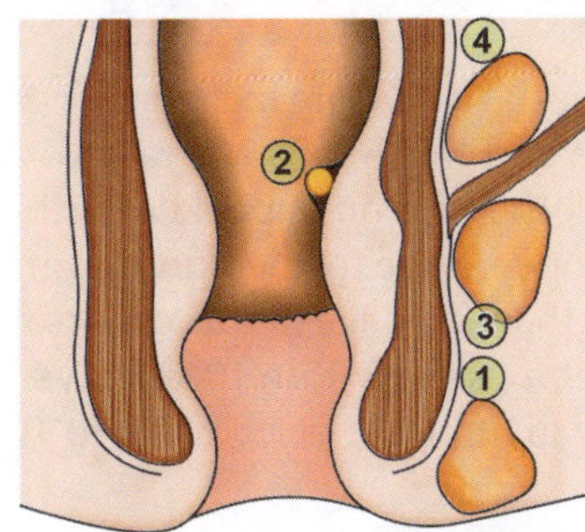

Fig. 49.69: Types of anorectal abscess (see text)

Treatment

Antibiotics, incision and drainage and excision of part of skin (roof).

2. *Submucous Abscess*

- Collection of pus under the mucous membrane of rectum or anal canal.
- It can also be due to infection of injected haemorrhoids. It can be drained using proctoscope.

3. *Ischiorectal Abscess*

- Collection of pus in the ischiorectal fossa, which is lateral to rectum and medial to pelvic wall.
- Bounded above by levator ani and inferiorly by pad of fat in the ischiorectal fossa.
- Ischiorectal fat is poorly vascularised. Hence, it is more vulnerable to infection.
- Abscess occurs due to spread of perianal abscess or due to blood-borne infection.
- Diabetes is the precipitating factor.

Clinical Features

- Severe throbbing pain is characteristic of ischiorectal abscess.
- Induration in the ischiorectal fossa
- Common in diabetic men
- Frank evidence of abscess such as fluctuation need not be seen and is a late sign (Key Box 49.17).
- High grade fever with chills and rigors.
- Per rectal examination is painful and bogginess can be appreciated on the side of the lesion.

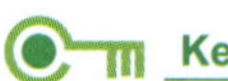 Key Box 49.17

Deep Abscess without Fluctuation

- Ischiorectal abscess
- Breast abscess
- Parotid abscess
- Prostatic abscess
- Midpalmar abscess

Treatment

Under anaesthesia, a cruciate incision (+) (Figs 49.70 and 49.71) is made and the 4 flaps are raised. All the pus is evacuated and the wound is packed with iodine roller gauze and left open. Edges of the skin are trimmed to leave an opening so that drainage of pus occurs freely. It heals with granulation tissue within 10–15 days. Appropriate antibiotics are given for a period of 5 to 10 days.

4. Pelvirectal Abscess

It is a pelvic abscess, which is drained through the rectum. The common causes are pelvic peritonitis, appendicitis, septic abortions, etc. The details of the causes, clinical features and the management are discussed on page 732. *See* Key Box 49.18 for summary of anorectal abscess.

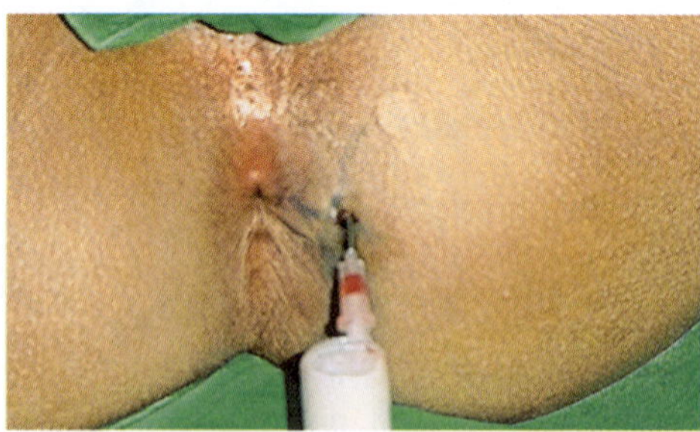

Fig. 49.70: Aspiration of ischiorectal abscess

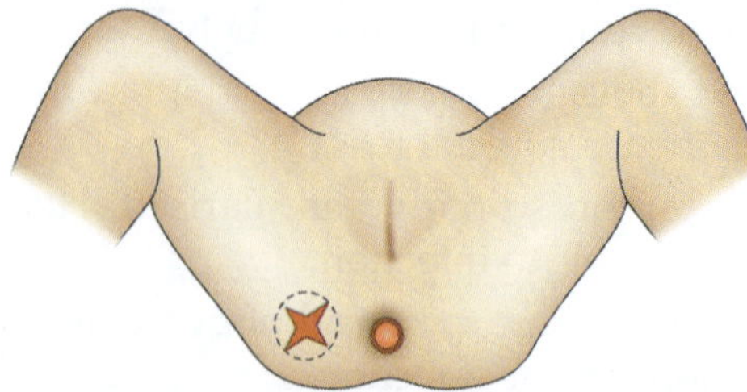

Fig. 49.71: Cruciate incision—drainage

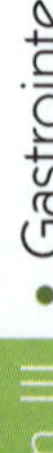

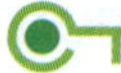 Key Box 49.18

Anorectal Abscess

- Common causes such as boil or infected sebaceous cyst has to be ruled out first.
- Remember other causes such as infection following haemorrhoidal injection or band ligation.
- Uncommon causes such as foreign body or penetrating trauma also can give rise to anorectal abscess.
- Last but not the least, AIDS and diabetes have to be ruled out in all cases of anorectal abscess.

FISTULA *IN ANO*

Competency

SU28.17.11: Describe aetiopathogenesis, clinical features and management of fistula *in ano*.

Abnormal communication between anal canal and rectum with exterior (perianal skin) is called fistula *in ano*. Even though multiple openings are seen in the perianal skin, **the internal opening is always single**.

Aetiopathogenesis

1. They occur due to **persistent anal gland infection,** which results in anorectal abscesses, rupture inside as well as outside resulting in a fistula. Once a fistula occurs, it persists because of infection and absence of rest to the part. As there are many anal glands, often, problem persists in spite of initial treatment of one fistula.
2. In India, **tuberculosis** is common. Patients with pulmonary tuberculosis have 1–2% chances of developing multiple anal fistulae. Whenever a patient presents with multiple anal fistulae, it is but natural to think of tubercular aetiology. Such fistulae are **not indurated and there is watery discharge without pus.**
3. In Western countries, **ulcerative colitis and Crohn's disease** are responsible for multiple anal fistulae.
4. **Colloid carcinoma of rectum** can present as multiple fistulae *in ano*. This type of carcinoma has worst prognosis. Rectal examination should be done in every patient with anal fistula.
   - Other causes of anal fistula are given in Key Box 49.19.

Classification

I. Standard Classification (Fig. 49.72)

1. Subcutaneous
2. Submucous

Key Box 49.19

Special Types of Fistula *In Ano*

- Fistula carcinoma
- Ileitis—Crohn's
- Schistosomiasis
- Tuberculosis
- Ulcerative colitis
- Lymphogranuloma venereum
- Anal fissure abscess

Students can remember as **FISTULA**

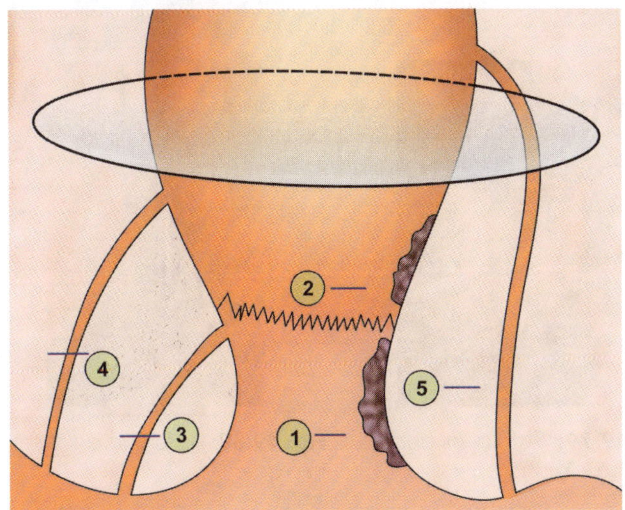

Fig. 49.72: Standard classification (see text)

3. Low anal
4. High anal
5. Pelvirectal

II. *Park's Classification* (Fig. 49.73)

1. Intersphincteric
2. Trans-sphincteric
3. Supralevator (internal opening is situated above the anorectal bundle).

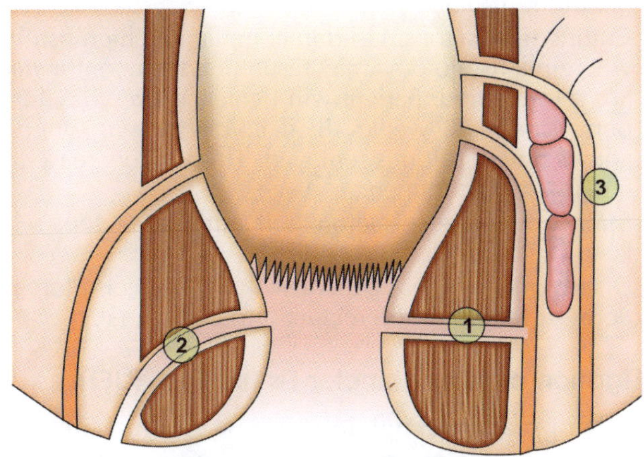

Fig. 49.73: Park's classification

Clinical Features

- Persistent seropurulent discharge, keeps the part always wet.
- Previous history of anal gland infection, with recurrent abscess.
- External opening can be single/multiple, with pouting granulation tissue, may discharge blood.
- Internal opening in carcinoma felt as a 'button hole' defect inside the rectum.
- **Goodsall's rule:** A fistula, with an external opening in the anterior half of anus within 3.75 cm tends to be direct type and in the posterior half, indirect type or curved and sometimes horseshoe type. It may communicate with the opposite side (Fig. 49.74).

Diagnosis

- External opening is found at the bottom of a depressed area or with granulation tissue or it is seen discharging pus.
- Internal opening may be felt on digital examination as **indurated** area or sometimes can be seen with proctoscopy or after sigmoidoscopy.
- The entire track may be palpable as indurated cord like structure.
- **Endorectal ultrasonography** and **MRI** seem to identify internal openings and fistula. However, they can be selectively used in deserving cases.
- Examination under general or regional anaesthesia.

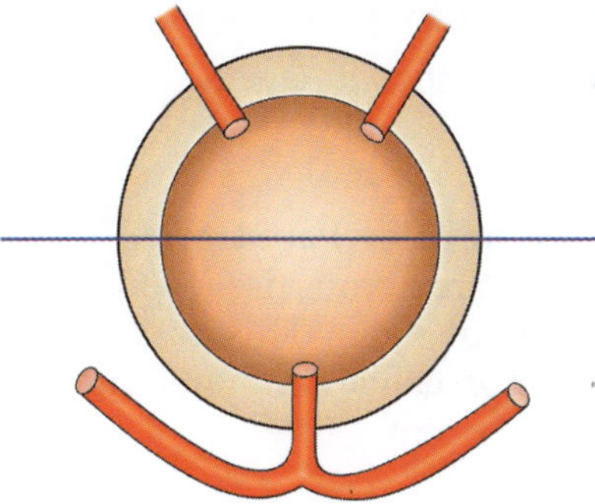

Fig. 49.74: Goodsall's rule

TREATMENT (Figs 49.75 to 49.80)

I. Fistulotomy

It is indicated in low fistula (internal opening below the anorectal bundle). A probe is passed through the external opening into the rectum and along the length of this tract the fistula is laid open. It is done under anaesthesia. The wound is left open and allowed to heal by granulation tissue developing from the floor of the fistula (marsupialisation). Intersphincteric and low trans-sphincteric fistulas of recent origin are treated by fistulotomy and marsupialisation.

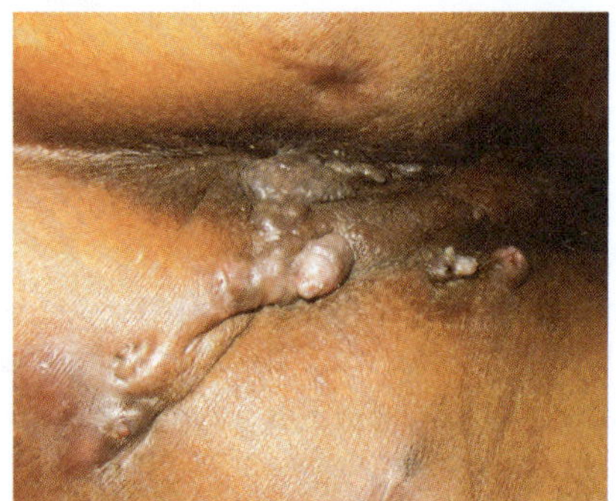

Fig. 49.75: Multiple recurrent fistula *in ano*—biopsy reported as tuberculosis

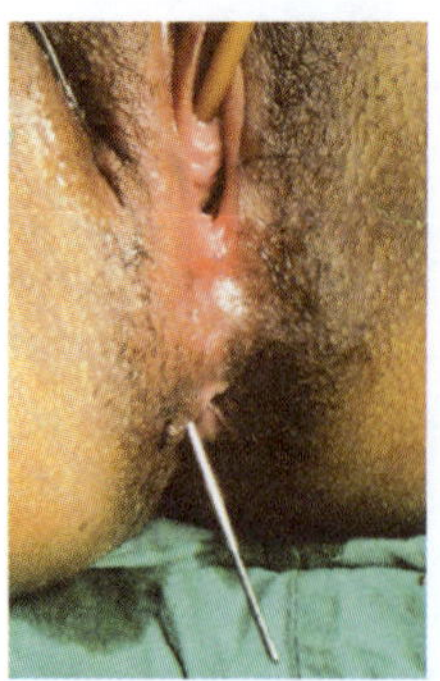

Fig. 49.76: Fistula—rectovaginal fistula

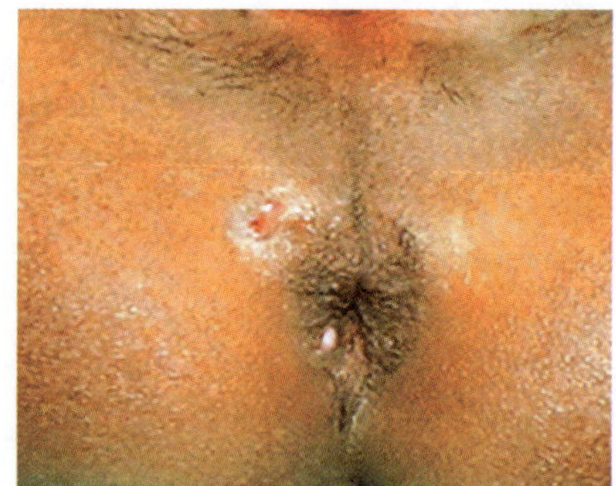

Fig. 49.77: Low fistula *in ano*

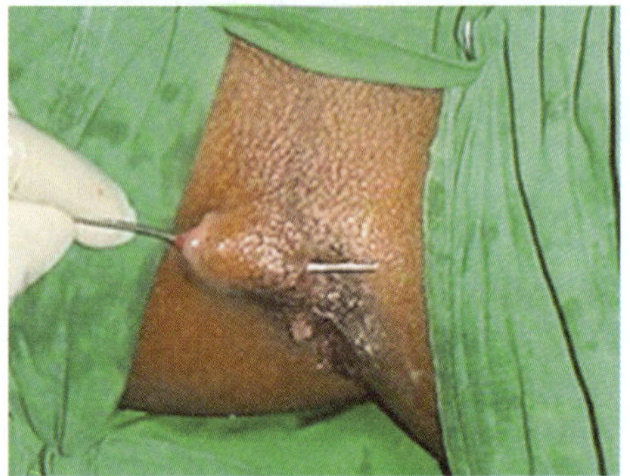

Fig. 49.78: Fistulotomy by passing a fistula probe

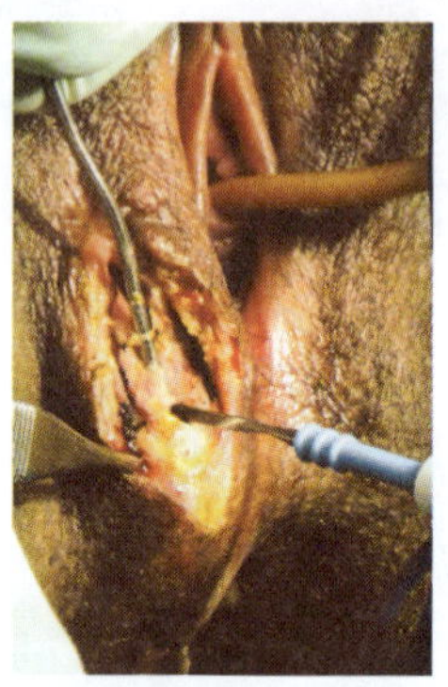

Fig. 49.79: Fistula *in ano*—excision is going on

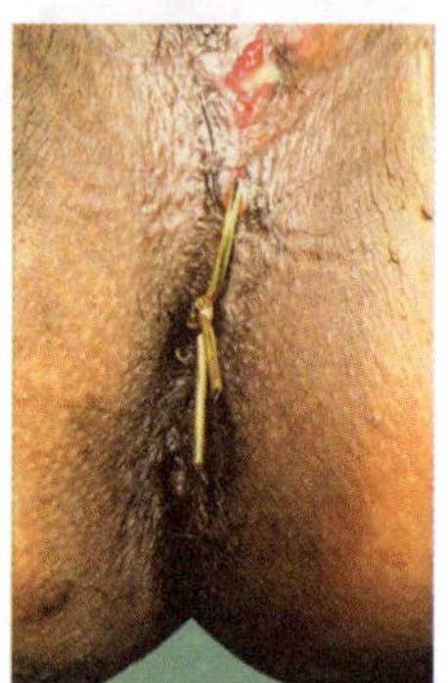

Fig. 49.80: Fistula *in ano,* seton in place

Advantages

- Least chances of recurrence
- Relatively easy procedure
- Minor degree of incontinence

II. Fistulectomy

All **chronic fistulae (low) are treated by fistulectomy** by excising the entire fibrous tissues and tract. Here also, the wound is kept open. This can also be done for **posterior semi-horseshoe and horseshoe** fistulae. Some incontinence can occur.

III. Fistulectomy with or without Colostomy

It is indicated in high fistula *in ano*. The internal opening is situated above the anorectal bundle. Hence, during fistulectomy, there is a chance of injury to the anorectal bundle and may cause incontinence. Temporary or permanent colostomy may be necessary. If there is a cause, treat the cause. Surgery of intersphincteric fistula and trans-sphincteric fistula may result in incontinence.

IV. Use of Seton or Medicated Thread (Ksharasutra)

Ksharasutra is an ayurvedic term. It is a medicated thread passed through the entire tract and both ends are tied and tightened once a week so that by 6 weeks it cuts through (Key Box 49.20).

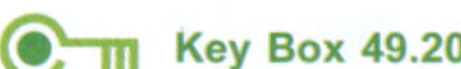

Key Box 49.20

Seton

- It is a Latin word. Seton means bristle—material such as thread, wire, or gauze that is passed through subcutaneous tissues.
- Varieties of materials used as setons—plastic tubes, infant feeding tubes, prolene suture material, medicated thread used in Ayurvedic method—Ksharasutra. Ksharasutra is a Sanskrit phrase in which Kshar refers to anything that is corrosive or caustic; while sutra means a thread.
- Loose setons for long-term palliation. Examples: Fistulae associated with Crohn's disease, complicated recurrent fistulae.
- Cutting tight setons: Used in complicated high fistulae wherein a fistulotomy may result in anal incontinence. So, seton is tied, patient will tighten it everyday for a period of 8–12 weeks till it comes down. Once it comes down, seton is removed. This will decrease the chances of incontinence.
- Main advantage of seton is it eliminates sepsis by keeping the track open.
- Disadvantage is that patient will always feel a foreign body sensation in the rectum and anal canal.

V. Ligation of Intersphincter Fistula Tact (LIFT)

Novel approach through intersphincter which involves ligation of tract close to internal opening and removal of the intersphincter tract.

See Key Box 49.21 for recent advances in fistula surgery. *See* Ten commandments for fistula *in ano*.

Key Box 49.21

Recent Advances in Fistula Surgery

1. **Biological agents:** The basic principle is to plug and seal the tract. It allows the ingrowth of healthy tissue. Thus initially fibrin glue was used but results are not good in long term. Porcine small intestinal mucosa or porcine dermal collagen also has been used. Results are not satisfactory.
2. **Video-assisted anal fistula treatment (VAAFT):** A novel sphincter-saving procedure for treating complex anal fistulae (more details on page 1304).
   - Visualisation of the fistula tract using the fistuloscope.
   - Aim is correct localisation of the internal fistula opening under direct vision.
   - A stapler or cutaneous-mucosal flap to close the internal opening after endoscopic treatment of the fistula.
   - Fistuloscopy is done under irrigation and followed by an operative phase of fulguration of the fistula tract.
   - Total closure of the internal opening and suture reinforcement with cyanoacrylate.

   You can remember as **VAAFT**

TEN COMMANDMENTS FOR FISTULA *IN ANO*

1. Should find out the internal and external openings.
2. Should try to define the type of the fistula in relation to sphincter.
3. Should define low or high fistula.
4. Should rule out special types of fistula.
5. Should conduct thorough examination again under anaesthesia before surgical procedure.
6. Should do MRI in difficult, recurrent and complicated fistula.
7. Should do fistulotomy in all intersphincteric fistulae and trans-sphincteric involving 30% of the voluntary musculature.
8. Should do fistulectomy in low fistula—it will open up the infected cavity better even though wound will be bigger than a simple fistulotomy wound.
9. Should use setons in high fistula or complicated fistula wherein a fistulotomy may result in recurrence or incontinence or when staged procedures are planned.
10. Should explain to the patient about possibility of some degree of incontinence and take consent for colostomy in high fistula.

FISSURE *IN ANO*

Competency

SU28.17.8: Describe aetiopathogenesis, clinical features and management of anal fissure.

Definition

Longitudinal tear in the lower end of anal canal results in fissure *in ano*. It is the **most painful condition** affecting the anal region. Commonly seen in young patients.

Aetiopathogenesis (Fig. 49.81 and Key Box 49.22)

- 90% of anal fissures occur in the **posterior part of anal** canal and 10% anteriorly. It is initiated by hard stool causing a crack. As a result of this, defaecation results in pain. Anal fissure is more common posteriorly in the midline because of relative ischaemia.
- **Due to pain, internal sphincter spasm** takes place which makes constipation worse resulting in a **chronic fissure**.
- **Anterior fissures** occur in elderly women secondary to repeated pregnancies. This is due to damaged pelvic floor and lack of support to anal mucous membrane. Acute fissure in females may occur after vaginal delivery.

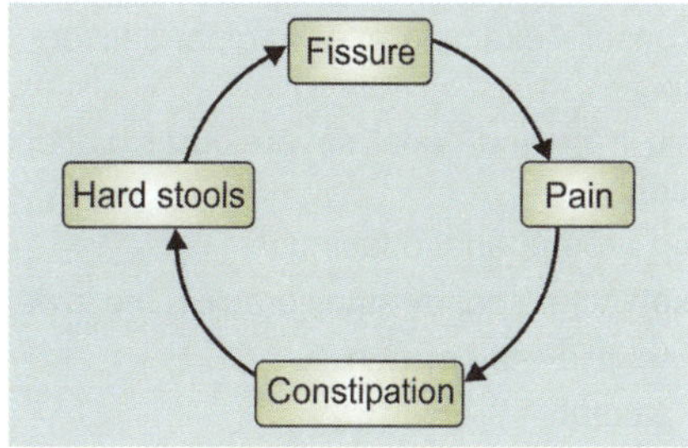

Fig. 49.81: Aetiopathogenesis of anal fissure

Key Box 49.22

Various Factors which Precipitate Anal Fissure

- Faeces—hard
- Ischaemia
- Surgical procedures—haemorrhoidectomy
- Sphincter hypertonia
- Underlying diseases—Crohn's, sexually transmitted diseases, etc.
- Repeated childbirth
- Enthusiastic usage of ointments and abuse of laxatives

Remember as **FISSURE**

Pearls of Wisdom

Fissure away from midline should raise the possibility of Crohn's disease, sexually transmitted diseases, etc.

Clinical Features

- Severe pain during and after defaecation, burning in nature, lasting for about ½ to 1 hour because of which defaecation is postponed.
- Severe constipation is present.
- Stools are hard, pellet like and there is a drop of blood or streaks of fresh blood.

Pearls of Wisdom

Drop of blood is due to anal fissure. Splash of blood is due to haemorrhoids, bloody slime is due to carcinoma.

- Sentinel pile refers to tag of skin at the outer end of the fissure.
- In some cases, fissure may be associated with a small perianal abscess resulting in worsening of pain.

Diagnosis (Table 49.5)

1. When the buttocks are spread apart, a longitudinal tear and a hypertrophied, thickened skin is seen near the lower end of fissure—**sentinel pile.**
2. Per rectal examination can be done (with lignocaine jelly application) and **sphincter spasm** can be appreciated.
3. Proctoscopy is contraindicated because the condition is very **painful**.

Treatment (Table 49.6)

I. *Conservative*

- Avoid constipation—encourage fibre diet, mild laxatives and not to postpone defaecation.
- Surface anaesthetic creams: Lignocaine jelly.
- Metronidazole and antibiotics
- Sitz bath

II. *Agents which Decrease Sphincter Pressure*

- **Glyceryl trinitrate** (0.2%) topical application: Significant headache and 50% recurrence are drawbacks. It reduces spasm, increases vascular perfusion.
- **Purified botulinum toxin** injection into internal sphincter: It inhibits presynaptic release of

Table 49.5 Difference between acute fissure *in ano* and chronic fissure *in ano*

Acute fissure	Chronic fissure
• Sudden onset—example after vaginal delivery or following hard stools • Acute pain in the anal canal, severe burning after defaecation with bleeding • No itching around anal opening • Severe sphincter spasm, small crack in the lower anal canal • No sentinel pile—tag of skin • PR very painful • Proctoscopes—better not try insertion • Usually responds to conservative treatment—local application of glyceryl trinitrate (GTN) 0.2% 3–4 times a day or diltiazem 2% twice a day • Emergency sphincterotomy may be required in a few patients	• A few months duration of symptoms • Chronic pain in the anal canal, burning after defaecation with bleeding—a few exacerbations • Itching is usually present due to ulcer or hypertrophied skin—sentinel pile • Sphincter spasm, chronic canoe-shaped ulcer in the lower anal canal • Sentinel pile—tag of skin • PR painful • Proctoscope—can be done with proper ligonocaine application to the anal canal • Responds to conservative treatment but effect is temporary, surgery is the treatment of choice • Lateral sphincterotomy or other procedures may be required

Table 49.6 Treatment of chronic fissure *in ano*

Pharmacological agents	Injection botulinum A toxin	Lateral sphincterotomy/flaps
• 0.2% **glyceryl trinitrate** ointment for local application • Headache is a complication • Still it is a popular treatment because it is simple • Drug releases NO (nitric oxide) at a cellular level and mediates relaxation of internal sphincter • **Oral nifedipine** 20 mg, twice daily. Topical nifedipine also helps	• Healing rate is 80% in chronic anal fissures • 6% recurrence in 6 months • Single injection, simple method, smooth recovery—chances of sepsis are present	• Gold standard • Manometry of anal sphincter can be done before procedure especially in women because 30–40% of patients develop incontinence following lateral sphincterotomy **Advancement flap** Women—postpartum fissure—poor anal tone

acetylcholine from cholinergic nerve endings and cause temporary paresis of striated muscle. Cost, perianal thrombosis and sepsis are drawbacks. Injection produces **prolonged but reversible effects,** thus avoiding **permanent injury** (Key Box 49.23).

- **Calcium channel blockers:** Nifedipine, diltiazem oral and topical applications **(2%)** also have been used.

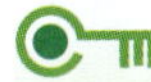
Key Box 49.23

Role of Botulinum Toxin Injection

- Achalasia cardia and other oesophageal motility disorders.
- Anal fissures
- Sphincter of Oddi dysfunction
- Frey syndrome

III. *Surgical Treatment*

1. **Lateral anal sphincterotomy of Notaras** (or dorsal) is **the best alternative procedure**. Here internal sphincter is divided away from fissure either in right or left lateral positions. The procedure can be easily done by using a bivalved speculum in the anal canal. This is the procedure of choice. **Sphincterotomy should be limited to the length of fissure to avoid incontinence.**
2. **Fissurectomy and local advancement flap:** This is indicated in **persistent, chronic, nonhealing fissure.** After excision of the fissure, the resulting defect in the anal canal is closed by a small (**rhomboid**) advancement flap. This should be considered not as a first line of treatment. Recovery from this operation takes much more time than other treatments for anal fissures.
3. **Lord's dilatation:** It is also called **blunt sphincterotomy**—a few fibres of internal sphincter are divided. It relieves the spasm and the fissure heals. Rarely, in female patients, it may result in incontinence. **It is not a recommended treatment nowadays.**

Pearls of Wisdom

Lateral sphincterotomy is very popular and gives good results.

PILONIDAL SINUS (JEEP-BOTTOM)

- Pilonidal sinus means **nest of hairs** in Greek. Also called **Jeep-bottom** because it was very common in jeep drivers.
- More common in dark people than fair people.
- It is an acquired condition, commonly found in hairy males.

It is acquired due to the following reasons:

- Appears between the age of 20 and 30 years.
- Hairy men are more affected.
- The **hair follicle is never demonstrated in the wall of the pilonidal sinus** but hair is the content of pilonidal sinus.

- Hair accumulates due to vibration and friction causing shedding of the hair. Thus, it accumulates in the gluteal cleft and enters the opening of the sweat glands.
- Pointed end of the dead hair is inside (blind end of the sinus).

Clinical Features

- External opening of the sinus seen just above the anal verge in the midline over the coccyx (Key Box 49.24).
- History of discharge of pus
- History of recurrent abscesses which rupture, discharging pus.
- Can be asymptomatic.

Key Box 49.24

Sites of Pilonidal Sinus

- Midline over the coccyx
- Umbilicus
- Interdigital in barbers

Diagnosis

Osteomyelitis of the coccyx is the only differential diagnosis for pilonidal sinus. Hence, X-ray of the coccyx should be taken.

Treatment (Figs 49.82 to 49.85)

- Inject methylene blue to demonstrate branches of the sinus followed by **excision of the sinus**. The patient is positioned prone with buttocks elevated (**Jack knife position)**.
- After excision, there are two methods to treat the wound—open and closed methods (Key Box 49.23).
- **Open method:** The wound is left open after excision followed by regular packing with iodine or eusol gauze pieces (Key Box 49.25).
- It may take 3–4 weeks for the healing of pilonidal sinus. Regular sitz bath is also given.
- This method carries the least recurrence.
- **Closed method:** The wound is closed by 'z' plasty. This method carries 10–20% chances of recurrence. Rhomboid flap (Limberg flap) can be raised to close the defect also.

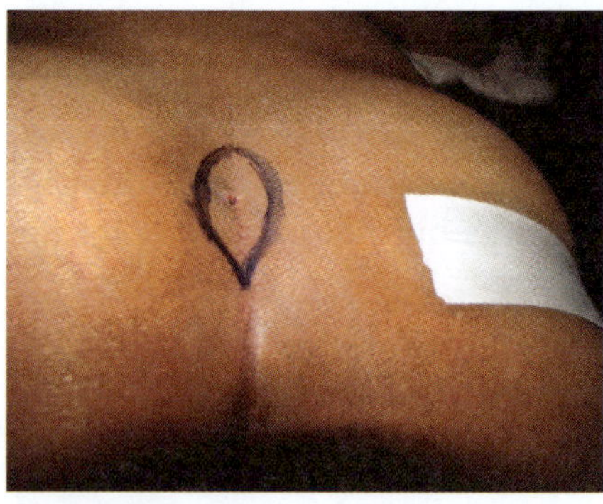

Fig. 49.82: A case of pilonidal sinus—methylene blue is first injected into the opening. The excision area is marked also with methylene blue

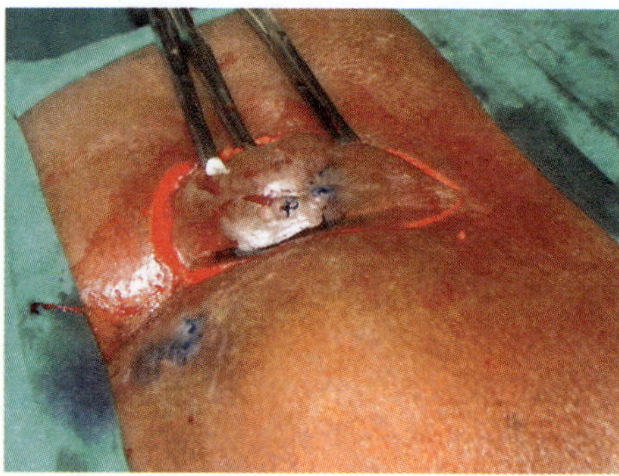

Fig. 49.83: Blue-stained tissues are dissected all around and removed

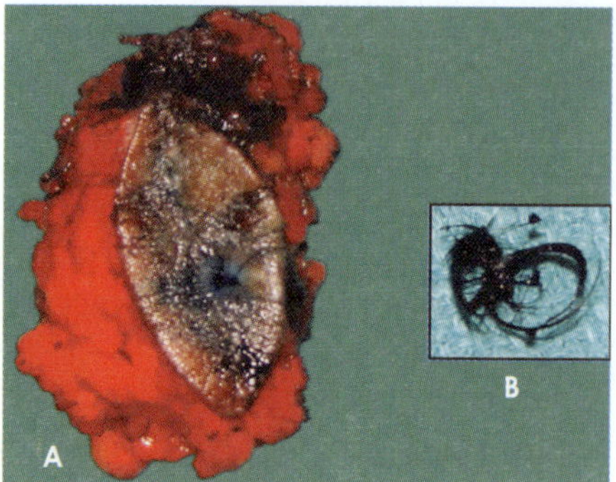

Figs 49.84A and B: (A) Specimen of excised tissue with sinus track, and (B) shows tuft of hair which was present within the sinus

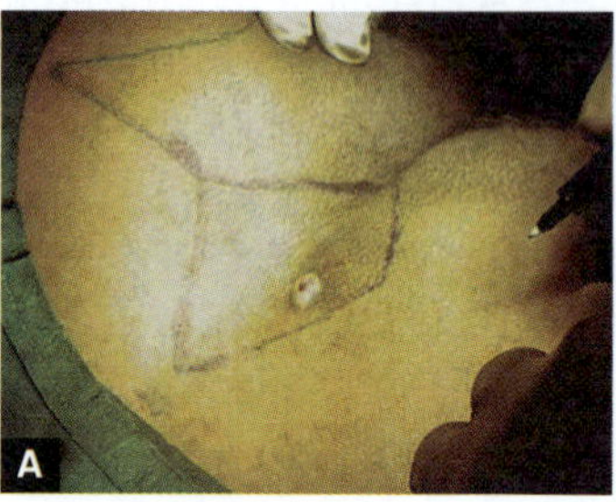

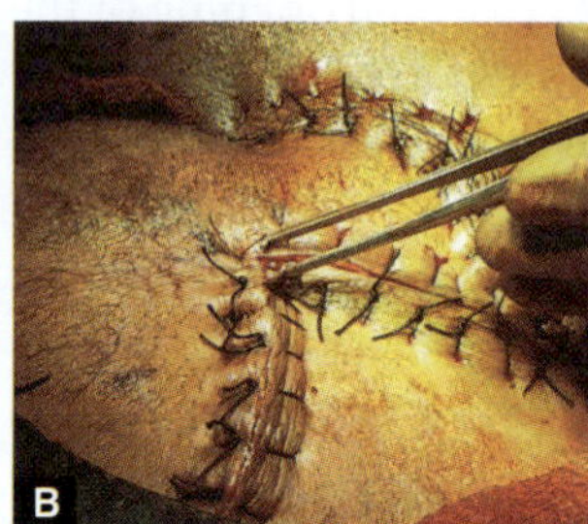

Fig. 49.85A and B: (A) Pilonidal sinus excision. Limberg flap—marking done; (B) After excision, you can see the suture lines. (*Courtesy*: Dr Dayananda Nooli, Consultant surgeon, Past Chairman ASI- Karnataka Chapter Chikkodi, Karnataka)

Key Box 49.25

Pilonidal Sinus

- It is acquired condition—popularly called Jeep-bottom
- Common in hairy men
- Multiple sinuses communicating with each other
- They open to the exterior by multiple openings
- The direction of the sinuses is cephaloid
- Recurrent abscesses which rupture are common
- Excision with or without marsupialisation, flap closure or z plasty are the treatment options.
- In spite of the adequate surgical procedures, recurrence is common.

- **Karydakis procedure:** Primary procedure is to remove all the sinus tracts and their branches till sacral bone. In this operation, semilateral incision is made around the sinuses and flaps mobilised to excise all the sinuses and their branches. Then tension free closure is done. Compared to elliptical incision, this incision and closure has decreased chances of skin necrosis.
- **Bascom's technique:** In this procedure, an incision is given laterally, not in the midline. After raising the flaps, wide excision of the infected sinuses and tracts is done followed by closure of the midline openings. Lateral wound is left open (in the conventional operation, midline wound is left open).

Pearls of Wisdom

Very, very rarely carcinoma can arise in a chronic pilonidal sinus.

SACROCOCCYGEAL TERATOMA

- It is a congenital condition affecting the sacrococcygeal region.
- In this region, totipotential cells persist for a longer period compared to rest of the area. Hence, it is the site of teratomas.

Clinical Features

- 20% of the cases are stillborn babies. It is common in a female child.
- Presents as a swelling in the sacrococcygeal region pushing the rectum anteriorly.
- The surface of the swelling ulcerates. Many cystic areas are present in the swelling.
- The swelling is fixed to the sacrum and coccyx from which it is impossible to separate/isolate.

Complications

- Ulceration
- Secondary infection
- Haemorrhage
- Teratocarcinomatous change occurs by one year of age.

Treatment

Excision of the teratoma with part of sacrum and coccyx.

MALIGNANT TUMOURS OF ANAL CANAL

Competency

SU28.17.12: Describe aetiopathogenesis, clinical features, diagnosis and management of carcinoma of anal canal.

- They are not uncommon tumours which present with bleeding per rectum, burning and itching in the anal region.
- The diagnosis is obvious in many cases once buttocks are separated or by digital examination.
- Tissue diagnosis is a must before radical treatment.

Types

1. **Squamous cell carcinoma:** Papillomas are the chief predisposing factors. Local excision or APR (abdominoperineal resection) is the treatment with external RT in appropriate cases (Fig. 49.86).
   - For sphincter preservation—chemoradiation can be used. It is called Nigri's regime.

   Refer also to Key Box 49.26.
2. **Basaloid carcinoma:** It is a highly malignant, non-keratinising, squamous cell carcinoma. Treatment is similar to squamous cell carcinoma.

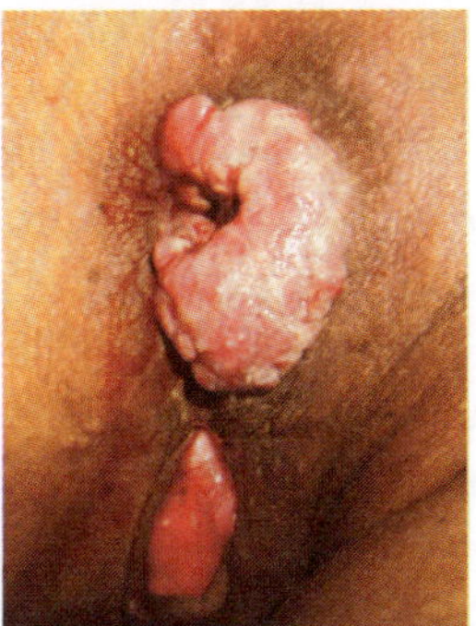

Fig. 49.86: Squamous cell carcinoma anal canal

Key Box 49.26

Anal Intraepithelial Neoplasia (AIN—Bowen's Disease)

- It is squamous cell carcinoma *in situ* of the anus.
- It is precursor to an invasive squamous cell carcinoma.
- It is associated with human papillomavirus type 16 and 18 (HPV 16,18).
- Anoscopy, biopsy to be done.
- Dysplasia is an indication for resection/ablation.

Pearls of Wisdom

Basal cell carcinoma is very rare in the anal canal.

3. **Melanoma:** Beware of a patient who comes with bilateral groin nodes which are bulky. The patient may be having malignant melanoma of anal canal—bluish/blackish ulcer in the anal canal. APR is potentially curable in early cases of melanoma. If metastasis is present, the prognosis is poor. So, only local excision is done so as to provide palliation but colostomy is avoided (Figs 49.87 to 49.90).

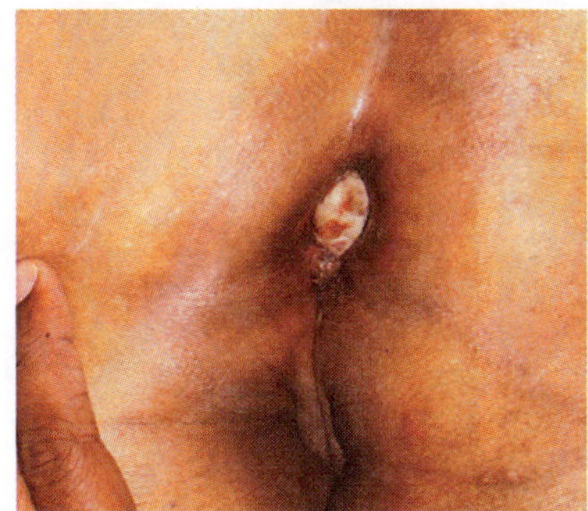

Fig. 49.87: Melanoma anal region

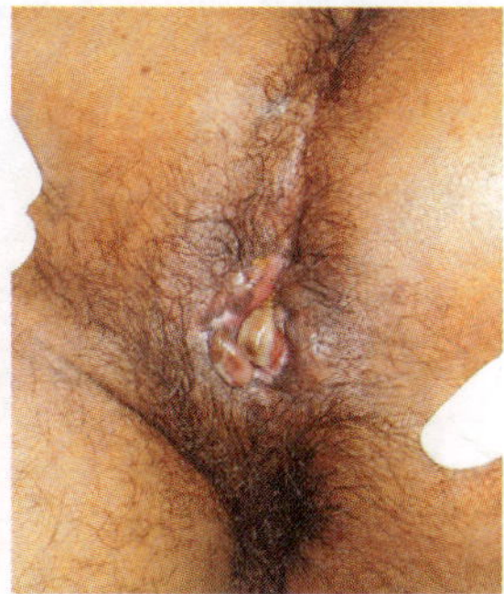

Fig. 49.88: Melanoma resembled prolapsed piles but pigmentation was evident on closer examination

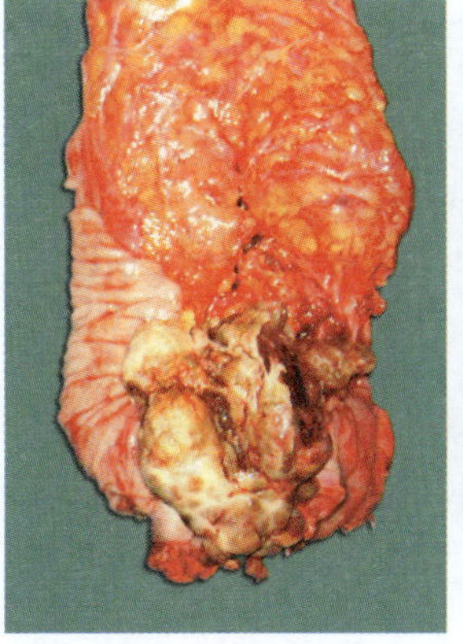

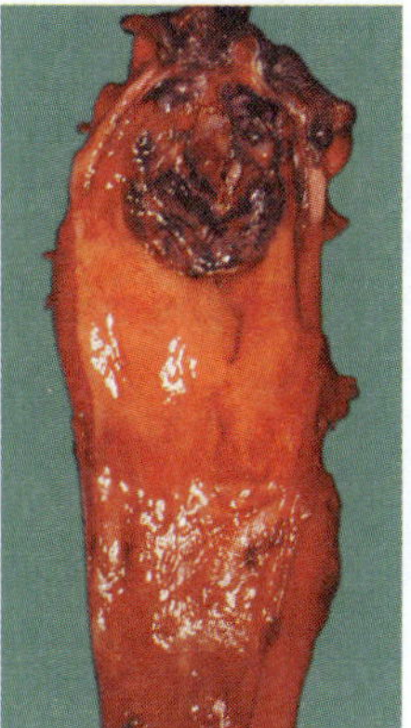

Figs 49.89 and 49.90: Malignant melanoma of the anal canal—APR specimens

4. **Adenocarcinoma** is rare. It can occur from the anal glands in pre-existing anal fistula. APR with 5-FU and radiation therapy is indicated.

Pearls of Wisdom

Please note that Bowen's disease, Paget's disease or verrucous carcinoma, squamous and basal cell carcinoma can also occur in the skin of anal margin.

STRICTURE OF ANAL CANAL AND RECTUM

Causes

1. **Postoperative:** Haemorrhoidectomy, pull-through operations, repeated diathermy fulguration of polyps.
2. **Irradiation:** It occurs one to two years after irradiation.
3. **Senile strictures**

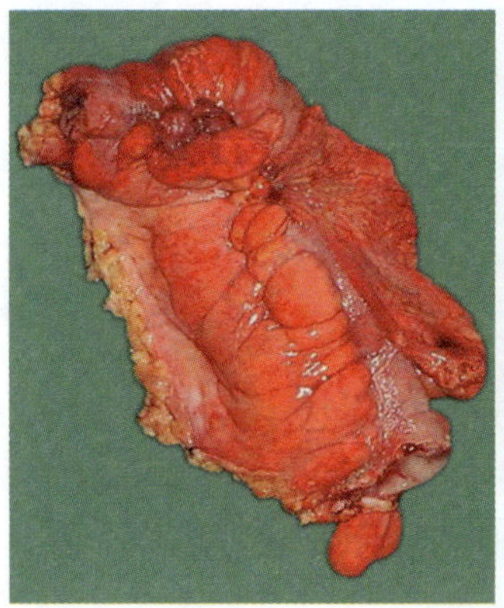
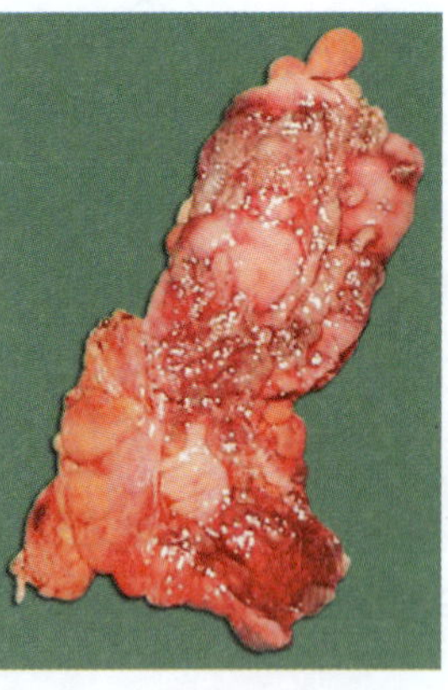

Figs 49.91 and 49.92: Rectal stricture due to CMV colitis (*Courtesy:* Dr Satyanarayana N, Dr Srinivas Pai, Dr Madhu, KMC, Manipal)

4. **Lymphogranuloma inguinale:** A sexually transmitted disease affecting both male and female patients. Initially pararectal lymph nodes are enlarged followed by development of multiple rectal strictures.
5. **Inflammatory bowel diseases:** Both ulcerative colitis and Crohn's disease result in rectal strictures (5–10%).
6. **Rare:** Congenital, amoeboma, carcinoid, endometriosis, tuberculosis, CMV colitis (Figs 49.91 and 49.92).

Clinical Features

Increasing constipation is the characteristic feature of stricture of the rectum. It may be associated with hard stools, bleeding and pain in some cases. Per abdominal examination may reveal loaded colon with scybalous masses. Rectal examination can detect a stricture.

Pearls of Wisdom

It is mandatory to rule out carcinoma rectum which is the most common cause of stricture.

Treatment

1. Conservative treatment includes bulk purgatives, a vegetable diet.
2. Regular dilatation may be necessary for the strictures situated low in the rectum and anal canal.
3. Intractable strictures need to be resected.
4. Treatment of the primary disease.

ANAL INCONTINENCE

Mechanism of Anal Continence

- Distension of rectum causes **tonic contraction of external sphincter**. This is controlled by cerebrum and the centre is in the **lumbosacral region of the spinal cord**.
- Faeces in contact with anal canal stimulates the specialised nerve endings. Nerve endings are also present in the puborectalis.
- **High pressure** in the anal canal (25–120 mmHg) and angle between rectum and anal canal (80°) are the important factors which maintain anal continence.

Anorectal Ring

- It marks the junction between the rectum and anal canal.
- It is formed by puborectalis, highest part of internal sphincter, longitudinal muscle and external part of sphincter.

Causes of Anal Incontinence (Key Box 49.27)

1. **Traumatic:** Injury to the anorectum due to sharp penetrating objects occurs due to accidents.
2. **Surgical procedures**
   - Damage to the internal and external sphincter can occur due to Lord's dilatation[1], a procedure done for fissure *in ano*. However, most of it is temporary.
   - Division of high fistula *in ano* may result in incontinence.
   - Following pull-through procedures done for anorectal anomalies, Hirschsprung's disease.
   - Haemorrhoidectomy—very large pile masses.
   - Extensive small bowel resection
   - Rectal excision
3. **Mass in the anorectum:** Prolapse piles, prolapse rectum and carcinoma rectum may produce temporary incontinence which subsides after surgical procedures.
4. **Neurological causes:** In females, **pudendal nerve neuropathy** which occurs due to chronic straining may result in incontinence. Spinal injuries, spina bifida, meningomyelocele are associated with anal incontinence.
5. **GI motility increase:** Inflammatory bowel diseases irritate bowel and produce temporary incontinence.

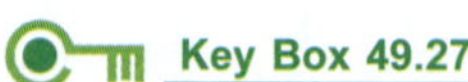

Key Box 49.27

Common Causes of Anal Incontinence

- **T**rauma
- **R**epeated pregnancies
- **A**nal surgery
- **U**nnatural sex—anal intercourse
- **M**egacolon—congenital or acquired
- **A**geing or senility

You can remember as **TRAUMA**

[1]Lord's dilatation or blunt sphincterotomy is no longer done.

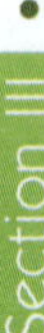

6. **Childhood/congenital causes:** Anorectal malformations, Hirschsprung's disease, spina bifida, abnormal behaviour.
7. **Miscellaneous:** Old age (senility), general debility and faecal impaction, Parkinson's disease, behavioural problem, etc.

Treatment

I. **Temporary incontinence:** Reassurance. Perineal exercises to improve the tone of internal and external sphincter.

II. **Permanent incontinence:**
1. Divided sphincter can be reunited, followed by overlapping of the remaining muscles.
2. Intersphincteric repair of puborectalis sling and plication of the external sphincter.
3. Gracilis muscle can be used to create a new anal sphincter by transposing it followed by electrical stimulation using a pacemaker.
4. Using artificial sphincter.

PROCTALGIA FUGAX

- This condition is characterised by attacks of severe cramp-like pain arising in the rectum.
- Anxiety status, straining at stools or ejaculation are a few precipitating factors.
- The pain may be unbearable, may recur at irregular intervals. It is possibly due to segmental cramp in the pubococcygeus muscle. The pain usually lasts for a few minutes and subsides (fleeting perianal pain).
- Symptomatic treatment in the form of analgesics are given.

PRURITUS ANI

Definition

This is intractable itching around the anus.

Causes

Perianal and anal discharge: Anal fissure, fistula *in ano*, prolapsed piles, polyps, genital warts are a few conditions which render the anus moist.

Pearls of Wisdom

Mucous discharge is an intense pruritic agent.

1. Poor hygiene, lack of cleanliness, excessive sweating and wearing tight and rough underclothing are common causes.
2. Parasitic causes—threadworms
3. Psychoneurosis
4. Allergy, diabetes are the other causes.

Pearls of Wisdom

Sexually transmitted diseases such as herpes, anal warts and HIV infection must be excluded.

Treatment (Key Box 49.28)

- Hygienic measures
- Prednisolone topical cream 1% with antifungal agent (miconazole nitrate 2%)
- Moisturising cream/lotion
- Antihistamine—promethazine hydrochloride 10–25 mg at night times.

Pearls of Wisdom

Pelvic floor dysfunction also referred to as nonrelaxing puborectalis syndrome is called ANISMUS. These patients present with constipation. It is a difficult problem to treat.

Key Box 49.28

Pruritus Ani—Avoid

- Toilet paper
- Soap
- Too tight underclothing
- Too many ointments
- Local anaesthetic cream

HIDRADENITIS SUPPURATIVA

Definition

It is a chronic recurrent suppuration of apocrine glands in the skin resulting in multiple abscesses which rupture causing multiple sinuses.

Sites

Axilla, groin, back, buttocks and anal regions are common sites.

Pathogenesis

- Occlusion of the gland ducts results in stasis, bacterial proliferation, abscess, rupture. Common organisms are *Staphylococcus aureus* and anaerobes (somewhat like breast abscess).
- Anogenital disease is more common in men. Hence, androgens may play a role in this condition.
- Obesity is another contributing factor.

Clinical Features

- Common after puberty till the age of 40 years.

- Typically, it is a folliculitis presenting as multiple boils which are painful.
- Pus formation, rupture and persisting sinuses are common.
- Interestingly, it neither affects above the level of dentate line nor sphincters.

Differential Diagnosis

All diseases resulting in multiple sinuses in and around perineum are the differential diagnosis such as Crohn's disease, tuberculosis, lymphogranuloma venereum, pilonidal sinuses, actinomycosis, etc.

Treatment

- When in doubt, rule out other causes mentioned above and if necessary, a good biopsy from the sinus tract and from the edge of the sinus.
- General measures such as weight reduction, antibiotics, antiseptic medicated soaps, washing the part with warm saline or water.
- Surgery includes laying open all the openings or wide excision with or without skin (radical excision) and direct closure or skin grafting of flap reconstruction are the other choices.

MISCELLANEOUS

Act of Defaecation (Key Box 49.29)

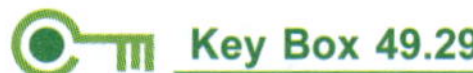
Key Box 49.29

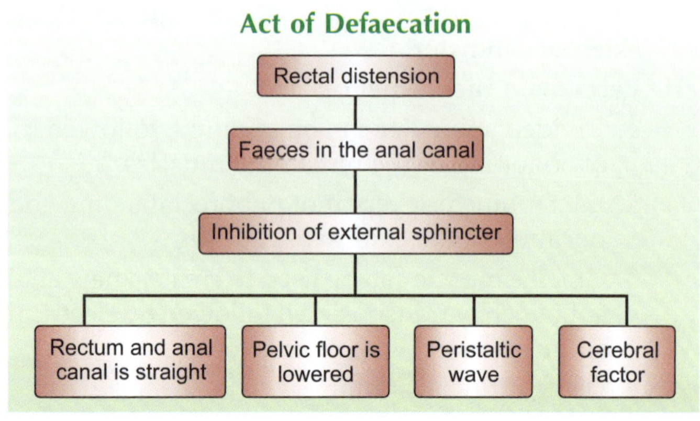

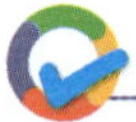

Multiple Choice Questions

1. **Splash in the pan is classically described for bleeding from which condition?**
   A. Carcinoma rectum B. Fissure *in ano*
   C. Haemorrhoids D. Polyp
2. **Which of the following are causes of anorectal fistulae in males *except*:**
   A. Crohn's disease
   B. Tuberculosis
   C. Ulcerative colitis
   D. Lymphogranuloma venereum
3. **Following are true about peritoneal coverings/fascia of the rectum *except*:**
   A. Upper one-third is completely covered
   B. Middle one-third is covered anterolaterally
   C. Lower one-third is covered anteriorly
   D. Waldeyer's fascia separates the rectum from sacrum
4. **About signet ring carcinoma rectum, following are true *except*:**
   A. It is seen in young patients
   B. Cells are filled with mucus and nucleus is displaced
   C. It carries bad prognosis
   D. Not an indication for chemotherapy
5. **Following are true for clinical features of carcinoma rectum *except*:**
   A. Can give rise to tenesmus
   B. Can present as bloody slime
   C. Can present as liver secondaries
   D. Can cause closed loop obstruction
6. **The ideal surgical treatment for growth at 8 cm from the anal verge is:**
   A. Abdominoperineal resection
   B. Abdominosacral resection
   C. High anterior resection
   D. Total mesorectal excision
7. **On-table lavage of the intestines for resection and anastomosis can be done via:**
   A. Enterotomy
   B. Colotomy
   C. Enema from rectum
   D. Appendicular stump

8. Local excision of malignant rectal tumour can be done, if:
A. The tumour is up to 6 cm size
B. Up to 60% of the rectal wall involvement
C. Lymphatic invasion is accepted
D. Tumour is well differentiated

9. Prolapse rectum is caused by several factors *except*:
A. Birth injuries to the nerve fibres
B. Defective collagen metabolism
C. It does not start as intussusception
D. Deep rectovesical pouch

10. Below the dentate line, squamous epithelium has:
A. No basal cells
B. Hair
C. Sweat glands
D. Pigment forming cells

11. Above the dentate line, lymphatic drainage goes to:
A. Para-aortic nodes
B. Superficial inguinal lymph nodes
C. Deep inguinal lymph nodes
D. Pudendal lymph nodes

12. Following are true for prolapsed piles *except*:
A. External sphincter grips the pile mass and cause gangrene
B. Thrombosis can occur
C. Portal pyaemia can be a complication
D. Requires hemorrhoidectomy

13. Which one of these precautions must be taken while applying band for haemorrhoids?
A. Bands are applied in grade 1 pile masses
B. Bands are applied in grade 4 haemorrhoids
C. Bands are applied below the dentate line
D. Bands should not be applied in patients who are taking anticoagulants

14. Anal stenosis is a complication of:
A. Stapler haemorrhoidopexy
B. Open haemorrhoidectomy
C. Too low application of the band
D. Cryosurgery

15. Following are true for injection line treatment of haemorrhoids *except*:
A. It is given perivascular
B. Given above the level of dentate line
C. It is painful
D. It is given in submucosal plane

16. Following are true for stapler haemorrhoidopexy *except*:
A. Recurrence rate is less
B. Less discomfort than open haemorrhoidectomy
C. Anal stenosis is not a complication
D. Ideal for 3rd or 4th degree haemorrhoids

17. In multiple fistula *in ano* and high fistula, which one of the following should not be done?
A. Biopsy of the track B. Colostomy
C. Fistulogram D. Multiple fistulotomy

18. Majority of the cases of fissure *in ano* are:
A. Anterior B. Posterior
C. Anterolateral D. Posterolateral

19. In lateral sphincterotomy:
A. Pecten fibres are ruptured
B. It is blunt sphincterotomy
C. External sphincter is divided
D. Internal sphincter is divided

20. In cases of pilonidal sinus:
A. Hair is demonstrated in the wall
B. It is congenital
C. It is known for recurrence
D. It undergoes malignant change

Answers

1. C	**2.** D	**3.** C	**4.** D	**5.** D	**6.** D	**7.** D	**8.** D	**9.** C	**10.** D
11. A	**12.** A	**13.** D	**14.** B	**15.** C	**16.** B	**17.** B	**18.** D	**19.** D	**20.** C

CHAPTER

50

Lower Gastrointestinal Bleeding

- Causes
- Clinical examination
- Investigations
- Exploratory laparotomy
- Haemobilia
- Angiodysplasia

Introduction

Lower gastrointestinal (LGI) bleeding refers to bleeding which occurs beyond the ligament of Treitz. Bleeding per rectum may be a manifestation of upper GI bleeding (UGIB), the causes of which have been discussed under haematemesis. In this chapter, bleeding per rectum due to lower GI causes will be discussed. LGI bleeding accounts for 1% of acute hospital admissions each year. Severe bleeding is that which continues for 24 hours after hospital admission or that which recurs 24 hours after resolution.

Pearls of Wisdom

In all, so-called the lower GI bleeding—rule out 3 important causes of upper GI bleeding, namely—oesophageal variceal bleeding due to portal hypertension, peptic ulcers—mainly duodenal ulcer bleeds and acute erosive gastritis or acute gastric mucosal lesions (AGML). Bleeding from these causes can be so massive, they result in fresh bleeding per rectum, thus adding confusion at the diagnosis. A **nasogastric tube lavage that yields blood or coffee-ground-like material confirms the diagnosis of upper GI bleeding.**

Definition

Competency

SU28.14: Describe the clinical features, investigations and principles of management of disorders of small and large intestines. (*Please note:* This chapter deals with GI tract bleeding. You will come across important causes of bleeding)

- **Haematochezia:** Bloody stools (LGIB or rapid UGIB).
- **Melaena:** Black tarry stools from digested blood. The duration of bleeding is more than 8 hours.
- **Massive GI tract bleeding:** The bleeding which requires more than 3 units of blood transfusions in 24 hours or **25% of intravascular blood volume loss.**
- **Obscure:** Bleeding which persists or recurs after initial evaluation has failed (with EGD and colonoscopy). Two types:
  A. *Obscure occult:* Iron deficiency anaemia, faecal occult blood positive, no visible bleeding. More than 80% resolve with **no treatment.**
  B. *Obscure overt:* Recurrent and visible bleeding, e.g. angiodysplasia.

Investigating a case of lower GI bleeding is like investigating a 'crime' by CBI officer. One should not jump to conclusions as soon as one cause of bleeding is found. There are innumerable examples of 'piles' being treated for bleeding, totally missing a growth above in the rectum (Table 50.1 and Key Boxes 50.1 to 50.3).

Table 50.1 Differential diagnosis of lower GI bleeding: Incidence

Colonic bleeding (90–95%)	Small bowel bleeding (5–10%)
Diverticular disease 30–40%	Angiodysplasia
Ischaemia 5–10%	Erosions or ulcers secondary to NSAID
Anorectal disease 5–15%	Crohn's disease
Neoplasia 5–10%	Radiation enteritis
Infectious colitis 3–8%	Meckel's diverticulum
Inflammatory bowel disease 3–4%	Neoplasia (adenocarci noma, lymphoma)
Angiodysplasia 3%	

Key Box 50.1

Common Causes of Lower GI Bleeding

- Most originate in the colon or rectum—haemorrhoids, polyps, carcinoma, and inflammatory bowel diseases are common causes.
- 10% from upper intestinal tract.
- Small intestinal haemorrhage is usually due to arterio-venous malformations (angiodysplasia), accounting for 70–80%.
- Jejunal diverticula, Meckel's diverticula, neoplasia, Crohn's disease, and aorto-enteric fistula following a previous aortic graft are other causes of bleeding from small intestines.

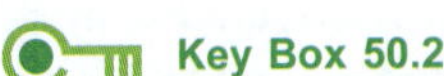

Key Box 50.2

Lower GI Bleeding—Types

Depending upon the source:

- Small bowel bleed—5%
- Colonic bleed—95%

Depending upon the clinical manifestation:

- *Melaena*: Passage of black tarry stools (altered blood) due to slow bleeding or more proximal source of bleed.
- *Haematochezia:* Passage of bright red stools with or without clots.

Key Box 50.3

Bleeding Per Rectum with Acute Abdomen

- Mesenteric ischaemia
- Intussusception
- Ischaemic colitis
- Necrotising enterocolitis

CAUSES

Depending on Aetiology

I. Congenital

- Polyps: Congenital polyp, Peutz-Jeghers syndrome, familial polyposis coli (FPC)
- Meckel's diverticulum
- Hereditary haemorrhagic telangiectasia (HHT)

Pearls of Wisdom

HHT is the most important inherited anomaly which produces bleeding.

II. Inflammatory

- Tubercular ulcers
- Enteric ulcers
- Crohn's ileocolitis
- Ulcerative colitis
- Necrotising enterocolitis
- **Dysentery**—amoebic, bacillary, strongyloides infestation

III. Neoplastic

- Papilloma of rectum
- Carcinoma colon, rectum
- GIST (*see* pages 585, 778)
- Lymphoma
- Carcinoma small bowel

IV. Vascular

- Angiodysplasia
- Ischaemic colitis
- Vasculitis—polyarteritis nodosa
- Haemangioma

V. Clotting disorders

- Haemophilia
- Thrombocytopaenia
- Leukaemia
- Warfarin therapy
- Disseminated intravascular coagulopathy

VI. Miscellaneous

- Piles, anal fissure
- Prolapse
- Injury to the rectum
- Diverticular disease

Depending on Site of Bleeding

I. Small intestine

- Peutz-Jeghers polyps
- Meckel's diverticulum
- Tubercular ulcers
- Crohn's ulcers
- Leiomyoma

II. Large bowel

- Angiodysplasia right colon
- Carcinoma colon
- Ulcerative colitis
- Dysentery
- Diverticular disease

III. Anorectal conditions

- Piles
- Prolapse rectum
- Fissure *in ano*

- Fistula *in ano* (rare)
- Injuries to the rectum

Most of the causes have been discussed in the respective chapters.

CLINICAL EXAMINATION

1. Age of the patient

- **Children and young boys:** Polyps, Meckel's diverticulum, necrotising enterocolitis.
- **Young age group:** Piles, tuberculosis, Crohn's, dysentery.
- **Middle and old age:** Carcinoma, piles, prolapse, diverticular disease.

2. Colour of blood

- **Bright red:** Piles, fissure, polyp.
- **Altered blood:** Carcinoma, tubercular ulcer, Crohn's colitis, dysentery.
- **Maroon colour:** Meckel's diverticulum.

3. Blood with mucus

- Intussusception
- Dysentery
- Inflammatory bowel diseases
- Carcinoma

4. Other special features

- Severe pain with bleeding: Anal fissure
- Splash in the pan: Piles
- Red currant jelly stools: Intussusception
- Streaks of blood: Anal fissure
- Bloody slime: Carcinoma rectum
- Blood with cherry-red mass coming out: Piles, polyps.

5. Palpable mass abdomen

- Hard mass in the colon: Carcinoma colon.
- Firm to hard mass in the right iliac fossa: Ileocaecal tuberculosis.
- Contracting mass: Intussusception.

6. Rectal examination (Fig. 50.1)

- Very painful: Anal fissure
- Pedunculated mass: Rectal polyp (juvenile polyps)
- Ulcerations in the rectum: Solitary rectal ulcer
- Indurated ulcer or growth: Carcinoma rectum (Fig. 50.2).

7. Evidence of bleeding tendencies

- Purpuric spots
- Haematoma

INVESTIGATIONS

1. Proctoscopy (Fig. 50.3)

- Cherry red to pink mucosal bulges: Haemorrhoids
- Bleeding ulcer or a growth: Cancer of rectum
- Single anterior ulcer: Solitary ulcer rectum.

2. Sigmoidoscopy (Fig. 50.4)

- Multiple small pinpoint ulcers: Ulcerative colitis
- Large deep flask-shaped ulcer: Amoebic ulcers
- Multiple small polyps: Hereditary polyposis coli.

3. Colonoscopy

- It is the gold standard investigation for lower GI bleeding. It can detect 3 important diseases: Carcinoma, inflammatory bowel diseases (IBDs) and diverticular diseases (Figs 50.5 to 50.18). It can also detect ischaemic colitis, polyps and angiodysplasia. It needs to be repeated. In massive bleeding, it can really tax an expert colonoscopist also.
- Colonoscopic adrenaline injections, snaring and coagulation (argon plasma coagulation) are therapeutic advantages.

4. Barium enema

- Irregular filling defect in the colon: Cancer colon.
- Contracted pipe-stem colon: Ulcerative colitis.
- Pincer ending: Intussusception.
- Saw-tooth appearance: Diverticular disease.

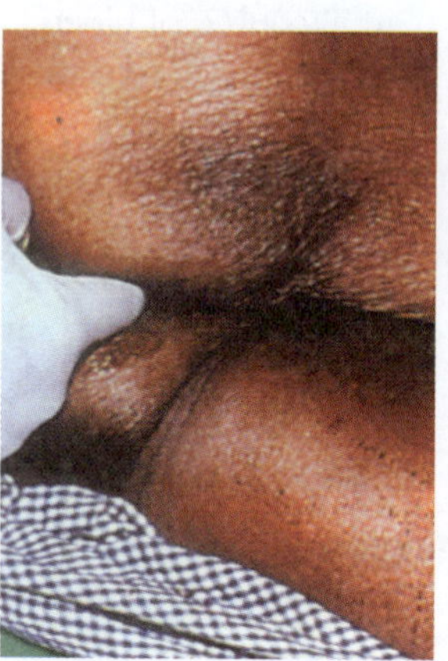

Fig. 50.1: Rectal examination

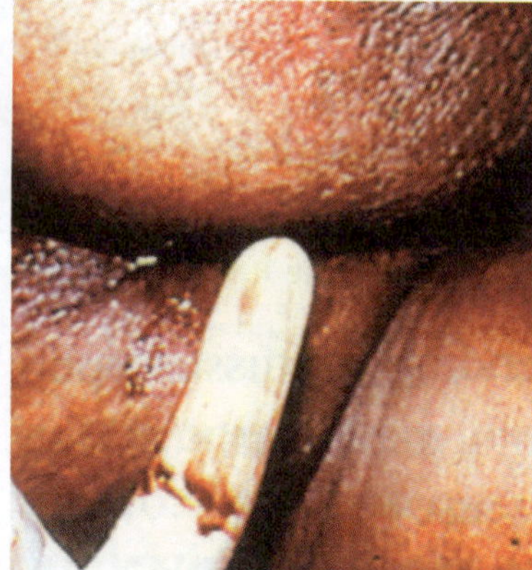

Fig. 50.2: Glove streaked with blood—carcinoma rectum

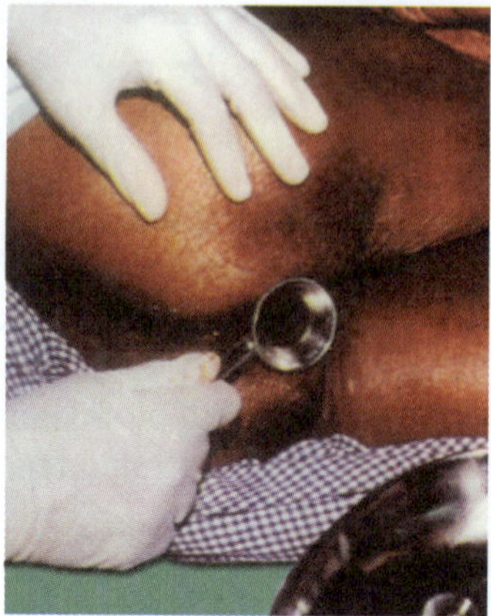

Fig. 50.3: Proctoscopy

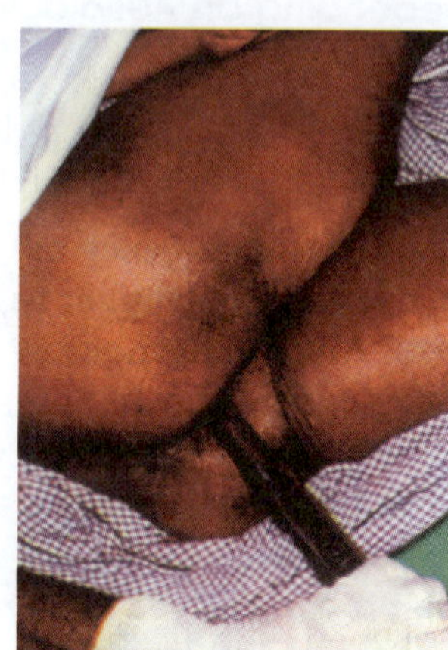

Fig. 50.4: Sigmoidoscopy

DIFFERENTIAL DIAGNOSIS OF LOWER GI BLEEDING (Figs 50.5 to 50.18)

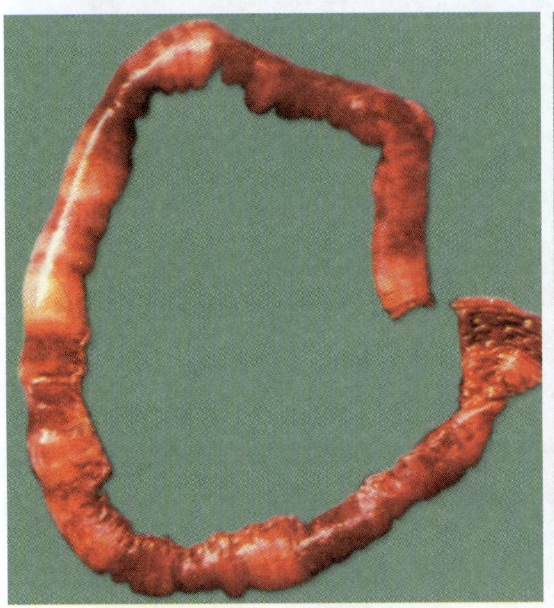

Fig. 50.5: Necrotising enterocolitis

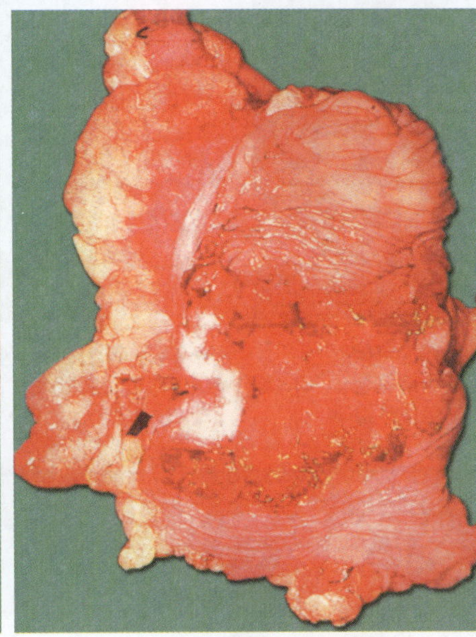

Fig. 50.6: Carcinoma colon

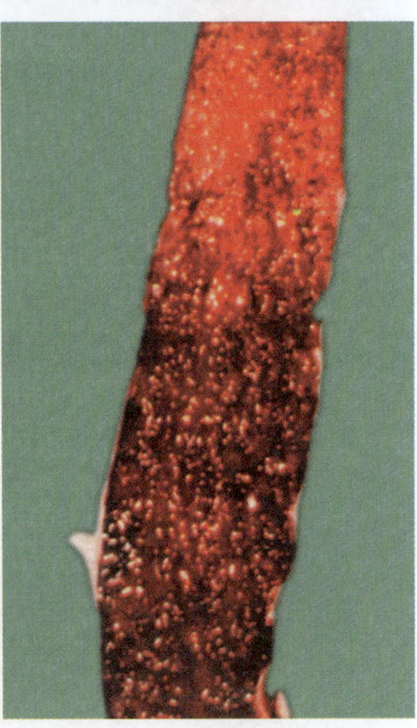

Fig. 50.7: Ulcerative colitis

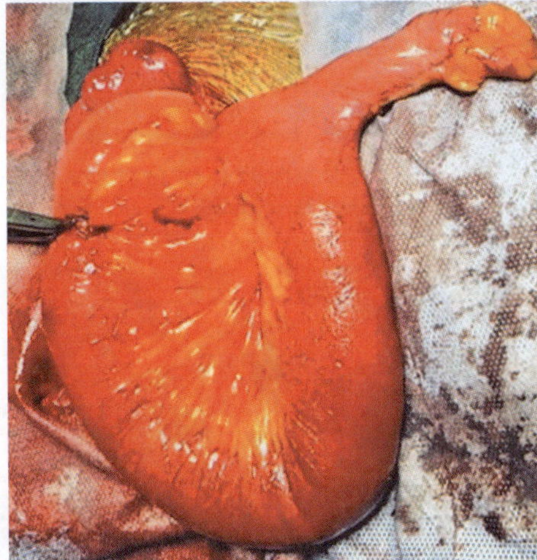

Fig. 50.8: Meckel's diverticulum (*Courtesy :* Dr Naaz Jahan sheik, Hospet, Karnataka)

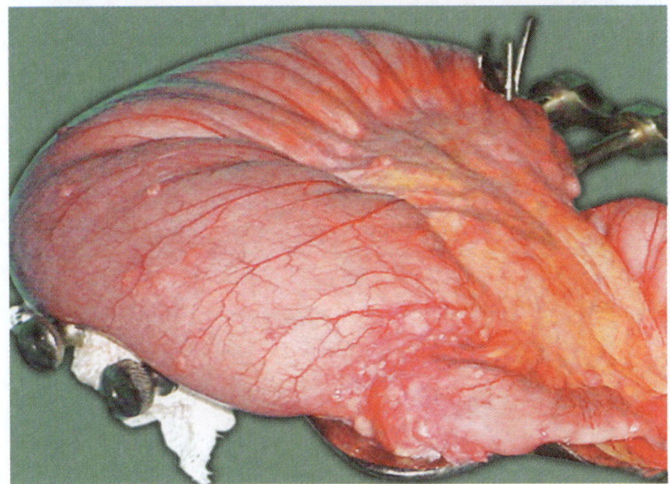

Fig. 50.9: Intestinal tuberculosis

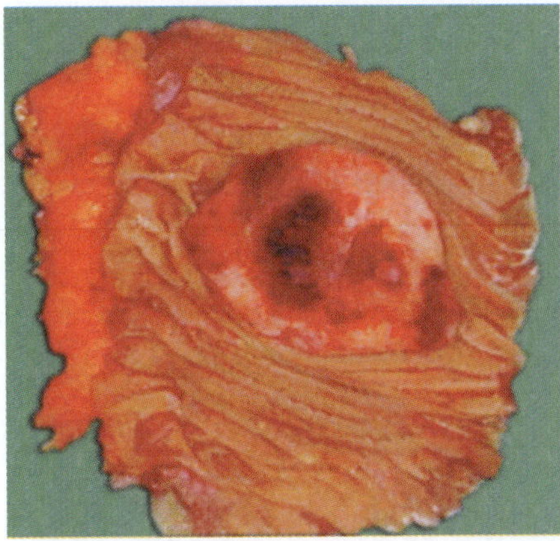

Fig. 50.10: Adenocarcinoma jejunum

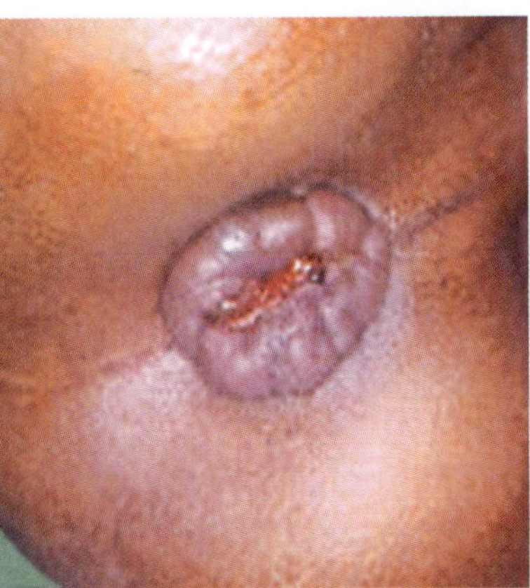

Fig. 50.11: Haemorrhoids

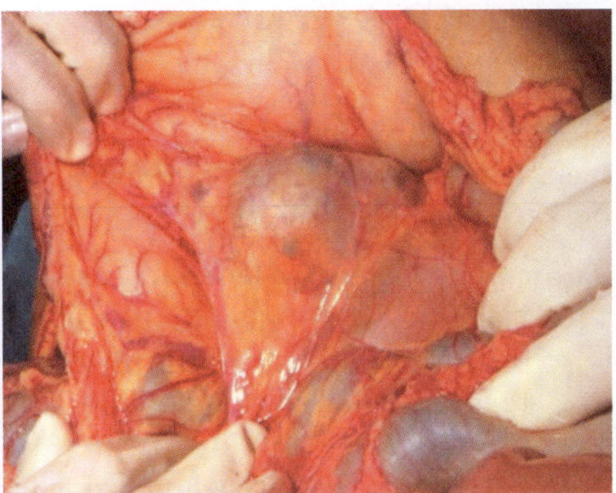

Fig. 50.12: Pancreatic pseudoaneurysm

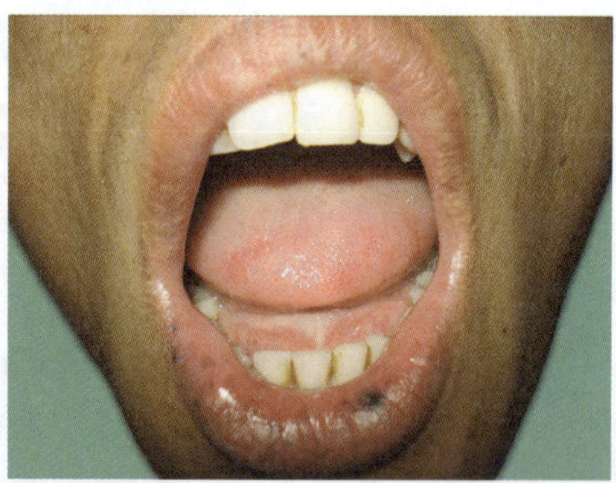

Fig. 50.13: Peutz-Jeghers syndrome (*Courtesy:* Dr Sreevatsa, Head, Department of Surgery, Dr Bharathi, Department of Surgery, MS Ramaiah Medical College, Bengaluru)

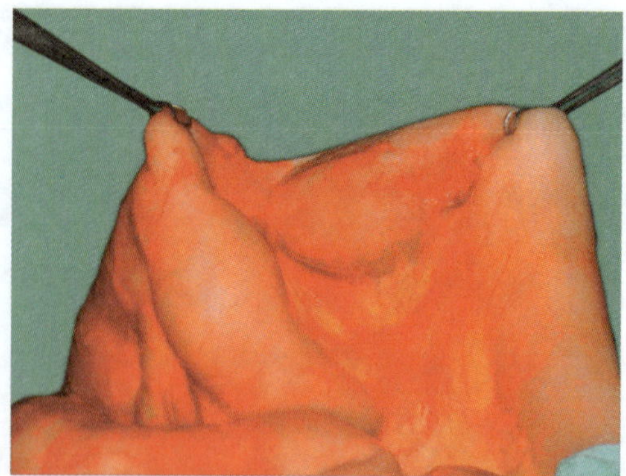

Fig. 50.14: Jejunal diverticulum from mesenteric border presented with occult blood in the stool—evaluation of anaemia, diagnosis was by enteroclysis

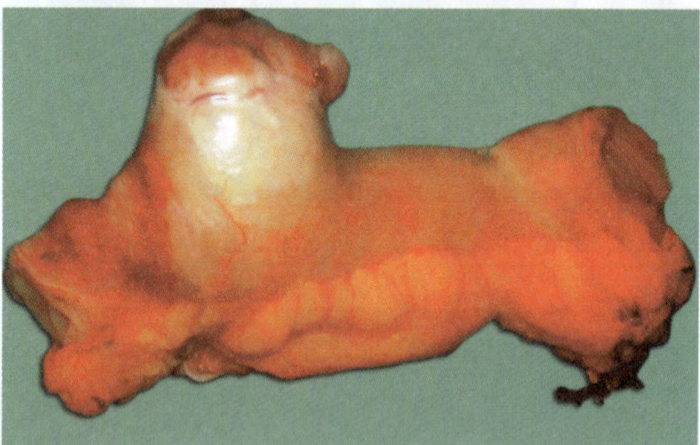

Fig. 50.15: Massive lower GI bleeding due to leiomyoma (GIST) of jejunum—resected specimen

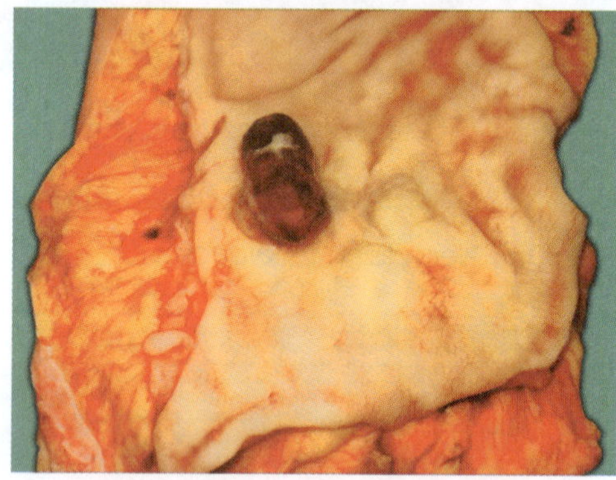

Fig. 50.16: Vascular malformation of rectum—misdiagnosed as solitary rectal ulcer with dysplasia

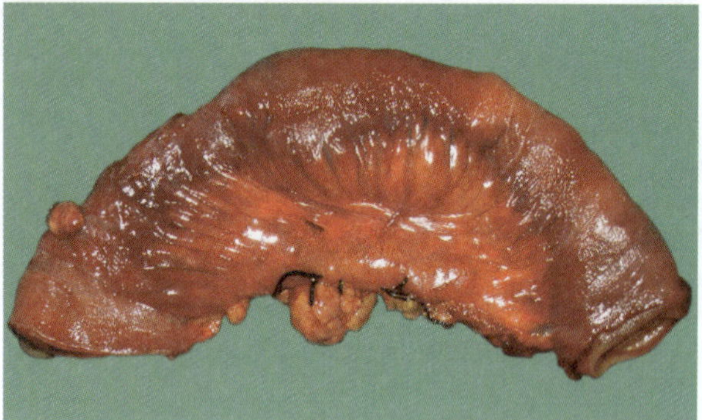

Fig. 50.17: Resected specimen of Crohn's disease

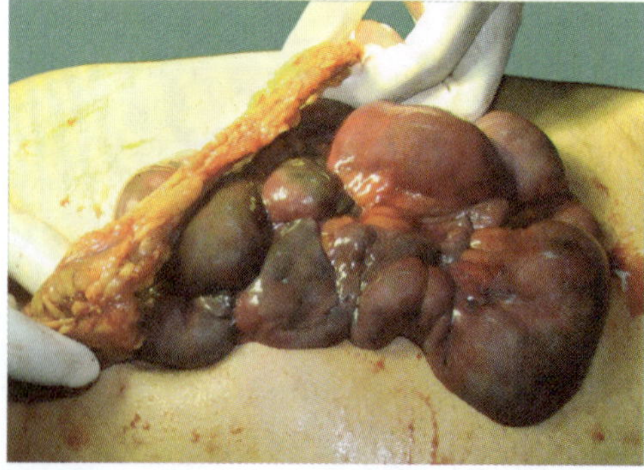

Fig. 50.18: Massive gangrene due to superior mesenteric arterial thrombosis

5. **Stool examination**
   - Amoebiasis, bacillary dysentery
   - Hookworm infestations.
6. **Small bowel enema (enteroclysis)**
   - Diverticulum in the terminal ileum is Meckel's diverticulum. Multiple ulcers and stricture terminal ileum can be due to tuberculous ulcer.
   - Barium studies have a little value in the presence of acute haemorrhage. They can be used in intermittent or chronic bleeding wherein endoscopy has failed to detect the cause.

Special Investigations

They are indicated when the diagnosis of lower GI bleeding cannot be made out. They are more useful where there is active bleeding or obscure bleeding.

A. Radionuclear Scanning

- ^{99m}Tc-labelled sulphur colloid or autologous red cells with ^{99m}Tc may be given which can detect the bleeding site. ***It is extremely sensitive, can detect as little as 0.1 ml/min of bleeding.***

- Less precise but less invasive with least complications. If ^{99m}Tc-tagged RBC scan is positive, then angiogram is used to localise the bleeding site.

B. Visceral Angiography (Fig. 50.19)

- All three vessels—coeliac, superior mesenteric and inferior mesenteric arteries are used.
- Extravasation of contrast into the bowel lumen is suggestive of a 'lesion'.
- Bleeding rate should be at least 0.5 ml/minute.
- Thus, Meckel's diverticulum, angiodysplasia, small bowel tumours, vasculitis, etc. can be diagnosed.

C. Capsule Endoscopy

Definition

- It is an investigation wherein a small camera pill is swallowed to study the entire GI tract, in particular, small intestines.
- This **'camera pill'** that is swallowed is disposable.
- It weighs 4 grams and is 26 mm × 11 mm in size.
- Parts: Video camera, lens, colour camera chip, 6 light emitting diodes. As it passes through the entire gastrointestinal tract, images are taken.
- Capsule endoscopy is useful to detect (observe) small intestinal bleeds that are missed by routine upper GI scopy and colonoscopy. The procedure takes very long time for detection of the lesions.

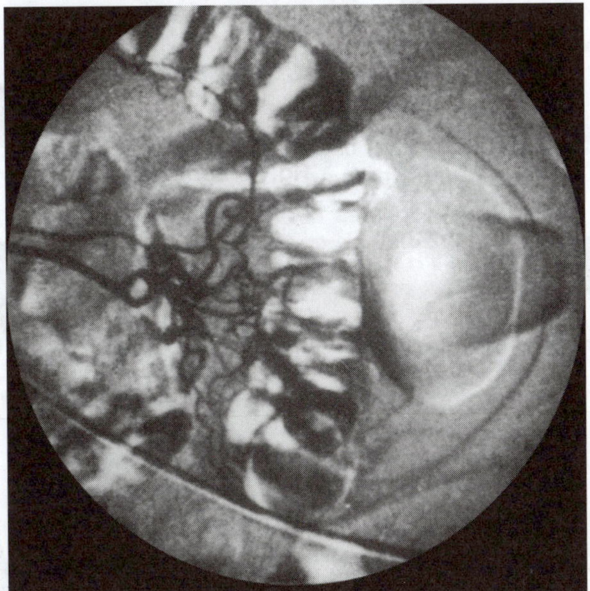

Fig. 50.19: Inferior mesenteric angiography showing leakage of dye into the lumen of sigmoid colon—sigmoid angiodysplasia

- Such bleeds are called '**obscure**' bleeds. These are very difficult problems to treat because they tend to recur.

Procedure

- Patient should be fasting overnight.
- Patient swallows the pill.
- Capsule camera sends signals and pictures—2 pictures/second are taken.
- Capsule gets deactivated in 8 hours and is passed out in stools.
- The receiver tied over patient's waist receives signals and 'endo' pictures. This is connected to computer software and pictures are obtained.

Drawbacks

- Biopsy of the lesion cannot be taken.
- It cannot detect motility disorders which are very important in GIT.
- Expensive, not available in many centres.
- **Capsule** retention resulting obstruction can occur (page 857).

Conclusion

- Thus it can detect polyps, inflammatory bowel disease (Crohn's disease), ulcers and tumours of the small intestine.
- Capsule endoscopy is an excellent tool in the patient who is haemodynamically stable but continues to bleed. Reported success rates as high as 90% in identifying small bowel pathology. It is usually well tolerated, although it is contraindicated in patients with obstruction or a motility disorder.

D. Push Enteroscopy (see Figs 50.29 and 50.30)

- It employs 400 cm scope which is 'pushed' (hence push enteroscope) through duodenum, through DJ flexure into intestines. It needs lots of skill and expertise. It can detect leiomyoma of jejunum, small intestinal diverticular bleed causing chronic anaemia, etc.
- Extended enteroscopy is the same as enteroscopy but may take 6–8 hours till the scope travels distally with peristalsis. Up to 70% small intestine can be visualised.

Pearls of Wisdom

A tagged red blood cell scan can detect bleeds as low as 0.1 ml/minute but does not provide anatomical details. Angiogram can detect bleed at 0.5 ml/min. Embolisation with metal coils can be done to correct bleed. Methylene blue can be injected to stain target segment of intestine.

ROLE OF COLONOSCOPY/ENTEROSCOPY

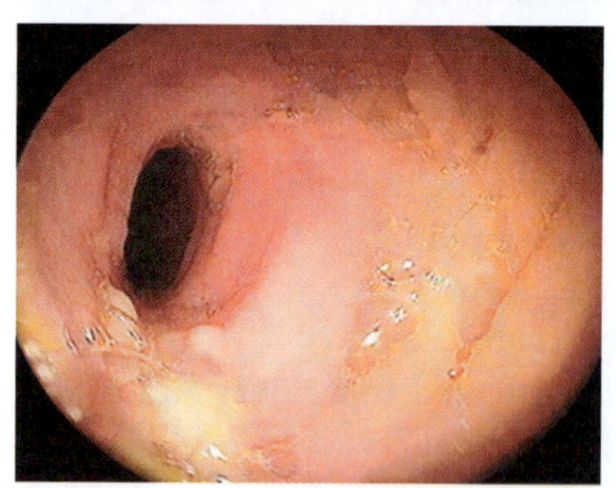

Fig. 50.20: Crohn's disease

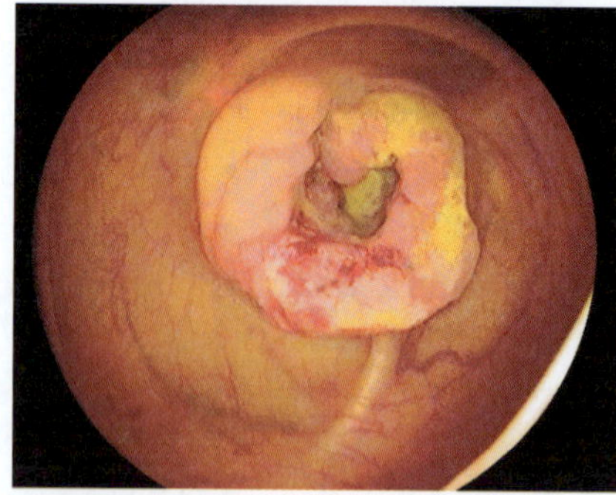

Fig. 50.21: Carcinoma caecum

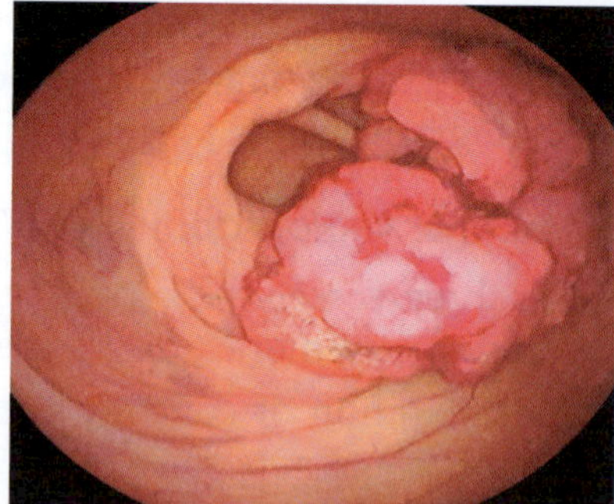

Fig. 50.22: Carcinoma sigmoid

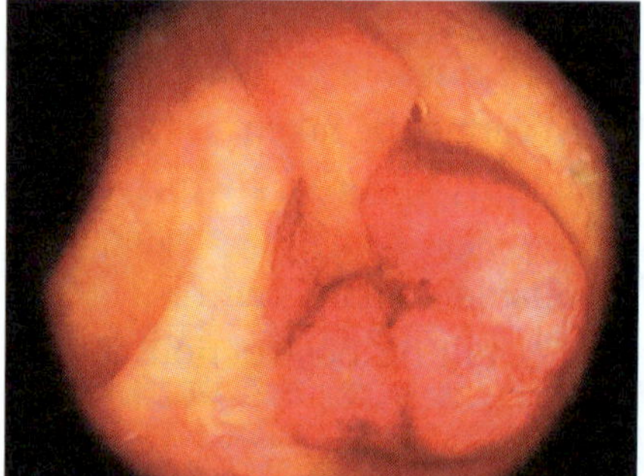

Fig. 50.23: Colonic polyps

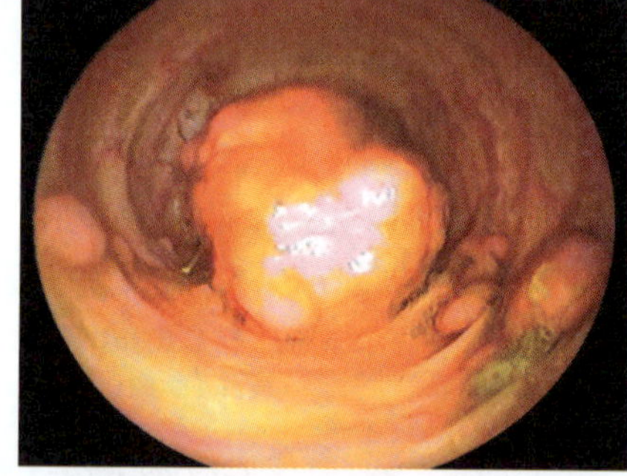

Fig. 50.24: Colonic polyposis

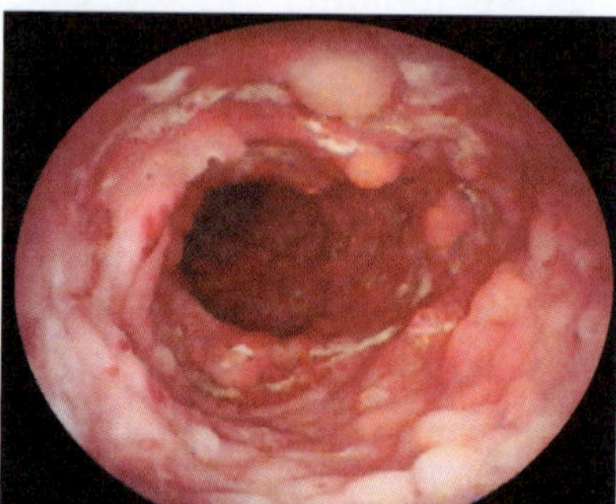

Fig. 50.25: Intestinal tuberculosis

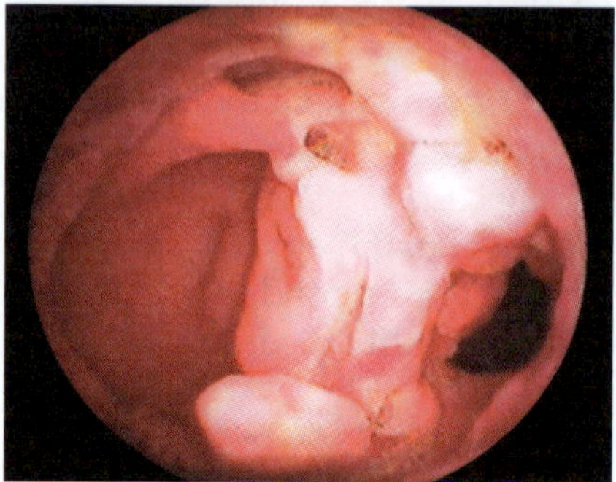

Fig. 50.26: Tuberculosis of the colon

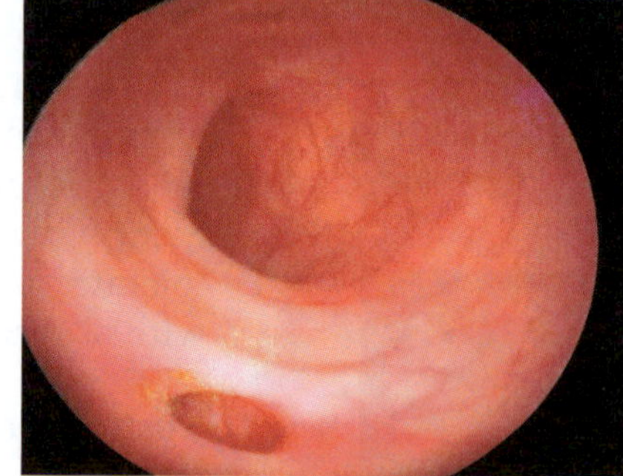

Fig. 50.27: Colonic diverticula

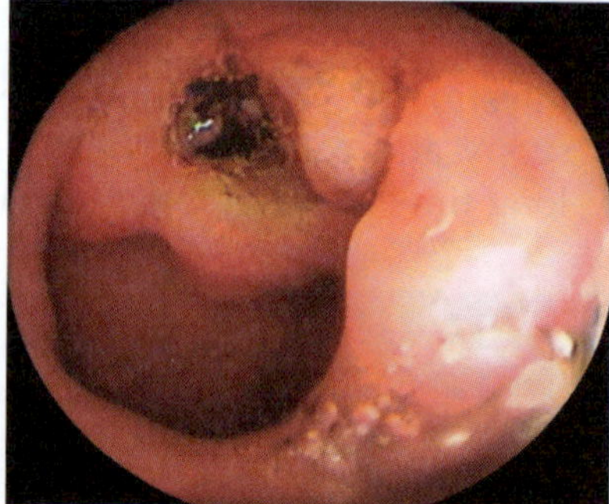

Fig. 50.28: Duodenal ulcer

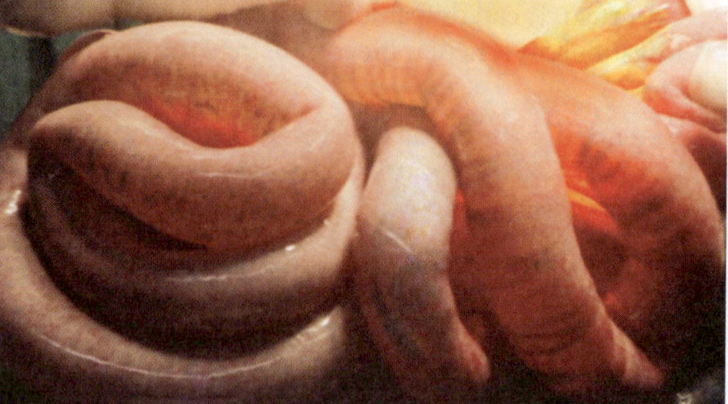

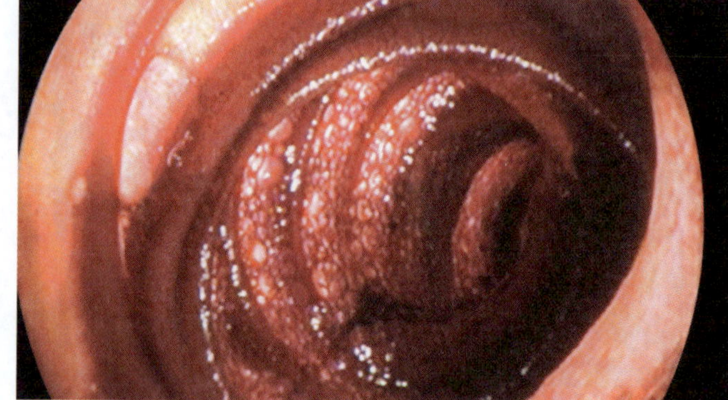

Figs 50.29 and 50.30: Enteroscopy done at laparotomy for suspected case of angiodysplasia of the jejunum—resected successfully. (*Courtesy:* For all the endoscopic pictures: Dr Filipe Alvares, Gastroenterologist, ex-KMC, Manipal)

MASSIVE LOWER GI BLEEDING

Massive lower GI bleeding is defined as haemorrhage distal to the ligament of Treitz that requires more than 3 units of blood in 24 hours (Fig. 50.31).

Common Causes

Diverticular disease, inflammatory bowel diseases, angiodysplasia, Meckel's diverticulum, haemobilia, etc.

Signs of hypovolemia:

- Mild to moderate hypovolemia: **Resting tachycardia.**
- Blood volume loss of at least 15%: **Orthostatic hypotension** (a decrease in the systolic blood pressure of more than 20 mmHg or decrease in diastolic pressure of more than 10 mmHg when moving from recumbency to standing).
- Blood volume loss of at least 40%: **Supine hypotension.**
- **Refer to page 62 for more details about haemorrhagic shock and details about resuscitation.**

Diagnosis

Diagnosis is established by colonoscopy, RBC tagged scan and angiography in most of the cases.

Treatment

- Initial aggressive resuscitation by fluids, blood transfusion and treatment of shock.
- Emergency colonoscopy and vascular malformations, if detected, can be treated by argon plasma coagulation or by cauterisation.
- Therapeutic ***vasopressin*** infusion 0.2 units/minute *via* ***angiographic catheter*** with or without embolization will stop or arrest the lower GI bleeds in more than 85% of cases.
- Unstable patient should be subjected to urgent laparotomy.

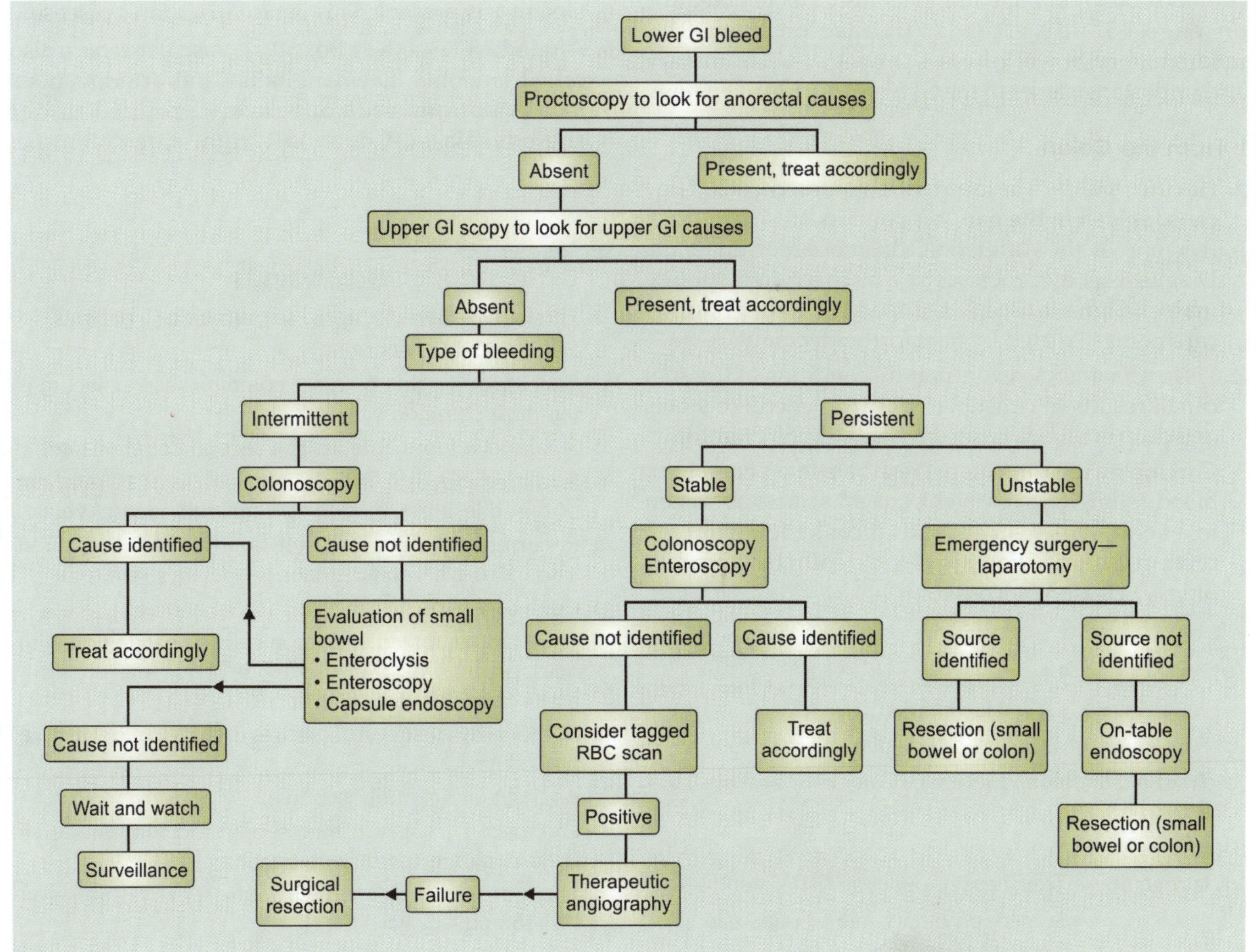

Fig. 50.31: Schematic representation of approach to lower GI bleeding (*Courtesy:* Dr Prasad S, Associate Professor, KMC, Manipal)

A Few Important Tips at Exploratory Laparotomy

- Midline incision is **preferred.**
- Careful inspection and palpation of entire small and large bowel.
- Empty small bowel. Then palpate for hidden lesions.
- Intraoperative enteroscopy, if no obvious lesion is found.
- Endoscopic evaluation of transilluminated gut wall.
- On-table colonoscopy *via* appendiceal opening after appendicectomy.
- Rarely, **blind right hemicolectomy/subtotal colectomy or blind resection of proximal jejunum** may be necessary in obscure bleeding (keeping in mind angiodysplasia).

DIFFERENTIAL DIAGNOSIS

All the topics related to GI bleeding have been discussed in the respective chapters. Example: Haemobilia (Key Box 50.4) on page 698, haemosuccus pancreatitis on page 657, diverticular disease on page 811, inflammatory bowel diseases on page 763. Summary and important causes of the GI bleeding are given here.

I. From the Colon

1. **Haemorrhoids:** These are the common causes. They cause **splash in the pan**. It is painless, fresh bleeding. It is one of the differential diagnoses for anaemia. Diagnosis is by proctoscopy—as cherry red spongy masses. Sigmoidoscopy is done to rule out proximal carcinoma. Treated by haemorrhoidectomy.
2. **Fissure *in ano*:** A severe painful condition of the anal canal, results in constipation, hard pellet-like stools and drop of blood. Treated by lateral sphincterotomy.
3. **Carcinoma rectum/colon:** Fresh bleeding per rectum, bloody slime, loss of weight, anaemia, mass abdomen in an elderly patient suggests it could be carcinoma rectum/colon. Diagnosis is by colonoscopy and biopsy. Treated by colectomy.

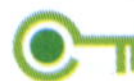 Key Box 50.4

Haemobilia

- Rare cause of UGI or LGI bleeding
- **Triad of Sandblom**: Melaena, biliary colic and obstructive jaundice
- External trauma
- Iatrogenic – Transhepatic puncture (PTC, stenting)
  – Surgery on biliary tree or pancreas
  – After dilatation of biliary strictures, etc.
- Endoscopy – Blood emerging from ampulla of Vater

4. **Diverticular disease of the sigmoid colon:** Common in Western patients, diet poor in fibre is mostly the cause. The diverticuli are acquired herniation of the mucosa, hence thin. Bleeding can be occult/intermittent or massive. Diagnosis is by colonoscopy. To visualise the bleeders, endotherapy can be done by injecting adrenaline into the bleeding vessel. In emergency situations, with massive lower GI bleeding, emergency colectomy is required.
5. **Inflammatory bowel diseases:** Commonly ulcerative colitis and less commonly Crohn's disease produces lower GI bleeding. Bleeding is intermittent with mucous diarrhoea, weight loss and malnutrition. Often patients are young. Diagnosis is by colonoscopy and biopsy. Initial treatment is always conservative—salazopyrines, steroids, etc. In massive bleeding to save the life—emergency total colectomy with or without pouch may be required. In Crohn's disease, the aim is always to conserve the segment of the intestine. Resection is required, only if massive bleeding is present. This is rare in Crohn's disease.
6. **Angiodysplasia** (Key Box 50.5): Vascular ectasia also called angioma, haemangiomas and arteriovenous malformations are collectively grouped under angiodysplasia. Commonly right side colon, i.e.

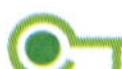 Key Box 50.5

Angiodysplasia

- They are acquired lesions, seen in elderly patients.
- Less rapid, but recurrent.
- Caecum and right colon are common sites—caecum is the most common site.
- Small bowel (proximal) is the second common site.
- Small red mucosal lesions between 2 and 10 mm, flat or raised lesions—dilated tortuous submucosal veins.
- Recurrent painless and self-limiting bleeding often associated with aortic stenosis—Heyde's syndrome.
- Colonoscopy is the investigation of choice.
- They can be treated endoscopically—coagulation with heat probe, bipolar electrode or laser, etc. but recurrence or failure can occur.
- Surgery by resecting the segment is a definitive procedure.
- Angiography is rarely positive.
- Enteroscopy, capsule endoscopy and intraoperative endoscopy are useful investigations.
- These lesions are seen in acute renal failure, von Willebrand's disease, HHT.
- Hormone treatment.
- Endoscopy directed resection.

caecum and ascending colon are affected. In the small intestines, jejunum is the most common site. Typically, elderly patients present with intermittent bleeding is cause of anaemia. Usual causes of lower GI bleeding are ruled out by colonoscopy and other investigations. Suspect angiodysplasia. A few cases present with massive bleeding—a difficult problem to treat. Repeat colonoscopy, capsule endoscopy, angiography, on-table enteroscopy are the taxing investigations—all may provide no results—emergency colectomy or intestinal resection of the suspicious segment may be required.

7. **Ischaemic colitis:** Elderly, hypertensive patients present with diffuse abdominal pain, severe in nature, with blood in stools—it is often massive, sometimes moderate. On examination, tenderness may be present on the left side of the colon. Plain X-ray abdomen supine will show **thumb printing sign** due to mucosal oedema and submucosal haemorrhage. CT scan—colonic wall thickening with posterior fat shadowing. Colonoscopy may reveal ulcers or a few changes in the splenic flexure region. If conservative measures fail such as blood transfusion, segmental colectomy may be required.
8. **Dysentery:** Various dysenteries such as amoebic, bacillary, Shigella, HIV related—all produce ulcerations in the colon resulting in blood and mucus in the stools. Gripping pain, acute in nature with or without fever and tenderness over the colon—in the right iliac fossa and in the left iliac fossa are suggestive. Diagnosis is by stool examination and colonoscopy. Treated with antiamoebic drugs or antibiotics.
9. **Irradiation proctitis or telangiectasia:** Usually occurs with pelvic radiotherapy, example—radiation given to treat carcinoma cervix. Most common site is rectum. Tenesmus, mucus and blood in stool are common. Proctoscopy reveals ulceration. Treated with stool softening agents, 5-ASA (aminosalicylic acid) topical or steroid enema. Acute irradiation injury occurs within six weeks of therapy. Chronic radiation procto-sigmoiditis has a more delayed onset. The first signs often occur at approximately 9 to 14 months following radiation exposure, but may develop after more than two years in some patients
10. **Adenoma, polyps, familial polyposis coli:** They are common in the colon. All are precursors for carcinoma colon. Often patients are young with lower gastrointestinal bleeding. Diagnosis is by colonoscopy and biopsy. Villous adenomas, polyps can be snared or excised. Always histological examination is a must.

II. From the Small Intestines

1. **Tubercular ulcers:** They are never massive bleeders. Patients are between 20 and 40 years old with blood and mucus in the stools, loss of weight, crampy abdominal pain, evening rise of temperature with or without pulmonary tuberculosis. On examination, mass may be palpable, if caecum is also involved (ileocaecal tuberculosis). Visible step ladder peristalsis indicates obstruction from a tubercular stricture or obstruction due to mass. Colonoscopy with visualisation of the terminal ileum and biopsy is the key to the diagnosis. Obstructed cases can be treated with stricturoplasty in a single stricture or resection in appropriate cases. Cases without obstruction are treated with antitubercular treatment.
2. **Crohn's ulcers:** Ileum is the commonest site—rest of the bowel can also be affected. Transmural inflammation, multiple ulcers, skip lesions are other features. Diagnosis is by CT scan, push enteroscopy and biopsy. Treatment is as for ulcerative colitis (for more details *see* page 762).
3. **Enteric ulcers:** High grade fever—enteric fever patient who has bleeding after 15 days of fever may be having enteric ulceration of the Peyer's patches with bleeding. In majority of the cases, bleeding is occult and usually stops once the disease is treated, rarely exploration and resection of the segment may be required in cases of massive bleeding cases.
4. **Meckel's diverticulum:** Children or young patients, often bleeds are intermittent, maroon coloured with or without abdominal pain. Peptic ulceration in the ectopic mucosal site in the Meckel's diverticulum causes bleeding. Colonoscopy is normal. RBC-tagged technetium scan is the investigation of choice. It can pick up as little as 0.1 ml/min of bleeding. Exploration and excision of the Meckel's diverticulum is the treatment of choice.
5. **Angiodysplasias:** Small intestines are the most common sites of angiodysplasia. They are the differential diagnoses for obscure bleeds. Angiogram and small bowel push enteroscopy, capsule endoscopy are the investigations. Diagnosis is by exclusion.
6. **Small bowel tumours:** They are uncommon causes of lower GI bleeding. They have to be kept in mind when the common causes described above are ruled out one by one. Adenocarcinoma, lymphoma and stomal tumours (GIST—gastrointestinal stomal tumours) are a few examples. GIST can affect small intestine. The mucosal ulcerations cause GI blood loss. Bleeding is not massive—can be intermittent and result in anaemia. **Palpable mass sometimes massive which is bosselated, anaemia and bleeding are the triad of GIST.** CT scan is the investigation of choice.

Resection almost cures the disease. Degree of malignancy is decided by the mitotic figures in pathology. Imatinib is the drug used in recurrent cases of GIST or GIST with metastasis. Patients with liver metastasis will live beyond 5–10 years with imatinib.

MISCELLANEOUS

Ischaemic Colitis

- Ischaemic colitis is a non-inflammatory condition affecting splenic flexure region resulting in ischaemia and lower GI tract bleeding.
- Elderly hypertensive patients are commonly affected.
- Often they are males.
- The splenic flexure region can have relative vascularity. The exact point is called **Griffith's point** (Fig. 50.32).

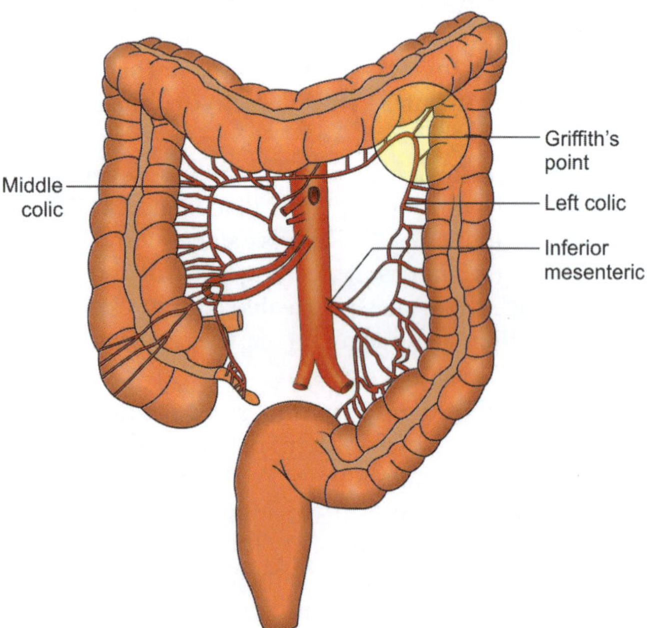

Fig. 50.32: Ischaemic colitis

- It is defined as the site of (a) communication of the ascending left colic artery with the marginal artery of Drummond, and (b) anastomotic bridging between the right and left terminal branches of the ascending left colic artery at the splenic flexure of the colon.
- Anastomosis at Griffith's point is present in 48%, poor or tenuous in 9%, and absent in 43%.

  Thus, it is important that in cases of ligation of inferior mesenteric artery, there is a possibility of ischaemia developing in that region.
- It can also be affected in "nonocclusive" ischaemic colitis.
- Three types have been classified—called Marston's classification:
  1. Gangrenous type
  2. Stricture type
  3. Transient type

Clinical Notes

A 28-year-old male patient had an urgency to pass stools early morning. He collapsed while passing stools, with a massive bleeding. He was brought to the hospital in a state of shock. He was resuscitated and blood transfusions were given. All investigations were normal. He had another bout of massive bleeding the next day, during which time, even an angiography could not detect the cause. Urgent laparotomy was done. A 4 cm small bowel tumour (haemorrhagic) was excised from jejunum and histology confirmed it as leiomyoma. Leiomyoma is called bleeding tumour of the small bowel. The case history highlights the importance of exploratory laparotomy. Leiomyomas are included under GIST.

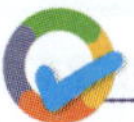

Multiple Choice Questions

1. Lower GI tract bleeding refers to bleeding:
A. Below ligament of Treitz
B. Below ampulla of Vater
C. Below Meckel's diverticulum
D. Distal to ileocaecal junction

2. Most important inherited anomaly which produces bleeding is:
A. Juvenile polyp
B. Meckel's diverticulum
C. Familial polyposis coli
D. Hereditary haemorrhagic telangiectasia

3. The ideal investigation for bleeding Meckel's diverticulum is:
A. CT scan
B. Colonoscopy
C. ^{99m}Tc-tagged RBC scan
D. Push enteroscopy

4. Following facts are true for angiodysplasia, *except*:
A. They are congenital lesions
B. Right colon is the common site
C. It is one of the causes of obscure bleeding
D. Small bowel is the second common site

5. Following are true about capsule endoscopy, *except*:
A. It is disposable pill
B. Ideal for small intestinal bleeds
C. Biopsy can be taken
D. Capsule retention can occur

6. Following are true for jejunal bleeding lesions, *except*:
A. Carcinoma
B. Meckel's diverticulum
C. Angiodysplasia
D. Hamartomatous polyp

7. Following are true for haemobilia, *except*:
A. It causes melaena
B. It causes biliary colic
C. Obstructive jaundice
D. Splenomegaly

8. Which one of the following is the cause for massive lower GI bleeding?
A. Carcinoma rectum
B. Crohn's colitis
C. Typhoid colitis
D. Diverticulitis of the colon

9. Which one of these causes bleeding with septic shock?
A. Carcinoma colon
B. Ulcerative colitis
C. Mesenteric ischaemia
D. Angiodysplasia

10. Which one of these causes painless and massive bleeding per rectum?
A. Angiodysplasia
B. Sigmoid volvulus
C. Necrotising enterocolitis
D. Mesenteric ischaemia

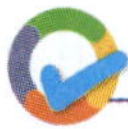

Answers

1. A **2.** D **3.** D **4.** A **5.** C **6.** B **7.** D **8.** D **9.** C **10.** A

CHAPTER

51

Appendix

- Development and anomalies
- Surgical anatomy
- Acute appendicitis
- Differential diagnosis
- Complications
- Appendicular mass
- Faecal fistula
- Neoplasm
- Mucocoele
- Valentino appendix
- Post-appendicectomy sepsis—a case report

Introduction

Acute appendicitis is the most common emergency encountered by the general surgeons. Men have slightly increased incidence of acute appendicitis compared to women. Incidence is 11 per 10,000 persons/year. Appendicectomy is a simple surgery, no doubt, but sometimes it can be very difficult and disappointing—sometimes one may not be able to find the appendix. Hence, appendicectomy should not be taken lightly. The choice of surgery today is laparoscopic appendicectomy—one advantage being one can look into all quadrants of the abdomen—not to miss other causes such as perforated duodenal ulcer (*see* later **Valentino appendix**), etc. and very helpful to detect subhepatic appendicitis.

Historical Events Related to Appendix

Claudius Amyand (1736)	Removed inflamed appendix from hernia sac
Reginald Fitz (1886)	Coined term Appendicitis
Charles McBurney (1889)	Described McBurney point
Kurt Semm	Did first laparoscopic appendicectomy
Santiaggo Horgan and Mark A Talamini	**Transvaginal removal of the appendix a procedure called NOTES—Natural Orifice Transluminal Endoscopic Surgery**

DEVELOPMENT AND ANOMALIES

Embryologically, the appendix and caecum develop as outpouchings of the caudal limb of the midgut loop in the sixth week of human development. By the fifth month, the appendix elongates into its vermiform shape, hence called vermiform appendix. At birth, the appendix is located at the tip of the caecum but due to unequal elongation of the lateral wall of the caecum, the adult appendix typically originates from the posteromedial wall of the caecum, caudal to the ileocaecal valve. A few anomalies are given below.

1. **Duplication of the appendix** is one anomaly which is further divided as follows:

   Type A: Single caecum—partial duplication

   Type B: Single caecum and 2 separate appendices

   Type C: Double caecum with each one having one appendix (Figs 51.1 and 51.2).
2. **Situs inversus:** In this condition, appendix is found on the left side. Adds confusion to the diagnosis of acute appendicitis.
3. **Subhepatic appendix:** It happens in malrotation of the gut. Patients with subhepatic appendicitis may complain of pain in the right lower quadrant. A McBurney incision is usually given only to find no appendix in that location. Laparoscopy has the advantage of looking into all quadrants of the abdomen.
4. **Congenital absence of the appendix** is rare.

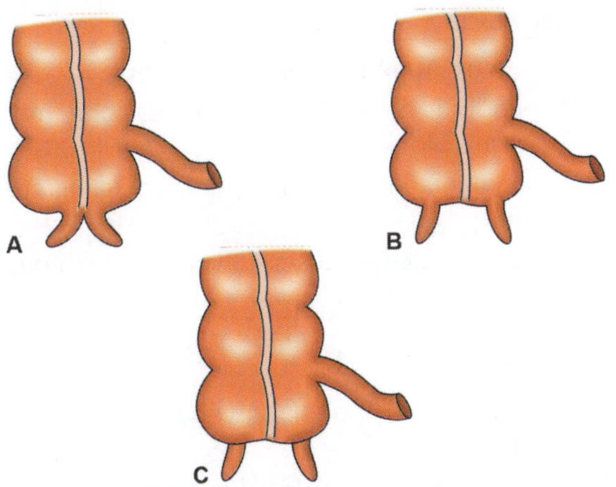

Fig. 51.1A to C: Anomalies of the appendix (see text for details)

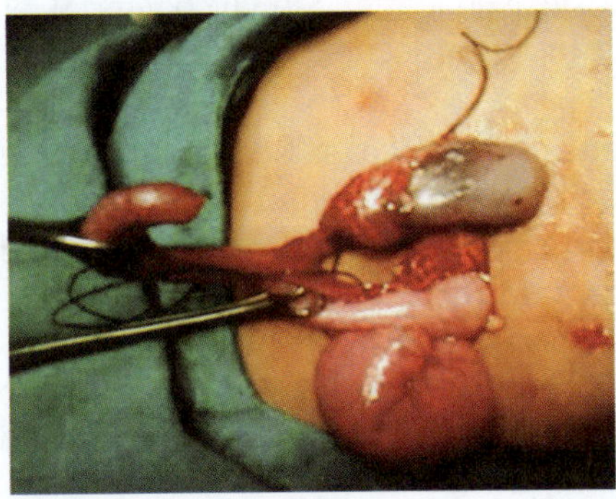

Fig. 51.2: Appendicular duplication and gangrene in one of the moieties

SURGICAL ANATOMY OF THE APPENDIX[1]

Competency

SU28.15.1: Describe applied anatomy of vermiform appendix.

- It is 8–10 cm long, may vary from 3 to 30 cm in length.
- It is situated 2 cm posteromedial to ileocaecal junction, at the point of convergence of the three taeniae coli.
- It is the primary cause of lower abdominal pain on the right side.

Positions of the Appendix (Fig. 51.3)

1. Retrocaecal in about 70% of patients (12 o'clock)
2. Pelvic in 20% of cases (4 o'clock)
3. Preileal and postileal (2 o'clock)
4. Subcaecal (6 o'clock)
5. Paracaecal
6. **Subhepatic appendix** is associated with subhepatic caecum. It occurs due to **malrotation of the gut.** (This position is not depicted in the figure.)

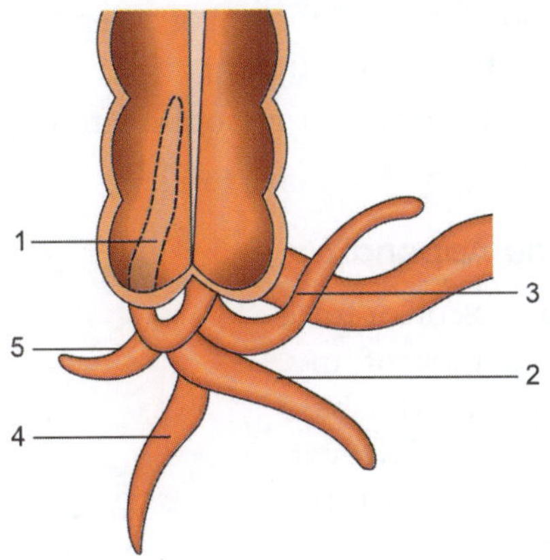

Fig. 51.3: Positions of the appendix (see text for numbers)

Layers of the Appendix

- Mesoappendix is the continuation of mesentery of the ileum above. It comes down carrying blood vessels in the mesoappendix.
- Appendix has a serosa and a mucosa lined by columnar epithelium (similar to intestinal mucosa) between which are the circular and longitudinal muscle fibres.
- **Submucosa has rich lymphoid follicles** (lamina propria). The lymphatic tissue decreases as age advances. Hence, incidence of **appendicitis is less after the age of 30 years**.
- Appendicular orifice is occasionally guarded by an indistinct semilunar fold of mucous membrane, known as ***valve of Gerlach***.

Blood Supply of the Appendix

- Appendicular artery is a branch of ileocolic artery. Accessory appendicular **artery of Seshachalam** (a branch of posterior caecal artery) is a branch of ileocolic artery, which runs in the mesoappendix (Fig. 51.4).
- Veins follow the artery and end in the superior mesenteric vein, thus draining into portal vein. This

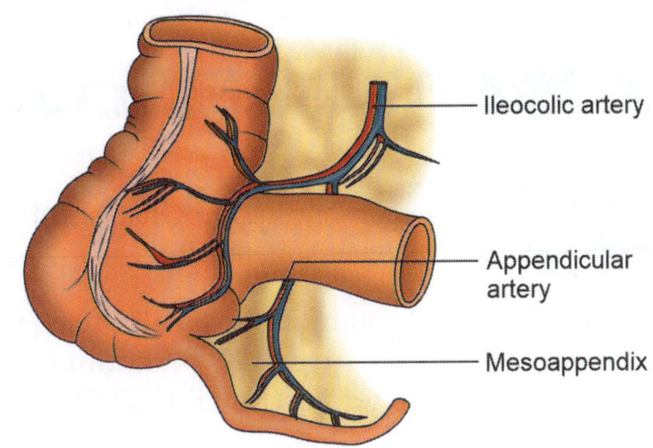

Fig. 51.4: Anatomy of the appendix

[1]Appendix secretes immunoglobulins particularly IgA. So, it is not considered as a vestigial organ anymore. However, appendicectomy is not associated with any immunological compromise.

is the reason for development of pylephlebitis in cases of suppurative appendicitis.
- Pylephlebitis means thrombophlebitis of portal veins or its branches.

Locating the Appendix

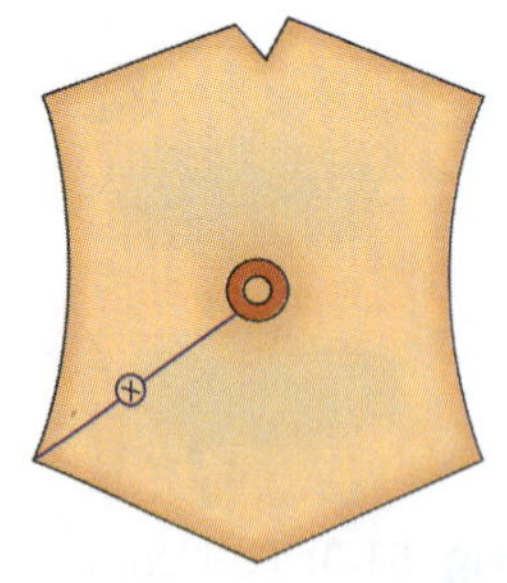

Fig. 51.5: McBurney's point

Trace the taenia coli or trace ileal loops at laparotomy. Taenia coli point to the base of the appendix. However, surface marking of the appendix is done as follows: Draw a line from anterior superior iliac spine to the umbilicus. The junction of lateral 1/3rd and medial 2/3rds of this line indicates the location of appendix. This is the point of maximum tenderness in appendicitis. This is called **McBurney's point** (Fig. 51.5).

Surgical Anatomy and Significance

1. **The area of the maximum tenderness** in acute appendicitis is called McBurney's point—corresponds to the site of appendix in vast majority of the cases. This is the site selected for incision in open method.
2. Appendicular artery must be ligated in open or laparoscopic method—**to free mesoappendix**.
3. Severe inflammation of the appendix can spread to portal vein via ileocolic vein and can result in **portal pyaemia,** a very dangerous condition.
4. **Malrotation of the gut**—appendix may be in subhepatic region—to be kept in mind in cases wherein appendix is not found in the right iliac fossa.

Lymphatics

The lymphatic channels which are 4 to 6 in number drain into ileocolic nodes, ileocaecal nodes and appendicular nodes in mesoappendix.

ACUTE APPENDICITIS

Competency

SU28.15.2: Describe etiology, pathogenesis, clinical symptoms and signs of acute appendicitis.

It is one of the most common surgical emergencies encountered by general surgeons. Sometimes acute appendicitis can be dangerous (Key Box 51.1).

Definitions

- **Acute appendicitis:** Sudden appearance of signs and symptoms of appendicitis.

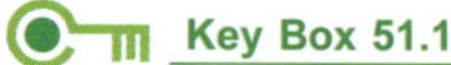

Key Box 51.1

Why Appendicitis is Dangerous?

- The appendix is a cul-de-sac (closed at one end) and can be easily blocked.
- The appendicular artery is an end-artery (gangrene can occur fast).
- Inflammatory oedema causes easy and early thrombosis of appendicular artery.
- The appendix has thin muscular coat. Hence, perforates easily.
- The lumen of the appendix is very narrow—1–3 mm in diameter.
- Closed loop obstruction: Intraluminal pressure builds up as the appendicular mucosa secretes fluid resulting in mucosal ischaemia. Slowly bacterial overgrowth and translocation occurs.

- **Recurrent appendicitis:** Recurrent attacks of acute appendicitis—incidence is 15 to 25%.
- **Grumbling appendicitis:** Low grade recurrent bouts of colics, vomiting with frequent admission, self-limiting cases.
- **Simple appendicitis:** If duration of symptoms is less than 48 hours or imaging does not show any abscess or phlegmon.
- **Complicated appendicitis:** Acute appendicitis with perforation or large abscess/phlegmon.
- **Pseudoappendicitis:** Acute ileitis mimics appendicitis following ***Yersinia* infection**. It can also be due to **Crohn's** disease.
- **Stump appendicitis:** It is the inflammation and infection of residual appendicular stump (postoperative cases). To avoid stump appendicitis, one should not leave appendicular stump **longer than 3 mm**.
  - Everybody should be aware of this condition.
  - Symptoms are similar to acute appendicitis.
  - More in laparoscopic appendicectomies because of lack of a three-dimensional perspective and absence of tactile feedback.
  - This can happen, if the exact junction of appendix with caecum is not clearly identified. CECT is the best investigation.
  - Rare cause of recurrent appendicitis after appendicectomy is duplicated appendicitis. It may require stump appendicectomy.
- **Prevention:** It is important to ligate and divide at the base of the appendix to avoid this complication (more so in laparoscopic appendicectomy).

Aetiology

1. Racial and dietary factors

- It is more common in White race than in coloured persons. Young males are affected more often.

- It may be related to **Westernization** of food—a diet rich in meat precipitates appendicitis and ***a diet rich in fibre (cellulose) protects the person from appendicitis.***

2. **Familial susceptibility:** It is related to having a ***long retrocaecal appendix*** in which case the blood supply is diminished to the distal portion and may precipitate appendicitis.
3. **Socioeconomic status:** Appendicitis is common in middle class and rich people. The exact reasons are not known.
4. **Obstructive theory:** Obstruction to the lumen of the appendix due to faecoliths, worms, ova and cysts. Obstruction *can also be due to lymphoid hyperplasia or neoplasm. Entamoeba* causes obstructive appendicitis. It is seen only in one-third of cases (Fig. 51.6).
5. **Non-obstructive theory:** It is due to bacteria such as *E. coli*, enterococci, Proteus, Pseudomonas, Klebsiella and anaerobes which produce diffuse inflammation of appendix and cause appendicitis. This seems to be more common cause than obstruction.

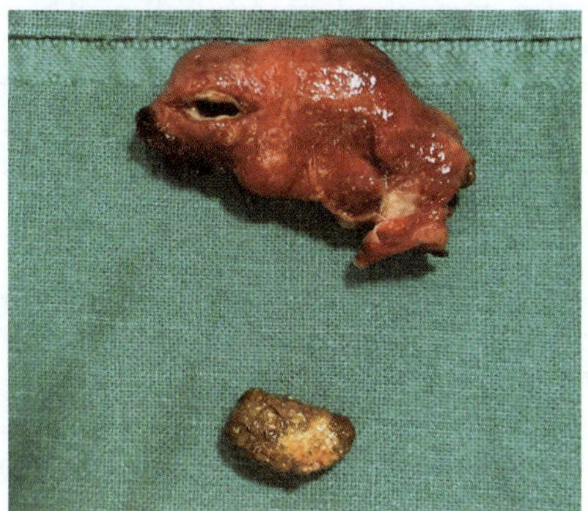

Fig. 51.6: Obstructive appendicitis due to large faecolith

Pathogenesis

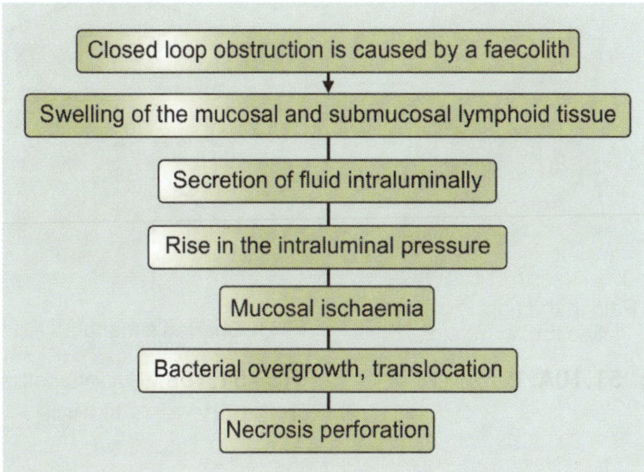

Fig. 51.7: Pathogenesis of appendicitis

Pathology

I. *In Non-Obstructive Cases (Catarrhal Appendicitis)*

- Process of inflammation is slow and gradual.
- A mild attack may completely resolve or mucosal and submucosal oedema can occur (Key Box 51.2).
- Ulceration of the appendix results in slow bacterial invasion of lymphoid tissue.
- Gangrene and perforation are rare.

II. *In Obstructive Cases*

- **Symptoms are abrupt, vomiting is more, pain is more and tenderness is more.**
- It is a more dangerous variety.
- Appendix looks inflamed, with congested blood vessels. The tip especially looks more inflamed. As the inflammation is more severe, the outer aspect looks dull and purulent exudates may be seen. Areas of blackening or green colour indicates gangrene or necrosis with perforation. In acute inflammation, neutrophils are dominant and in cases of gangrenous appendicitis, vascular thrombosis is a feature. The important pathological events can be summarized as follows—due to obstruction, the contents get infected fast and the tension increases. The appendix becomes a closed loop, which results in septic thrombosis of vessels. Gangrene of appendix, perforation, peritonitis, followed by a local abscess can occur (Fig. 51.7).
- In **children, greater omentum is very thin.** Hence, it cannot localize the infection. In adults, omentum is like a fatty apron which localizes the infection.
- In **aged patients,** because of atherosclerosis, **gangrene** occurs **very fast** resulting in peritonitis. Obstruction is caused by faecoliths, worms and bands which cause tenting. ***Obstructed appendicitis is one of the examples for closed loop obstruction.*** Other causes are volvulus, carcinoma hepatic flexure with competent ileocaecal valve.

Key Box 51.2

Nonobstructive Theory in Acute Appendicitis

- This is seen in two-thirds of the cases. Hence, it is more common than obstructive theory.
- Bacterial or viral infection is the cause.
- It causes mucosal ulceration.
- This is followed by bacterial invasion.
- The decrease in the incidence of enteric fever in the Western world has decreased incidence of acute appendicitis—a support for infective theory.
- In many cases of appendicitis, the appendix is not dilated (against obstructive theory).

- Common bacteria encountered in acute appendicitis are *Bacteroides fragilis, Escherichia coli, Clostridium perfringens, Streptococcus faecalis, Pseudomonas aeruginosa*, etc.

Clinical Features

The peak incidence is in the second and third decades. Very uncommon before the age of two.

Symptoms

- **Pain** is severe, colicky type, initially felt in the umbilical region and it is due to ***distension of appendix.*** This is a visceral pain. After a few hours, the pain localizes to the right iliac fossa. It is a ***somatic pain*** which is due to ***inflammation of parietal peritoneum.*** This type of pain is called ***shifting pain of acute appendicitis*** (Fig. 51.8) or ***migratory pain—most reliable symptom of acute appendicitis***.
- Normal appendix is mobile. So, the site of maximum pain and tenderness can vary.
- **Vomiting** occurs once or twice due to reflex pylorospasm. It contains **stomach contents**. However, it is never frequent such as in intestinal obstruction.
- Appendicitis is unlikely in patients with normal appetite. Usually, patients have **anorexia**.
- **Fever** is of low grade (around 100°F) and indicates bacterial inflammation.

Pearls of Wisdom

Pain first, followed by vomiting and then by fever is called Murphy's[1] triad of symptoms of acute appendicitis (Murphy's syndrome).

- **Haematuria** is uncommon and it is due to inflammation of retrocaecal appendix which irritates the ureter in the retroperitoneum.
- **Constipation** is the usual feature, except in pre- and post-ileal appendicitis, where they produce diarrhea due to irritation of ileum.

Competency

SU28.15.9: Demonstrate the signs of acute appendicitis.

Signs

1. ***Cough tenderness*** **(Dunphy's sign—Fig. 51.9)** indicates inflammation of parietal peritoneum. This is an important physical sign which differentiates acute appendicitis from right-sided ureteric colic.
2. ***Tenderness and rebound tenderness*** are present at McBurney's point. Rebound tenderness is called **Blumberg sign.** It is due to inflammation of the parietal peritoneum. This physical sign can be elicited in all cases of peritonitis.
3. ***Guarding and rigidity*** are present in the right iliac fossa **in complicated appendicitis**. However, guarding and rigidity of back muscles (erector spinae) indicates retrocaecal appendicitis.
4. ***Rovsing sign:*** Palpation of left iliac region of abdomen produces pain in the right iliac region. It is because of displacement of colonic gas and small bowel coils impinging upon the inflamed appendix (Fig. 51.10A).
5. ***Hyperaesthesia*** in the Sherren's triangle (Fig. 51.10B): Sherren's triangle is formed by anterior superior iliac spine, umbilicus and pubic symphysis. It is due to irritation of lower abdominal nerves.
6. ***Cope's psoas test:*** Seen in retrocaecal appendicitis. There will be irritation of psoas major which produces flexion at the hip. If any attempt is made to extend the hip, it produces pain.
7. ***Cope's obturator test:*** Seen in pelvic appendicitis due to irritation of the obturator muscle. Flexion and medial rotation produce pain.
8. ***Features of generalised peritonitis*** are seen only when there is a rupture. Gangrene and perforation

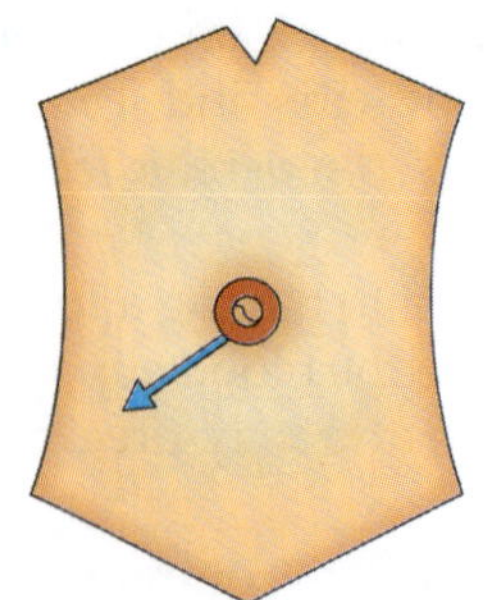

Fig. 51.8: Shifting pain (migratory pain)—most reliable symptom

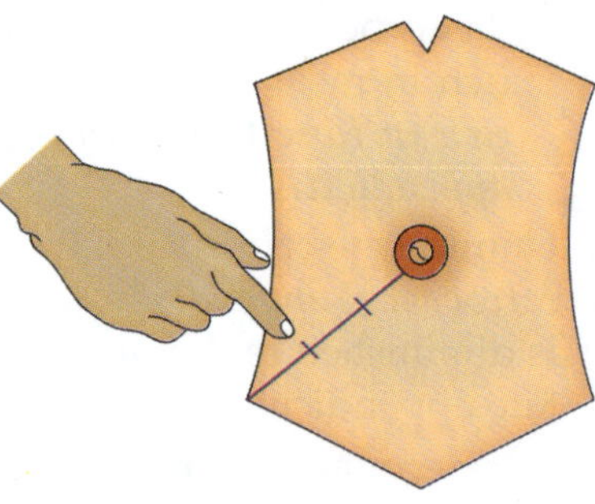

Fig. 51.9: Cough tenderness (Dunphy's sign)

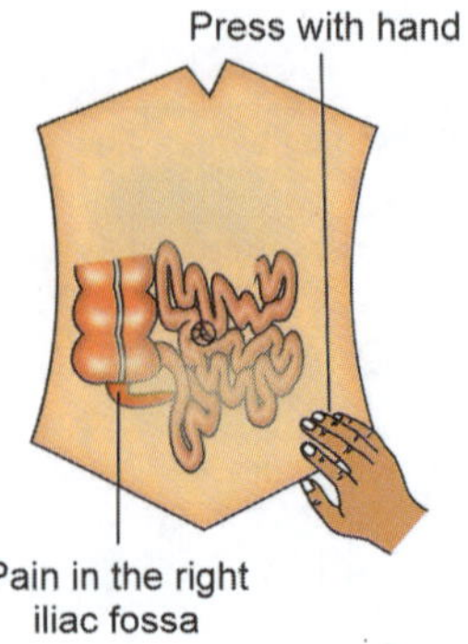

Fig. 51.10A: Rovsing sign

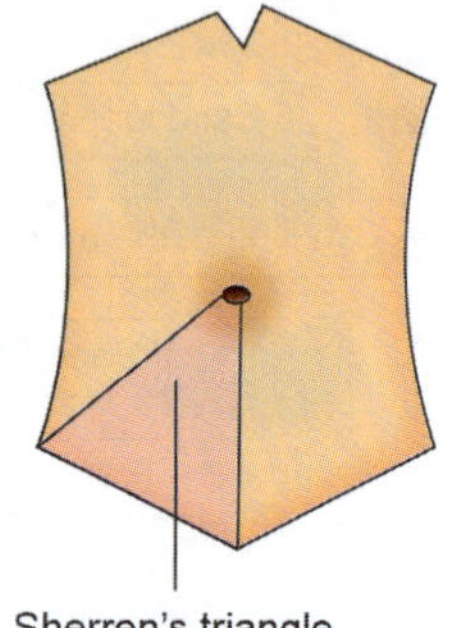

Fig. 51.10B: Hyperaesthesia in the Sherren's triangle

[1]Can you find out what is Murphy's sign and Murphy's punch test?

is more common in elderly patients because of atherosclerosis. In infants, omentum is very thin without much of fat. Hence, diffuse peritonitis occurs very fast.

9. *Rectal examination:* There is tenderness in the right rectal wall—**differential tenderness**.
10. *Per vaginal examination:* Presence of ovarian mass, tenderness on **movement** of cervix, adnexal tenderness may suggest obstetric pathology.
    - Signs and symptoms vary depending upon the location (Key Box 51.3).

Key Box 51.3

Variations in Acute Appendicitis

1. **Retrocaecal:** Silent (no rigidity in the right iliac fossa).
2. **Pelvic:** Causes diarrhoea.
3. **Postileal:** Causes diarrhoea—called missed appendix.
4. **Subhepatic:** Manifests as pain in the right iliac fossa, very difficult to remove from gridiron incision.
5. **In pregnancy:** The location of the pain is shifted higher up and laterally.

Pearls of Wisdom

Pregnancy testing is mandatory in women of childbearing age.

Investigations

Competency

SU28.15.3: Describe complications and principles of management of acute appendicitis.

1. **Total WBC count** is almost always increased above 10,000 cells/mm^3, in most of the patients (95%).
    - A very high white blood cell count (>20,000/mm^3) suggests complicated appendicitis with gangrene or perforation.
2. **Urine examination** is mainly to rule out urinary tract infection, haematuria and sometimes pyuria. In suspected patients, pregnancy test can also be done.
3. **C-reactive protein** is elevated in any inflammatory condition such as appendicitis. Elevated in the first 12 hours of any acute inflammation and is very nonspecific. However, if total counts and CRP levels are not elevated, probability of acute appendicitis is almost nil.
4. **Plain X-ray abdomen erect** is taken to rule out other causes of acute abdomen such as perforation of hollow viscous (Free gas under the diaphragm) and intestinal obstruction (multiple air fluid levels). In appendicitis, one or two dilated small bowel loops may be seen in right lower region due to ileus. If a radio-opaque stone in the direction of ureter is found, it suggests ureteric colic. Presence of faecolith is highly suggestive of acute appendicitis in plain X-ray.
5. **Abdominal ultrasound** to rule out other causes including gynaecological causes. Ultrasound can demonstrate a non-compressible, aperistaltic tubular organ with a thick wall. It can be used to elicit probe tenderness (sensitivity of 85%, specificity of 90%).

Advantages

- It is a simple bedside investigation.
- Economical
- Can confirm acute appendicitis in about 50% of the patients.
- Appendicolith, pericaecal fluid collection or inflammation can be diagnosed—indirect features of acute appendicitis (Figs 51.11A and B).
- More sensitive and specific in children—thin abdominal wall.

Disadvantages

- It is operator-dependent
- It is not a choice in fatty obese patient
- Gas within the dilated intestine may obscure the appendix

6. **CECT: Contrast enhanced CT scan is the investigation of choice** (sensitivity of 90 to 100%, specificity of 90%), **especially** when diagnosis is not established or in atypical cases. All the findings mentioned in the ultrasound can also be defined by CT scan (Fig. 51.12).

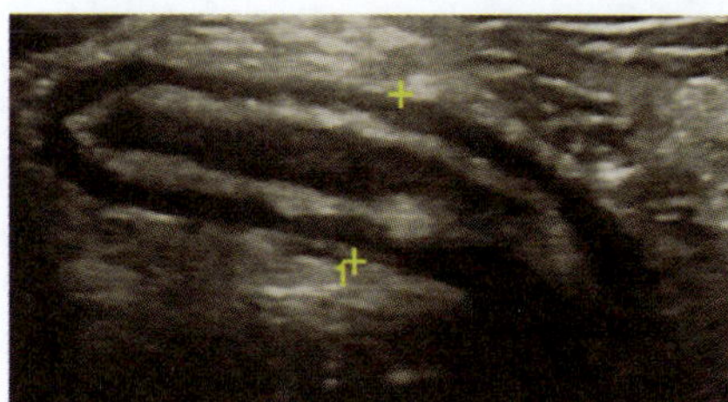

Fig. 51.11A: Ultrasound of appendix showing thickened appendix suggestive of acute appendicitis.

Fig. 51.11B: At Surgery, you can see inflamed and thickened appendix.

(*Courtesy*: Dr Naaz Jahan Shaikh, Consultant Surgeon, Hosapete, Karnataka)

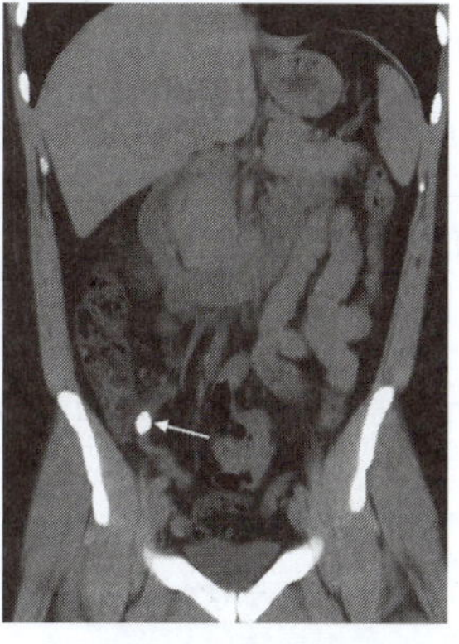

Fig. 51.12: CT scan in acute appendicitis—showing a faecolith

Typical CT findings

1. Appendix is more than 7 mm in diameter
2. Thick inflamed wall
3. Mural enhancement (target sign)
4. Periappendicular fluid or air

Advantages

- More objective.
- Sensitivity and specificity is almost about 95%.
- Helps to rule out carcinoma caecum, duodenal perforation, acute pancreatitis, etc.
- Can detect anomaly as in subhepatic appendicitis.

Disadvantages

- Pregnant woman—it is contraindicated.
- In children—better to avoid it for the fear of radiation exposure and risk of cancer developing at a later date.
- Expensive, long time for the contrast to reach the site.
- Low fat, sensitivity is less.
- Allergy to contrast and contrast nephropathy (dehydration, high creatinine, diabetics precipitating factors).
- The importance of CT scan is highlighted in the clinical notes given later.

7. **MRI:** Ideal in pregnant women.

Clinical Notes

A 65-year-old lady was examined for feature of acute appendicitis of 8 hours duration. On examination, she had McBurney tenderness but a vague mass was palpable. It is unusual for an appendicular mass to appear within 8 hours following appendicitis. Ovarian pathology was considered, and gynaecological opinion was requested. It was normal. CT scan was done. It revealed mucocoele of the appendix (8 cm size). She underwent lower midline laparotomy and it was removed. CT scan gave a correct diagnosis, and it guided the treatment policy.

SCORING SYSTEM

Competency

SU28.15.7: Describe components, advantages and disadvantages of scoring systems applied in diagnosis of acute appendicitis.

To avoid negative appendicectomies, many scoring systems have been developed considering signs, symptoms and investigations. Most commonly used **Alvarado scoring system** is given in Table 51.1.

Score less than 5	:	Not sure
Score 5–6	:	Compatible
Score 6–9	:	Probable
Score more than 9	:	Confirmed

Table 51.1 Alvarado scoring system

Features	*Score*
Symptoms:	
Migrating RIF pain	1
Anorexia	1
Nausea, vomiting	1
Signs:	
Tenderness RIF	2
Rebound tenderness	1
Elevated temperature	1
Laboratory:	
Leucocytosis	2
Shift to left	1
Total	**10**

- Even though Alvarado scoring is highly suggestive of appendicitis, it is only a simple and cost-effective scoring system. This can be applied when sophisticated investigations such as ultrasonography and CT scan are not available.

Surgical wisdom: Symptoms, signs (tenderness in McBurney point) and rebound tenderness with increased total counts, you often do not need any **sophisticated imaging** tests. However, ultrasound being an extended surgical arm, it should be done.

DIFFERENTIAL DIAGNOSIS OF ACUTE APPENDICITIS

Competency

SU28.15.4: Describe the differential diagnosis of appendicitis in children, adult, and elderly individuals.

Innumerable conditions may mimic some signs of appendicitis. A few important conditions have been considered here.

In Children (Fig. 51.13A to D)

A. **Enterocolitis** is common in children. It presents with severe diarrhoea with blood and mucus in the stools.

B. **Meckel's diverticulitis** can present with abdominal pain, vomiting, fever—signs and symptoms are similar to acute appendicitis (difficult to differentiate clinically).

C. **Worm ball** is common in children in the developing countries. However, features of intestinal obstruction will be present.

D. **Acute iliac/mesenteric lymphadenitis**—non-shifting pain and rebound tenderness are absent. It is viral in origin and self-limiting. Neck nodes will give clue to the diagnosis.

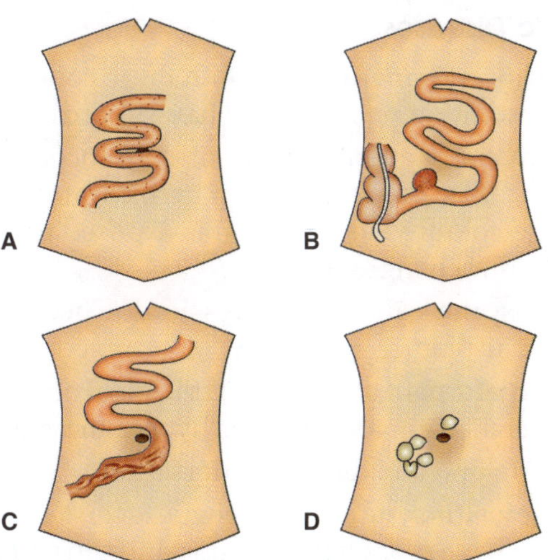

Fig. 51.13A to D: In children (see text)

In Young Adults (Fig. 51.14A to D)

A. **Right-sided ureteric colic:** Haematuria, severe pain from loin to groin, absence of cough tenderness help in excluding acute appendicitis.

B. **Amoebic typhlitis** is associated with diarrhoea, blood in the stools and tenderness in left iliac fossa (Manson Barr's amoebic point of tenderness).

C. **Torsion of undescended testis:** Absence of testis in the scrotum clinches the diagnosis.

D. **Meckel's diverticulitis**

E. **Yersinia ileitis:** Acute, self-limiting inflammation of the ileum caused by *Yersinia pseudotuberculosis*.

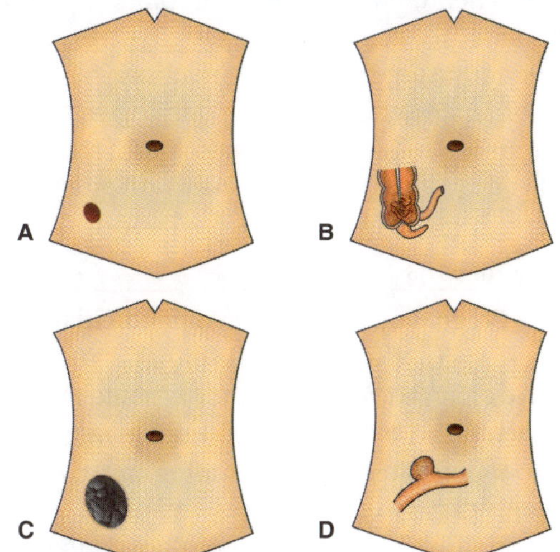

Fig. 51.14A to D: In adults (see text)

In Middle Age (Fig. 51.15A to D)

A. **Acute pancreatitis:** Inflammatory exudate collects and gravitates in the right iliac fossa resulting in pain, guarding and rigidity in the right iliac fossa. History of alcohol intake, severe backache and tenderness in the epigastrium help in diagnosing acute pancreatitis.

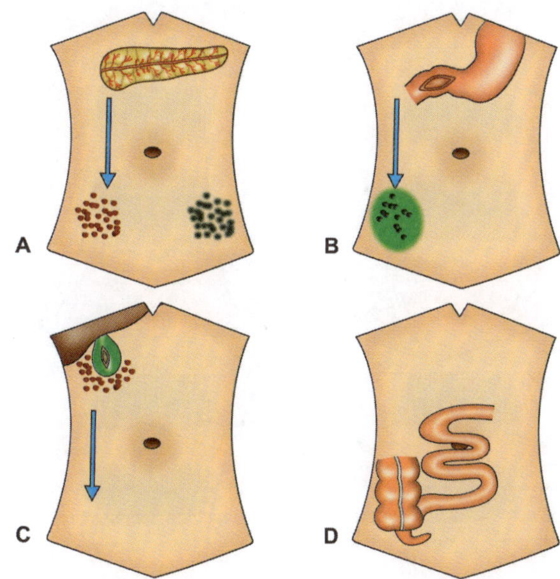

Fig. 51.15A to D: In middle age (see text)

B. **Perforated duodenal ulcer** can present with pain in the right side of the abdomen due to similar causes mentioned above.

C. **Acute cholecystitis** can also present with features of acute appendicitis. However, it is common in elderly females.

D. **Pain** in the right iliac fossa and tenderness is due to dilated intestinal loop peristalsis as in ileocaecal tuberculosis or carcinoma caecum. Presence of an irregular and hard mass suggests carcinoma caecum.

In Females (Fig. 51.16A to D)

A. **Ruptured ectopic gestation:** Missed periods, features of haemorrhagic shock (pallor), and extreme tenderness on movement of cervix during *per vaginal* examination clinch the diagnosis.

B. **Pelvic inflammatory diseases:**
- These are group of inflammatory conditions affecting young women.
- Tubo-ovarian sepsis, salpingitis and endometriosis are grouped under this.
- Bilateral pelvic pain, high degree fever, and absence of anorexia are some of the features.
- Tenderness is present in both iliac fossae on deep palpation—no cough tenderness.
- Vaginal discharge helps in the diagnosis.
- Culture for *Chlamydia trachomatis* and *Neisseria gonorrhoeae* must be obtained.

C. **Midmenstrual** (mittelschmerz) rupture of ovarian follicle occurs about 14th to 16th day and can produce abdominal pain.

D. **Torsion of ovarian cyst** produces very severe abdominal pain with a mass.

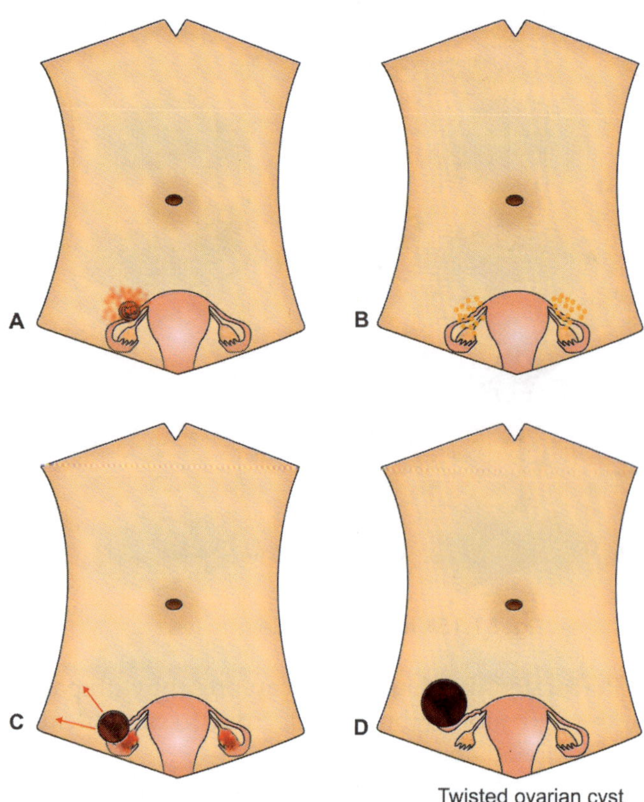

Fig. 51.16A to D: In females (see text)

Clinical Notes

- A 30-year-old lady was diagnosed to have acute appendicitis with classical features—pain, fever, vomiting and tenderness in the McBurney's point. A gynaecological examination revealed pelvic infection. An infected copper T was removed which was the cause of abdominal pain.
- A 22-year-old man underwent appendicectomy for right-sided abdominal pain. At laparotomy, appendix was normal. However, it was removed. He continued to have abdominal pain. An ultrasound of the abdomen revealed torsion of the undescended testis. Nobody had examined his external genitalia!
- A 36-year-old male who had previous history of abdominal pain underwent appendicectomy for tenderness and rebound tenderness in the right iliac fossa. Operative surgery notes said that the appendix was slightly inflamed and seropurulent fluid was present in the right iliac fossa. After 2–3 days, greenish fluid (bile) started draining out through the tube. The condition of the patient deteriorated and on re-exploration this time, by midline incision revealed perforated chronic duodenal ulcer!!

Pearls of Wisdom

Any female patient with right-sided lower abdominal pain should undergo a gynaecological examination to rule out the causes mentioned above, before subjecting to appendicectomy.

Systemic Diseases

1. **Pleurisy** and **pneumonia:** Both these conditions can have radiating pain and can have guarding.
2. **Porphyria:** Violent intestinal colic occurs due to spasm. It is precipitated by barbiturates. Urine is orange-coloured and when it is exposed to sunlight, the colour changes to amber.
3. **Pott's spine** causes compression of nerve roots—radicular pain.
4. **Preherpetic pain** of 10th and 11th dorsal nerves is located over the same area. Marked hyperesthesia is present.
5. **Purpura** and bleeding disorders.
6. **Polyserositis syndromes:** Dengue fever, leptospirosis, etc. can have peritoneal irritation and can secrete fluid in the peritoneal cavity. Ultrasound may even reveal probe tenderness. Doing an appendicectomy can be dangerous in these patients. It may worsen pre-existing condition including pneumonia, etc. may result in ARDS.

A Few Special Situations

One should be careful and be firm in decision making of appendicectomy in these cases (Key Boxes 51.4 to 51.6).

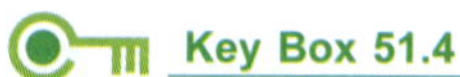

Key Box 51.4

Children and Acute Appendicitis

- Appendicitis is rare under 2 years of age because lymphatic tissue is not yet developed by that time.
- Signs are not very well located.
- Greater omentum is very thin. Perforation peritonitis is common.
- Hence, early surgery is recommended.
- Open or laparoscopic method is followed.
- Remember to rule out acute mesenteric lymphadenitis (viral), Yersinia ileitis and Meckel's diverticulitis.

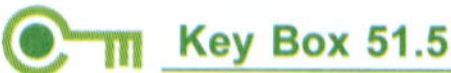

Key Box 51.5

Pregnancy and Acute Appendicitis

- Most common cause of abdominal pain and **non-obstetric** emergency in pregnancy is acute appendicitis.
- Incidence may be 1 to 1.5/1000 pregnancies.
- Symptoms of nausea and vomiting are confused for morning sickness.
- Migration of pain need not be present. Leukocytosis is seen in pregnancy cases—it is normal occurrence.
- Tenderness is shifted because appendix is displayed superiorly and laterally.
- Ultrasound is the investigation of choice. When in doubt MRI is useful investigation.
- Treatment is by laparotomy and appendicectomy.
- **Fetal loss** is 3% but with perforation, it is 30%.
- Maternal mortality rate in perforated appendicitis is 4%.

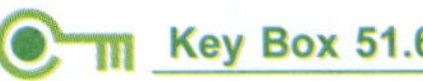

Key Box 51.6

Acquired Immunodeficiency Syndrome (AIDS) and Appendicitis

- Incidence of acute appendicitis is more common in AIDS patients: 4-fold than non-AIDS patients
- Pain is chronic than acute
- Diarrhoea is more common
- Leukocytosis is not common
- Delay in the presentation may be present especially patients with low CD count
- Interestingly, outcome or results are surprisingly good after surgery

COMPLICATIONS OF ACUTE APPENDICITIS

1. **Appendicular mass** (Figs 51.17A and B): Following an attack of acute appendicitis, infection is sealed off by greater omentum, caecum, terminal ileum, etc. which results in a tender, soft to firm mass in the right iliac fossa. **Presence of a mass** is a **contraindication for appendicectomy** because it is very difficult to remove appendix from such a mass. An attempt to remove it may result in a faecal fistula.

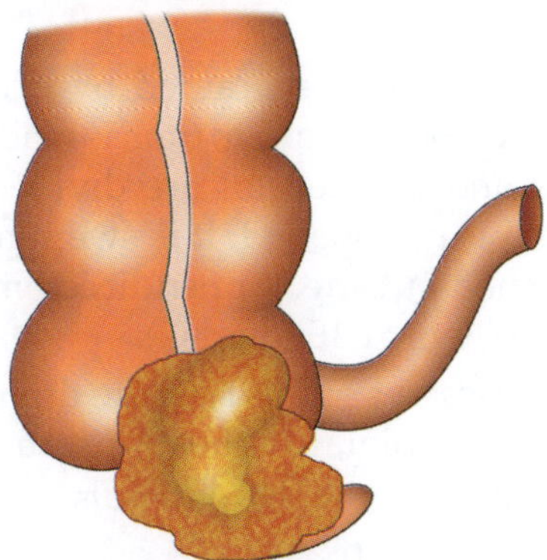

Fig. 33.17A: Appendicular mass—tender, diffuse mass

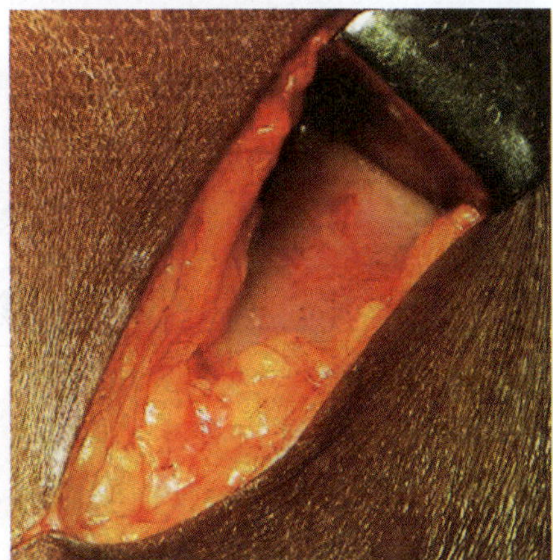

Fig. 33.17B: Appendicular mass: Laparotomy done for appendicectomy but could see the mass. Abandoned the procedure

Pearls of Wisdom

If appendicitis is more than 2 days old and one cannot assess mass clinically due to guarding, always palpate right iliac fossa after general anaesthesia is given, to rule out mass. This can prevent unnecessary exploration.

Competency

SU28.15.5: Describe management of appendicular mass.

Appendicular mass is treated by **Ochsner and Sherren regime**.

- **A**spiration with Ryle's tube to give rest to the gut, only if vomiting is present.
- **B**owel care—purgatives should not be used (may cause perforation).
- **C**harts—temperature, pulse, respiration, diameter of the mass. Swinging temperature, and increase in size of mass indicates an appendicular abscess.
- **D**rugs to cover all the organisms—gram-positive, gram-negative and anaerobic organisms.
- **E**xploratory laparotomy should not be done. However, when the condition of the **patient is not improving,** there is a suspicion of an abscess (Fig. 51.17B) and when doubtful of the diagnosis, exploration is indicated (see the clinical notes).
- **F**luids (Table 51.2): Patient is kept nil orally for one or two days. During this time, intravenous fluids are given to correct dehydration.
- After 3–4 days, the abdomen becomes soft, tenderness decreases and once stools are passed, Ryle's tube is removed. Clear oral fluids followed by soft diet is given. By one week, the patient is back to normal. **After 6–8 weeks**, patient is advised **elective appendicectomy**.
- Interval appendicectomy is not done nowadays until and unless patient has recurrent symptoms of appendicitis or there is faecolith.

Clinical Notes

A 60-year-old lady was diagnosed to have appendicular mass and was undergoing conservative management. On the fourth day, she developed features of early septic shock. As the patient was not improving, laparotomy was done. It was a case of volvulus of the caecum.

2. **Perforated appendicitis**

- Incidence is about 8–10%.
- More common in children and elderly patients.
- Delay in seeking medical treatment is the main factor.
- Other factors which precipitate perforation are diabetes mellitus, AIDS, faecolith.
- The pain usually localizes to the right lower quadrant, if the perforation has been walled off by surrounding intra-abdominal structures including the omentum.

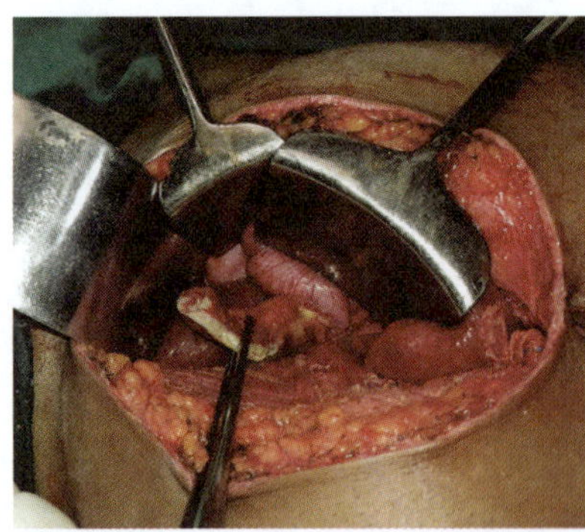

Fig. 51.18: Perforated appendicitis at surgery—22-year-old boy presented with septic shock

- Perforated appendicitis can also give rise to generalised peritonitis and septic shock (Fig. 51.18).
- Rigors and chills with fever of 102°F (38.9°C) or above.
- As a complication of perforation peritonitis, portal pyaemia (pylephlebitis) can develop, it can be very dangerous.
- Emergency laparotomy, appendicectomy, drainage of pus, peritoneal lavage, and antibiotics are main principles.
- It causes generalised peritonitis with 10–20% mortality rate. Mortality depends upon various factors including age, performance status and delay is presentation to the hospital. Mortality is due to uncontrolled sepsis and multiorgan failure.

Perforated appendicitis: Principles of surgery

- Careful handling of appendix, gentle separation of bowel loops.
- Crushing of base is not required. Appendicectomy is done in the usual manner.
- Drainage of abscess cavity/pus. Always drain the peritoneal cavity.
- Wound is closed but skin is not closed (prevents wound infection).
- Continue antibiotics for 4 to 7 days. Enteral nutrition (oral) to be started once paralytic ileus settles down.

3. **Appendicular abscess** (Fig. 51.19A): If the infection is not controlled properly following an attack of appendicitis, an abscess can occur in relation to the appendix. They are (A) retrocaecal, (B) postileal and preileal, (C) pelvic, (D) subcaecal abscesses. Clinically, it presents with high-grade fever with chills and rigors and a tender boggy swelling in the right iliac fossa or in the right lumbar region. Pelvic abscess presents with diarrhoea. Diagnosis is by late presentation to the hospital (3–4 days) and high-grade fever with chills and rigors (Key Box 51.7).

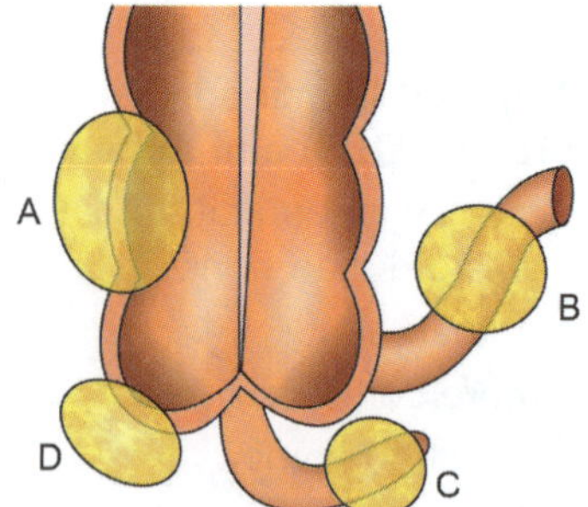

Fig. 51.19A: Appendicular abscess (*see* text for A to D)

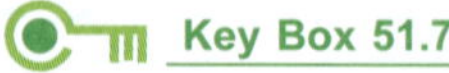

Key Box 51.7

Appendicular Abscess

- Ultrasound/CT scan is done to assess the size and location of abscess.
- Abscess greater than 4–6 cm in size needs to be drained by guided percutaneous aspiration or drainage through rectum or vagina.
- Ongoing inflammation may force a surgeon to do appendicectomy (open/laparoscopic) at the same admission.
- Those who improve require appendicectomy after 6 weeks.

A. **Retrocaecal abscess** is drained by extraperitoneal approach. An incision of 5 to 6 cm is made in the right iliac fossa and all muscles are divided. However, peritoneum is not opened. It is swept medially and pus is drained outside. Appendicectomy is done at a later date (Figs 51.19B and C).
   - Most of abscesses of this type are drained by ultrasound guided pigtail catheter insertion.

B. **Preileal and postileal abscesses** also can be drained by a pigtail catheter.

C. **Pelvic abscess** is drained *via* the rectum (*see* page 723).

D. **Subcaecal:** May require extraperitoneal drainage.

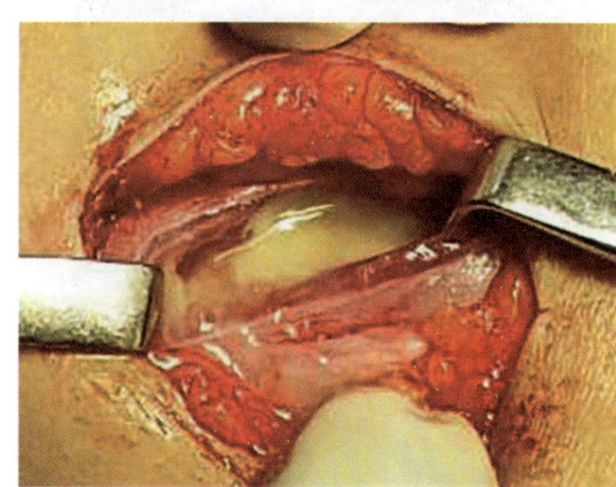

Fig. 51.19B: Appendicular abscess is drained by extraperitoneal route (*Courtesy:* Dr Jyothi, Head, Department of Surgery, GIMS, Gadag, Karnataka)

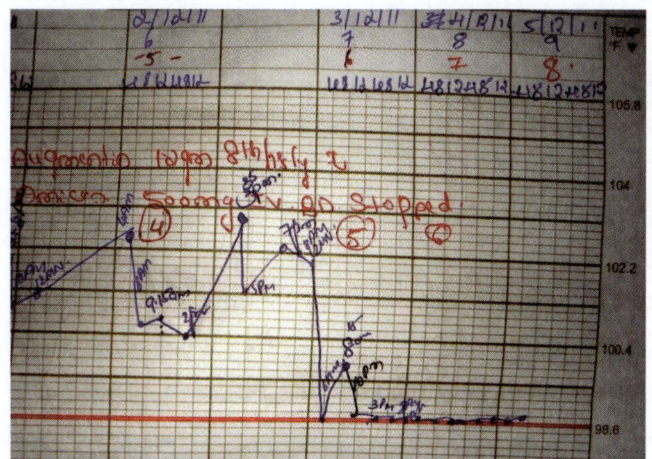

Fig. 51.19C: Appendicular abscess—once drained, fever touched the base

4. Few cases can have spreading necrotizing fasciitis of the lateral abdominal wall including inguinal region and scrotum. They require more aggressive approach of treatment with antibiotics, debridement, appendicectomy, drainage of pus, etc.

Treatment of Acute Appendicitis

Preoperative Resuscitation

- Once diagnosis of acute appendicitis is suspected, the patient is admitted to the hospital.
- IV fluids—isotonic saline or Ringer lactate is given.
- Electrolytes are corrected especially in late cases of acute appendicitis/perforation peritonitis, etc.
- Ryle's tube is not necessary in simple appendicitis but is definitely required in complicated cases (peritonitis).
- Fluroquinolones second generation cephalosporins along with metronidazole is given.
- Informed consent is taken.
- **Laparoscopic emergency appendicectomy:** Emergency appendicectomy is offered when patient comes within 24 to 48 hours of abdominal pain. It is very important to rule out or detect a mass, especially if a decision is made to operate around 2nd or 3rd day. If a mass is palpable, it is better not to operate at that time (please refer to operative surgery, appendicectomy). A few important steps are given here (Figs 51.20 to 51.22).
- The appendix is identified by tracing *Taenia coli* which converges onto the base of the appendix. Mesoappendix is divided in between ligatures. A purse-string suture is applied all around the appendix in the caecum. The appendix is divided in between ligatures, the stump is invaginated and the purse-string is tightened. The abdomen is closed in layers.

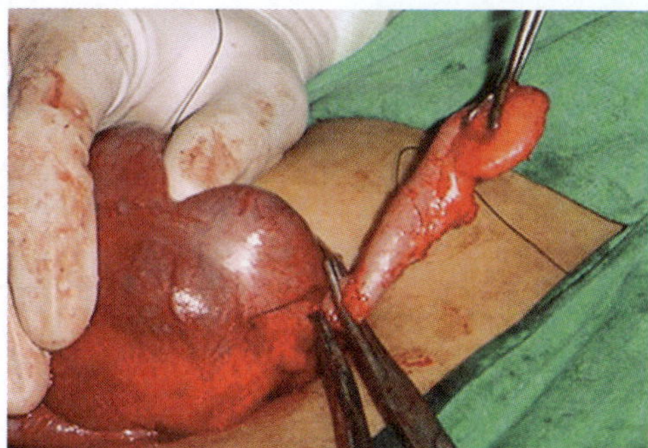

Fig. 51.20: Emergency appendicectomy—appendix is identified, isolated by dividing and freed till the base. The base is crushed and divided in between 2 artery forceps

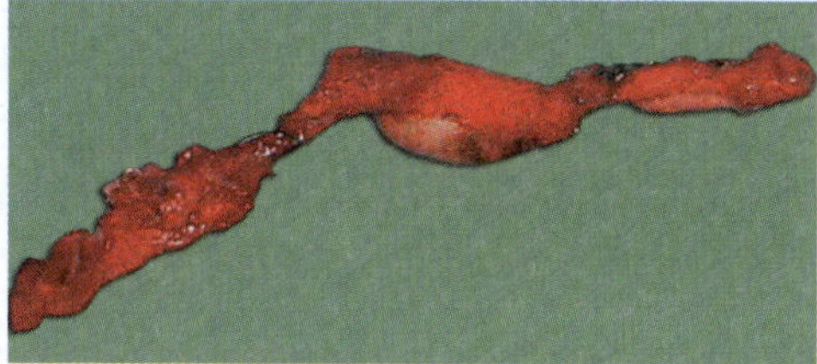

Fig. 51.21: Large faecolith resulting in acute appendicitis

- **Laparoscopic appendicectomy** has become more popular nowadays because of less postoperative pain, speedy recovery. Benefit is maximum in obese, women and elderly patients. (*see* Chapter in Operative Surgery).

Pearls of Wisdom

- Early uncomplicated appendicitis is increasingly being managed conservatively nowadays by some experts.
- When you trace Taenia coli and you do not find appendix, it means you are holding and tracing Taenia of the sigmoid colon. (It can be found on the right side sometimes).

Algorithm of treatment of appendicitis is shown in Fig. 51.22.

Problems Encountered during Appendicectomy

1. **The incision is small:** Location is higher up—one can extend the incision to about 2–3 cm in cases of slightly higher placed appendix. However, if it is sub-hepatic, never hesitate to close the incision and give a midline incision and do appendicectomy. An attempt to remove the appendix with McBurney incision, with traction and limited exposure may result in injury to ileum or colon and may result in faecal fistula.
2. **Normal appendix is found:** Look for Meckel's diverticulitis, intestinal obstruction, stricture, etc. If bile is found, it means perforated duodenal ulcer—most common (Valentino appendix—page 929). Close the incision and do laparotomy. If mesenteric nodes are enlarged, do lymph node biopsy.
3. **Sometimes you will find some other pathologies** (Table 51.2).

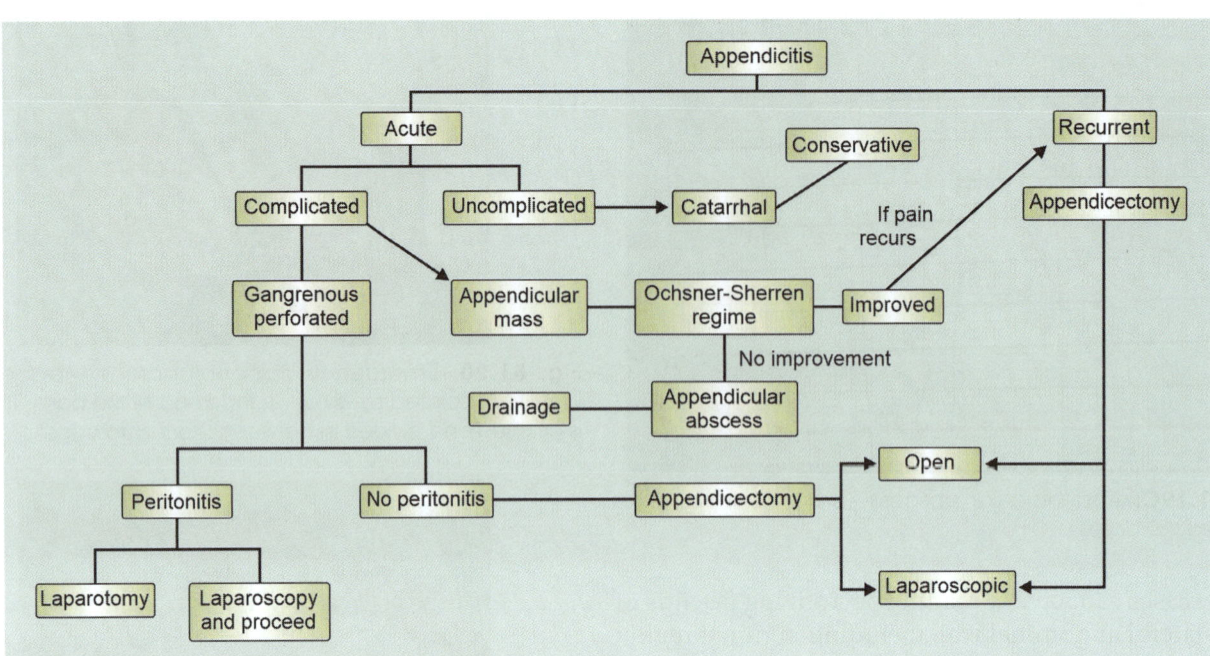

Fig. 51.22: Treatment of appendicitis (*Courtesy:* Dr Amith Jain, Professor of surgery, SRR Medical College, Bengaluru, Karnataka)

Table 51.2 Wisdom/mistakes/surprises for surgeon while conducting appendicectomy—4 scenarios

1. Observes straw-coloured fluid	2. Observes bile-coloured fluid	3. Observes 'foul' fluid	4. Observes haemorrhagic fluid
Completes appendicectomy Closes the wound Realises 3 days later, it was acute pancreatitis **How could it have been avoided?** Serum amylase and lipase were not sent. A preoperative ultrasound was not done	Completes appendicectomy Puts a drain Closes the wound Postoperative biliary fistula Asks for contrast CT, **realises duodenal ulcer perforation**, explores, sutures the perforation He had not done a simple chest X-ray or plain X-ray abdomen erect preoperatively in this case	Completes appendicectomy Postoperative faecal fistula Re-explores by midline incision Perforated Meckel's diverticulum Resection, anastomosis	Completes appendicectomy Ignores fluid Patient continues to have pain OBG consultation given Twisted ovarian cyst Laparotomy and ovariectomy
Surgical wisdom: If these investigations were done before surgery, they could have helped the surgeon. Luckily, the patient recovered from this unnecessary, avoidable surgery	**Surgical wisdom:** He had not taken history properly (valentino syndrome)	**Surgical wisdom:** Surgeon had not examined the terminal 2 feet ileum during appendicectomy	**Surgical wisdom:** Surgeon had not done ultrasound and gynaecological consultation was not requested before surgery

Pearls of Wisdom

During open appendicectomy, after opening the peritoneum, if the appendix pops out immediately, then it is called "goodmorning appendix".

1. Creeping fat: Crohn's disease
2. Ileum: Meckel's diverticulum
3. Mesentery: Lymph nodes
4. Peritoneum: Tubercles
5. Ovaries: Tubo-ovarian mass
6. Sigmoid colon: Diverticulitis (redundant colon)
7. Bile: Perforation of duodenal ulcer

Incidental appendicectomy should not be done because appendix may actually have a role in the maintenance of healthy colonic flora.

4. **Gangrenous appendix involving base:** Problem one can face here is that the purse-string can be applied but invagination of the stump is not possible. Risk of faecal fistula is also present. Appendicectomy, wash and a drain is kept.
5. **Difficult to isolate the appendix which is gangrenous but pus is present:** Limited ileocecectomy can be done.

6. **The appendix cannot be found:** First mobilise the caecum and look for subcaecal or retrocaecal sites. Look also into preileal or postileal sites. Then mobilise the ascending colon also. Agenesis of the appendix is very rare.
7. **Surprise findings of carcinoma caecum** (Fig. 51.23): If suspicion of a carcinoma is high, hemicolectomy should be done. Otherwise take a biopsy—do appendicectomy.

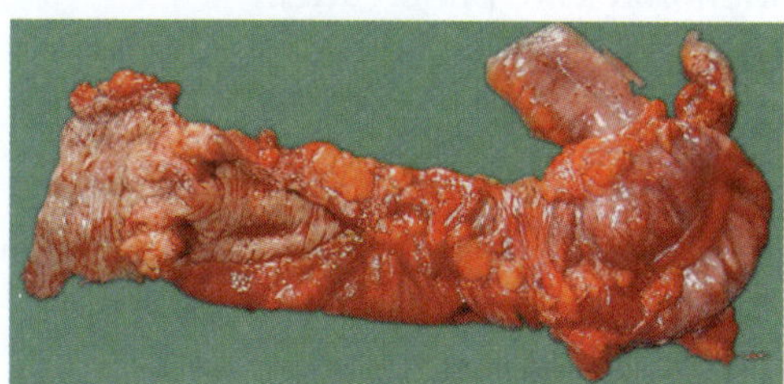

Fig. 51.23: Carcinoma colon with appendicitis

Pearls of Wisdom

Today because of imaging and laparoscopy majority of such wrong diagnosis/mistakes/problems encountered in an appendicectomy is largely eliminated or can be solved or treated with ease. Just to prove again evidence based science.

Incidental Appendicectomy

It means removal of normal appendix at laparotomy for another condition. Examples: When you do Laparotomy and ileal resection for stricture and anastomosis. (Can we do appendicectomy?)

Ovarian cyst: Torsion (right) ovary is removed. (Can we add appendicectomy?)

Since benefits of appendicitis/appendicectomy are more in young patients, if patient is under 30 years, it may be justifiable to do incidental appendicectomy provided it can be removed through same incision, without much difficulty. The patient should be stable to tolerate the procedure.

Contraindications for Incidental Appendicectomy

- Crohn's of caecum
- Radiation treatment of caecum
- Immunosuppression
- Vascular grafted patient (aortoiliac, etc.)

  Chances of infection are high in this group of patients. The result will be faecal fistula—difficult to treat.

POST-APPENDICECTOMY FAECAL FISTULA

Competency

SU28.15.6: Describe surgical management and post-operative complications of acute appendicitis. (For more details, refer to page 1288 in operative surgery chapter.)

- It can occur after appendicectomy especially when gangrene of the appendix extends to base of the caecum. It can also occur, if purse-string suture is not properly applied, or injury to the terminal ileum or caecum, etc. Tuberculosis is one of the important causes of faecal fistula in Indian patients to be kept in mind. Actinomycosis is a rare cause of faecal fistula following appendicectomy, discharge of faeculent contents or faecal matter after appendicectomy suggests faecal fistula (Key Box 51.8).
- Usually discharge stops after a few days provided there is no distal obstruction.
- Cases which do not respond to conservative treatment: Fistula with long tracks, complex fistula, some diseases such as tuberculosis are managed by resection of the diseased portion of the caecum or ascending colon.

Key Box 51.8

Faecal Fistula—can Occur

- After drainage of appendicular abscess
- After appendicectomy—if purse-string sutures are not properly applied
- If the caecum is also involved by inflammation
- If the cause of appendicitis is carcinoma
- If chronic diseases develop or are present—tuberculosis, Crohn's disease or actinomycosis
- If appendicitis is associated with carcinoma caecum

Pearls of Wisdom

The important causes for faecal fistula are carcinoma caecum and ileocaecal tuberculosis in India and Crohn's disease in the West.

Clinical Notes

- A 23-year-old girl presented to the hospital with faecal fistula following appendicectomy of 6 months duration. It was a low output fistula. She had a colostomy bag applied to 4 × 2 cm oval opening at the incision site in the right iliac fossa.
- CT fistulogram showed two irregular contrast-filled tracts connected to caecum, ascending colon and retroperitoneum.
- Exploratory laparotomy and limited right colectomy were done. Tubercles were noted in the peritoneum. Biopsy was taken (Fig. 51.24).
- Final histopathology report was tuberculosis.
- She was put on ATT for 6 months. She recovered well.

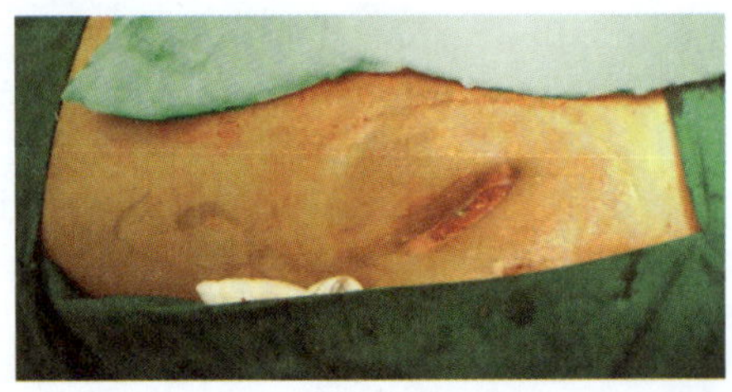

Fig. 51.24: Post-appendicectomy faecal fistula due to tuberculosis

NEOPLASM OF THE APPENDIX

Competency

SU28.15.8: Describe tumours of appendix and clinical features, management of them.

1. Neuroendocrine Tumour

(more details on page 779)

- It is the most common neoplasm of the appendix (Fig. 51.25), less aggressive, majority are benign and cured with simple appendicectomy.
- Goblet cell carcinoid tumour—it is more aggressive, requires right hemicolectomy. If the tumour is more than 2 cm, has more than 2 mitosis per high power field and lymphovascular invasion, it is adenocarcinoma of the appendix.

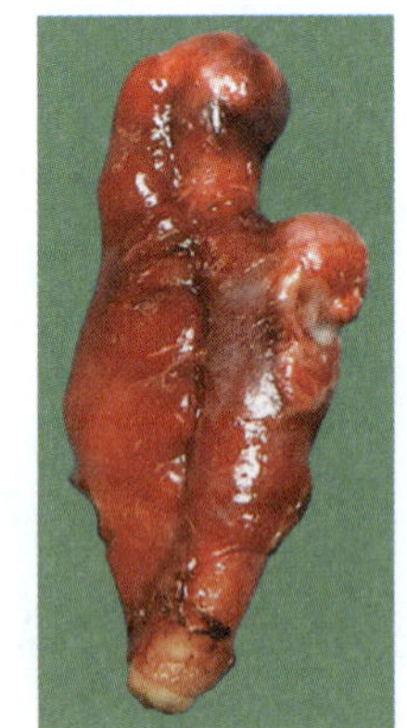

Fig. 51.25: Neuroendocrine tumour of the appendix

2. Carcinoma

- It is very rare.
- Often it is colonic type. Other type is mucinous adenocarcinoma.
- Can present as acute appendicitis due to obstruction caused by the tumour.
- Mucinous variety has better prognosis.
- Colonic variety should be treated by right hemicolectomy.

3. Cystic Neoplasm of the Appendix

- Rare occurrence.
- Simple cyst (non-neoplastic mucocoele) and mucinous cystadenoma (like pancreatic).
- Can attain large size.
- Diagnosis is by ultrasound/CT scan.
- Appendicectomy is the treatment of choice.
- It can rupture into peritoneal cavity resulting in pseudomyxoma peritonei.

MUCOCOELE OF THE APPENDIX

Definition: It means accumulation of mucus within the lumen of the appendix.

Causes: It can be a simple retention cyst due to blockage by foreign body or mucosal hyperplasia. It can also be due to a mucinous adenocarcinoma (Fig. 51.26).

Pathology (Figs 51.26 to 51.28)

- The majority of epithelial tumours of the appendix are mucin rich, thus results in gross distension.
- Mucocoeles resulting from non-neoplastic occlusion (simple retention cysts) rarely exceed 2 cm in diameter.
- Mucinous neoplasms of the appendix are by far the most common cause of mucocoeles.
- Mucocoeles larger than 2 cm are more likely to represent benign neoplasms.

Diagnosis

- It is impossible to differentiate clinically mucocoele of the appendix and acute appendicitis when they

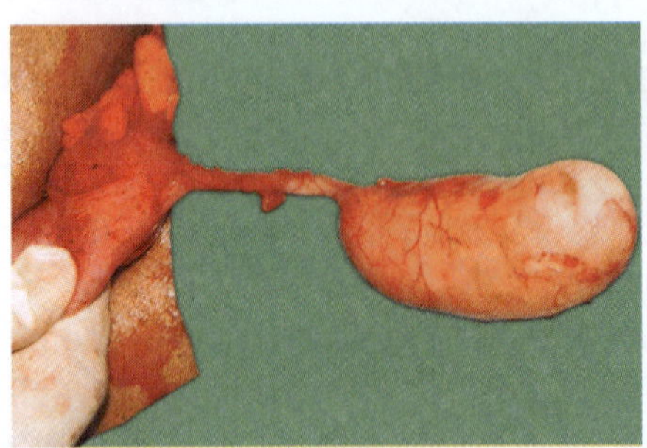

Fig. 51.26: Mucocoele of the appendix (*Courtesy:* Dr Raghunath Prabhu, KMC, Manipal)

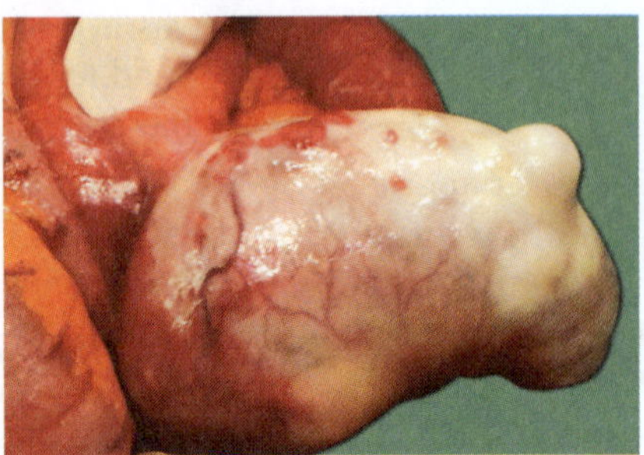

Fig. 51.27: Mucocoele (*Courtesy:* Dr Rajesh Sisodia, KMC, Manipal)

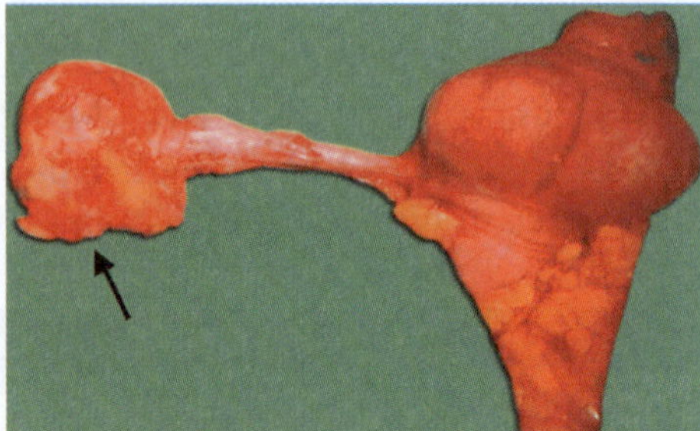

Fig. 51.28: Appendicular tumour arising from the tip has been removed—reported as carcinoid (*Courtesy:* Dr Raghunath Prabhu, KMC, Manipal)

present with abdominal pain. If a mass is palpable, it can be confused with appendicular mass.

- CT scan is the investigation of choice. The anatomic relationship between the elongated cystic mass and the caecum is usually more clear at CT scan than at ultrasound.

Complications

1. **Gross enlargement** and can present as mass abdomen.
2. **Rupture** will result in pseudomyxoma peritonei (more details are given in Chapter 45, Peritonitis).
3. **Secondary infection:** Can result in 'empyema' of the appendix.

Pearls of Wisdom

Rule out adenocarcinoma of the base of the appendix causing mucocoele.

Treatment: Appendicectomy.

MISCELLANEOUS

VALENTINO APPENDIX

Rudolf Valentino was an Italian actor acting in Hollywood who was operated for right iliac fossa pain with features of peritonitis in the early 20th century. Following a few days of surgery, he died of sepsis. The actual disease was perforated duodenal ulcer. This is a typical case scenario that holds true even today. The contents from upper abdomen after perforation or pancreatitis, gravitate down along right paracolic gutter. The symptoms and signs mimic appendicitis. CT scan is the investigation needed to rule out other causes.

POST-APPENDICECTOMY SEPSIS (A CASE REPORT)

A 32-year-old man presented to casualty with septic shock after 5 days after appendicectomy. It was a difficult appendicectomy. Gangrene of the appendix was almost involving the base. On examination, he was having paralytic ileus and jaundice. Abdomen was distended—guarding was present, more in the right iliac fossa. He was admitted to the hospital.

Investigations

- Total counts were 20,000 cells/cu mm: Indicate sepsis
- Urea: 51 mg%, creatinine 1.1 mg%—dehydration, pre-renal failure
- $[K^+]^-$ 3.2 mmol/l, $[Na^+]^-$ 129 mmol/l
- Total Bilirubin: 19 mg%, Direct bilirubin: 16.6 mg%
- AST: 189 IU/l, ALT: 100 IU/l, ALP: 167 IU/l
- ***Plain X-ray*** chest revealed free gas under the diaphragm (Fig. 51.29).

Remarks: It showed he was in sepsis—counts were elevated, urea was high—renal failure set in slowly, increased bilirubin levels—sepsis with cholestasis.

CT scan: Done after hydration—showed pneumoperitoneum and liver cyst (incidental) and free fluid in the peritoneal cavity (Fig. 51.30).

Conclusion

He was in sepsis. The probable reason was that the appendicular base (stump) had given way.

Exploratory Laparotomy

- Faecal peritonitis
- One litre of frank purulent pus in the peritoneal cavity.
- Gangrene of lateral wall of caecum with sloughing of caecal wall.
- Appendix not seen—post-appendicectomy
- Ileum normal

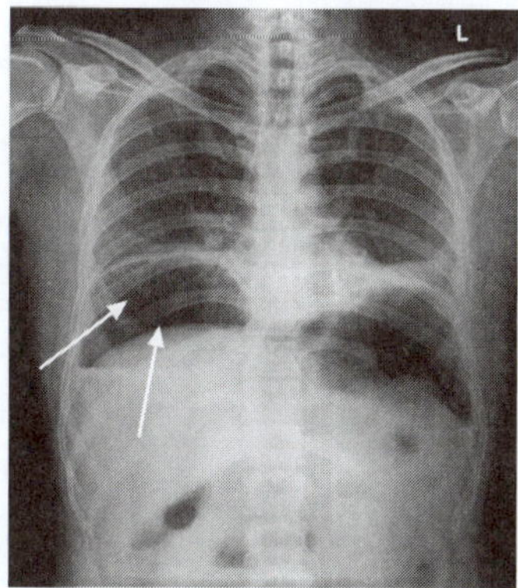

Fig. 51.29: Free gas under the right dome of the diaphragm

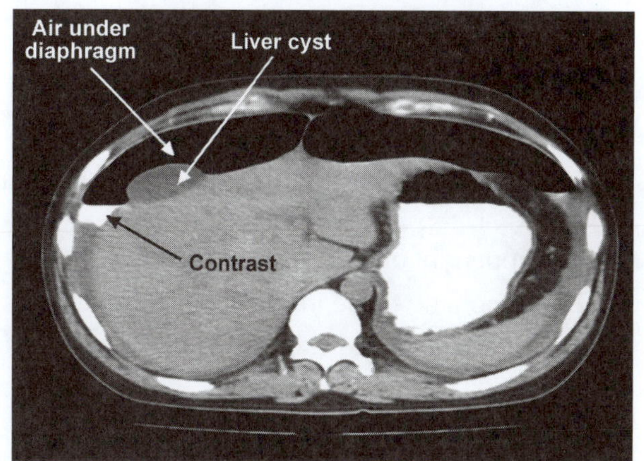

Fig. 51.30: Free gas under the right dome of the diaphragm pneumoperitoneum and liver cyst

- Cystic lesion on anterior surface of right lobe of liver
- Rest of viscera was normal.

Procedure

- Limited resection of ileocaecal segment and end-toend ileo-ascending colon single layer anastamosis
- Peritoneal lavage
- Drains in the pelvis and subhepatic space
- Skin not closed (wound infection is very common)

Postoperative

6th Postoperative Day

- Patient had greenish discharge from the right DT.
- Anastomotic leak and enterocutaneous fistula was suspected.
- Patient was passing flatus.
- RS: Basal crepitations
- Managed conservatively
- TPN was given for 5 days.
- Discharge subsided by 5 days.

8th Postoperative Day

- Breathlessness
- Fever
- Hypoxia: SpO_2: 85%
- Chest X-ray—pneumonia
- Intubated, ventilated for 5 days, appropriate antibiotics
- By 20th day, he was discharged from the hospital—leak had stopped.
- This case report has been given here for the following message:
  1. Acute appendicitis can be dangerous.
  2. Leak should be suspected, if a patient who underwent appendicectomy does not improve in the postoperative period.
  3. High total count, increased bilirubin, oliguria suggest sepsis.
  4. CT scan is the best investigation in such cases. When in doubt re explore. Danger lies in delay, not in resurgery.

INTERESTING 'MOST COMMON'

- Most common surgical emergency encountered by a general surgeon is acute appendicitis.
- Most common emergency surgery is appendicectomy.
- Most common non-obstetric surgical disease of the abdomen during pregnancy is acute appendicitis.
- Most significant symptom of acute appendicitis is migratory pain.
- Most significant sign of acute appendicitis is rebound tenderness in the McBurney's point.
- Most prominent scoring system to diagnose acute appendicitis is Alvarado score.
- Most common anaerobic bacteria in acute appendicitis is *Bacteroides fragilis* and aerobic bacteria is *Escherichia coli*.
- Most common complication after appendicectomy is wound infection.
- Most common age group for acute appendicitis is below 40 years.
- Most common neoplasm of the appendix is carcinoid tumour.

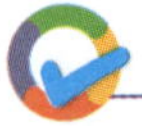

Multiple Choice Questions

1. The most common position of the appendix is:

A. Subhepatic B. Subcaecal
C. Retrocaecal D. Pelvic

2. The incidence of appendicitis is less after 30 years because:

A. The appendix undergoes involution
B. The lymphatic tissue in the appendix decreases
C. Most people would have had their appendices removed
D. The vascularity reduces

3. The name Seshachalam is associated with which of the following arteries?

A. Accessory appendicular artery
B. Appendicular artery
C. Ileocolic artery
D. Posterior caecal artery

4. Appendicular orifice is occasionally guarded by an indistinct semilunar fold of mucous membrane called:

A. Valve of Gerlach B. Valve of Heister
C. Valve of Kerckring D. Valve of Houston

5. The most common scoring system used for appendicitis is __________ scoring system.

A. Child-Pugh B. Furtado
C. Murray D. Alvarado

6. Palpation of left iliac region of abdomen produces pain in the right iliac region in appendicitis because of:

A. Sympathetic reaction
B. Displacement of colonic gas and small bowel coils
C. Sigmoid colon is also affected
D. Ileocolic reflex

7. Cope's psoas test is positive in:

A. Retrocaecal appendicitis
B. Pelvic appendicitis
C. Preileal appendicitis
D. Subcaecal appendicitis

8. Rebound tenderness in acute appendicitis is called:

A. McBurney's sign B. Blumberg's sign
C. Rovsing's sign D. Sherren's sign

9. The most common cause of non-obstetric emergency with abdominal pain in pregnancy is due to:

A. Acute appendicitis B. Acute cholecystitis
C. Acute gastritis D. Acute hepatitis

10. Contraindications for incidental appendicectomy include all of the following *except*:

A. Crohn's of caecum
B. Radiation treatment of the rectum
C. Immunocompetent individuals
D. Previous vascular reconstruction in the abdomen

11. The following statement is TRUE about appendicular abscess:

A. Abscess greater than 4–6 cm in size needs to be drained by laparotomy
B. Appendicectomy must be done along with laparotomy for appendicular abscess
C. Can present with diarrhoea
D. Conservative management is advised till inflammation settles down.

12. Most common aerobic bacterium involved in acute appendicitis is:

A. *Salmonella typhi*
B. *Streptococcus*
C. *Escherichia coli*
D. *Clostridium perfringens*

13. The following statement is FALSE about occurrence of faecal fistula following appendicectomy:

A. Faecal fistula can occur if the cause of appendicitis is carcinoma caecum
B. Faecal fistula can occur if chronic diseases such as tuberculosis is present
C. Faecal fistula can occur if purse string sutures are not applied properly
D. It is always due to actinomycosis

14. The most reliable symptom of acute appendicitis is:

A. Fever B. Migratory pain
C. Right iliac fossa pain D. Vomiting

15. Appendicular perforation is common because of the following reasons *except*:

A. Appendix is a cul-de-sac
B. It has blood supply with profuse collaterals
C. It has a narrow lumen
D. The muscle coat of appendix is thin

16. Appendicular mucosa contains following *except* (predominantly):

A. Columnar epithelium B. Neuroendocrine cells
C. Goblet cells D. Paneth cells

17. About Paneth cells following are true *except*:

A. They are found mainly in colon
B. Found just below crypts of Lieberkühn
C. Have antibacterial property
D. They produce lysozymes

18. Following precautions have to be taken to treat appendicitis in a pregnant lady in the 2nd trimester *except*:

A. Initial evaluation should be by ultrasound imaging
B. MRI is the most ideal imaging
C. Gadolinium contrast should be used
D. Open (Hasson) technique is used in laparoscopic appendicectomy.

Answers

1. C	**2.** B	**3.** A	**4.** A	**5.** D	**6.** B	**7.** A	**8.** B	**9.** A	**10.** C
11. C	**12.** C	**13.** D	**14.** B	**15.** B	**16.** D	**17.** A	**18.** C		

CHAPTER

52

Hernia

- Anatomy of the inguinal region
- Inguinal defence mechanism
- Classification of hernia
- Aetiology of hernia
- Indirect hernia, direct hernia
- Clinical examination of a case of hernia
- Complications of hernia
- Recurrent hernia
- Special hernias
  - Giant hernia
  - Sliding hernia
  - Sportsman hernia
- Femoral hernia
- Umbilical hernia
- Incisional hernia
- Management of massive abdominal wall hernia
- Epigastric hernia
- Interparietal hernia
- Spigelian hernia
- Lumbar hernia
- Obturator hernia
- Perineal hernia
- Parastomal hernia

INTRODUCTION

- Hernia is not a disease but manifestation of a disease. Several factors may contribute for development of a hernia. (They have been discussed later.)
- Hernia is a common condition affecting patients, especially inguinal hernia in males and incisional hernia in females. Even though several types of surgery have been described for hernias, mesh hernioplasty remains the gold standard treatment. Majority of the hernias require surgical treatment leaving apart small asymptomatic direct hernias in the elderly. Today, laparoscopic hernia is becoming gold standard. Obstructed hernia is an emergency and late cases carry significant mortality. As far as students are concerned, hernia is the most common case in the examination. Hence, detailed clinical examination of hernia, complications, various types of hernias and their treatment have been described in this chapter.
- Hernia means to bud, protrude or rupture (Latin).

DEFINITION

Abnormal protrusion of a viscus or a part of it through a weak point in the body (opening) is known as a hernia. Inguinal hernia occurs either through the deep inguinal ring (indirect hernia) or through the posterior wall of the inguinal canal (direct hernia).

ANATOMY OF THE INGUINAL REGION (Fig. 52.1)

Competency

SU28.1.1,2,3,9,10: Describe applied anatomy of abdominal wall and its weaknesses in pathophysiology of abdominal hernias.

Inguinal Ligament (Poupart's Ligament) (1)

- It is the ligamentous portion of the external oblique aponeurosis which folds inwards and extends from anterior superior iliac spine to the pubic tubercle.
- The midpoint between these two structures is called midpoint of the inguinal ligament.

Lacunar Ligament (Gimbernat's Ligament)

- Some fibres of inguinal ligament pass posteriorly to attach to superior pubic ramus lateral to the tubercle and form lacunar ligament.

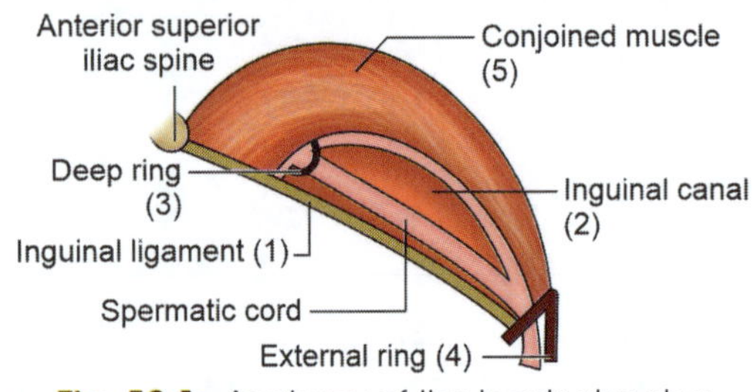

Fig. 52.1: Anatomy of the inguinal region

- The midpoint between the anterior superior iliac spine and pubic symphysis is called midinguinal point.

Inguinal Canal (2)

It is 4 cm in length extending from the deep inguinal ring to the superficial inguinal ring.

Deep Ring (Internal Ring) (3)

It is a U-shaped defect in the fascia transversalis which forms the posterior wall of the inguinal canal. It lies 1.25 cm above the midpoint of the inguinal ligament.

External Ring (Superficial Ring) (4)

Superficial ring is a triangular defect in external oblique aponeurosis. It is bounded by the lateral and medial crura formed by the external oblique aponeurosis and the base of the triangle is formed by the pubic crest.

Boundaries of Inguinal Canal

- **Anterior:** External oblique aponeurosis and a few fibres of the **conjoined muscle** (especially of internal oblique) laterally.
- **Superior:** Arched fibres of the **conjoined muscle** (5).
- **Inferior:** Inguinal ligament and the lacunar ligament on the medial side (Gimbernat's ligament).
- **Posterior:** Fascia transversalis and the conjoined tendon medially. Thus, the inguinal canal is strong in the lateral part anteriorly and the medial part posteriorly.

Contents of Inguinal Canal

1. Spermatic cord (Key Box 52.1)
2. Ilioinguinal nerve (Key Box 52.2)
3. Genital branch of genitofemoral nerve
4. Round ligament in females
5. Vestigial remnant of processus vaginalis sac

Myopectineal Orifice of Fruchaud[1] (Fig. 52.2)

- This weak area is the site of all groin hernias according to Fruchaud.

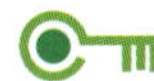
Key Box 52.1

Contents of the Spermatic Cord

- Vas deferens
- Testicular artery
- Artery to the vas
- Cremasteric artery
- Pampiniform plexus of veins
- Lymphatics
- Sympathetic nerves
- Genital branch of genitofemoral nerve
- Processus vaginalis

Key Box 52.2

Ilioinguinal Nerve

- The ilioinguinal nerve is a branch of the first lumbar nerve (L1). It separates from the first lumbar nerve along with the larger iliohypogastric nerve.
  It pierces the transversus abdominis and internal oblique muscles to enter the inguinal canal from the side
- Ilioinguinal nerve does not pass through the deep inguinal ring. It only travels through part of the inguinal canal.
- After going through inguinal canal, it pierces the internal oblique muscle, distributes nerve fibres to it, and then accompanies the spermatic cord through the superficial inguinal ring.
- Divides into anterior scrotal nerve/anterior labial nerve.
- Supplies the skin of the upper and medial part of the thigh, scrotum/vulva.
- Entrapment or injury to the ilioinguinal nerve is one of the causes of post-herniorrhaphy pain.
- Hence, a few recommend division of ilioinguinal nerve during hernia surgery.

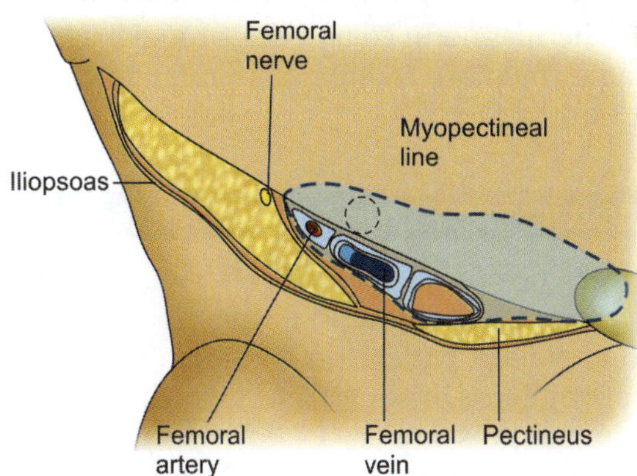

Fig. 52.2: Myopectineal line and anatomy

- It is the area between inguinal ligament anteriorly and iliopubic tract posteriorly.
- **Iliopubic tract:** It is the thickened inferior margin of the transversalis fascia which appears as a fibrous band running parallel and posterior (deep) to inguinal ligament. It inserts into superior pubic ramus to form lacunar ligament.
- **Boundaries of myopectineal orifice of Fruchaud:**
  Superiorly: Arched fibres of internal oblique
  Laterally: Iliopsoas muscle
  Medially: Lateral border of rectus abdominis muscle
  Inferiorly: Pubic pecten—Cooper's ligament—bony margin of the pelvis

[1]Henri R Fruchaud, 1956: The surgical treatment of inguinal or femoral hernia must not be closure of inguinal canal or femoral ring but deep reconstruction of abdominal wall in the whole groin region

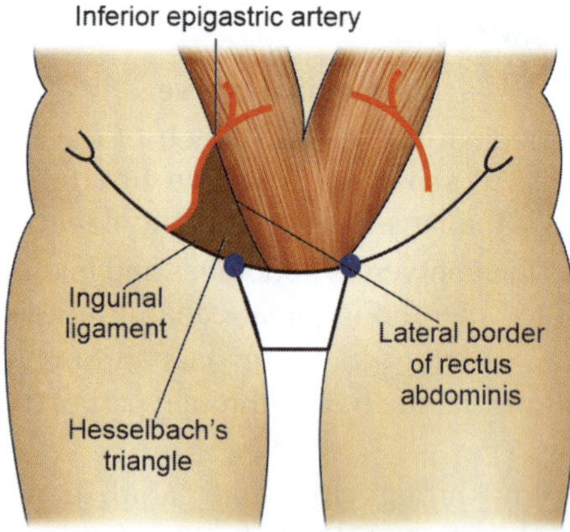

Fig. 52.3: Hesselbach's triangle

- **Surgical importance of iliopubic tract:** Recognition of this is a part of laparoscopic repair (initial step)—visualising from within. This structure reinforces posterior wall and floor of inguinal canal as it bridges structures traversing subinguinal space. Hesselbach's triangle (Fig. 52.3).
- It is bounded medially by lateral border of rectus abdominis muscle, laterally by inferior epigastric artery and inferiorly by inguinal ligament.
- Direct hernias occur commonly through Hesselbach's triangle (medial), indirect hernia lateral to inferior epigastric artery.

AETIOLOGY OF HERNIA: WHAT CAUSES HERNIA?

- Indirect hernia occurs largely due to persistent processus vaginalis sac. Manifestations of this can be seen in elderly patients in whom an indirect hernia can be triggered by some factors which increase intra-abdominal pressure.
- Direct hernia occurs mainly due to weakness of transversalis fascia in Hesselbach's area. However, increase in abdominal pressure due to chronic cough, constipation or difficulty in passing urine, development of ascites (portal hypertension, nephrotic syndrome), etc. can precipitate development of hernia.
- Collagen and hernia: Few studies involving studying fibres of transversalis fascia have proved that few cases of primary inguinal hernias and recurrent hernias occur due to intrinsic and inherent weakness in the tissue. Type I Collagen: It is characteristic for mature scars or fascial tissues. Type III Collagen: It is mechanically instable, less cross-linked collagen synthesized during the early days of wound healing. For adequate strength and function of transversalis fascia, presence of collagen in adequate amount is important. The decreased tensile strength of collagen type III plays a key role in the development of incisional hernias.
- Collagen disorder: In prune-belly syndrome, collagen fibre disorder causes development of not only hernias but also interstitial hernias, bilateral hernias, etc. Hernia occurs due to inherited imbalance in the types of collagens.

RISK FACTORS

It can be classified as patient related and external factors.

I. Patient related: A patent processus vaganalis sac. Chance of developing a hernia in males about 20–25%.

- Some other factors responsible are failed obliteration of the processus vaginalis (PV) sac, persistent smooth cells and insufficient calcitonin gene-related peptide from spinal nucleus of genitofemoral nerve. Smooth cells help in propelling testis into scrotum.
- Hernias are more common on right side in children because right PV sac is obliterated later than left PV sac.

II. External factors:

- Smoking causes increased collagen degradation and decreased synthesis. This is due to the effect of nicotine, which weakens the abdominal wall.
- Increased abdominal pressure caused by coughing, jumping, lifting of the load have been mentioned.
- Constipation has a doubtful relationship.

Summary of various factors for development of hernis has been summarized in Key Box 52.3.

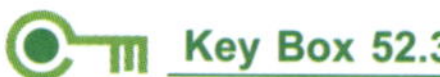 **Key Box 52.3**

Aetiology/Causes of Hernia

1. **Congenital:**
   Persistent processus vaginalis sac: Chief cause of indirect hernia.
2. **Collagen fibre disorder**
   - Prune-belly disorder—congenital
   - Smoking: Acquired collagen deficiency
3. Corpulence obesity
4. Chronic causes of increased intra-abdominal pressure
   - Chronic cough, chronic constipation, straining at micturition, ascites
5. Conjoined tendon weakness/rupture of a few fibres following:
   - Lifting heavy weight
   - Postappendicectomy—injury to ilioinguinal nerve.
   - Chronic illness/debilitating disease causing weakness of transversalis fascia in the Hesselbach's area.

INGUINAL DEFENCE MECHANISMS

1. Obliquity of inguinal canal (in children, it is straight).
2. During straining or coughing, the conjoined tendon contracts, and since it forms the anterior, superior and posterior boundaries, it closes the inguinal canal—**shutter or sphincter-like effect**.
3. Increased intra-abdominal pressure produces plugging effect at the external ring. The deep ring is pulled upwards and laterally because it is adherent to the posterior surface of **transversalis muscle**. This occludes the ring and prevents herniation—**Ball valve** effect.

CLASSIFICATION OF HERNIA

I. Anatomical classification: (1) Indirect hernia, (2) direct hernia.

II. Nyhus classification: This classification is based **primarily on the defect**, which helps in planning an appropriate repair.

Type 1: Indirect hernia with normal deep ring—normal posterior wall

Type 2: Indirect hernia with dilated deep ring—normal posterior wall

Type 3: Based on posterior wall defect: (a) Direct hernia, (b) pantaloon, sliding—enlarged deep ring, (c) femoral

Type 4: Recurrent hernia—direct, indirect femoral, combined.

III. The European Hernia Society classification

- Primary (P), Recurrent (R)
- Lateral (L), Medial (M), Femoral (F)
- Defect size assumed to be 1.5 cm

  Thus, primary direct hernia with 3 cm defect size is written as PM2.

IV. Gilbert's classification (Table 52.1)

- It is based on the defect in the posterior wall (direct hernia) or defect in the internal ring (indirect).
- Depending upon the defect, the suggested repair is given below. However, basic principles are the same.
- The last two types—type VI and type VII are modifications by Robbin.

Algorithm showing classification of inguinal hernia

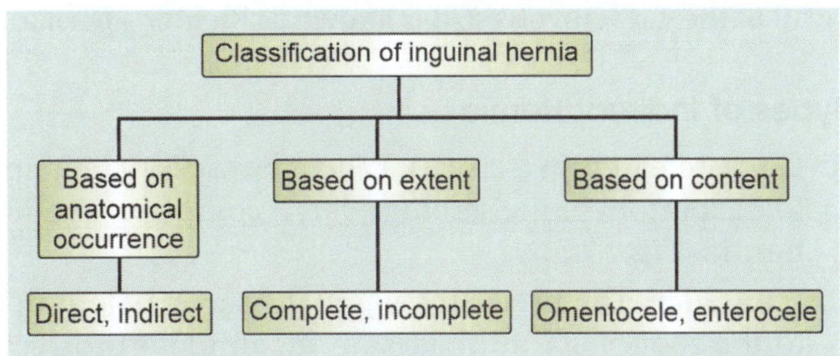

INDIRECT HERNIA

It is a herniation of abdominal contents through the deep ring into the inguinal canal. **Indirect hernia occurs due to persistent processus vaginalis sac.** It is the most common type of hernia in the body. The preformed sac passes through the deep ring, traverses the inguinal canal and may extend into the scrotum through the external ring. As it comes into the inguinal canal, it is invested by the following coverings:

1. External spermatic fascia derived from external oblique aponeurosis.
2. Cremasteric fascia derived from internal oblique.
3. Internal spermatic fascia from fascia transversalis.

Table 52.1 Gilbert's classification and suggested repair

Types	Classification	Repair
I.	Snug internal ring Preperitoneal indirect sac Does not admit one finger	Herniorrhaphy or hernioplasty
II.	Moderately enlarged internal ring Bubonocoele Admits one finger	Herniorrhaphy or hernioplasty
III.	Large defect—2 or 3 finger-breadths internal ring. May be sliding hernia	Preperitoneal mesh by slitting transversalis fascia
IV.	Large direct hernia with full blow out defect Internal ring is normal	Mesh repair
V.	Direct hernia with punched out hole/defect in the transversalis fascia The internal ring is intact	Plug the defect or purse-string closure of the defect followed by mesh repair
VI.	Pantaloon hernia	Mesh repair
VII.	Femoral hernia	Femoral hernia repair

Parts of the Hernia (Fig. 52.4)

Hernial sac is part of the peritoneum which is dragged into the inguinal canal. The mouth of the sac is in the peritoneal cavity. The neck is the narrowest portion (deep ring). The actual hernial sac has a body and a fundus. Depending upon the contents, it can be named as follows: Omentum—omentocoele, intestine— enterocoele.

Littre's hernia—hernia containing Meckel's diverticulum. It may also contain ovary or appendix. **When part of the wall of the gut is involved, it is known as Richter's hernia.**

Types of Indirect Hernia

1. **Complete hernia** (scrotal): When the sac is patent up to the bottom of the scrotum, it is a **complete scrotal hernia** (Fig. 52.5).
2. **Funicular:** The processus vaginalis sac is patent up to the root of scrotum, it is an **incomplete indirect hernia** (Figs 52.6 and 52.8).
3. **Bubonocoele:** Processus vaginalis sac is confined to the inguinal region or the inguinal canal only. Such hernias are seen in young patients (Fig. 52.7).

Coverings of the Indirect Inguinal Hernia from Outside to Inside

1. Skin
2. Two layers of superficial fascia: Fatty and membranous (Camper's and Scarpa's fascia respectively).

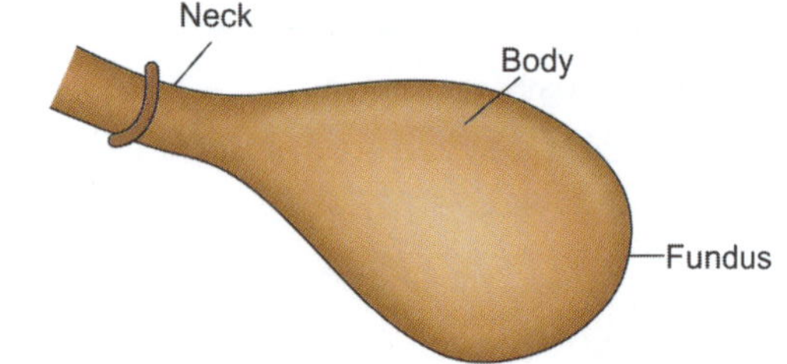

Fig. 52.4: Parts of the hernial sac

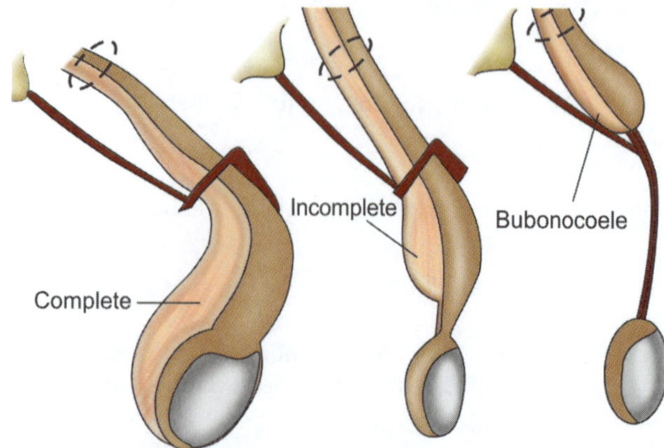

Figs 52.5 to 52.7: Three types of indirect hernia

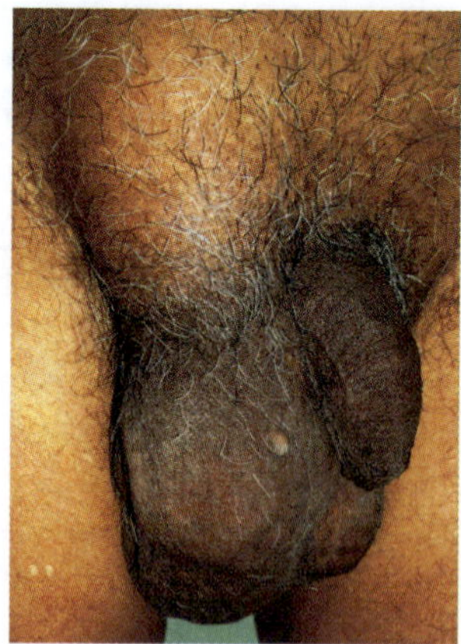

Fig. 52.8: Incomplete hernia bulge is seen

3. External spermatic fascia, a continuation of the external oblique aponeurosis.
4. Cremaster muscle and fascia, a continuation of the internal oblique.
5. Internal spermatic fascia: Derived from the fascia transversalis.
6. Extraperitoneal fat
7. Peritoneum

DIRECT HERNIA

It is always acquired (Fig. 52.9). It occurs through ***Hesselbach's triangle,*** a weakness in the ***posterior wall*** of the inguinal canal (transversalis fascia). Chronic cough and benign prostatic hypertrophy (BPH) are the common risk factors. Other risk factors mentioned earlier such as smoking also apply here.

Boundaries of ***Hesselbach's triangle***

- Medially: Lateral border of the rectus abdominis
- Laterally: Inferior epigastric artery
- Below: Inguinal ligament

Coverings of the Direct Inguinal Hernia from Outside to Inside

1. Skin
2. Two layers of superficial fascia
3. External oblique aponeurosis
4. Conjoined tendon
5. Fascia transversalis
6. Peritoneum

Pearls of Wisdom

As the direct hernia pushes through the posterior wall, it is very unusual for it to descend into the scrotum. It can descend into the scrotum if few fibres of transversalis fascia are missing (congenital).

Ogilvie Hernia

This is a type of direct hernia wherein the hernial sac appears through a circular defect (congenital) in the conjoined tendon.

CLINICAL EXAMINATION OF A CASE OF HERNIA

Competency

SU28.1.4: Describe clinical presentation, examination findings, and role of radiological investigations in diagnosis and management of hernia.

History

- Swelling in the inguinal region which is gradually increasing in size. To start with, the swelling disappears on lying down and increases on straining, walking, etc. Later it cannot be reduced (due to adhesions).
- History of dragging pain indicates omentocoele.
- Since the omentum is attached to the stomach above and supplied by T10, the pain is referred to the umbilical region.
- Sudden, severe pain in the hernia, vomiting and irreducibility indicates 'obstructed hernia'.
- History of chronic cough, constipation, difficulty in passing urine should be asked. If present, it may suggest the cause of hernia.
- **History of appendicectomy:** Division of ilioinguinal nerve during appendicectomy may cause denervation of fibres of the right transversus abdominis, which forms U-shaped ring, resulting in weakness of the abdominal wall.

Clinical Examination: In the standing position

Inspection (a Model Case of Incomplete Hernia) (Figs 52.9 to 52.11)

Direct hernia pops out as soon as patient stands (Fig. 52.9).

- There is a swelling in the inguinal region extending to the root of the scrotum measuring about 6 × 3 cm.

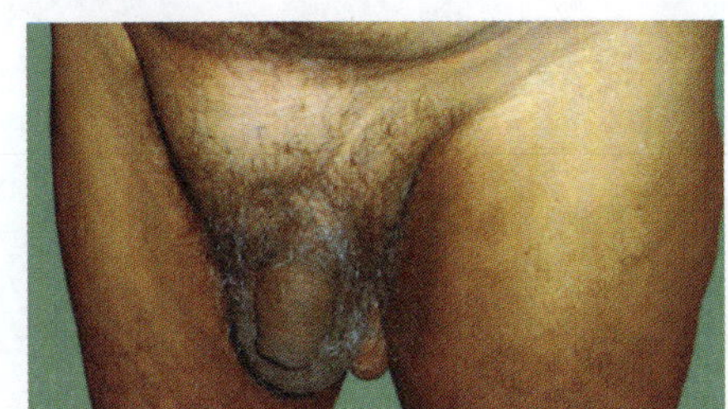

Fig. 52.9: Direct hernia pops out when patient stands

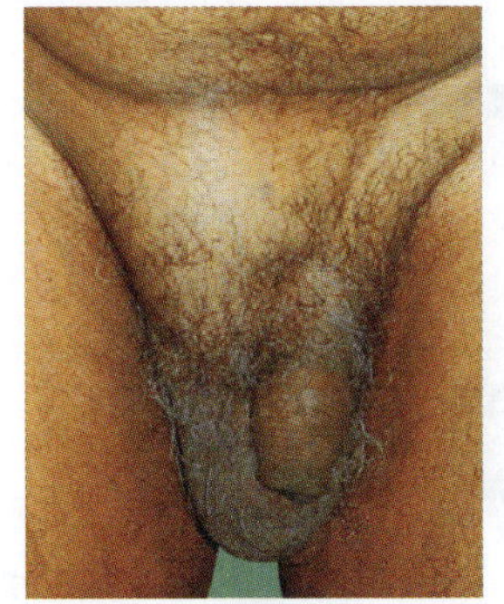

Fig. 52.10: Incomplete indirect hernia

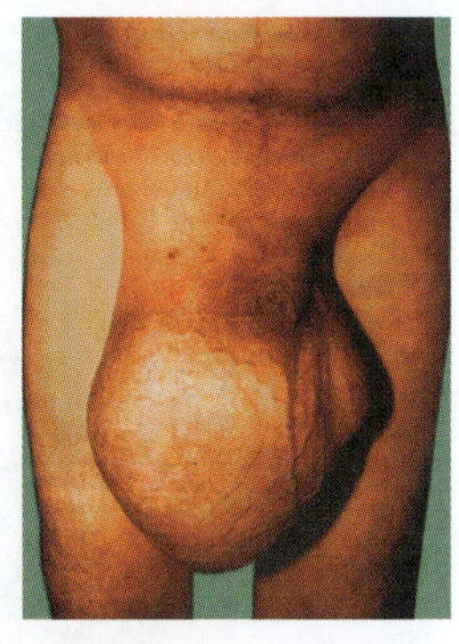

Fig. 52.11: Complete indirect hernia—scrotal hernia

Key Box 52.4

Expansile Impulse on Cough

- Hernia
- Meningocoele
- Dermoid cyst with intracranial communication
- Laryngocoele
- Lymphatic cyst in children
- Empyema necessitans

Its surface is smooth, borders are round, skin over the swelling is normal and it is pyriform in shape.

- Ask the patient to cough—**expansile impulse on cough is present**. If peristalsis is present, it indicates an enterocoele. Expansile impulse on cough is diagnostic of hernia (Key Box 52.4).
- Presence of scar indicates a recurrent hernia. Ragged scar indicates infection.
- Direct hernia pops out as soon as the patient stands and often it is bilateral.

Palpation

- Inspectory findings should be confirmed. Swelling is soft, and gurgles, if it is an enterocoele.
- It may be firm or granular, if it is an omentocoele.

1. **Ask the patient to cough**—expansile impulse is felt at the root of scrotum.
2. **Getting above the swelling**[1] should be done in the standing position (Fig. 52.12).
   - At the root of scrotum, the spermatic cord is palpated between the finger and the thumb. In cases of complete indirect hernia, spermatic cord cannot be felt as a naked structure because it is covered anterolaterally by the sac. This is called as **getting above the swelling not possible** (negative).

[1]This test has no meaning or usefulness in bubonocoele. It is a test to differentiate scrotal swelling from inguinoscrotal swelling and assumes significance in complete hernias.

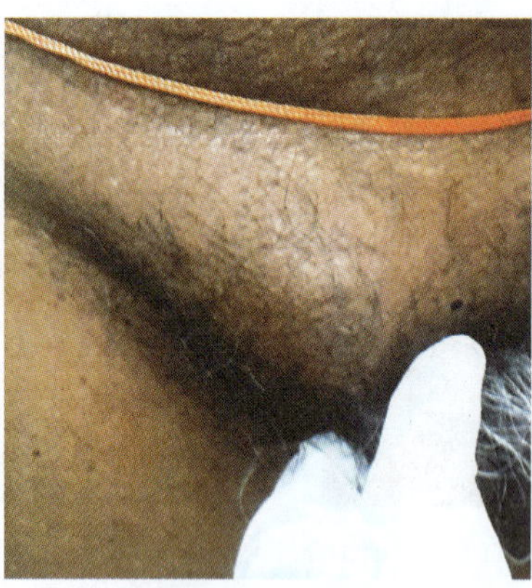

Fig. 52.12: The swelling is palpated at the root of the scrotum. Getting above the swelling is not possible. A case of incomplete hernia

Pearls of Wisdom

Getting above the swelling is a test to differentiate scrotal swellings from inguinoscrotal swellings.

3. **Reducibility**—ask the patient to lie down.
   - If the swelling becomes smaller or disappears, it is a hernia (hydrocoele is not reducible).
   - **Omentocoele:** Initially, reduction is easy but later, becomes difficult (due to adhesions). If it is difficult to reduce, ask the patient to reduce it. Otherwise, flex and medially rotate the hip and try to reduce it, a method called ***taxis***.
   - If in spite of this, the swelling is not reduced, it is called an irreducible hernia.
4. **Internal ring occlusion test** (deep ring occlusion test): Reduce the swelling first (Fig. 52.13).

   Locate the deep ring above the midpoint between anterior superior iliac spine and symphysis pubis. Occlude the deep ring with the thumb and ask the patient to cough.

   a. If impulse and the swelling are seen, it is a direct hernia because it occurs in the Hesselbach's triangle (medial to deep ring).

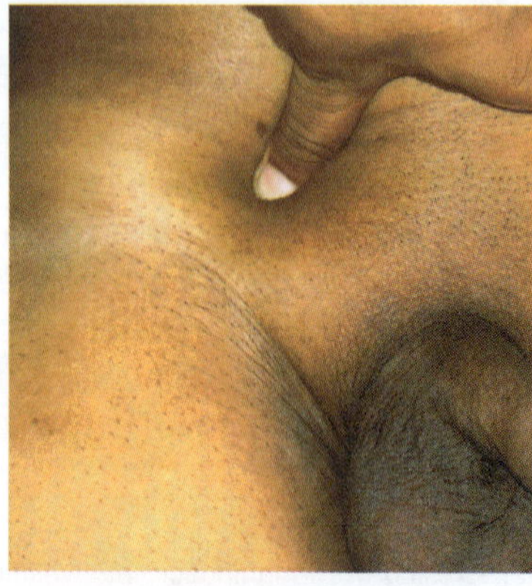

Fig. 52.13: Deep ring occlusion test

   b. If the swelling is not seen, it is an indirect hernia. Deep ring occlusion test can be done with the patient in standing and supine position.

   Problems of deep ring occlusion test:

   a. If occlusion is not done properly, results may vary.
   b. Pantaloon hernia (Romberg hernia, saddlebag hernia, dual hernia). It is a direct hernia having indirect component.
5. **Zieman's method** (Figs 52.14A and B): Three-finger method.

   Keep index finger at deep ring, middle finger on the posterior wall above and lateral to the external ring and ring finger at femoral ring. Now ask the patient to cough. Depending upon the type of hernia, impulse is felt. It is not necessary to perform this test in incomplete or complete indirect hernias.
6. **Leg raising test** or head raising test (Fig. 52.15):
   - Weakness of oblique muscles is manifested by Malgaigne's bulgings above the medial half of inguinal ligament. ***It is an absolute indication for hernioplasty.***
   - **Malgaigne's bulgings indicate weakness of the oblique muscles of the abdominal wall.**

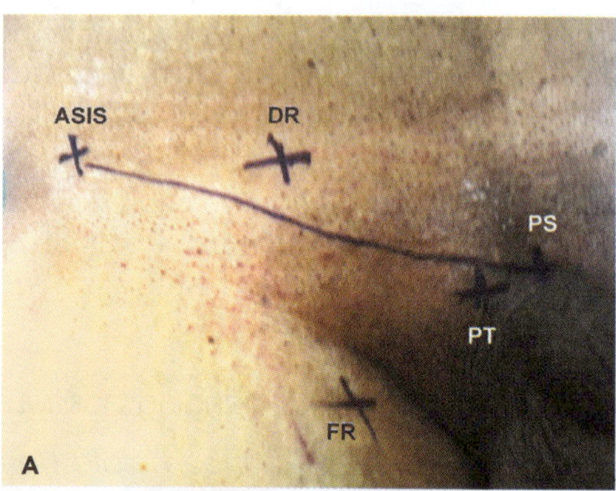

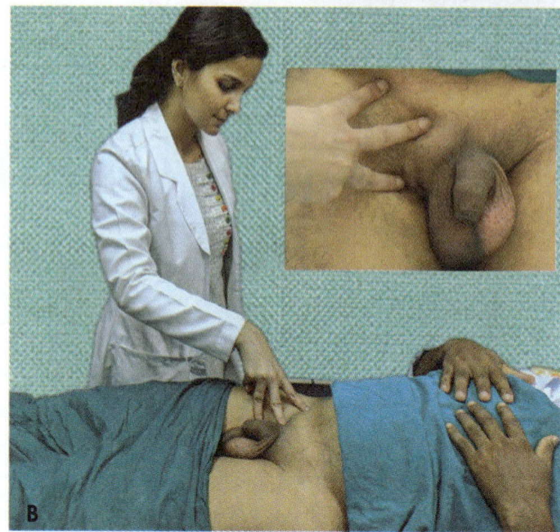

Figs 52.14A and B: Zieman's method: Anterior superior iliac spine (ASIS), deep ring (DR), pubic symphysis (PS), pubic tubercle (PT) and femoral ring (FR) have been marked for doing Zieman's test

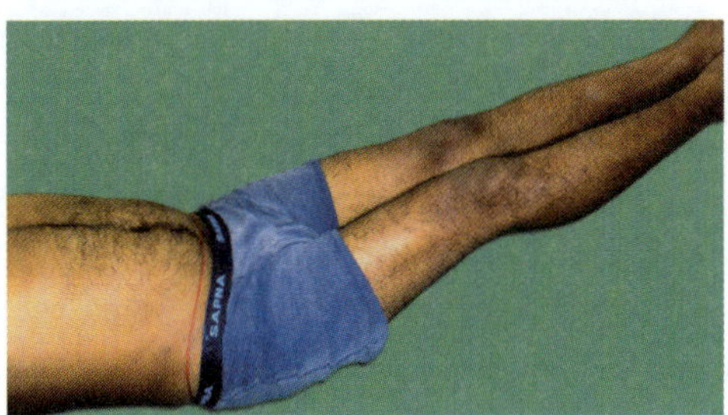

Fig. 52.15: Leg raising test

7. **Per abdomen:** To rule out any mass (colonic).
8. **Look for phimosis/stricture urethra:** Young patients having urinary complaints with hernia may be suffering from stricture urethra. Lift the scrotum and feel for any strictures in the bulbar urethra. Retract skin of prepuce and rule out phimosis.
9. **Per rectal examination** should be done in elderly patients to rule out prostatic enlargement.
10. **Examination of respiratory system** is done to rule out chronic bronchitis, tuberculosis, etc.

Pearls of Wisdom

Examine the opposite side and all hernial sites such as femoral, umbilical and incisional hernia sites.

Clinical Examination of a Hernia in a Child

- Swelling may not be visible at first as it may be covered by thick pad of fat. Examine when a child strains (cry), or after child's play (jumping, etc.). Examine the root of scrotum—may find hernial sac (thickening).
- **Gornall's test:** By gentle compression on child's abdomen (hold the child on its back), hernia may become apparent.
- Invagination test is almost impossible. Hence, it is better not to do it.

Diagnosis *(One Example)*

Right side, indirect, incomplete, uncomplicated, reducible omentocoele. Refer to Table 52.2 for differences between direct and indirect hernia and Table 52.3 for differences between hernia and hydrocoele.

DIFFERENTIAL DIAGNOSIS OF A GROIN SWELLING

Competency

SU28.1.11: Describe differential diagnosis of inguinal and inguinoscrotal swellings.

Groin refers to the junction of lower abdomen with the thigh. Hence, swellings in the inguinal region and upper thigh (femoral region) close to the inguinal ligament are included under groin swellings.

1. **Inguinal hernia** (Fig. 52.16).
2. **Femoral hernia:** The main sac is below and lateral to pubic tubercle (Fig. 52.17).

Table 52.2 Differences between direct and indirect hernia

	Direct hernia	Indirect hernia
1. Age	Common in elderly	Can occur in any age group
2. Aetiology	Weakness of posterior wall of inguinal canal	Preformed sac
3. Precipitating factors	Chronic bronchitis, enlarged prostate	—
4. On standing	Pops out	Does not pop out
5. Side	Usually bilateral	Unilateral (30% bilateral)
6. Internal ring occlusion test	Swelling is seen	Swelling is not seen
7. Malgaigne's bulgings	May be present	Absent
8. Complications	Not common because neck is wide	Common, neck is narrow—obstruction and strangulation
9. Relationship of sac to the cord	Sac is posterior to the cord	Sac is anterolateral to the cord
10. Direction of the sac	It comes out of Hesselbach's triangle	Sac comes through the deep ring

Table 52.3 Clinical differences between hernia and hydrocoele

	Indirect complete hernia	Vaginal hydrocoele
1. Standing position	Swelling of scrotum and inguinal region	Swelling confined only to scrotum
2. Impulse on coughing	Present	Absent
3. Getting above swelling	Not possible	Possible
4. Reducibility	Usually present unless complicated	Not reducible
5. Consistency and transillumination	Soft, gurgling, no transillumination	Soft, fluctuant, transillumination is present

3. **Vaginal hydrocoele:** Fluctuation and transillumination tests are usually positive and getting above swelling is possible. (Please note that in infantile hydrocoele and hydrocoele *en bisac*, getting above swelling is not possible) (Fig. 52.18).
4. **Retractile testis:** It can present as a firm swelling in the inguinal region. Scrotum is empty (Fig. 52.19).
5. **Saphena varix:** The patient can present with a swelling in the thigh. Swelling is usually about 2.5 cm below the pubic tubercle. **A swelling that disappears on elevation of the leg is characteristic of a swelling of venous origin** (Fig. 52.20).
6. **Funiculitis:** A funiculitis can occur with or without acute epididymoorchitis. Severe pain in the inguinal region, tender swelling, high grade fever with chills and rigors are characteristic. Spermatic cord is thickened and swelling is not reducible (Fig. 52.21).
7. **Inguinal lymphadenitis:** Pain and nodular swelling below inguinal ligament is a feature. It is not reducible and some source of infection in the lower limb is usually present (Fig. 52.22).
8. **Lipoma of the cord:** It presents as a soft, lobulated but irreducible swelling in the inguinal region (Figs 52.23A and B).

Investigations

Hernia is a clinical diagnosis. Except for small direct hernia in very elderly patients above 80 years, almost all inguinal hernias should be treated. In the vast majority of the cases, no investigations are required specific to the diagnosis of hernia. However, in appropriate cases imaging can be done.

- First advice in a smoker with hernia is to stop smoking at least 3 to 6 weeks before surgery. If a patient is high-risk patient, he should stop smoking at least 6 months before surgery.

1. **Ultrasound:** In apparently occult cases wherein patient has groin pain but clinically not evident, ultrasound can detect a sac—however it is operator dependent. In large hernias including sliding hernias, ultrasound can identify structures such as urinary bladder or colon, thus giving useful information to the surgeon. Ultrasound is also useful in cases of postoperative swelling in the groin to rule out haematoma/seroma/recurrence.

Pearls of Wisdom

Hernia is a clinical diagnosis. If you are asked to give one investigation to confirm hernia (may be in early cases), it is ultrasound.

2. **Computed tomography (CT)** scan is ideal in cases of giant hernias, sliding hernias or special types such as obturator hernia, perineal hernia, etc.
3. **Routine investigations** such as complete blood picture (CBP) and urine examination are done. In elderly patients, chest X-ray, electrocardiography or even pulmonary function tests may be necessary. Patients with urinary complaints are evaluated for prostatic enlargement and stricture urethra.

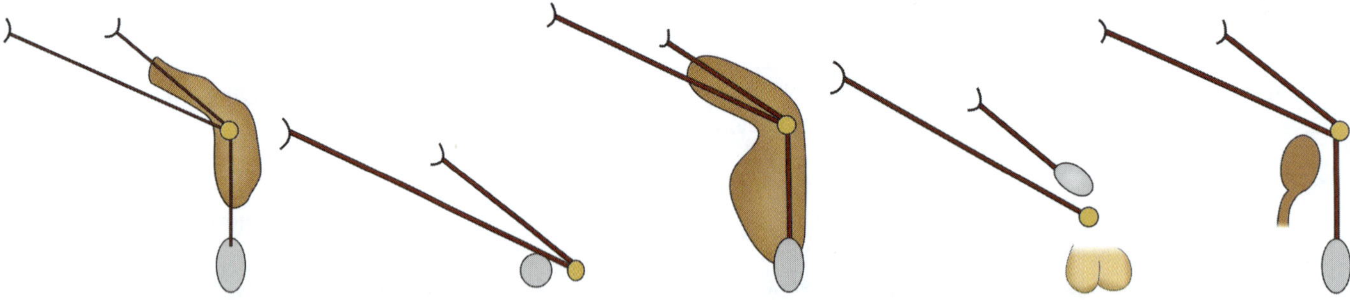

Fig. 52.16: Inguinal hernia **Fig. 52.17:** Femoral hernia **Fig. 52.18:** Infantile hydrocoele **Fig. 52.19:** Retractile testis **Fig. 52.20:** Saphena varix

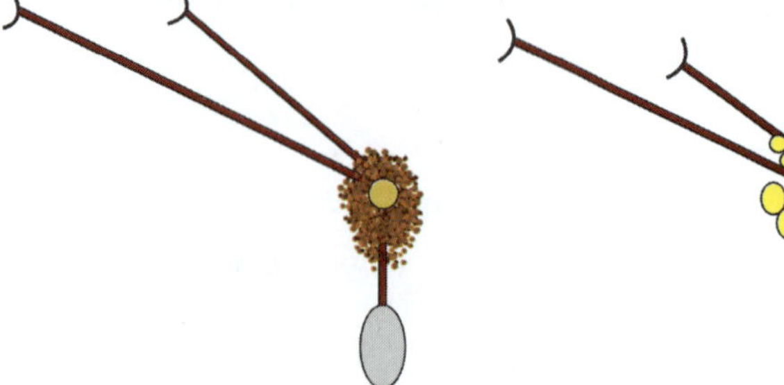

Fig. 52.21: Funiculitis **Fig. 52.22:** Inguinal lymphadenitis

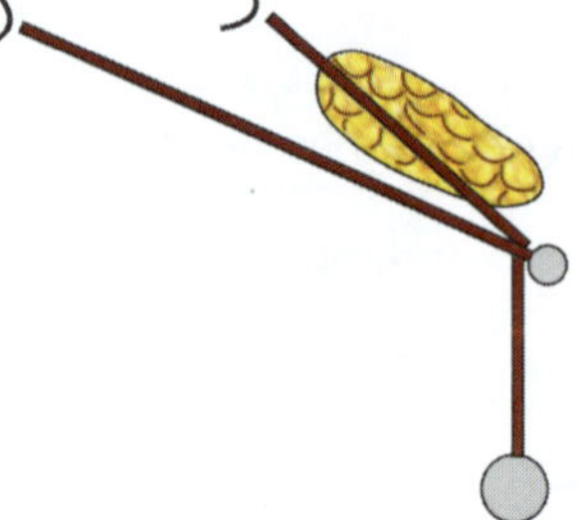

Fig. 52.23A: Lipoma of the cord

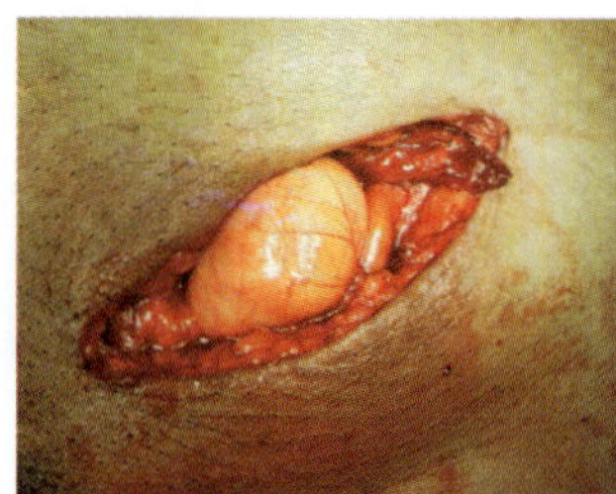

Fig. 52.23B: Left inguinal lipoma of the cord

4. **Magnetic resonance imaging (MRI):** Ideal in sportsmen who complain of groin pain, to differentiate between hernia, to rule out muscle sprain or any other orthopaedic disorders. Refer to Gilmore groin–page 949.

Preoperative Preparation

- A patient with chronic bronchitis and bronchial asthma should be properly treated with bronchodilators, antibiotics, mucolytic agents, etc. Cigarette smoking should be stopped at least 3 weeks before the surgery.
- Elderly patients with bilateral hernia mostly suffer from benign prostatic hypertrophy. **Prostatectomy should be considered first followed** by repair of hernia, in such cases. Recent history of constipation and appearance of a hernia should arouse the suspicion of carcinoma colon. Investigate by colonoscopy/fibre-optic sigmoidoscopy before the treatment of hernia.
- Often patients are smokers with chronic obstructed pulmonary diseases.
- Young adults with difficulty in passing urine may have a stricture urethra. They should undergo proper treatment for the stricture. Now it is rare to find a patient with hernia having a stricture urethra.

Treatment (Flowchart 52.1)

Competency

SU28.1.6: Describe general principles of management of abdominal wall hernias and the basic operative approach.

1. **Herniotomy:** Excision of hernial sac. No repair is required. It is done only in children.
2. **Hernioplasty:** Strengthening of posterior wall—mostly by prolene mesh is the most popular surgery called **Lichtenstein repair**. Details of hernioplasty are given below. It can be done by open or laparoscopic method. Details are also available in the operative surgery chapter.
3. **Herniorrhaphy:** Approximation of conjoined tendon to inguinal ligament by using nonabsorbable sutures is called Bassini's herniorrhaphy. It is not done nowadays because of high chances of recurrence. Hence it is not discussed here.

Pearls of Wisdom

Herniotomy, herniorrhaphy and hernioplasty are the three "key" operations for inguinal hernia. Mesh hernioplasty is the gold standard for inguinal hernias.

Flowchart 52.1: Algorithm showing type of hernia surgeries

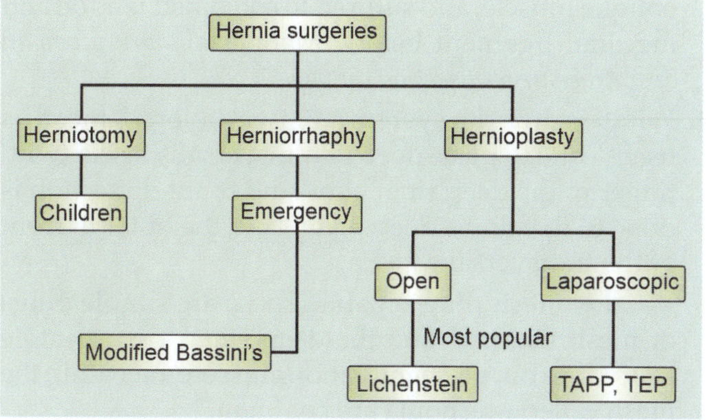

HERNIOPLASTY

There are two types of hernioplasties.

A. **Lichtenstein repair:** The posterior wall **(Lichtenstein repair)** (Fig. 52.24, Key Boxes 52.5 and 52.6) of inguinal canal is strengthened by a prolene mesh or Marlex mesh. The fibroblasts and capillaries grow over the mesh, converting it into a thick fibrous sheath and strengthening the posterior wall. The mesh is fixed inferiorly to lacunar and inguinal ligaments, medially to overlap rectus sheath and fixed to fascia over the pubic bone. A few interrupted sutures are put to fix it to the transversalis fascia. **Laterally, an artificial deep ring is created by crossing of both upper and lower leaves of the mesh.** To attain this, a slit is given on one side of mesh. (Lacunar ligament is that portion of the inguinal ligament which extends backwards and upwards to the pectineal line and forms the medial margin of the femoral ring).

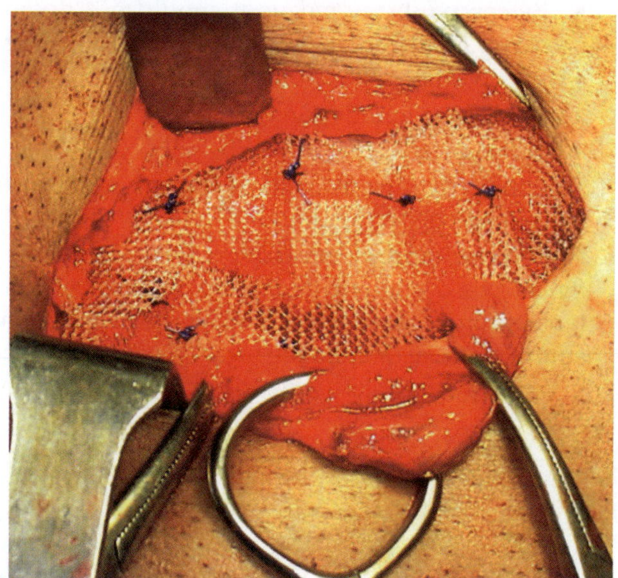

Fig. 52.24: Lichtenstein repair is the most popular type of open hernia repair

Key Box 52.5

Lichtenstein Repair*

- Polypropylene mesh is used (Fig. 52.24).
- 8 × 16 cm mesh is tailored to patient's requirement.
- **Preparation of mesh:** Corners can be cut so as to give a round shape. A slit is given on the lateral border of the mesh at the junction of lower one-third and upper two-thirds, to allow spermatic cord to pass through. The two tails (slit-ends) are overlapped.
- **Suturing:** Medially, the mesh overlaps the pubic tubercle and is sutured over the tissue of symphysis (avoid pubic bone to prevent osteitis pubis). Laterally, the two tails are placed beyond deep ring and sutured. Inferiorly, it is sutured to inguinal and lacunar ligaments and superiorly to conjoined tendon.

****Dr Irving Lichtenstein—Linchtenstein repair: The tension-free repair 1989. Los-Angles***

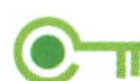

Key Box 52.6

Advantages of Polypropylene Mesh

- High tensile strength
- Biocompatible, nonabsorbable
- Monofilament strong, elastic and transparent mesh
- Ideal porosity for high visibility and colonisation
- Strong mechanical reinforcement
- Encourages rapid ingrowth of connective tissue
- Cheaper
- Flexible for any anatomic placement

Advantages of Light Weight and Large Pores Mesh

- Less shrinkage of mesh, more flexible, better tissue integration, better comfort.

Characteristics of the ideal mesh

- Biocompatibility means it should not do any harm, should be chemically and physically inert.
- Risk of infection should not be there.
- Handling should be good.
- Economical
- Longevity (also refer to biological mesh given in next page).

B. **Prolene (polypropylene) nylon darning:** Suturing the conjoined tendon to the inguinal ligament without tension in a criss-cross manner by using prolene suture material (handmade mesh). This is preferred in direct and indirect hernias described by Maloney.

Biological Mesh

These are sterilised sheets of connective tissue derived from human or animal dermis or porcine intestinal submucosa:

- They are decellularised
- Like the mesh, they provide scaffold for connective tissue to grow and collagen deposition.
- Enzymatic reaction takes place in the host followed by fibrous tissue formation.
- Advantages: Chronic inflammation and foreign body reaction, stiffness and fibrosis, and mesh infection are uncommon—usually do not occur.
- They can be used in presence of infection.
- They are very expensive.

Other Surgeries for Inguinal Hernia

1. **Shouldice repair**
   - It is the most popular tensionless method wherein only local tissues are used.
   - After opening the inguinal canal, herniotomy is done.
   - Transversalis fascia, which forms the posterior wall, is incised from the internal ring till pubic tubercles.
   - Then, upper and lower flaps of transversalis fascia are sutured in a double-breasting manner by using nonabsorbable sutures such as 34 gauge stainless steel wire, polyamide or polypropylene. This is the **first layer** of Shouldice repair.
   - The **second layer** is like Bassini's, wherein conjoined tendon is sutured to the inguinal ligament by using nonabsorbable sutures.
   - The **third layer** is completed by suturing upper flap of external oblique aponeurosis to the inguinal ligament.
   - The results have been good in Shouldice's hands. The operation needs **expertise**.
2. **Nyhus repair:** Ideally indicated in bilateral direct hernia or recurrent hernia, wherein a broad mesh is kept in the preperitoneal space. It requires a single large incision covering both groins. However, same surgery now can be done by laparoscopically by keeping a mesh in the extraperitoneal space.
3. **Dasarda technique:** In this operation, a strip of external oblique aponeurosis is prepared isolated but still connected medially and laterally to the external oblique muscle, and sutured to conjoined tendon and inguinal ligament below. *More details are given in operative surgery section on page 1291.*
4. **What is hernia system?** A two-layered mesh is used—one to place deep to transversalis fascia (with finger in the deep ring, blind and blunt dissection is done to develop a deep plane) and the other in front of the transversalis fascia.
5. **What is mesh plug repairs?** These are simple plugs of mesh inserted into the deep ring. It is a simple procedure but mesh migration and seroma within the mesh called Meshoma are common.

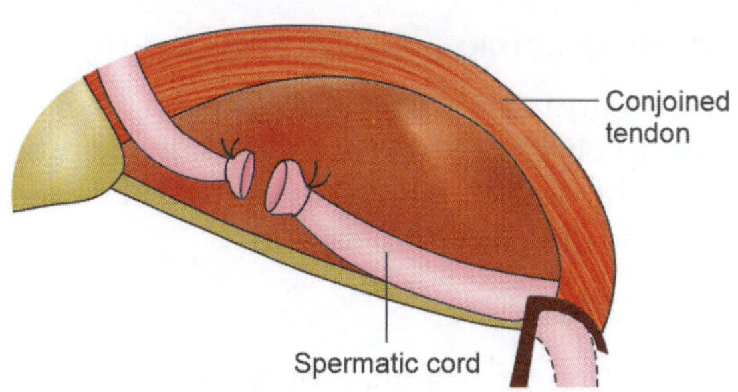

Fig. 52.25: Kuntz operation

Rare/uncommon surgeries

1. **Kuntz operation** (Fig. 52.25): In this operation, the spermatic cord is divided at the deep ring and it is removed along with the testis, so that the deep ring can be permanently closed, and hernia never recurs. It is indicated in elderly patients with recurrent hernia and poor abdominal muscle tone. Hamilton Bailey's operation—cord is divided but testis is retained.
2. **Stoppa repair:**[1] **The Stoppa repair is a tension-free type** of hernia repair. It is performed by wrapping the lower part of the parietal peritoneum with prosthetic mesh and placing it at a preperitoneal level over Fruchaud's myopectineal orifice. This operation is also known as giant prosthetic reinforcement of the visceral sac (GPRVS).

Pearls of Wisdom

"Hernia is a complex disease with many complications and surgeries and every effort should be made to understand and treat it in as simple effective way as possible".

—Prof Amit Jain

COMPLICATIONS OF HERNIA SURGERY

These are common complications after surgery. Often they are mild and not so worrisome. However, some of the complications can be serious which require immediate attention and treatment.

1. **Complications during surgery**
   - **Injury to the iliac vessels:** The most serious but rare complication is injury to iliac vessels. It can happen in thin patients when suturing of the inguinal ligament is done from lateral to medial side. The sudden jet of fresh red blood indicates that the bite has been taken through the artery. It is better to call the vascular surgeon, extend the incision, have a proximal control, suture directly or do a resection and end to end anastomosis. They have to be anticoagulated with low molecular weight heparin followed by oral anticoagulants.
   - **Injury to the urinary bladder:** This can happen when anatomy is not clear as in few giant or scrotal hernias, perineal hernias or distortion due to previous surgery. Sudden finding of clear fluid with urinary smell means bladder injury. Immediate repair with 2–0 vicryl followed by urinary catheter placement for 3 weeks is the treatment.
2. **Early postoperative period**
   - **Pain:** Pain is common due to the incision in the skin and some degrees of retraction of structures such as inguinal ligament downwards and conjoint tendon upwards. The pain can be decreased by local anaesthetic infiltration, e.g. bupivacaine 0.25%—20 ml.
   - **Bleeding:** Perfect haemostasis is the aim of all surgeries. In spite of this, a few bleeders may open up, mostly venous blood—may be pampiniform plexus veins or arterial blood from inferior epigastric artery. The bleeding may stop with compression bandage. Otherwise, exploration and ligation of bleeders needs to be done in the operation theatre.
   - **Urinary retention is common, more so in males:** Pain, spinal or epidural anaesthesia, sedatives, lack of privacy are contributing factors. Provide analgesia, privacy and hot fomentation to suprapubic region. If all of these fail, catheterise bladder as a last step.
   - **Abdominal distension:** This is not common. It can happen when large intestinal contents of the hernia sac are reduced or handled as in scrotal hernias or sliding hernias. It is also important to realise that omentum is attached to stomach and colon above. One should see that bleeders from injured arteries of the omentum are ligated properly. Some intraperitoneal blood may add to paralytic ileus.
3. **Intermediate—between 3 and 7 days**
   - **Seroma** is due to inflammatory response to mesh or suture materials. It causes swelling and anxiety that it may be a recurrence. When in doubt, get an ultrasound examination first. Seroma needs to be aspirated. Seroma is more common after laparoscopic hernia repairs.
   - **Surgical site infection:** Hernia is a clean surgery. Infection should not occur. However, poor handling of the tissues, haematoma, seroma and diabetes may precipitate wound infection. Patients with skin disease or co-morbid factors are given injection cefazolin 1–2 g intravenously 30 minutes before the incision or clindamycin, if patient is allergic to cefazolin. If infection is suspected, open the sutures, drain the pus and use appropriate antibiotics. Persistent wound infection may prompt removal of the mesh. A few cases of tuberculosis have been reported. This is due to improper sterilisation of the mesh used.

[1]It was first described in 1975 by Rene Stoppa.

4. **Late:** Late complications are not all that common. One complication which bothers a few patients is chronic pain called inguinodynia. It is seen in about 10% of post-hernioplasty pain. It is defined as persisting pain more than 3 months after surgery.

- **Inguinodynia:** The chief factor is injury to the following nerves: Iliohypogastric, ilioinguinal and genital branch of genitofemoral nerve. Injury can be in the form of entrapment of the nerves, traction injury, cauterisation, transection, etc. These are more common after mesh repair because of entrapment of the nerves or perineural fibrosis and adhesions between mesh and the nerves. Clinical features include dull aching or dragging pain in the groin, genitalia, suprapubic region. Some may complain of diminished sensation or even hyperaesthesia. Treatment usually includes reassurance, simple analgesics, nerve blocks with anaesthetic agents and injection of steroids. Neurolysis by inguinal exploration or neurectomy may be required in appropriate cases.

Ischaemic orchitis and testicular atrophy

- It occurs due to thrombosis of veins of pampiniform plexus within spermatic cord. It is more common in direct hernias where handling of the spermatic cord while separating it from the long-standing sac may result in thrombosis.
- It can also be due to injury to testicular artery.
- Venous congestion results in ischaemic orchitis causing pain in the testis.
- It is treated with anti-inflammatory drugs.
- Ischaemic orchitis is more common after recurrent hernia surgeries.

COMPLICATIONS OF HERNIA

Competency

SU28.1.5: Describe complications of abdominal hernias.

1. Irreducibility (Key Box 52.7)

It occurs due to adhesions formed between omentum, sac and the contents. Irreducibility produces dull aching pain.

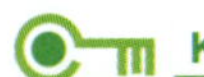 **Key Box 52.7**

Diagnosis of Irreducible Hernia

- Hernia is tense
- Tender
- Irreducible
- No impulse on cough
- Recent increase in size of swelling

2. Obstructed Hernia (Key Box 52.8 and Fig. 52.26)

Irreducible hernia + obstruction to the lumen of the gut gives rise to obstructed hernia. Clinically, it produces severe colicky abdominal pain, abdominal distension, vomiting and step ladder peristalsis.

Treatment

Urgent division of the neck of the sac followed by hernioplasty.

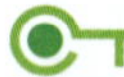 **Key Box 52.8**

Factors Responsible for Obstructed Hernia

- Narrow neck
- Irreducibility
- Sudden straining
- Too many contents
- Long duration of hernia
- Sliding hernia

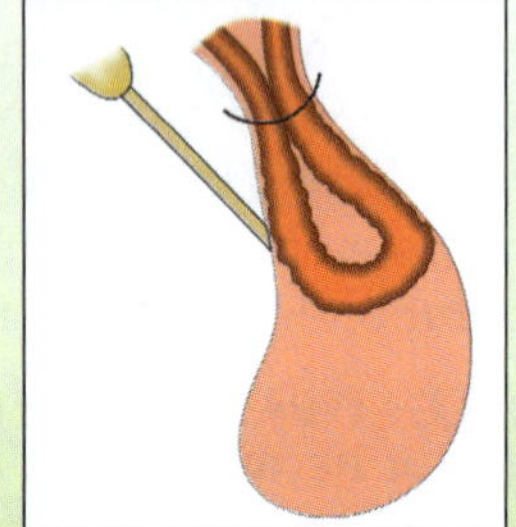

Fig. 52.26: Obstructed hernia

3. Strangulated Hernia

Irreducibility + obstruction + impairment of blood supply to intestine.

Pathology

- Strangulation commonly occurs in femoral hernia, obturator hernia and in indirect hernia.
- Initially the venous return is occluded, the part gets congested, and mucosal ulceration and haemorrhage occurs into the gut wall. It also results in oedema due to capillary exudation.
- If the obstruction is not relieved, constriction of the artery takes place resulting in gangrene of bowel. If this happens, there is a proliferation of bacteria.
- Gangrene appears at the ring of constriction first. Later it develops in the antimesenteric border (Fig. 52.27).

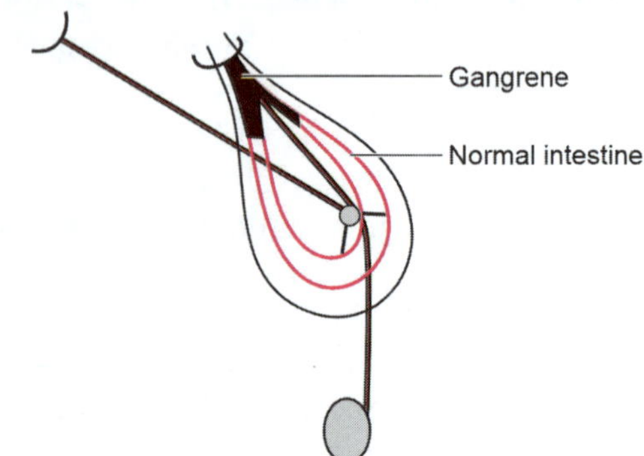

Fig. 52.27: Gangrene appears at ring of constriction first and then progresses

- Such a gangrenous segment contains decomposed blood in which gram-negative organisms multiply. They produce endotoxins resulting in endotoxic shock. If the gangrene extends into the intra-abdominal segment of the bowel, peritonitis can occur.
- The deep ring and the external ring are the common constricting sites.

Clinical Features

- Sudden, severe, prolonged pain with some features of shock are indicative of strangulation.
- **Clinical examination of such hernia reveals** (Fig. 52.28):
  - Tense (hernial sac is tense—differentiates it from obstructed hernia)
  - Tender
  - No impulse on cough
  - Irreducible
  - Recent increase in the size of the swelling
- General condition of the patient is poor:
  - Feeble pulse, hypotension, rebound tenderness, absent bowel sounds, toxic look.

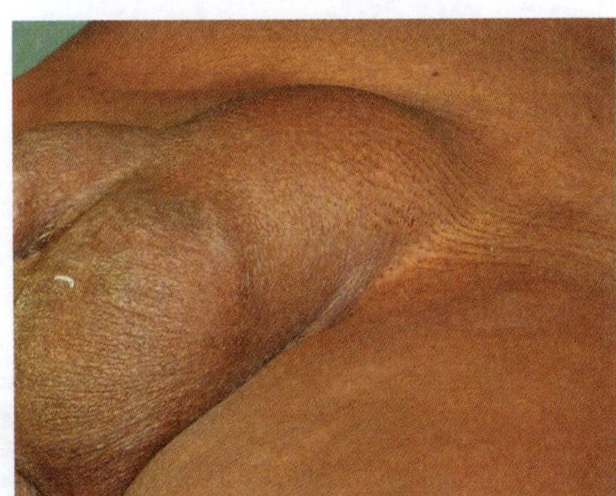

Fig. 52.28A: Strangulated hernia

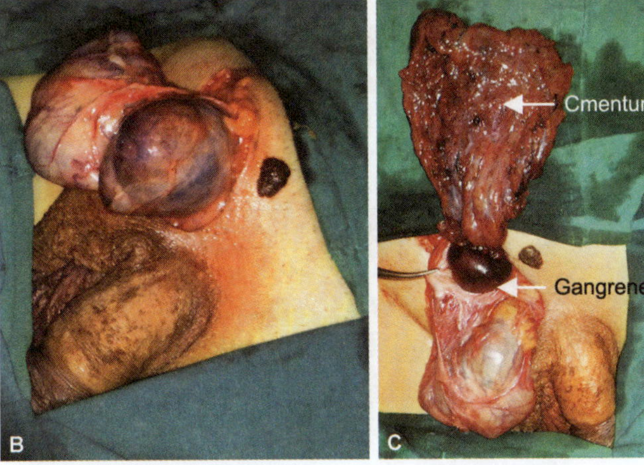

Figs 52.28B and C: Strangulated hernia with gangrene

Treatment

I. General measures

- The patient is hospitalised. The foot end of the bed is raised so that an irreducible hernia may reduce by gravity. However, if there is a suspicion of gangrene, this step is not recommended.
- A Ryle's tube is introduced to decompress the stomach, thus preventing vomiting and reducing abdominal distension.
- Intravenous fluids are given to correct dehydration and to prevent renal failure.
- Narcotic analgesics are required to reduce the pain.
- An attempt should be made to reduce the swelling when there is no gangrene by the following measures:
  A. Good sedation
  B. Patient's thigh is flexed, adducted and medially rotated.
  C. With the right hand, the sac is gently squeezed by applying pressure over the scrotum. At the same time with the left hand, the proximal portion of the sac is guided into the inguinal canal. This procedure is described as taxis. **Taxis is contra-indicated, if there is gangrene**.
  D. **Complications of forced reduction** include contusion of intestinal wall, rupture of the sac at the neck and reduction *en masse*, i.e. the entire sac with the contents are reduced into the abdominal cavity but the intestine still remains strangulated.
- The patient is prepared for surgery and blood is grouped and cross-matched.

II. Surgery (Key Box 52.9)

- With broad-spectrum antibiotic coverage, the hernia is explored by an inguinoscrotal incision and hernia sac is defined. At this stage, ***the constricting ring should not be divided.*** First all the toxic fluid from the sac is aspirated. The constriction is then divided using a grooved director or hernia bistoury. **While dividing the constricting ring, the inferior epigastric vessels which are situated medially may be**

Key Box 52.9

Surgery for Strangulation

- Generous inguinal incision, identify the sac
- First aspirate toxic fluid
- Divide constricting agent
- Check for viability
- Resection of gangrene
- Repair of hernia—without mesh
- Broad-spectrum antibiotics

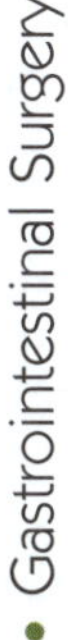

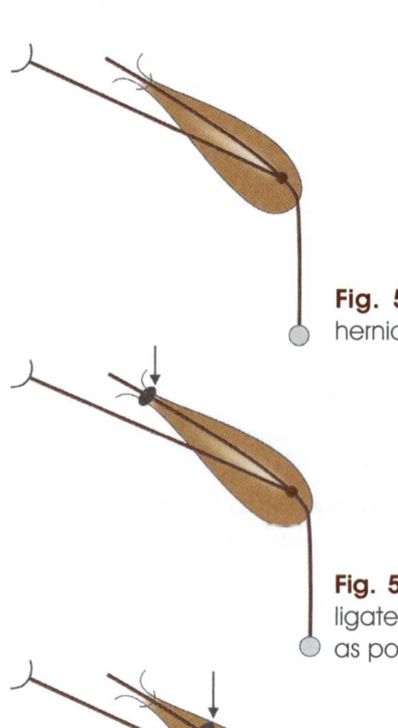

Fig. 52.29: Indirect incomplete hernia

Fig. 52.30A: High ligation—sac is ligated as close to the deep ring as possible

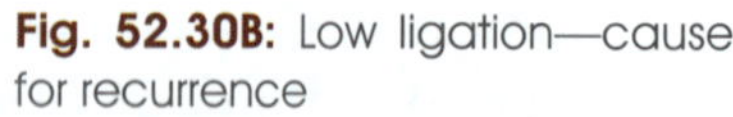

Fig. 52.30B: Low ligation—cause for recurrence

damaged. Therefore, care has to be taken to protect these vessels. High ligation of the sac should be done (Figs 52.29 and 52.30A). Low ligation (Fig. 52.30B) should not be done because it causes recurrence.

- If the bowel is gangrenous, resection of gangrenous segment and anastomosis is done. Closure of incision includes placement of tube drain, which is brought out through a separate incision.
- Mesh should not be used in this situation. A simple darning or herniorrhaphy can be done.
- If viability of the bowel is doubtful, the intestinal loops are covered with warm wet mops for a period of 5–10 minutes and 100% oxygen is given to the patient (request the anaesthetist). Return to pink colour, peristalsis of bowel and pulsations in the mesentery indicate viability.
- If the general condition of the patient permits, repair of the hernia may also be done.
- If evidence of peritonitis is present or if gangrene is spreading within, laparotomy should be done.

4. Incarcerated Hernia

It is an obstructed hernia due to obstruction caused by faecal matter. It generally occurs in a sliding hernia. ***(Nowadays incarcerated hernia has been renamed as obstructed hernia).***

5. Inflamed Hernia

It occurs when the contents of hernia get inflamed, e.g. appendicitis in a hernial sac, Meckel's diverticulitis in hernial sac. Thus, complications of hernia can be dangerous (Key Box 52.10). It may range from a simple obstruction to a life-threatening strangulation. Hence, early diagnosis and early treatment are necessary in all cases of indirect hernia. In a few selected cases of direct hernia, wherein the defect is big, the chances of strangulation are less. However, if there are no medical contraindications, surgery has to be advised. Following are a few examples of strangulations without obstruction. They have diarrhoea and bleeding per rectum rather than constipation (Key Box 52.11).

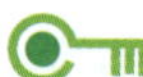 **Key Box 52.10**

Summary of Complications of Hernia

- Irreducibility
- Obstructed hernia
- Strangulation
- Incarcerated hernia
- Inflamed hernia

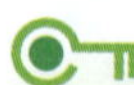 **Key Box 52.11**

Strangulation without Obstruction

- Omentocoele (Fig. 52.31)
- Richter's hernia
- Littre's hernia (Fig. 52.32)

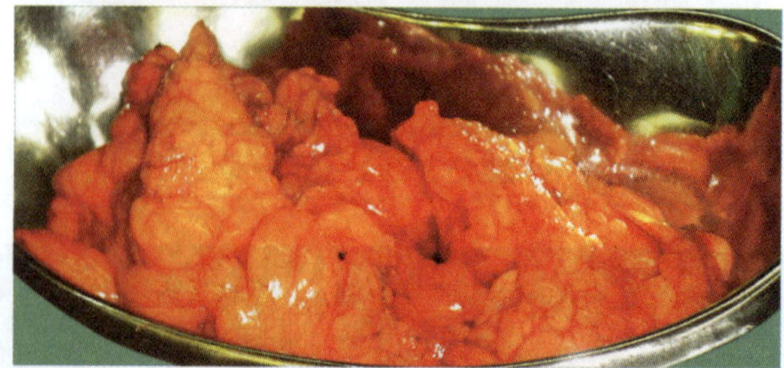

Fig. 52.31: Excised omentum in the kidney tray

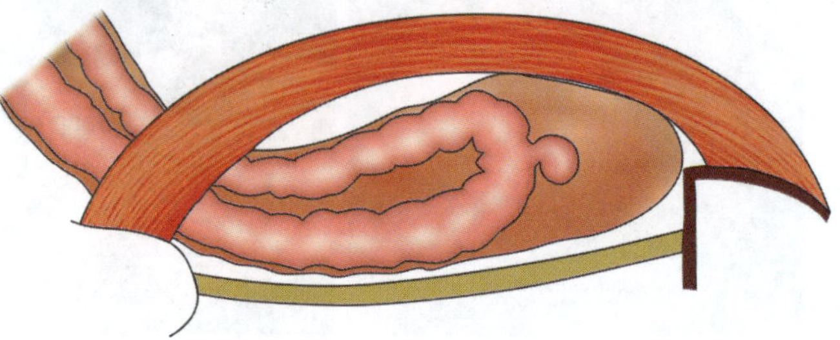

Fig. 52.32: Littre's hernia

RECURRENT HERNIA

Incidence of 10% recurrence is common medially.

Causes

I. Preoperative

1. Chronic cough
2. Weak muscle tone
3. Straining while passing urine, constipation
4. Obesity, ascites, anaemia.

II. Intraoperative

1. **Improper excision of the sac:** The sac should be ligated at the level of deep ring (neck). This is called **high ligation of the sac**. Very often, the sac is seen as soon as the inguinal canal is opened. If it is ligated at the fundus or body (low ligation), it invariably results in recurrence. A missed indirect sac can be a cause of recurrence (Figs 52.31 and 52.32).
2. **Absorbable sutures** such as catgut have lifespan of 2–3 weeks. If they are used for reconstruction, they invariably result in recurrence.
3. **Bleeding:** At the end of the surgery, small bleeding points should be coagulated by using diathermy or ligatures. Haematoma formation predisposes to infection, which can be the cause of recurrence.
4. **Tension** between suture lines can cause strangulation and fibrosis of muscle fibres. Hence, care and gentleness are important while suturing conjoined tendon to the inguinal ligament.

III. Postoperative

1. **Persistent postoperative cough** weakens the suture line.
2. **Haematoma** can get secondarily infected resulting in pus formation. The sutures give way leading to recurrence. Hence, if there is a significant haematoma, it should be drained.
3. **Infection:** Even though hernia is a clean surgery, chances of infection are present specially in diabetics, alcoholics and immunocompromised patients. Prophylactic antibiotics such as 2nd generation cephalosporin should be given. If infection occurs, it should be treated accordingly.
4. **Exertion:** Too much exertion in the postoperative period, in the form of lifting heavy weights or carrying heavy weights on the shoulder, may weaken the suture line, resulting in hernia.

   Most of the recurrences occur within one year. Incidence of recurrent hernia may vary from 2 to 8% even in experienced hands. In a case of recurrent hernia, it is difficult to say whether it is a direct hernia or indirect hernia. From the management point of view, it does not matter.

Treatment

- If the sac is present due to incomplete excision at the previous surgery, it should be completely excised up to the level of deep ring, followed by hernioplasty.
- Meshplasty is the surgical treatment for a recurrent hernia. However, if mesh cannot be placed either due to infection or due to nonavailability, prolene darning can be done.
- Tuberculosis must be ruled out in cases of persisting infection.
- In all these cases, precipitating factors if any, should be treated first.
- The only way to totally prevent recurrence is by closure of the deep ring. This can be done only after dividing the spermatic cord (Kuntz procedure). It is indicated in elderly patients who have multiple recurrences.

SPECIAL HERNIAS

1. **Giant hernia:** Sac extends up to mid-thigh (Fig. 52.33).

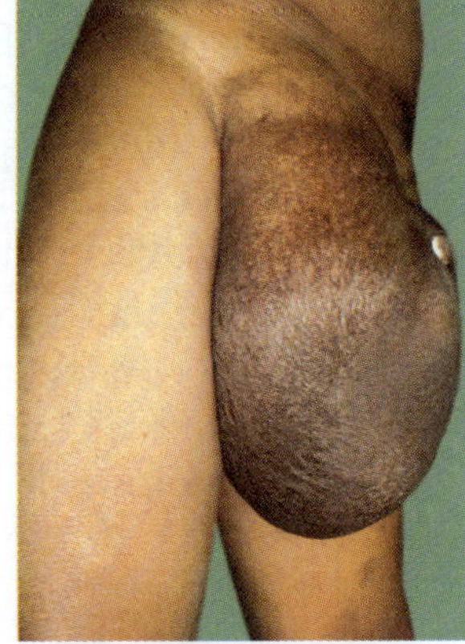

Fig. 52.33: Giant hernia

Definition: A giant inguino-scrotal hernia is defined as a hernia that extends below the midpoint of the inner thigh in the standing position.

Clinical features

- Most patients would have had their hernia for several years.
- The contents often include colon, small intestines and bladder.
- A few of these are also sliding inguinal hernias.
- Hence, more prone for complications such as incarceration, intestinal obstruction and scrotal ulceration. The last complication is due to pressure necrosis or due to friction while walking or moving.
- Differential diagnosis includes scrotal elephantiasis.
- A few precautions to be taken during surgery are:
  – Preoperative chest physiotherapy.
  – Catheterise the bladder. This will decrease the incidence of urinary bladder injury.
  – Bowel wash before surgery.
  – Dissect the sac carefully all around.
  – Perfect haemostasis.

- Omentectomy and rarely colectomy may be required (Fig. 52.31).
- If bowel is not resected, mesh can be placed safely.
- In cases of emergency and patient with co-morbid factors including cardiac problems, take consent for orchidectomy—the best option will be to divide the cord at the level of deep ring and close the deep ring during orchidectomy.

2. **Dual hernia:** It has two sacs, one direct and another indirect, connected by an isthmus which is behind the inferior epigastric artery. It is also known as saddlebag hernia, **pantaloon hernia**, dual hernia or Romberg hernia.

Significance

- Deep ring occlusion test: The inference of the test may not be correct.
- It is the cause of recurrence, if one sac is not treated properly.

3. **Prevesical hernia:** It is also called **funicular direct hernia**. It is a hernia containing portion of the bladder with prevesical fat through the defect in the conjoined tendon on the medial side. History of the swelling becoming less prominent after micturition may be present. Due to narrow neck, it is prone for strangulation.
4. **Littre's hernia** (Fig. 52.32): It is referred to a hernia containing Meckel's diverticulum. When the diverticulum gets infected, such hernias are called inflamed hernias. Infection may be precipitated by partial obstruction to the diverticulum by constricting agents.
5. **Maydl's hernia (Hernia-en-W)** (Fig. 52.34)
   - It is a **W** hernia wherein the intra-abdominal bowel loop segment becomes gangrenous very early but in the scrotum, there are no signs of gangrene.

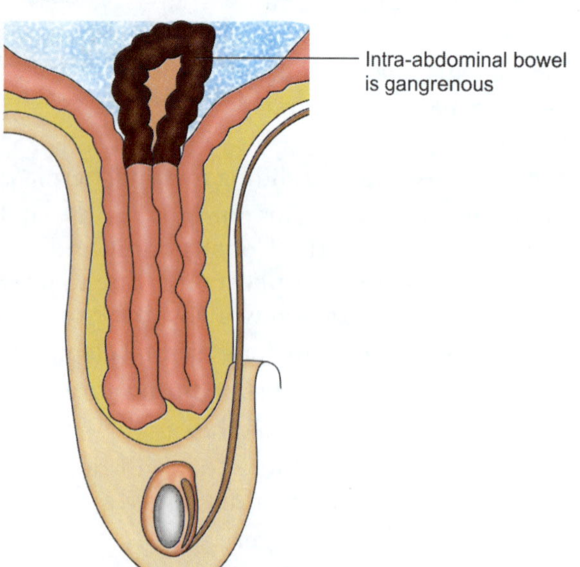

Fig. 52.34: Maydl's hernia

   - The patient presents with obstructed hernia and at operation, the inguinoscrotal segment has no gangrene. The intra-abdominal segment must be examined and the gangrenous portion should be excised. It can also be called retrograde strangulation. Clinically, there is tenderness above the inguinal ligament.

6. **Richter's hernia** (Fig. 52.35)
   - When only part of circumference of bowel becomes strangulated, it is called Richter's hernia.
   - It may spontaneously reduce

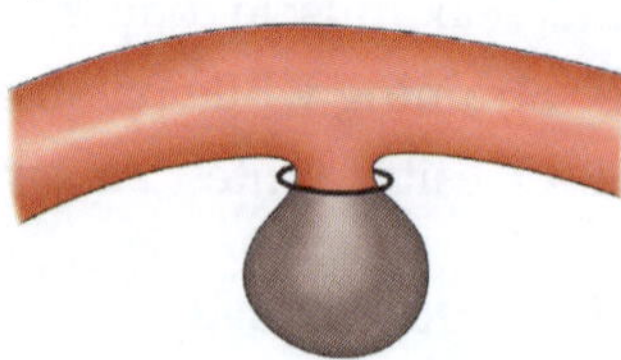

Fig. 52.35: Richter's hernia

   - Thus, gangrene may be overlooked at operation
   - Even though the patient has features of intestinal obstruction, there will be diarrhoea and often blood in stools.
   - Femoral hernia and obturator hernia are a few examples of hernia which can sometimes present as **Richter's hernia**.

7. **Sliding hernia** (Hernia-en-glissade) (Figs 52.36A to C)
   - Incidence: 1–3%
   - Always acquired hernia
   - It occurs as a result of the slipping of posterior peritoneum along with the retroperitoneal viscus. As a result of which, the caecum, on the right side and the sigmoid colon on the left side, form the posterior wall of the sac.
   - **If the caecum and appendix are the contents of the hernial sac, it is not a sliding hernia.**
   - However, a true hernial sac containing omentum or intestines exists.
   - Weakness of the abdominal wall at the deep ring lateral to inferior epigastric vessels is also a contributing factor.
   - Urinary bladder can also be the content of the hernial sac (Fig. 52.36A).

Clinical features

- It almost always occurs in males.
- It commonly affects elderly patients.
- It can be suspected when there is a large hernia descending down into the scrotum.
- Left-sided is more common than right-sided hernia.
- It practically always occurs in long-standing cases of inguinal hernia.
- They are not completely reducible.
- It can be direct hernia and indirect hernia also.

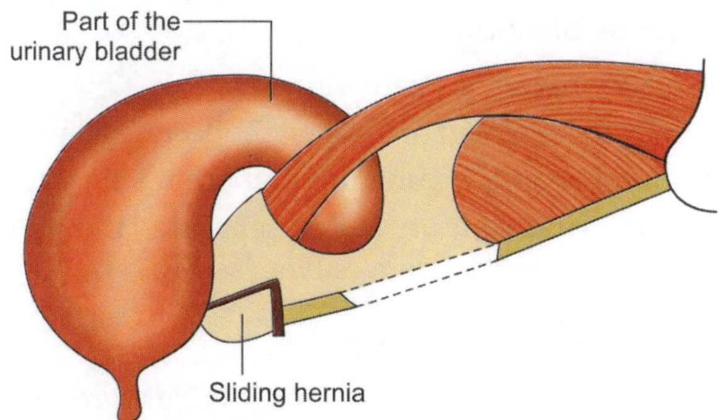

Fig. 52.36A: Sliding hernia

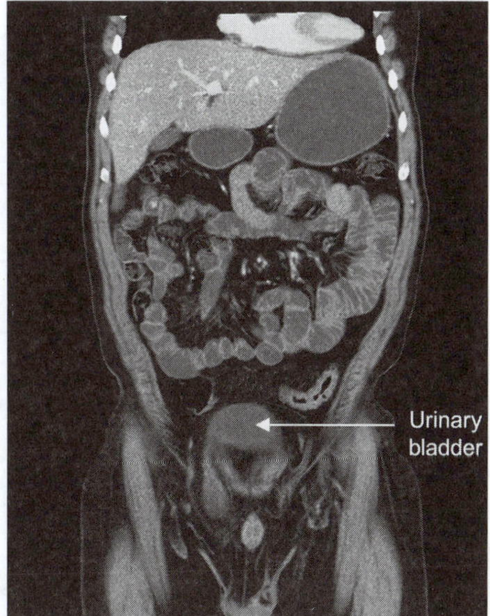

Fig. 52.36B: CECT scan: Sliding hernia showing part of the urinary bladder. (*Courtesy:* Prof. SS Prasad, Dr Rajendra, Dr Vijayendra, Associate Professors, Department of Surgery, KMC, Manipal)

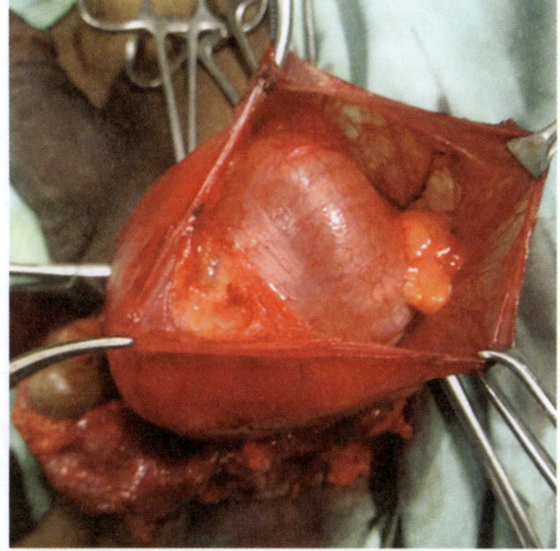

Fig. 52.36C: Sliding hernia. Note that sigmoid colon is forming wall of the sac, (*Courtesy:* Dr Amit Jain, Brindhavvan Areion Hospital, Bengaluru)

Complications: These hernias can easily strangulate and since its wall contents include the large intestine, the mortality and morbidity increases.

Treatment

- Truss is absolutely contraindicated.
- Once the hernial sac is opened, the sac **should not be twisted**.
- A purse-string suture is applied within to avoid injury to caecum/sigmoid colon.
- The sac is removed and the repair of the hernia done.
- In elderly patients, orchidectomy is advised to give a permanent cure for hernia.

Sliding hernia—key points

- Always acquired
- Always (almost) in males
- Always occur in long-standing hernias
- Always irreducible
- Always colon or urinary bladder forms the wall of the sac
- Always requires a repair
- Always technical difficulties are encountered by junior surgeons while operating on these patients

8. Sportsman's hernia

- This is common in men who play rugby or football wherein injury due to the ball may occur.
- Pain is in the groin radiating to scrotum and upper thigh.
- On examination, there may be tenderness in the inguinal region.
- Orthopaedic disorders must be ruled out first by MRI or CT scan. They are soft tissue injury in the groin, pubic bone diastasis, adductor spasm, etc.
- If hernia is due to tearing of muscles **(Gilmore's groin)**—it should be repaired in the usual manner.

FEMORAL HERNIA

Competency

SU28.1.15: Describe anatomy, pathophysiology, required investigations for diagnosis of femoral hernia and the surgical techniques in management of femoral hernia.

Herniation of intra-abdominal contents through the femoral canal is described as femoral hernia (Key Box 52.12). Women are more often involved, as compared to men with the ratio being 2:1, which is doubled in parous women. However, it should be remembered that **in women, inguinal hernias are the most common type of hernia, followed by incisional hernia.** Femoral hernia is the third most common type of hernia.

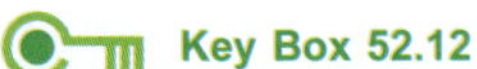
Key Box 52.12

Femoral Hernia: Coverings

- Sac
- Fat and lymphoid tissue
- Transversalis fascia
- Cribriform fascia
- Superficial fascia
- Skin

Commonly the hernia is unilateral, the right side being affected more often than the left side. It is bilateral in about 15–20% of the patients.

Anatomy of Femoral Canal and Femoral Ring (Fig. 52.37)

- The femoral canal extends from the femoral ring to the saphenous ring. It is 1½ inches below and lateral to the pubic tubercle. It is the innermost compartment of femoral sheath.
- It is similar to a truncated cone **which is narrow at the femoral ring**.
- **Contents of femoral canal are:**
  - Fat
  - Fascia
  - Lymphatics: Lymph node of Cloquet
- Femoral vein is in the middle compartment of the femoral sheath and femoral artery is in the lateral compartment.
- Femoral nerve is outside the femoral sheath.
- Femoral sheath: Fascia transversalis is continued downwards behind the inguinal ligament as the anterior layer of the femoral sheath. Fascia iliaca continues behind the femoral vessels as the posterior layer of the femoral sheath.

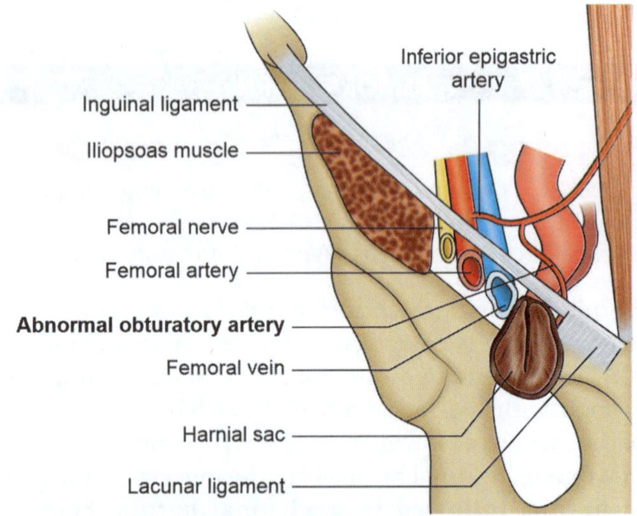

Fig. 52.37: Femoral hernia: Anatomy

Boundaries of Femoral Ring

- *Anterior:* Inguinal ligament.
- *Posterior:* Ligament of Cooper, iliopectineal ligament.
- *Medial:* Lacunar ligament (Gimbernat's ligament).
- *Lateral:* Thin septum which separates the femoral canal from femoral vein (silver fascia).

Causes for Femoral Hernia

1. **Pregnancy:** As the gravid uterus compresses the external iliac vein, the empty femoral sheath on the medial side allows the femoral vein to expand within femoral sheath. Thus, increased abdominal pressure due to repeated pregnancies is one of the chief factors responsible for femoral hernias. The maximum incidence is around 30–40 years of age.
2. **Wide femoral canal:** This is due to the narrow insertion of iliopubic tract into the pectineal line of the pubis and may be responsible for a few cases of femoral hernia.

Pearls of Wisdom

Femoral hernia is never congenital.

Course of the Hernial Sac

As the hernia comes into the femoral canal, it is an oblong swelling due to the rigid femoral canal. When it comes out through the saphenous opening, it expands and becomes retort shaped because Scarpa's fascia is attached to the deep fascia of thigh below the saphenous opening.

Clinical Features of Femoral Hernia

- Females between the age of 20 and 40 years are commonly affected.
- **Gaur sign:** Dilatation of superficial epigastric/circumflex iliac veins due to compression.
- Right side is more commonly affected because of the dominant nature of right side of the body.
- To start with, there is a small swelling below the inguinal ligament, which goes unnoticed very often.
- Expansile impulse is often not present due to the narrow canal.
- Reducibility may be present.
- Typically, the swelling is below and lateral to the pubic tubercle (inguinal hernia is above and medial to pubic tubercle) (Fig. 52.38).
- Many (30–80%) present with strangulation.

Treatment (Key Box 52.13)

1. **Low operation of Lockwood:** Incision is placed directly over the swelling in the thigh. The sac is

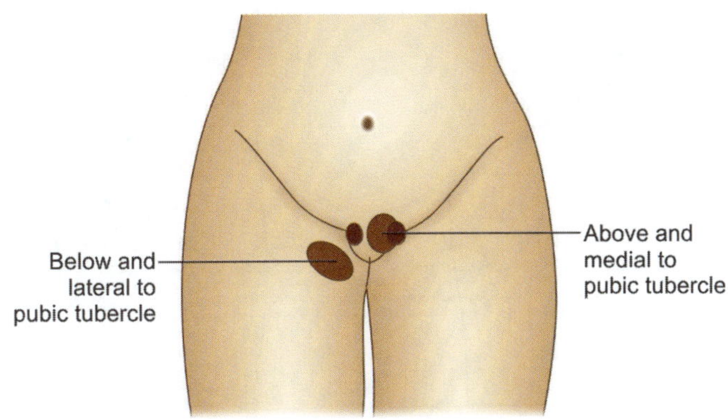

Fig. 52.38: Femoral hernia (R) and indirect hernia (L)

Key Box 52.13

Surgery of Femoral Hernia

- Should be done as early as possible, once the diagnosis is made.
- For elective repair, low (femoral) approach: Incision directly over the swelling is ideal. Injury to abdominal obturator artery can occur in this route (found on lateral side in 20% of cases).
- Transinguinal (Lothiessen): Can use it when there is gangrene. However, it may weaken inguinal canal.
- Combined: High approach is the choice for strangulated femoral hernias. Approximate inguinal ligament and pectineal ligament.

carefully dissected out without damaging the femoral vein. The sac is ligated at the neck, excised and the hernia is repaired—the **inguinal ligament is sutured to Cooper's ligament** (iliopectineal ligament) thus obliterating the femoral ring. Nonabsorbable suture such as prolene or ethilon is ideal. Low approach is indicated in uncomplicated hernia. It is very difficult to manage a gangrenous loop of bowel with this approach.

Abnormal obturator artery

Normal obturator artery is a branch of the internal iliac artery. It gives a pubic branch which anastomoses with pubic branch of the inferior epigastric artery. Occasionally, this anastomosis is large and obturator artery then appears to be a branch of the inferior epigastric. Usually it passes lateral to the femoral canal in contact with the femoral vein. Occasionally, the abnormal artery may lie along the medial margin of the femoral ring, i.e. along the free margin of the lacunar ligament. This artery is in danger during surgery for obstructed femoral hernia.

2. Inguinal operation

- Through an **inguinal incision,** the inguinal canal is opened. The transversalis fascia is incised. Hernial sac is visualised. This is followed by excision of the sac. The high approach is preferred when there is a strangulated femoral hernia. This offers a very good view of the abnormal obturator artery from above, if it is present.
- Repair is done by suturing the conjoined tendon to iliopectineal line.

3. **Combined approach: High operation of McEvedy:** Inguinofemoral approach: A vertical incision is made over the swelling and extended above the inguinal ligament, and the sac can be dissected from both above and below (look for abnormal obturator artery—see below). This approach has the advantages of both operations mentioned above.
4. **Henry's approach:** Lower midline for bilateral hernia.

Complications of Femoral Hernia

1. As the femoral ring and the neck of the sac are narrow, obstruction and strangulation are very common.
2. Richter's hernia
   - Commonly seen in femoral hernias and obturator hernias, which have narrow necks.
   - This occurs when a **portion of the circumference of the bowel** is caught within the hernial sac and which is constricted by the narrow ring. Signs and symptoms of intestinal obstruction are absent, even though it is an obstructed hernia, because the lumen is not obstructed.
   - The hernia is tense, tender, irreducible and has no cough impulse.
   - As the lumen is patent, there may be bloody diarrhea rather than constipation. Gangrene can occur soon.
   - **Treatment:** Combined or inguinal approach to deal with gangrene.

Summary of Femoral Hernia (Key Box 52.14)

Rare Types of Femoral Hernia

1. **Lacunar hernia (Laugier's hernia):** In this case, the hernia passes through a small defect in the lacunar ligament.
2. **Prevascular hernia (Narath's femoral hernia):** In this case, the hernial sac is located behind the femoral

Key Box 52.14

Femoral Hernia

- Rarely occurs in males (5–10%)
- Commonly associated with Richter's hernia
- Fatty female with small swelling under a big belly usually goes undetected.
- Dangerous because of early strangulation
- Cannot be controlled by a truss
- Surgical repair is a must

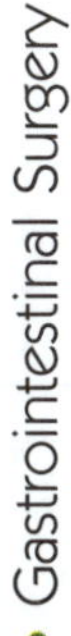

vessels and the inguinal ligament. It may be associated with congenital dislocation of the hip (Narath's hernia).

3. **Pectineal hernia:** In this case, the hernia passes between the pectineus muscle and its fascia, behind the femoral vessels. It is also called Cloquet's hernia.
4. **External femoral hernia:** It is a hernia lateral to the femoral artery (Hesselbach's hernia).

Differential Diagnosis of Femoral Hernia

1. **Inguinal hernia:** An inguinal hernia is above and medial to pubic tubercle. The femoral hernia is below and lateral to pubic tubercle (Fig. 52.39).
2. **Saphena varix:** It is the dilated, saccular, upper end of long saphenous vein with varicosity. It disappears on lying down because of gravity. Thrill may be felt on coughing (Fig. 52.40).
3. **Lipoma:** Soft and lobular, slips under palpating fingers (Fig. 52.41).
4. **Femoral artery aneurysm** is rare. It presents as a pulsatile swelling in the groin with a continuous murmur. Peripheral pulses are often weak (Fig. 52.42).
5. **Enlarged femoral lymph nodes** are firm and round. They can be enlarged in lower limb infections, abrasions, wounds in the perineum and also in carcinoma penis (Fig. 52.43).

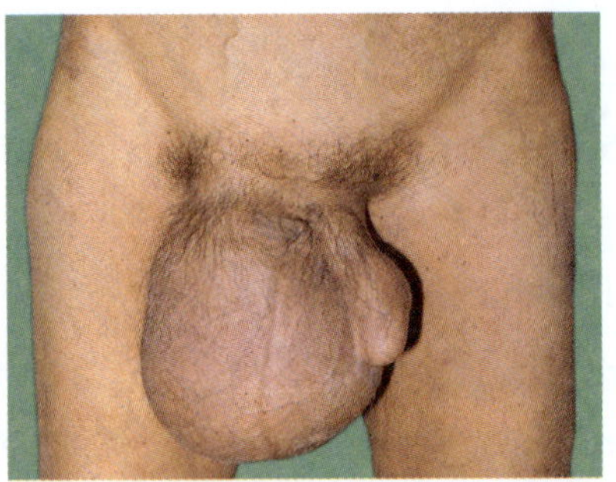

Fig. 52.39: Large direct hernias

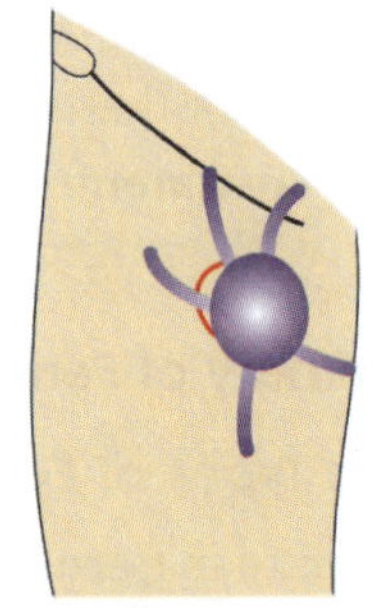

Fig. 52.40: Saphena varix

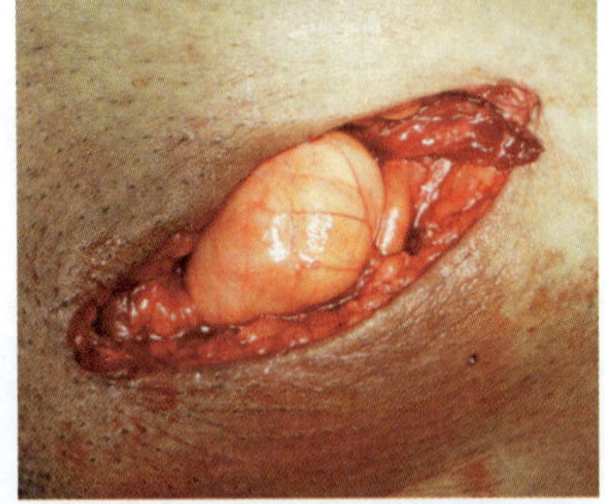

Fig. 52.41: Left inguinal lipoma of the cord

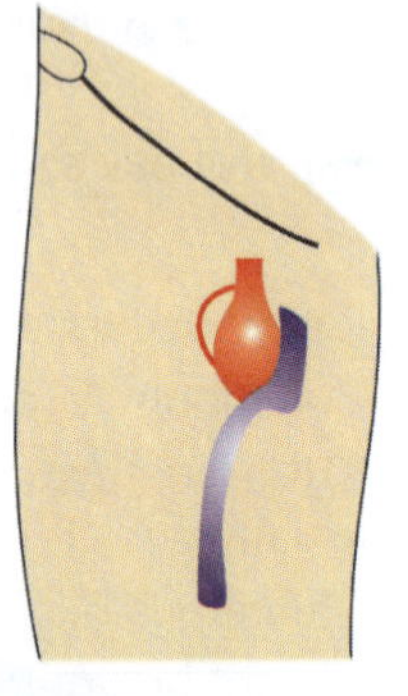

Fig. 52.42: Femoral artery aneurysm

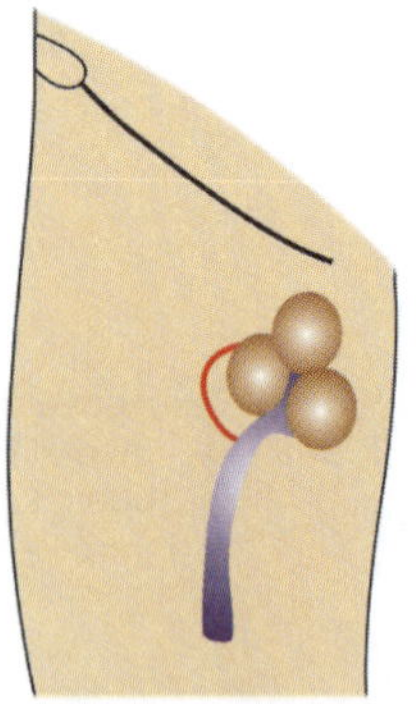

Fig. 52.43: Lymphadenitis

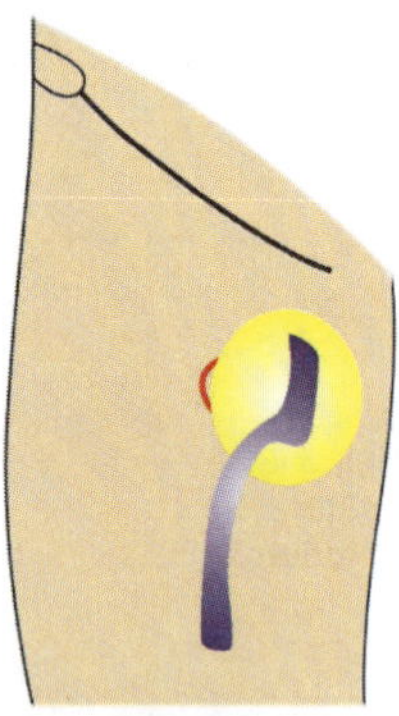

Fig. 52.44: Psoas bursa

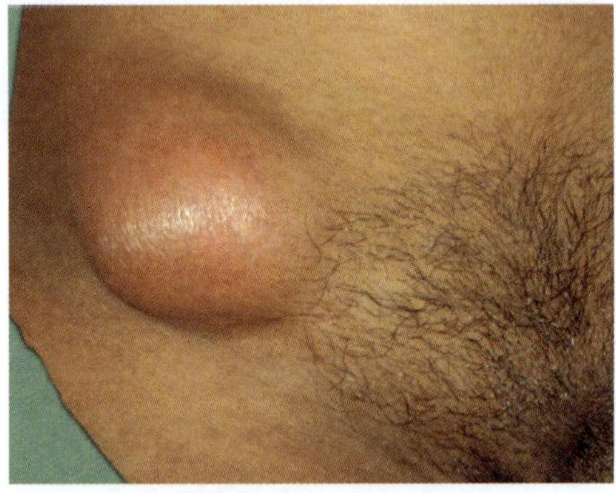

Fig. 52.45: Iliopsoas abscess

6. **Psoas bursa:** Osteoarthritis of the hip can produce distension of psoas bursa, which disappears on flexing the hip. Tuberculosis spine can present as iliopsoas abscess (Fig. 52.44).
7. **Psoas abscess:** It is an iliopsoas abscess due to tuberculosis of spine. There are two swellings, one above and one below the inguinal ligament. Cross fluctuation can be elicited between these two swellings. Tenderness over the spine and X-ray of the spine help in arriving at a diagnosis (Fig. 52.45).

UMBILICAL HERNIA

It can be discussed under three headings:

I. Umbilical hernia of newborn
II. Umbilical hernia of infants and children
III. Umbilical hernia of adults.

UMBILICAL HERNIA OF NEWBORN

- It is called *omphalocoele—exomphalos*.
- It is found 1 in 6000 live births.
- Failure of midgut as a **whole or part** to return into coelomic cavity during embryonic life results in exomphalos.

- It is also associated with weakness of abdominal musculature (few fibres may be absent). Two types have been recognised.

1. Exomphalos Minor (Fig. 52.46A)

- In this condition, the umbilical cord is attached to the summit of the sac.
- Sac is small and defect less than 5 cm.
- It is treated by twisting the cord and ligating the sac. Care should be taken to avoid damage to the intestine. For example, nursing the child preoperatively in prone position can damage intestines.

2. Exomphalos Major (Fig. 52.46B)

- In this condition, the umbilical cord is attached to the inferior aspect of the sac, containing intestines, abdominal structures, e.g. liver, bowel.
- Many children are stillborn.
- This type of hernia is usually associated with absent abdominal musculature.
- The operation should be done before the rupture of the sac as the morbidity increases greatly in the event of a rupture of the sac.
- During the operation, skin flaps are raised on both sides to cover the defect. A true repair is necessary and is done at a later date.
- *See* also Figs 52.47 and 52.48.

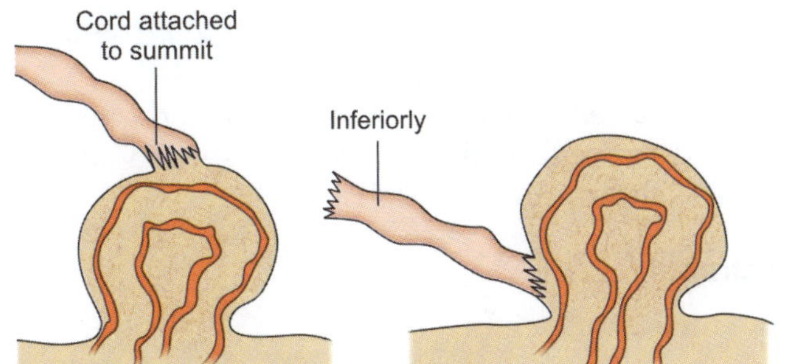

Fig. 52.46A: Exomphalos minor **Fig. 52.46B:** Exomphalos major

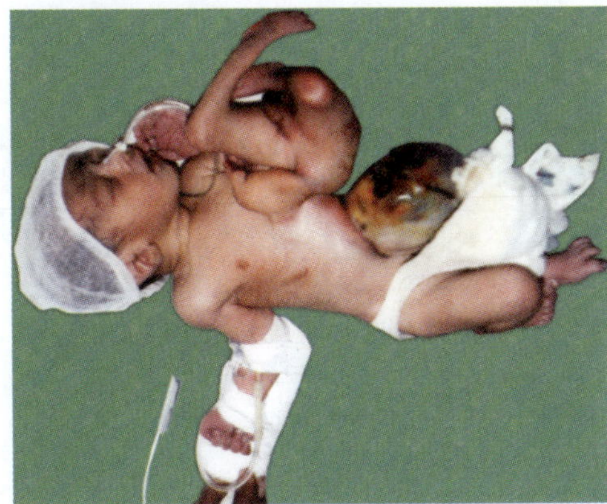

Fig. 52.47: Epigastric heterophagus with exomphalos major

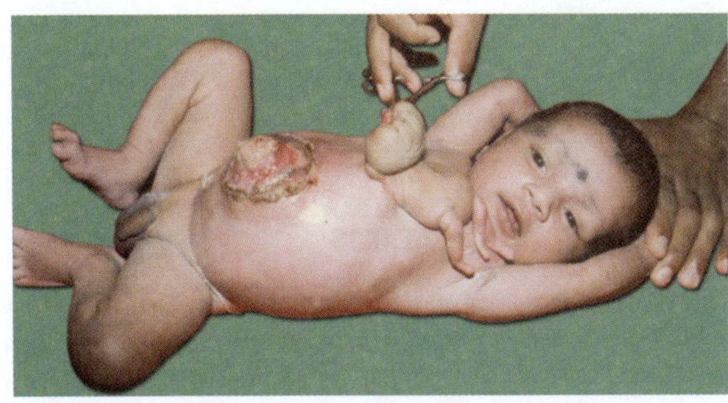

Fig. 52.48: Same child on the 21st postoperative day. The repair is done by rotating flaps from gluteal region of the parasitic baby. (*Courtesy:* Prof Vidyadhar Kinhal, Late Prof RS Channagiri, Dr Channanna, Department of Surgery, Vijayanagar Institute of Medical Sciences, Bellary, Karnataka)

UMBILICAL HERNIA OF INFANTS AND CHILDREN

- It occurs as a complication of umbilical sepsis, which weakens the umbilical scar.
- It is a true umbilical hernia containing either omentum/intestines.

Clinical Features

- Common in male children
- The child is brought with the complaint of swelling in the umbilical region whenever the child cries.
- Most of the cases are symptomless. Parents are anxious about the swelling.
- Strangulation is rare (Fig. 52.49).

Treatment

- **Reassurance** is the most important advice given to the parents.
- **No treatment is required** other than **strapping** the abdominal wall by keeping a pad in front of umbilicus.

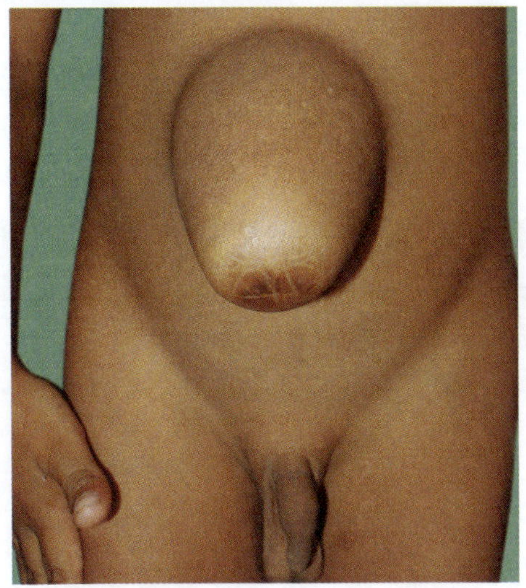

Fig. 52.49: Umbilical hernia in a child

- Majority of the hernias get corrected by 2 years of age (90%).
- If the hernia does not correct itself, repair is necessary to close the defect in the linea alba.

UMBILICAL HERNIA OF ADULTS

- It is not a true umbilical hernia but it is a para-umbilical hernia in which the hernia occurs either above, below or to the side of the umbilicus, through the linea alba.
- The contents are the greater omentum, transverse colon or small bowel. Due to adhesion, it is often irreducible.

Aetiology

- Females in the 5th decade are commonly affected. Male:female ratio is 1:5.
- **Obesity** with flabby abdominal muscle predisposes to paraumbilical hernia.
- Repeated **pregnancies** also weaken the abdominal wall.
- Ascites may precipitate hernia specially in cirrhotic patients.

Clinical Features

- Patient presents with a swelling in the umbilical region, which increases on straining or coughing.
- On asking the patient to cough, **expansile impulse** is present (Fig. 52.50).
- They may also have inguinal hernia.
- **Reducibility can be present.**
- **Dragging pain** is usually due to omentum which is felt as a firm or granular mass. If gurgling is present, it is indicative of small intestines in the hernial sac.
- After reducing the swelling, the **defect** can be felt in the linea alba.

Refer to Table 52.4 for comparison between umbilical hernia in infants and adults.

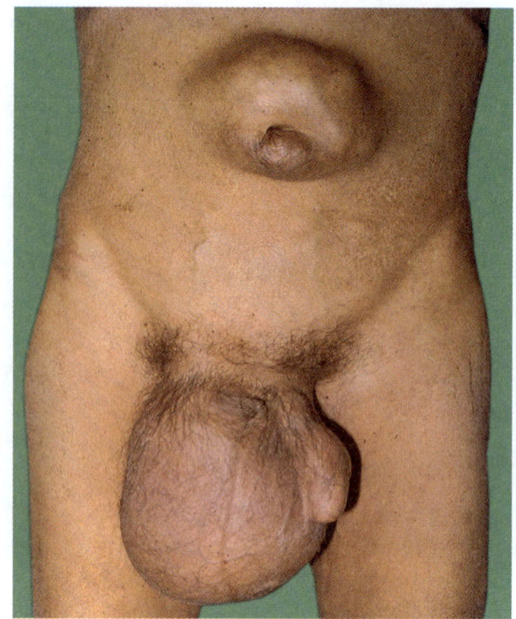

Fig. 52.50: Large direct hernia with umbilical hernia

Complications

1. **Irreducibility** is common due to adhesions between omentum and the sac.
2. **Obstruction** presents with colicky abdominal pain and vomiting. Distension follows soon. Untreated cases develop strangulation. Very often, these patients present with **incarcerated** hernia due to the presence of transverse colon in the sac. They require urgent intervention, failing which gangrene will set in.
3. As the sac enlarges, due to its weight and gravity, it sags down resulting in friction of the skin and this causes **intertrigo** (Fig. 52.51).

Treatment

1. Reduction of weight.
2. **Anatomical repair:** Small defects can be closed with nonabsorbable sutures such as nylon or prolene (Fig. 52.52).

Table 52.4 Comparison between umbilical hernia in infants and adults

Features	Infants	Adults
Age in years	0–3	50–60
Sex	Common in male child	Common in females
Causes	Neonatal sepsis	Obesity, weak muscles, pregnancy
Defect	A small defect in the umbilical scar	Above or below the umbilicus
Symptoms	Symptomless	Symptoms are present
Strangulation	Rare	Very common
Treatment	Conservative (strapping), surgery (rare)	Mayo's repair

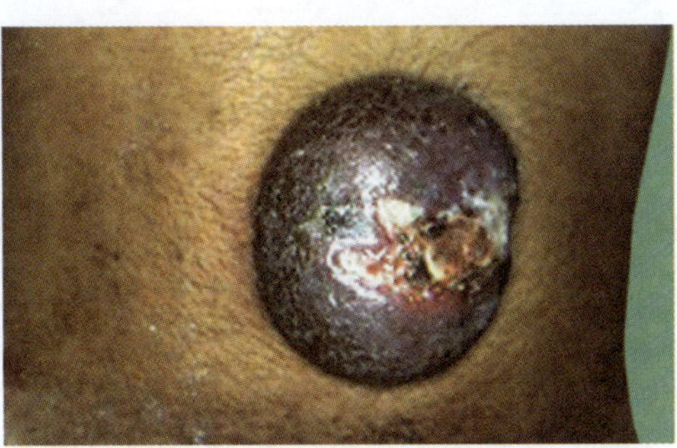

Fig. 52.51: Umbilical hernia in a cirrhotic patient with skin changes and ulceration

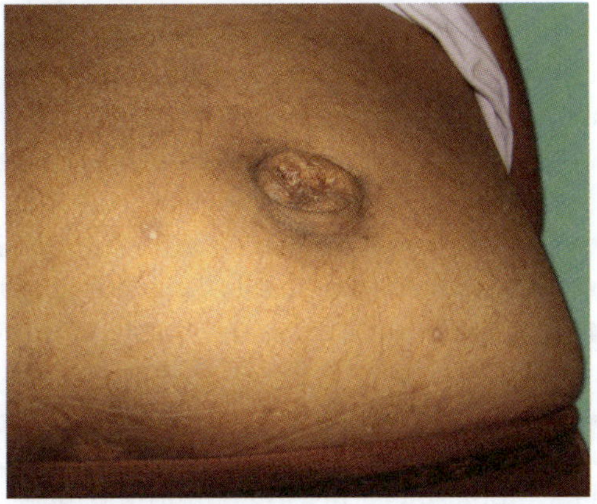

Fig. 52.52: True congenital umbilical hernia in an adult can be repaired by simple closure of the defect by non-absorbable sutures

3. **Most favoured** surgery for umbilical hernia is laparoscopic **mesh repair**—IPOM (intraperitoneal onlay mesh repair). It is a tensionless repair. It can also be done by **laparoscopic method** which is popular today. However, cost of the mesh and tackers for laparoscopic repair is a limiting factor especially in unaffordable patient.
4. ***Mayo's repair*** (surgical treatment, Fig. 52.53 and Key Box 52.15). Not done nowadays. In case of obstruction or strangulation, some surgeons may do this whereas others prefer anatomical closure.

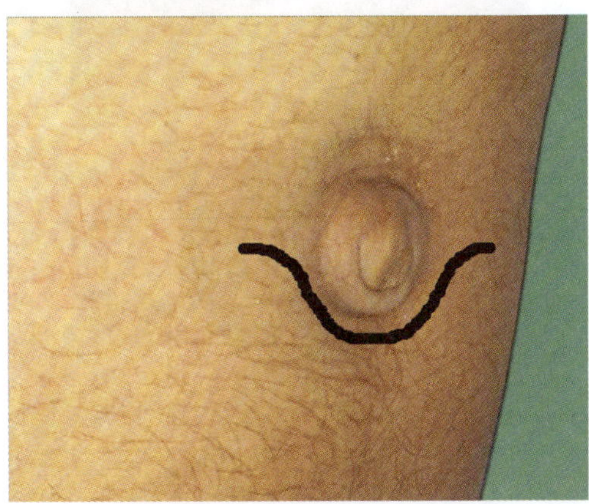

Fig. 52.53: Curvilinear incision

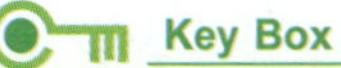

Key Box 52.15

Mayo's Umbilical Herniorrhaphy

- Excision of umbilicus
- Reduction of contents and excision of the sac
- Double breasting of the fibrous aponeurotic layer
- Haemostasis, suction and obliteration of dead space
- Additional lipectomy and umbilicoplasty

INCISIONAL HERNIA

Competency

SU28.1.16: Describe classification of ventral hernias and clinical presentation and indications for surgical management of various ventral hernias.

It is also called **ventral hernia** or postoperative hernia. It is a hernia that occurs through a weak scar. Very common in females.

ABDOMINAL WALL—SURGICAL ANATOMY

Contents

It consists of **skin, muscles, aponeurosis, linea alba, sheaths, ligaments, openings—rings**, blood vessels and nerves. Anatomically weak areas are the rings, junctions, empty spaces and where blood vessels pierce abdominal wall.

Formation of Rectus Sheath (Fig. 52.54)

A. Above the costal margin, only external oblique with aponeurosis contributes for rectus sheath.

B. Between xiphisternum and umbilicus, external oblique is in front. Internal oblique splits to enclose the rectus muscles. The transverse abdominis is behind the internal oblique. All fuse to form linea alba in the midline. Hence, this is the strong midline area.

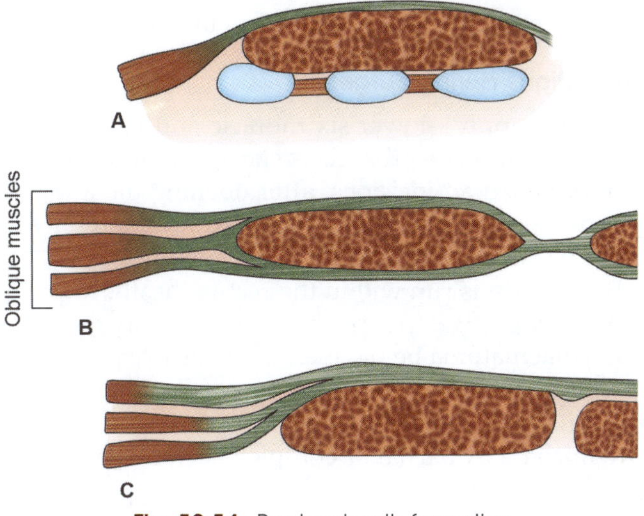

Fig. 52.54: Rectus sheath formation

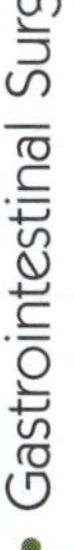

C. Below semilunar line: All 3 aponeuroses are anterior to the muscles and fuse in the midline to form linea alba.

Significance

- Rectus sheath—posterior rectus sheath is absent below semilunar line. Incisional hernia and spigelian hernia are common below the umbilicus.
- Linea alba—white, relatively avascular, broad above and narrow below. It is the strongest layer of the abdominal wall. Hence, during the closure of the midline incisions, it is important to include good bites through linea alba.
- Umbilicus—strong fibrous ring. Umbilical hernias are common in children due to childhood umbilical infections, in obese patients due to weak muscles and in multiparous woman due to stretching of the muscles due to repeated pregnancies.

MUSCLES OF THE ANTEROLATERAL ABDOMINAL WALL—OBLIQUE MUSCLES

- The anterolateral abdominal wall is made up mainly of muscles. On either side of the midline, there are four large muscles. These are the *external oblique*, the *internal oblique*, the *transversus abdominis* and the *rectus abdominis*. Two small muscles, the *cremaster* and the *pyramidalis* are also present. The external oblique, the internal oblique and the transversus abdominis are large flat muscles placed in the anterolateral part of the abdominal wall. Each of them ends in an extensive aponeurosis that reaches the midline. Here the aponeuroses of the right and left sides decussate to form a median band called *linea alba*. The rectus abdominis runs vertically on either side of the linea alba. It is enclosed in a *sheath* formed by the aponeuroses of the flat muscles named above.
- Tendinous intersections—rectus sheath haematoma will be confined within the sheaths as it is prevented from spreading due to tendinous intersections.

Precautions during Surgery

- Nerve supply—lower six thoracic and first lumbar nerves. They enter the rectus sheath laterally. In cases of paramedian incisions, after opening the anterior rectus sheath, rectus should be retracted laterally to define and incise the posterior rectus sheath.
- Blood vessels run within the rectus sheath. Rupture of inferior epigastric artery is a known entity resulting in a haematoma below the umbilicus (*see* page 975). Differential diagnosis includes spigelian hernia.
- Weak muscles—interstitial hernias—prune-belly syndrome: A partial or complete lack of abdominal muscles. There may be wrinkly folds of skin covering the abdomen. An undescended testicle in males can also be the problem.

FACTORS WHICH PRECIPITATE INCISIONAL HERNIA

(Key Box 52.16)

1. **Infection:** Cases operated for peritonitis such as perforated duodenal ulcer, gangrene of the intestines, etc. usually develop incisional hernia. The drainage tubes which are placed inside the peritoneal cavity help in reducing the postoperative incisional hernias, by draining peritoneal contents outside.
2. **Anatomical site:** The midline[1] is especially weak in the lower abdomen because of absence of posterior rectus sheath below the arcuate line or semilunar line.
3. **Obesity with weak muscle tone** predisposes to incisional hernia.
4. **Faulty technique** of closure of the abdomen or **faulty sutures** are also responsible for incisional hernia.
5. **Ascites, distension and persistent postoperative cough** further weakens the incision.
6. **Wrongly placed incisions** wherein nerves of the abdominal muscles are cut, precipitate incisional hernia. Lumbar incisions, lower midline incisions and large transverse incisions often give rise to incisional hernias (Figs 52.55 to 52.59).

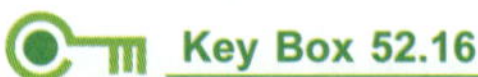

Key Box 52.16

Causes of Incisional Hernia

- Infection uncontrolled
- Incision wrongly placed
- Improper suture material
- Increased intra-abdominal pressure

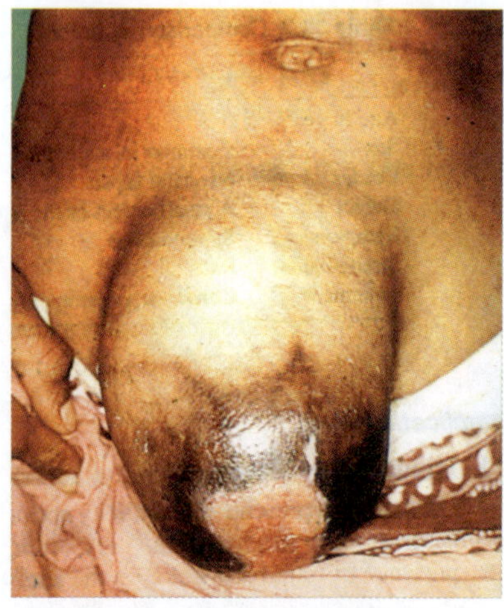

Fig. 52.55: Incisional hernia with decubitus ulcer due to obesity and weak muscle tone

[1]Is that the reason why we see many cases of incisional hernia after gynaecological operations?

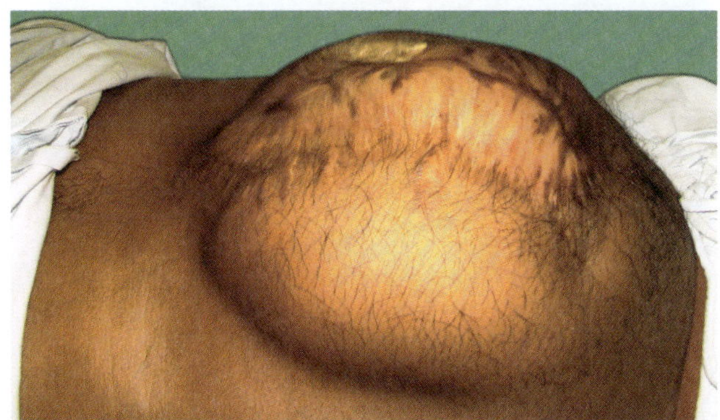

Fig. 52.56: Incisional hernia following laparotomy for perforated duodenal ulcer. He had stormy postoperative period

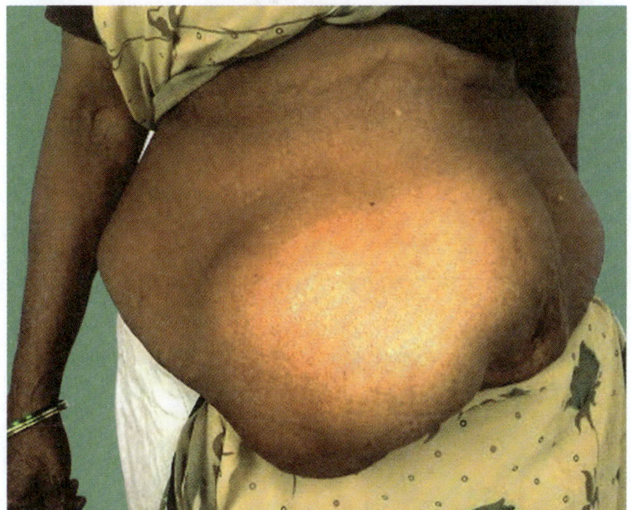

Fig. 52.57: Incisional hernia—large. (*Courtesy:* Late Dr Manjunath Shenoy, Professor, Department of Surgery, JSS Medical College and University, Mysuru)

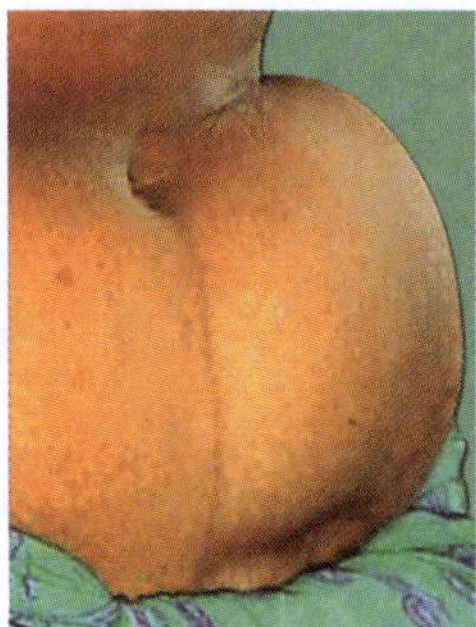

Fig. 52.58: Incisional hernia—sac towards left side

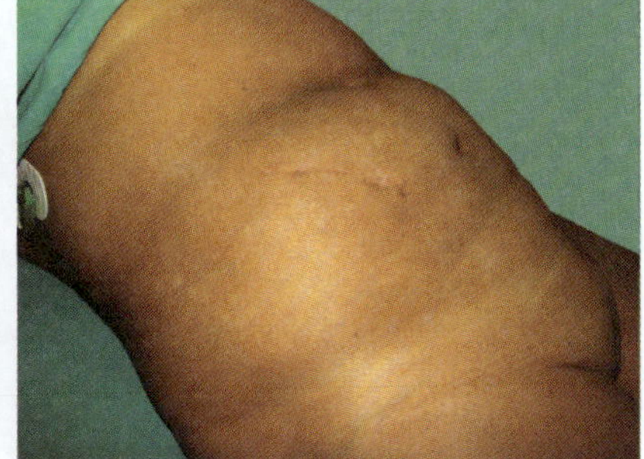

Fig. 52.59: Appendicectomy—incisional hernia

7. **Incisions** wherein nerves are cut, the chances of incisional hernias are more. Examples: Subcostal incision for removal of gallbladder.

Clinical Features

- Serosanguineous discharge on the 4th postoperative day through the main suture line is a signal of development of partial or total wound dehiscence. Such cases later develop an incisional hernia.
- History of infection during the first surgery, postoperative cough is usually present.
- There is a bulge/swelling in relation to the scar.
- Scar is thin and evidence of secondary healing in the form of irregular scar may be present.
- Expansile impulse on cough and reducibility may be present.
- After reduction of the contents, a defect can be palpated through the scar. Defect depends upon number of stitches that have given way.

Treatment

- Surgical treatment is necessary if the **defect is narrow,** if there is **discomfort** to the patient or if there is a **danger** of obstruction (Figs 52.60 to 52.62).
- Preoperative preparation includes reduction of weight, control of cough, etc.
- There are various operations for the treatment of incisional hernia depending upon the size of the defect, anatomical location of the incision and presence of precipitating factors.

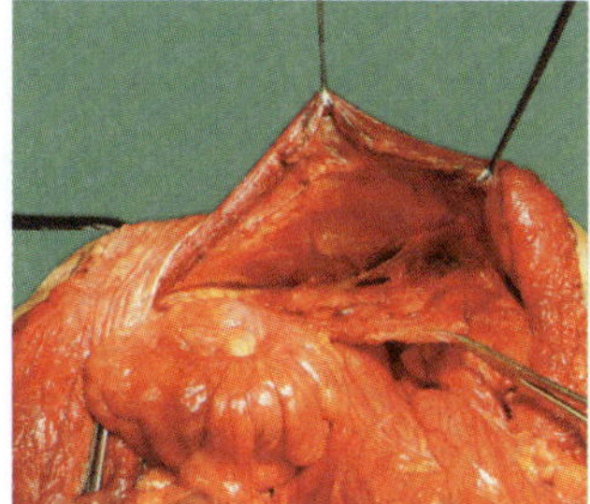

Fig. 52.60: Anatomical repair

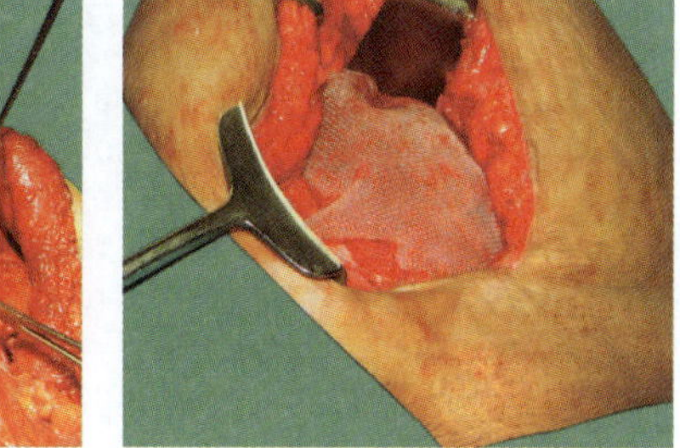

Fig. 52.61: Incisional hernia mesh repair

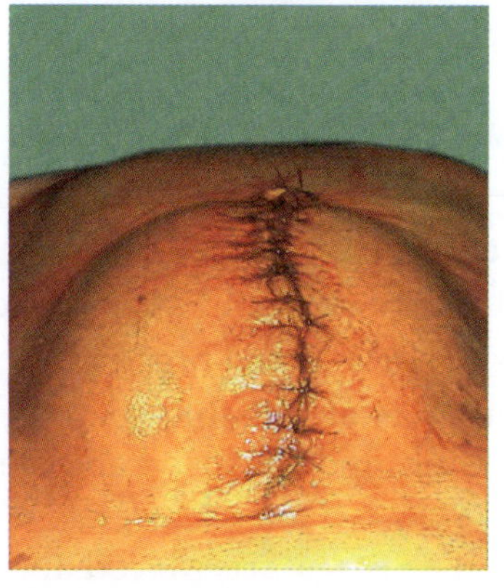

Fig. 52.62: Seroma after incisional hernia

1. Anatomical Repair

In this operation, all the anatomical layers such as peritoneum, posterior rectus sheath, linea alba and the subcutaneous tissue are identified. Closure is done layer by layer by using nonabsorbable suture material.

2. Mesh Repair (Fig. 52.64 and refer to Principles also)

- As most of the incisional hernias are due to a large defect in the main incision and the majority of it occurs in obese women, repair using mesh has become the most popular method. **Mesh repair is considered as the best repair, especially in obese, multiparous female patients with poor muscle tone.**
- In this operation, the sac is opened, greater omentum is excised, the contents are reduced followed by closure of the peritoneum. A mesh is then placed. Prolene mesh or Marlex mesh is commonly used. **In all these repairs, tensionless, nonabsorbable suture repairs are done.** Seroma is a common complication (Fig. 52.62).

Principles

- Previous incision is opened to full length and the scar is excised
- Flaps are raised on both sides
- The edges of rectus abdominis muscles are defined
- The sac is identified, dissected, freed from surrounding structures
- It is opened, contents reduced, may have to excise omentum
- Redundant sac is excised
- Peritoneum is closed
- Placement of the mesh: Onlay means subcutaneous. It is a simple procedure. Mesh should overlap at least 5 cm all around the defect. Alternately, plane is created between posterior rectus sheath and rectus muscle, mesh is placed in that location and anterior rectus sheath is sutured. This is called retromuscular sublay mesh repair. This may not be possible below the arcuate line because there is no posterior rectus sheath there.

3. Laparoscopic Mesh Repair

This is the procedure of choice today.

- It is increasingly used nowadays.
- Major advantage is minimal scars, minimal pain, early recovery.
- It gives an excellent exposure from within.
- One can define all the defects properly.
- Reduce all the contents and a broad sac.
- Defect can be sutured and broad mesh is placed.
- Mesh which has absorbable surface will face the peritoneal cavity and nonabsorbable surface will face abdominal wall.
- Transfascial sutures are placed to fix the mesh (Figs 52.63 to 52.67).

Major disadvantage is cost of mesh and tackers

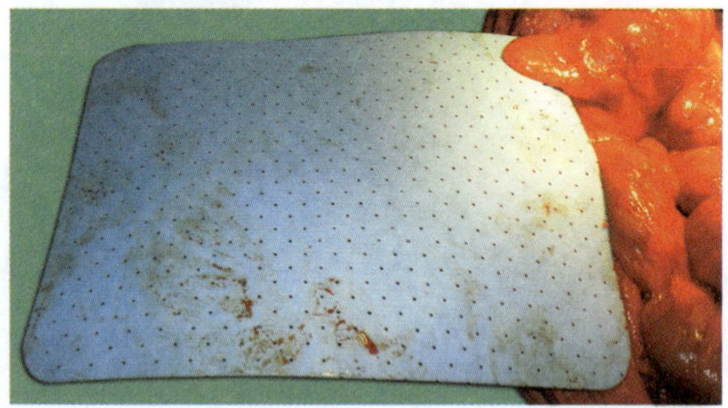

Fig. 52.63: Dual mesh

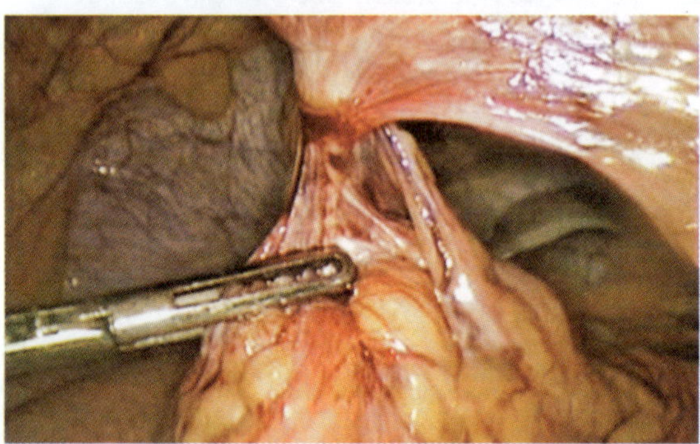

Fig. 52.64: Laparoscopic release of omentum from the hernial sac

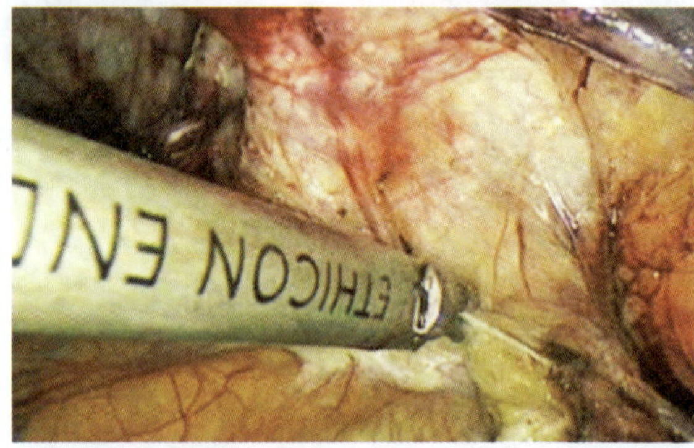

Fig. 52.65: Laparoscopic mobilisation of the sac

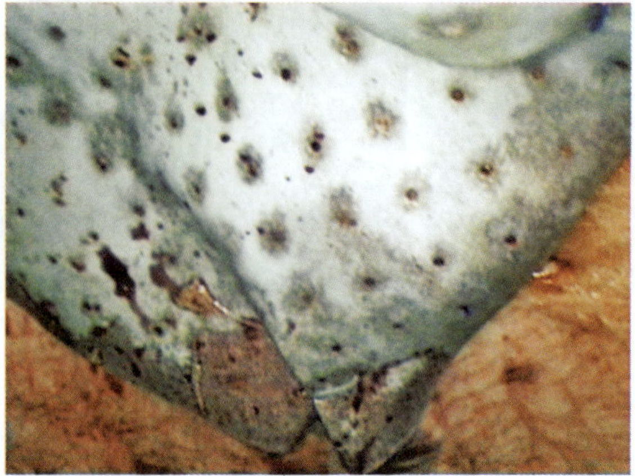

Fig. 52.66: Laparoscopic dual mesh has been kept in place and sutured

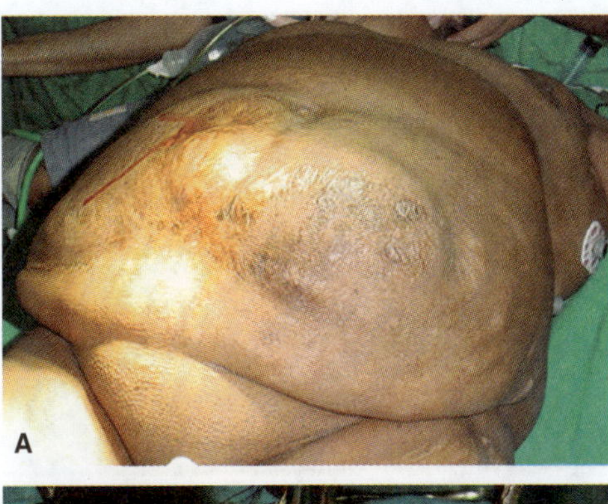

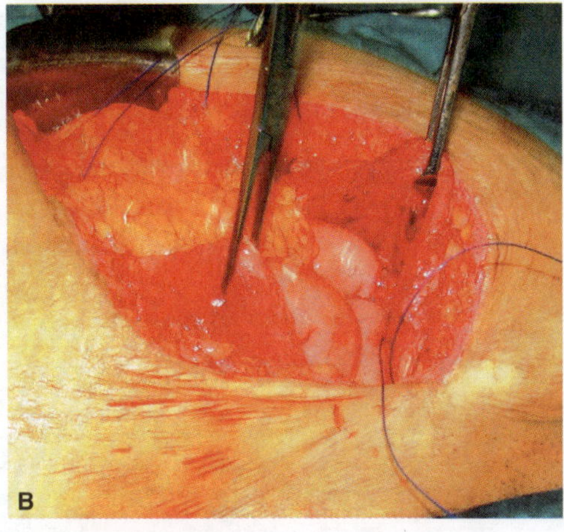

Figs 52.67A and B: Three times operated case of incisional hernia, repair is being done

Following advice or techniques are followed before taking up these cases:

1. Fitness for surgery
2. Chest physiotherapy
3. Reduction of weight
4. Deep vein thrombosis prophylaxis by using low molecular weight heparin.
5. Progressive pneumoperitoneum over weeks.
6. Additional lipectomy, removal of colon, omentectomy may have to be done.
7. *Ramirez component separation technique*: In this, relaxing incisions are given in the external oblique aponeurosis or rectus sheath so that they can be brought together and stitched together because in these cases, muscles are widely separated.

MANAGEMENT OF MASSIVE ABDOMINAL WALL HERNIAS

Massive or giant ventral hernia poses a challenge to the surgeon in appropriate management and to the patient by incapacitating him to live with poor quality of life. There is no consensus on standard definition but most surgeons agree that giant or massive ventral hernias are those having more than 10 cm defect size with loss of domain. Giant ventral hernias can arise due to:

1. Primary hernias which are left unattended for a long time.
2. Recurrence after one or more failed hernia repairs.
3. Result of open abdomen or laparostomy. The contents in such cases may be multiple bowel loops or other viscera which protrude outside the abdominal cavity causing "second abdomen" due to muscle retraction on either side of the defect.

In such a clinical scenario, the standard repair becomes an impossible proposition. Closing the abdomen with tension is not an option because it causes cardiorespiratory embarrassment and later, lateral recurrence of hernia due to disruption of linea semilunaris.

The most critical issue in the management is to optimize these patients before posting them for surgery and to do a good counselling about the difficulties involved in such cases. The patient needs a thorough clinical examination not only of the hernia but rest of the abdomen and the whole body. Putting the abdominal muscles into contraction by head raising and leg raising test, asking the patient to cough in lying down position and again examination in standing position will give a fair knowledge of the loss of domain, reducibility and defect size. Loss of domain (LOD) means a significant amount of viscera has herniated through the abdominal wall into the sac and more viscera may be outside than inside the abdominal cavity. Imaging by CT scan is essential to assess the defect size, status of viscera, abdominal wall musculature and any other intra-abdominal pathology. If the surgeon is inexperienced or the center is not well equipped to manage such patients, then the patient needs to be referred to a higher centre.

Such patients should stop smoking for at least 3 months prior to surgery and any remote infections should be treated. Diabetic patients need good glycemic control with HbA1c around 6.5% and they should not have any chronic liver disease. If there are any precipitating factors such as chronic cough, constipation or difficulty in passing urine, they should be corrected before surgery. Incentive spirometry and breathing exercises must be commenced prior to planned surgery.

If the patient is morbidly obese, the BMI needs to be reduced to around 35 kg/m^2. Some patients will require bariatric surgery (e.g. sleeve gastrectomy) as a first step and later definitive surgery for ventral hernia once the patient attains acceptable BMI.

There are two methods to optimize patients with loss of domain so that the capacity of the abdominal cavity increases and they do not develop cardiorespiratory embarrassment when the contents are pushed in during repair of ventral hernia.

1. Botulinum toxin (type A) injection to abdominal wall muscles.
2. Preoperative progressive pneumoperitoneum.

Botulinum toxin injected 4 weeks prior to surgery under ultrasound guidance on either side to abdominal wall muscles in anterior axillary line will cause temporary flaccid paralysis making midline closure possible. Similarly, progressively distending the abdomen with air for 10 to 14 days through an indwelling catheter inserted to abdominal cavity will facilitate reinsertion of bowel loops into abdominal cavity.

Once the abdominal cavity is sufficiently expanded by above methods and contents from the sac have returned to abdominal cavity, the patient is ready for definitive procedure. This can be confirmed by CT scan.

The aim of surgery is to correct the abdominal wall weakness by moving tissues medially by redistributing the abdominal muscles. A dynamic and durable repair is obtained with midline closure and reinforcement of abdominal wall with a large polypropylene mesh. Every precaution to prevent mesh infection is mandatory.

Most commonly performed surgery in massive ventral hernias is the open posterior component separation technique (PCST) or also known as transverse abdominal muscle release (TAR) which may be done on one side or on both sides for a tension-free midline closure. This can also be performed by robotic or laparoscopic (eTEP-TAR) method. Anterior component separation technique (ACST) is another way to achieve midline closure in massive ventral hernias. During emergency situations such as obstruction or gangrene, a staged repair strategy is adopted to deal with the emergency in first surgery and plan for hernia repair after a few months (Figs 52.68 to 52.70).

To conclude, the management of massive or giant ventral hernia requires a carefully planned approach with adequate optimization prior to surgery and a tension-free midline closure by component separation technique with reinforcement by a nonabsorbable mesh to achieve good results.

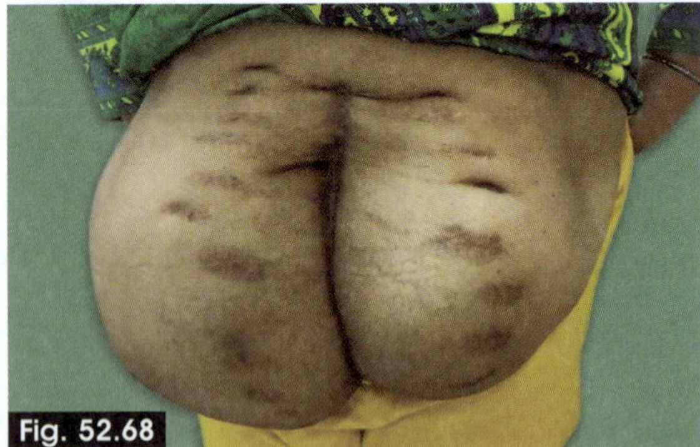

Fig. 52.68

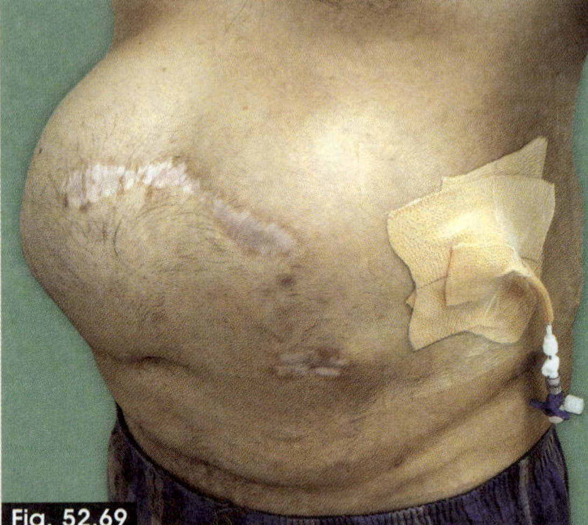

Fig. 52.69

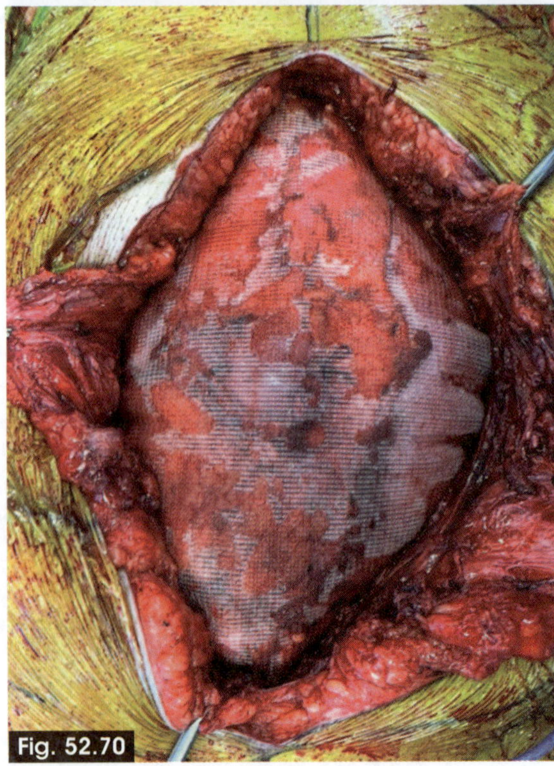

Fig. 52.70

Figs 52.68 to 52.70: Massive incisional hernia repaired by component separation and mesh repair. (*Courtesy:* Dr HV Shivaram, Consultant Surgeon, Aster Hospital, Bangalore, Karnataka)

EPIGASTRIC HERNIA

- It is also called **fatty** hernia of the linea alba.
- This type of hernia occurs in the epigastrium through the linea alba which extends between the xiphoid process and umbilicus.

Precipitating Factors

Sudden straining or heavy exercise results in the tearing of a few fibres of linea alba and is responsible for precipitating an epigastric hernia. Initially there is a small protrusion of extraperitoneal pad of fat. Rarely, if it enlarges, it is due to the dragging of the peritoneal sac. The opening is very narrow. Hence, the hollow viscus cannot enter the sac. Diastasis of rectus muscles which results in a wide linea alba can also precipitate an epigastric hernia.

Clinical Features

- Common in muscular men, manual labourers.
- Typically the swelling is situated in the upper abdomen midway between xiphoid process and umbilicus. Often, it contains only an extraperitoneal protrusion of fat (Fig. 52.71).
- An expansile impulse on cough is rare.
- Dull aching pain is due to the fatty contents which are partially strangulated. However, tenderness is an important feature of epigastric hernia (Key Box 52.17).
- Many cases are associated with peptic ulcer disease.
- On head-raising, it becomes more prominent (Fig. 52.72).

Treatment

A small incision is made over the swelling and the fatty tissue is isolated. It is ligated and excised because usually a tiny blood vessel enters the pad of fat. If a hernial sac is present, it is opened, the contents are reduced and the defect is closed using nonabsorbable sutures (Fig. 52.73).

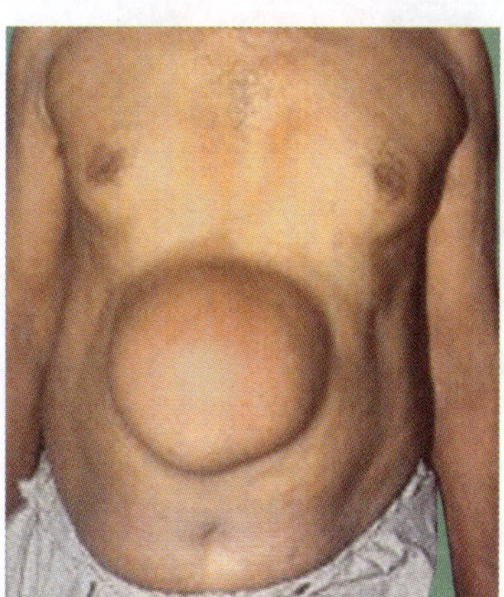

Fig. 52.71: Epigastric hernia

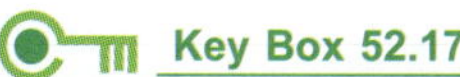

Key Box 52.17

Peculiarities of Epigastric Hernia

- Common in muscular men
- Hernial sac is uncommon
- Hollow viscus in the sac is rare
- Impulse on cough is rare
- Reducibility is rare
- Tenderness is an important feature

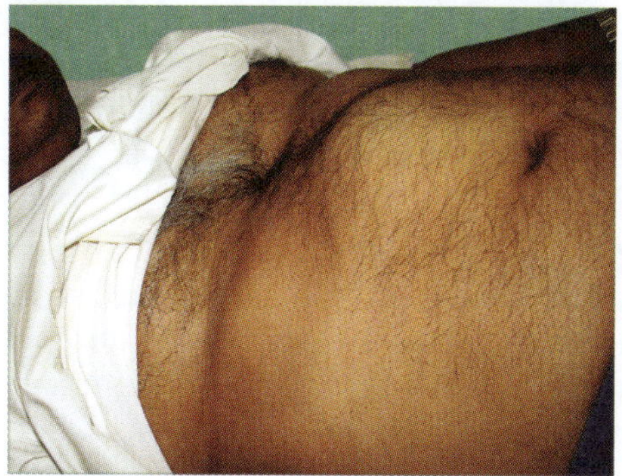

Fig. 52.72: Epigastric hernia: On head-raising, it becomes more prominent (head-raising test)

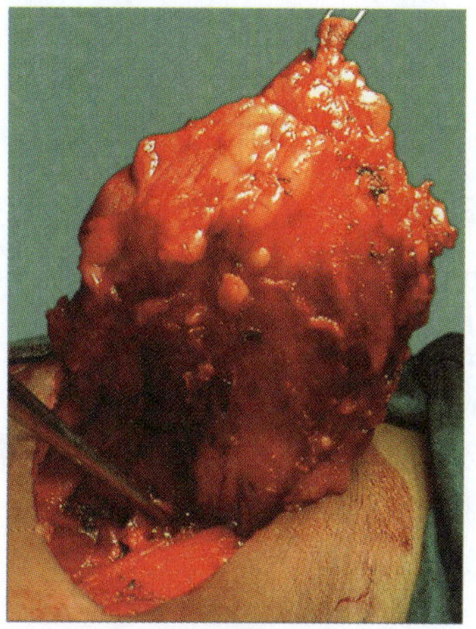

Fig. 52.73: Epigastric hernia sac

RARE EXTERNAL HERNIAS

Competency

SU28.1.17: Describe special hernias—spigelian, lumbar, obturator, perineal, sciatic and paranormal hernias and etiology, clinical presentation, various surgical approaches and techniques in their management.

INTERPARIETAL HERNIA

- It is also known as interstitial hernia.
- Basically, they are inguinal hernias. However, the processus vaginalis sac instead of following the normal route into the scrotum, traverses between various layers of the abdominal wall (parietes) resulting in interstitial hernias.
- Patients with Down's syndrome and prune-belly syndrome are commonly affected.

Types

1. **Preperitoneal:** In this variety, the hernial sac lies between the transversalis fascia and peritoneum. It is seen in about 20% of patients. The sac is like a small diverticulum.

2. **Interparietal:** It is also called intermuscular type. It is the commonest variety wherein the sac passes between the external oblique and internal oblique muscles. The swelling caused by the hernial sac causes discomfort to the patient. Sometimes, this can be a bilocular sac.
3. **Extraparietal:** It is also known as inguino-superficial variety. In this variety, the hernial sac passes exterior (superficial) to the external oblique aponeurosis beneath superficial fascia of the abdominal wall. It is commonly associated with undescended testis or ectopic testis.
   - Majority of such cases present with features of intestinal obstruction.
   - They are treated by identifying the sac, excision followed by closure of the defect or repair by using nonabsorbable sutures.

SPIGELIAN HERNIA[1]

- It is an interstitial hernia which occurs through the Spigelian fascia. This is a thin strip of fascia which runs parallel to the outer border of rectus sheath from the tip of the 9th costal cartilage to the pubic tubercle.
- Since it is very wide in the region of umbilicus/arcuate line, Spigelian hernias occur commonly at this level.
- Spigelian fascia contributes a few fibres to form rectus sheath.

Spigelian belt

- It is a 6 cm horizontal transverse zone located within umbilicus and the two anterior superior iliac spines.
- Starts as a direct protrusion behind rectus abdominis.
- They are intramural; sac penetrates across transverse muscles and lies behind external oblique muscles.

Precipitating Factors

Repeated pregnancies, advancing age, obesity, muscular degeneration, sudden strain due to coughing, weight lifting, etc. give rise to Spigelian hernias.

Clinical Features

- Seen in both sexes equally around 50 years of age.
- A round, soft, reducible swelling situated just below and lateral to the umbilicus—located typically at the junction of the arcuate line and lateral border of rectus abdominis. Sometimes, it is tender.
- The swelling gives rise to an expansile impulse on cough.
- As the hernia enlarges, it insinuates between external and internal oblique muscle. Hence, it is an example for interparietal hernia (Figs 52.74 to 52.77).

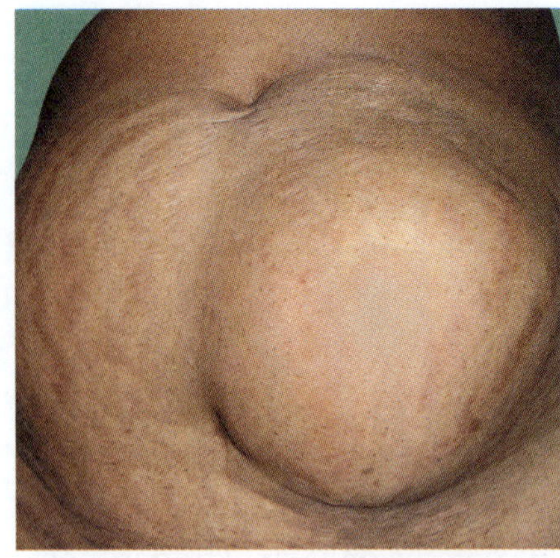

Fig. 52.74: Obstructed Spigelian hernia in a 70-year-old lady— first presentation to the hospital

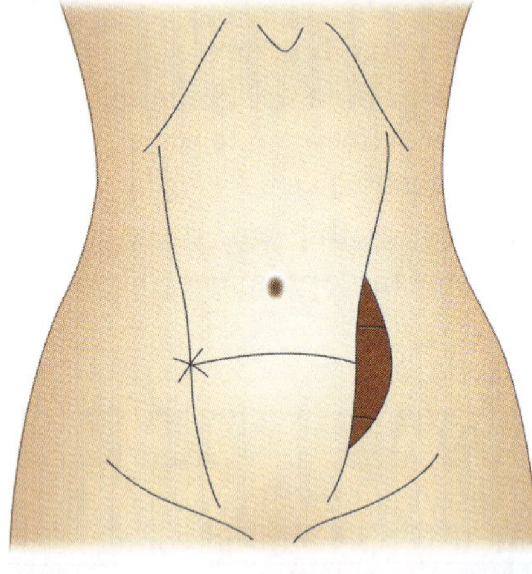

Fig. 52.75: Spigelian fascia and the site of hernia

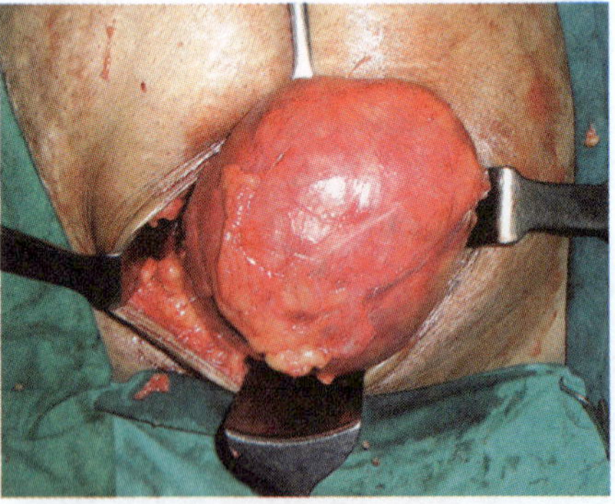

Fig. 52.76: Delivery of the sac

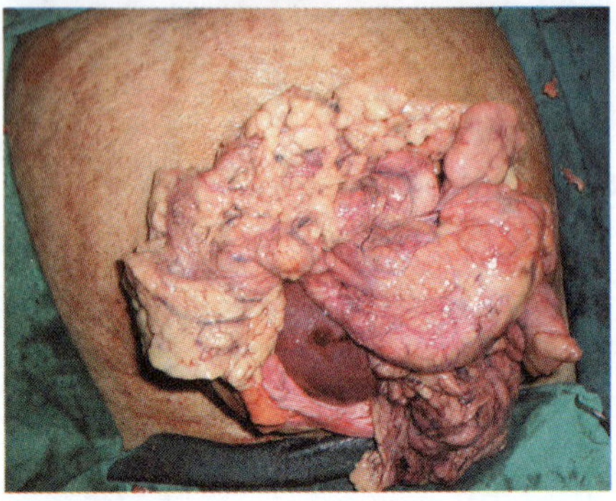

Fig. 52.77: Contents of the sac

(*Courtesy:* Prof MG Shenoy and Dr Prasad, KMC, Manipal, Figs 52.76 and 52.77)

[1]Prof Spigel, Professor of Anatomy and Surgery, not only described Spigelian fascia but also the caudate lobe of the liver.

Investigations

1. An ultrasound can define the defect in the semilunar line.
2. X-ray abdomen, lateral view shows coils of bowel outside the peritoneal cavity.

Differential Diagnosis

- Haematoma within the rectus sheath. However, it will not give rise to impulse on cough. It occurs suddenly and it will be a tender swelling.
- Pyogenic or pyaemic abscess can occur in the abdominal wall, more so, in diabetic patients. Tenderness and high temperature clinches the diagnosis.

Complication

Strangulation is common due to the rigid fascial ring surrounding the hernial sac. Richter's hernia also can occur here.

Treatment

An incision of about 5 to 6 cm is made over the swelling and abdominal wall muscles are split or cut. The sac is excised after reducing the contents and the defect is repaired. Recurrence occurs in about 5% of the patients.

LUMBAR HERNIA

Two types of lumbar hernia are well-recognised. They are as follows:

1. **Primary** which occurs through an anatomical defect:
   - **Through the inferior lumbar triangle of Petit.** Its boundaries are:
     Inferiorly: Iliac crest
     Laterally: External oblique
     Medially: Latissimus dorsi
   - **Through the superior lumbar triangle of Grynfeltt.** Its boundaries are (Fig. 52.78)
     Above: 12th rib
     Medially: Sacrospinalis
     Laterally: Internal oblique
2. **Secondary** to a renal operation done through a loin incision. It is an example of a *lumbar incisional hernia*, which occurs due to either infection or weakness of loin muscles. The operation done for tuberculosis of spine through a loin incision, very often gives rise to a secondary lumbar hernia (it is an incisional hernia) (Fig. 52.79).

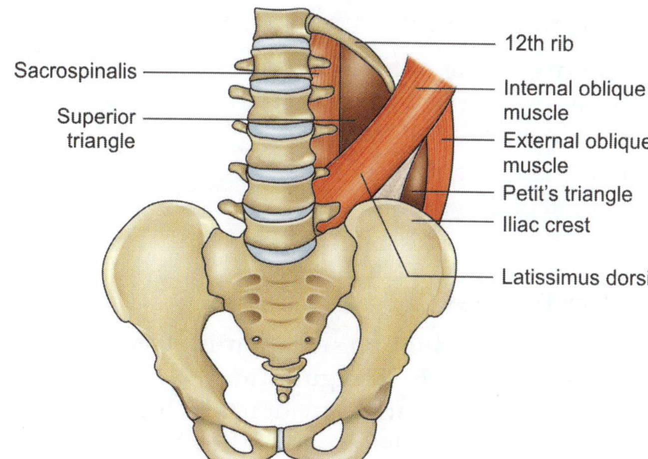

Fig. 52.78: Petit's triangle

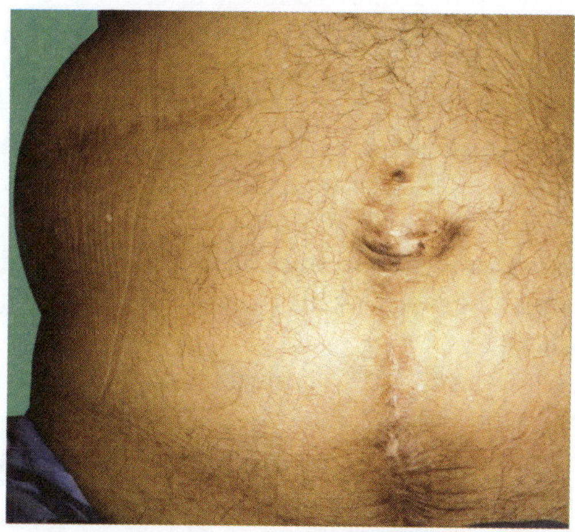

Fig. 52.79: Lumbar hernia

Differential Diagnosis

1. **Lipoma** is common in the lumbar region (loin). It is soft, lobular, and slips under the palpating fingers.
2. **Cold abscess** secondary to tuberculosis of the spine gives rise to a nontender swelling in the paravertebral space. Tenderness is present over the spine which gives a clue to the diagnosis. Patients may have deformity of the spine in the form of gibbus.

Treatment

Small defects can be closed with simple sutures. Large defects need to be closed with or without mesh.

> *Pearls of Wisdom*
>
> Primary lumbar hernias are very rare.

OBTURATOR HERNIA

- This hernia occurs through the obturator canal which is bounded above by the superior ramus of pubis and below by the sharp edge of the obturator membrane.
- As the hernia is covered by the pectineus muscle, it is often overlooked.

Precipitating Factors

- In females, the **obturator foramen** is wider in the transverse direction (it is triangular in shape in females and oval in males).
- Repeated pregnancies
- Loss of body weight
- Chronic lung diseases

Clinical Features

- The **most common presentation** is acute intestinal obstruction **with strangulation** (80%). Recurrent attacks of intestinal obstruction which get resolved spontaneously is also common (Key Box 52.18).
- This hernia causes more pain than any other type of hernia. Pain often radiates along the obturator nerve and may even be referred to the knee *via* its geniculate branch called ***Howship-Romberg sign.*** The leg is usually kept in the *semiflexed position* and movement of the limb gives rise to pain. If the limb is flexed, abducted and rotated outwards, the hernia becomes prominent. Patients are usually over 60 years of age and women are more frequently affected than men.
- Due to strangulation and blood in the hernial sac, bruising is seen below the medial edge of the inguinal ligament.
- A few patients (20%) complain of palpable ***hernia mass*** in the groin.
- Per vaginal examination can reveal a tender lump on the lateral side of the vault.

Treatment

The constricting agent in case of obstruction is the **obturator fascia,** which needs to be divided. Nerves and vessels are posterolateral to the hernial sac. Since majority of the cases present with intestinal obstruction and strangulation, a lower laparotomy is done. A grooved director is used to divide the obturator fascia.

- The contents are reduced or if there is gangrene, the affected bowel is resected.
- Closure of the obturator opening is done by stitching the broad ligament over the opening or by using monofilament nylon.

Key Box 52.18

Obturator Hernia

- The most common presentation is not a swelling but acute intestinal obstruction
- Can present as only pain in the knee—(Howship-Romberg sign)
- Vaginal examination: Tender mass can be felt on the lateral side
- Very high chance of strangulation

PERINEAL HERNIA

These are very rare hernias which confuse many clinicians and present in different varieties. Hernia protrudes through muscles and fascia of the perineal floor.

1. **Anterolateral perineal hernia:** This occurs in women and presents as a swelling of the labium majus. Often, the patient is examined by a gynaecologist and Bartholin's cyst is diagnosed (Figs 52.80 and 52.81).
2. **Posterolateral perineal hernia:** This type of hernia passes through levator ani and enters ischiorectal fossa.
3. **Median sliding hernia** is nothing but complete prolapse of rectum.
4. **Postoperative hernia** through perineal scar, e.g. after abdominoperineal resection wherein rectum is removed.
   - It is also used to occur following perineal prostatectomy.

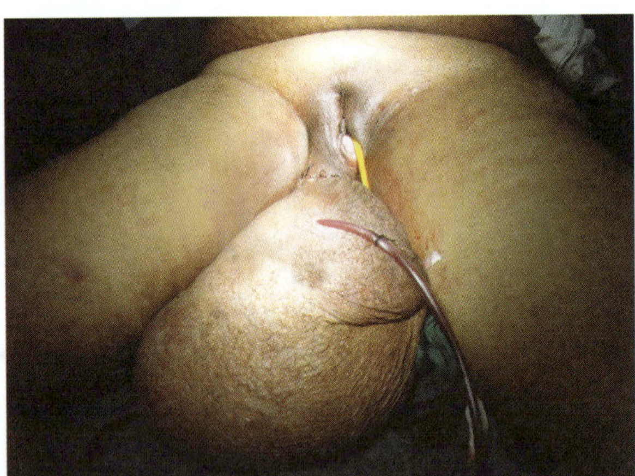

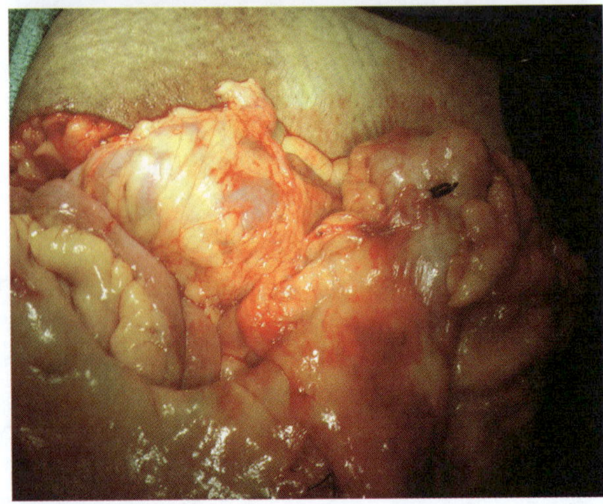

Figs 52.80 and 52.81: A 40-year-old lady with large perineal hernia was diagnosed to have a Bartholin's cyst and was explored by a gynaecologist. To his surprise, it had 3 feet of small intestine and portions of large intestines. It started bleeding and he kept a drain and referred the patient to our hospital

Clinical Features

They can present as asymptomatic swelling, pain, dysuria, bowel obstruction or perineal ulceration and bleeding.

Diagnosis

- Ultrasound can detect loops of bowel/fluid.
- CT scan/MRI can clearly define the course of hernia, its relationship with urinary bladder/ureter and its descent into the pelvis.

Repair

It can be very difficult in large hernias. Often a combined approach, both perineal and abdominal, may be necessary. Mesh repair with adequate fascial and muscular perineal repair is required (Fig. 52.82).

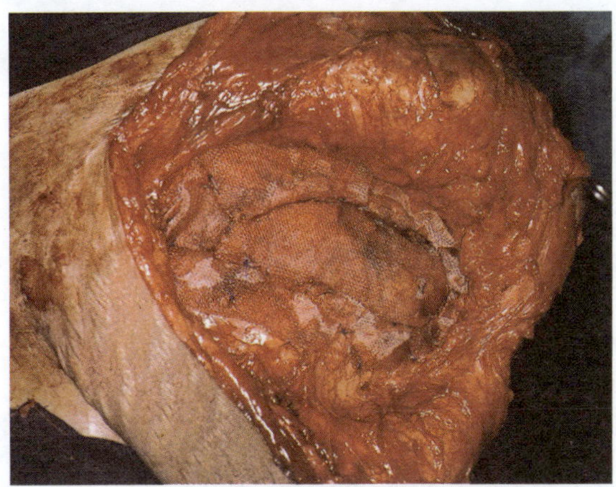

Fig. 52.82: Contents were reduced, sac was excised, a large mesh could be placed in the defect and sutured all around. Postoperatively she had urinary fistula. CT cystogram revealed bladder injury. It healed after two weeks

PARASTOMAL HERNIA (Fig. 52.83)

- It is an acquired condition/iatrogenic
- It is a complication of ileostomy/colostomy
- Herniation occurs from the side of colostomy/ileostomy and hence called parastomal hernia.

Devlin's Classification

1. **Subcutaneous:** It is the most common variety. It takes more time for obstruction.
2. **Interstital:** In this variety, herniation happens through intermuscular plane—between transversus abdominis and internal oblique muscles, etc.

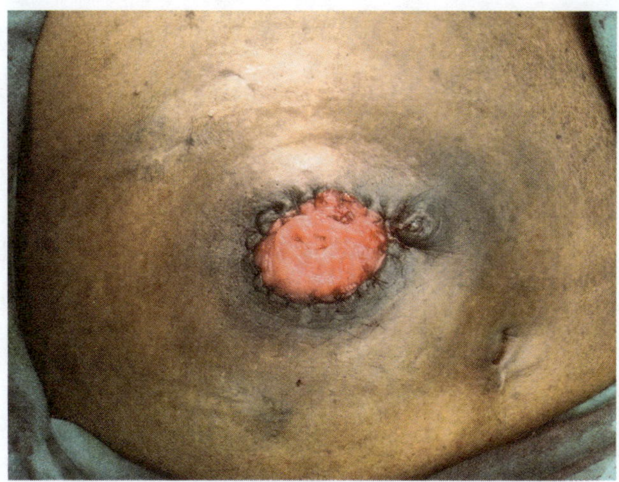

Fig. 52.83: Parastomal hernia. (*Courtesy:* Dr Vipin Goel, Surgical oncologist Indo American Cancer Hospital, Hyderabad)

3. **Intrastomal:** Here, the herniation occurs between emerging and everting part of the stoma.
4. **Perstomal:** In this variety, herniation occurs between layers of prolapsed stoma.

Clinical Features

- Patient complains of swelling on her side of ostomy, which increases/prolapses on coughing/straining, decreases at rest.
- Pain, irreducibility indicates obstruction.
- Tense and tender abdomen, pain indicates obstruction.

Diagnosis

CECT abdomen provides accurate diagnosis of the type of hernia.

Treatment

Contents are reduced, defects identified, broad mesh is placed over the intraperitoneal and parastomal defects and sutured by nonabsorbable sutures, and extraperitoneal meshes applied.

INTERNAL HERNIAS

These hernias occur intra-abdominally wherein the bowel protrudes through peritoneal or mesenteric aperture or foramen. They may cause obstruction. Examples are hiatus hernia and Petersen's hernia (occurs in space posterior to gastrojejunostomy).

Multiple Choice Questions

1. Length of inguinal canal is:
A. 4 cm B. 6 cm
C. 8 cm D. 10 cm

2. Which of the following is not a boundary of the Hesselbach's triangle?
A. Rectus abdominis
B. Inguinal ligament
C. Inferior epigastric artery
D. Testicular artery

3. Following are true about external ring *except*:
A. It is not a ring
B. It is a defect in the internal oblique aponeurosis
C. Invagination test is done through external ring
D. It transmits spermatic cord

4. About deep inguinal ring, which one of the following is true?
A. It is a defect in the external oblique aponeurosis
B. It is a defect in the internal oblique aponeurosis
C. It is a defect in the transversalis fascia
D. It is a defect in the cremasteric fascia

5. Following are true for deep inguinal ring *except*:
A. Deep ring is a defect in the transversalis fascia
B. Indirect hernial sac comes out lateral to the deep ring
C. Pantaloon hernia can be on both sides of deep ring
D. It is closed at the end of hernia repair to prevent recurrence

6. The ideal surgical treatment for sliding inguinal hernia will be:
A. Herniotomy B. Bassini's herniorrhaphy
C. Marsey's repair D. Lichtenstein's repair

7. Following are contents of the spermatic cord *except*:
A. Vas deferens
B. Testicular artery
C. Genital branch of genitofemoral nerve
D. Ilioinguinal nerve

8. About sliding inguinal hernia following are true *except*:
A. Urinary bladder can be the part of hernial sac
B. It can be both direct or indirect type
C. The hernial sac should be twisted as in indirect hernia treatment
D. Often it is irreducible

9. Richter's hernia refers to:
A. Hernia containing intestines
B. Strangulated hernia
C. Only a part of circumference of the intestine is caught in a hernial sac
D. Hernia containing urinary bladder

10. Immediate structure anterior to direct hernial sac is:
A. External oblique aponeurosis
B. Internal oblique aponeurosis
C. Transversalis facia
D. Posterior rectus sheath

11. Femoral hernia has following features *except*:
A. It is more common in women
B. It is below and lateral to pubic tubercle
C. It is known for strangulation
D. It can be managed by hernia truss

12. Diagnostic feature of a saphena varix is:
A. It is transilluminant
B. It is soft and reducible
C. It is below the pubic tubercle
D. Disappears on elevation of the leg

13. Which one of the following hernias is called Littre's hernia?
A. Hernia containing Meckel's diverticulum
B. Hernia containing urinary bladder
C. Hernia containing sigmoid colon
D. Hernia containing ovary

14. Which one of the following is the most important step in preventing recurrence of hernia?
A. Complete excision of cremasteric muscle
B. Reconstruction of the external ring
C. Reconstruction of the internal ring
D. High ligation of the sac

15. Following are true for strangulated inguinal hernia *except*:
A. It will be tense
B. Tender
C. Irreducible
D. Impulse on cough is present

16. Following are true for anatomy of the femoral canal *except*:

A. Femoral canal is the outermost compartment of femoral sheath

B. Femoral canal extends from femoral ring to saphenous ring

C. Femoral canal is below and lateral to pubic tubercle

D. Femoral canal contains lymph node of Cloquet

17. In obstructed femoral hernia, at surgery which of the following steps should not be done?

A. Best done with low approach through incision directly over the swelling

B. Closure of the ring is done by prolene suture material

C. Abnormal obturator artery should be looked for

D. Urinary bladder may be in danger

18. Following hernias are known for high chances of strangulation *except*:

A. Femoral hernia

B. Obturator hernia

C. Spigelian hernia

D. Direct hernia

19. In which condition femoral hernia occurs behind the femoral vessels?

A. Prune-belly syndrome

B. Poliomyelitis

C. Congenital dislocation of the hip

D. Defect in the lacunar ligament

20. In cases of epigastric hernia, all are true *except*:

A. It is more common in muscular men

B. Impulse on cough is common

C. Sac is uncommon

D. It is tender

21. Spigelian hernia, is an example for:

A. Direct hernia B. Indirect hernia

C. Interstitial hernia D. Type of femoral hernia

22. In Spigelian hernia swelling is seen:

A. Below and lateral to umbilicus

B. Below the umbilicus

C. Around the umbilicus

D. Just above the umbilicus

23. Differential diagnosis of lumbar hernia includes the following *except*:

A. Lipoma B. Cold abscess

C. Haematoma D. Meningocoele

24. Following are true for obturator hernia *except*:

A. Hernia is covered by pectineus muscle

B. Pain is radiated to the knee

C. Cannot be felt by vaginal examination

D. Patients keep their leg semiflexed

25. The most common presentation of obturator hernia is:

A. Groin swelling

B. Intestinal obstruction

C. Bruising below inguinal ligament

D. Tender mass on vaginal examination

Answers

1. A	**2.** D	**3.** B	**4.** C	**5.** D	**6.** D	**7.** D	**8.** C	**9.** C	**10.** C
11. D	**12.** D	**13.** A	**14.** D	**15.** D	**16.** A	**17.** A	**18.** D	**19.** C	**20.** B
21. C	**22.** A	**23.** D	**24.** A	**25.** B					

CHAPTER

53

Umbilicus and Abdominal Wall

- Classification of umbilical diseases
- Umbilical inflammation
- Umbilical fistulae
- Umbilical neoplasms
- Umbilical hernia
- Umbolith
- Abdominal dehiscence
- Divarication of recti
- Rectus sheath haematoma
- Meleney's gangrene
- Desmoid tumour
- Endometriosis

UMBILICUS—SURGICAL ANATOMY AND EMBRYOLOGY

Definition: The umbilicus is the normal scar in the anterior abdominal wall formed by the remnants of the root of the *umbilical cord.*

The position of the umbilicus is variable. In healthy adults, it lies in the anterior median line, at the level of the disc between the third and fourth lumbar vertebrae. It is lower in infants and in persons with a pendulous abdomen (Fig. 53.1, Tanyol's sign). It can be displaced upwards as in ovarian tumours (Fig. 53.2).

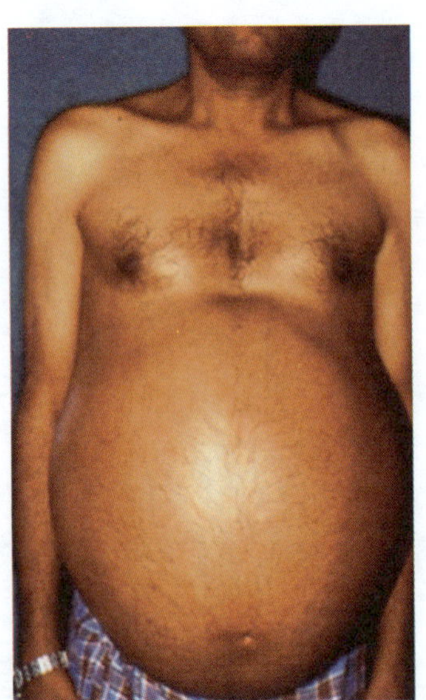

Fig. 53.1: Tanyol's sign

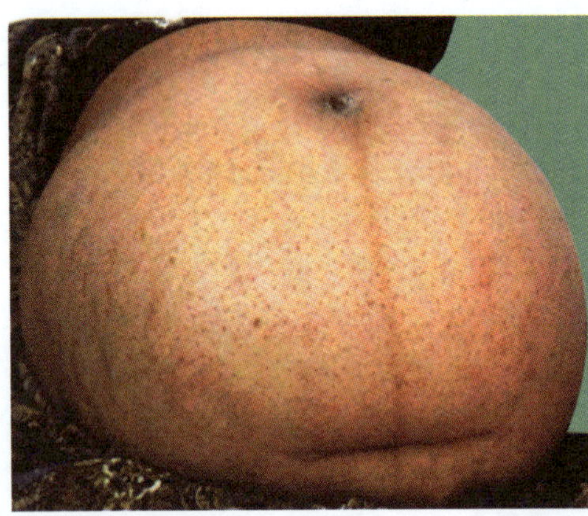

Fig. 53.2: Large ovarian tumour displacing umbilicus upwards

Apart from its embryological importance, there are several facts of interest about the umbilicus. These are given below.

Anatomical Importance

1. With reference to the lymphatic and venous drainage, the level of the umbilicus is a *watershed.* Lymph and venous blood flow upwards above the plane of the umbilicus; and downwards below this plane. These do not normally cross umbilical plane.
2. The skin around the umbilicus is supplied by segment T10 of the spinal cord.
3. The umbilicus is one of the important sites at which tributaries of the portal vein anastomose with

systemic veins (*portocaval anastomoses*). In portal hypertension, these anastomoses open up to form dilated veins radiating from the umbilicus called the *caput medusae.* However, the blood flow in the dilated veins is normal, and does not break the barrier of the watershed line.

Embryological Importance

1. Umbilicus is the meeting point of the four (two lateral, head and tail) folds of embryonic plate.
2. This is also the meeting point of three systems, namely the digestive (vitellointestinal duct), the excretory (urachus), and vascular (umbilical vessels).

CLASSIFICATION OF UMBILICAL DISEASES

- I. Inflammation
  - A. Omphalitis
  - B. Granuloma
  - C. Dermatitis
  - D. Pilonidal sinus
- II. Fistulae
  - **A. Faecal**
    1. Patent vitellointestinal duct (Key Box 53.1)
    2. Carcinoma transverse colon
    3. Tuberculous peritonitis
  - **B. Urinary:** Patent urachus
  - **C. Biliary**
- III. Neoplasms
  - **A. Benign**
    1. Adenoma: Raspberry tumour
    2. Endometrioma
  - **B. Malignant**
    1. Primary carcinoma
    2. Secondary carcinoma from: Stomach, colon, ovary, and breast
- IV. Umbilical hernia
- V. Umbilical calculus (umbolith)

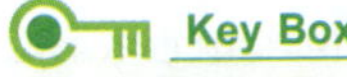
Key Box 53.1

Umbilical Cord Structures

In foetal life
- Umbilical vein
- Right and left umbilical arteries
- Urachus

In embryonic life
Vitellointestinal duct and structures mentioned above

UMBILICAL INFLAMMATION

A. Omphalitis

- Inflammation of the umbilical cord due to *Staphylococcus aureus* and streptococci occurs in the neonatal period 3–4 days after birth. The incidence is increased in hospital births.
- Rarely, gram-negative organisms and *Clostridium tetani* can cause omphalitis,[1] if strict aseptic precautions are not taken. If infection is not controlled, it can result in further complications.
  1. **Abscess of the abdominal wall:** Pus can be seen coming out of umbilicus. It may need drainage with antibiotic cover. Gentle squeezing will help, followed by antiseptic dressings and systemic antibiotics.
  2. **Extensive ulceration of the abdominal wall,** similar to Meleney's ulcer, is a rare complication (subcutaneous synergistic gangrene) of omphalitis.
  3. **Septicaemia** can occur due to organisms entering the umbilical vein and then into portal vein. This results in pylephlebitis with jaundice, fever, chills and rigors.
  4. **Neonatal jaundice** due to intrahepatic cholangitis.
  5. **Portal vein thrombosis** resulting in extrahepatic portal hypertension (prehepatic).
  6. **Umbilical hernia** can occur due to a weak scar produced by sepsis.

B. Granuloma

Granuloma indicates persisting inflammation underneath. It is a cause of great concern and worry to the patients. This can be destroyed by **application of copper sulphate or silver nitrate solution**.

C. Dermatitis

Dermatitis more often occurs in adults wherein chronic infection of the umbilicus sets in with foul smelling discharge.

D. Pilonidal Sinus

Umbilicus is a low area compared to the surface of abdominal wall. Hence, hairy men may shed their hair which accumulates in the umbilicus and may result in pilonidal sinus. It may need removal of sinus along with tuft of hair or rarely the umbilicus itself.

UMBILICAL FISTULAE

A. Faecal

1. **Persistent vitellointestinal duct** is an uncommon congenital anomaly. Many a time the intestinal

[1]Application of cowdung to the umbilical cord is still prevalent in a few places in our country. In addition to causing omphalitis, it can also cause neonatal tetanus.

opening is so small that only mucoid contents come out of umbilicus. Rarely, if the opening is big, omphaloenteric faecal fistula results.

2. **Internal hollow viscus malignancies,** especially carcinoma of the transverse colon can erode through umbilicus resulting in a faecal fistula.
3. **Tuberculous peritonitis** induces dense adhesions, strictures and perforations. A perforation which is sealed off by coils of matted bowel and omentum results in local abscess which may perforate through a weak point, i.e. umbilicus resulting in a faecobiliary fistula. If a diagnosis can be proved by wall biopsy of the sinus/fistula, antituberculous treatment can cure the disease. Laparotomy is extremely difficult in such cases. One may end up creating more holes in the bowel and is better avoided.

Pearls of Wisdom

One innocent disease (VI DUCT), one prevalent disease (TB) and one malignant disease (carcinoma bowel) are the causes of umbilical faecal fistula.

B. Patent Urachus (Fig. 53.3 and Key Box 53.2)

- The ventral urogenital sinus which forms the urinary bladder is continued cranially as urachus which extends into the umbilical cord—allantoic stalk. If this portion persists, patent urachus forms which connect umbilicus with urinary bladder. If it is fibrosed, as it occurs normally, it is called **median umbilical ligament**.

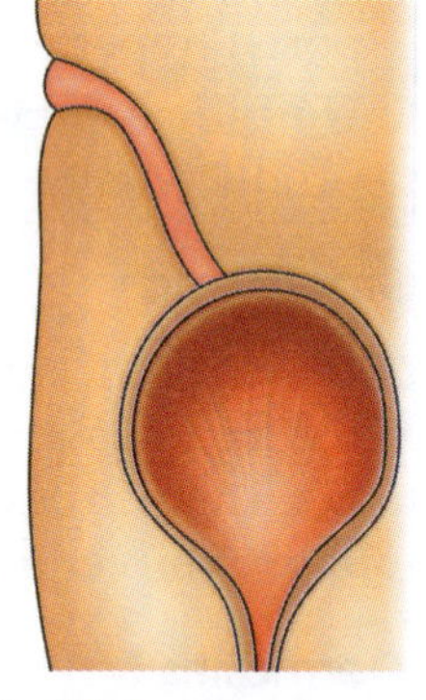

Fig. 53.3: Patent urachus

- A patent urachus may manifest as urinary discharge from umbilicus. It manifests usually in childhood and early adult life. In most cases, there will be some kind of obstruction to the normal passage of urine. Entire urachus is excised after correcting distal obstruction.

C. Biliary Fistula

Rarely, perforation of gallbladder due to severe form of cholecystitis may result in local abscess which may rupture through umbilicus resulting in biliary fistula. Instances are recorded wherein stones have come out of umbilicus.

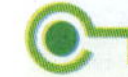 **Key Box 53.2**

Abnormalities of Urachus

- Patent urachus
- Urachal sinus
- Urachal cyst
- Urachal diverticulum

UMBILICAL NEOPLASMS

1. **Umbilical adenoma** is a pedunculated swelling having raspberry colour. Hence, the name **Raspberry tumour**.
   - It is due to unobliterated vitellointestinal duct.
   - Mucosa of the persistent duct prolapses through umbilicus and produces this adenoma.
   - It is moist with mucus and tends to bleed (columnar epithelium rich in goblet cells).

   Treatment
   - If the tumour is pedunculated, a ligature is tied around it and by a few days, the adenoma drops off.
   - If tumour reappears, excision of umbilicus is advised.
2. **Endometrioma** of umbilicus is rare but patients have a typical history to tell, i.e. it bleeds during menstruation.
3. **Malignant:** Secondary carcinomatous nodule in and around umbilicus reflects advanced malignancy commonly from stomach and colon. Ovary, uterus, breast are other causes. The nodule is tender, fixed and reddish in colour (Fig. 53.4). Figures 53.5 to 53.9 show some interesting diseases of umbilicus.

UMBILICAL HERNIA

Umbilicus is one of the weak points in the body. Hence, it is one of the sites of hernia. All the details of umbilical hernia have been discussed on page 953.

UMBOLITH

- It is composed of desquamated epithelium which becomes inspissated and gets collected in the umbilicus. With secondary infection, there will be blood-stained discharge. It is treated by controlling infection, debridement and, if necessary, removal of umbilicus.
- This umbolith or umbilical calculus is black in colour.

ABDOMINAL WALL

Introduction

Abdominal wall consists of skin, muscles, aponeurosis, linea alba, sheaths, ligaments, openings, rings, blood vessels and nerves. Thus it is complex structure. Anatomical weak areas are rings, junctions, empty spaces, blood vessel piercing, etc. Weakness of these structures results in hernias.

SOME INTERESTING DISEASES OF UMBILICUS

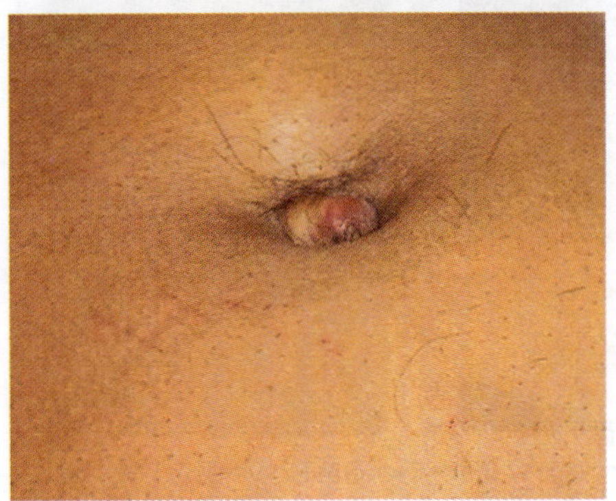
Fig. 53.4: Sister Mary Joseph's nodule

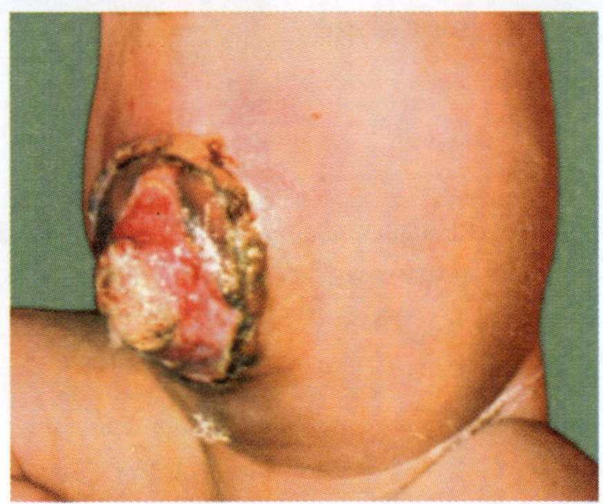
Fig. 53.5: Exomphalos major

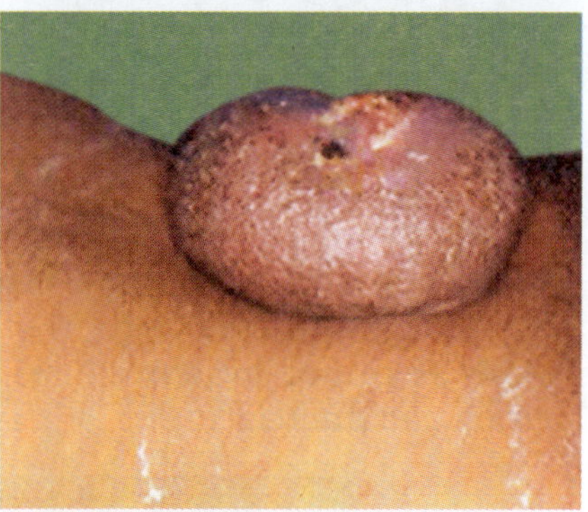
Fig. 53.6: Irreducible umbilical hernia in a cirrhotic patient

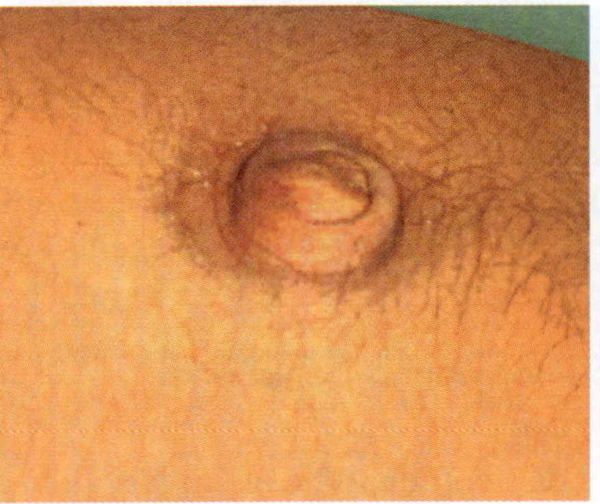
Fig. 53.7: Umbilical hernia

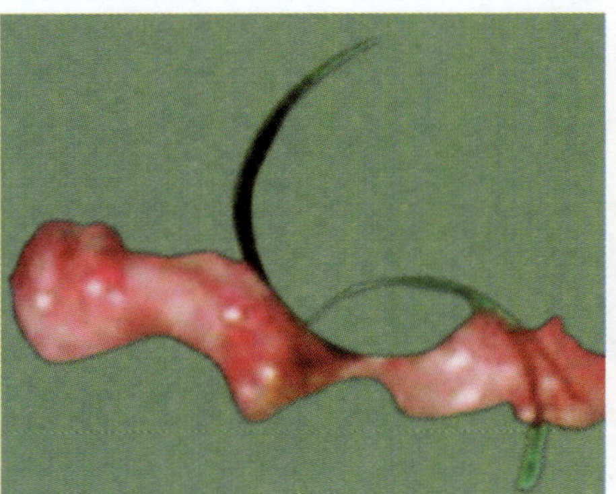
Fig. 53.8: Pilonidal sinus

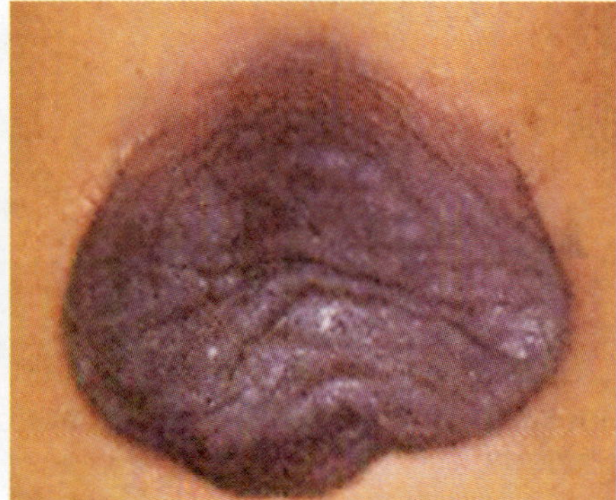
Fig. 53.9: Observe skin of umbilical hernia in cirrhosis of liver, resembling scrotal skin

- Weakness of muscles can also be due to damage to nerves, e.g. as in surgeries such as appendicectomy wherein ilioinguinal nerve may get damaged resulting in inguinal hernia. Empty spaces next to arteries are for expansion of veins but that may cause hernia. Example: Femoral hernia through medial empty space in femoral sheath.
- **Boundaries:** Roof is formed by diaphragm. Pelvis forms the inferior boundary with perineum which is the central muscular portion. Laterally, 3 abdominal muscles each having separate sheath run across towards midline and form rectus sheath (details later). Rectus sheath covers strong rectus abdominis muscles that extend from ribs to pelvis.

Formation of Rectus Sheath (Details are given in Chapter 52: Hernia)

Anatomical Significance

- **Rectus sheath:** Posterior rectus sheath is absent below semilunar line. More chances of hernia.
- **Linea alba:** White, relatively avascular, broad above and narrow below—surgical incision in the midline can be made without any blood loss. Hernia of the linea alba occurs through the opening pierced by blood vessel.
- **Umbilicus:** Strong fibrous ring can also be the site of infections and weakness causing umbilical hernias.
- Tendinous intersections in the rectus sheath and branches of superior and inferior epigastric arteries run within rectus sheath, posteriorly—rectus sheath haematomas are always confined within.
- Nerve supply comes from lateral side. Hence, traction or retraction of rectus should be done laterally so as to avoid traction injuries to nerve fibres.
- Blood vessels like superior and inferior epigastric arteries run within the rectus sheath, posteriorly. Haematoma can occur due to rupture but it is confined within the rectus sheath.
- Weak muscles—interstitial hernias—Prune-Belly syndrome—a partial or complete lack of abdominal muscles. There may be wrinkly folds of skin covering the abdomen and undescended testicles in males.

- Ramirez component separation or slide operation is based on making relaxing incisions over the lateral muscles and slide them medially so as to cover large abdominal wall defects.

PYOGENIC ABSCESS (Fig. 53.10)

Abdominal wall is one of the sites of pyogenic abscess especially in diabetic patients. It is a part of pyaemia. Localised tenderness suggests an abscess. Diagnosis can be confirmed by ultrasound and it is treated by incision and drainage.

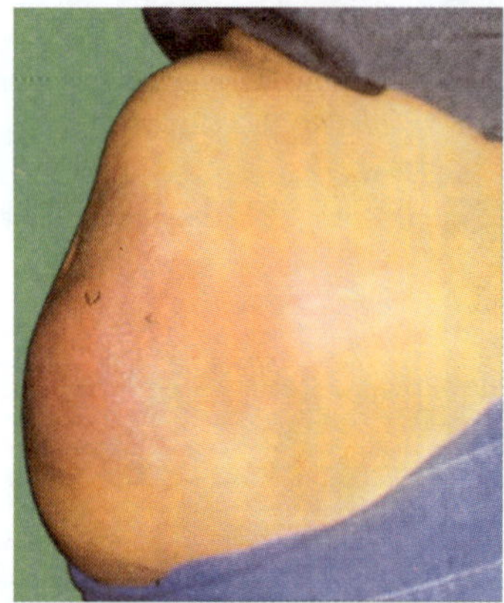

Fig. 53.10: Abdominal wall abscess in a diabetic patient (see clinical notes)

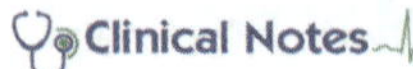

Clinical Notes

A 60-year-old diabetic, male patient had a large pyaemic abscess on the abdominal wall below and to the right of umbilicus. An incision and drainage of the abscess was done. Within 2 hours of surgery, the surgeon was called to see this patient who had hypotension and blood was pouring out of the incision. Exploration of the wound revealed large 'clots' and bleeding from inferior epigastric artery, which was ligated. Probably, while breaking all the loculi of the abscess cavity, the vessel was injured.

ABDOMINAL WALL VEINS

- Veins are seen in portal hypertension. In relation to umbilicus, they are called **caput medusae**. Direction of the veins are important which can be demonstrated by emptying the vein and filling (Fig. 53.11).
- In cases of inferior vena caval obstruction, veins are seen on the flank. These veins are called inguino-axillary veins (Fig. 53.12).

BURST ABDOMEN: ABDOMINAL DEHISCENCE

A soundly healed abdominal scar can withstand any amount of intra-abdominal pressure. However, 1–2% of the abdominal wounds (incisions) give way resulting in prolapse of intra-abdominal contents outside.

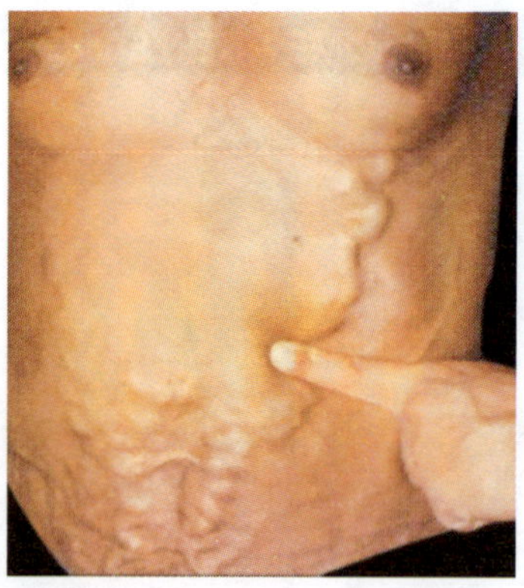

Fig. 53.11: Dilated tortuous veins due to portal hypertension—caput medusae

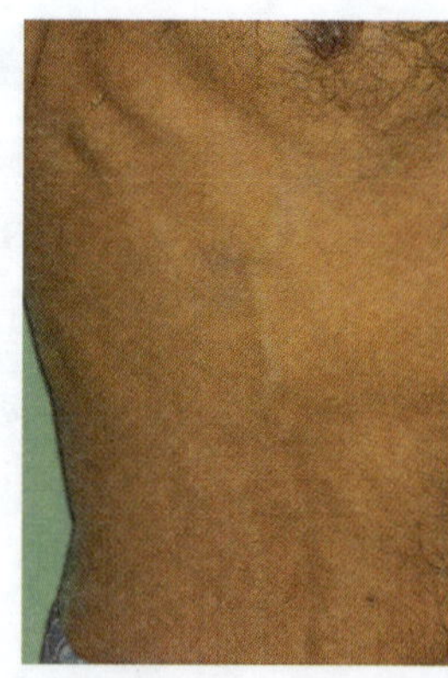

Fig. 53.12: Veins on the lateral abdominal wall suggestive of inferior vena caval obstruction

This causes great concern, or anxiety to the patient, and more so for relatives. It is said that the anxiety and worry caused by the intestines prolapsing out is much more than that is caused by emergency re-explorations for open cardiac surgery. It is not possible to prevent wound dehiscence totally because causative agents are multifactorial.

Factors Responsible for Wound Dehiscence (Key Box 53.3)

1. **Surgery:** It depends upon the type of surgery done. Surgery done for grossly contaminated cases such as peritonitis, biliary fistula or faecal fistula have a high incidence of wound dehiscence (Fig. 53.13).
2. **Sepsis:** Uncontrolled infection (sepsis) can digest the suture material used and will result in burst abdomen.
3. **Suture material used:** Absorbable sutures, such as catgut, give rise to increased incidence of wound dehiscence than nonabsorbable sutures.
4. **Surgeon-related factors:** Meticulous dissection, haemostasis, gentle handling of tissues, a good tensionless tight closure, carefully judged incisions will have reduced incidence of burst abdomen. Midline vertical incisions have decreased chance of wound dehiscence than paramedian incision.

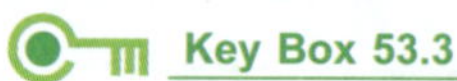

Key Box 53.3

Burst Abdomen: Factors

- **S**urgery → Peritonitis
- **S**epsis → Uncontrolled infection
- **S**utures → Absorbable—catgut
- **S**urgeon → Poor quality
- **S**ick patient → Malignancy, diabetes, uraemia, jaundice
- **S**training → Coughing, vomiting

Remember the causes of burst abdomen as ***6 Ss***

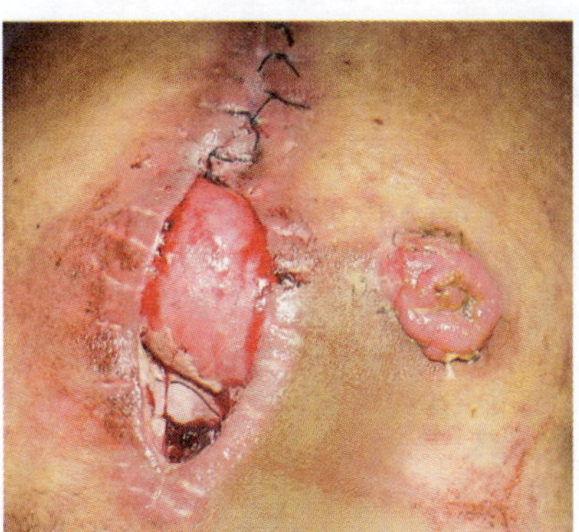

Fig. 53.13: Wound dehiscence in a case of APR (abdominoperineal resection)—probably due to placement of colostomy closer to the suture line

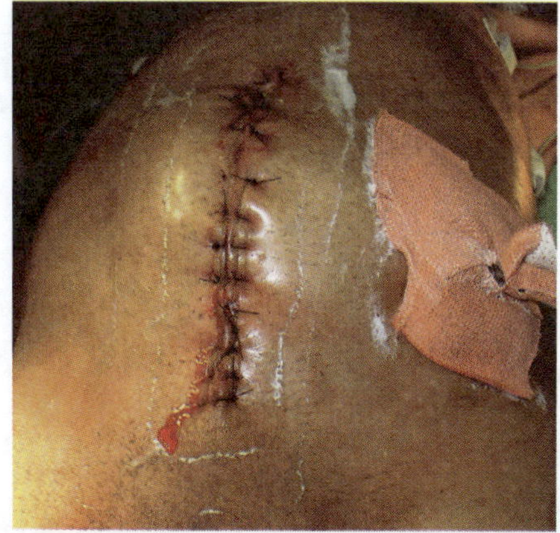

Fig. 53.14: Wound dehiscence—pink discharge

5. **Sick patient:** Patients with malignancy, jaundice, obesity, anaemia, hypoproteinaemia, uraemia have poor wound healing.
6. **Straining:** In the postoperative period, violent cough, persistent vomiting, abdominal distension due to paralytic ileus predispose to burst abdomen.

Clinical Features

- Patients who are recovering reasonably well in the postoperative period suddenly complain of pink- or brownish-coloured serosanguinous discharge. It is the pathognomonic sign of burst abdomen.
- It usually occurs on the 6th to 8th postoperative day.
- If skin sutures are removed, omentum or small bowel coils will be seen outside.

Pearls of Wisdom

Interestingly, it is a painless, shockless disruption (with) full of apprehension.

Treatment

- Reassurance
- The bowel or the contents are covered with pads and bandage.
- Emergency surgery and closure is done.

Principles of Surgery

1. Adequate exposure
2. Bowel is washed with saline and gently replaced into the peritoneal cavity.
3. Edges of the wound/incision are trimmed.
4. A single layer closure of the abdominal layer, by taking suture bites through whole thickness of the abdominal wall is done.
   - A few tension sutures (Figs 53.14 to 53.17) tied over a rubber or a plastic tube are placed and are removed after 2 weeks.

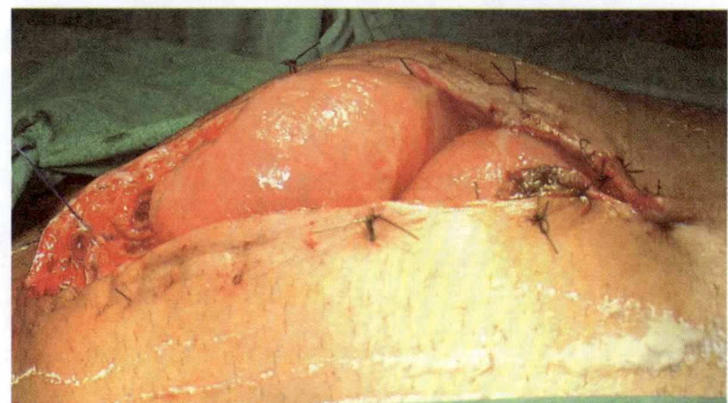

Fig. 53.15: Sutures opened. Distended bowels are seen

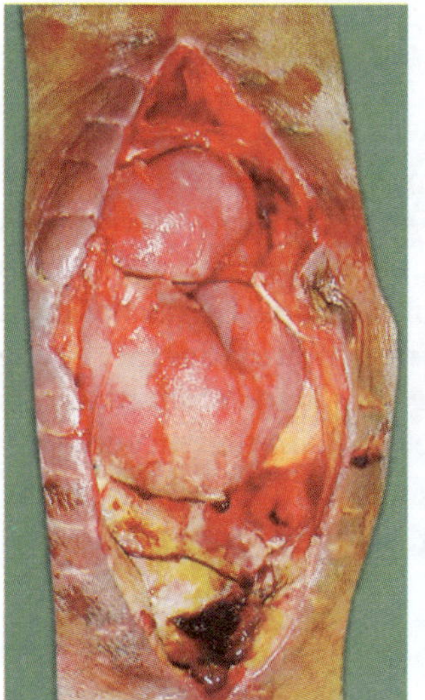

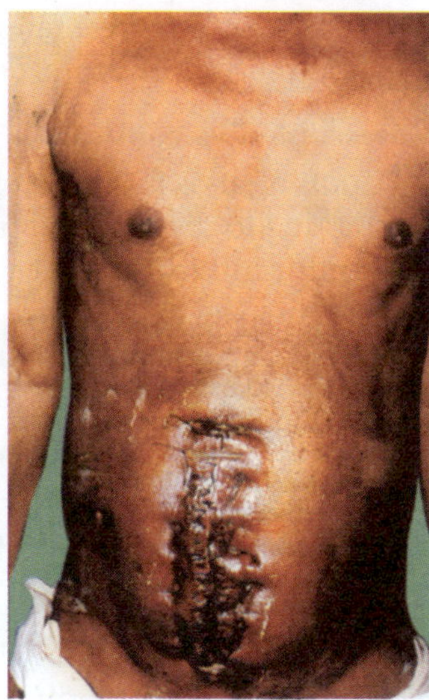

Figs 53.16 and 53.17: Wound dehiscence due to gangrene of the intestine—laparotomy was done, resection followed by closure of the abdomen with tension sutures

   - It should be remembered that **secondary wound healing is better than primary wound healing** and infection rarely occurs.
5. **Closer of midline incision:** In all cases of midline incision, it is the linea alba with or without anterior fascial layer is approximated to the corresponding fascia on the other side.

- 'Fascia' usually refers to the anterior rectus fascia, the fascia above the rectus muscles. This fascia holds the abdomen together and is the most important layer of closure.
- The fascia can extend beyond the muscles and bind to other fascia.
- An extension of the fascia is called an aponeurosis.

Complications of Wound Closure

I. **Early complications:**
- Infection
- Dehiscence

II. **Late complications:**
- Incisional hernia
- Suture sinus
- Wound pain

Prevention of Incisional Hernia

Competency

SU14.3: Describe the materials and methods used for surgical wound closure.

Suturing techniques:
- There should be 1 cm interval between 2 suture bites.
- Length of suture material and length of wound should be 4:1 or more, definitely not less.

Interrupted vs continuous technique:
- Continuous is faster, accommodates wound lengthening due to distension, bursting strength of wound is significantly higher. It minimizes number of knots and thus lower incidence of incisional hernia has been found. **A continuous suture also provides** more type 1 collagen and thus has higher wound strength. Thus continuous sutures are better than interrupted.
- **Disadvantages:** Wound security depends on single strand of suture and limited number of knots.

Mass closure:
- Incorporate all layers of abdominal wall (except skin) as 1 structure and suturing is called mass suture. However, increased chances of hernia and dehiscence can occur following mass closure.
- Layered: Peritoneum, musculo-aponeurotic layer, skin. Adhesions, longer surgery time, compromises adequacy of subsequent layer closure.

Aponeurosis only:
- Good approximation of the edges of aponeurosis. No separation of wound edges. No soft tissue necrosis.
- Not necessary to suture peritoneum in midline incisions. A good closure of linea alba is all that is required. Peritoneum heals on its own by epithelialisation of mesothelium.

Absorbable vs non-absorbable:
- Non-absorbable sutures are associated with more pain and suture sinuses but less chances of incisional hernias. Example: Polypropylene.
- Equally good results are found with slowly absorbable sutures—**slowly absorbing like polydioxanone (PDS) sutures.**
- Fast absorbing sutures are related to higher rate of incisional hernias. Examples: Catgut or polygalactin (Vicryl).

Antibacterial (PLUS) sutures to prevent SSI:
- Presence of suture material may increase the risk of infection.
- Bacterial growth on suture material appeared to have the characteristics of biofilm formation. Suture with antiseptic may help in reducing complications related to infection of the suture material such as inflammation, pus discharge, etc.
- Technical details about sutures and measures to prevent incisional hernia are given in Key Boxes 53.4 and 53.5.

Key Box 53.4

Surgeon's Role in Preventing Incisional Hernia

- Continuous *vs* interrupted sutures
- Knotting technique—secure knots
- Suture length/wound length ratio
- Bite size
- Mass closure vs aponeurosis only
- Tensionless sutures
- Suture material—nonabsorbable
- Anti-SSI (surgical site infection) measures—prophylactic antibiotics

Key Box 53.5

Continuous Sutures

- Continuous suturing is faster
- Accommodates wound lengthening due to distension
- Bursting strength of wound is significantly higher
- Minimises number of knots—equivalent or lower incidence of incisional hernia
- Disadvantages (theoretical): Wound security depends on single strand of suture and limited number of knots

DIVARICATION OF RECTI

- In this condition, the two rectus abdominis muscles are widely separated (not in the midline).
- Repeated pregnancy in quick succession is the most important cause. Chronic constipation or over-

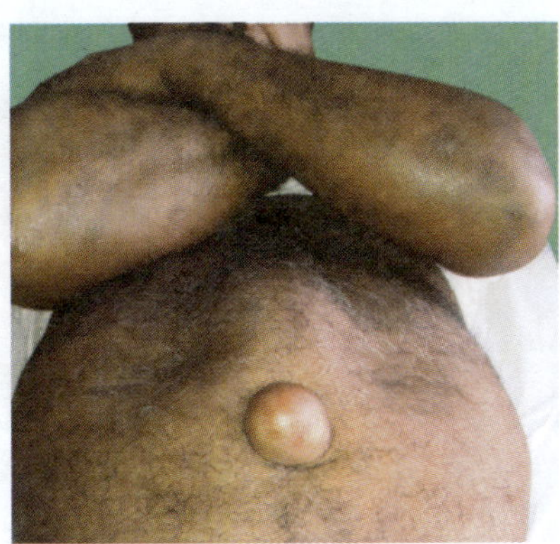

Fig. 53.18: Divarication of recti with umbilical hernia

straining may be another factor. Obviously women are commonly affected.

- Exercises and abdominal corset are helpful.
- Symptomatic cases are operated—divaricated recti are brought towards midline (Fig. 53.18).
- Mesh repair may be required.

RECTUS SHEATH HAEMATOMA

Collection of blood in relation to rectus sheath and muscles occurs due to tearing of one of the branches of inferior epigastric artery. A parietal haematoma occurs usually at the level of the arcuate line. It is an uncommon condition. However, the causes can be as follows:

1. **Trauma:** A sudden blow to the abdominal wall.
2. **Straining:** Sudden straining such as violent cough or vigorous exercise in a muscular man can cause haematoma.
3. **Pregnancy:** Rarely, the cause of haematoma can be pregnancy, in late trimester. The exact cause is not known.

Clinical Features

- History of sudden straining or coughing, etc.
- A tender lump develops just below and to the side of umbilicus at the level of arcuate line where posterior rectus sheath is absent.
- Nausea, vomiting, and pyrexia are the other features.

Differential Diagnosis

Spigelian hernia (it is rare).

Treatment

- The condition is self-limiting. With antibiotics and analgesics, a haematoma subsides within 5–7 days.
- If it persists or progresses or if there is a doubt about the diagnosis, exploration and evacuation of haematoma should be done and the bleeding vessels are ligated. The results and recovery are excellent.

MELENEY'S PROGRESSIVE POSTOPERATIVE SYNERGISTIC GANGRENE

This dangerous complication is rare nowadays, thanks to the good pre- and postoperative antibiotics.

Aetiopathogenesis

- It is caused by synergistic action of microaerophilic non-haemolytic Streptococcus and *Staphylococcus aureus*.
- Surgical operations which have increased risk of Meleney's gangrene include perforated appendix, biliary tract surgery, colectomy, etc.
- Atherosclerosis, and diabetes are the other precipitating factors.
- Starts as cellulitis with reddish skin and postoperative fever.
- The spread may occur within 3–5 days, with extensive gangrene and sloughing of the skin of the abdominal wall with purulent discharge.

Clinical Features

- Postoperative patient with cellulitis of abdominal wall.
- Fever of moderate degree, an extremely tender abdominal wall and purulent discharge.
- Toxicity and deterioration of general health may follow soon.

Treatment

1. **At the stage of cellulitis:** Broad-spectrum antibiotics to cover not only the organisms mentioned above but to cover anaerobic organisms also. Thus, a combination of benzylpenicillin, gentamicin and metronidazole is used.
2. **At the stage of gangrene:** Emergency aggressive debridement is the treatment. Dead skin and subcutaneous tissue are excised, pus drained and the slough is removed.
3. **Hyperbaric oxygen** may be very useful.
4. Skin grafting is done, once the wound is healed with granulation tissue.

FIBROMATOSES: DESMOID TUMOUR

Classification

- *Superficial or deep.* **Deep** fibromatoses, also called ***aggressive fibromatoses and desmoid tumours,*** are **uncapsulated fibromas** which occur in the abdominal wall.
- They arise from muscles and aponeurotic layer of the abdominal wall.

Incidence

- In children, most desmoid tumours are extra-abdominal with a female predominance.
- In young adults, desmoid tumours almost always occur in the abdominal wall (of women). ***Hormonal effects and pregnancy*** are believed to influence the growth of this tumour.
- Some tumours express hormone receptors (oestrogen and progesterone), and therefore ***tamoxifen*** and other hormonal modulators are among the adjuvant therapies for this tumour.

Aetiopathogenesis

- Childbirth, trauma or operative scars are the possible aetiological factors.
- Desmoid tumour is one of the components of Gardner's syndrome.
- It is benign but has a tendency to infiltrate the muscles. Some fibromas exhibit dysplastic changes. The cut surface is compared to an onion—whorled fibroma with spindle-shaped cells.
- Sarcomatous changes and metastasis do not occur.

Clinical Features

- **Abdominal fibromatosis** is far less prone to recurrences than desmoid tumours in other sites.
- It usually occurs in the abdominal wall of women of childbearing age during or after pregnancy.
- Clinically, the lesions present as deep-seated, firm, nonencapsulated, slow-growing, locally invasive and painless masses.
- It typically manifests as a slow-growing, progressive mass that becomes more prominent on abdominal muscle contraction. Mass is in the abdominal wall and is firm to hard in consistency.
- **Mesenteric fibromatosis**, probably the commonest among the group, usually presents as a slow-growing mass that involves small bowel mesentery or retroperitoneum.
- The recurrence rate of mesenteric fibromatosis seems to be substantially higher in patients who have Gardner's syndrome than in patients who do not have this syndrome.

Treatment

- Simple excision results in recurrence. Hence, **wide excision with 2–3 cm** of normal **healthy margins** is necessary with reconstruction of the abdominal wall (Figs 53.19 and 53.20).
- In spite of adequate surgery, 10–20% chances of recurrence occur (Key Box 53.6).

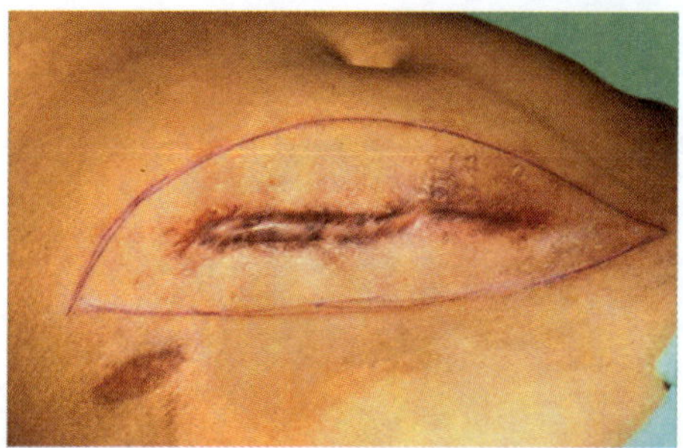

Fig. 53.19: Wide excision of recurrent desmoid tumour in the abdominal wall

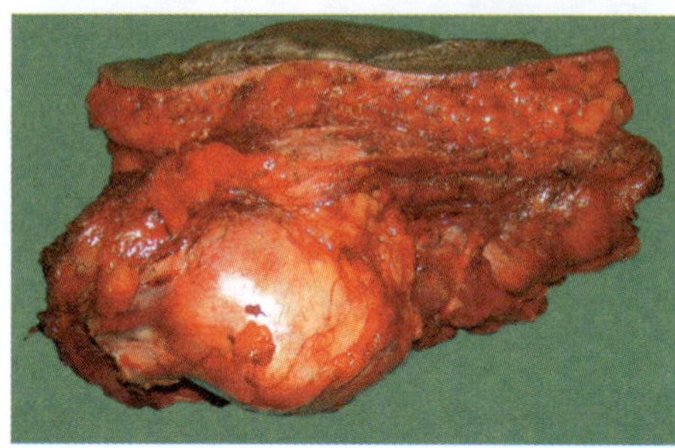

Fig. 53.20: Specimen of desmoid tumour which is removed along with normal tissue

Key Box 53.6

Peculiarities of Desmoid Tumour

- Uncapsulated fibroma
- Infiltrates muscles, even though benign
- Does not change into sarcoma
- It may be a part of Gardner's syndrome
- Simple excision results in recurrence
- Wide excision is recommended

ENDOMETRIOSIS OF THE ABDOMINAL WALL

Drugs like sulindac and tamoxifen have also been used here, with some success.

- It occurs due to mechanical implantation of endometrial cells during surgery (sites—Key Box 53.7 and Fig. 53.21).
- Painful, palpable swelling, more symptomatic at the time of menstruation are characteristic features.
  - Perimenstrual cyclical bleeding can occur.
- Oral contraceptive pills may control the symptoms.
- Otherwise, excision of the nodule has to be done (Fig. 53.22).

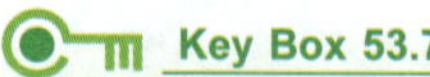

Key Box 53.7

Sites of Endometriosis

- Laparoscopic port – Umbilicus
- Gynaecological surgery – Abdominal incision
- Episiotomy – Perineum

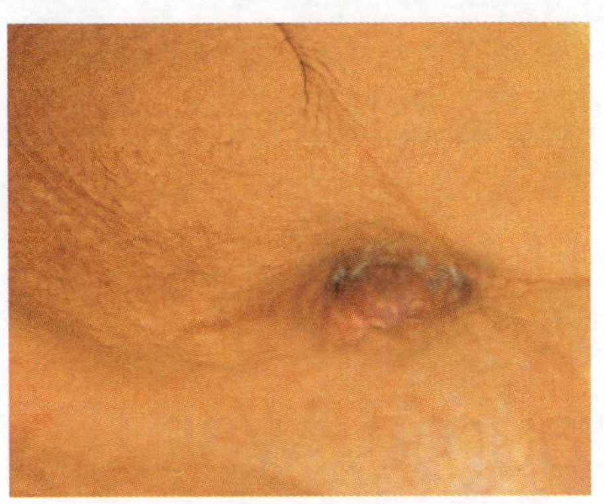

Fig. 53.21: Scar endometriosis

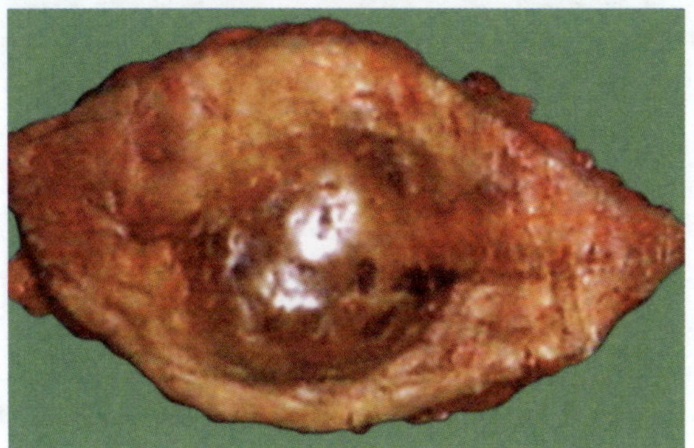

Fig. 53.22: Wide excision of scar endometriosis

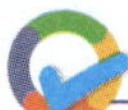

Multiple Choice Questions

1. The following is *not* a cause of umbilical faecal fistula:
   A. Persistent vitellointestinal duct
   B. Tuberculosis
   C. Carcinoma
   D. Raspberry adenoma

2. The following statement is true about burst abdomen:
   A. It is very painful
   B. It is associated with shock
   C. Straining can produce it
   D. Conservative management is the choice

3. About desmoid tumour:
   A. Is a capsulated fibroma
   B. Infiltrates muscles
   C. Often changes to sarcoma
   D. Simple excision is recommended

4. The following is true of Meleney's postoperative synergistic gangrene *except*:
   A. Is progressive
   B. Can occur after appendicectomy
   C. Starts as cellulitis
   D. Is painless

5. The following is true about rectus sheath haematoma *except*:
   A. It can occur with pregnancy
   B. Sudden straining can precipitate it
   C. Presents as painless lump above umbilicus
   D. Nausea, vomiting and fever are other features

6. The principles of surgery for burst abdomen include all of the following *except*:
   A. Layer by layer careful suture
   B. Adequate exposure
   C. Tension sutures
   D. Trimming of edges

7. The pathognomonic sign of burst abdomen is:
   A. Shock
   B. Pink or brown serosanguinous discharge
   C. Pain
   D. Occurs on the second postoperative day

8. Umbilical adenoma:
   A. Sessile swelling
   B. Is a premalignant condition
   C. Can be treated with ligature
   D. Occurs due to persistent umbilical vessels

9. Pilonidal sinus is known to occur in the following places *except*:
   A. Internatal cleft B. Umbilicus
   C. Interdigital cleft D. Axilla

10. Meleney's gangrene is a synergistic gangrene caused by:
   A. *Streptococcus* and *Staphylococcus*
   B. *E. coli* and *Klebsiella*
   C. *Clostridium* and *Pseudomonas*
   D. *Salmonella typhi* and *paratyphi*

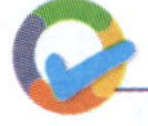

Answers

1. D **2.** C **3.** B **4.** D **5.** C **6.** A **7.** B **8.** C **9.** D **10.** A

CHAPTER

54

Trauma—Initial Management, Blunt Abdominal Trauma, War and Blast Injuries and Triage

- Initial management of trauma victims
- Blast injuries
- Warfare injuries
- Missile wounds of abdomen
- Blunt abdominal trauma
- Triage
- Liver injuries
- Small bowel injuries
- Colonic injuries
- Duodenal injuries
- Pancreatic injuries
- Renal injuries
- Retroperitoneal haematoma
- Medicolegal aspects of wound healing and gunshot wounds
- Vascular trauma
- Chest injuries

INITIAL MANAGEMENT OF TRAUMA VICTIMS

INTRODUCTION

Trauma originates from the Greek word meaning ***wound.*** This occurs due to physical force exerted on a person. Trauma constitutes a large proportion of the number of lives lost, especially in the productive age group. The most effective way of reducing trauma-related deaths is by prevention which involves building safer roads and educating the masses on observation of road discipline. Wearing of protective gear such as helmets for two-wheeler drivers and riders, seat belts for four-wheeler drivers and passenger must be made mandatory. Trauma can also be due to earthquakes, wars, major accidents involving trains, etc. So much has been learnt from various wars including World War I and II, Korean wars, Vietnam wars, etc. It is said—*those who cannot remember the past are condemned to repeat it (George Santayana)*—really hold good for trauma.

Once trauma occurs, all efforts will need to be made to reduce morbidity and mortality. Trauma-related deaths have a trimodal distribution: First, mortality that occurs at site or on transfer due to severity of trauma injuries. These deaths cannot be prevented and only a behavioural change can reduce them. The victim's injuries are so severe resulting in massive exsanguination or severe head injuries such that saving the life of that trauma victim is impossible. The second phase of deaths, usually due to hypovolaemia and other trauma-related injuries are often avoidable and treatable. Timely and appropriate intervention at this stage can reduce the effects of trauma and prevent morbidity secondary to the injury. The third phase includes those patients who die of complications of trauma such as infection, embolism, sepsis, acute respiratory distress syndrome and septic shock. A well-managed second phase is likely to reduce the incidence of the third phase.

When a patient/patients sustain trauma, it is a natural tendency in India for onlookers, police or fire personnel to load them into the first available vehicle and transfer them to the nearest available hospital. Although their intentions are good, they may actually cause more harm. Many of these patients may have sustained cervical spine injuries which may be undisplaced at first but get displaced, if careful attention to prevention of neck movements is not given during transfer. In view of this, the salient features of trauma care must be widely publicised among the lay public.

Doctors and other medical personnel get involved in patient care only after the patient reaches the hospital. They too may not be trained to deal with trauma and it is common to find trauma care area in chaos, especially when multiple patients arrive in a short span. A systematic approach to victim/victims of trauma is very necessary to ensure best outcome.

PREHOSPITAL PHASE

Scene Safety

Every rescuer must always ensure that the scene is safe for oneself before proceeding to help a trauma victim. A liquid petroleum leak, radiation exposure, floods, landslides are a few examples. When unsure, it may be more prudent to enquire from the fire personnel and then approach the victim.

Trauma Triage

Modern medical triage was invented by Dominique Jean Larrey, a surgeon during the Napoleonic wars, **Triage** is derived from the French word ***trier***, meaning **to sort**. When there are multiple victims, the philosophy of trauma triage will need to be adopted. This is a method of sorting out injured patients, during mass casualties depending on the severity of injury. If you are the first on the scene, first priority is to get expert help (call up fire services, regional trauma centre, etc.).

Triage is a skilled activity by a trauma team, wherein there is a leader (usually senior-most doctor/surgeon) and there are many assistants. The leader sorts out patients (people) depending upon their severity of injury. The term ***'multiple casualties'*** is used when there are more than two trauma victims but the number does not overwhelm the facilities available at the treating centre. The term ***'mass casualties'*** is used when there are more than two trauma victims but the number overwhelms the facilities available at the treating centre.

Colour Coding

When there are multiple or mass casualties, rescuers use universal colour codes to mark each victim based on the severity of injuries to help decide on the treatment priority to be given to each patient. The colour codes are as follows:

CODE BLACK (EXPECTANT): These patients have very severe injuries and may not be expected to survive very long with the available care.

CODE RED (IMMEDIATE): These patients may have life-threatening injuries to the airway, breathing or circulation which are potentially reversible with immediate care.

CODE YELLOW (DELAYED): These patients are relatively stable and would not be expected to become unstable in a few hours. They too can have a threat to life but not immediate.

CODE GREEN (MINOR): These patients have injuries but can be seen in due course. The 'walking wounded' belong to this group.

Thus, in the event of a large number of patients arriving at the trauma centre and they have been coded, all patients with 'red' code must be attended to immediately followed by the 'yellow' coded patients. The 'green' coded patients can be seen in the outpatient department, whereas the 'black' coded ones can be given attention when possible.

Communication

All ambulance drivers must be instructed to store the telephone numbers of the contact person in the referral hospitals. It is essential that advance information is given to the trauma centre ahead of arrival of trauma victims to optimize care.

Pearls of Wisdom

The leader assesses the patient—flags and moves forward and it is his assistant who carries out the necessary resuscitation. The leader should not resuscitate any patient. There are others waiting for his expert help.

A Common Scheme or a Quick Assessment

1. **Can the patient walk?**

   Yes: Delayed (green), No—check for breathing.

2. **Is the patient breathing?**

   No: Open the airway—Are they breathing (ventilating) him?

   Yes: Immediate (red) , No—DEAD (white).

   Yes: Count or estimate respiratory rate (over 15 sec).

   <10 to >30 per minute—immediate (red).

   10–30 per minute—check the circulation.

3. **Check the circulation**

   Pulse >120/min (capillary refill >2s)—immediate (red).

   Pulse <120/min (capillary refill <2s)—urgent (yellow).

- If any regional trauma centre is well equipped and nearby, one has to transport all the injured patients to hospital (scoop and run), where expert help is available. Meanwhile trauma centre can be alerted about the arrival of casualties. If expert help is far away, then one may have to treat the patients at the accident site (stay and play). Resuscitation is done as per ATLS guidelines.
- During these exercises, do not forget to take care of your own safety, in burning vehicles, burning or falling buildings, etc.

Pearls of Wisdom

An initial quick evaluation of the patient for anaemia, level of consciousness, if necessary volume replacement, application of cervical (C) collar to the neck, etc. are done.

TRAUMA CENTRE PREPARATION

Plan in Advance

Every trauma centre must be in a state of constant preparedness to receive trauma victims. The trauma centre must be manned by dedicated personnel and must have the necessary equipment which is checked on a daily basis and rechecked after every use.

Trauma Care Personnel

The core group responding to trauma cases include nurses, trauma technicians, qualified doctors (general surgeon, orthopaedician or emergency physician) and a set of doctors on call to deal with referrals (neurosurgeon, cardiothoracic vascular surgeon).

Trauma Care Area

The trauma care area must be a dedicated area called the **'resuscitation bay'**. All personnel caring for the patient must wear **personal protective equipment** including goggles, gown, gloves and shoe covers. The patient must be received on a trolley bed and each bed must have a **multimodal monitor** including pulse oximeter, noninvasive blood pressure and electrocardiogram. An **oxygen source** and **suction apparatus** also must be available with each bed.

Resuscitation Equipment

Resuscitation equipment will include **airway equipment** such as airways, endotracheal tubes, laryngoscopes, laryngeal mask airways, infraglottic airways, Magill's forceps and a stethoscope. *Cervical collar of different sizes must also be available.* **Equipment for circulatory resuscitation** include intravenous fluids (isotonic saline, Ringer lactate), intravenous cannulae, pressure bags, body and fluid warmers, syringes, **medications** including vasopressors, inotropes, anticholinergics, analgesics, etc.). An ultrasound machine must be available for focused abdominal sonography in trauma **(FAST)**. A portable X-ray machine must also be available to obtain the basic X-rays (neck, chest, pelvis).

Competency

SU17.1: Describe the principles of first aid to trauma patients.

APPROACH TO TRAUMA

The approach to trauma must be done in the following steps: **Primary survey and resuscitation, secondary survey and definitive care.**

Primary Survey and Resuscitation

The purpose of this step is to very quickly evaluate for any life-threatening emergency and deal with it immediately. Often an obvious external trauma, such as fracture femur diverts the attention of the caregivers, but a life-threatening injury is missed. The evaluation must be performed in the following order: **A, B, C, D and E. However, when bleeding is obvious and external, it can be easily controlled. Thus, now it is being referred as cABCDE.**

A—Airway with cervical spine control
B—Adequate breathing
C—Circulation with haemorrhage control
D—Disability assessment, and
E—Exposure and environment control.

Control of bleeding: When an external bleeding is visible and massive, control of bleeding is more important than airway. Often in a trauma, source of bleeding may be in the limbs—muscle or arterial bleeding. Immediate first aid involves pressure packing principle. If an arterial bleeding is visible, a hemostat is used to control it. Hemostatic dressing is applied.

If a tourniquet is available, rubber or better one pneumatic—it should be used. Tourniquet time is noted and immediate transfer to referral centers should be done.

- **An obvious fracture lower limb due to a fall is common in elderly patients**. A posterior slab is given for immobilization.
- **Simple wounds which are bleeding are thoroughly cleaned and sutured.**

Survey

A very quick way of evaluating airway, breathing and circulation is to address the patient and elicit a response (e.g. ask the patient's name). If he replies appropriately, it is evident that the patient's airway is patent, breathing is optimal and circulation to his brain is adequate. If the patient does not respond to call, a painful stimulus is given and the response is quickly graded on the *AVPU scale, where A = Alert, V = Responds to verbal commands, P = Responds to pain and U = Unresponsive.* **Quick primary survey and actions are given below in the form of ABCDE of primary survey.**

1. Airway with cervical spine immobilization: *All patients sustaining trauma, especially to the head and who have an altered sensorium must be assumed to have cervical spine injury until proved otherwise.* The mechanism of injury would provide a clue to the possibility of cervical trauma. The neck must be immobilised in a rigid cervical

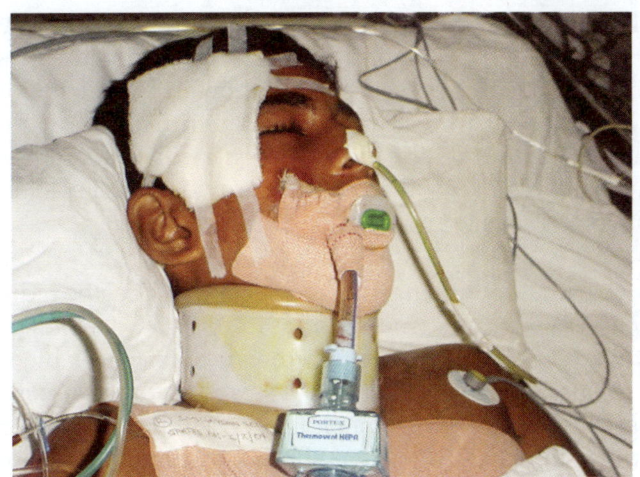

Fig. 54.1: Management of a polytrauma patient in an intensive care unit—cervical collar has been applied and patient is being ventilated

collar (Philadelphia cervical collar or similar) as early as possible. Rapid assessment of signs of obstruction should be looked for—foreign body, laryngeal and facio-maxillary fracture, fallen back tongue (Fig. 54.1).

If the airway is not patent or the patient's ability to maintain his airway is questionable, the airway must be secured. Signs of compromised airway include snoring, stridor, agitation, active accessory muscles of ventilation/paradoxical chest movements and cyanosis.

*Open the airway first with a jaw thrust, **oral airway** or a **nasopharyngeal airway*** (Key Box 54.1). An oral airway is preferred, if the patient is unconscious and is suspected to have sustained base of the skull fracture. A nasopharyngeal airway is chosen, if the gag reflex is intact and the patient is semiconscious. Insertion of a nasopharyngeal airway in a patient with base of skull fracture is risky as it can enter the brain through the fracture. Provide oxygen using face mask and ventilate as necessary.

Indications for **endotracheal intubation** or **tracheostomy** for securing the airway include obstructed airway, apnoea, hypoxia, severe head injury, maxillofacial injury, penetrating neck trauma with expanding haematoma and chest trauma.

Key Box 54.1

Quick Reminder Mnemonic at Treatment Centre

- **L**ift jaw
- **I**ntubation: Airway
- **F**allen tongue/foreign body to be checked
- **T**racheostomy/cricothyrotomy/oropharyngeal or nasopharyngeal throat suction
- **J**aw fractures to be ruled out

Remember as **LIFTJAW**

Endotracheal intubation provides the most definitive airway. It is required in patients who are unconscious, not able to maintain their own airway, who have sustained extensive faciomaxillary injuries or airway burns. A rapid sequence induction and intubation is preferred. The level of sedation required for intubation would depend on the level of consciousness and haemodynamic stability. Generally, midazolam or etomidate is used for sedation and succinyl choline as the muscle relaxant for intubation.

The cervical collar is used to limit neck movements but it often also limits mouth opening and increases the difficulty of securing airway. Hence, it is recommended that *the cervical collar is removed during endotracheal intubation and the neck immobilized manually.* The collar is reapplied after airway is secured.

If endotracheal intubation is difficult, the airway can be maintained using **supraglottic airway** adjuncts such as laryngeal mask airway or laryngeal tube. If these are inadequate, a **cricothyrotomy** (infraglottic airway) may need to be performed. This should be followed by a regular **tracheostomy.** Cricothyrotomy is advocated as the initial choice as it can be done very quickly. Time is of essence in a hypoxic emergency.

2. Breathing—look, listen and feel: Inspect (look) at the chest for the respiratory rate, depth and pattern. If the patient's breathing is inadequate as evidenced clinically (rate and depth) or if the patient is cyanosed/oxygen saturation is low (<93%), breathing must be assisted and oxygen supplementation given as required. Look for presence of flail chest, open chest wounds and use of accessory muscles of respirations.

Palpate (feel) for tracheal shift, broken ribs and subcutaneous emphysema. **Percuss** for diagnosis of haemothorax and pneumothorax.

Auscultate both sides of the chest for equality of breath sounds and for any added sounds. Rule out endobronchial intubation, if an endotracheal tube is already in place.

If breath sounds are unequal, inspect the neck for any distended veins, tracheal position and then percuss the chest. If neck veins are distended, trachea is deviated and the chest is resonant to percuss on the side of reduced air entry, suspect tension pneumothorax. The patient may require needle thoracostomy. A large bore (16–18 G cannula) is inserted in the fifth intercostal space slightly anterior to the anterior axillary line (ATLS 10th edition). In children, an appropriately large bore needle or cannula must be placed in the second intercostal space in the midclavicular line. If air hisses out, decompression of chest would have been achieved. Chest tube insertion can follow later during secondary survey.

Pearls of Wisdom

Tension pneumothorax is a clinical diagnosis. Do not delay the treatment while waiting for chest X-ray.

Cardiac tamponade: It is a serious condition which results due to collection of blood/fluid in the pericardial cavity.

Causes: Gunshot injuries, penetrating injuries, ruptured aortic aneurysms, invasive and interventional procedures including central venous catheter insertions, angiograms can also cause cardiac tamponade.

Pathophysiology: **The distended pericardial cavity compresses all chambers of the heart.** As a result of this, venous return is impeded, ventricular filling is impaired resulting in hypotension, and hypoperfusion. **Ventricles cannot contract effectively and leads to cardiovascular collapse and cardiac arrest.**

Clinical features: **Hypotension, tachycardia, low volume pulse, cold peripheries, chest pain, breathlessness, syncope and cardiovascular collapse.** The neck veins may be distended. **The Beck's triad** includes hypotension, **elevated systemic venous pressure**, often with jugular venous distention; muffled heart sounds. This can occur with sudden intrapericardial haemorrhage. The Kussmaul sign—a paradoxical elevation in jugular venous pulse (JVP) during inspiration is sometimes seen in cardiac tamponade.

Diagnosis: **It is a medical emergency.** The gold standard investigation is ultrasound examination. The extended focussed abdominal sonography in trauma (E-FAST) obtained in patients with trauma includes evaluation for presence of cardiac tamponade. Echocardiography can confirm the presence of pericardial effusion and determine its size. It can also reveal compromise of cardiac function (right ventricular diastolic collapse, right atrial systolic collapse, plethoric IVC). A chest X-ray may show an enlarged heart. CT chest can diagnose pericardial effusion. However, if the cardiac tamponade is significant, one should not wait for chest X-ray or CT chest but proceed with pericardiocentesis using point-of-care ultrasound.

Treatment: In case of urgency, a needle pericardiocentesis is performed at the bedside using ultrasound-guided needle placement from a subxiphoid window. If ultrasound is not available, the patient is on the verge of collapse and there is a strong suspicion of cardiac tamponade, the traditional landmark technique may need to be adopted. A large bore needle is inserted from the subxiphoid point into the pericardial cavity by directing it inwards, superiorly and towards the left shoulder with continuous aspiration. Support airway, breathing and circulation as necessary. Supplementing oxygen, positive pressure ventilation and leg elevation also will help these patients depending upon the severity of the tamponade. Standard cardiac life support measures (ACLS) will need to be provided, if the patient develops cardiac arrest.

3. Circulation with haemorrhage control: Feel the radial pulse for its rate, rhythm, quality (strong, feeble and thready) and equality with opposite side. Check blood pressure. *The commonest cause of shock in trauma is hypovolaemia.* Neurogenic shock is a possibility in cases of spinal injury. Obstructive shock can occur in tension pneumothorax and cardiac tamponade. Septic shock is unlikely but not impossible in early trauma.

If the pulse is feeble, irregular and the patient is hypotensive, rule out the possibility of a pericardial tamponade by looking at neck veins. If the neck veins are distended, radial pulse is not felt, heart sounds are faint and needle thoracostomy has not treated the condition, perform a pericardiocentesis. Ultrasound of the heart (FAST) is very useful to confirm the diagnosis and guide the procedure. If ultrasound is not available, it is reasonable to proceed with landmark-guided drainage of the pericardium.

The possible sites of bleeding can be remembered as ***blood on the floor and four more****. The blood on the floor refers to external and obvious bleeding. The four other sites are the thorax, abdomen, pelvis and long bones.* Look very quickly for any obvious bleeding from any part of the body. If present, apply pressure and stop the bleeding. Application of a tourniquet is not advisable unless absolutely necessary. If applied, it should be removed as early as possible to avoid injury to tissues.

An intravenous line should be secured and intravenous fluids, preferably around 40°C (crystalloids—saline, Ringer lactate or plasmalyte), infused very quickly to restore volume. Initial bolus of 2 litres of crystalloid solutions.

Dextrose containing solutions are not recommended. Two large peripheral lines are preferred for the initial resuscitation. Insertion of central lines is not recommended (unless done by skilled personnel) as it takes much longer to insert, requires expertise and can be associated with complications. If a peripheral intravenous access is not available, intraosseous needle can be inserted and fluids infused into the bone marrow. *All infusions that can be given intravenously can also be given intraosseously. External jugular venous access is another option for quick transfusion of large amounts of fluids and blood products.*

Obvious bleeding sites in the upper limb or lower limb in cases of soft tissue injuries with or without fractures should be inspected, if necessary, immediate tourniquet to be applied and even can be stopped by an artery forceps depending upon the severity.

Pearls of Wisdom

The immediate goal is to arrest bleeding rather than replacing the blood.

Check the abdomen and pelvis. Abdominal trauma can be penetrating or nonpenetrating. Inspect and then palpate the abdomen for any distension, abrasion or contusion. Spring the pelvis to rule out pelvic instability due to fracture. Perform a focused abdominal sonography in trauma **(FAST)** to rule out liver and splenic injuries. If any abdominal injury with haemorrhage is suspected, the patient will need an urgent life-saving laparotomy.

'Damage control surgery/laparotomy' should be done as soon as possible in patients with evidence of abdominal trauma and maintaining a systolic BP at 80–90 mmHg with fluid resuscitation is unsuccessful. The aim of this laparotomy is to stop the bleeding, often only packing, after which the mid-line incision is temporarily closed within 30 minutes with towel clamps. *This laparotomy is described as not a surgery, but a resuscitative procedure.* In polytrauma, when multiple organs are involved, to conduct the complete repair of all the injuries will require many hours. These patients develop coagulopathy, hypothermia, acidosis and thus they succumb. In such situations, packs are used to stop the bleeding and these packs need to be removed after 48 hours. Thus, laparotomy wound is closed only at the skin level. If intestine is transected, staple the intestine thus to avoid contamination. One can go in after 48 hours for a definitive repair. In presence of sepsis, instead of doing an anastomosis, it is better to exteriorize and definitive repair is done at a later date.

The American College of Surgeons Classification of hypovolemic shock can be used as a quick guide to gauge the amount of blood lost. If the patient is tachycardic (heart rate >120/min) and hypotensive (systolic blood pressure is <90 mmHg), the patient has Class III shock or higher where the patient has lost >30–40% blood volume. Such patients will also require transfusion of blood products (packed cells and fresh frozen plasma). It may be necessary to activate massive transfusion protocol (when available at the hospital) if the patient is bleeding profusely. Replacing the lost volume along with hemorrhage control is important to restore perfusion and prevent tissue damage.

In cases where the hemostasis is insecure or not definitive, volumes should be controlled to maintain systolic BP at 80–90 mmHg till the bleeding can be stopped. This is called *'hypotensive fluid resuscitation' or 'permissive hypotension'*. Small boluses of IV fluids—250 ml of O negative blood or normal saline can be given till blood is available. It is important to maintain the patient warm through the resuscitation as hypothermia impairs coagulation, increases bleeding, depresses respiration and circulation as well as increases chances of infection.

The pelvis should be examined by springing the pelvis. This should be done only once and if any instability is noted, the pelvis should be immobilized by application of pelvic binder and later on with an external fixator to stop bleeding.

Role of tranexamic acid in trauma:

- It is an anti-fibrinolytic drug to be used in trauma patients with bleeding.
- Given 1 g IV over 10 minutes followed by next dose of 1 g over 8 hours.
- Tachycardia with pulse rate more than 110/minute or systolic blood pressure less than 110 mmHg.
- Ideally should be administered within 3 hours of trauma.

Special Patient Groups

Trauma can affect a person of any age. Older patients on multiple medications may not manifest blood loss. Often, they may not show a tachycardia or hypertension. Children tend to have high heart rates, whereas trained athletes may have low heart rates making these signs unreliable in these patients.

Disability

The patient's Glasgow Coma Scale (GCS) must be assessed as also the pupillary response to light must be recorded. Observe for neurologic deterioration. The patient must be turned to lateral position using log rolling technique and the spine is examined (Key Box 54.2).

Key Box 54.2

Disability: AVPU system

- Awake
- Open eyes to Voice
- Open eyes to Painful stimulus
- Unarousable

Exposure

The patient's whole body must be exposed and every orifice must be examined. Quick examination of all orifices. Examples: Look for bleeding from the ear, nose, oral cavity, rectum, vagina, and urethra. A per rectal examination must be done after examination of the spine to rule out urethral injuries. Hypothermia must be avoided. A pregnancy test must be obtained in every female patient in the reproductive age group.

Adjuncts to Primary Survey

Monitors: The patient's vitals are monitored using a pulse oximeter, noninvasive blood pressure and electrocardiogram. Arterial blood gases and capnography are extremely useful and must be made available in dedicated trauma centres.

Tubes and catheters: The patient is then placed supine. Tubes and catheters are inserted and X-rays obtained. A nasogastric tube and urinary catheter are inserted, X-rays of the neck, chest and pelvis and ultrasound abdomen are obtained at this stage.

Secondary Survey and Definitive Care

Once the life-threatening emergencies are ruled out or dealt with, secondary survey involving a more detailed head-to-toe examination of the patient is performed. All through the secondary survey, if there is any change in patient condition the primary survey starting with A, B and C will need to be performed. If the patient is being treated in a smaller hospital without facility to treat that trauma, the patient must be transferred to a higher centre after stabilization of vital signs. The transfer itself must be well-planned with well-delegated tasks for each personnel and the transfer communicated to the referral hospital. More details are given under abdominal trauma.

BLAST INJURIES

- Bursting of bombs or shells rupture their casing and impart high velocity to resulting fragments. These fragments cause more devastating injuries than blast wave.
- **The two main components are: Blast pressure wave** (dynamic overpressure) with positive and negative phase and mass **movement of air (blast wind).**
- Positive phase of blast wave lasts few milliseconds (close to the explosion it may be over 7000 kN/m^2) (tympanic membrane ruptures at 150 kN/m^2).
- Like sound waves blast, pressure waves flow over and around an obstruction and affect persons sheltering behind a wall. The pressure affecting such a person is known as incident pressure (pressure at 90° to direction of travel of blast shock front).
- Person standing in front of a wall facing an explosion is subject to added effect of reflected pressure. Mass movement of air displaces air at supersonic speed. This disrupts environment, hurting debris and people. Blast wave under the water travels at great speed and to greater distance. Injuries tend to be complex and severe.

Pearls of Wisdom

Structures injured by primary blast wave are ears, lungs, heart and gastrointestinal system.

- Most will have combination of blunt, blast and thermal injuries. Deafness, lung contusion, capillary leakage and haemorrhage into alveoli and ARDS precipitated by over transfusion are the features. Perforation of the intestines and penetration injuries to the eye are the other features.
- Management consists of resuscitation in a well-equipped trauma unit, blood transfusions, intensive care monitoring, antibiotics and appropriate surgical procedures.

WARFARE INJURIES

Penetrating missile wounds, injuries from blast phenomena and burns are typical features of modern conventional war. The most common wounding agent in surviving casualties is a fragment wound and not a bullet wound as many erroneously believe. The aim in modern war is to incapacitate and **not to kill**. Hence, a large number of surviving casualties is a major financial and logistic burden on a nation engaged in war.

Wound Ballistics and Mechanisms of Injury

Bullets fired from handguns are propelled at low velocity, have low available energy and result in low velocity transfer wounds (100–500 J), whereas those from assault rifle have high velocity and have high available energy (2000–3000 J) and they cause high energy transfer wounds. **Low energy** transfer wounds leave injury confined to wound tract. **High energy** transfer wounds cause local laceration, crush injury and also cause remote injury from wound tract due to temporary cavitation phenomena.

Management

- Entrance and exit wounds do not indicate considerable damage that may have occurred to deeper structures.
- Resuscitate as per ATLS guidelines.
- Record the wounds in case sheets, take photographs, if necessary.
- Under anaesthesia, excise skin around entry and exit wounds, give liberal longitudinal incision through skin and deep fascia, which allows proper visualisation of underlying structures.

- Debride (cut till healthy tissues are seen) all dead tissues—dead muscle does not bleed or contract, looks dusky.
- Identify neurovascular bundles and examine them.
- Dissect and mark injured nerves for possible future repair.
- Repair arteries and veins, if injured.
- Give thorough wash and let out all the dirt.
- Injured tendons are trimmed and tied for easy identification at future surgery.
- Fix bones by appropriate methods.
- Cover the wound with absorbable dressing.
- Appropriate antibiotics and injection tetanus toxoid are given.
- Amputation may be necessary, if limb is grossly mutilated.
- Delayed primary closure is done (4–6 days later) once the wound starts healing.

MISSILE WOUNDS OF ABDOMEN

- Every penetrating and perforating missile wound of the abdomen should be explored by laparotomy. A full midline incision from xiphisternum to pubis is recommended and it may be extended to thorax, if necessary.
- The rest of the treatment depends on the nature of injury. Bleeding mesenteric vessels are ligated, injured small bowel is repaired by suturing or by resection and anastomosis. In colonic injuries, simple closure or closure with protective colostomy is necessary depending upon the nature of the colonic injury and contamination.
- Liver, splenic, pancreatic and renal injuries have been discussed in respective chapters.

Competency

SU5.4: Describe medicolegal aspects of wound healing and gunshot wounds.

The process of wound healing will have following medicolegal implications:

1. **Formation of scar tissue:** Scar tissue over specific areas like face may cause disfigurement. If that scar formation is due to injury sustained as a result of trauma, then it is an example for grievous hurt as per section 320 IPC.

   Scar formation may result in contractures. If it involves a joint, then there will be restriction of movements leading to disability. Then the injury caused may be classified as grievous as per section 320 IPC.
2. **Child abuse (battered baby syndrome):** Presence of healing wounds of different duration indicates the possibility of repeated physical abuse of the child. This has to be kept in mind while examining a child with injury in paediatric outpatient department (OPD).
3. **Elder (geriatric) abuse:** Presence of healing wounds of different duration indicates the possibility of repeated physical abuse of the elderly. This has to be kept in mind while examining a geriatric age group person with injury in outpatient department (OPD).

Gunshot Wounds

Gunshot wounds are high energy injuries that can result in extensive damage to soft tissues, viscera, bone, etc. Depending upon the site of entry and exit points, damage can occur. Lucky are a few where on bullet enters and exists missing major vascular structure or viscera as it may happen in the abdomen.

Damage caused by a bullet is directly related to its kinetic energy. It is due to various factors such as passage of missile, cavitation and secondary shock wave. Cavitation refers to the damage caused by bullet to the surrounding tissue due to fragmentation, shearing forces and turbulence.

Kinetic energy is mass and velocity to the power of 2 divided by 2.

The basic principles of the management of gunshot wounds are control of haemorrhage, preventing infection, and reconstruction. The extent to which a gunshot wound needs to be surgically explored can be difficult to determine sometimes. The aim is not to remove the bullet which may be visible in an X-ray or CT scan but to see the effects of tissue destruction such as bleeding, intestinal perforations, mesenteric tear or soft tissue and vascular injuries in the neck.

If fractures occur and fragmentation of bullet occur means wound severity is more and, therefore, a requirement for more surgical exploration, followed by debridement of dead and crushed tissues.

Gunshot wounds should never be closed primarily; the full range of reconstruction from secondary intention to free tissue transfer may be required.

Treatment

As an urgent measure, if active bleeding is visible, apply pressure and try to stop the bleeders. Bleeders can be from vessels or from muscles. Temporary tourniquet can be applied to buy some time and proceed to shift the patient to the operation theatre for corrective measures. Dressings are applied and antibiotics to be started. Tetanus toxoid injections are given. Wound debridement should be thorough with saline irrigation. Fractures are treated initially by immobilisation/stabilisation. Patient may require one more debridement or delayed exploration depending upon the situation.

Exploratory laparotomy is done in abdominal gunshot wounds—perforations are sutures, transacted intestines are resected, and anastomosis is done. Bleeding liver and spleen are sutured to stop the bleeding. Shattered spleen requires splenectomy. Bleeding mesenteric vessels are ligated. Look for intestinal ischaemia in such cases. Non-viable intestines need to be respected.

Penetrating Trauma of the Abdomen

Today all penetrating injuries of the abdomen need not be explored by laparotomy. Good physical examination of the patient, entry and exit point, and haemodynamic status of the patient followed by investigations such as ultrasonogram and CT scan will guide the decision for laparotomy (Key Box 54.3).

Advanced trauma life support—ATLS is essential in the early hour of trauma. It is ideal that every surgeon/ doctor has studied ATLS manual.

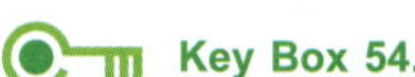
Key Box 54.3

Indications for Laparotomy

- Tenderness, guarding, rigidity
- Unexplained shock
- Evisceration of contents
- Positive investigations
  - Positive DPL
  - Gas under diaphragm
  - IVP, cystoscopy, cystogram
  - Ultrasonogram
  - CT scan

Management

Primary survey cABCDE and resuscitation is done as described earlier.

Competency

SU17.3: Describe principles in management of mass casualities.

Management of Mass Casualities

Introduction: In this modern world, terrorist attacks and bombings are largely responsible for mass casualties. When hundreds of patients are brought to the casualty, we need to quickly triage them in such a way that attention first should be given to treat moderate to severe injures patients who are likely to survive than severely injured patients who are unlikely to survive.

Definition: Any number of casualties that exceed the resources normally available from local resources has been described as mass casualties. Examples of mass casualties are terrorist attacks, bombings, railway accidents, etc. In cases of multiple casualties, full resources can be brought to treat each individual patient.

Mass casualty level: Depending upon number of patients who are brought to the casualty, a classification has been developed which is given below.

- Level 1—mass casualty incident resulting in less than 10 surviving victims.
- Level 2—mass casualty incident resulting in 10 to 25 surviving victims.
- Level 3—mass casualty incident resulting in more than 25 surviving victims.
- Level 4—mass casualty incident resulting in a number of surviving victims that could necessitate an inter-region response and/get ready for an additional disaster plan.

Four steps in mass casualties

1. **Mitigation:** Mitigation includes variety of measures which are taken before an event that occurs which may result in illness or loss of lives or property. Basically, in hospital in anticipation of a mass casualty or disaster, certain beds are year marked or a team of doctors are made available with the help of group messages or to arrange for many ventilators, etc.
2. **Preparedness:** This may vary from place to place depending upon resources available including staffing. Few important considerations are given for safety measures, security of the hospital and to treating doctors, arranging for quick radiological investigations, etc.
3. Response
4. Recovery.

Health risk in mass casualty: In the year 2001, earthquake happened in Gujarat. Around 20000 people died and about few thousands were injured. The organs which most commonly injured were lower extremity (56%), spinal and pelvic (17%), upper extremity (13%), and chest and/or abdomen (<2%). What one can observe here is many of such patients can be saved provided a good triaging is done and treatment is started immediately before shock and multiorgan failure develops.

Responsibilities of a surgeon

- Surgeons must be prepared for especially complex and difficult wounding patterns that are not typically seen in routine practice, and that greatly increase morbidity and mortality, such as blast lung, and multiple penetrating injuries from both destructive shrapnel increasingly used in bombs and from automatic firearms.
- Surgeon should be trained in managing mass casualties, disasters at local and community level.

- Surgeon should avoid over triaging—means patients who are likely to die should not be treated.
- We also should recognize small minority of patients with urgent and salvageable life-threatening injuries at immediate risk of death (undertriage).
- Ideally triage should be done outside the hospital.
- At operation theatre, damage control should be the principle till the influx to the operation theatre ends.
- All intensive care unit beds should be made available for accommodating these patients whenever it is possible.
- Every attempt is made to decrease mortality rate.

BLUNT ABDOMINAL TRAUMA

INTRODUCTION

Blunt abdominal trauma (BAT) is one of the common surgical emergencies encountered by general surgeons. Increasing number of vehicles, high speed and poor maintenance of the roads are the contributing factors. Blunt injury abdomen with polytrauma is one of the commonest causes of death in the younger population. Thus, it is important for a house officer to recognise a polytrauma patient, to diagnose and to suspect intra-abdominal injury, so that urgent resuscitation and treatment can be offered to the patient at the proper time, at the proper hospital and by a proper surgeon. Major systems involved are given in Key Boxes 54.4 and 54.5.

Key Box 54.4

Common Viscera Involved in Blunt Injury

Spleen	Significant bleeding
Liver	Significant bleeding
Kidney	Significant bleeding
Intestines	Perforation—peritonitis
Mesentery	Bleeding
Pancreaticoduodenal injuries	Usually missed—bleeding
Diaphragm	Missed—tachypnoea
Urinary bladder	Urinary peritonitis

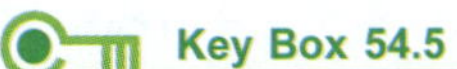

Key Box 54.5

Major Systems Involved

- Craniospinal
- Chest
- Abdomen
- Pelvis
- Skeletal

Craniospinal and chest injuries are discussed in their respective chapters. Pelvic and skeletal injury is beyond the limits of this book. In this chapter, blunt injury of the abdomen is discussed.

Causes of Blunt Injury Abdomen

1. Rail and road traffic accidents (most common)
2. Fall from a height and dashing against an object
3. Seat belt syndrome
4. Assault

Regions/Anatomy of the Abdomen (Fig. 54.2)

1. **Anterior abdomen** means it involves 9 regions, namely right and left hypochondrium, epigastrium, right and left lumbar regions, umbilical region, right and left iliac fossa and hypogastrium.
2. **Thoraco-abdomen:** This area is inferior to nipple line anteriorly and infrascapular line posteriorly and superior to costal margins. Liver, spleen and diaphragm are the important organs here.
3. **Flank:** It is between the anterior and posterior axillary lines from the 6th intercostals space to the iliac crest. Covered by thick muscles which often protects renal injuries from penetrating wounds.
4. **Back:** Again there are thick muscles such as erector spinae, quadratus lumborum, etc. Back is an area from the tip of the scapulae to the iliac crests, posterior to posterior axillary lines. These areas contain retroperitoneal structures which are usually missed sites in trauma of the abdomen. The organs include duodenum, posterior parts of the descending and

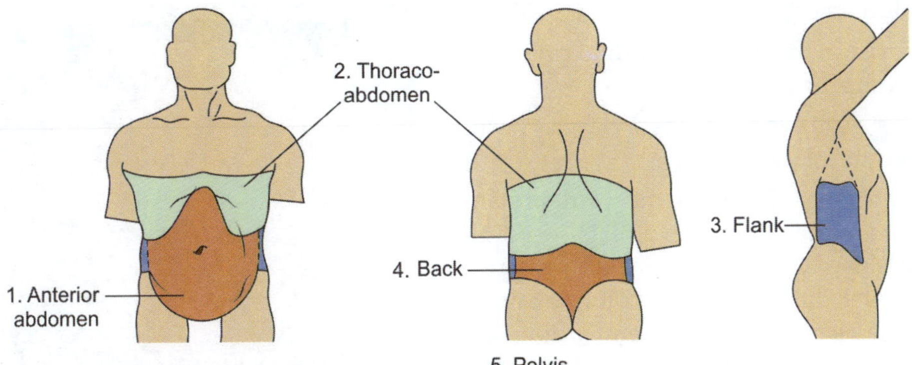

Fig. 54.2: Regions of abdomen for trauma assessment

ascending colons, pancreas, kidney and ureters, vascular structures such as aorta and inferior vena cava. Diagnostic laparoscopy, focussed assessment sonography in trauma (FAST), diagnostic peritoneal lavage will not be of help. CT is the best investigation of choice.

5. **Pelvic cavity:** It contains some very important structures such as rectum, urinary bladder, reproductive organs, iliac vessels, etc. It is also the extension of retroperitoneal and intraperitoneal spaces. Pelvic fractures and injuries may result in significant bleeding which can be life-threatening.

Mechanisms of Injury/Pathophysiology

They can be broadly classified into blunt abdominal trauma (BAT) or penetrating abdominal trauma. Following are various mechanisms of abdominal trauma.

- **Direct blow or crush:** This can be from lower rim of steering wheel or from the door of a motor vehicle results in crushing injuries of both solid and hollow viscera. Transverse colon is one of the hollow viscera in this type of injuries.

  Crushing effect: Here solid viscera are crushed between anterior abdominal wall and vertebral column or posterior thoracic cage.
- **Shearing:** These injuries will occur when a restraint device is worn improperly, e.g. lap belt.
- **Deceleration injuries** are the one in which differential movement of fixed and nonfixed parts of the body occurs. Examples being liver, spleen and small bowel injuries.

  It causes differential movement among adjacent structures. Shearing forces are created; they cause solid, visceral organs and vascular pedicles to tear at relatively fixed points of attachment. Examples:
  - Renal pedicle injury
  - Injury to distal aorta than proximal mobile aorta as former is attached to thoracic spine.
- **Bursting:** Acute tracheoaesophageal burst injuries are reported from blunt chest trauma.

  Sudden dramatic rise in the intra-abdominal pressure due to external compression
  - Hollow viscus ruptures (in accordance with principles of **Boyle's law**).
- **Penetration:** Penetrating injuries are the result of stab wounds, gunshot wounds or due to pellets (used to shoot wild bore). Most commonly involved structures are liver, small bowel, diaphragm and colon. In cases of gunshots and pellets, injuries depend upon the speed of the shot, cavitation effect and bullet fragmentation.
- Vehicular trauma is by far the leading cause of blunt abdominal trauma.

ASSESSMENT HISTORY—AT CASUALTY/TRIAGE

- *Exact nature of the accident*—collision, penetrating trauma, fall from height, shotgun, pellet injuries explosion. In addition to high-speed vehicle accidents, polytrauma is also common in India due to fall form height due to coconut plucking from coconut tree or from construction site fall.
- History of loss of consciousness initially followed by recovery may be the indication of extradural haemorrhage—to be kept in mind.
- History of medications specially beta-blockers and anticoagulants should be elicited, if present to be recorded. Even if a patient is not in hyovolaemia, there can be bradycardia, if patient is taking propranolol.

Physical Examination–Primary Survey

ABCDE (ATLS protocol)	**AMPLE** (History)
Airway	**A**llergy
Breathing	**M**edication
Circulation	**P**ast medical illness
Disability	**L**ast meal
Exposure	**E**vents leading to incident

Secondary Survey and Definitive Care

- Inspection, palpation, percussion and auscultation should be done in the usual manner. Patient should be exposed full length—entire chest, abdomen and pelvis—both anterior and posterior.
- Tachycardia and hypotension are the early features of ongoing bleeding. Patient who is lying down without any pain but anxious may be having bleeding and one who is not moving but with pain may be having hollow viscus perforation. ***Restless patients have often head injuries.***
- Abdominal distension (Fig. 54.3) is quite often due to solid viscus bleed from liver or spleen. It is also

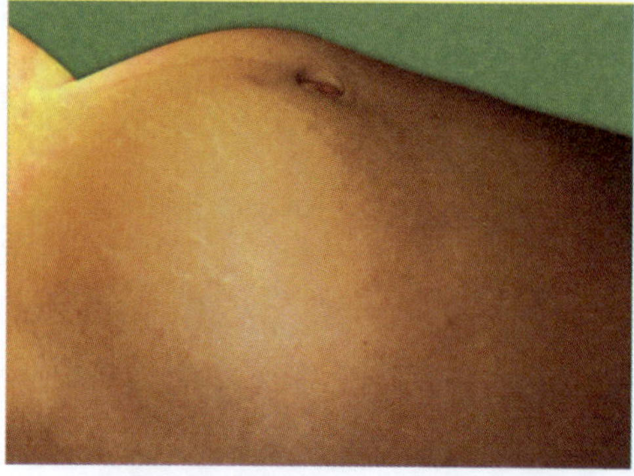

Fig. 54.3: Abdominal distension

due to perforation of a viscus and retroperitoneal injuries resulting in paralytic ileus.

- Abrasions, echymosis, lacerations over the abdominal wall, stab injuries, foreign bodies, evisceration of omentum or intestines to be recorded.
- Lapbelt injuries sign: If these are present they indicate underlying injuries.
- Saree sign: *See* page 998.

Indian women—vulnerability: The Saree and Churidar are traditional Indian dresses. One end of the Saree is tied around the waist and the other draped freely along the shoulder. If care is not taken, the free end often gets caught in the mill belt and causes injuries around the waist (blunt abdominal trauma) due to the drag created. The impression created on the abdomen is by the Saree and not the mill belt. The Shawl of the Churidar (has two free ends) can get caught in a belt or a wheel to cause injuries around the neck. The drag may be sufficient to cause even strangulation. The author remembers a case of scalp avulsion due to long hair of a woman getting caught in a mill belt.

- **Cullen sign, Grey Turner sign:** Discolouration around umbilicus and flanks respectively indicate retroperitoneal bleeding.
- **London sign:** If you see some pattern of the tyre, seatbelt, it indicates a severe compression and invariably there will be underlying intra-abdominal injury.
- Entry- and exit-bullet wounds.

PALPATION, PERCUSSION, AUSCULTATION

- Tenderness is a feature of peritonitis. It may be minimal in cases of bleeding. Superficial tenderness results due to abdominal wall muscle injures and deep tenderness is the sign of peritonitis. Palpation of high riding prostate is the sign of significant pelvic fracture.
- Percussion is done to elicit peritoneal irritation.
- Bowel sounds are absent in cases of peritonitis.

Pearls of Wisdom

No time should be wasted in doing unnecessary percussion to find out the fluid because it will be detected later by FAST. Once examination is completed, patient should be covered with warm blankets to **prevent** hypothermia. Because hypothermia results in coagulopathy and ongoing bleeding.

ASSESSMENT OF PELVIC STABILITY

- **Pelvic fracture** should be suspected when hypotension is present in a conscious patient who has no obvious injuries. Blood at the urinary meatus, high riding prostate, scrotal haematoma, (rupture urethra), limb length discrepancy suggest pelvic fracture.
- Gentle pressure over iliac bone in a downward and medial direction is applied. Laxity and instability suggests pelvic fracture. Only one attempt to test the pelvis should be done. Frequent tests may result in more bleeding and even dislodge the clot.
- **It is better to avoid this test in patients with hypotension.**

Examination of Pelvic Organs and Gluteal Region

- **Urethra:** Blood at meatus and scrotal a haematoma suggests urethral injury. Catheterisation should not be done in such cases.
- **Rectal examination** to look for bleeding, loose sphincter and high riding prostate. In cases of rupture of membranous part of urethra, prostate will not be palpable as it is displaced upwards. It is called high riding prostate also described as **Vermooten's sign.**
- **Vaginal examination** to be done when you suspect vaginal injuries as in presence of perineal lacerations and pelvic fractures.

  Gently turn the patient like a logwood and examine the back and gluteal region. Gunshots or stab injuries may cause gluteal injuries. It may involve intra-abdominal injuries and rectum also.

Signs of pelvic fracture can be remembered as PELVIS

- **P**rostate—high riding
- **E**xternal meatus—drop of blood
- **L**imb discrepancy
- **V**aginal tear
- **I**liac vessels—hypotension
- **S**crotal haematoma

Tertiary Survey

Repeat primary survey, secondary survey and repeat laboratory/imaging studies for wisdom lines in blunt abdominal trauma.

Investigations

1. **Complete blood count,** coagulation studies, grouping and cross-matching. Fall in haemoglobin is an indication of on-going haemorrhage—especially while managing a patient with liver/splenic injury on conservative line of management.
2. **Serum electrolyte** analysis
3. **Serum amylase/lipase**
   - May be elevated because of **pancreatic ischaemia due to hypotension**

- **Persistent elevation** may be indication of **pancreatic injury.**

4. **Plain X-rays** (Fig. 54.4)
   - **Chest X-ray:** If it shows pneumoperitoneum, cresenteric air shadow under the right dome of the diaphragm, it suggests perforation of the hollow viscus. Look for pneumothorax (Fig. 54.5). Fundic, stomach (air bubble in thorax as in diaphragmatic injury, retroperitoneal air—duodenal perforation).
   - Pelvic fractures.
5. **Role of ultrasound** (Fig. 54.6)

   FAST: Focussed assessment with sonography for trauma.
6. **Diagnostic peritoneal lavage (DPL)**

   It is indicated in BAT in the following situations:
   - Multiple injuries and shock
   - Spinal cord injury
   - Obtunded patient with possible abdominal injury
   - Intoxicated patient

   Also *see* splenic trauma (*see* page 703).

Types

- **Open:** Infraumbilical skin incision and open peritoneum.
- **Semiopen:** Infraumbilical skin incision deepen up to linea alba.
- **Closed:** Blind insertion of needle.

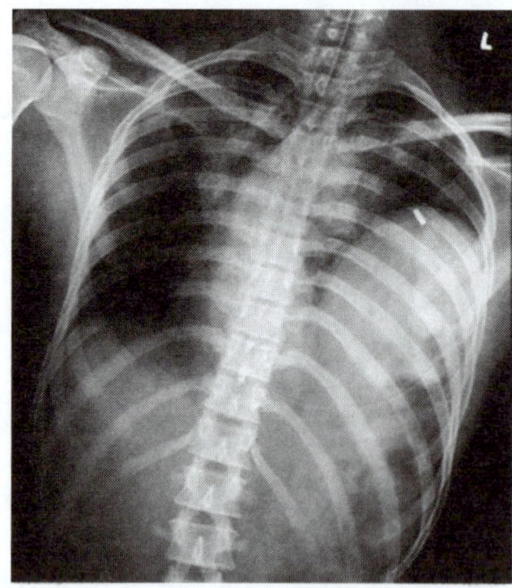

Fig. 54.4: Chest X-ray showing diaphragmatic hernia on the left side

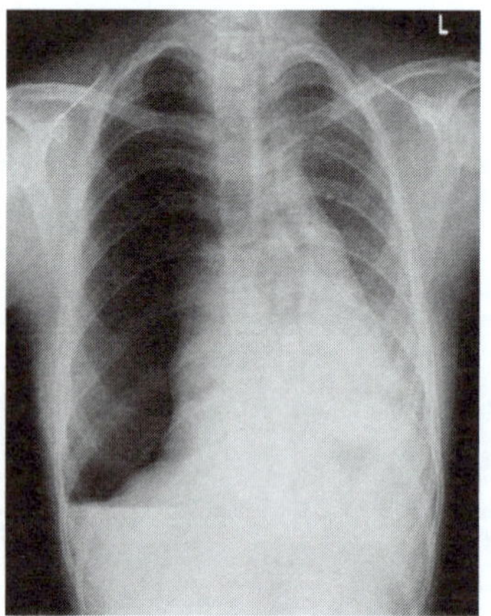

Observe **5 Ts** of pneumothorax
- **T**achypnoea
- **T**achycardia
- **T**ympanic note
- **T**otal absence
- **T**racheal shift

Fig. 54.5: Pneumothorax

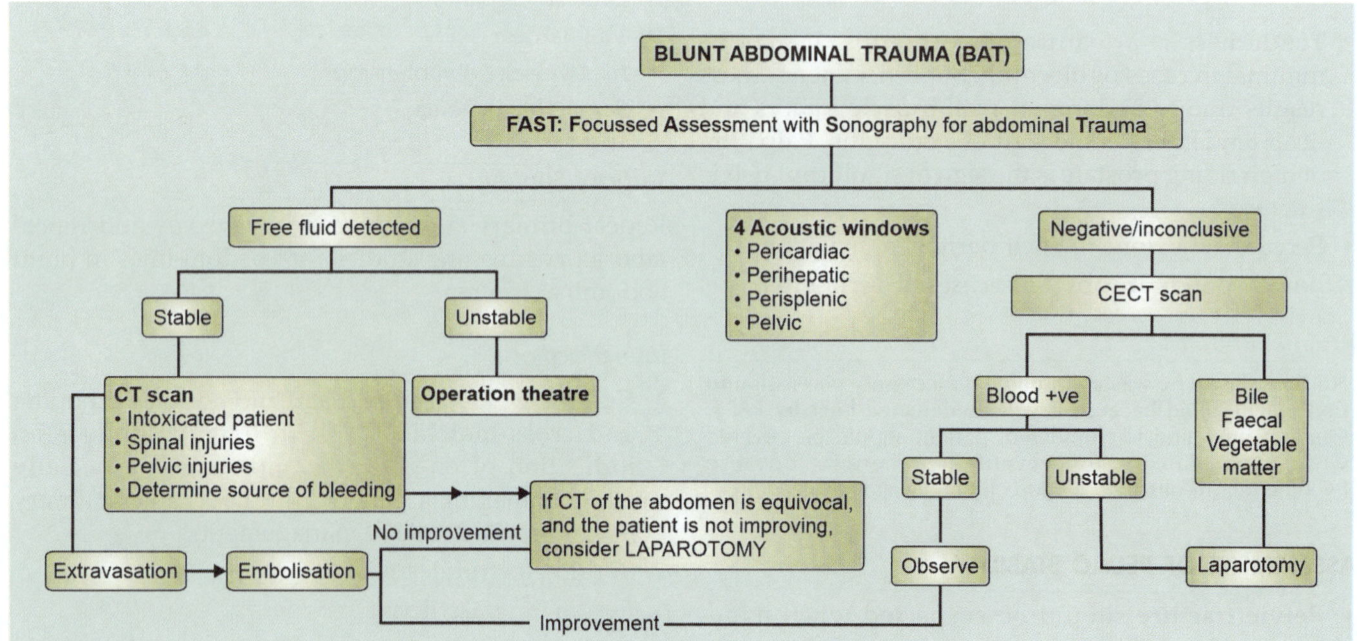

Fig. 54.6: Algorithm of investigations in BAT (*see* FAST)

Precautions

- Foley's catheter to empty bladder
- Ryle's tube to empty stomach
- X-ray pelvis to detect pelvic fracture.

Positive DPL

- 10 ml of gross blood aspirate before infusion of lavage fluid.
- More than 100,000 RBC/ml
- More than 500 WBC/ml
- Bile and bacteria are demonstrated
- Vegetable matter

Pearls of Wisdom

Positive DPL means intraperitoneal injury is present. It does not mean that the patient should be shifted to operation theatre immediately.

7. **CT scan** (Fig. 54.7)
   - Gold standard for solid organ injuries
   - CT also can reveal other associated injuries such as vertebral or pelvic fractures.
   - CT can also pick up **diaphragmatic injury** (CT chest).
   - It can detect **source of haemorrhage**.
   - CT is an excellent scan for pancreas, duodenum, etc.
8. **Diagnostic laparoscopy:** Done when CT scan is negative, suspicion of diaphragmatic injury is present (Fig. 54.8).

Pearls of Wisdom

Stable patients with solid organ injuries are managed more often by nonsurgical methods with close monitoring.

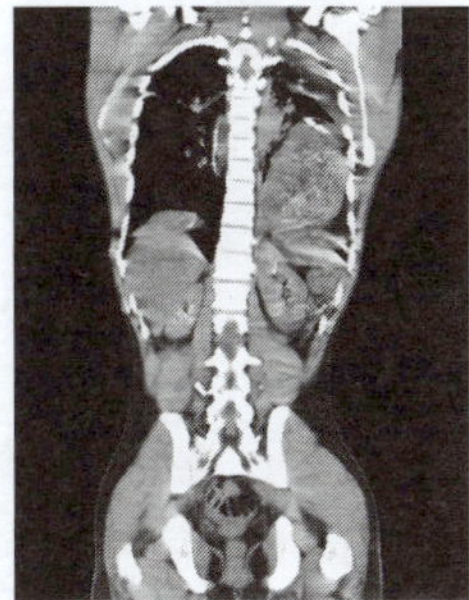

Fig. 54.7: Diaphragmatic hernia—CT scan (*Courtesy:* Dr Yashdeep Sharma, Associate Professor, KMC, Manipal)

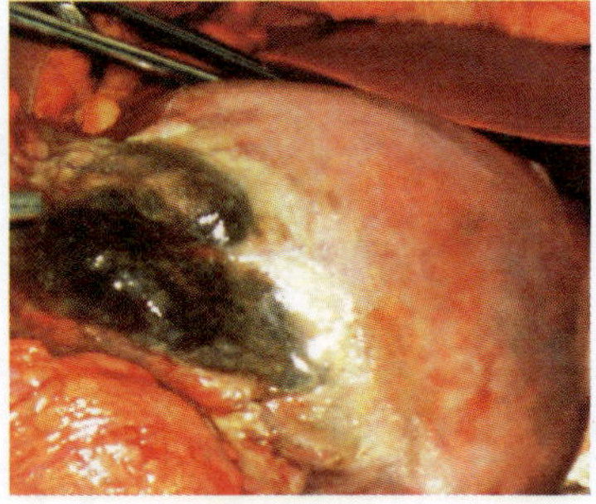

Fig. 54.8: Diaphragmatic hernia with gangrene of the stomach

Remarks

With the availability of FAST and CT scan, role of DPL is now limited to unstable patients whose FAST results are negative or inconclusive.

ADJUNCTS TO PHYSICAL EXAMINATION—TUBES AND CATHETERS

- **Nasogastric (Ryle's) tube:** Vast majority of cases, tube is passed through nose—nasogastric. Confirm it is in place by auscultation of the abdomen and by pushing air. In cases of skull base fractures, the tube may enter the cranial cavity hence better to pass the tube through oral cavity, orogastric. When in doubt an X-ray abdomen can confirm the tube in the stomach. Blood in the aspirate suggests esophagogastric injuries. Nasogastric tube insertion will decrease the abdominal distension, prevents vomiting and thus aspiration. **One of the life-saving uses of nasogastric aspiration is for acute gastric dilatation (AGD) which is a potentially dangerous condition often seen following blunt trauma abdomen.** Passive air sucking by negative intragastric pressure and a flaccid lower esophageal sphincter have been proposed as causes of AGD in trauma patients. Aerophagia in confused, agitated trauma patients, reflex gastric ileus due to visceral and somatic nerve stimulation and gastric atony due to excessive potassium and chloride losses have also been suggested as causes of AGD in trauma patients.
- **Urinary catheter:** Firstly, one should not introduce a Foley catheter, if you suspect urethral injuries. For example: Blood at the urinary meatus. Once urethral injury is ruled out, catheterization is done by using all aseptic measures and a proper lubrication. It will help in relieving retention—distended bladder (may help for DPL later), help in monitoring urinary output. Significant bleeding will indicate renal tract injuries, namely kidney and urinary bladder.

Indications for Laparotomy

- BAT with hypotension and intraperitoneal bleeding and positive FAST
- Hypotension following stab injuries or penetrating wounds
- Evisceration (Fig. 54.9)
- Peritonitis—diffuse tenderness and rebound tenderness
- Free air, diaphragmatic rupture, retroperitoneal air
- Contrast CT with evidence of hollow viscous perforation, renal pedicle or splenic pedicle injury, intraperitoneal bladder injury.

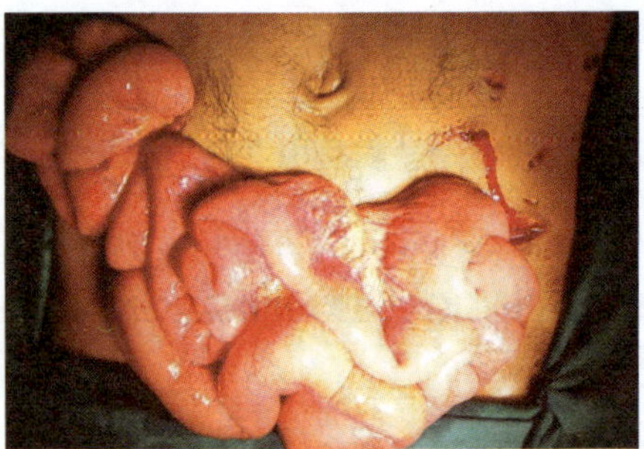

Fig. 54.9: Evisceration following stab injury

Competency

SU28.10: Describe the applied anatomy of liver. Describe the clinical features, investigations and principles of management of live abscess, hydatid disease, injuries and tumours of the liver.

LIVER INJURIES

Liver injury should be suspected when a patient with suspected blunt injury abdomen is brought with the following features:

- Right lower ribs fracture.
- Injury marks on the lower chest or upper abdomen.
- Patient with persistent hypotension or patient who had shock following blunt injury abdomen.
- A child can have liver injury without fracture of ribs because of elastic nature of the rib cage.

Clinical Presentation

- The most common presentation is features of intraperitoneal haemorrhage, which includes hypotension, thready pulse, abdominal distension. Peritoneal signs are minimal as early bleeding does not produce much peritoneal irritation.
- However, massive lacerations of the liver including stellate fractures present with rapidly developing hypotension and shock, which are life-threatening.

Investigations

- Ultrasonography and more precisely CT scan should be done in all patients who are haemodynamically stable with or without support (Figs 54.10 to 54.13 and Key Box 54.6).

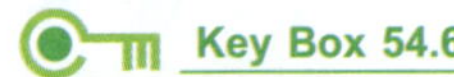

Key Box 54.6

CT Scan with IV Contrast

- It can grade the liver injury.
- It can guide a conservative or operative treatment.
- It also rules out other injuries.
- Grade I and Grade II injuries can be managed by non-operative treatment.
- Free contrast in and around the liver is indicative of active bleeding.

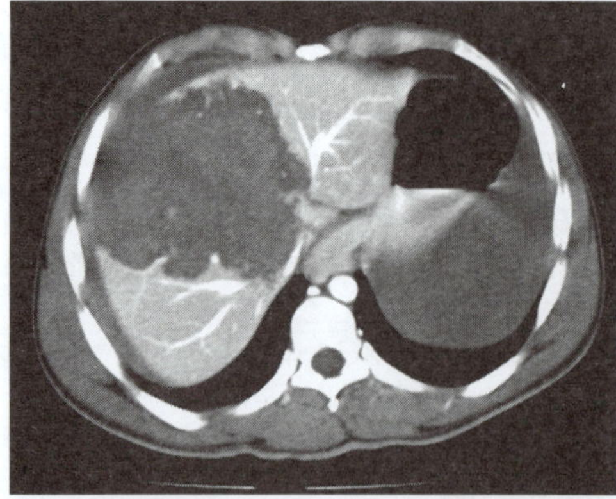

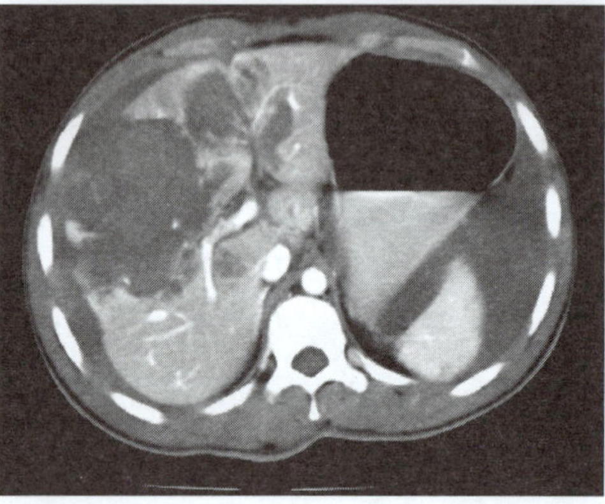

Figs 54.10 and 54.11: CECT arterial phase—Grade IV laceration of the liver with haemoperitoneum—interestingly patient was stable, managed conservatively, got discharged on 10th day

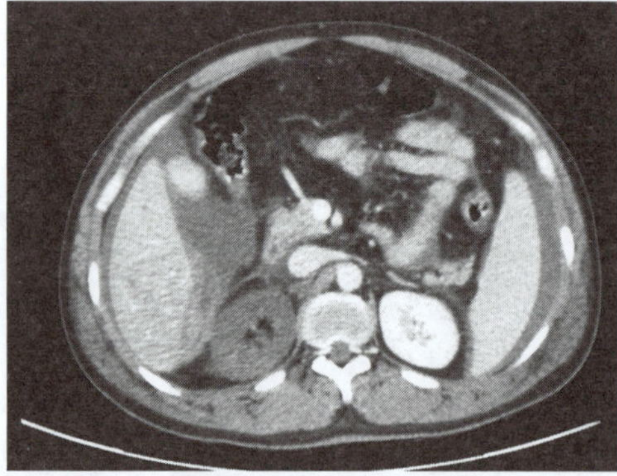

Fig. 54.12: Coronal section liver and kidney injury

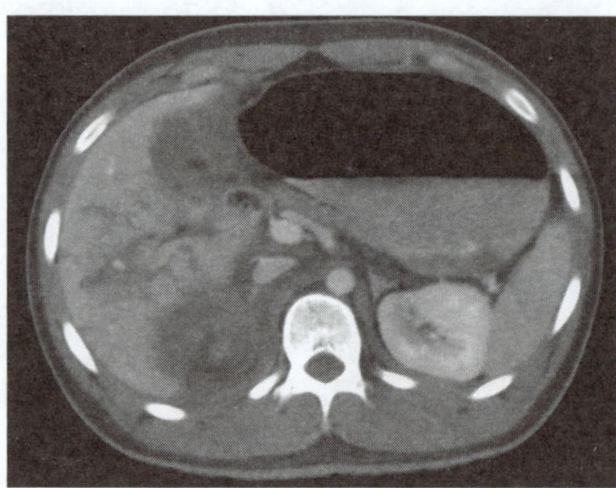

Fig. 54.13: Liver injury Grade II

Table 54.1 Liver injury scale

Grade	Injury	Description
I	Haematoma	Subcapsular haematoma; <10% surface area
	Laceration	Capsular tear, <1 cm parenchymal depth
II	Haematoma	Subcapsular, 10–50% surface area; intraparenchymal extension <10 cm diameter
	Laceration	<10 cm long; 1–3 cm parenchymal depth
III	Haematoma	Subcapsular, >50% surface area; expanding intraparenchymal haematoma of >10 cm or expanding
	Laceration	>3 cm, intraparenchymal depth
IV	Laceration	Parenchymal disruption of 1–3 Couinaud's segments within a single lobe
V	Laceration	Parenchymal disruption >3 Couinaud's segments within a single lobe
	Vascular	Retrohepatic vena cava/central major hepatic veins
VI	Vascular	Hepatic avulsion

- Also *see* Table 54.1.

Treatment (Key Boxes 54.7 and 54.8)

1. **Simple lacerations which are not bleeding at laparotomy:** A drain is kept in the liver bed, blood and clots are sucked out and peritoneal wash is given.
2. **Simple laceration with bleeding:** It is sutured by interlocking horizontal mattress sutures by using special liver suturing needle. If too much tension is applied while suturing, cutting through can occur. Omentum can be used as a **Plug** in between the laceration (Fig. 54.14). Absorbable sutures are used.

Key Box 54.7

Haemostatic Techniques at Surgery

- Liver suture
- Perihepatic packing
- Resection
- Argon beam coagulator followed by fibrin glue and sheet of Surgicel (haemostatic agent)
- Selective arteriography and embolisation in arterio-venous fistula or haemobilia

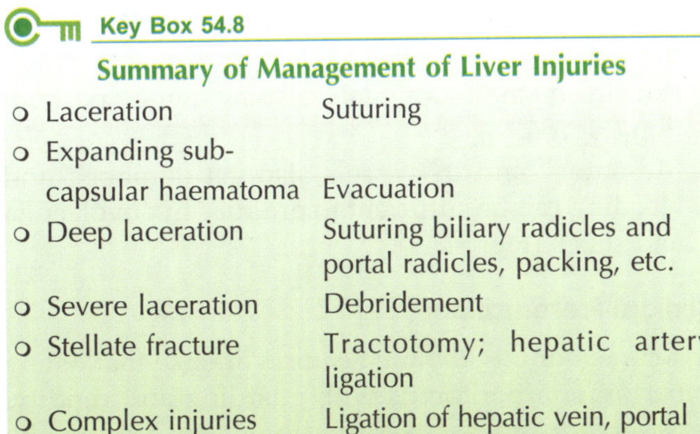

Key Box 54.8

Summary of Management of Liver Injuries

Laceration	Suturing
Expanding subcapsular haematoma	Evacuation
Deep laceration	Suturing biliary radicles and portal radicles, packing, etc.
Severe laceration	Debridement
Stellate fracture	Tractotomy; hepatic artery ligation
Complex injuries	Ligation of hepatic vein, portal vein branches or lobectomy, etc.

3. **Subcapsular haematoma:** If present, should be evacuated.
4. **Deep laceration with bleeding:** In such situations, wound should be opened. Dead liver parenchyma is removed, bleeding vessel at depth and biliary radicle are ligated. It is described as **tractotomy**.
5. **Severe lacerations:** These injuries present with massive bleeding (Fig. 54.15). Temporary control is

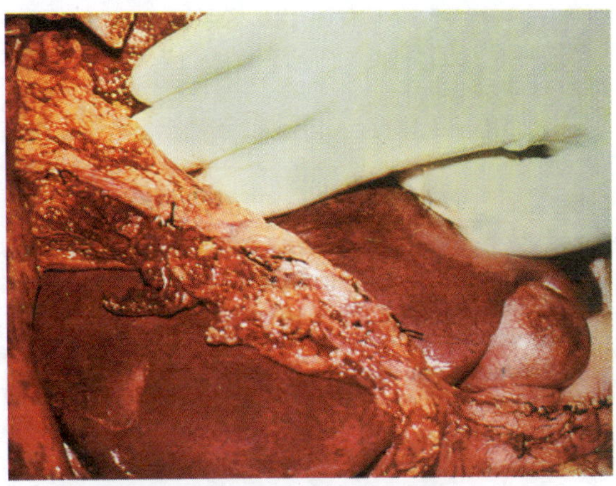

Fig. 54.14: Liver injury—use of omentum

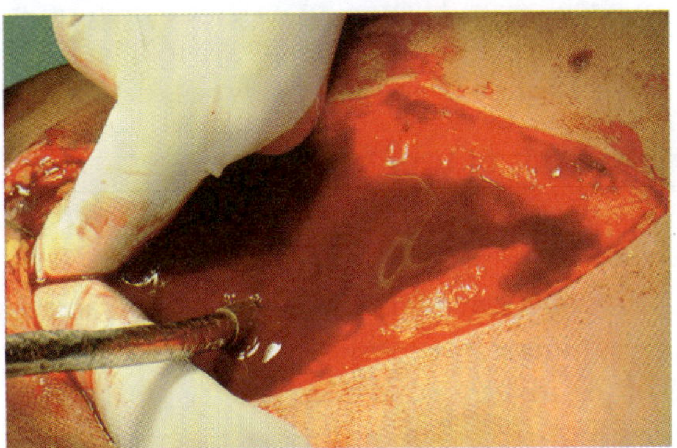

Fig. 54.15: Massive bleeding—challenging task (*Courtesy:* Dr Sunil Krishna, Associate Professor, KMC, Manipal)

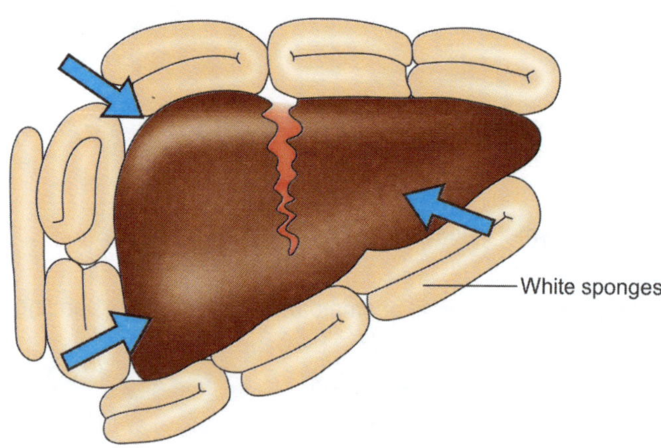

Fig. 54.16: Perihepatic packing

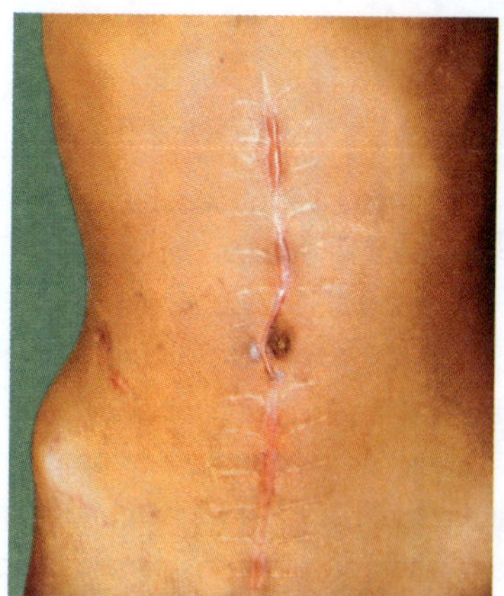

Fig. 54.17: Laparotomy scar in a patient who had liver laceration that was sutured. He presented with massive haematemesis later—**a case of haemobilia**

obtained by compression of portal vein and hepatic artery in gastrohepatic omentum in front of **foramen of Winslow (Pringle manoeuvre)**. If bleeding stops, portal veins or branches of hepatic artery are damaged. If bleeding continues, hepatic veins are the source of bleeding. Visualisation of source of bleeding with debridement of avascular liver tissue is done by finger fracture method. **Perihepatic packing can be used to compress the liver as a temporary measure to buy time for resuscitation, to explore rest of the abdomen or as a definitive treatment when other measures fail.** Pack is usually removed after 24–48 hours (Fig. 54.16).

- Nonanatomical resection may have to be done, in a few cases.

6. **Complex liver injuries:** These injuries involve hepatic veins, retrohepatic vena cava or branches of portal vein resulting in massive haemorrhage. This type of massive injury can be managed by a large thoracoabdominal incision or abdominosternal incision by doing sternotomy. Division of the right triangular ligament helps in visualising bleeding from hepatic veins.
   - **Schrock shunt:** Failure of Pringle manoeuvre means juxtahepatic and retrohepatic vena caval injuries. In such cases, Heaney manoeuvre clamping both infra- and suprahepatic vena cava followed by atriocaval shunt or venovenous bypass can be done.

Complications of Liver Injuries

1. Massive bleeding, hypovolaemia and cardiac arrest.
2. Haematoma can get infected resulting in an **abscess**.
3. Haematoma can rupture into the peritoneal cavity resulting in leakage of bile—biliary peritonitis.
4. **Haemobilia** refers to rupture of the haematoma into the bile duct—it may result in massive haematemesis or melaena.

Clinical Notes

- A 24-year-old male patient was operated for blunt injury abdomen by laparotomy. Liver laceration was found. It was sutured (Fig. 54.17).
- After 15 days, he came to our hospital with haematemesis. Initially it was diagnosed as erosive gastritis. Ultrasonography revealed a pseudoaneurysm of one of the branches of middle hepatic artery. CT angiography and embolisation was tried but not successful. He had another bout of haematemesis. He underwent exploratory laparotomy and ligation of branches of middle hepatic artery. Bleeding stopped. Now since 6 months, no further attacks of haematemesis.
- It was a case of haemobilia.

SMALL BOWEL INJURIES

- The shearing injuries produce either disruption or laceration of the bowel between fixed and mobile points, i.e. at the **duodenojejunal flexure or at ileocaecal junction**. These are the most common sites of small bowel injuries.
- Injury to the small bowel can also occur due to crush injury between spine and a steering wheel or handle bars, etc.
- Bruising on the abdominal wall may suggest perforation (Fig. 54.18).
- Mesentery and its vessels also get damaged and bleeding can be sufficient to produce hypovolaemia and shock (Fig. 54.19).

Clinical Presentation

1. **Acute abdominal pain:** Features are like that of any perforation peritonitis with guarding and rigidity. Erect abdominal X-ray shows gas under the diaphragm.

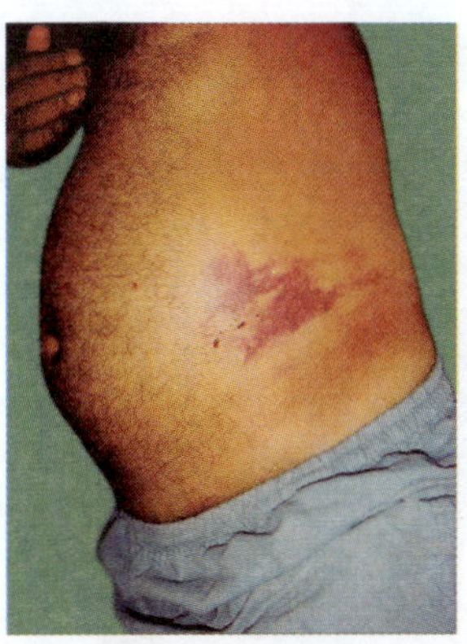

Fig. 54.18: Observe London's sign: Bruising (imprint abrasion) over the abdominal wall signifying hollow viscus perforation

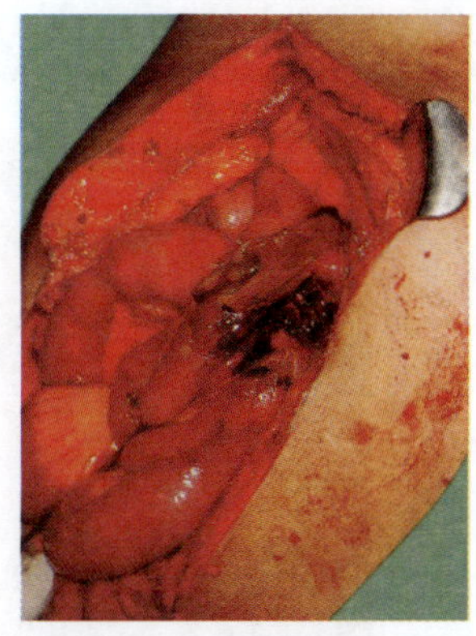

Fig. 54.19: Gangrene of the jejunal loop due to injury to mesenteric blood vessels in the same patient as in Fig. 54.18

2. **Features of peritonitis** with haemoperitoneum are the result of bowel injury with bleeding from the mesentery.
3. **Occult or hidden perforation:** A small perforation gets sealed off by coils of bowel and omentum. Most of these patients present with abdominal pain. However, very often, features of peritonitis are missed as a result of other associated injuries such as fracture pelvis or retroperitoneal haematoma. After 3–4 days, a localised abscess may form and rupture into the peritoneal cavity, resulting in peritonitis. This is aggravated by intake of oral fluids which stimulate peristalsis. **Repeated examination is the most honoured, most fruitful investigation in blunt injuries of the abdomen** (*see* clinical notes).

Investigation

- X-ray abdomen, erect or lateral decubitus (Fig. 54.20), demonstrates free gas under the right dome of the diaphragm in majority of cases. Four-quadrant tap or diagnostic peritoneal lavage is also useful.

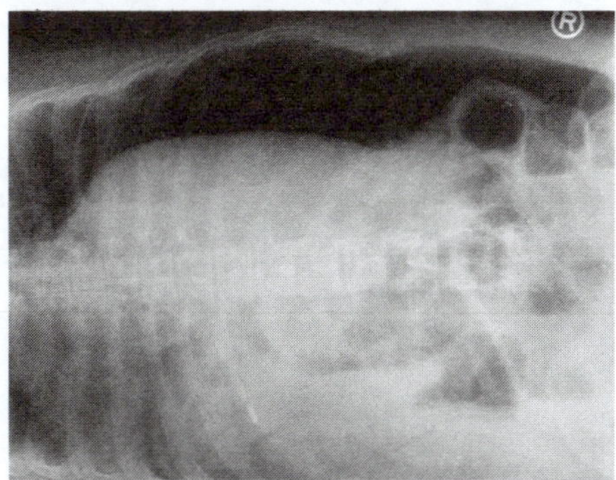

Fig. 54.20: Lateral decubitus picture is extremely useful in polytrauma cases when patient is unable to stand due to fractured limbs. However, **CT scan is the best investigation in blunt abdominal trauma** because it not only detects pneumoperitoneum but also other injuries

- When in doubt, CT scan of abdomen should be requested to diagnose hollow viscus perforation and bleeding.

Clinical Notes

- A 23-year-old male with fracture femur and pelvic fracture was admitted to the hospital after 12 hours of injury. A general surgeon was consulted to rule out an intra-abdominal injury. Pulse rate was 100/min and on deep palpation, there was tenderness in the right iliac fossa. Keeping in mind associated pelvic injury, it was decided to treat him conservatively. X-ray abdomen left lateral decubitus (Fig. 54.20) (erect film could not be taken as patient could not stand) film did not show free intraperitoneal air (gas). Ultrasound revealed a retroperitoneal haematoma of 8 cm × 3 cm.
- The patient was treated conservatively with Ryle's tube for 3 days. On the 4th day, oral fluids were started, as patient passed stools once. On 7th day morning, patient had tachypnoea. Pulse was 120/min, BP was 90/60 mmHg. Previous 24 hours urine output was only 450 ml. Abdominal examination revealed guarding and rigidity in the right iliac fossa. It was decided to do a laparotomy. At laparotomy, there was a small 2 cm perforation in the ileum with bilioma surrounded by intestinal loops and gross contamination of peritoneal cavity. The perforation was closed and the peritoneal cavity was drained. The patient made a good recovery from septicaemia, thanks to early antibiotics and surgery.

Treatment

Golden time to operate is within 6 hours.

- **Perforation:** Single or multiple, have to be closed, after trimming the edges by using non-absorbable sutures such as silk (Fig. 54.21).
- A **lacerated** or a macerated bowel has to be resected.
- Bleeding mesenteric vessels have to be ligated, haematoma must be evacuated and bowel should be inspected for any ischaemia. Food particles and bile should be evacuated (Figs 54.22 and 54.27).
- A perforation of ileum **close to the ileocaecal junction** is treated by **ileocolectomy** rather than simple closure for the fear of enterocutaneous fistula, due to suture line leakage.

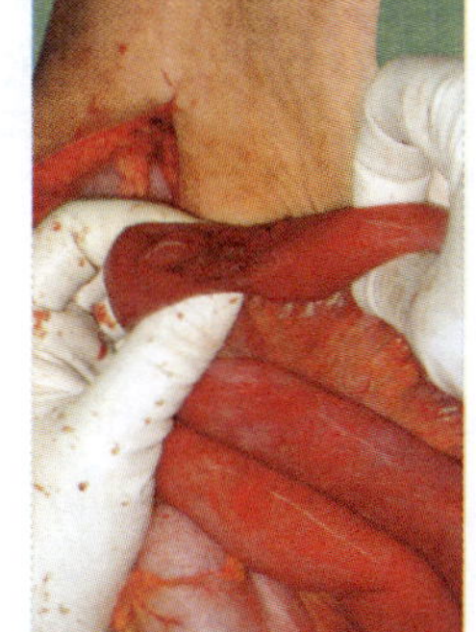

Fig. 54.21: Peritonitis following ileal perforation. Golden time to operate is within 6 hours of perforation

PHOTOGRAPHS OF SMALL INTESTINAL PERFORATION (Figs 54.22 to 54.26)

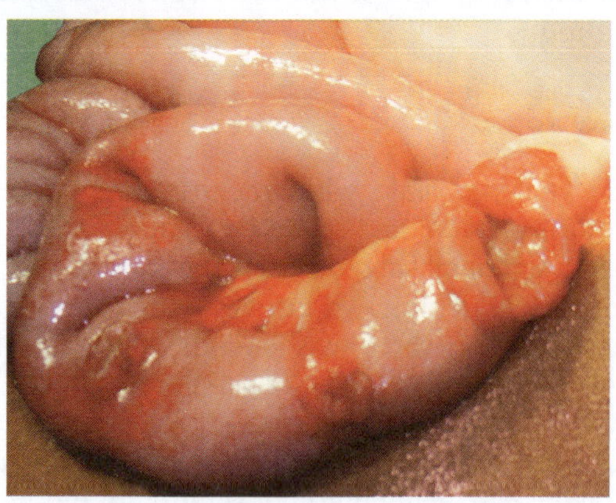

Fig. 54.22: Jejunal transection—6 cm away from DJ flexure. It is better to resect and anastomose in this type of cases (*Courtesy*: Dr Saurabh Aggarwal, Associate Prof, KMC, Manipal)

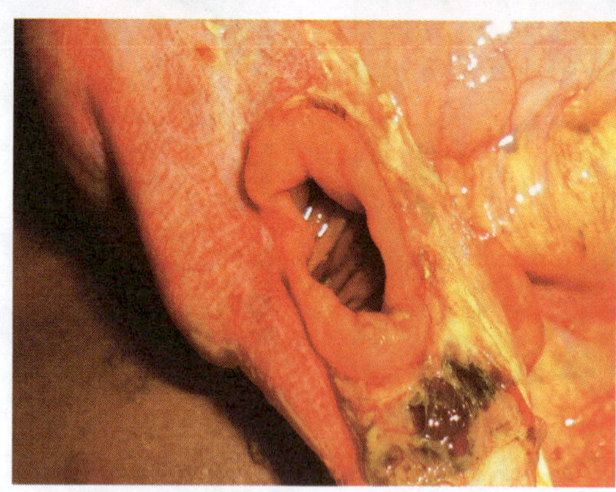

Fig. 54.23: 72 hours old perforation close to ileocaecal junction. Limited colectomy done

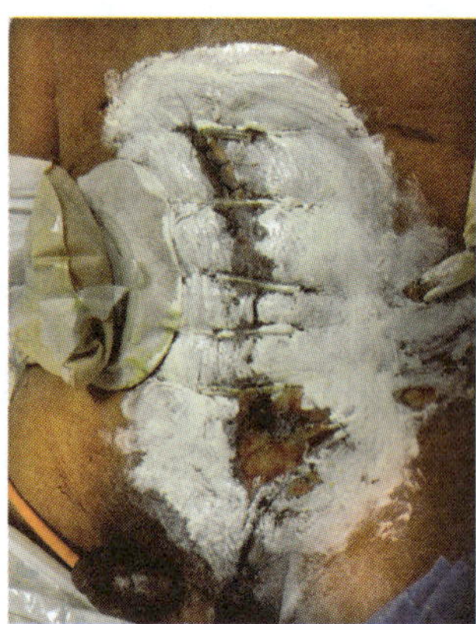

Fig. 54.24: Anastomotic leak following limited colectomy. Ileostomy done. It was closed after 8 weeks. You can see the wound infection

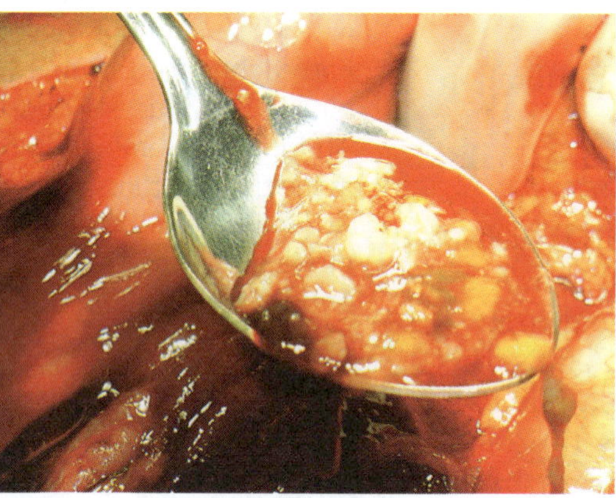

Fig. 54.25: Food particles—definite indication, if found in DPL for laparotomy

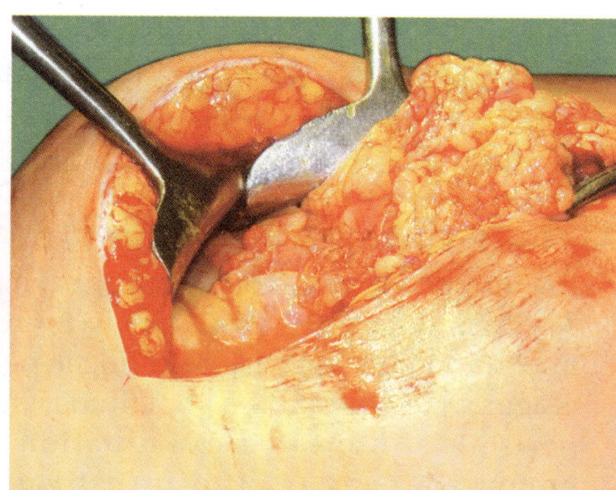

Fig. 54.26: Bile and blood in the peritoneal cavity

COLONIC INJURIES

- Blunt injury of the colon is not uncommon.
- Mobile sigmoid is more prone to injury than fixed parts.
- Steering wheel injury can directly crush the transverse colon and can cause perforation.
- Bruise or laceration of the colon can undergo ischaemic necrosis and it can present after 5–7 days with signs of peritonitis/sepsis (Figs 54.27 and 54.28).
- Diagnosis is by clinical examination/contrast enhanced CT scan.
- Depending upon the contamination, contusion or laceration and duration of injury, treatment can be resection and anastomosis within 6–8 hours of the injury or simple suturing or diversion colostomy, if gross contamination is present (Fig. 54.29).
- Even in penetrating injury, primary closure can be done.

DUODENAL INJURIES

- Retroperitoneal duodenum is commonly injured.
- Steering wheel, belt or a blow in the epigastrium may injure the duodenum as it is crushed against the spine.

Clinical Features

- Peritonitis features are not common as it is the retroperitoneal duodenum (part II and part III) that is injured.
- Tenderness is present on deep palpation.
- Being retroperitoneal, these injuries manifest late with abscess formation or fluid in lesser sac, etc.

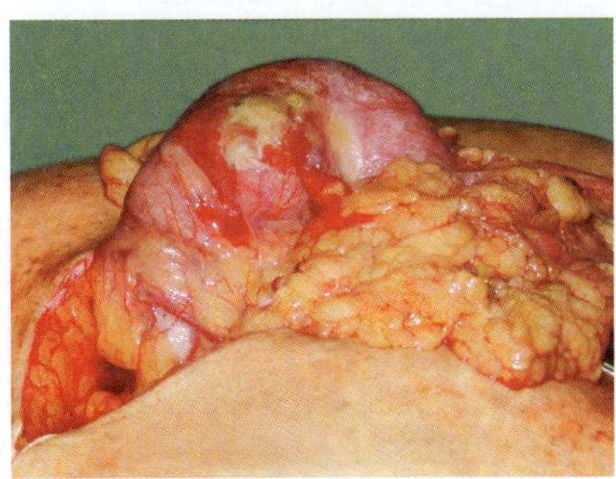

Fig. 54.27: Colonic perforations. The patient presented 7 days later with abdominal distension and early sepsis—steering wheel injury to the transverse colon

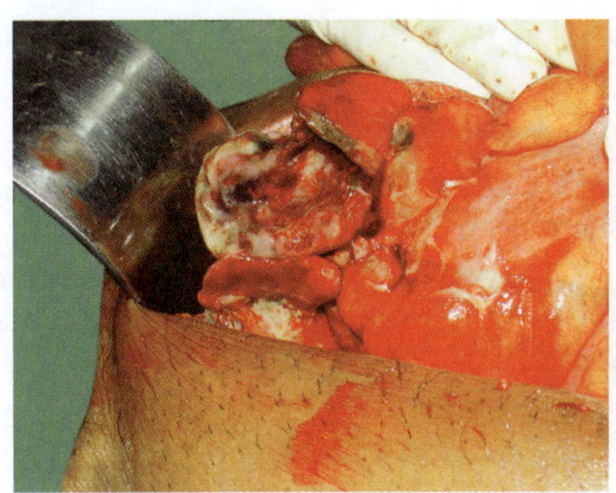

Fig. 54.28: Sigmoid perforation

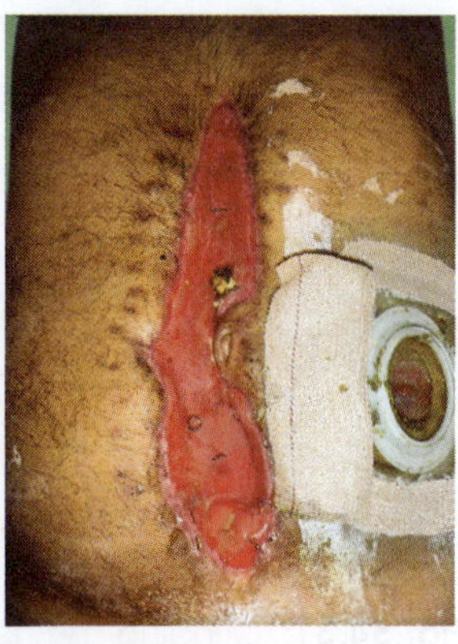

Fig. 54.29: Traumatic faecal fistula

Investigations

- X-ray abdomen
  - Obliteration of psoas shadow
  - Air outlining the kidney—Chilaiditi's sign (Fig. 54.30)
  - Absence of air in the duodenum
- Raised serum amylase is one of the biochemical parameters that should arouse a suspicion of pancreatic injuries along with duodenal injury.

Treatment

- Golden time to operate is within 6 hours.
- When in doubt, about narrowing of lumen, duodenojejunostomy may be indicated.
- When in doubt regarding duodenal fistula, tube duodenostomy is done.
- Duodenal haematoma is managed conservatively.
- Better to add a feeding jejunostomy

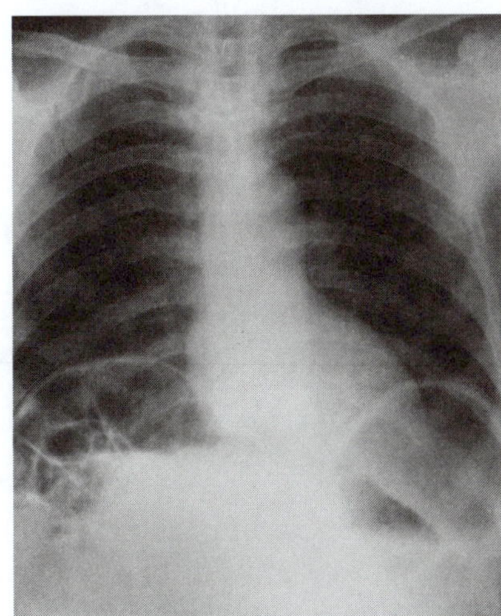

Fig. 54.30: Air outlining small portion of the kidney and air pockets under the diaphragm—Chilaiditi's sign

PANCREATIC INJURIES

Because of anatomical close approximation of pancreas with vertebral column, blunt injury abdomen in the epigastrium, kicks or **seat belt injuries** crush the pancreas against **the vertebral column** (Key Boxes 54.9 and 54.10).

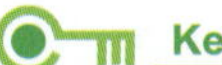

Key Box 54.9

Pancreatic Injuries

- Anatomically hidden
- Very often, injuries missed
- Peritonitis features are not seen
- Dangerous because of enzymatic activation
- Can manifest as pleural effusion

Key Box 54.10

Pancreaticoduodenal Injuries

- Diagnosed late
- Peritonitis features are minimal
- Shock is very rare
- At laparotomy, they are missed
- Surgical treatment needs more skill and experience.
- Feeding jejunostomy is very useful
- Mortality and morbidity around 50%

Mill belt: Saree or *churidar* cloth may be caught in the belt of a running conveyor belt and result in compression force in the centre of the abdomen (Figs 54.31 to 54.34 and clinical notes).

Diagnosis

- Pancreatic injury alone is diagnosed when patient presents with a pseudocyst of the pancreas 2–3 weeks following an injury.

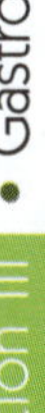

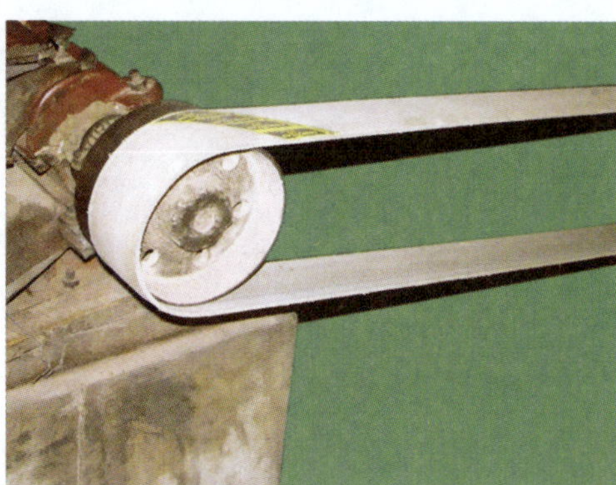

Fig. 54.31: Grinding mill having a conveyor belt (*Courtesy:* Dr Rakesh Hegde, Associate Professor, Department of Surgery, KMC, Manipal, 2006–2009)

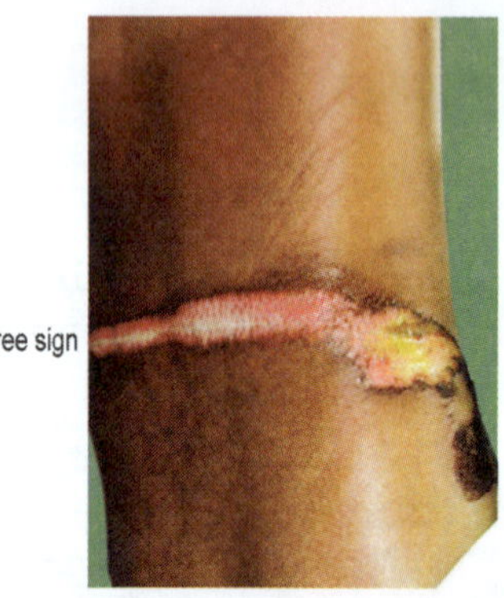

Fig. 54.32: Impression of the saree all around waist in a lady who was dragged by the conveyor belt when her saree got caught

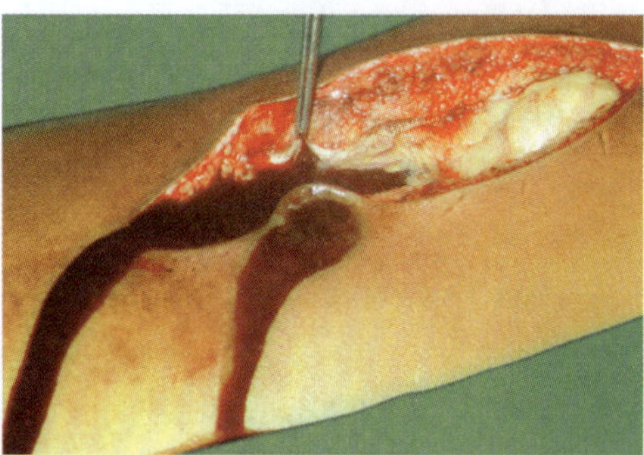

Fig. 54.33: On laparotomy, blood gushing out (*Courtesy:* Dr Raghunath Prabhu, Associate Prof, KMC, Manipal)

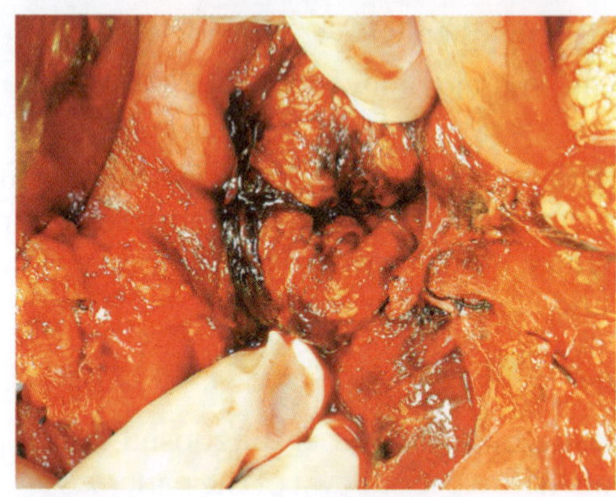

Fig. 54.34: Pancreas split into 2 parts

- Very often, laparotomy is done for haemorrhage or perforation. In such situations, retroperitoneal bleeding, collection of bile or collection of fluid in the lesser sac arouses suspicion of pancreatic injuries.

Treatment

- **Pseudocyst** following blunt injury abdomen invariably requires **surgical drainage,** e.g. **cystogastrostomy** because of injury to pancreatic duct, fistula will remove for a long period.
- Injury to body and tail require **subtotal pancreatectomy** with splenectomy.
- Rarely, **pancreaticoduodenectomy** may be required for significant injury to the head of pancreas with injury to the duodenum.

Complications

- Pancreatic fistula
- Pancreatic pseudocyst
- Pleural effusion

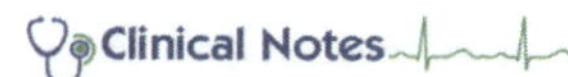

Indian women—vulnerability (Figs 54.31 to 54.34). The Saree and Churidar are traditional Indian dresses. One end of the Saree is tied around the waist and the other draped freely along the shoulder. If care is not taken, the free end often gets caught in the mill belt and causes injuries around the waist (blunt abdominal trauma) due to the drag created. The impression created on the abdomen is by the saree and not the mill belt. The Shawl of the Churidar (has two free ends) can get caught in a belt or a wheel to cause injuries around the neck. The drag may be sufficient to cause even strangulation. The author remembers a case of scalp avulsion due to long hair of a woman getting caught in a mill belt.

RENAL INJURIES

Types (Fig. 54.35)

I. **Minor injuries:** Subcapsular haematoma, minor laceration and renal contusions.

II. **Major injuries:** Bleeding into renal pelvis from laceration of medulla, corticomedullary rupture, hilar injury.

Clinical Features

- **Haematuria** is the most important (80–90%) sign of renal injury. It may be mild, or sometimes can be massive depending upon the extent of injury. It may be absent in renal pedicle avulsion.
- **Loin bulge** due to perinephric haematoma

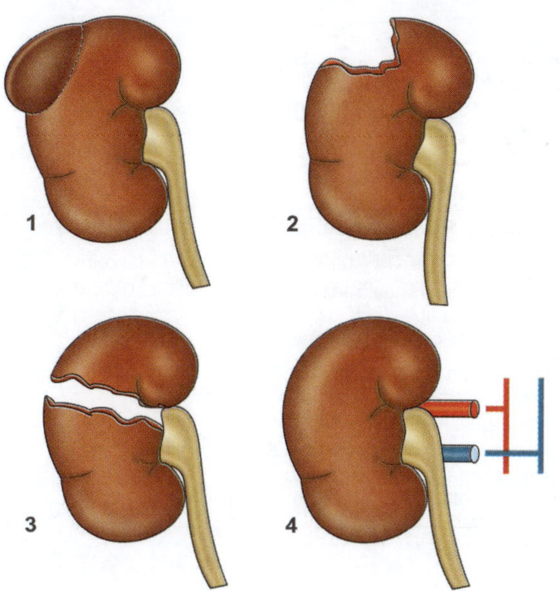

Fig. 54.35: Closed renal trauma: (1) Subcapsular haematoma, (2) laceration, (3) avulsion of one of the poles and (4) avulsion of renal pedicle

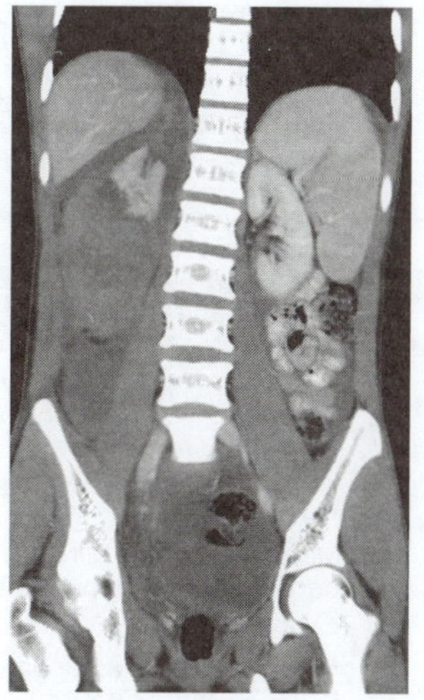

Fig. 54.36: Renal trauma: Right kidney is transected and upper pole is displaced by a large haematoma. Left kidney is normal (*Courtesy:* Dr Padmaraj Hedge, Professor and Head, Department of Urology, KMC, Manipal)

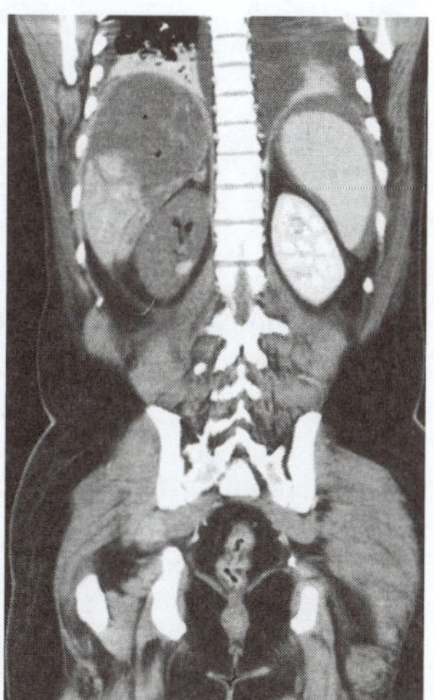

Fig. 54.37: Liver and kidney injury. It is not uncommon to get liver and kidney injuries in a blunt abdominal trauma. Always look for urine microscopy/haematuria while treating liver injury cases

- **Bruising** of soft tissue in the loin
- Retroperitoneal haematoma compressing on splanchnic nerves (meteorism) results in paralytic ileus, which causes **abdominal distension.**
- Associated injuries such as fractures of the transverse process of lumbar spine may be present.

Investigations

1. **Intravenous pyelography can demonstrate:**
   - Intrarenal extravasation
   - Extrarenal extravasation (pararenal pseudohydronephrosis due to extravasated blood and urine, slowly occluding pelviureteric junction).
   - Function of injured kidney
   - Function of opposite kidney
2. **Ultrasound and CT scan** are other investigations which are useful when there is an expanding haematoma (Figs 54.36 and 54.37).

Treatment

1. **Conservative:** Minor injuries are managed conservatively with close monitoring of vital signs such as pulse, blood pressure, temperature and respiration, Hb% and PCV.
   - Sedation and analgesics are also given.
2. **Surgical exploration**
   - **Small laceration** sutured over gel foam or by using detached muscle.
   - **Major laceration** involving one pole—a partial nephrectomy is done.
   - **Major multiple lacerations**, avulsions, require nephrectomy.

RETROPERITONEAL HAEMATOMA

- It is quite common because of accidents, fall from height.
- Fracture vertebrae, fracture pelvis, injury to retroperitoneal veins give risk to RPH
- Bleeding from vena cava and aorta can be fatal.
- Haematomas which are not expanding should not be disturbed.

  Diagnosis and management of retroperitoneal haematoma as shown in Fig. 54.38.

Pelvic Fractures and Retroperitoneal Haematoma

- Pelvic fractures are also an important cause of retroperitoneal haematoma.
- The most frequent mechanisms causing pelvic fractures are motor vehicle accidents, motorcycle accidents, falls and accidents involving pedestrians. Associated injuries to urethra in males should be ruled out first. Per rectal examination should be done to evaluate the position of the prostate. CT scan is done to assess pelvic fracture and also to assess retroperitoneal haematoma.
- Retroperitoneal bleeding can be arterial, venous, or osseous in origin. Unstable pelvic fractures are generally associated with increased blood loss. Posterior fractures with involvement of the sacroiliac

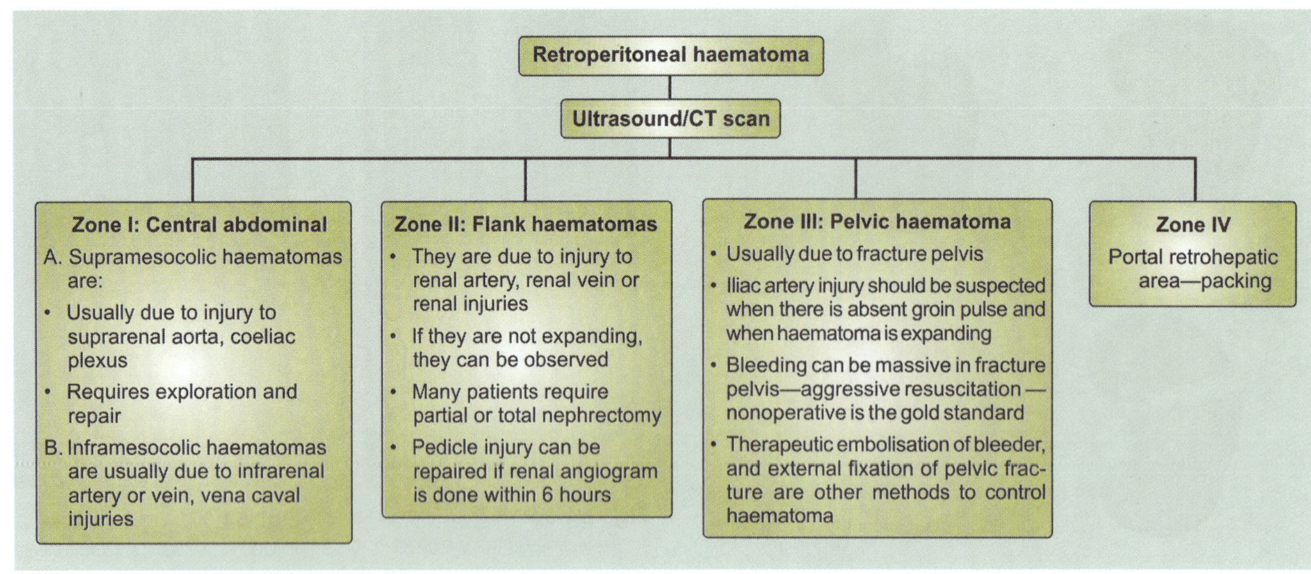

Fig. 54.38: Diagnosis and management of retroperitoneal haematoma

joint are frequently associated with arterial bleeding, which can be controlled by embolisation of the bleeding vessel, usually branches of the internal iliac artery. Unstable fractures should be fixed by external fixation. Expanding haematoma should be explored. Control the bleeders, otherwise pack the pelvis. Nonexpanding haematoma should not be explored. Wait and watch.

GENERAL PRINCIPLES IN A BLUNT INJURY ABDOMEN

- A patient should be admitted to the hospital and carefully monitored if there is a slight doubt regarding blunt injury abdomen.
- **Repeated examination,** careful monitoring of pulse rate, temperature and blood pressure, chest X-ray, estimation of Hb%, frequently help in many cases of silent blunt injuries.
- Most of the cases today are **polytrauma** cases, hence all systems should be examined. Among all these, priority should be given to life-threatening, salvageable injuries such as **extradural haematoma, haemothorax, splenic injuries, liver injuries**.
- It is easier to make a diagnosis of fracture[1] (revealed injuries) which can be treated later. FRACTURE CAN WAIT BUT NOT RUPTURE. Concealed injuries should be carefully looked for.
- Undoubtedly, **diagnostic peritoneal lavage, ultrasound** (CT scan is the immediate noninvasive investigation) help in diagnosis of more than 90% of cases of blunt injury abdomen.
- Adequate blood, appropriate antibiotics, aggressive resuscitation before surgery to treat hypovolaemia and shock are the major factors which decide the outcome of surgery.
- In a major accident involving many patients and limited resources, quick decision should be taken regarding **triage**—who can be saved, who cannot be saved (Fig. 54.39).

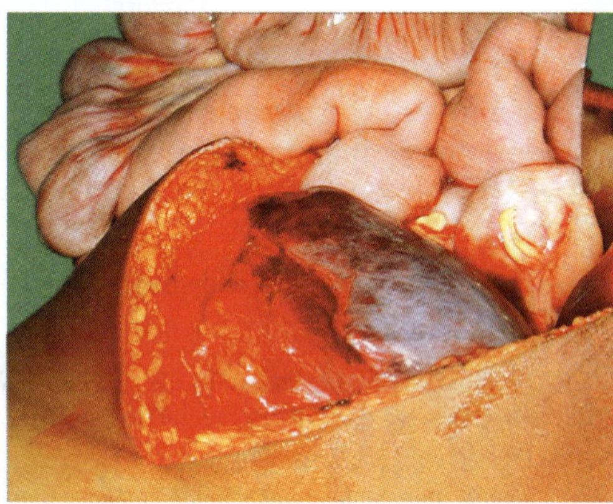

Fig. 54.39: Splenic haematoma—initially managed by conservative method. However, patient was developing hypotension—importance of careful monitoring of the patient in intensive care unit

SOFT TISSUE INJURIES

Competency

SU17.7: Describe the clinical features of soft tissue injuries. Chose appropriate investigations and discuss the principles of management.

Soft tissue injury term is used to describe injuries occurring to muscle, tendons or ligaments. They are common in clinical practice especially in sport events (like football, cricket or rugby), falls/slips or during exercises. One of the most commonly involved joint is the knee joint that gets affected.

Strains, sprains and contusion are examples of soft tissue injuries. Other types include tendinitis and bursitis.

Injury to muscle or tendon is referred to as strain whereas injury to ligament is referred to as sprain. Common areas for strain are ankle, knee and wrist.

Common symptoms include swelling, pain and weakness. Examination often reveals oedema, tenderness, inability to move the affected part.

Diagnosis is often through history and thorough clinical assessment. Radiographs are taken to rule out bony injuries. Ultrasound and MRI can be used for diagnosis of sprain or strain.

Treatment consists of rest to the affected area, ice application that aims to decrease pain and inflammation, compression to decrease swelling and elevation to drain the accumulated fluid. NSAIDs are used to decrease pain.

Prevention is important strategy in soft tissue injuries. Wearing appropriate athlete shoes, warming up before activity, slow stretching and adequate rest are essential in preventing injuries

Remember **RICE** for soft tissue injury management (this is a known published pneumonic in old journals)

R—Rest
I—Ice
C—Compression
E—Elevation

VASCULAR TRAUMA

Although any blood vessel can be injured in a traumatic event, injuries of extremities account for 80% of cases. Traumatic event can be blunt trauma or penetrating injury.

Mechanism of Injury

1. **Blunt trauma:** Compression and crushing of blood vessels.
2. **Penetrating trauma:** Compression and direct tissue separation by sharp object.

Clinical Presentation

1. Tissue ischaemia distal to site of injury
2. External bleeding
3. Occult bleeding in body cavities or tissue planes with or without hypovolaemic shock
4. Pulsatile Haematoma

Clinical features are divided into soft and hard signs to triage and guide further treatment of patients in accident and emergency department.

Soft signs	Hard signs
1. History of significant haemorrhage	1. Pulsatile external haemorrhage
2. Diminished distal pulses	2. Absence of distal pulses
3. Neurologic deficit in affected limb	3. Ischaemic limb
4. Injury near area of major vessel	4. Pulsatile haematoma
	5. Bruit or thrill

Types of arterial injuries

1. Partial laceration
2. Complete transection
3. Contusion leading to thrombosis
4. Pseudoaneurysm may have bruit or thrill
5. Traumatic arteriovenous fistula
6. External compression by haematoma or fractured bone

Treatment (Fig. 54.40)

Endovascular

1. Transcatheter embolization
2. Covered stents

Operative

Principle

1. Incision along line of vessel
2. Obtain proximal and distal control before approaching site of injury
3. Debride till normal arterial wall
4. Proximal and distal embolectomy to remove clot
5. Heparinization

Type of repair: Repair depends upon extent of vascular damage.

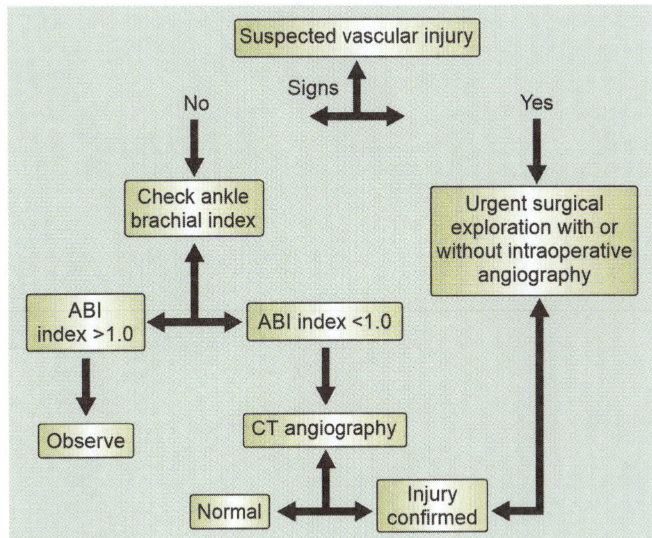

Fig. 54.40: Algorithm of management of vascular trauma

1. Ligation of injured vessel can be considered at sites where good collateral flow is present, e.g. forearm and leg.
2. End-to-end anastomosis, if vessel can be sufficiently mobilized to ensure tension free anastomosis.
3. Interposition graft is used in majority of cases.

Vascular Grafts

1. Autologus saphenous vein

- Harvested from uninjured leg
- Used in reverse direction because of venous valves
- Best patency rates
- Small vein can lead to size discrepancy with injured artery

2. Prosthetic graft

- Used, if autologous vein is not sufficient or poor quality.
- Various sizes are available, so can be used for most of vessels.

A. Expended polytetrafluoroethylene (ePTFE)

- Inferior to autologous vein but better than Dacron for infrainguinal or upper limb revascularization.
- More needle hole bleeding during surgery
- Resistant to infection compared to Dacron

B. Dacron

- It can be woven or knitted depending on textile technique used.
- Woven graft has less porosity and less bleeding.
- Knitted grafts are more porous and need pre-clotting before implantation.
- Mainly used for thoracic or abdominal aortic surgeries, rarely used for limb vascularization.

Complications

1. Irreversible limb ischaemia and necrosis, if repair delayed beyond 6–8 hours
2. Infection
3. Pseudoaneurysm
4. Graft thrombosis
5. Reperfusion injury
6. Rhabdomyolysis and myoglobinuria leading to renal failure

Please Note:

Remember following mnemonics in blunt injury abdomen:

- AMPLE : *See* page 988
- ABCDE : *See* page 988, 990
- FAST : *See* page 990
- LIFT JAW : *See* page 981
- AVPU : *See* page 983

FURTHER READING

Ann Surg. 2004 Mar; 239(3): 319–321.

Multiple Choice Questions

1. The most common bedside investigation done for suspected blunt abdominal trauma for bleeding is:
A. CT scan
B. MRI scan
C. Diagnostic peritoneal lavage
D. Ultrasound

2. Which one of the following is a definite indication for laparotomy in blunt injury abdomen?
A. Splenic injury
B. Pancreatic injury
C. Liver injury
D. Aspiration of bile in the peritoneal aspirate

3. If air bubble like picture is found within the thorax following blunt injury abdomen what do you suspect?
A. Splenic rupture
B. Liver injury
C. Injury to the stomach
D. Diaphragmatic injury

4. How do you rule out a head injury with factors given below?
A. Hypotension responding to fluid
B. CSF rhinorrhoea
C. Fracture skull
D. Hypertension and bradycardia

5. Which is an important sign of hollow viscus perforation?
A. Cullen's sign B. Grey Turner's sign
C. Mallet Guy sign D. London sign

6. The following are true for conservative management of liver injury *except*:
A. Hollow viscus injury should not be there
B. Free contrast in and around liver in CT scan
C. Grade I and Grade II injury
D. Haemodynamically stable patient

7. Pringle manoeuvre refers to:
A. Compression of left gastric artery to stop the bleeding from giant gastric ulcer
B. Compression of hepatic artery to stop the bleeding during liver resection
C. Compression of hepatic artery and portal vein in front of foramen of Winslow
D. Compression of gastroduodenal artery during Whipple's procedure

8. The salvage procedure to buy time in massive bleeding from liver include following:
A. Pringle manoeuvre
B. Plug by omentum
C. Perihepatic packing
D. Portovenous shunt

9. Perforation within 4 cm of the ileocaecal junction following blunt injury is better treated by:
A. Suturing and drainage
B. Resection and anastomosis and drainage
C. Suture and bypass
D. Exteriorisation

10. Which of the following is not a feature of retroperitoneal duodenal perforation?
A. Can occur with steering wheel injury
B. Chilaiditi sign may be present
C. Free gas under diaphragm
D. Guarding and rigidity is minimal

11. Initial third of resuscitation in haemorrhagic shock in blunt abdominal trauma is:
A. Ringer lactate B. Saline
C. Dextrose D. Plasma

12. Death triad in blunt abdominal trauma is:
A. Hyperthermia, acidosis, coagulopathy
B. Hypothermia, acidosis, coagulopathy
C. Hypothermia, alkalosis, coagulopathy
D. Hyperthermia, alkalosis, coagulopathy

Answers

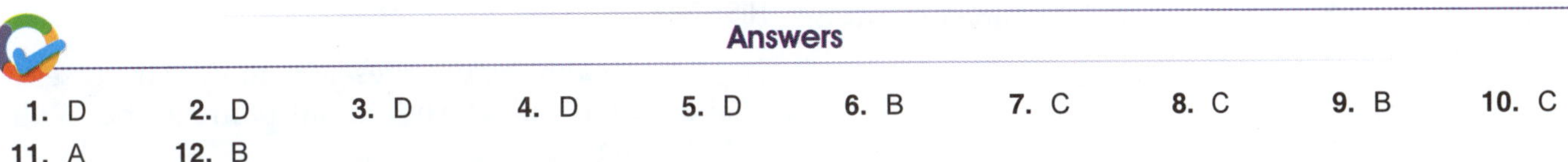

1. D **2.** D **3.** D **4.** D **5.** D **6.** B **7.** C **8.** C **9.** B **10.** C
11. A **12.** B

CHAPTER

55

Abdominal Mass

- Clinical examination of abdominal mass
- Mass in the right iliac fossa
- Firm to hard nodular mass in the umbilical region
- The cystic mass in the abdomen
- Mass in the epigastrium
- Mass in the right hypochondrium
- Mass in the right lumbar region

INTRODUCTION

The abdomen is like Pandora's box. However, a student who is examining a case of abdomen is like an investigating CBI officer. He has to collect information at every level of examination, i.e. history, past history, general examination and abdominal examination. An attempt has been done here to highlight the importance of history and clinical examination. **Ten points** in the history, if taken and analysed properly may give a definite **clue** in majority of cases. After getting this **clue**, clinical examination of the mass may become easy.

CLINICAL EXAMINATION OF ABDOMINAL MASS (CLINICS)

REGIONS IN THE ABDOMEN

- Abdomen is divided into nine regions (quadrants) by two horizontal lines and two vertical lines.
- Upper horizontal line or transpyloric line is midway between xiphisternum and umbilicus.
- **Lower horizontal line (transtubercular line)** is the line joining iliac crest tubercles of each side, about 5 cm behind anterior superior iliac spine.
- The vertical lines are drawn on either side through midpoint between anterior superior iliac spine and symphysis pubis. Following are the nine regions of the abdomen (Fig. 55.1).
  1. Right hypochondrium
  2. Epigastrium
  3. Left hypochondrium
  4. Right lumbar region
  5. Umbilical region
  6. Left lumbar region
  7. Right iliac fossa
  8. Hypogastrium
  9. Left iliac fossa

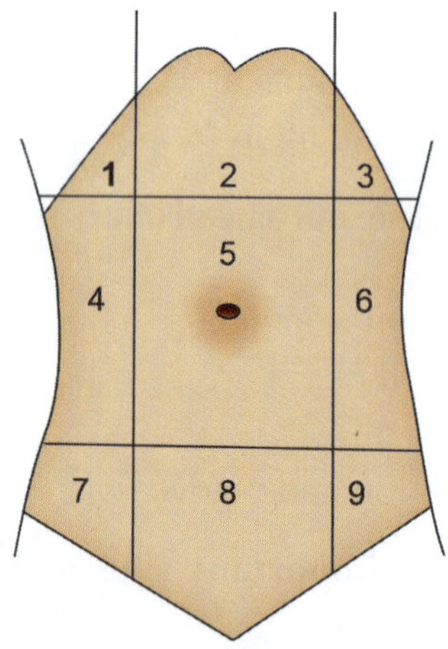

Fig. 55.1: Regions of the abdomen (see text)

More details have been given in Manipal Manual of Clinical Methods in Surgery, First Edition

Do not forget to examine 10th and 11th regions to lumbar regions and 12th region—external genitalia in males

HISTORY

1. **Abdominal pain:** It is present in most of the cases of abdominal mass. Abdominal pain can be of the following types:

A. *Dull aching pain:* It suggests a solid organ enlargement. It is a continuous pain felt in the anatomical location of the swelling. Patients often describe it as a discomfort rather than pain.

Examples

- Liver enlargement: Pain in the right hypochondrium. It occurs due to stretching of **parietal capsule** (Glisson's) (Fig. 55.2A)
- Splenic enlargement: Pain in the left hypochondrium
- Renal enlargement: Pain in the back and costal region or costovertebral pain (Fig. 55.2B)
- Enlarged lymph nodes (para-aortic), pancreatic tumours: Backache

B. *Colicky pain* suggests hollow viscus obstruction. This pain is due to hyperperistalsis. It is severe and intermittent (comes and goes). Each attack may last for 5–10 minutes. The patient bends on himself, holds the abdomen and puts pressure on the abdomen which gives some kind of relief. Being visceral type of pain, it is not very well localised. Following are a few examples:

- Mass in the right iliac fossa (carcinoma caecum or ileocaecal tuberculosis). Initially there may be a vague discomfort. However, when partial obstruction occurs, it results in a colicky abdominal pain which is centrally located and sometimes unbearable.
- Ureteric colic and biliary colic (Fig. 55.2C).
- Carcinoma pyloric antrum or pyloric stenosis produces colicky upper abdominal pain with gastric peristalsis. However, this type of pain is not an unbearable one.

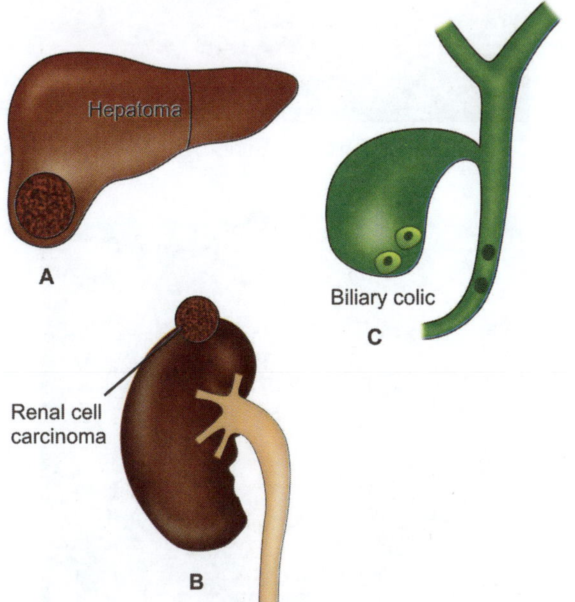

Figs 55.2A to C: Source of the pain

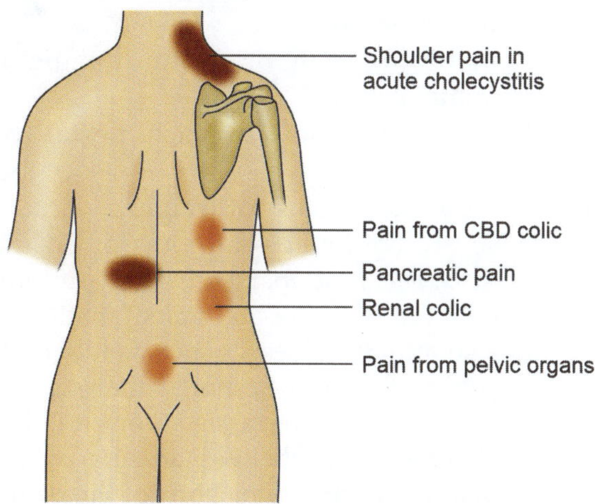

Fig. 55.3: Referred pain (posterior view)

C. *Referred pain:* Tuberculosis of spine is a common problem in India. Often patients present with iliopsoas abscess. Patients can complain of referred pain in the lower abdomen (Fig. 55.3).

Pearls of Wisdom

Recent backache in elderly male may be due to carcinoma prostate and in females may be due to carcinoma breast.

2. Sensation of fullness/early satiety

- Carcinoma of the stomach and pyloric obstruction. Also hepatoma or large pancreatic tumours can cause extraluminal compression on the stomach resulting in sensation of fullness in the abdomen.
- Early satiety is due to loss of receptive relaxation of stomach due to malignant infiltration of muscle layer.

3. Vomiting

- Persistent, profuse, projectile and nonbilious vomiting suggests pyloric stenosis. Chronic duodenal ulcer and carcinoma stomach are the common causes of pyloric obstruction (pain is absent/negligible).
- Persistent, profuse, projectile, bilious vomiting—intestinal obstruction. For example, ileocaecal tuberculosis, stricture of the small bowel, adhesions (pain is severe and colicky).

4. Haematemesis

- Epigastric mass suggests carcinoma stomach.
- Splenomegaly may be an indication of portal hypertension.

Pearls of Wisdom

History of gastrojejunostomy and vagotomy done a few years back presenting with severe pain abdomen, epigastric mass and haematemesis could be due to retrograde jejunogastric intussusception.

5. **Bleeding *per* rectum**
   - Fresh blood with or without melaena—carcinoma rectum
   - Melaena—carcinoma stomach, portal hypertension
6. **Loss of appetite and loss of weight**
   - These are common symptoms of GI malignancies. Please note that these two symptoms are seen not only in intra-abdominal malignancies but also in many diseases such as tuberculosis. However, it should be noted that one of the **earliest signs of carcinoma stomach is loss of appetite. Severe weight loss is an early and important feature of carcinoma body of the pancreas.**
   - Significant weight loss refers to loss of 10 kg or more in the last 6 months.
7. **Bowel habits**
   - Fresh bleeding *per* rectum: Carcinoma rectum
   - Blood and mucus (bloody slime): Carcinoma rectum
   - Alternate constipation and diarrhoea: Carcinoma colon
8. **Jaundice**
   - Progressive, persistent, pruritic jaundice: Periampullary carcinoma or carcinoma head of pancreas. However, in periampullary carcinoma, fluctuation can occur if growth ulcerates.
   - Mild recurrent jaundice: Haemolytic anaemia.
   - Intermittent jaundice, pain, fever: **Charcot's triad**—stone in the common bile duct.
9. **Haematuria:** Fresh bleeding/clots: Renal cell carcinoma.
10. **Fever**
    - **High-grade fever**, with chills and rigors: Stone in common bile duct
    - **Low-grade fever**: Hepatoma, renal cell carcinoma, lymphoma. Fever is due to some pyrogens released into circulation or due to tumour necrosis.
    - In a **tropical country** like India, **hepatomas with fever** are often diagnosed as **amoebic liver abscess and mistreated.**
11. **Abdominal distension:** The only chief complaint can be abdominal distension, most often due to ascites. In surgical wards, the common cause of ascites in young patients is tuberculous ascites, in middle-aged men is due to cirrhosis (alcohol is the most common cause) and in elderly patients malignancy. Large pseudocysts, retroperitoneal tumours, and in females ovarial tumours can present with abdominal distension. In the absence of any of these, distension can be caused by retroperitoneal tumours.

Pearls of Wisdom

- After taking all this history, when nothing is pointing towards any specific site of involvement of intra-abdominal organs, think of retroperitoneum.
- Distension is what patient says, protuberant is what the patient's abdomen can be.

ON EXAMINATION

Inspection

- The patient is asked to breathe well with mouth open.
- Students should spend a few minutes watching the abdomen carefully.

1. **Shape of the abdomen**
   - **Scaphoid** in normal cases
   - **Protuberant** in fatty abdomen (Figs 55.4 and 55.5).
   - Generalised distension with **fullness in the flanks** is usually due to **ascites.**
   - Localised distension can be due to a mass
   - Presence of **step ladder peristalsis** indicates **small bowel obstruction,** visible gastric **peristalsis indicates pyloric stenosis** and **right to left peristalsis** indicates **colonic obstruction** (Fig. 55.6).
2. **Restricted movement** of any one region of the abdomen indicates an inflammatory pathology.

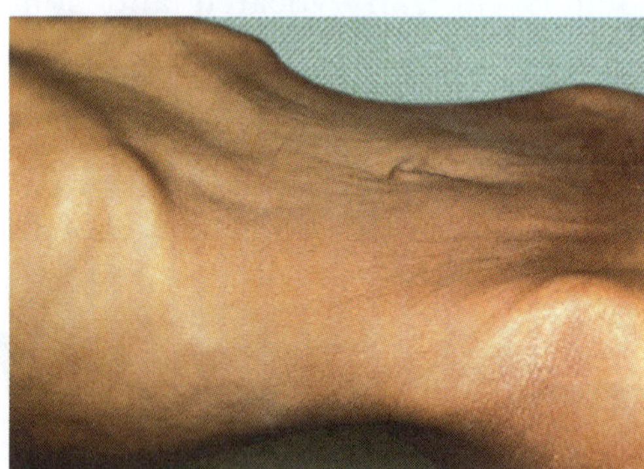

Fig. 55.4: Normal scaphoid abdomen

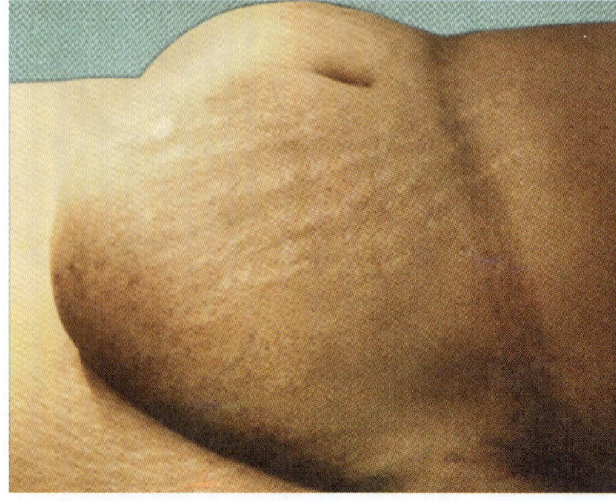

Fig. 55.5: Protuberant abdomen due to central obesity

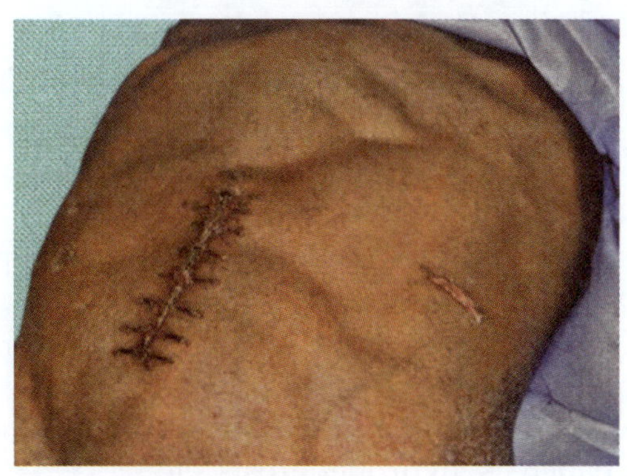

Fig. 55.6: Step ladder peristalsis due to terminal ileal obstruction. Patient was misdiagnosed as acute appendicitis and appendicectomy was done—a case of ileocaecal tuberculosis

3. **Umbilical nodule (Sister Joseph's)** indicates intra-abdominal malignancy (carcinoma of stomach, colon, pancreas).
4. **Details about the mass** such as size, shape, surface, borders, movement with respiration have to be mentioned if mass is visible. If the details about the mass cannot be appreciated or if mass is not clear on inspection, **it is better to say "there is fullness"** rather than trying to manipulate the details about the mass.
5. **Inspection of male genitalia:** If scrotum is empty, it could be a case of undescended testis[1,2].

Palpation

Methods of Palpation

Following are the methods of palpation available to the clinician and done depending upon the merits of the case:

a. **Superficial palpation:** Gentle superficial palpation of the abdomen gains confidence of the patient. It can detect superficial lesion of the abdominal wall such as lipomatosis, neurofibromas or fibromas, etc. It can also detect an area of tenderness, so that clinician is careful while doing deeper palpation. Superficial palpation is done with the flat of the hand or fingers.

b. **Deep palpation:** These are important requirements for deeper palpation:
   - Patient should be well-relaxed, with flexion of the knee for about 45°.
   - The patient's face should be turned to the opposite side and he is asked to breathe comfortably with open mouth.
   - **Deep palpation** should be started from the **quadrant situated diagonally opposite** to the site of pain.
   - Palpation should **cover not only the 9 quadrants of the abdomen,** but also **2 more quadrants, i.e. the 2 renal angles** and **12th quadrant—external genitalia in males[3].**
   - Deep palpation is carried out with the palmar surface of the fingers and some degree of angulation depending upon the depth of palpation.

Tests

1. **Movement with respiration:** This test is done by placing the fingers (hand) over the lower border of the swelling and the patient is asked to take a deep breath. Movement with respiration is positive when there is "up and down" movements not anteroposterior movement. Any structure in contact with diaphragm moves with respiration (Key Box 55.1). For example:
   - Liver, stomach, spleen, gallbladder move very well with respiration.
   - Splenic flexure growth, due to contact with the lower pole of the spleen and hepatic flexure growth due to contact with liver move with respiration.
   - Renal swelling moves with respiration because kidney is enclosed by fascia of Gerota which is attached above the diaphragm.
2. **Size, shape and surface**
   - An egg-shaped mass or globular mass suggests gallbladder lesion (Fig. 55.7A).
   - A horseshoe shape may indicate a horseshoe kidney (Fig. 55.7B) with pathology, e.g. hydronephrosis.
   - Reniform-shape suggests a renal swelling (Fig. 55.7C).

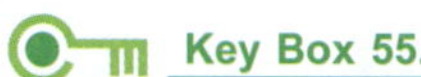

Key Box 55.1

Movement with Respiration

- Liver, spleen and stomach masses move freely with respiration
- Gallbladder mass also moves freely with respiration because of its proximity to liver
- Mass arising from hepatic flexure and splenic flexure of colon also have some mobility because it is in contact with liver and spleen
- Renal masses exhibit minor degree of movement with respiration because of indirect attachment to diaphragm

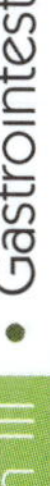

[1]A case of mass abdomen diagnosed to be soft tissue sarcoma or lymphoma of the para-aortic node region by U/S proved to be a seminoma in an undescended testis. Patient said that 6 months back his right testis was removed by a 'groin' incision.

[2]Inspection and palpation of external genitalia is important in males only, **NOT TO BE DONE in females, unless indicated.**

[3]Don't forget the 12th man in a cricket match. He is also an important player.

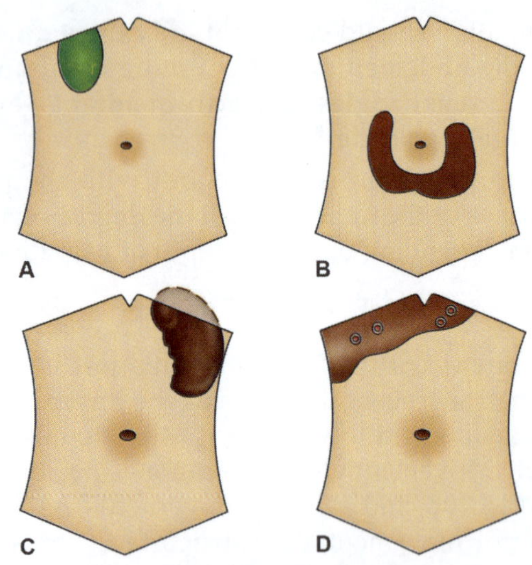

Figs 55.7A to D: Shapes of the intra-abdominal mass

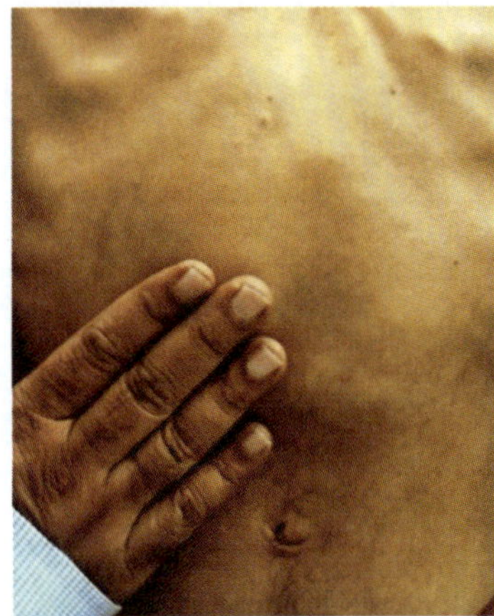

Fig. 55.8: Secondaries in the liver (nodular liver)

- **Large nodular surface** is seen in the following conditions (Fig. 55.7D):
  - Polycystic kidney (Fig. 55.8)
  - Secondaries in the liver
  - Group of lymph nodes

Pearls of Wisdom

Tensely cystic swellings may feel firm. Examples: Tense distended gallbladder in cases of obstructive jaundice due to periampullary carcinoma.

- **Smooth surface** usually indicates a benign lesion.
  - Splenomegaly, hydronephrosis, ovarian cyst, gallbladder swelling.
- **Irregular surface** is an important feature of malignancy such as carcinoma of the stomach, carcinoma caecum.

3. **Consistency**
   - **Hardness** is a feature of malignant lump. Thus, hepatoma, carcinoma stomach, pancreatic carcinoma present as hard lump. However, it should be remembered that often the malignant lump is firm and not hard.
   - **Firm** consistency is found in ileocaecal tuberculosis, nodes of lymphoma.
   - A peculiar **doughy** feel is described for tuberculous abdomen.
   - It is difficult to elicit fluctuation test for intra-abdominal swellings, and often tensely cystic swellings feel firm on palpation, e.g. pseudocyst of pancreas, hydronephrosis, etc.
   - Indentation or pitting on pressure can be found in a colon loaded with faeces.
   - Temporary contraction of a stomach (visible gastric peristalsis) should not be confused as a **mass**.
4. **Margins or borders** (Fig. 55.9)
   - **Upper border** cannot be made out in liver, splenic and renal swellings.
   - **Lower border** is not appreciated in pelvic masses, e.g. uterine fibroid, ovarian cyst (pelvic).
   - A **characteristic notch** is felt in the anterior border of splenic swelling.
   - Lower border is **sharp** as in a malignant liver swelling.
5. **Finger insinuation test:** This test has relevance in an upper abdominal mass.
   - Liver and spleen are under right and left costal margins, respectively. Hence, it is not possible to get the upper margin, or upper border of these organs. An attempt to invaginate between the costal margin and these masses is not possible. On the other hand, finger invagination under the costal margin is possible in a stomach mass (Fig. 55.10).
6. **Intrinsic mobility test** (Key Box 55.2)
   - An intra-abdominal mass can be mobile if it has loose attachments or if it is not within the bony cage. Thus, liver, spleen, uterine mass are not mobile because of their location within bony cage.

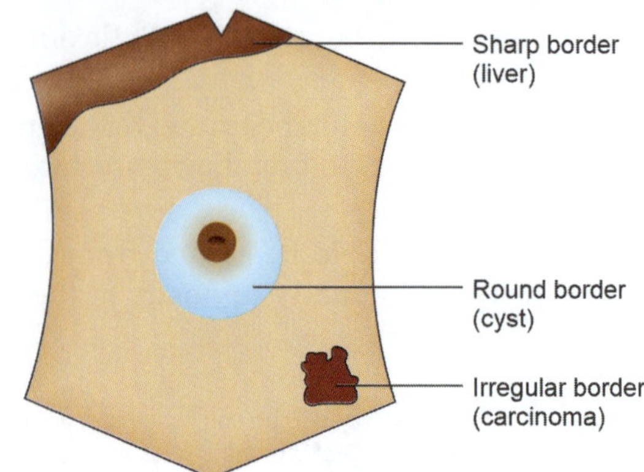

Fig. 55.9: Various types of borders

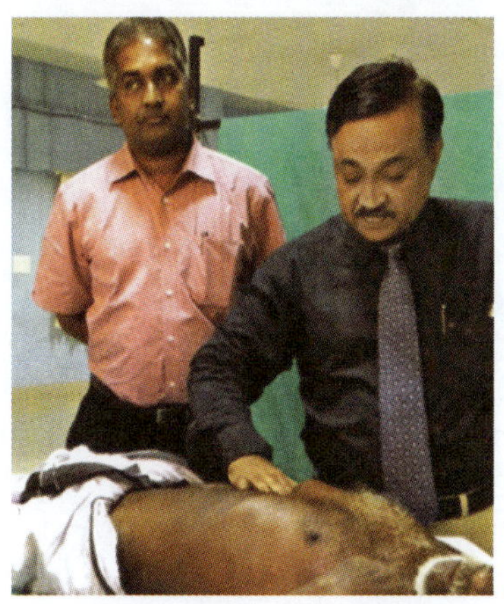

Fig. 55.10: Checking for finger insinuation test (CME, Calicut Medical College, 2014)

Key Box 55.2

Intrinsic Mobility—Mass

- Side-to-side — Gallbladder
- Vertical — Transverse colon
- All directions — Ovarian cyst
- Right angle to the direction of mesentery — Mesenteric cyst
- Push back to renal — Kidney pouch
- Tree top mobility — Pancreatic cystadenoma

Pearls of Wisdom

Check for intrinsic mobility in different positions.

- Carcinoma pyloric antrum can exhibit movements in different positions—left lateral, right lateral or even in the sitting position.
- Pancreatic carcinoma, advanced malignancies and lymph nodal masses also may not have intrinsic mobility.
- However, there are a few swellings which have characteristic mobility.

Examples

A. **Ovarian cyst** is a freely mobile swelling which can be moved in all directions (Fig. 55.11A).

B. **Mesenteric cyst** moves at right angles to the direction of the line of mesentery (Fig. 55.11B).

C. **Pseudopancreatic cyst** may have a minimal side-to-side mobility (Fig. 55.11C).

D. **Carcinoma transverse colon** has vertical mobility unless it is advanced (Fig. 55.11D).

E. **Pancreatic masses:** Even though they do not exhibit mobility, a cystadenoma of the pancreas because of the size and a narrow base, will exhibit **tree top mobility** (Fig. 55.11E). Any big mass abutting the undersurface of the diaphragm also moves with respiration.

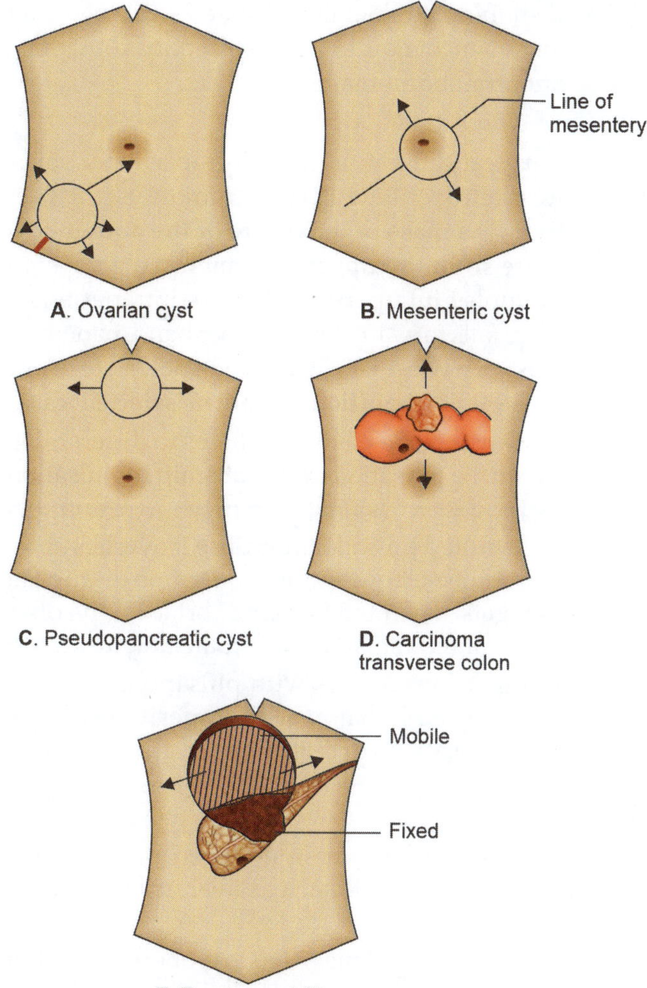

Figs 55.11A to E: Different types of intrinsic mobility

F. Renal mass comes down during inspiration. As it comes down, it can be held back and can be pushed back to the renal pouch.

7. Plane of the swelling

A. Leg raising test or head raising test

- The purpose of this test is to contract rectus abdominis muscles (also other abdominal wall muscles). Intra-abdominal swellings become less prominent. On the other hand, abdominal wall swellings become more prominent, e.g. fibroma, neurofibroma, or lipoma in the abdominal wall.
- This test is done by asking the patient to raise his legs without bending at the knee (extended legs) or by raising the shoulders from the bed with arm folded over the chest.

B. Nose blowing test or straining test

- This test can be done by asking the patient to blow through the nose with mouth closed. **The lateral abdominal muscles are more contracted with this test.**

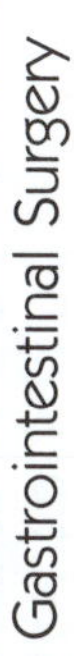

- It should be remembered that a swelling or the mass which moves with respiration is obviously an intra-abdominal mass.

C. Knee-elbow test

- This test differentiates an intraperitoneal mass from retroperitoneal mass. It is more useful when there is a **mass in the centre of the abdomen—more so in the upper abdomen**. To give a few examples, intraperitoneal cyst or intraperitoneal mass falls forward. On the other hand, pancreatic mass or a lymph node mass will not fall forward. **The test has significance only in 'selected' cases.**
- However, knee-elbow test helps to differentiate expansile pulsation from transmitted pulsation.
- Examples: A pseudocyst of pancreas will give transmitted pulsations because it overlies aorta. In the knee-elbow position, pulsation disappears as it gets separated from the aorta. On the other hand, aneurysms exhibit expansile pulsations.
- Intraperitoneal mass with pulsations over it is likely to be hepatoma. Retroperitoneal mass with pulsations over it is pancreatic mass.

Special Tests

1. **Bimanual palpation:** Grossly enlarged swellings may be bimanually palpable such as liver, spleen, kidney (Fig. 55.12).
2. **Ballotability:** 'Ballot' means to toss about. To ballot, the swelling should be bimanually palpable and there should be a gap or space between hands which are kept anterior and posterior to the mass. Typically, renal swellings are **ballotable**. This test is done when the patient is in supine position, by keeping one hand anteriorly in the lumbar region over the swelling and the other hand posteriorly in the renal angle. A gentle push is given from behind and the swelling touches the hand which is placed anteriorly and it goes back. **Ballotability is because of perirenal pad of fat and due to 'pedicle'.**

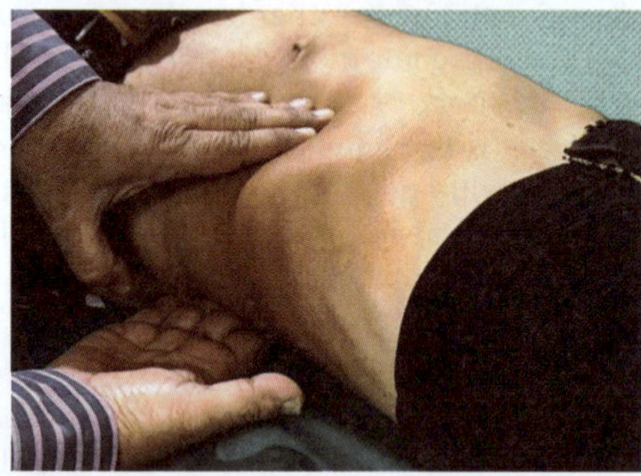

Fig. 55.12: Bimanual palpation and ballotability

Renal Ballotability

- **P**osterior enlargement is more—thus space for movement anteriorly
- **P**laced peripheral—thus can be felt by both hands
- **P**edicled organ—free movement possible
- **P**erirenal pad of fat—thus cushion effect

4 Ps to remember

3. **Splenic dullness:** It is elicited in the 9th intercostal space in the left midaxillary line and it is continuous with splenic mass.

Traube's space is a semilunar space between the lower edge of the left lung, the anterior border of the spleen, the left costal margin and the inferior margin of the left lobe of the liver. Anatomically superiorly bounded by left sixth rib, laterally by the left midaxillary line and inferiorly by left costal margin. Stomach which is posterior to this space, hence gives tympanitic note normally but gives dull note when spleen is enlarged.

Percussion

1. To demonstrate mild ascites, the patient is put in a knee-elbow position and percussion is done around umbilicus. It gives a dull note if minimal fluid is present (normally area around the umbilicus is resonant).
   - Significant or moderate fluid in the abdomen is demonstrated by percussion of the centre and flanks of the abdomen in the lying down position and in the left or right lateral position.
   - In the supine position, flanks give a dull note due to fluid. However, in the lateral position, fluid shifts down and coils of bowel float up.
2. Liver dullness is elicited in the 5th intercostal space and the dullness is continuous with the mass, if it is arising from the liver.
3. Splenic dullness is elicited in the 9th intercostal space in the left midaxillary line.
4. **Percussion** over the mass (Key Box 55.3):
   - Splenic and liver masses classically are **dull** to percuss.

Key Box 55.3

Percussion

○ Dull note	:	Liver, spleen, renal angle
○ Resonant	:	Bowel anterior to the mass (e.g. retroperitoneal mass)
○ Impaired	:	Stomach mass
○ Shifting dullness	:	Ascites

- Retroperitoneal masses may give **resonant** note because of intestines anterior to it. However, when they attain large size, e.g. sarcomas, they push the bowel to one side and hence, they are dull to percuss.
- Stomach mass may give **impaired resonant** note because of solid growth and due to the presence of air in the stomach.
- **Renal angle percussion:** In cases of enlargement of kidney, there will be a band of resonance anteriorly due to the colon but posteriorly it gives a dull note.
- **Hydatid thrill:** It is demonstrated by placing 3 fingers over the swelling and percussing the middle finger. Due to the fluid in the cyst, the fluid thrill (after-thrill) is felt by the other two fingers. This clinical sign is rarely demonstrable.

Auscultation (Fig. 55.13)

1. Loud noisy sounds **(borborygmi)** with or without peristalsis may indicate subacute obstruction. Such patients may be having ileocaecal tuberculosis or carcinoma caecum. This should be done at right iliac fossa to listen bowel sounds.
2. Auscultation over the liver mass may reveal a **bruit** as in a rapidly growing hepatoma.
3. **Succussion splash** is a splashing sound in cases of pyloric obstruction either due to carcinoma or due to chronic duodenal ulcer.
4. Perisplenitis and perihepatitis give rise to **friction rub** as in sickle cell anaemia due to repeated infarction and adhesions.
5. Aortic aneurysm will give a **continuous murmur** in the upper abdomen.
6. **Auscultopercussion** or auscultoscraping test is done to assess lower border of the stomach or greater curvature of the stomach.

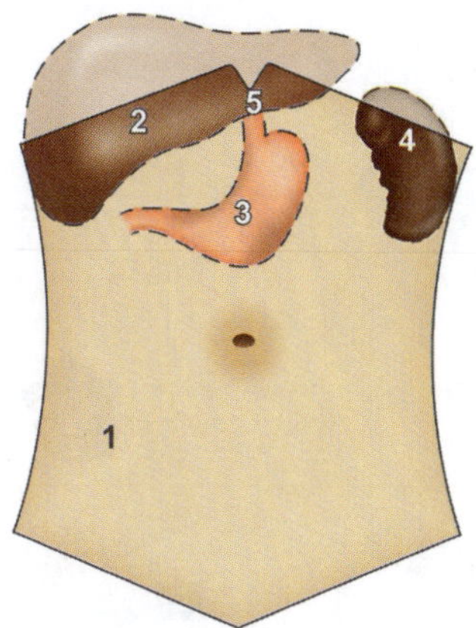

Fig. 55.13: Auscultation sites: 1–5 (see text above)

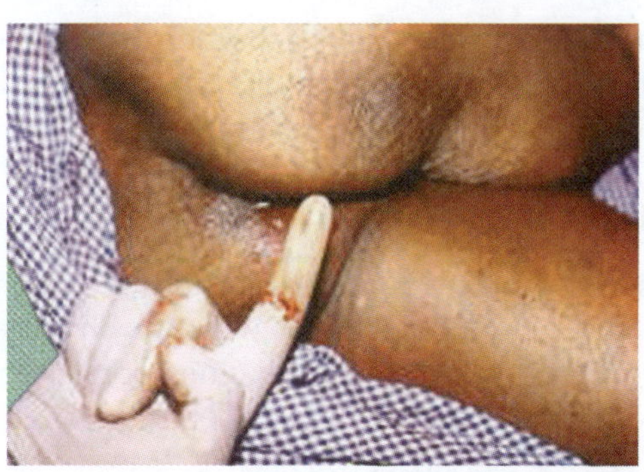

Fig. 55.14: Per rectal examination: Glove stained with blood

Rectal Examination

Should be done in a case of intra-abdominal mass.

- It can detect a carcinoma or a growth in the rectum in a case of secondaries in the liver.
- It can detect secondaries in the rectovesical pouch. **Blumer's shelf**—as hard, nodular mass and rectal mucosa is free during digital examination (Fig. 55.14).

Vaginal Examination

Should be done to rule out carcinoma cervix or to detect lymph nodes in the pouch of Douglas.

Bimanual Examination

This should be done in cases of pelvic masses. One hand (left) is placed over the mass in the hypogastrium and right index finger or fingers inserted in the vagina or rectum in virgin females and the left hand is pressed downwards and backwards above the pubic symphysis. By this manoeuvre, details of the pelvic mass, solid or cystic, uterine or ovarian, free or fixed can be made out.

Examination of Lymph Nodes

In cases of abdominal masses arising from lymph nodes, a thorough search of the body should be done to rule out other group of lymph nodes such as axillary, iliac, inguinal, neck nodes (lymphoma).

Significance

- **Left supraclavicular nodes** (Virchow's) are enlarged very often in visceral malignancies mainly from gastrointestinal tract. It indicates "inoperable" nature of the disease. Entire gastrointestinal lymph drains into the thoracic duct which joins the point of confluence of internal jugular vein and subclavian vein on the left side. This explains the significance of enlargement of Virchow's node. In 20% of cases, thoracic duct is single and 10–15% of cases, it is double.
- **Significance of right supraclavicular node:** The lymphatics from the right mediastinal lymph trunk,

and from the posterior right thoracic wall which form the right upper lymph trunk drain into the commencement of the right brachiocephalic vein.

SYSTEMIC EXAMINATION

Systemic examination should include respiratory system and cardiovascular system. Evidence of tuberculosis of the chest gives a clue about the mass in the abdomen, which may be a tubercular mass.

Differential diagnosis: Students are requested to refer clinical books for details. However, mass arising from five different quadrants are discussed below.

MASS IN THE RIGHT ILIAC FOSSA

Parietal Swelling

A. Parietal wall abscess
B. Desmoid tumour

Intra-Abdominal Swelling

A. Arising from normal structures
B. Arising from abnormal structures

From Normal Structures

I. Intestines
1. Appendicular mass
2. Appendicular abscess
3. Ileocaecal tuberculosis
4. Carcinoma caecum
5. Amoeboma
6. Intussusception
7. Actinomycosis

II. Lymph nodes
1. Acute lymphadenitis
2. Lymphoma
3. Secondaries

III. Retroperitoneal structures
1. Sarcoma
2. Aneurysm
3. Iliopsoas abscess
4. Chondrosarcoma

IV. In females
1. Ovarian cyst
2. Fibroid
3. Tubo-ovarian mass

From Abnormal Structures

1. Undescended testis: Seminoma
2. Unascended kidney

DIFFERENTIAL DIAGNOSIS OF MASS IN THE RIGHT ILIAC FOSSA

I. Parietal swelling: They are extra-abdominal. On head or leg raising test, they become more prominent. They are uncommon swellings.

A. Parietal wall abscess: It is a pyogenic abscess which can occur in a haematoma, or a pyaemic abscess which can occur as a part of pyaemia as in diabetic patients. Such abscesses are very tender, with warm surface and are associated with fever, chills and rigors.

B. Desmoid tumour: It is an unencapsulated fibroma occurring in the abdominal wall.

- Occurs in multiparous females. Repeated stretching of abdominal layers (due to pregnancy) is supposed to initiate formation of tumour.
- It can also occur following abdominal wall injury including laparotomy.
- It is a firm to hard swelling.
- It has no capsule. Hence, it should be treated with wide excision.
- It does not undergo sarcomatous change.
- After wide excision, the abdominal wall has to be reconstructed by using mesh.

II. Intra-abdominal swelling

A. Arising from structures normally present in the right iliac fossa

1. **Appendicular mass** (Fig. 55.15A): It is a tender, soft to firm mass which develops 48–72 hours following acute appendicitis. It is nature's attempt to limit the spread of infection by forming a mass consisting ***of omentum, terminal ileum, caecum with pericaecal fat and inflammatory oedema.*** It is managed conservatively by Oschner-Sherren's regime because an attempt to remove the appendix may result in faecal fistula. 6–8 weeks later, an elective appendicectomy can be done.

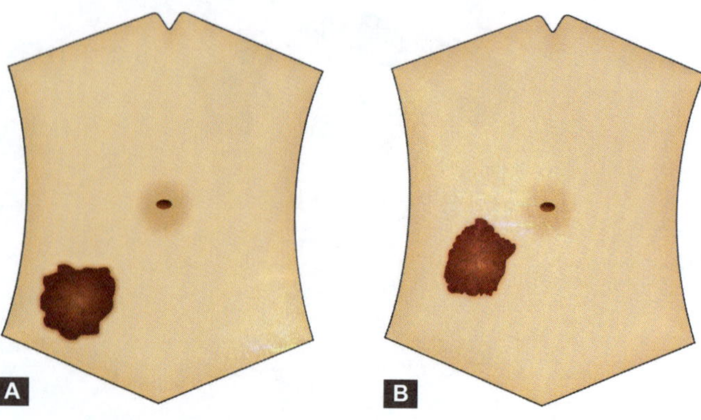

Figs 55.15A and B: Mass in the right iliac fossa

2. **Appendicular abscess:** It will be a very tender, firm, fixed mass. Such patients will have fever with chills and rigors.
3. **Ileocaecal tuberculosis** (Fig. 55.15B): Hyperplastic variety of tuberculosis forms a chronic cicatrising granulomatous reaction involving terminal ileum, caecum and part of ascending colon resulting in a mass in right iliac fossa. It is a chronic, nontender, firm, nodular mass, may have mobility, situated slightly (lumbar) on the higher side. Features of tuberculosis are usually present. It is treated by limited resection followed by ileocolic anastomosis.
4. **Carcinoma caecum** (Figs 55.16 to 55.20):
   - More common in females, around 40–50 years of age.
   - It produces bleeding per rectum, severe anaemia, etc.
   - Hard, irregular mass in right iliac fossa with fixity or restricted mobility is a usual feature. Psoas spasm indicates infiltration into psoas muscle. It is treated by right radical hemicolectomy.
5. **Amoeboma:** Can be acute or chronic. It follows an attack of amoebic typhlitis (inflammation of the caecum). Amoeboma is tender and soft to firm. It is not common to find amoebomas nowadays because of effective treatment of amoebiasis with metronidazole, tinidazole, etc.
6. **Intussusception:** Acute or chronic intussusception can give rise to a mass in the right iliac fossa which is tender and soft to firm. When acute intussusception occurs in children, it is described as idiopathic intussusception. Chronic intussusception may disappear spontaneously.

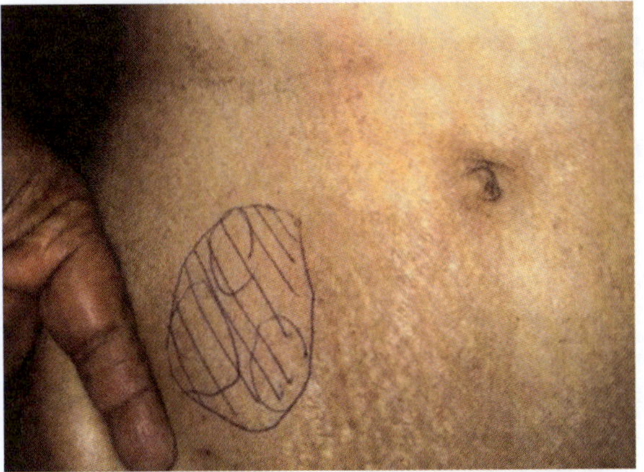

Fig. 55.16: Clear space between lower border of the mass and iliac bone and inguinal crease. It rules out ovarian tumour

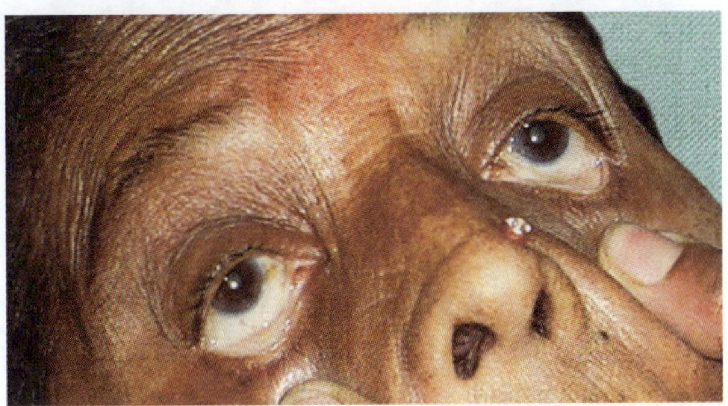

Fig. 55.17: Gross pallor in 60-year-old lady

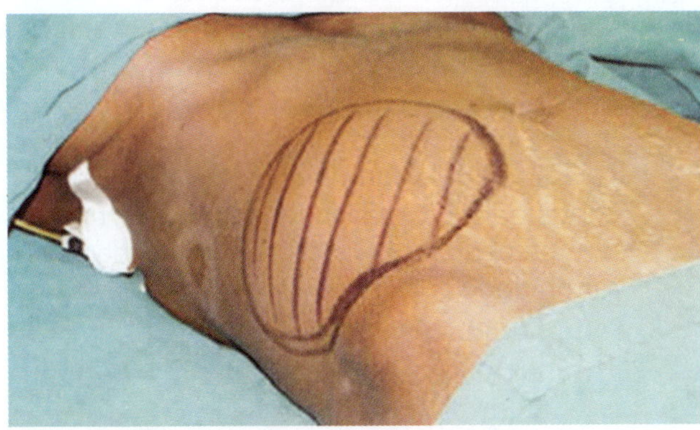

Fig. 55.18: Surface marking of the mass abdomen

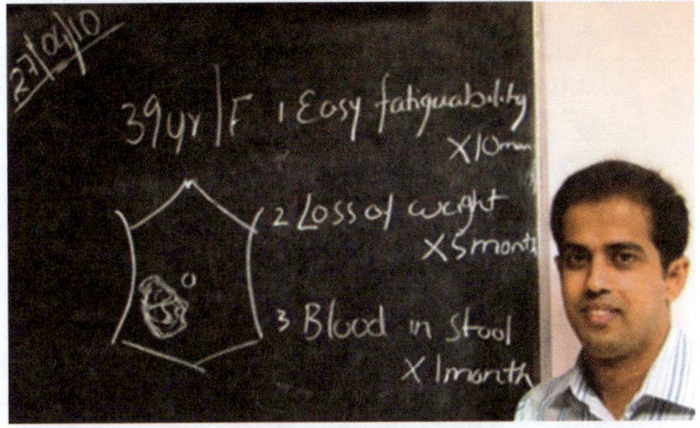

Fig. 55.19: Blackboard sketch (*Courtesy:* Dr Sunilkrishna, postgraduate student, year 2010, KMC, Manipal)

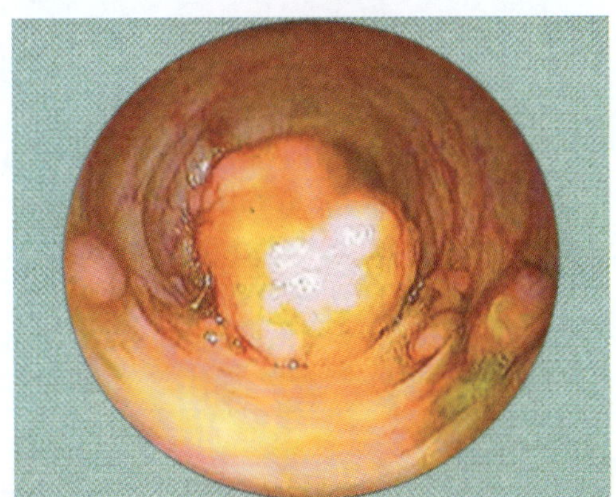

Fig. 55.20: Colonoscopy showing multiple polyps and growth

7. **Actinomycosis:** This is a rare mass in the right iliac fossa which usually develops 2–3 months after appendicectomy. A woody hard, indurated tender mass with multiple sinuses is characteristic of this condition. Sinuses discharge sulphur granules which can trickle down. Unlike tuberculosis, narrowing of lumen of the gut and lymph node enlargement does not occur.
8. **Lymph node mass**
   - Acute mesenteric lymphadenitis is common in children. It produces tender, nodular and firm mass in right iliac fossa. The child usually has fever. Acute lymphadenitis can also involve external iliac nodes as in filariasis.
   - Lymphoma involving external iliac nodes, nodular, firm to hard mass with involvement of other nodes, liver, spleen, etc.
   - Secondaries in lymph nodes (external iliac) from carcinoma ovary, cervix, etc. Nodes are hard and fixity is a feature.
9. **Retroperitoneal sarcoma** (Fig. 55.21)
   - Common in young patients
   - Huge, nodular, fixed lump involving lumbar, umbilical and right iliac fossa. Recent increase in size draws the attention of the patient.
   - Fixed to posterior abdominal wall
   - Later, obstruction of inferior vena cava results in oedema of legs.
   - Pressure on the ureter can give rise to hydronephrosis.
   - Liposarcoma is the commonest and may arise from pre-existing lipoma.
   - Fibrosarcoma, haemangiosarcoma, leiomyosarcoma are other sarcomas.
   - It is treated by wide excision followed by radiotherapy.
   - Chemotherapy is also helpful, when it is not possible to remove the entire mass.
   - Debulking even if it is an advanced case is recommended.
10. **Aneurysm:** Iliac artery aneurysm is rare and occurs in old-aged patients. It produces a soft, pulsatile swelling in the right iliac fossa. Bruit or thrill is usually present.
11. **Iliopsoas abscess** (Fig. 55.22)
    - It is the result of tuberculosis of thoracolumbar spine. It should be suspected when a young patient complains of pain in the back referred to abdominal wall.
    - Spine movements are limited.
    - Gibbus is present.
    - Initially, it forms paravertebral abscess and later it gravitates down beneath the medial arcuate ligament and forms psoas abscess. Psoas abscess burrows into the thigh under inguinal ligament and forms iliopsoas abscess.
    - Fluctuation is present on both sides of the inguinal ligament. It is described as cross-fluctuation test (Fig. 55.23).

Fig. 55.22: Iliopsoas abscess

12. **Chondrosarcoma of the iliac crest:** It is a hard, fixed tumour which cannot be separated from the bone.

In females

13. **Ovarian cyst:** To start with, the cyst develops in the pelvis and gives rise to discomfort in the lower abdomen. As the cyst grows, it comes out of the pelvis and forms a mass in right iliac fossa. It has smooth surface, round borders, is cystic,

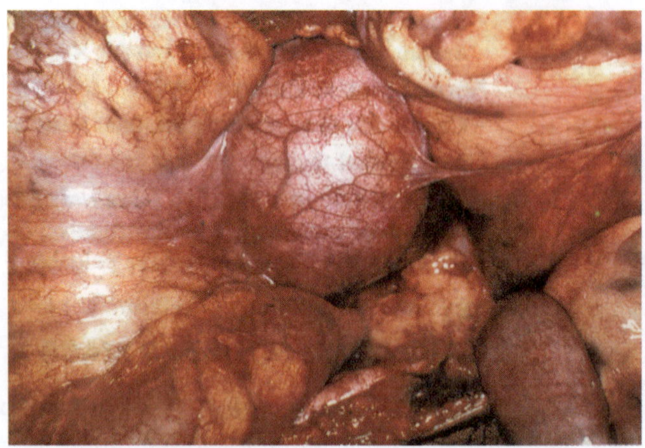

Fig. 55.21: Retroperitoneal sarcoma

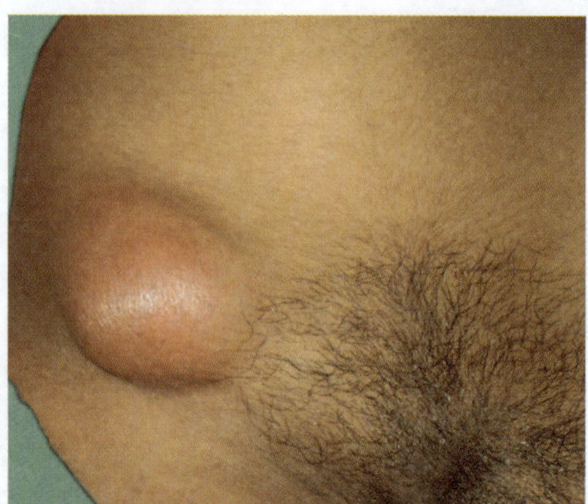

Fig. 55.23: Cold abscess—the swelling was partly above and partly below the inguinal ligament

freely mobile and can be pushed back into the pelvis. Sometimes, the cyst can attain huge size. Such freely mobile ovarian cysts have a long pedicle. Per vaginal examination gives the clue to the diagnosis.

14. **Fibroid of the uterus:** It presents as a firm to hard nodular mass in the suprapubic region and in the right iliac fossa.
15. **Tubo-ovarian mass**
    - It is usually tender
    - Pelvic infection is present
    - It is soft to firm
    - It can be bilateral

B. Arising from structures which are not normally present

1. **Unascended kidney:** It can be either in the pelvis or in the iliac fossa. Such kidney is usually not very well-developed. It presents as a lobular mass.
2. **Normal mobile kidney:** It can be felt in lumbar region, iliac fossa and can be pushed back into the loin.
3. **Undescended testis:** It is palpable in right iliac fossa *only* when it is involved by Seminoma. It is an intra-abdominal testis and is hard, irregular, fixed mass. *Absent testis* in the scrotum clinches the diagnosis. Patient may have palpable para-aortic nodes, supraclavicular nodes, etc. (Fig. 55.24).

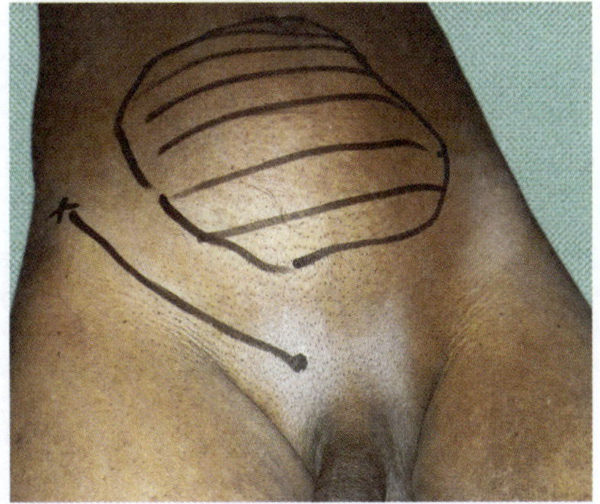

Fig. 55.24: Large testicular tumour arising in undescended testis

FIRM TO HARD NODULAR MASS IN THE UMBILICAL REGION

1. Mass Arising from Lymph Nodes

a. **Metastasis or secondaries** is one of the common lymph node masses in the abdomen. Mass can be due to para-aortic nodes from testicular tumour, melanoma, carcinoma of ovary, carcinoma of penis, carcinoma of rectum, colon, stomach in late cases.

- A para-aortic lymph node mass has the following features:
  1. Fixed
  2. Does not move with respiration
  3. No intrinsic mobility
  4. Does not fall forward
  5. Coils of bowel can be felt over the mass
  6. Percussion may be resonant because of intestinal coils (Fig. 55.25).

b. **Lymphoma:** The mass is enlarged para-aortic group of lymph nodes. It has all features of nodes mentioned above. Presence of lymph nodes in the neck along with palpable liver and spleen clinches the diagnosis.

c. **Tuberculosis** can affect para-aortic nodes. However, it is uncommon.

2. Retroperitoneal Sarcoma (Fig. 55.26)

- Common in young patients
- Rapidly growing, enlarging mass in the abdomen of short duration.
- It is firm, hard, nodular, fixed, does not fall forward and has intestinal coils anterior to it.
- Large sarcomas can cause compression on inferior vena cava or on the ureter. Therefore, pedal oedema and hydronephrosis can occur.

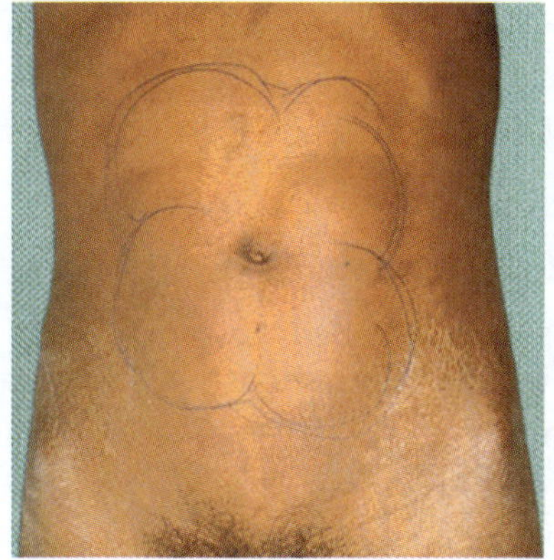

Fig. 55.25: Para-aortic lymph node mass due to seminoma

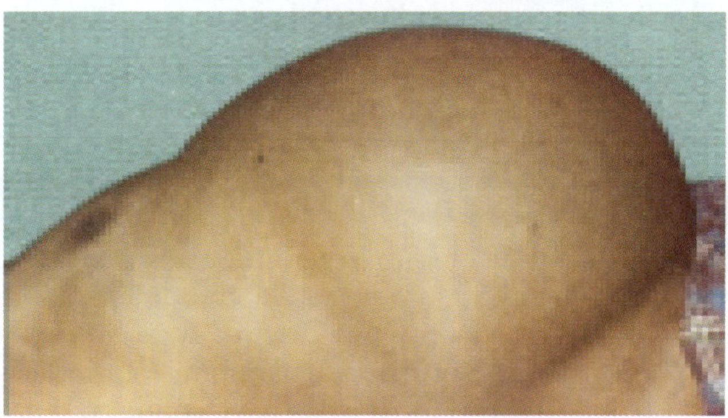

Fig. 55.26: Retroperitoneal liposarcoma

- Liposarcoma and fibrosarcoma are common.
- Radical surgery should be attempted and it is the only hope of cure. (Many cases may require debulking and follow-up with radiotherapy and chemotherapy.)

3. Carcinoma Body of Pancreas (Fig. 55.27)

- Cystadenocarcinoma of pancreas can attain a huge size. Otherwise, it is uncommon to get a large nodular pancreatic mass. However, carcinoma pancreas presenting as a palpable nodular mass indicates nonresectability. Presence of **pulsations over the mass** (transmitted) clinches the diagnosis.
- Men in the 6th decade are usually affected.
- Severe backache, loss of weight, recent development of diabetes suggest pancreatic pathology.
- Jaundice does not occur unless and until liver secondaries develop.
- It has all the features of retroperitoneal mass.
- These cases are advanced with ascites, rectovesical deposits, etc.

4. Carcinoma Transverse Colon (Fig. 55.28)

- Elderly patients present with constipation and bleeding per rectum.
- Firm to hard nodular mass occupying umbilical region may be found.
- It may have vertical mobility and being intra-abdominal, it falls forward.
- Caecum may be distended. Right to left peristalsis may be visible.

5. Tuberculous Abdomen (Figs 55.29 and 55.30)

- The mass can be rolled up omentum, with lymph nodes and coils of intestines which are matted.
- This is common in children and also occur in young adults in India.
- History of evening rise in temperature, loss of weight, loss of appetite, emaciation and improper digestion gives the clue to the diagnosis.
- Ascites is present in almost all cases.
- Features of subacute intestinal obstruction can also be present.

Mass in the umbilical region

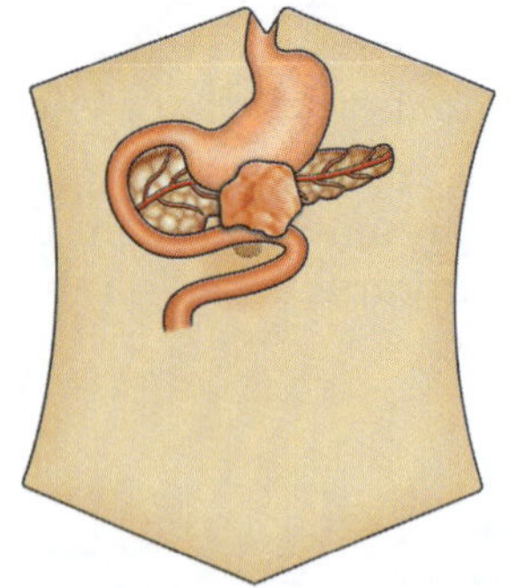

Fig. 55.27: Carcinoma body of pancreas

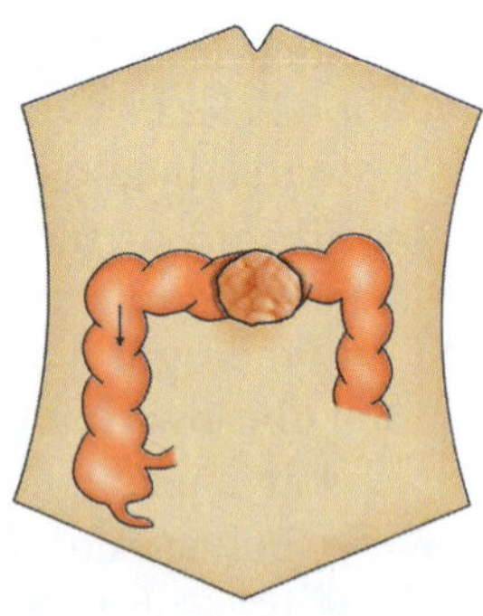

Fig. 55.28: Carcinoma transverse colon

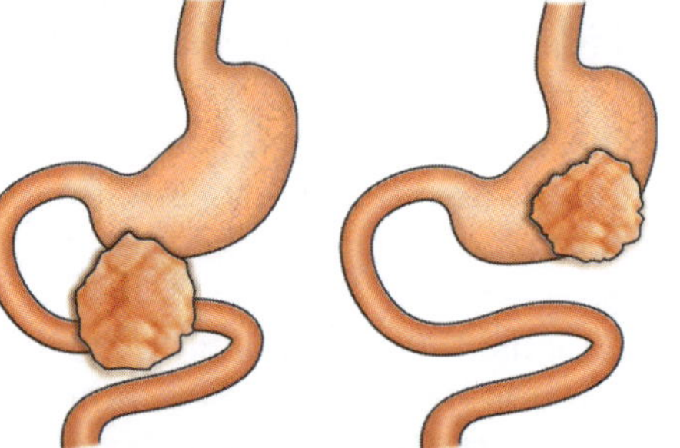

Fig. 55.29: Omental mass

Fig. 55.30: Carcinoma stomach

Fig. 55.31: Pseudocyst pancreas

THE CYSTIC MASS IN THE ABDOMEN

Intra-abdominal cystic swellings are interesting swellings. They occur in young children, adults, middle-aged persons. There are many cases of cystic swellings which have given a surprise at laparotomy (notoriously so in females). In children cysts have confused many competent paediatricians!! Being intra-abdominal cysts, it is not possible to elicit fluctuation and very often they are firm due to increased tension. The details of important cystic swellings are given below.

1. Pseudocyst of Pancreas (Figs 55.31 and 55.32)

Tensely cystic upper abdominal mass may feel firm and tender, and does not move with respiration (*see* page 677 for details). Getting above the swelling is possible. Transmitted pulsations of the aorta can be felt over the mass which disappears on knee-elbow position. History of acute pancreatitis or blunt injury abdomen gives the clue to the diagnosis (Fig. 55.32).

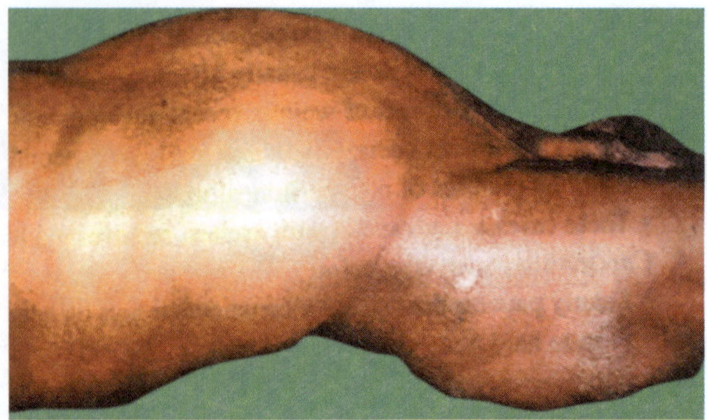

Fig. 55.32: Pseudocyst of pancreas (large)

Section III • Gastrointestinal Surgery

2. Hydatid Cyst of Liver (Fig. 55.33)

This swelling is of long duration, is symptomless or with dull pain in the upper abdomen. The cyst is spherical with smooth surface, rounded borders and feels firm. Since it is a mass arising from liver, it moves with respiration and getting above the swelling is not possible. Classical hydatid thrill, mentioned in the books, is rarely appreciated. Simple cyst of the liver can also present as a cystic mass (Fig. 55.34).

3. Mesenteric Cyst (Fig. 55.35)

These are congenital cysts, enterogenous or chylolymphatic, manifests in young children or during adolescence. Typically, the cyst is located in the umbilical region which moves at right angles to the direction of mesentery.

Types of Mesenteric Cyst (Key Box 55.4 and Figs 55.36 to 55.38, *see page 744 also*)

A. **Chylolymphatic cyst** is a lymphatic cyst arising from mesentery of ileum. It is a thin-walled cyst with clear fluid or chyle. It has a separate blood supply. Hence, enucleation is the treatment without sacrificing the bowel.

B. **Enterogenous cyst** is a duplication cyst from the intestine or due to diverticulum of the mesenteric

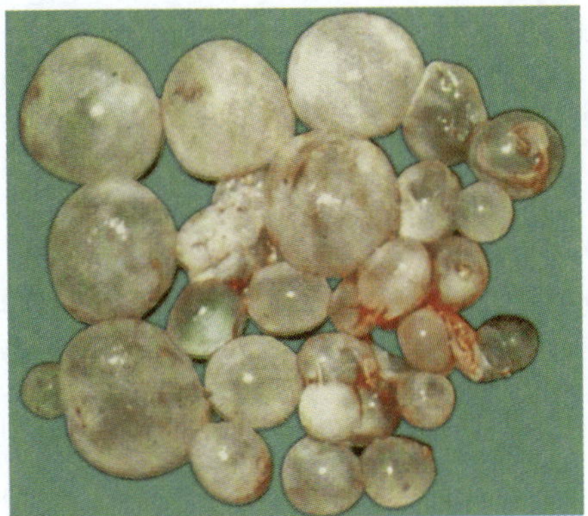

Fig. 55.33: Hydatid cyst

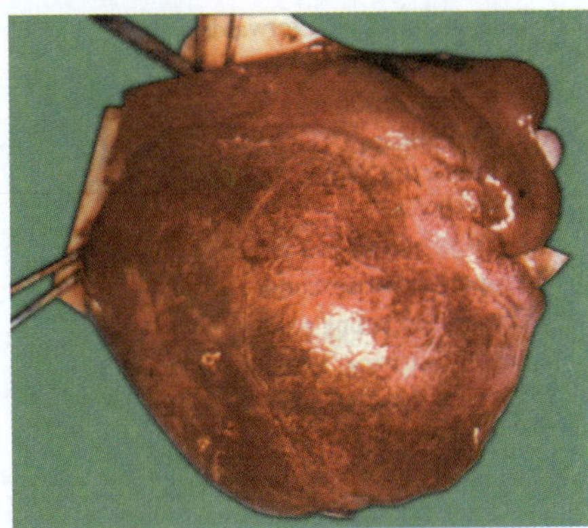

Fig. 55.34: Intra-abdominal cyst: Serous cyst in the liver

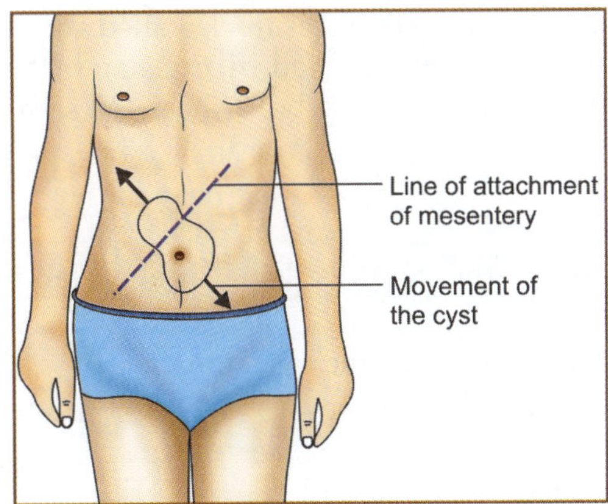

Fig. 55.35: Line of mesentery and classical movement of mesenteric cyst

Key Box 55.4

Mesenteric Cyst—Types

- Chylolymphatic cyst
- Enterogenous cyst
- Urogenital remnant
- Teratomatous dermoid cyst

Tillaux's triad

1. Fluctuant swelling near the umbilicus.
2. Movement perpendicular to the line of mesentery.
3. It is dull surrounded by a zone of resonance and traversed by band of resonance.

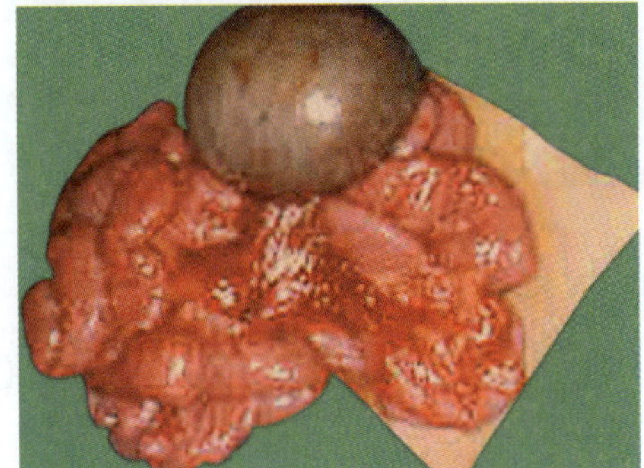

Fig. 55.36: Enterogenous cyst at surgery

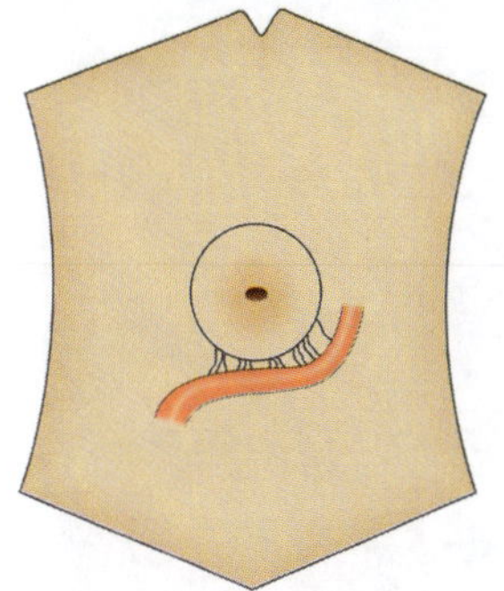

Fig. 55.37: Chylolymphatic cyst—it can be excised without resection of the bowel

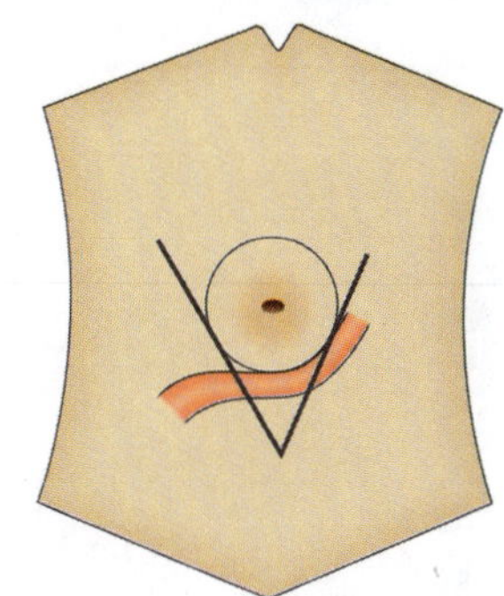

Fig. 55.38: Enterogenous cyst—it requires excision of intestine also along with the cyst

border of the intestine. It is thick walled and contains mucus. This cyst is treated by excision of cyst with bowel segment because both share the same blood supply.

Complications

- Torsion of the cyst resulting in acute abdominal pain.
- Rupture of the cyst due to trauma.
- Haemorrhage into the cyst.

4. Hydronephrosis

Large hydronephrosis can attain a huge size without producing any symptoms. Bulk of the swelling is confined to one side of abdomen, with prominent bulge in the loin. It is difficult to elicit fluctuation in a tensely cystic intra-abdominal mass. Bimanual palpation and ballotability give the clue to the diagnosis. One of the large cysts of polycystic kidney can present as a large renal cyst.

5. Ovarian Cyst

It is a freely mobile, firm or soft mass in any quadrant of the abdomen. Such ovarian cysts, once they come out of pelvis will have free mobility. On pushing **the mass upwards there will be traction** on the pedicle, which may result in pain (Fig. 55.39). In any female patient who presents with lower abdominal mass, ovarian mass has to be considered first, and only then consider other possibilities.

6. Retroperitoneal Lymphatic Cyst

Retroperitoneal cyst is one of the commonest of lymphatic cysts, which grows slowly to attain large size. Typically it is painless, seen in young patients and is tensely cystic. The bowel loop may be felt over the mass (retroperitoneal mass), or bowel loops may be pushed to the side.

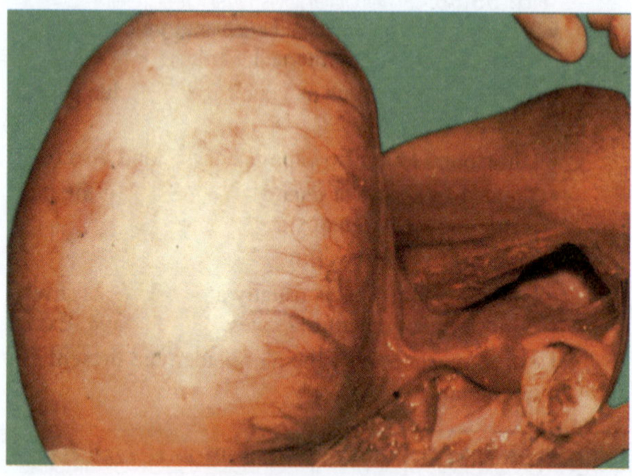

Fig. 55.39: Ovarian cyst

7. Encysted Ascites

This consists of ascitic fluid loculated by many loops of intestine along with omentum. Loss of weight, fever, anorexia, emaciation are the other features.

8. Abdominal Aortic Aneurysm (AAA)

- Majority of cases are due to atherosclerosis and most of the aortic aneurysms are infrarenal. Hence, they present with a swelling in the umbilical region or epigastric region and are associated with backache (Key Box 55.5).

Key Box 55.5

Aortic Aneurysm

- Elderly males >60
- Hypertensive
- Expansile pulsation +
- Anterior rupture: 20%—haemoperitoneum
- Posterior rupture: 80%—retroperitoneal haematoma
- >6 cm size—dangerous

- Often they contain clotted blood. Hence, they feel firm, not compressible, fixed and tender.
- Characteristic feature of an abdominal aortic aneurysm is **expansile pulsation**. This can be appreciated by palpating the swelling gently all around. In the knee-elbow position, the pulsations do not disappear. (Transmitted pulsations disappear in the knee-elbow position.)
- The **femoral pulses** may be normal unless there is thrombosis or rupture of the aneurysm, giving rise to features of acute ischaemia.
- Pressure effects such as **venous oedema** due to pressure on the inferior vena cava or erosion of vertebrae may be found.
- Ultrasound to confirm the aneurysm and also to rule out suprarenal aneurysm.
- It is treated by repair of aneurysm, by incising the aneurysm and suturing a dacron graft end to end, inside the aneurysmal sac.

9. Rare Cystic Swellings in the Abdomen (Fig. 55.40)

- **Omental cyst:** This is usually a lymphatic cyst which occurs in children and can attain a huge size. Sudden enlargement indicates haemorrhage. Excision is easy.
- **Large mucocele** of the gallbladder can present as a tense cystic, slightly tender mass in the upper abdomen.

Pearls of Wisdom

One should not forget distended bladder in the lower abdomen as a cause of cystic swelling.

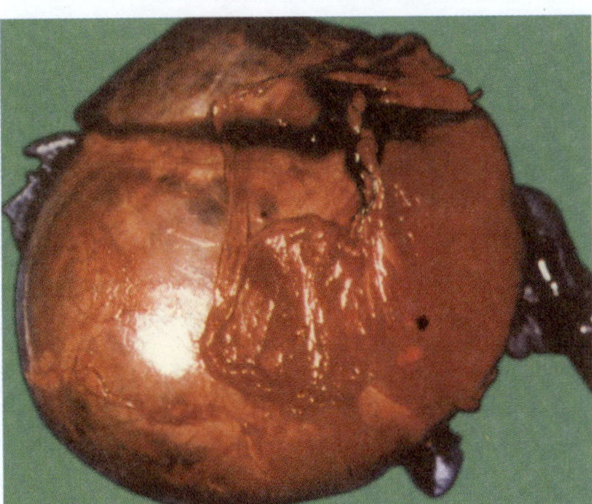

Fig. 55.40: Large lymphatic cyst arising from omentum

Clinical Notes

A female child, aged 6 years, was examined by a paediatrician for generalised abdominal distension. All the investigations were normal. The child was put on antituberculous treatment, as the treating paediatrician diagnosed this case as tuberculous ascites. Child was brought back after 9 months with no improvement and having abdominal pain since 2 days due to sudden increase in the size of the swelling. A paediatric surgeon was consulted, who palpated the abdomen and said she does not have ascites but has a cyst and that the wall of the thin cyst can be felt. At exploration, a large cyst arising from the omentum and occupying all the 9 quadrants of the abdomen, was excised. Histopathological report was lymphatic cyst (Fig. 55.40).

MASS IN THE EPIGASTRIUM

Mass in the epigastrium is one of the common long cases kept in the examination. Students should consider mass arising from liver and stomach first. Other possibilities must be considered later because common cases are common.

I. MASS ARISING IN THE ABDOMINAL WALL

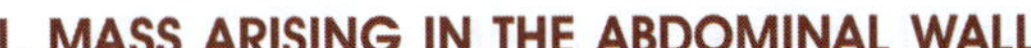

- First do the head raising test. If the mass becomes more prominent, it is extraperitoneal (abdominal wall).
- Lipoma, neurofibroma or desmoid tumour arising from the rectus sheath can present as a mass in the epigastrium.
- Also note epigastric hernia occurs in this region. It is a hernia, not a mass.

Pearls of Wisdom

Any hard subcutaneous swelling in the abdominal wall of recent origin can be a metastasis.

II. INTRAPERITONEAL MASS

1. Mass Arising from the Liver

A. **Hepatoma** (Fig. 55.41): Liver is enlarged, hard, irregular, and nontender. However, rapidly growing hepatomas are tender, firm and even a bruit is heard over the swelling. Rapid deterioration of health in a cirrhotic patient is usually due to the development of a hepatoma.

B. **Secondaries in the liver** (Fig. 55.42): Usually both lobes are enlarged, have nodular surface without a bruit. Jaundice is a late feature in secondaries of the liver. The primary may be obvious as a colonic mass, a stomach mass or a testicular tumour, etc. (*see* page 685).

C. **Hydatid cyst** (Fig. 55.43): It is a benign swelling. History of contact with a dog is usually present. Epigastric swelling is due to enlarged liver which is smooth or irregular, nontender with rounded borders. Classical hydatid fremitus and thrill are rarely elicited. General health of the patient is usually good.

D. **Simple cyst** (Fig. 55.44): It is not a clinical diagnosis but is mentioned here only for discussion. It is a serous cyst. Single big cyst can also be a part of polycystic disease of the liver.

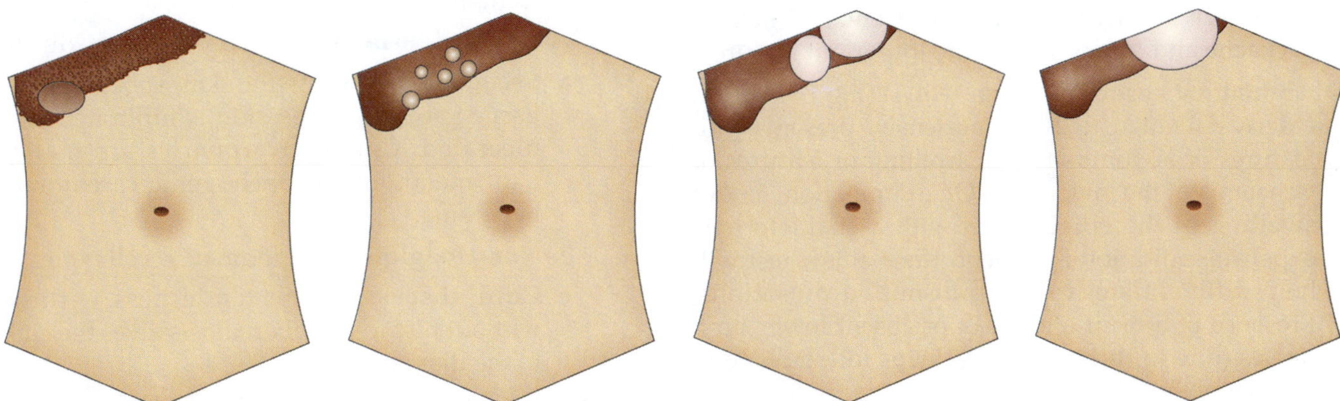

Fig. 55.41: Hepatoma **Fig. 55.42:** Secondaries in the liver **Fig. 55.43:** Hydatid cyst **Fig. 55.44:** Simple cyst

2. Mass Arising from the Stomach

For all practical purposes, the only mass arising from the stomach in the epigastrium is carcinoma stomach. It is hard, irregular and moves with respiration. Usually the patient is a male with loss of appetite and weight. Vomiting is a feature. If there is a growth in the pyloric antrum, visible gastric peristalsis can be seen in the epigastrium. (Students are hereby requested **not to offer lymphoma of the stomach or GIST** of the stomach as a **clinical diagnosis unless asked for by the examiner,** for a differential diagnosis.)

3. Omental Mass

- Omentum gets involved in tuberculosis as a firm, nodular mass (Fig. 55.45) or in secondaries from intra-abdominal malignancies as a hard, nodular mass (Fig. 55.46). Classically it moves with respiration.
- Rarely, omental cyst can present as a tensely cystic mass in the epigastrium.

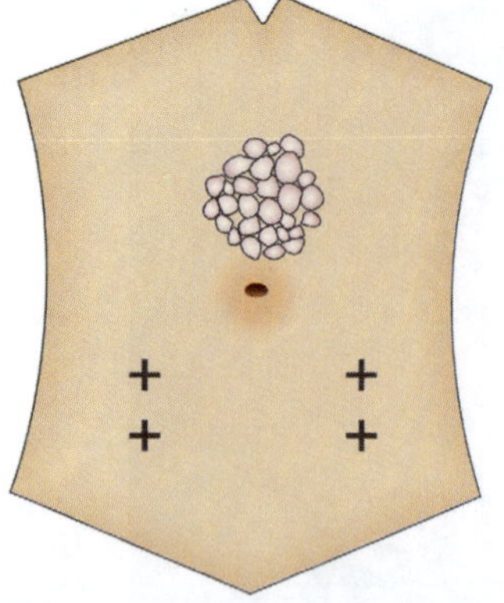

Fig. 55.45: Tuberculous abdomen—ascites and rolled up omentum

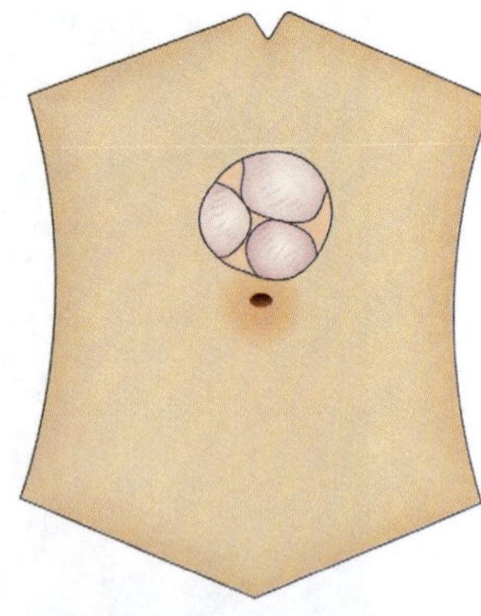

Fig. 55.46: Mass of lymph nodes—nodular, fixed and hard

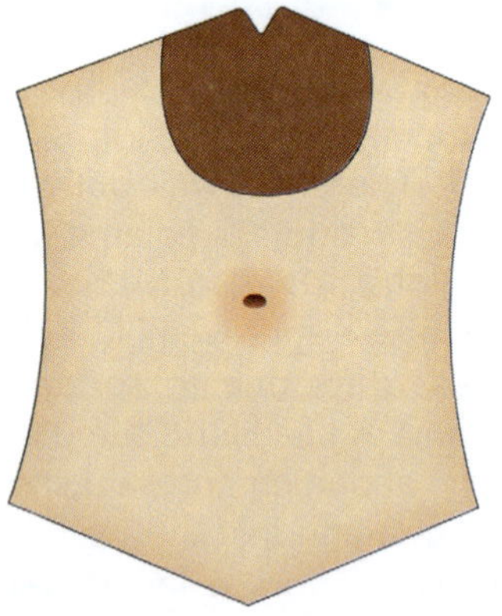

Fig. 55.47: Pseudocyst of pancreas: Large enough— in contact with diaphragm

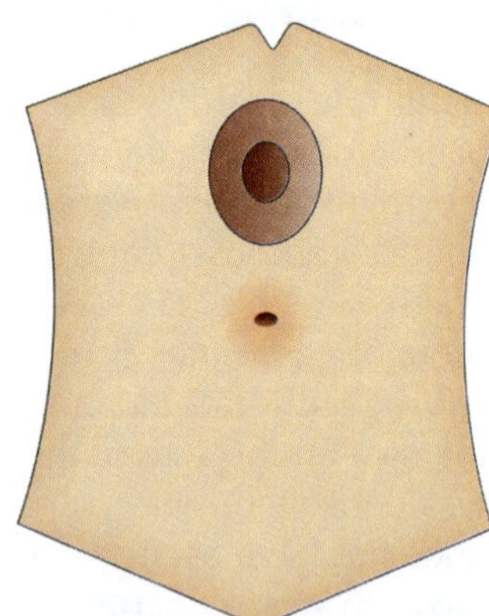

Fig. 55.48: Abdominal aortic aneurysm: Pulsatile firm mass

III. RETROPERITONEAL MASS

A. **Pseudopancreatic cyst** (Fig. 55.47): It forms a tense cystic mass, felt as firm mass in the epigastrium. Its upper border can be made out. It does not usually move with respiration. It has smooth surface and round borders. History of acute pancreatitis or blunt injury abdomen is usually present. Pulsations over the mass (transmitted) suggest that it is a mass close to the aorta. In such a case, it is a pseudocyst. Gurgle heard anteriorly suggests distended stomach.

B. **Cystadenoma:** Cystadenomas of pancreas are benign and can attain huge sizes. It can present as a mass in the epigastrium, left hypochondrium or umbilical region. They exhibit what is described as 'tree top mobility'.

C. **Carcinoma body of pancreas** can present as a mass in the lower part of epigastrium or upper umbilical region. The mass is hard, irregular, fixed and does not move with respiration. Presence of severe backache and loss of weight are important features.

D. **Abdominal aortic aneurysm (AAA)** (Fig. 55.48): An elderly patient, usually a hypertensive presents with features of abdominal pain, swelling or features of ischaemia of the lower limb. On examination, tender swelling in the epigastrium with a characteristic expansile pulsation is present. Knee-elbow test will help differentiate it from transmitted pulsations. Presence of a bruit and weak or absent lower limb pulses (due to thrombus) also helps in establishing the diagnosis.

E. **Lymph node mass** (Fig. 55.46).

MASS IN THE RIGHT HYPOCHONDRIUM (Fig. 55.49)

I. *Parietal:* On head raising test, the lump becomes more prominent.

  A. **Lipoma, neurofibroma:** They can be part of multiple lipomatosis or multiple neurofibromatosis. If pain and pigmentation are present, it is neurofibroma.

  B. **A hard nodule in the parietal wall** can be due to

    a. **Secondary deposit** in the skin/subcutaneous tissue specially when skin is infiltrated and ulcerated. Common primaries are malignant melanoma, bronchogenic carcinoma, hepatoma.

    b. **Non-Hodgkin's lymphoma:** 'T' cell type.

    c. **Cold abscess:** Spine tenderness with or without history of tuberculosis gives the clue to the diagnosis.

II. *Intra-abdominal swellings:* On head raising test, the lump becomes less prominent.

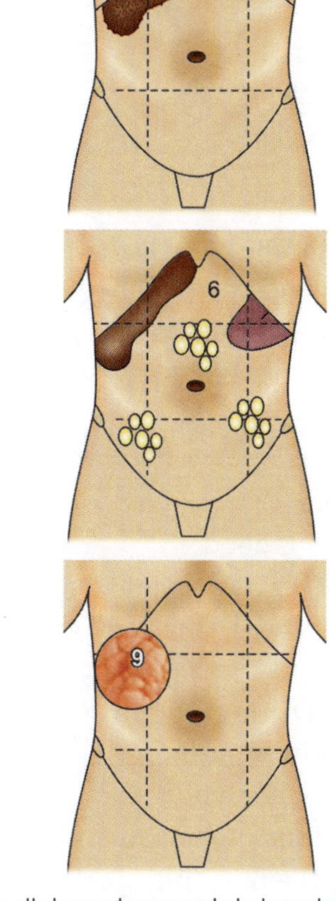

Fig. 55.49: Differential diagnosis of mass in the right hypochondrium: (1) Smooth hepatomegaly in lymphoma or due to medical causes, (2) secondaries in the liver—hard and nodular, (3) hepatoma—irregular, hard or firm, (4) polycystic disease of the liver—firm and nodular with round borders, (5) with splenomegaly—could be portal hypertension, (6) hepatomegaly, splenomegaly, para-aortic lymph nodes and iliac nodes—Hodgkin's lymphoma, (7) carcinoma ascending colon—hard irregular mass, (8) palpable gallbladder—smooth, round borders, and (9) renal mass

1. Liver: Only chronic masses are discussed.

A. Secondaries in liver (Fig. 55.50 and Key Box 55.6)

- Entire liver is enlarged (both lobes)
- Nodular surface
- Sharp border
- Hard in consistency

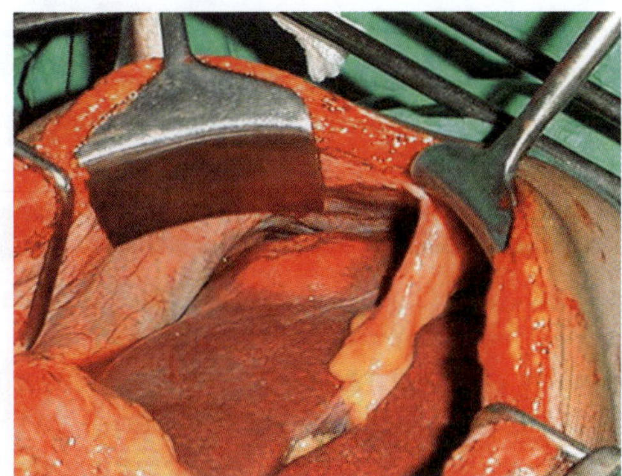

Fig. 55.50: Large secondary in the liver from carcinoma stomach

Key Box 55.6

Anatomic Features of Liver Mass

- Location: Hypochondrium (right and left) and epigastrium
- Moves with respiration
- Finger—insinuation between costal margin and mass is not possible
- No intrinsic mobility and dullness
- Dull note over the liver which will continue with the mass

- Rare umbilication sign, evidence of primary, emaciated patient, poor health, loss of appetite and weight are other features.

B. Hepatoma (Key Box 55.7)

- One lobe is enlarged
- Firm to hard, irregular
- Very tender liver
- Bruit/thrill may be present

Key Box 55.7

Tender Liver Mass

- Hepatoma
- Amoebic liver abscess
- Suppurative pylephlebitis
- Congestive cardiac failure
- Infected hydatid cyst

- Evidence of chronic liver disease such as serum hepatitis or cirrhosis is usually present.

C. Polycystic disease of the liver

- Both lobes are enlarged
- Nodular
- Nontender
- Round borders
- General health is good

The patient would have presented to the hospital with pain due to haemorrhage in a cyst.

D. Hydatid cyst

- One or both lobes are enlarged
- Smooth or nodular surface
- Round borders, nontender
- General condition of the patient is good
- **Hydatid thrill—rare 'physical sign'** may be present.

E. Cirrhosis of liver

- Liver may be enlarged: Firm and irregular in pre-cirrhotic cases. Splenomegaly, ascites will help in the diagnosis.
- Other features of liver cell failure such as gynaecomastia, spider naevi, palmar erythema may be present.

F. Lymphoma

- Liver is palpable, one or two finger-breadths, firm or hard, smooth or irregular, nontender.
- Splenomegaly and lymphadenopathy will help in the diagnosis.

G. Congenital Riedel's lobe: It is a tongue-shaped projection from the inferior border of liver. It is on the right side, can be mistaken for gallbladder.

2. Gallbladder mass (Key Box 55.8)

Causes of gallbladder enlargement

- **Back pressure:** Distal obstruction periampullary carcinoma. Such gallbladder is firm, smooth and associated with jaundice.
- **Carcinoma gallbladder:** Hard, irregular, fixed
- **Acute cholecystitis:** Tender, vague, well-defined mass.

Key Box 55.8

Clinical Features of a Gallbladder Mass

a. It is oval, e.g. egg-shaped swelling
b. It is tense. Hence, feels more firm in consistency
c. Moves freely up and down with respiration—better seen in thin patients
d. May have slight side-to-side mobility
e. It is felt slightly posterior to (step deep) inferior border of the liver

- **Mucocele:** Nontender, palpable gallbladder without jaundice
- **Empyema:** Very tender, gallbladder mass

3. Colonic mass

A. Carcinoma hepatic flexure

- Firm to hard irregular mass
- Restricted mobility
- Moves with respiration because of its contact with liver
- Resonant or impaired resonant note on percussion (liver is dull on percussion)
- Caecum may be distended, if there is obstruction.

B. Large ileocaecal tuberculosis with pulled up caecum may also be palpable. Such masses may be bimanually palpable but not ballotable.

4. Renal mass

- Importantly renal mass is palpable mainly in the **lumbar region, loin** and in the right hypochondrium.
- Carcinoma kidney is hard and irregular
- Upper border is usually not palpable—it is under cover of the 12th rib.
- Hydronephrotic kidney will be firm and smooth

5. Suprarenal mass

- Clinically they have all features of a renal mass
- Hence, symptoms of the patient may have to be correlated. A few examples are given here:
  - Cushing's syndrome
  - Phaeochromocytoma

MASS IN THE RIGHT LUMBAR REGION

1. Renal mass (Figs 55.51 and 55.52): Renal masses are the most common masses in the lumbar region followed by colonic masses. Kidney is present in the loin and it is a posterior structure. Hence, in majority of the cases, enlargement is more obvious posteriorly. However, uniform enlargement causes the kidney to enlarge anteriorly thus making it bimanually

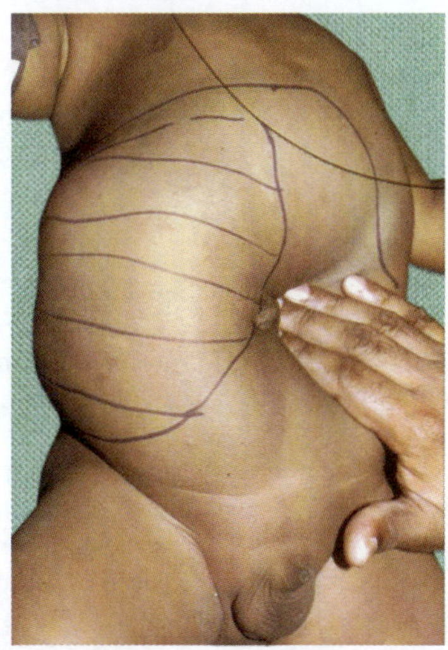

Fig. 55.51: Wilms' tumour in a two-year-old child (*Courtesy:* Dr Vijay Kumar, Dr Sandeep PT, Department of Paediatrics Surgery, KMC, Manipal)

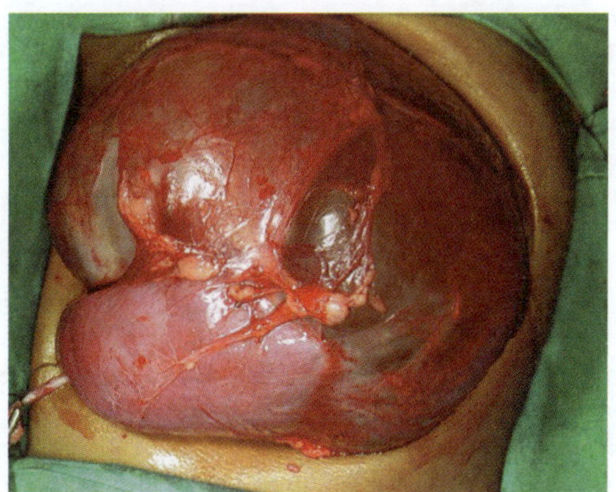

Fig. 55.52: Renal cell carcinoma

palpable. One characteristic feature of a renal mass is ballotability. Kidney ballots because it has a pedicle and a cushion of perirenal pad of fat surrounding it. Ballotability is demonstrated by the following method. One hand is kept posteriorly close to the abdominal wall and the other hand anteriorly. A push (ballot means to toss) is given with posterior hand. The mass tosses and touches hand, anteriorly placed and goes back. Thus, following features of a kidney help to say that mass is arising from kidney.

- Kidney is present in the lumbar region and it has reniform shape.
- It enlarges in superoinferior direction.
- It moves with respiration because it is enclosed by fascia of Gerota which blends with diaphragm above.
- It is bimanually palpable and ballotable.
- It is possible to insinuate the fingers between the upper border of the mass and the costal margin.
- Normal resonant note posteriorly in the loin (colonic) gets obliterated because as the kidney enlarges, it displaces the colon.

CECT scan is the most common useful investigation to differentiate renal masses (Figs 55.53 and 5.54). The most common renal masses which are palpable in the lumbar region—renal cell carcinoma, polycystic disease and hydronephrosis have been compared in Table 55.1.

Various causes of hydronephrosis have been given in Fig. 55.55.

2. **Liver mass:** A large liver mass is easily palpable in the lumbar region. In these cases, you have to present

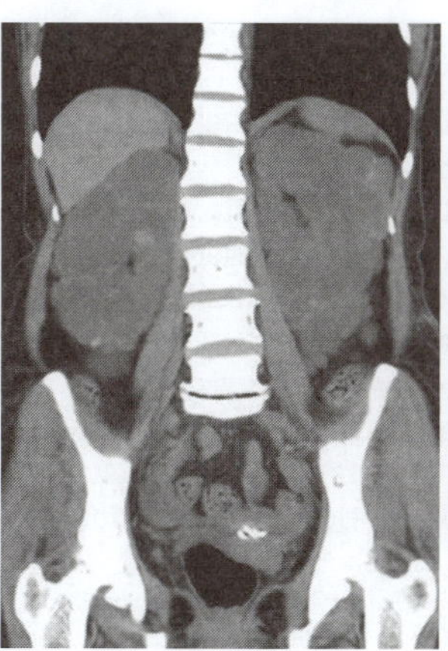

Fig. 55.53: CT scan showing cysts

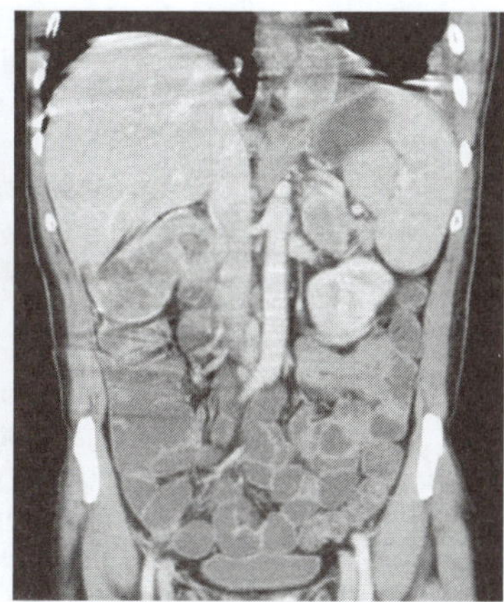

Fig. 55.54: CT scan—renal cell carcinoma affecting the upper pole of the right kidney

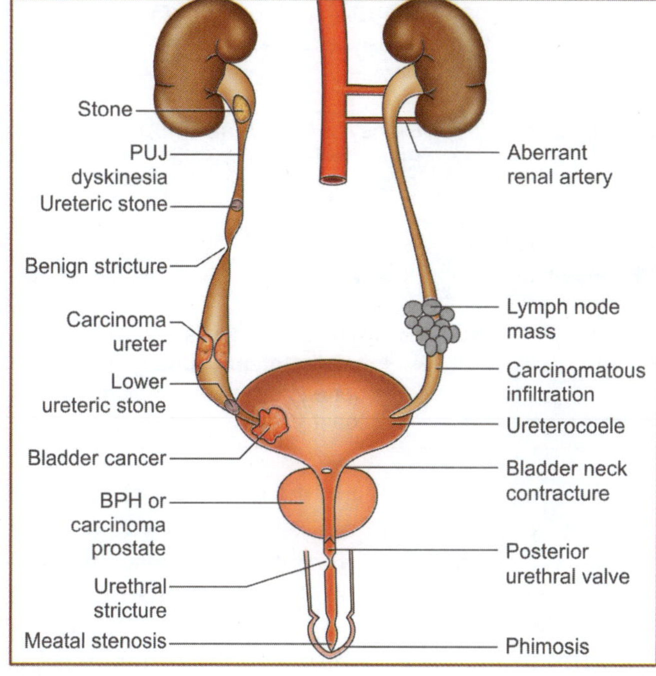

Fig. 55.55: Diagrammatic representation of hydronephrosis

Table 55.1 Three common masses arising from kidney

Feature	Polycystic kidney disease	Hydronephrosis	Renal cell carcinoma
Age	30–40 years	**Congenital—young 20–30 years** **Acquired—elderly**	40–60 years
Incidence	Females > Males	Females > Males	Males > Females
Clinical features Renal mass **Upper border cannot be made out when the kidney is enlarged**	• **Mass per abdomen** – Bilateral – Massive enlargement – Nodular/Bosselated surface – Firm to hard, sometimes cystic – Not fixed, nontender	• **Mass per abdomen** – Unilateral/bilateral enlarged kidney(s) – Smooth surface – Firm, tensely cystic – Not fixed, nontender	• **Mass per abdomen** – Unilateral enlarged kidney – Irregular, nodular surface – Hard, ballotable, bimanually palpable – Fixity +/–, nontender
Other features	• Dull aching pain in loins—dragging pain • Micro-/macroscopic haematuria • Hypertension • Features of renal failure: Thirst, vomiting, abdominal distension, anuria, uremic smell, coated tongue, anaemia • Infection—pyelonephritis • Acute pain: If there is haemorrhage into or infection of a cyst; colicky pain—due to blood clot in ureter	• May be asymptomatic, or • Abdominal distension • Abdominal pain—dull aching pain in loin • Previous history of calculus disease in the ureter and symptoms—colicky radiating abdominal pain, haematuria • Elderly male—it is BPH, hence history of hesitancy and frequency of micturition	**Triad of RCC** 1. Pain-dragging/intermittent 2. Intermittent haematuria 3. Palpable mass **Other features** • Pathological fractures • Anaemia • Fever • Hypertension • Liver dysfunction
Investigations	• Urea, creatinine: Rule out renal failure • Plain X-ray KUB: Enlarged kidney • *Abdominal USG/CT scan*: Confirm Dx; multiple hypodense areas without enhancement • IVU—spider leg deformity of calyces Biopsy is not done—no role for FNAC	• Urea, *creatinine*: Rule out renal failure • *Plain X-ray KUB*: Enlarged kidney, stones • *Abdominal USG*: Detect enlarged kidney and the cause. *CT scan*: Investigation of choice; dilated pelvicalyceal system with uniform filling of contrast • *IVU*: Gross dilation of pelvicalyceal system—not done if we do contrast CT No role for biopsy or FNAC	• *Urine exam*: Look for malignant cells if haematuria is present • *Plain X-ray KUB*: Enlarged kidney • *Abdominal USG*: Enlarged kidney, locate tumour, size, extent • *CECT scan*: Investigation of choice for staging • *IVU*: Irregular calyces
Treatment	1. *Asymptomatic*: Regular follow-up 2. Symptomatic, dialysis plus renal transplantation if uncontrolled hypertension or renal failure is present	*Congenital*: Anderson Hyne's pyeloplasty *Acquired*: Treat the cause, e.g. BPH with hydronephrosis = TURP	Radical nephrectomy with or without other treatment

the case as a mass is felt in the right hypochondrium and it extends into lumbar region. Once you confirm it is liver, common differential diagnoses include hepatoma, secondaries in the liver, hydatid disease of the liver, etc.

3. **Gallbladder mass:** A large gallbladder mass is palpable in the lumbar region but it starts from the right hypochondrium, Shape is oval with smooth surface and tensely cystic. The usual cause is mucocele. Mucocele of the gallbladder is due to a stone blocking the cystic duct and causing massive enlargement of the gallbladder. These patients do not have jaundice. Other causes of enlargement have been already discussed.

4. **Ascending colonic mass**

   a. ***Ileocaecal tuberculosis*** is felt as an irregular or nodular firm mass in the right iliac fossa and in the lumbar region. The mass is due to thickened caecum and ascending colon. **The caecum is higher in position because it is pulled up. Younger age of the patient, fever, weight loss, loose stools and colicky abdominal pain are the symptoms. (More details under mass in the right iliac fossa).**

   b. ***Carcinoma ascending colon:*** Typically, a patient is around 50–60 years of age who presents with change in bowel habits—mucus in the stools and bleeding per rectum. Anaemia, loss of weight and weakness are the features. On examination, the mass is palpable in the lumbar region which is firm to hard, irregular with restricted mobility. Gurgling is elicited due to presence of air in the lumen, thus it differentiates from solid organ enlargement. **Large tumours can be bimanually palpable** but they are not ballotable. Colonoscopy to confirm the diagnosis followed by ultrasound and CT scan to know the metastasis and resectability are the investigations. Right radical hemi-colectomy or extended hemicolectomy depends upon whether the hepatic flexure is involved or not is the treatment of choice (Fig. 55.56).

   c. ***GIST:*** Patients with gastrointestinal stromal tumour are between 20 and 50 years of age. These tumours attain a large size. They grow outside the lumen and hence do not produce obstruction. However, a mucosal ulceration results in bleeding.

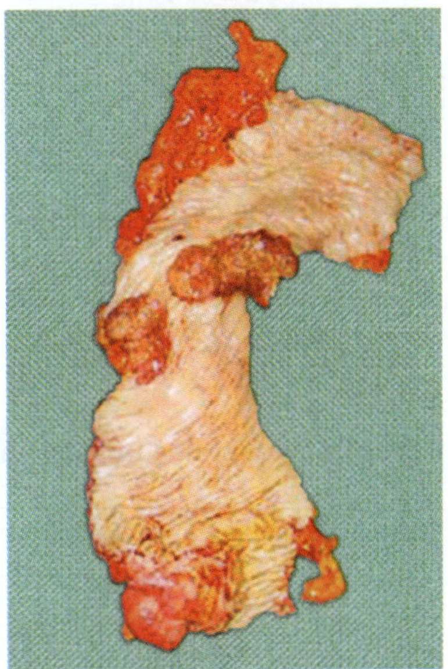

Fig. 55.56: Carcinoma ascending colon

   The stomach is the commonest site of GIST. GIST arising from intestines can present in the lumbar region. This should be the exclusion diagnosis. If you suspect a bowel mass think of colonic malignancy first, followed by tuberculosis as second and chronic intussusception as third. When all 3 are ruled out, if features of GIST are present, then offer the diagnosis of GIST.

   d. ***Chronic intussusception:*** It is usually a firm gurgling mass with regular borders which may contract during palpation. Recurrent or intermittent abdominal pain for one or two years may be present. Chronic intussusception is non tender. When the intussusception reduces, all symptoms will disappear. Percussion will reveal a resonant note. Most of the patients are young. If intussusception is the diagnosis in elderly, it is usually ileocolic or colocolic and invariably a colonic malignancy is the cause. These intussusceptions are called secondary intussusceptions. The common causes of secondary intussusception or chronic intussusception are polyps, purpura, submucosal lipoma, Meckel's diverticulum, carcinoma, carcinoid, etc. Ultrasound followed by CECT scan is done to confirm the diagnosis followed by resection of the bowel and anastomosis.

5. **Retroperitoneal mass:** Typically retroperitoneal masses are liposarcomas. They occur in young patients. They can attain huge size before they become clinically palpable. They present with painless, progressive, massive enlargement of the abdomen. Compression on the iliac veins will result in unilateral limb oedema. Inferior vena caval obstruction may cause bilateral limb oedema and dilated veins in the flank (inguinoaxillary veins). Examination will reveal a large, firm, irregular mass with all borders felt and with restricted mobility. On percussion a resonant note is felt because of intestines over the surface of the mass. Liposarcoma is the commonest retroperitoneal sarcomas followed by fibrosarcoma or epithelioid sarcomas. CT scan is done to locate the tumour and to find out the vascular invasions and to find out the infiltration of the surrounding structures. Resection of the tumour is the best form of treatment. All other modalities such as chemotherapy and radiotherapy are palliative.

Pearls of Wisdom

Offer renal mass as diagnosis. When asked for differential diagnosis, mention suprarenal mass.

Multiple Choice Questions

1. **The most diagnostic sign of a renal mass is:**
   A. Moves with respiration
   B. Upper pole cannot be felt
   C. It enlarges downwards
   D. Ballotability

2. **Which one of the following lower horizontal lines divides abdomen into regions?**
   A. Transpyloric line
   B. Transcolic line
   C. Transtubercular line
   D. Transanterior superior iliac spine line

3. **Which of the following masses does not move with respiration?**
   A. Kidney
   B. Hepatic flexure
   C. Tail of the pancreas
   D. Para-aortic lymph node mass

4. **Notch is a diagnostic sign of which mass?**
   A. Spleen B. Liver
   C. Kidney D. Adrenal gland

5. **Which of the following does not have intrinsic mobility?**
   A. Fibroadenoma breast B. Ovarian cyst
   C. Mesenteric cyst D. Multinodular goitre

6. **The following are true for renal masses *except:***
   A. It is bimanually palpable
   B. It is ballotable
   C. It does not move with respiration
   D. Upper border is usually not felt

7. **Blumer's shelf refers to:**
   A. Rectouterine pouch B. Rectovesical pouch
   C. Rectosacral pouch D. Rectoprostatic pouch

8. **Following tumours can occur in the abdominal wall *except:***
   A. Desmoid tumour B. Endometriosis
   C. Dermoid tumour D. Fibromatosis

9. **Following appendicectomy, after 2 months, if woody indurated mass develops in the right iliac fossa with sinuses, what is the diagnosis?**
   A. Tuberculosis
   B. Crohn's disease
   C. Amoeboma
   D. Actinomycosis

10. **Acute intussusception mass has the following features *except:***
    A. Mass is tender
    B. Mass is felt in the umbilical region
    C. It is a sausage-shaped mass
    D. In the right iliac fossa caecum gurgles

11. **Which of the following masses does not have cross-fluctuation?**
    A. Iliopsoas abscess B. Plunging ranula
    C. Collar stud abscess D. Branchial cyst

12. **Following are true for retroperitoneal sarcoma *except:***
    A. Common in young patients
    B. Mass does not move with respiration
    C. It can attain a hard and large mass
    D. Free fluid is usually present in the abdomen

13. **The diagnostic feature of mesenteric cyst is:**
    A. It is present in the umbilical region
    B. It is dull to percuss
    C. It falls forward
    D. Moves at right angle to the direction of mesentery

14. **Which of the following masses is nontender?**
    A. Hepatoma
    B. Appendicular mass
    C. Carcinoma stomach
    D. Cholecystitis

15. **Murphy's triad of symptoms include the following *except:***
    A. Pain B. Vomiting
    C. Fever D. Jaundice

Answers

1. D	2. C	3. D	4. A	5. D	6. C	7. B	8. c	9. B	10. A
11. D	12. D	13. D	14. C	15. D					

Section

IV

Urology

56. Investigations of the Urinary Tract
57. Kidney and Ureter
58. Urinary Bladder and Urethra
59. Prostate and Seminal Vesicles
60. Penis, Testis and Scrotum
61. Haematuria and Urinary Tract Infections

CHAPTER

56

Investigations of the Urinary Tract

- Urine examination
- Blood test
- X-ray KUB
- Retrograde pyelography
- Renal arteriography
- Cystourethrography
- Urethrography
- Ultrasonography
- Computerised tomography
- Radioisotope scanning
- Endoscopy
- Urethroscopy
- MR urography

Competency

SU29.1: Describe the causes, investigations and principles of management of haematuria. Also refer to page 1114.

Please note: This chapter is the basic chapter which deals with investigations of the urinary tract for all diseases, hence read this chapter first and apply the knowledge when you are answering other questions.

URINE EXAMINATION

Urinalysis can be accorded the status of "liquid renal biopsy." It gives many clues to diseases affecting the urinary tract.

Specific gravity: It varies from 1.005 to 1.040 according to the patient's state of hydration. In chronic renal failure, the concentrating ability of the kidneys is lost, and the specific gravity remains fixed at 1.010. This is called isosthenuria.

pH: The urinary pH normally ranges from 4.5 to 8. It varies depending on serum pH. Urine pH influences the type of stone formed (e.g. alkaline urine—infection by urea-splitting organisms resulting in infection stones, acidic urine—uric acid and cystine stones).

Normally, urine is devoid of blood, protein, and sugar.

Proteinuria: It is defined as protein excretion >150 mg/day. Protein, especially albumin, appears in urine following exercise, glomerulonephritis, and nephrotic syndrome.

Sugar: It appears in urine in diabetes mellitus. Transient postprandial glycosuria may be seen when serum glucose levels exceed the renal threshold.

Blood: This is seen as the presence of red blood cells (RBCs) in urine. The presence of >3 RBCs/hpf is considered significant. In haematuria, urine will be reddish, while in haemoglobinuria and myoglobinuria, urine will be brownish black.

The causes of haematuria may be glomerular or non-glomerular. Glomerular causes are nephritis, analgesic nephropathy, IgA nephropathy, and connective tissue disorders. Non-glomerular causes are stones or tumours that involve the urinary tract (e.g. renal cell carcinoma, urothelial carcinomas). More details are given in Chapter 61.

Ketones: Ketone bodies, namely acetoacetic acid , beta-hydroxy butyric acid, and acetone are seen in the urine in cases of diabetic ketoacidosis, starvation, and pregnancy.

White blood cells (WBCs): Presence of WBCs in the urine is called pyuria (>5 cells/hpf). Causes include urinary tract infection, stones, glomerulonephritis, foreign bodies, tuberculosis (sterile pyuria), and malignancies (sterile pyuria). In practice, the most common cause of sterile pyuria is unconfirmed infection treated empirically with antibiotics.

Casts and Crystals

Casts: Tamm-Horsfall protein is a mucoprotein from renal tubular cells. It forms the nucleus of all casts by entrapping RBC/WBC/epithelial cells. Hyaline casts do not have cells and are normal.

Crystals: Different types of crystals are formed in acidic and alkaline urine and act as precursors for stone formation. Calcium phosphate and struvite crystals form in alkaline urine. Calcium oxalate, uric acid, and cystine crystals form in acidic urine. While most of the crystals mentioned here can be seen in normal subjects, cystine crystals (hexagonal or benzene ring-shaped) are truly pathological.

Urine Cytology

Urine cytology refers to the microscopic examination of urinary samples for exfoliated cellular elements. For enhancing diagnostic yield, freshly voided specimens are essential. If positive, it indicates transitional cell carcinoma of bladder. Cytology is not useful for detecting other types of carcinoma, such as squamous cell or adenocarcinoma.

24-hour Urinary Studies

These are indicated for the metabolic evaluation of stone disease (identifies various abnormalities of electrolyte homeostasis) and the evaluation of recurrent pyelonephritis in children and diabetic nephropathy (degree of proteinuria).

BLOOD TESTS

- **Prostatic surface antigen (PSA):** A glycoprotein that liquefies semen, an essential step in reproduction, is elevated in prostatic diseases. Its estimation is used to screen for carcinoma prostate, but is not specific for this condition. Normal levels are 0–4 ng/ml. Carcinoma should be suspected if levels exceed 4 ng/ml (*see* page 1086).
- **Testicular tumour markers**
  - ***Alpha-fetoprotein (AFP):*** Elevated in embryonal carcinoma, yolk sac tumour.
  - ***β-human chorionic gonadotrophin (β-hCG):*** Very high levels in choriocarcinoma.
  - ***Lactate dehydrogenase (LDH):*** Elevated in embryonal carcinoma and seminoma. It indicates bulk of the disease or tumour burden.
- **Sex hormones:** Hormonal assays are useful in specific situations. Pre- and post-treatment estimation of serum testosterone is useful when androgen deprivation is used to treat prostatic cancer. Similarly, a rise in serum androgens is seen in boys with precocious puberty due to Leydig cell tumors.

X-RAY KUB (KIDNEY, URETER, BLADDER)

- Plain X-ray KUB is a baseline investigation in suspected cases of calculous disease. The majority of urinary stones are radio-opaque, which facilitates their visibility on a plain X-ray.
- It should be taken in the supine position and cover the pubic symphysis and lower two ribs.
- Patients should take a fat-free, low residue diet, dimol 2 tablets, or any suitable anti-flatulence medication 3 times daily for 2–3 days prior to the X-ray.
- Stones appear as a white shadow when radio-opaque, and depending on the calcium content, the higher the calcium, the denser is the shadow! (images are given in Renal Stones, *see* pages 1042 to 1044).

IMAGING

Physical findings are often meagre in afflictions of the urinary tract; hence, imaging is relied on. Advances in imaging technology today have made renal imaging (Fig. 56.1) the most important part of urinary tract investigations. Some important investigations are given below.

Iodinated Contrasts

Ionic: Diatrizoate, metrizoate, ioxaglate (more side effects, cheaper).

Nonionic: Iopamidol, iopromide (fewer side effects, costly).

INTRAVENOUS PYELOGRAPHY (IVP) AND INTRAVENOUS UROGRAM (IVU) (Figs 56.1–56.5)

Aim

- To study renal function
- To detect any pathology in the kidneys, ureters, and bladder
- To study any anatomical variations of the renal system.

Procedure

- A fat-free, non-residue diet is given for 2–3 days prior to the procedure to avoid intestinal gas shadows.
- Dimol 2 tablets, 3 times daily for 2–3 days prior to the procedure to expel the gas.
- The patient should not take oral fluids 6 hours before the procedure.
- Radiological contrast dye: 45% sodium diatrizoate, 20–40 ml is injected through the median cubital vein.

Requirements before IVP

1. Normal renal function is a prerequisite for IVU. Serum creatinine is reliable, but not urea because of

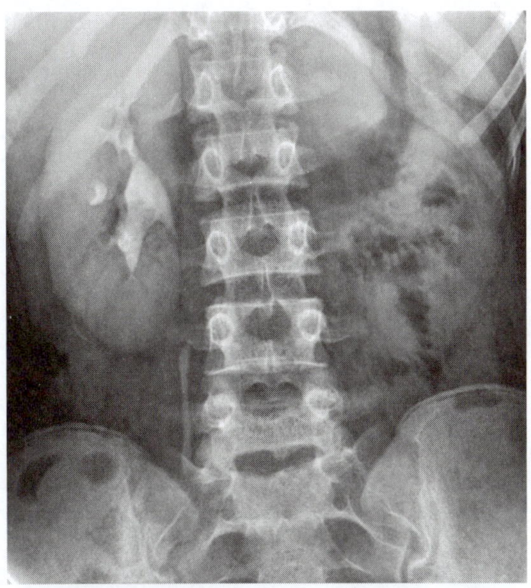

Fig. 56.1: IVU after 5 minutes

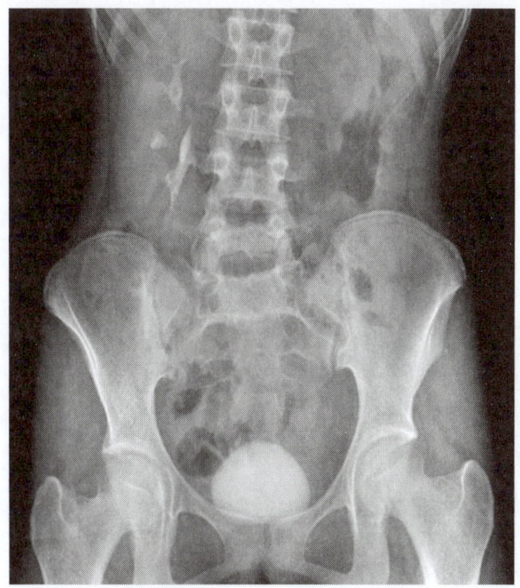

Fig. 56.2: IVU after 20 minutes

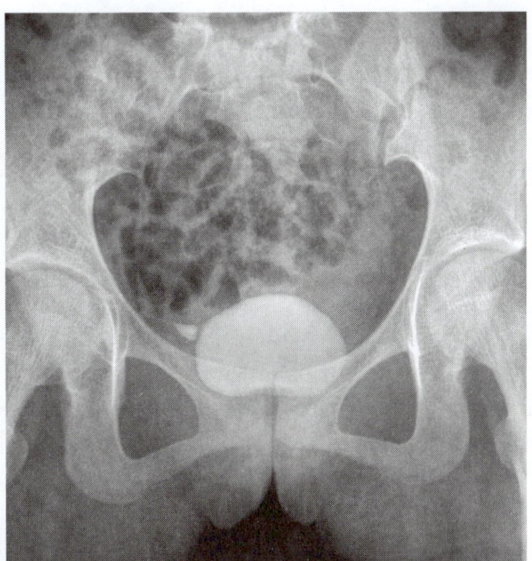

Fig. 56.3: Observe bowel gas, inadequate preparation

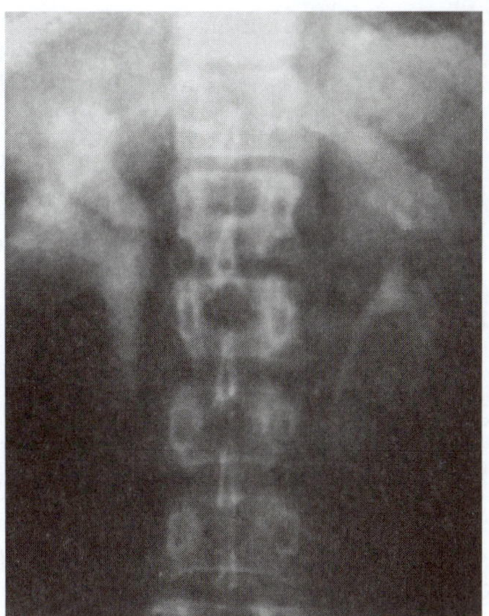

Fig. 56.4: IVU showing hydronephrosis

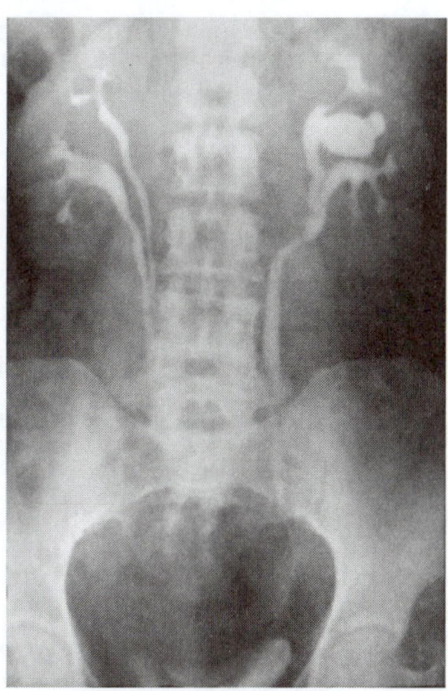

Fig. 56.5: IVU showing double ureter

variations in urea levels based on hydration. The normal value of serum creatinine is 0.5–2 mg%.

2. Plain X-ray KUB region to look for a renal stone—90% of renal stones are radio-opaque (only 10% of gallstones are radio-opaque).
   - To distinguish between renal stones and gallstones on plain abdominal X-ray, take lateral film. Opacities anterior to the vertebral column are gallstones, and those overlying the spine are renal stones.

Precautions while Injecting the Dye Contrast Medium

1. The dye should be given very slowly.
2. The dye should not extravasate.
3. If bronchospasm occurs, hydrocortisone 100 mg and an antihistaminic should be administered IV in addition to inhalation of bronchodilator.
4. In cases of urticaria and skin rashes, an antihistaminic should be given.

Radiography

1. Early films taken after 2 or 5 minutes demonstrate the kidney outline (nephrogram).
2. 5 minutes later, pelvicalyceal system is visualised (Fig. 56.1).
3. 15–20 minutes later, the ureter and bladder can be visualised (Fig. 56.2).

4. A post-voiding picture is taken to demonstrate any residual contrast in the urinary bladder. At times, a voiding phase is also included to study the urethra non-invasively. However, such a study is not useful to study vesicoureteral reflux, which calls for standard micturating cystourethrography (vide infra).

- Abdominal compression should be applied to better demonstrate pyelograms.

Contraindications for IVU

1. **Idiosyncrasy to iodine:** Test dose should be given beforehand.
2. **Renal failure:** Kidneys fail to excrete the drug.
3. **Multiple myeloma:** The contrast medium precipitates myeloma proteins, blocks the ureter and kidney, and causes anuria.
4. **Hyperuricaemia:** Uric acid crystals deposit in the renal tubules.
5. **Sickle cell anaemia:** Precipitates sickle cell crisis.
6. Dehydration.

Uses of IVU

1. To diagnose congenital abnormalities, such as polycystic kidney, horseshoe kidney, single kidney, and duplication of kidneys and ureters.
2. To diagnose hydronephrosis, hydroureter (Fig. 56.4).
3. To diagnose obstruction to the pelviureteric junction, ureters, primary obstructed megaureter.
4. To diagnose renal, ureteric stones and bladder stones.
5. To diagnose renal tuberculosis, tumours.

Intraoperative One-shot IV Pyelogram

In ureteral injuries, when delayed contrast images are not possible because of haemodynamic instability, an intraoperative one-shot (2 mg/kg IV contrast material given 10 min before flat plate abdominal X-ray) IV pyelogram (IVP) is recommended for patients with hypotension or a history of significant deceleration, despite the absence of gross haematuria.

RETROGRADE PYELOGRAPHY (RGP) OR RETROGRADE URETEROGRAPHY (RGU)

Indications

1. When the kidney is not visualised by IVU
   a. Gross hydronephrosis (Fig. 56.6)
   b. Very high blood urea
2. To selectively collect a urine sample from renal pelvis (e.g. renal tuberculosis)

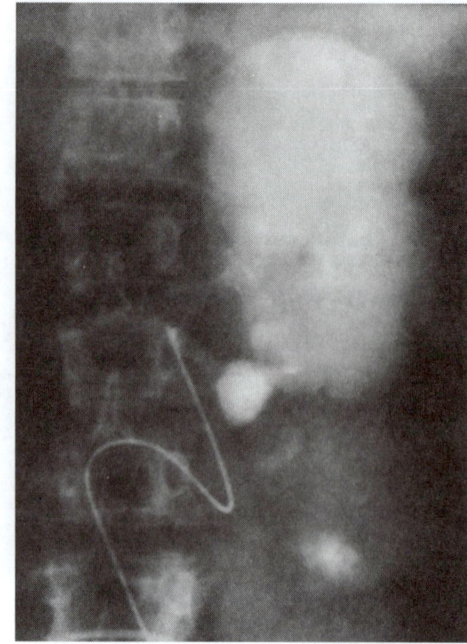

Fig. 56.6: RGP: Retrocaval ureter with hydronephrosis

3. History of allergy to IV contrast materials. Caution should be exercised in such situations to avoid intravasation of contrast by forcible injection, which may precipitate an allergic reaction and rarely cause fatality.
4. Prior to ureteroscopy.

Procedure

- A cystoscopy is performed first.
- Ureteric orifices are identified and cannulated by a flexible catheter, which is introduced up to the pelvis of the kidney, and the contrast medium is injected. X-rays are taken at 5 minutes, 15 minutes, and 30 minutes.

Uses

1. Anatomical evaluation of the pelvicalyceal system.
2. Early diagnosis of renal tuberculosis.
3. Since the contrast medium is injected directly into the pelvis, the pelvicalyceal system can be identified better, helping to diagnose early transitional cell carcinoma of kidney.

Complications of RGP

1. It is an invasive procedure; hence, urinary tract infection can occur. Prophylactic antibiotics are given prior to the procedure.
2. Chances of bladder or ureter perforation are rare. Retrograde ureteropyelogram using a bulb-tipped ureteric catheter lodged in the ureteric orifice eliminates the risk of inadvertent injuries due to retrograde catheterisation of the ureter.

RENAL ARTERIOGRAPHY: ANGIOGRAPHY

Technique

The technique used now is digital subtraction angiography (DSA). There are two methods:

1. **Retrograde arteriography** using Seldinger technique. Selective renal angiography can be performed using a catheter over a guidewire passed into renal artery.
2. **Translumbar aortography** wherein the aorta is punctured with a needle from behind, above the renal arteries, at the level of 1st lumbar vertebra.

Dose

For aortography, 30 ml of contrast (hypaque), and for selective renal angiography, 6–8 ml are used.

Uses (Key Box 56.1)

1. To demonstrate pathological anatomy of the renal artery when renal artery stenosis or aneurysm is suspected.
2. In renal cell carcinoma, tumour vascularity and extension of the tumour into the renal vein can be diagnosed during the venous phase.
3. Bleeding from the kidney due to trauma, post-percutaneous nephrolithotomy (PCNL) bleeding, or arteriovenous malformation.
4. Therapeutic application:
   - Transluminal angioplasty can be done by inflating the balloon in cases of renal artery stenosis.
   - Embolization of bleeding vessels, aneurysms (Fig. 56.7).

Key Box 56.1

Repair in Tidy Wound

- Tubular necrosis of the kidney
- Paraplegia due to spasm of spinal arteries
- Haematoma
- Thromboembolism

MICTURATING CYSTOURETHROGRAPHY (MCU)

In this procedure, the contrast medium is injected into the urinary bladder via an indwelling catheter, and X-rays are taken when the patient passes urine.

Indications

1. In children, to demonstrate vesicoureteric reflux
2. Posterior urethral valve
3. Vesical trauma
4. Vesicovaginal or vesicocolic fistula.

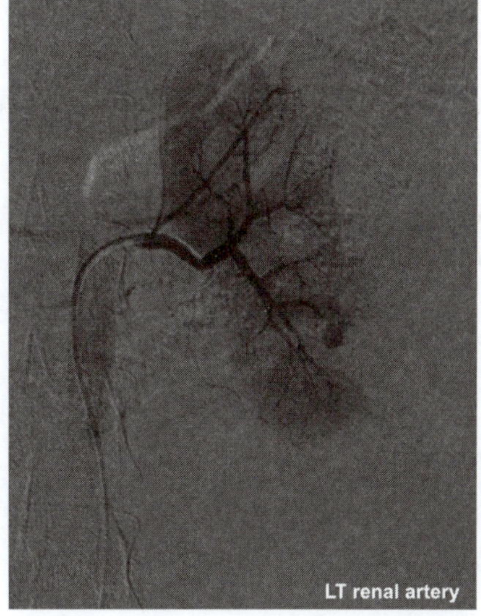

Fig. 56.7: Renal angiogram—aneurysm

Procedure

A catheter is passed into the urinary bladder, and the dye is injected. The catheter is removed, and the child is screened for vesicoureteric reflux during voiding of urine (Fig. 56.8).

Films

Filling phase, full bladder, voiding, and post-voiding phase films are taken.

Newer

Direct or indirect radionuclide cystography using isotopes, which can even pick up minute reflux.

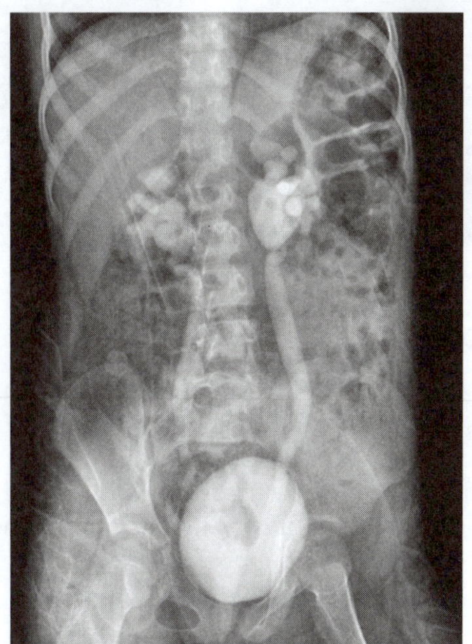

Fig. 56.8: MCU voiding phase: Observe the ureter due to reflux

Complications

Due to the invasive nature of the procedure, urinary tract infection may occur. Hence, prophylactic antibiotics should be used.

ASCENDING URETHROGRAPHY (ASU) OR RETROGRADE URETHROGRAPHY (RUG)

Urethrography is used in the diagnosis of urethral stricture, to know the length of stricture, proximal dilatation, or diverticulum. (Fig. 56.9).

Indications

- Evaluation of urethral injury
- Investigation of urethral stricture

Contraindication

Urethral haemorrhage, active urethral bleeding.

Precaution

Barium and medium containing oil such as lipiodol should not be used due to the risk of oil embolism with a urethral mucosal tear or breach. Conray 280 is injected slowly into the urethra. In acute settings, RGU is best done under cine control by trickling the contrast in increments.

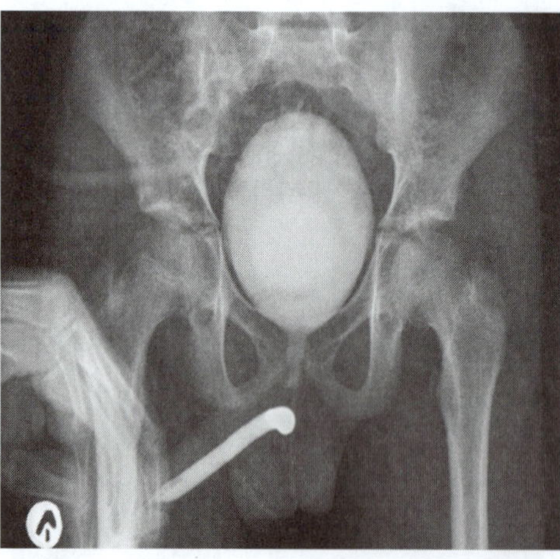

Fig. 56.9: ASU and MCU—stricture urethra

ULTRASONOGRAPHY (USG) (Fig. 56.10)

This is a non-invasive investigation, that uses ultrasonic waves (sound waves with frequency >20,000 Hz). These waves cannot be heard by the human ear but are reflected or absorbed by tissues to various degrees that help diagnose different conditions. Ultrasound can be used through different approaches:

- Transabdominal
- Transrectal (Key Box 56.2)
- Transvaginal (used mostly by gynaecologists).

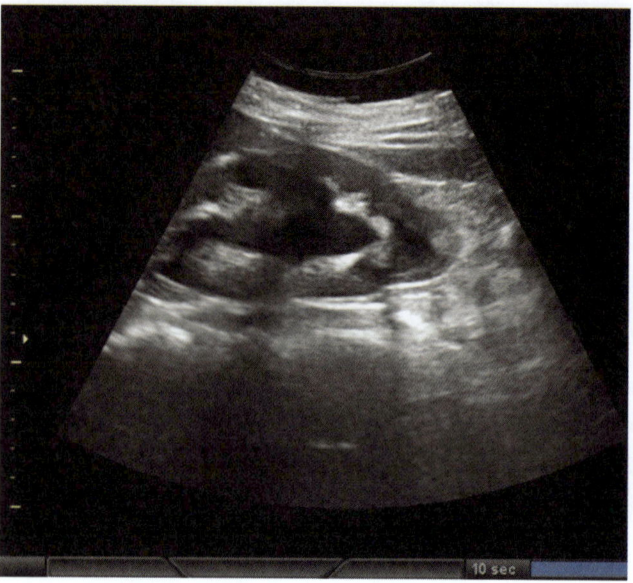

Fig. 56.10: USG showing hydronephrosis

Key Box 56.2

Transrectal Ultrasonography in Carcinoma Prostate

- Disruption of the echo architecture
- Invasion of the capsule
- Biopsy—ultrasonography-guided

Limitations of USG

- Operator-dependent
- Air precludes adequate imaging: Bowel gas may prevent satisfactory imaging of the pancreas/ kidneys.
- Obesity: Poor visualisation.

Uses of USG

A. Fluid can be differentiated from solid tissue. Hence, cystic swellings can be made out.

B. Stones can be diagnosed. Stones appear as hyperechoic lesions and postacoustic shadowing.

C. In an enlarged kidney with a thick cortex, disruption of the echo architecture can be made out, as in hydronephrosis.

D. Residual urine in the bladder can be identified, which may be an indication of enlarged prostate.

E. The volume of the prostate can be measured.

Ultrasonography has become the investigation of choice to diagnose foetal hydronephrosis due to various reasons. This is advantageous because the management of the disease causing hydronephrosis can be planned at the early stage, thereby preventing damage to the kidney. Moreover, intrauterine interventions are also possible, if the need arises.

COMPUTERISED TOMOGRAPHY (CT) SCANNING

- CT can be done with or without contrast (Fig. 56.11).
- CT without contrast (plain CT) is the investigation of choice for evaluating renal/ureteric colic.
- CT scan can visualise most urinary tract calculi, even radiolucent stones not seen on plain X-ray KUB or IVU. The rare exception is indinavir stones.
- Contrast CT gives information about kidney function, similar to IVU. However, unlike IVU, which gives information only about the renal parenchyma and collecting system, CT can provide valuable information about perinephric events (e.g. urinoma, abscess, lymph nodes compressing ureters causing hydronephrosis).
- CT angiography is replacing conventional angiography for the diagnostic evaluation of renal vascular anatomy.
- It is more useful than arteriography to assess and display images of the body at selected levels.
- To diagnose of kidney tumour and its extent, spread, and infiltration.
- To stage cancer of prostate, bladder, kidney, testicular tumours, and renal trauma (Figs 56.12 and 56.13).

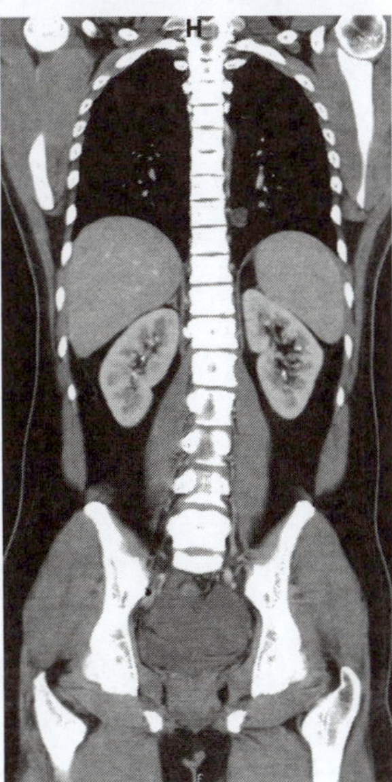

Fig. 56.11: CT scan showing normal kidneys

Pearls of Wisdom

Presently, CT with contrast is fast supplanting IVU for evaluating the urinary tract because of its advantages.

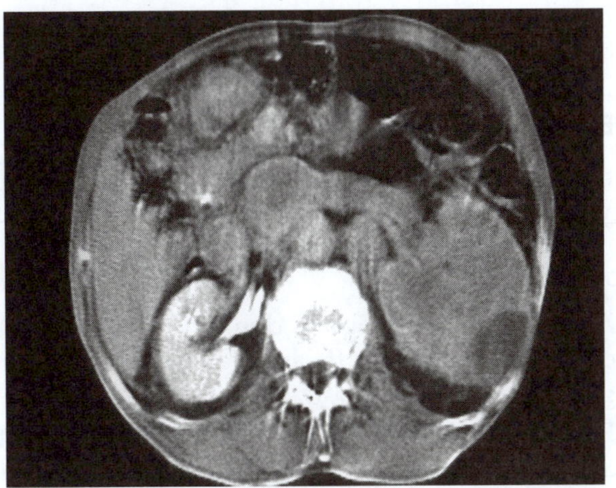

Fig. 56.12: CT scan showing left renal cell carcinoma

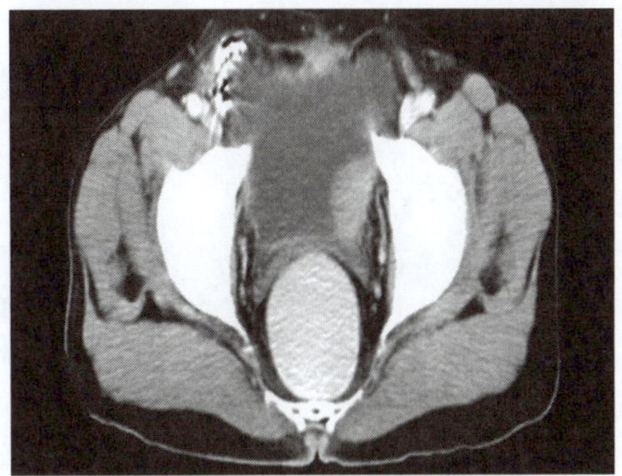

Fig. 56.13: CT scan showing bladder carcinoma

RADIOISOTOPE SCANNING

Gamma camera screening following the injection of technetium 99m gives information about proximal tubular function. To assess differential renal functions, diethylenetriamine penta-acetic acid (^{99m}Tc DTPA) or dimercaptosuccinic acid (^{99m}Tc DMSA) is used, which is filtered and secreted into the tubular lumen.

^{99m}Tc DTPA: Diethylenetriaminepenta-Acetic Acid

This scan is done to determine the relative functions of both kidneys; it also tells about the total GFR and what percentage of total GFR is contributed by each kidney. A relative function of 45 ±2% is considered acceptable for each kidney. The main indication for DTPA is long-term hydronephrosis. Examples are newborn with antenatally diagnosed hydronephrosis, children with posterior urethral valves, etc. This scan is also useful to assess the improvement in relative function of the kidney after surgery for the above conditions. The yield of DTPA scan can be improved by injecting IV lasix. This is known as diuretic renography and will unmask marginal pelviureteric junction obstruction (Fig. 56.14).

^{99m}Tc DMSA: Dimercaptosuccinic Acid

It is primarily used for cortical imaging. It shows details of the renal parenchyma. It is particularly useful when looking for segmental abnormalities of kidney (e.g. renal scarring secondary to conditions like chronic pyelonephritis and renal tumours) (Fig. 56.15 and Key Box 56.3).

Key Box 56.3

Radioisotope Scanning in Urology

- ^{99m}Tc DTPA : Renal function, drainage
- ^{99m}Tc DMSA : Renal parenchyma
- ^{99m}Tc Methyl diphosphonate (MDP) : Bone secondaries
- ^{131}I MIBG : Phaeochromocytoma
- ^{99m}Tc Sestamibi : Parathyroid adenoma

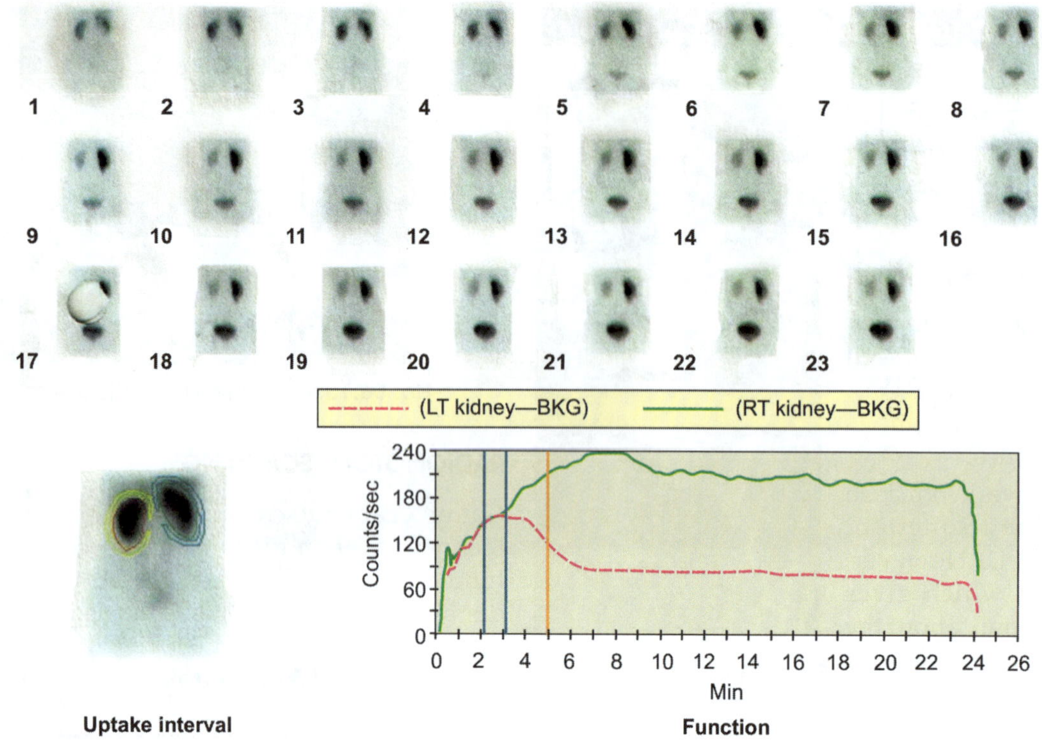

Fig. 56.14: DTPA scan showing sluggish clearance of contrast in the right kidney. Left kidney is normal in clearance and function

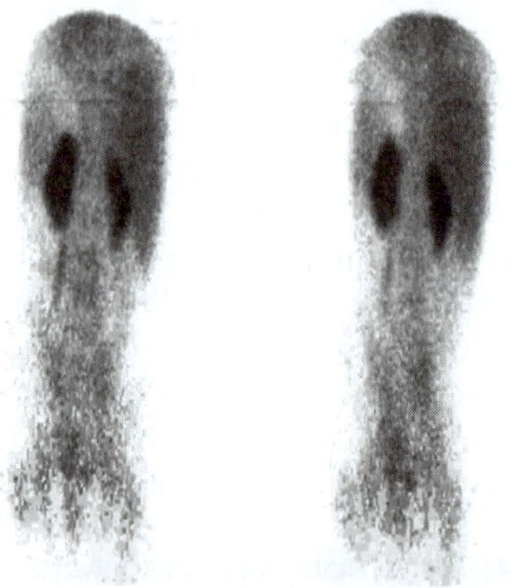

Fig. 56.15: DMSA scan

ENDOSCOPY

Cystourethroscopy: The bladder and urethral mucosa can be visualised.

- The procedure is done under surface anaesthesia.
- **Preparation:** The external genitalia are cleaned with soap solution or an antiseptic agent, and 1% lignocaine jelly is injected into urethra to provide lubrication and anaesthesia. This should be left in place for 10 minutes for its action.

Uses of Cystoscopy

1. Diagnosis of bladder cancer, papilloma, cystitis
2. Position and character of ureteric orifices—in tuberculosis involving the urinary bladder, the ureteric orifices are shifted upwards; gaping in golf hole ureter.
3. Indigo carmine test: 7 ml of 0.4% dye is injected IV. Observe the ureteric orifice through the cystoscope. Unilateral delay in dye appearance suggests obstruction. If there is bilateral delay, it indicates impaired renal function.
4. As a preliminary step for RGP.
5. To rule out bladder involvement in gynaecological cancer (e.g. cancer cervix).
6. To remove bladder stones (cystolitholapaxy)
7. For transurethral resection of bladder tumour in early bladder cancers.

URETHROSCOPY

It refers to the visualisation of the urethra by introducing a cystoscope.

Types of Urethroscopy

1. Anterior urethroscopy is done in urethral stricture or chronic urethritis. It can rule out strictures due to granuloma.
2. Posterior urethroscopy: To visualise prostatic urethra and verumontanum
   - Verumontanum is red in cystoprostatitis.

- In chronic prostatitis, prostatic ducts may be seen discharging pus.
- When the lateral lobes are enlarged, they bulge into the prostatic urethral lumen and occlude it in the midline. In trilobar enlargement, the median lobe can be made out at the bladder neck, which juts into the vesical lumen.

MAGNETIC RESONANCE (MR) UROGRAPHY

MRI of the genitourinary system is useful in many situations. It is more expensive compared to other investigations.

Uses of MR Urography

- For accurate evaluation of the inferior vena cava, thrombus in renal cell carcinoma.
- Extrinsic causes of ureteric obstruction causing hydronephrosis (e.g. retroperitoneal fibrosis, pelvic tumours).
- MR urethrography for accurate delineation of urethral injuries.
- MR is a poor method for visualizing stones and calcification.

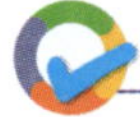

Multiple Choice Questions

1. When do you say there is significant haematuria?
A. Presence of >2 RBCs/hpf
B. Presence of >3 RBCs/hpf
C. Presence of >1 RBC/hpf
D. Presence of RBCs in the urine

2. Which of the following can be detected by urine examination?
A. Transitional cell carcinoma
B. Squamous cell carcinoma
C. Adenocarcinoma
D. Adenosquamous cell carcinoma

3. When do you suspect carcinoma prostate?
A. If the patient has urgency of micturition
B. Rectal examination reveals grade 2 enlargement of prostate
C. If PSA levels are > 4 ng/ml
D. If the patient has recurrent urinary tract infection

4. Spider leg deformity in intravenous pyelography (IVP) is a diagnostic sign of which disease?
A. Hydronephrosis B. Polycystic kidney
C. Horseshoe kidney D. Carcinoma kidney

5. Which of the following is a contraindication for IVP?
A. Staghorn calculi B. Renal tuberculosis
C. Horseshoe kidney D. Multiple myeloma

6. The following are advantages of retrograde pyelography over IVP *except*:
A. A urine sample can be selectively collected from the renal pelvis
B. Can be done when the kidney is not visualised by IVP
C. Intravenous contrast need not be given
D. It is an invasive procedure

7. The investigation of choice in foetal hydronephrosis is:
A. CT scan B. MRI scan
C. Ultrasound D. DTPA scan

8. The investigation of choice for renal parenchymal/ cortical function or damage is:
A. IVP
B. Contrast enhanced CT scan
C. DTPA scan
D. DMSA scan

9. The investigation of choice for renal function/ drainage is:
A. CT scan B. MRI scan
C. DTPA scan D. DMSA scan

10. Indigo carmine test is done to study:
A. Ureteric obstruction B. Prostatic obstruction
C. Urethral obstruction D. Renal obstruction

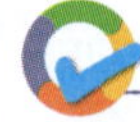

Answers

1. B 2. A 3. C 4. B 5. D 6. D 7. C 8. D 9. C 10. A

CHAPTER

57

Kidney and Ureter

- Surgical anatomy of kidney
- Polycystic kidneys
- Horseshoe kidney
- Renal stones
- Ureteric stone
- Hydronephrosis
- Renal tuberculosis
- Renal neoplasm
- Wilms' tumour
- Renal cell carcinoma
- Pyonephrosis
- Perinephric abscess

SURGICAL ANATOMY OF KIDNEY

- Kidneys are bean-shaped retroperitoneal organs placed one each on either side of vertebral column. Kidneys are often referred to as reniform (kidney-like), implying no parallels in their contour.

  Owing to the presence of the liver, the right kidney is 1–2 cm lower than the left kidney. The right kidney extends from L1 to L3, and the left kidney extends from T12 to L3.
- Anatomical relations of the kidneys (Table 57.1, Fig. 57.1) are important, as they may get injured during kidney operations and may get directly involved by the local spread of renal malignancies.

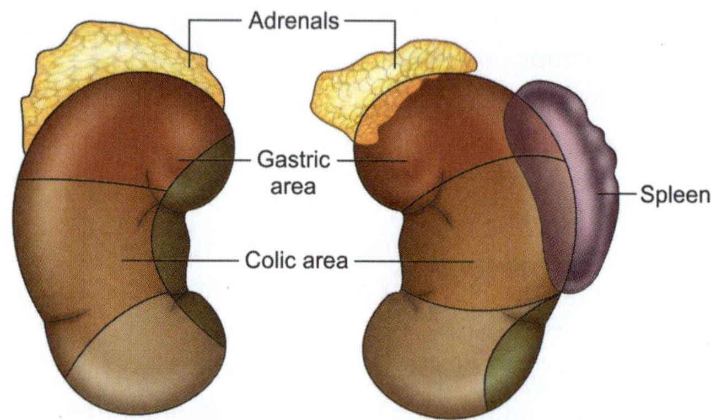

Fig. 57.1: Anterior relations of the kidney

Table 57.1 Relations of kidneys

	Right	*Left*
Anterior (Fig. 57.1)	Below: Hepatic flexure of colon Medial: 2nd part of duodenum	Below: Splenic flexure, pancreas and splenic vessels, below the pancreas is jejunum, above the pancreas are stomach and spleen
Medial	Above: Adrenal, liver, IVC	Above: Adrenal, duodenojejunal flexure, inferior mesenteric vein, ureter
Lateral	Below: Ascending colon Above: Liver	Below: Descending colon Above: Spleen
Posterior	Same in both kidneys. Each kidney rests upon four muscles: Psoas, transversus abdominis, quadratus lumborum, diaphragm	

Fascial Attachments

The kidneys and ipsilateral adrenal glands are tightly wrapped by a fibrous capsule (perirenal fat and the Gerota's fascia). Both these covers can be surgically lifted off the kidneys. This cover has a distinct yellowish brown hue which helps distinguish it from peritoneal fat, which is yellow in colour.

- Perinephric fat and the renal pedicle are responsible for the classical ballotability of renal swellings.
- The kidneys possess intrinsic anteroposterior mobility as they are suspended from the great vessels upon their pedicles and held in position within pliant perinephric fat contained within the anterior and posterior sheaths (laminae) of the Gerota's fascia (renal fascia). This anatomical feature is responsible for the classical clinical sign of ballotability (Italian word that means tossing a ball) of renal swellings.

Superiorly

The anterior and posterior sheaths of the Gerota's fascia fuse at the superior limits of the adrenal gland only to blend further with the intrinsic fascia of the diaphragm. This anatomical arrangement allows the kidneys, which are retroperitoneal, to move with respiration (which is otherwise a feature of intraperitoneal structures).

Medially

The anterior sheath or lamina (also called fascia of Toldt) blends with its counterpart from the other side anterior to the aorta. The inferior vena cava is closely related to the overlying peritoneum, while the posterior sheath or lamina (also called fascia of Zuckerkandl) gets attached to the ventral surface of the vertebral bodies.

Inferiorly

Gerota's fascia remains an open potential space that contains the ureter and gonadal vessels.

- Gerota's fascia forms an important anatomical barrier and tends to confine pathological processes that originate from the kidney.
- However, because of its deficiency inferiorly, a collection within Gerota's fascia may track down and extend into the pelvis.

Some Points to Remember

- The entire renal arterial system comprises end arteries (without anastomosis and collateral circulation). Occlusion of any branches of the renal artery within the kidney (known as segmental arteries) results in infarction of the area supplied by it.
- In contrast, the renal parenchymal veins anastomose freely with each other and the perinephric veins.

Competency

SU29.2: Describe the clinical features, investigations and principles of management of congenital anomalies of genitourinary system. Also refer to page 1068 and 1102.

POLYCYSTIC KIDNEYS (CONGENITAL CYSTIC KIDNEYS)

Congenital cystic disease of the kidneys is broadly of two types—genetic and non-genetic.

Two entities under the genetic type are important—autosomal dominant polycystic kidney disease (ADPKD) and autosomal recessive polycystic kidney disease (ARPKD).

Examples of non-genetic cystic lesions are multicystic dysplastic kidney and multilocular cystic nephroma.

Types

- **ADPKD: A**utosomal **D**ominant **P**olycystic **K**idney **D**isease (Figs 57.2 and 57.3).
- **ARPKD: A**utosomal **R**ecessive **P**olycystic **K**idney **D**isease.

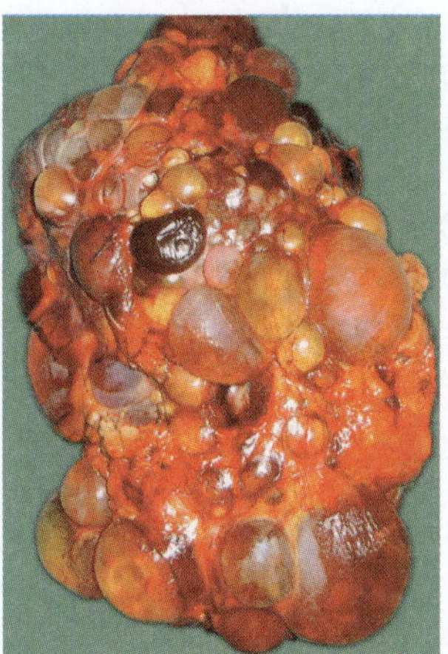

Fig. 57.2: Autosomal dominant polycystic kidney disease

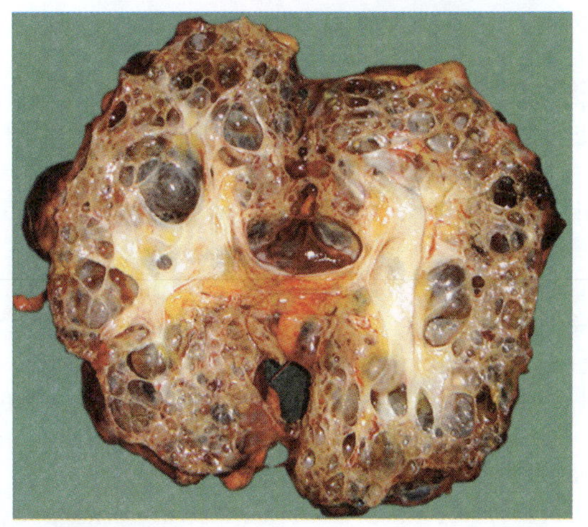

Fig. 57.3: Autosomal dominant polycystic kidney disease: Cut section

Autosomal Dominant Polycystic Kidney Disease (ADPKD)

- It is the most common inherited cystic disease of the kidneys with an incidence of 1 in 1000.
- Both sexes are equally affected.
- It typically presents in adulthood, but earlier presentation may occur.

Associated Lesions

- Cysts of the liver (most common—33%)
- Berry aneurysms (30%)
- Cysts of the pancreas (10%)
- Cysts of the spleen (<5%)
- Mitral valve prolapse
- Cysts in the seminal vesicles (30%)
- Cysts in the testis and prostate (extremely rare)
- Ovarian cysts

Pathology

During development, some of the uriniferous tubules fail to join with the collecting ducts and develop into cysts. PKD1 gene on chromosome 16 and PKD2 gene on chromosome 4 are the culprit genes. The important pathological features are as follows:

- Both kidneys are affected.
- They often enlarge to 3–4 times the normal size.
- Cysts are distributed evenly throughout the cortex and medulla.
  - The contents of the cysts vary but do not contain urine.
- The kidneys are studded with multiple large cysts.
- When a cyst ruptures into the pelvis of the kidney, it results in haematuria.
- As the disease progresses, cysts progress in size, leading to pressure atrophy of the functional renal parenchyma and renal failure.

Clinical Features

- Even though it is congenital, it manifests around 40 years of age.
- Dull-aching (dragging) pain in both loins is due to stretching of the renal capsule.
- Microscopic or macroscopic haematuria occurs in 70–80% cases.
- Secondary hypertension (75%) is due to renal ischaemia, which stimulates the juxtaglomerular apparatus to secrete renin. It may also be related to a separate genetic factor.
- Bilateral renal mass: Both kidneys are enlarged, have a nodular or bosselated surface, are firm to hard consistency, and are sometimes cystic.
- Features of renal failure: Thirst, vomiting, abdominal distension due to paralytic ileus, anuria, uraemic smell, coated tongue, and anaemia. Renal failure is the most common cause of death.
- Infection, pyelonephritis.
- Acute pain occurs if there is haemorrhage into or infection of a cyst. Colicky pain is due to a blood clot in the ureter.

Diagnosis

1. Serum urea and creatinine to rule out renal failure. Normal creatinine levels: 0.8–1.6 mg%. Normal urea: 20–40 mg%.
2. Abdominal USG/CT scan to confirm the diagnosis (Figs 57.4 and 57.5).
3. IVU: Spider leg deformity of the calyces (Swiss cheese appearance).

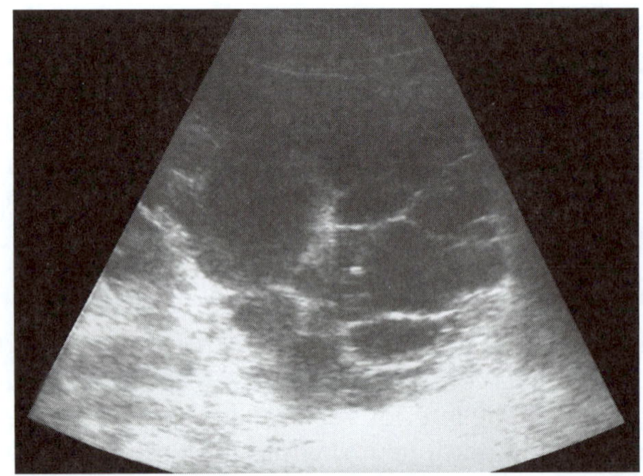

Fig. 57.4: USG image of autosomal dominant polycystic kidney disease

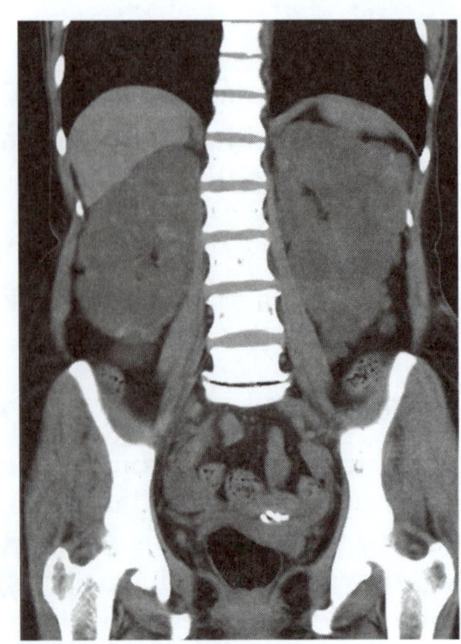

Fig. 57.5: CT image of autosomal dominant polycystic kidney disease

Treatment

- Asymptomatic polycystic kidney does not require any treatment other than regular follow-up.
- **Polycystic kidney with hypertension:** Control hypertension with drugs. If hypertension is uncontrollable, bilateral nephrectomy followed by renal transplantation is done.
- **Infected cyst or if pyelonephritis develops:** Appropriate antibiotics are given, and if necessary, the cyst is aspirated under ultrasound guidance.
- **Polycystic disease with renal failure:** Emergency dialysis followed by renal transplantation is the treatment of choice. The related donor should be screened for polycystic trait.

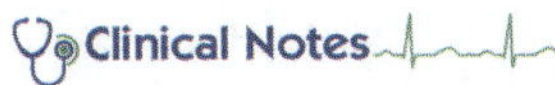

My MS Exam Case, June 1986, Wenlock Hospital, KMC, Mangalore.

A 45-year-old lady with an abdominal mass was allotted as my long case. She had undergone open cholecystectomy 3 months prior (ultrasound was not available at that time). She had a vague renal mass in her right loin. I was not sure. When I recorded her BP, it was 200/110 mmHg. I was able to palpate a renal mass on the opposite side. The diagnosis became evident. It was polycystic kidney. In fact, one of the examiners was a surgeon who had previously operated on this patient for open cholecystectomy, at which time he noticed her enlarged kidneys. The patient was asymptomatic.

Autosomal Recessive Polycystic Kidneys

This occurs in 1 in 10,000–40,000 cases and presents during infancy or childhood (hence, referred to as 'infantile polycystic kidneys'). Oligohydramnios with large echogenic foetal kidneys on prenatal ultrasound suggests a more severe form of this disorder. Large renal masses may cause obstructed labour and neonatal mortality. Those diagnosed in the neonatal period, infancy, or early childhood have a poor course due to immature lungs and congenital hepatic fibrosis, which are invariable associations of this disorder. These children may also have facial and limb abnormalities. Almost all succumb to fatal uraemia and portal hypertension. Very few reach adulthood and become candidates for renal transplantation.

There is no cure for this condition. Only palliative treatment can be offered.

HORSESHOE KIDNEY

- It is the most common renal fusion abnormality. Prior to the 6th week of intrauterine life, the metanephric blastema, which are bilateral structures that give rise to the definitive kidneys, are very close to one another in the pelvis. If the caudal ends of these fuse in the midline around this time (Theory: Overcrowding in the pelvis by large umbilical arteries), normal rotation and ascent is prevented, resulting in horseshoe kidney—the most common fusion anomaly (Fig. 57.6).

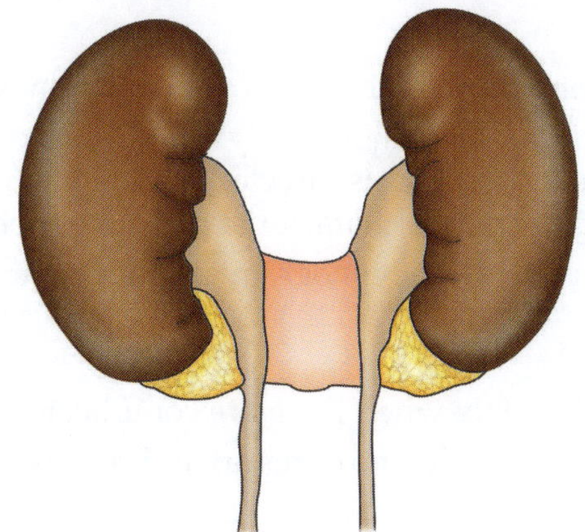

Fig. 57.6: Horseshoe kidney

- Rarely, upper polar fusion may occur, giving rise to reverse horseshoe kidney.
- The inferior mesenteric artery crosses the isthmus at the level of L3–L4. Hence, horseshoe kidney cannot ascend fully. It is felt lower down in the abdomen.

Associated anomalies are mentioned in Key Box 57.1.

Key Box 57.1

Associated Anomalies

- Spina bifida
- Congenital hemivertebra
- Turner's syndrome
- Cleft lip and cleft palate

Clinical Features

- Horseshoe kidney occurs once in 500 live births with a male preponderance (M : F—2 : 1).
- It may be asymptomatic for many years.
- A palpable mass below and to the right and left of the umbilicus or umbilical region may be a horseshoe kidney.
- Recurrent urinary tract infection (UTI) is common because the ureters are angulated over the kidney isthmus.
- They are more prone to hydronephrosis due to angulation of the ureters.
- **Rovsing's sign:** Hyperextension of the spine results in abdominal pain, nausea, or vomiting due to stretching of the capsule.

Diagnosis

1. Ultrasonography (USG) to locate the kidney.
2. IVU: Upper and middle calyx are directed laterally but the lower calyx is directed medially where there is fusion, which is characteristic of horseshoe kidney.
3. CT scan or isotope renogram are confirmatory.

Treatment

- Indicated only when there are complications.
- Removal of the stone or repair and reconstruction of hydronephrosis are done in a standard manner.
- For aortic aneurysm repairs, the isthmus may need to be divided.

Competency

SU29.5: Describe the clinical features, investigations and principles of management of renal calculi.

RENAL STONES

Aetiopathogenesis

Lithogenesis involves complex physical–chemical interactions *in vivo*. These are summarized as follows:

1. **Infection:** Organisms such as Proteus, Pseudomonas, and Klebsiella produce recurrent UTI. These organisms produce the enzyme urease, which splits urea into ammonium and carbon dioxide. Ammonium renders the urine alkaline, which facilitates the precipitation of phosphates. Triple phosphate stones (also called struvite stones) are formed in this manner. The nucleus of the stone may harbour these bacteria (Fig. 57.7).
2. **Hot climate** causes dehydration, which results in the production of highly concentrated urine laden with precipitable solutes, namely calcium and oxalate, which lead to the formation of calcium oxalate stones.

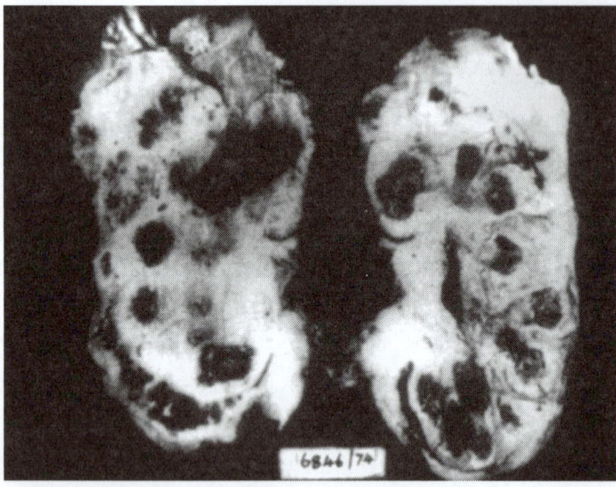

Fig. 57.7: Chronic pyelonephritis with calculi (*Courtesy:* Prof Sasidharan, Head, Dept of Urology (2002–2008), KMC, Manipal)

3. **Dietary factors**
   - Diets rich in red meat, fish, and eggs may give rise to aciduria (purine-rich diet causes uric acid stones).
   - Diets rich in calcium—tomatoes, milk, spinach, rhubarb—produce calcium oxalate stones.
   - Diets lacking vitamin A cause desquamation of the urothelium and cellular debris, providing a nidus for crystal aggregation around it.
4. **Metabolic causes**
   - Hyperparathyroidism increases serum calcium levels by parathormone-induced hypercalciuria which complexes with oxalate crystals to form renal stones.
   - Gout increases uric acid levels and causes multiple uric acid stones. Any cause of hyperuricaemia (increased uric acid levels in the serum) can cause aggregation of uric acid crystals to form uric acid stones. Common causes of hyperuricaemia include dietary excess, gout, and increased cellular destruction as in chemotherapy.
5. **Immobilisation:** Immobilisation, as in bedridden patients, leads to extensive bone demineralization. This in turn causes hypercalciuria, which increases the risk of stone formation. Such stones are called "recumbency stones."
6. **Decreased urinary citrate:** Citric acid (300–900 mg/24 hours) keeps the urinary pH low. When citric acid levels decrease, it promotes the precipitation of urinary calcium. Citrate excretion is under hormonal control. Citrate is a naturally occurring stone-inhibiting substance.
7. **Urinary stasis:** Urinary stasis due to resistance to urinary flow (horseshoe kidney, ectopic kidneys, congenital pelviureteric junction obstruction, congenital vesico-ureteric junction obstruction, etc.) increases the risk of infections and stone formation.
8. **Randall's plaques:** Randall's observation of submucosal whitish-yellow precipitations of crystalline substances at the tips of renal papillae—well-known as Randall's plaques—supports the "fixed particle theory" of lithogenesis. The fixed plaque initiates nucleation, the first step in stone formation. Nucleation can be induced by a variety of substances—free crystals (free particle theory), proteinaceous matrix, foreign bodies (suture material), crystals in clogged lymphatics (Carr's hypothesis), and particulate tissue.

Types of Renal Stones

1. *Calcium Oxalate Stones*

- They are the most common variety (85%) of urinary calculi.

- Two subtypes: Relatively friable calcium oxalate dihydrate (Weddelite) and harder calcium oxalate monohydrate (Wewellite).
- They are radio-opaque.
- They are called mulberry stones as they resemble the mulberry fruit.
- Their thorny surface (Fig. 57.8) can abrade the urothelium and cause haematuria, which in time imparts a brownish hue to these stones (acid hematin forms by the breakdown of haemoglobin in acidic urine).
- Small spiky stones cause intense pain, especially when they travel down the ureters.
- In infected urine, they exist as mixed stones (calcium oxalate and calcium phosphate).
- Citrate deficiency is often found in patients with this type of stone.

2. *Uric Acid Stone* (Fig. 57.9)

- Comprise 5–10% of all stones
- Pure uric acid stones are radiolucent.
- Usually multiple with a smooth surface and yellowish hue.
- Acidic pH and dehydration favour their formation.
- May occur as a mixed stone with calcium oxalate, which is visible on X-ray KUB.
- Common in those who eat red meat.
- Amenable to medical management by alkalanization.
- Suitable for extracorporeal shockwave lithotripsy (ESWL).

Lesch-Nyhan syndrome is a rare inherited disorder, wherein high levels of uric acid production result in uric acid stones. High levels of uric acid in the blood can form needle-like crystals in a joint and cause episodes of severe and sudden pain, tenderness, redness, and swelling (gout).

3. *Phosphate Stone* (Figs 57.10–57.12)

- Pure calcium phosphate stones are rare and are more common in women than in men.

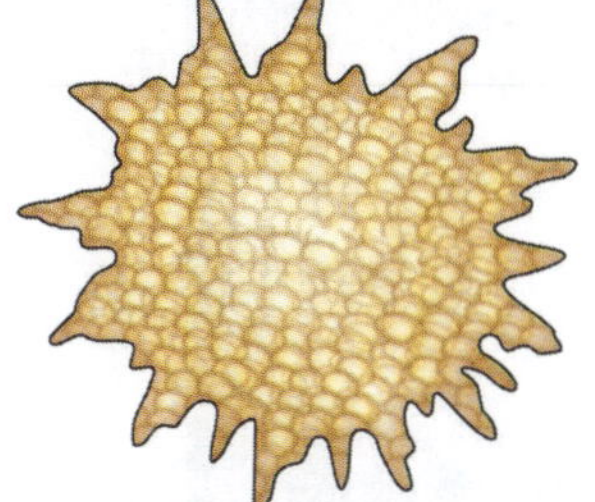

Fig. 57.8: Oxalate stone—thorny surface

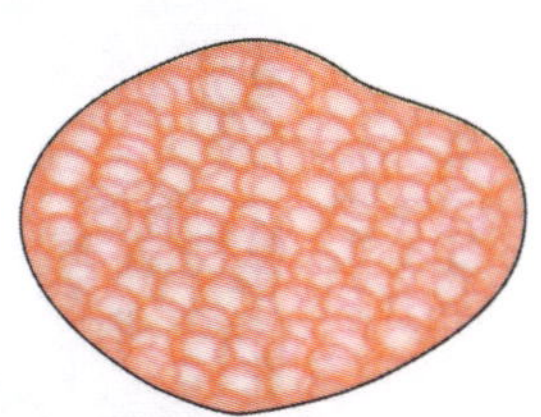

Fig. 57.9: Uric acid stone

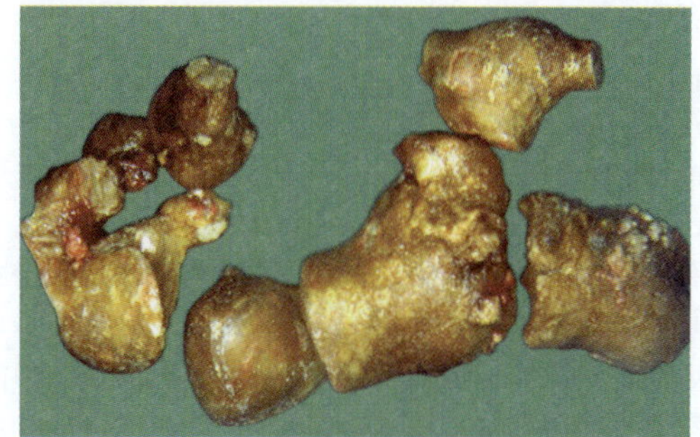

Fig. 57.10

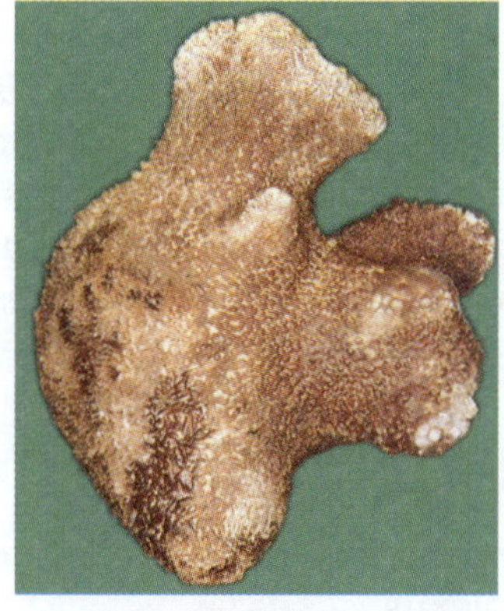

Fig. 57.11

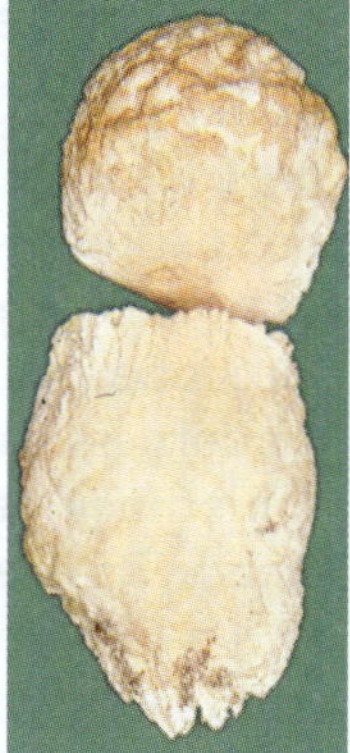

Fig. 57.12

Figs 57.10–57.12: Staghorn calculi and phosphate calculi

- They usually occur as triple phosphate stones (calcium, magnesium, and ammonium—struvite).
- With growth, they tend to fill the collecting system and become its cast. Such configuration resembles the branched horn of a stag, hence called 'staghorn calculus' (Fig. 57.13).
- Alkaline urine facilitates their formation (infections due to urea-splitting bacteria typically render the urine alkaline, hence called infection stones).
- Infection stones may cause recurrent urinary tract infection and in the long run cause renal parenchymal damage.

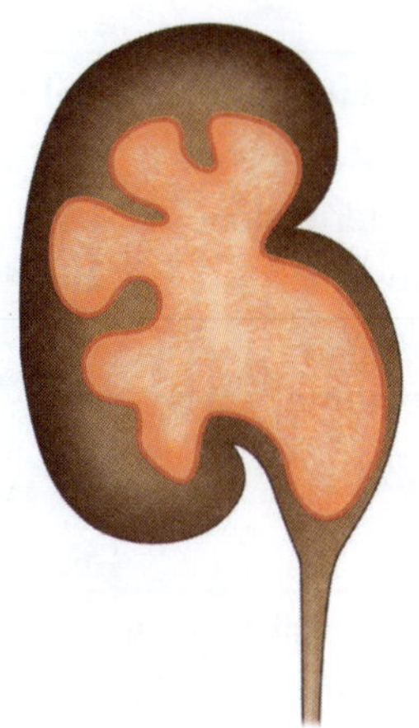

Fig. 57.13: Staghorn calculi

4. *Cystine Calculus*

- Cystinuria is an inborn error of metabolism that occurs due to decreased reabsorption of cystine from the renal tubules.
- Occurs in young girls at puberty.
- Increased excretion of cystine in the urine results in cystine calculus.
- Stones are hard and radio-opaque due to sulphur.
- Benzene/hexagonal crystals in the urine.
- D-pencillamine is administered to dissolve the stones.

Clinical Features

- **Renal pain:** Dull-aching to pricking type of pain is present posteriorly in the renal angle formed by the sacrospinalis and the 12th rib. Pain is the most common symptom and is not related to the size of the stone. Murphy's kidney punch test demonstrates tenderness at the renal angle. The same pain may sometimes be felt anteriorly in the costal margin. Hence, it is described as costovertebral pain. Nausea and vomiting are due to intense sympathetic stimulation caused by stretching of the renal capsule mediated by the coeliac plexus.
- **Ureteric colic:** When the stone is impacted in the pelviureteric junction or anywhere in the ureter, it causes severe colicky pain originating in the loin and radiating to the groin, testicles, vulva, and medial side of the thigh. This may be associated with strangury. The referred pain is due to irritation of the genito-femoral, ilioinguinal, and iliohypogastric nerves.
- **Haematuria** is common with renal stones because the majority of stones are oxalate stones. The quantity of blood loss is small, but it is fresh blood (Key Box 57.2).
- **Recurrent UTI:** Fever with chills and rigors, burning micturition, pyuria, and increased frequency of micturition.
- **Guarding and rigidity** of the back and abdominal muscles during severe pain.

Key Box 57.2

Causes of Haematuria: Renal Conditions

1. Polycystic kidney disease
2. Renal stone, ureteric stone
3. Renal tuberculosis
4. Carcinoma kidney
5. Urothelial carcinoma
6. Renal infarction

Pearls of Wisdom

Acidic urine: Calcium oxalate, cystine, uric acid

Alkaline urine: Calcium phosphate, struvite (magnesium, ammonium, phosphate)

Complications

1. **Calculous hydronephrosis** occurs due to back pressure producing renal enlargement. Stretching of the renal capsule results in pain. In such cases, an associated palpable kidney mass suggests hydronephrosis.
2. **Calculous pyonephrosis:** Infected hydronephrosis wherein the kidney is converted into a bag of pus.
3. **Renal failure:** Bilateral staghorn calculi may not be symptomatic until they present with uraemia and renal failure.
4. **Squamous cell carcinoma:** Long-standing stones increase the risk of carcinoma.

Investigations

1. **Blood urea and creatinine to rule out renal failure.**
2. **Plain X-ray KUB** (Figs 57.14 and 57.15)
   - To diagnose stones. 90% of renal stones are radiopaque.
   - Enlarged renal shadow can be seen.

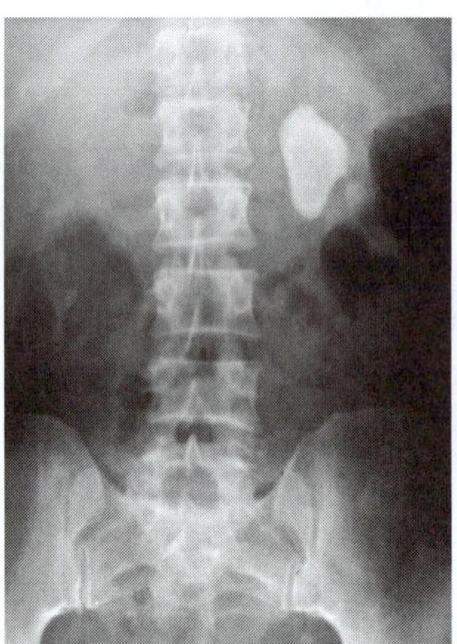

Fig. 57.14: Plain X-ray KUB showing a large stone in the renal pelvis

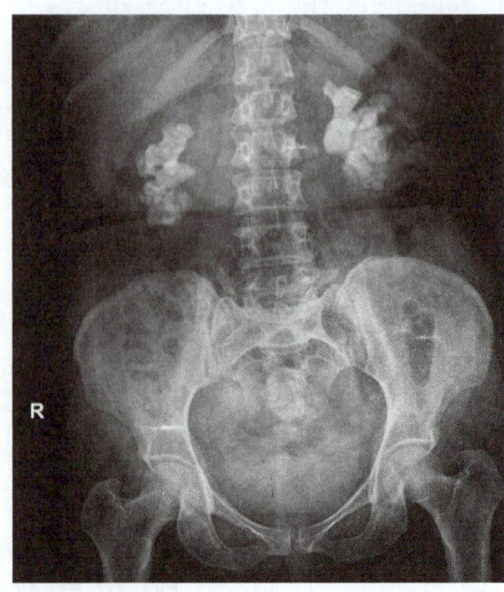

Fig. 57.15: Plain X-ray KUB showing bilateral staghorn calculi

3. **USG**
   - Presence of the stone can be confirmed.
   - Exact size and location of the stone can be evaluated.
4. **Noncontrast CT scan:** It is the gold standard investigation.
5. **Intravenous urogram (IVU)**
   - To accurately locate the stone within the collecting system of the kidney (pelvicalyceal system and ureter) and to assess renal function. A nonradiopaque stone can be seen as a filling defect. Hydronephrosis and hydronephroureterosis may be seen.
   - CT scans are used to more accurately detect causes of abdominal colic.
6. **Urine for culture and sensitivity.**
7. **Metabolic workup** is done in young patients with stones, recurrent stones, nephrocalcinosis, and struvite stones—serum uric acid, ionized calcium, etc.

Treatment

The treatment of renal stones can be divided into nonoperative treatment and operative treatment.

I. *Nonoperative Treatment*

1. **Conservative:** Small stones < 5 mm in size and stones in the lower ureter may pass off with a copious amount of fluid intake and at times with forced diuresis. Intravenous hydration followed by intravenous frusemide may help to spontaneously pass the stones.
2. **Extracorporeal shock wave lithotripsy (ESWL):** It is indicated for stones <2 cm in size. It causes stone fragmentation by focusing externally generated shock waves on the stone within the renal collecting system through intact skin and across the body wall. There are three methods of shock generation: Electromagnetic, piezoelectric, and electrohydraulic. The lithotripters depend on either ultrasound or fluoroscopy for stone localization. ESWL is performed *in situ* when the stone burden is <1 cm and after cystoscopically placing a DJ stent for a larger stone burden (Fig. 57.16) because there may be obstructive columnation of stone fragments in the ureter. The fragments that result after ESWL are passed naturally (Key Box 57.3).

   Hard stones like cystine and calcium oxalate monohydrate are refractory to treatment by ESWL.

II. *Operative Treatment*

1. Endoscopic procedures
2. Open surgical procedures

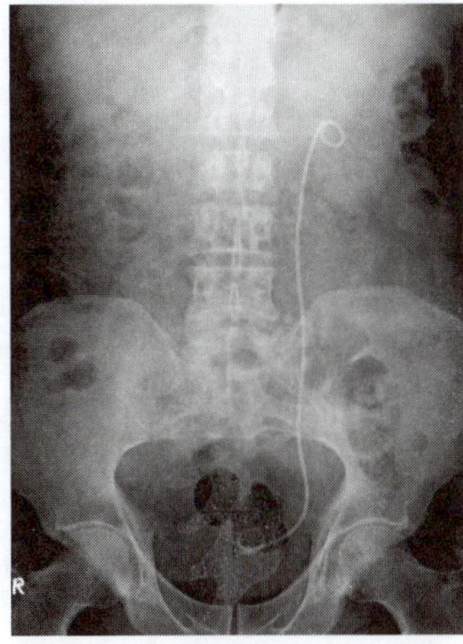

Fig. 57.16: After clearance, DJ stent in place

Key Box 57.3

ESWL

Advantages	**Disadvantages**
○ No incision	○ Cost factor
○ No pain	○ Availability

1. *Endoscopic Procedures*

Percutaneous nephrolithotomy (PCNL): It is indicated for stones > 2 cm in size. Retrograde pyelography (RGP) is done when the stone is located in the pelvis of the kidney. With a small 1 cm incision in the loin, the PCNL needle is passed into the pelvis of the kidney and confirmed by fluoroscopy. A guidewire is passed through the needle into the pelvis of the kidney. The needle is withdrawn, with the guidewire is left within the pelvis. Dilators are passed over the guidewire, and a working sheath is introduced into the pelvis. A nephroscope is passed into the pelvis, and if the stone is small, it can be removed. If it is big, it may have to be crushed using ultrasound probes, after which the fragments are removed. Ultrasound or pneumatic energy is used for fragmenting. Holmium-Yag laser may also be used to fragment the stones. Laser fiber may be introduced through the operating nephroscope to achieve this. The method of fragmenting renal stones using different energies introduced through endoscopes is called intracorporeal lithotripsy.

Complications of PCNL

- Injury to the colon/sepsis
- Injury to the blood vessels
- Urinary leak may persist for a few days.

2. *Open Surgical Procedures*

Depending on the stone's location, various procedures are done.

A. **Pyelolithotomy:** When there is extrarenal pelvis.

B. **Nephrolithotomy:** When there is intrarenal pelvis, the stone has to be removed by incising the kidney parenchyma.

C. **Extended pyelolithotomy:** By retracting the kidney parenchyma from the collecting system, the incision over the pelvis can be extended to the calyx to remove a stone present there. Even a large staghorn calculus can be removed.

D. **Pyelonephrolithotomy:** The stone is extracted through an incision in the pelvis and the renal parenchyma.

E. **Partial nephrectomy:** When the stone is impacted in polar calyces and causes segmental atrophy (polar scarring).

F. **Nephrectomy:** Significant functional loss (poorly functioning kidney) which is not expected to recover even after stone removal. This is done in patients with recurrent infections.

Special Situations

A. **Bilateral renal stones:** Dealing with bilateral stone disease is a matter of clinical judgment. In most instances, the time interval between interventions for both sides is 1–2 weeks. Hence, the symptomatic or obstructed side is dealt with first. If both kidneys are obstructed or are causing symptoms, any one side is destoned (rendered stone-free) in the first phase with concurrent drainage (DJ stenting or percutaneous nephrostomy) for the other side, which is dealt with after 1–2 weeks. In bilateral disease, if the patient is uremic, urgent bilateral drainage either by DJ stenting or nephrostomy is performed. Definitive intervention is done once functional recovery takes place. Kidneys with better function should be operated first. The opposite side can be operated 1–2 weeks later.

B. If there is pyonephrosis with high-grade fever, pain, and tenderness, percutaneous nephrostomy is done under ultrasound guidance in which a tube drain is placed in the pelvis of the kidney to drain the pus and urine. Once the pus clears, renal function is reassessed. If the kidney is nonfunctioning, nephrectomy is done. If the kidney is functioning, ESWL/PCNL/open procedure is done.

Pearls of Wisdom

Open procedures for managing stone disease have become obsolete and are found in old surgery textbooks.

URETERIC STONE

Stones come down from pelvis of the kidney and may get impacted at any site of anatomical narrowing of the ureter, namely:

1. Pelviureteric junction
2. Crossing of the iliac artery
3. Crossing of the vas deferens or broad ligament
4. Site of entry into the bladder wall
5. Ureteric orifice

If left untreated, it may lead to hydroureteronephrosis, renal parenchymal atrophy, infection, and/or pyonephrosis.

Clinical Features

- Pain in the loin radiating to the groin: Pain is severe, colicky, intolerable, and lasts for a few hours. When the stone descends into the lower ureter, pain radiates to the testicles, labia majora, and the upper portion of the thigh due to irritation of the genitofemoral nerve. Colic lasts for 4–6 hours and is relieved by antispasmodics, narcotics, and NSAIDs. This is the most common clinical presentation of ureteric stones.
- Microscopic haematuria invariably accompanies acute ureteric colics. Some patients have gross haematuria. At times, it may present with fever and chills, suggestive of UTI when pyuria is also present.
- Guarding and rigidity of the abdominal wall, if present on the right side, may be confused for acute appendicitis.

Investigations

Same as for renal stone.

Treatment

1. Most ureteric stones pass naturally (urine). The patient is asked to consume a lot of water and take antispasmodics. Oral administration of alpha-blockers (example: Tamsulosin) with or without deflozacort may be used to achieve stone expulsion (medical expulsive therapy).
2. **Flushing therapy:** About 2 L of IV fluid, with 20–40 mg Inj. frusemide (Lasix). It may be repeated for a few days.
3. **Stone in the upper ureter:** ESWL is the ideal treatment. Retrograde intrarenal surgery (RIRS) is done for ureteric, renal, and calyceal stones. Flexible ureteroscopy with laser fragmentation may also be done.
4. **Middle ureteric stone:** ESWL, ureteroscopy basketing, or open surgery (ureterolithotomy).

5. **Lower ureteric stone:** Ureteroscopic removal. With the use of a ureteroscope, direct visualisation and manipulation of the stone (even if it is impacted) can be done. A laser or ultrasonic lithotripter can be used to disintegrate the stone.
6. **Vesicoureteric junction:** Ureteroscopic removal or endoscopic meatotomy of the vesicoureteric junction. For a stone impacted at the ureterovesical junction, cystoscopy is performed. The ureteric orifice is identified, and a cut is given at its mouth. Under fluoroscopic monitoring, the stone can be manipulated and basketed out using a dormia basket or other type of basket.
7. An impacted stone which is not amenable to ESWL, fluoroscopic, or ureteroscopic manipulation has to be extracted by ureterolithotomy (open surgical method).

Prevention of Stone Disease

1. Metabolic work-up of urine and blood to identify metabolic causes. Example: Hyperparathyroidism should be suspected when serum calcium is high. It should be followed-up with parathormone assay as a confirmatory test.
2. Fluid management: 1.5 L/day
3. Dietary adjustment: Red meat (rich in uric acid) to be avoided.
4. Drug treatment
   - Allopurinol, sodium bicarbonate: Uric acid stones
   - Potassium citrate: Calcium stones
   - Thiazides small dose: Calcium stones
   - D-penicillamine: Cystine stones
   - Urease inhibitors (e.g. acetohydroxamic acid): Infection stones

Competency

SU29.4: Describe the clinical features, investigations and principles of management of hydronephrosis.

HYDRONEPHROSIS

Definition

Aseptic dilatation of the pelvicalyceal system due to intermittent total or continuous partial obstruction to urine outflow across the PUJ.

If there is concomitant dilatation of the ureter, the term hydroureteronephrosis is used.

Causes of Unilateral Hydronephrosis/ Hydroureteronephrosis (Fig. 57.17)

I. *Intraluminal (within the lumen)*

Stones, sloughed papillae (as in diabetics and those with analgesic nephropathy), sloughed urothelial cancer, organized blood clots, chylous balls, fungal bezoars, and

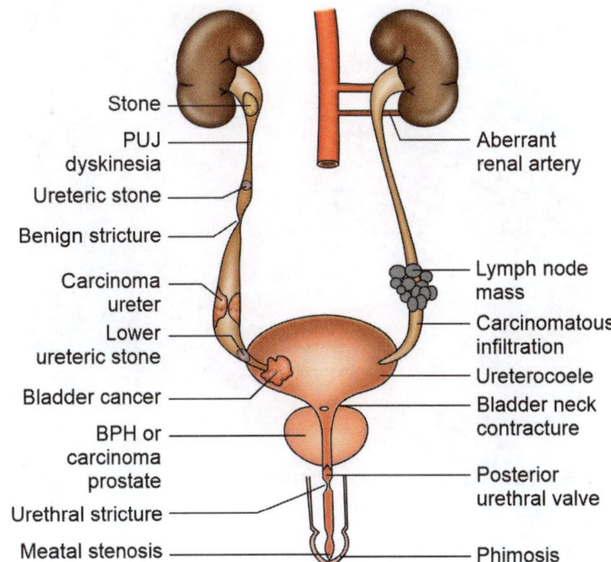

Fig. 57.17: Causes of hydroureteronephrosis

inflammatory synechiae may obstruct the lumen to varying degrees.

II. *Intramural (in the wall)*

1. Congenital

- PUJ obstruction (PUJ dyskinesia or achalasia of PUJ) is a congenital lesion where hydronephrosis occurs due to failure of transmission of neuromuscular impulses across the PUJ. It may also be bilateral. Male: Female ratio is 2:1. It is more common on the left side. PUJ obstruction may be seen in ectopically placed kidneys as well as in horseshoe kidneys.
- Ureterocele (cystic dilatation of the terminal ureter), congenital obstructive megaureter (functional obstruction at the level of the vesicoureteric junction, pathology is akin to that which occurs in PUJ obstruction)—both cause hydroureteronephrosis.

2. Acquired

- Carcinoma of the ureter or carcinoma of the bladder involving the ureteric orifice.
- Stricture of the ureter secondary to stone: After dislodgement of the stone, there may be inflammatory stricture of the ureter.
- Tuberculosis of the ureter and bladder.

III. *Extramural*

1. Malignant infiltration of the ureter (from cancers of the uterine cervix, rectum, urinary bladder), obstructive encasement as in retroperitoneal tumours, and compression by enlarged lymph nodes (metastatic or primary).

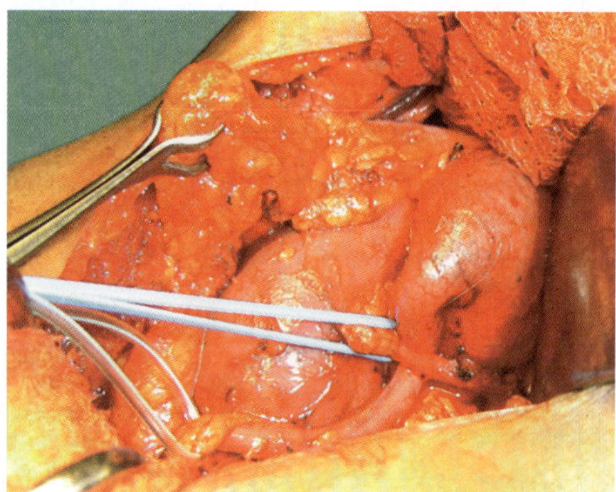

Fig. 57.18: PUJ obstruction with an aberrant crossing vessel

2. Obstruction by aberrant vessels (Fig. 57.18): Aberrant renal artery going to the lower pole of the kidney may cause ureteric obstruction.
3. Retrocaval ureter
4. Idiopathic retroperitoneal fibrosis

Causes of Bilateral Hydronephrosis/ Hydroureteronephrosis (Fig. 57.17)

Obstruction below the bladder neck due to any cause may cause bilateral hydroureteronephrosis (infravesical causes). Any cause of unilateral ureteric obstruction when operational on both sides simultaneously may cause bilateral hydronephrosis (supravesical causes). Idiopathic retroperitoneal fibrosis (Ormond's disease) may cause fibrous encasement of the ureters, which is a rare supravesical cause of bilateral hydroureteronephrosis.

The flow of urine is unidirectional and always towards the bladder from the upper urinary tracts. At times, this is reversed, and there is retrograde propulsion of the ureter from the bladder into the ureters. This is called vesico-ureteric reflux (VUR). In severe grades of VUR, there may be bilateral or unilateral hydroureteronephrosis.

Common Causes

I. *Causes in Children*

1. Phimosis
2. Meatal stenosis
3. Posterior urethral valve
4. Bilateral vesicoureteric reflux

II. *In young adults*

- Stricture urethra was commonly due to gonococcal urethritis. Iatrogenic strictures following instrumentation of the urethra and those which develop following rupture urethra are becoming more common.
- Bilateral aberrant vessels: Quite often, these may be the branches of the renal artery and vein which cross the ureters.

III. *Causes in middle age and above*

- Benign prostatic hypertrophy (BPH)
- Bladder neck contracture
- Idiopathic retroperitoneal fibrosis (Ormond's disease)

IV. *Physiological: Pregnancy*

Compression due to a growing gravid uterus and the relaxant effect of progesterone on ureteric smooth muscle.

Pathogenesis

The back pressure effect depends on the type of pelvis (Figs 57.19 and 57.20).

1. In patients with an intrarenal pelvis, the kidney gets damaged very early. As time goes on, the urine in the collecting system gets diluted. All the salts are absorbed and replaced by a watery type of fluid having a specific gravity of 1.010.
2. Patients with an extrarenal pelvis have minimal damage to the renal parenchyma for a long time.
3. Even with complete obstruction, glomerular filtration occurs to an extent, resulting in the production of some amount of urine. This is opposed by the rising pressures in the pelvis. To maintain filtration and protect the renal parenchyma from harmful pressure effects, several back flow mechanisms are pressed into service. The important decompression mechanisms are pyelosinus, pyelovenous, pyelolymphatic, pyelotubular and pyelointerstitial back flows. Back flows occur across the epithelial membranes between two anatomical structures through microscopic discontinuities called 'back flow breaks'.

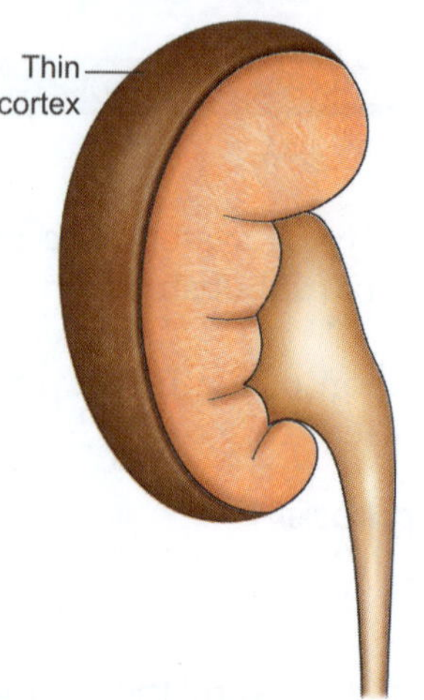

Fig. 57.19: Kidney with an intrarenal pelvis

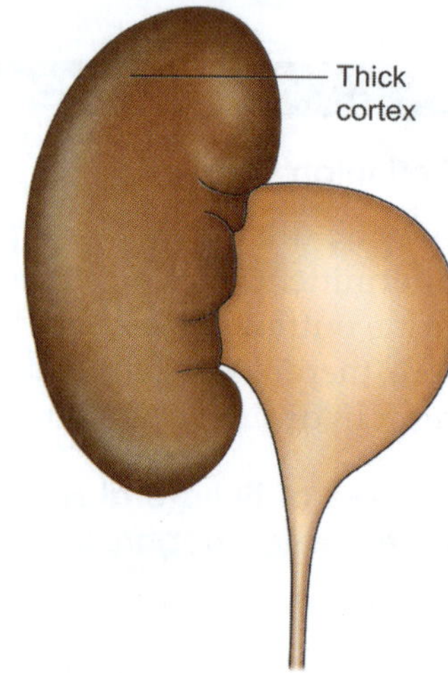

Fig. 57.20: Kidney with an extrarenal pelvis

- Further progression of the disease leads to a nonfunctional kidney.
- Acute bilateral obstructions present with symptoms of uremia, and untreated bilateral obstructions lead to chronic kidney disease (CKD) over time.

Clinical Features

1. Painless enlargement of the kidney. A renal mass is felt in the loin. It has a smooth surface and is firm in consistency (tensely cystic).
2. Dull-aching pain in the loin.
3. Previous history of calculus disease.
4. Hypertension and haematuria are rarely seen.
5. **Dietl's crisis:**
   - It is a clinical phenomenon of intermittent hydronephrosis.
   - It is common in calculous hydronephrosis.
   - Following an attack of renal colic, ureteric obstruction occurs due to a stone, which results in enlargement of the renal pelvis felt as a palpable mass in the loin. After a few hours, the mass disappears due to the passage of a large quantity of urine due to reflux polyuria or due to slippage of the stone.
6. The symptoms of the primary cause may be evident in the history (e.g. colicky radiating abdominal pain due to stones and haematuria).

Investigations

1. **Plain X-ray KUB**
   - Enlarged renal outline can be made out
   - Demonstration of stone
2. **USG** can detect enlarged kidneys and the cause of hydronephrosis in most cases.
3. **CT scan** is the investigation of choice. It can assess the anatomy and function more accurately than IVU (Fig. 57.21).
4. **Intravenous pyelography (IVP)** (Fig. 57.22)
   - Normally, the calyces are concave.
   - They become flat and later convex/club-shaped followed by dilatation of the pelvis and ureter depending on the level of obstruction.
   - In hydronephrosis with gross impairment of renal function, contrast may not be visible for a few hours on X-ray. In such cases, high doses of contrast (100–200 ml) may have to be used, and the pictures may have to be taken even after 24 hours. Such a situation is seen in PUJ dysfunction.

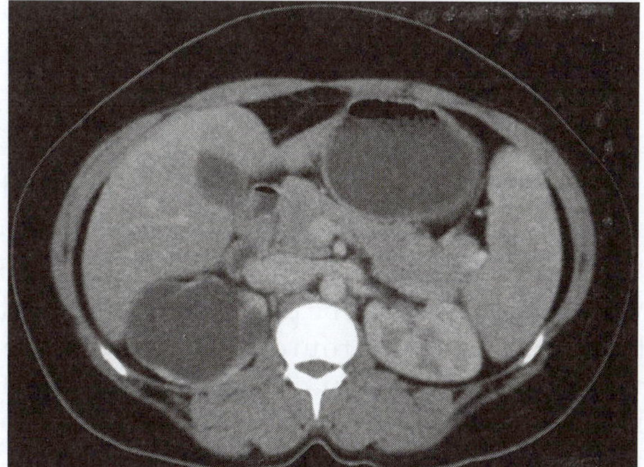

Fig. 57.21: CT—right hydronephrosis. Normal left kidney.

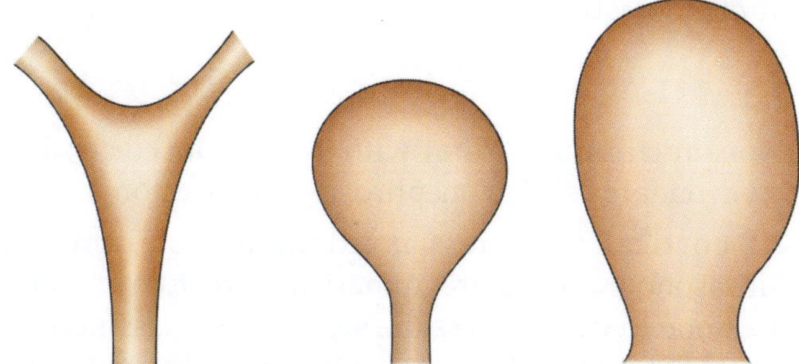

Fig. 57.22: Normal, flattened, and club-shaped calyx

5. **Isotope renography:** Technetium 99m-labelled DTPA (diethylene triamine penta-acetic acid) scan using a Gamma camera. The above Gamma radiation emitter is injected intravenously. It can be detected in the urinary tract above the level of obstruction and does not get washed off even after giving frusemide injection.
6. **Retrograde pyelography (RGP)**
   - When IVP fails to demonstrate the kidneys, RGP is a useful investigation. It can be done just prior to definitive surgery to confirm the site of obstruction.
   - Less quantity of contrast material is required, and better configuration of calyces can be made out.
7. **Blood urea and creatinine** are estimated to rule out renal failure.

Treatment of Hydronephrosis

I. *Hydronephrosis Secondary to a Cause*

Treat the cause.

a. **Stones:** Pyelolithotomy, ureterolithotomy.
b. **Stricture:** Strictureplasty or excision and end-to-end anastomosis.
c. **Aberrant vessel:** Transection of the ureter and anastomosis in front of the vessel.

d. **Phimosis:** Circumcision.
e. **Meatal stenosis:** Meatoplasty.
f. **Posterior urethral valve (PUV):** Transurethral fulguration of the valve.
g. **Benign prostatic hypertrophy (BPH):** Transurethral resection of the prostate (TURP).
h. **Carcinoma of the prostate:** Bladder outlet obstruction (infravesical cause) can be palliated by transurethral channelization. Hydroureteronephrosis can be managed by short-term or long-term DJ stenting along with the institution of options appropriate to the stage (hormonal treatment, radiation therapy, and cytotoxic drugs).
i. **Stricture urethra:** Visual internal urethrotomy or urethroplasty.

Principles of Surgery

1. **Nonfunctioning kidney** with thinned out cortex and hydronephrosis/pyonephrosis—nephrectomy.
2. If cortical thickness is adequate (0.5 cm) by ultrasonography, a preliminary nephrostomy should be done to decompress the system. Reassessment of renal function is done after a few days. If renal function improves, definitive surgery for hydronephrosis can be done. If it remains a nonfunctioning kidney and the opposite kidney is normal, nephrectomy is done.
3. In bilateral hydronephrosis, the better functioning kidney should be operated first. An exception to this principle is when the relatively poor functioning kidney is a seat of sepsis, for which some means of drainage by either DJ stenting or percutaneous nephrostomy should be done before definitive correction of the better functioning side.

II. Patients with Congenital Hydronephrosis—Pelviureteric Junction (PUJ) Dysfunction

Congenital hydronephrosis needs special mention here. With the increasing use of obstetric ultrasound, the incidence of antenatally detected foetal hydronephrosis is on the rise. Antenatal detection of foetal hydronephrosis has become the most common mode of presentation of congenital hydronephrosis.

Congenital hydronephrosis is defined as the anteroposterior diameter of the renal pelvis > 10 mm at > 20 weeks of gestation. PUJ obstruction is the main cause (Fig. 57.23). These foetuses undergo serial ultrasound monitoring during the rest of pregnancy. Based on the increase or decrease in the pelvic diameter during this period, postnatal management can be planned even before the child is born.

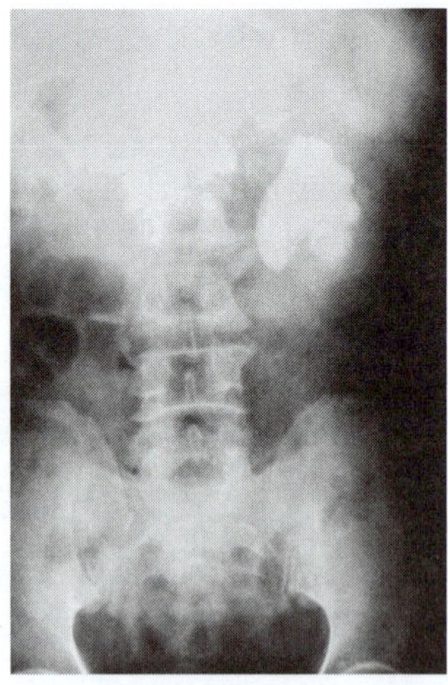

Fig. 57.23: Gross hydronephrosis due to PUJ obstruction

Indications for Surgery (Key Box 57.4)

Key Box 57.4

Indications for Surgery in Hydronephrosis

Pain
Atrophy of the kidney (damaged)
Infection
Nephrosis—hydronephrosis
Remembered as **PAIN**

Grades of Renal Pelvic Diameter and Management

I Mild	11–20 mm
II Moderate	21–35 mm
III Severe	> 35 mm

- Grade I hydronephrosis can be managed conservatively by serial monitoring of the pelvic diameter by ultrasound and of renal function by DTPA scan. These kidneys improve over a period of time.
- Grade II hydronephrosis: Majority (almost 80–90%) may be managed conservatively. However, close monitoring of the patient is required to detect any deterioration in renal function, which is an indication for surgical intervention. In this group, 10–20% of patients benefit from early surgery (patients with renal function of the involved kidney < 40%).
- Grade III hydronephrosis: All these patients should be operated early—modified Anderson-Hynes pyeloplasty to prevent permanent damage to the kidney.

Types of Pyeloplasty (Modified Anderson-Hynes)

This is the most popular type of dismembered pyeloplasty (Figs 57.24A and B).

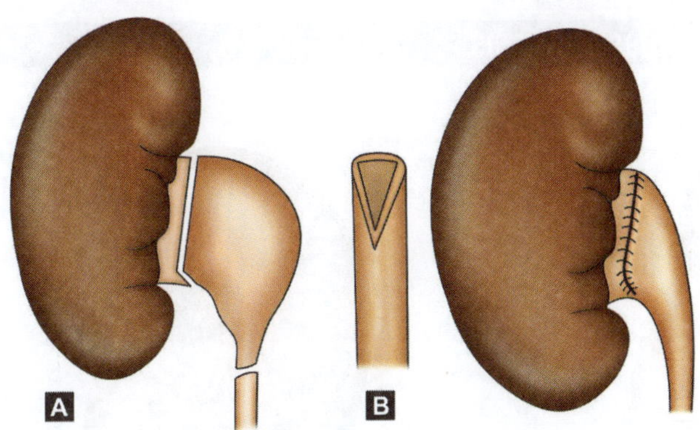

Figs 57.24A and B: Anderson-Hynes reduction pyeloplasty. (A) Excision of the redundant pelvis along with PUJ. (B) Completed ureteropelvic anastomosis.

1. *Dismembered Pyeloplasty—Anderson-Hynes Pyeloplasty*

Principles (Foley Criteria)

A. Excision of the redundant pelvis (pelvic reduction)
B. Excision of the dysfunctional PUJ segment.
C. New ureteropelvic anastomosis is done in such a way that urine drains by gravity.
D. Watertight anastomosis.

2. *Nondismembered Pyeloplasty*

- Foley's Y-V plasty or flap pyeloplasty, in which the PUJ is not transected, are not very popular.

3. *Endoscopic Pyeloplasty*

It can be done if the stricture is < 2 cm.

RENAL TUBERCULOSIS (TB)

- This is secondary to pulmonary TB/lymphatic TB. The primary focus is often difficult to identify.
- Common in males aged 20–40 years.
- Infection is always haematogenous. One may not find any active lesion in the lung or lymph nodes.
- Usually unilateral.

Pathology (Figs 57.25–57.33)

1. Tubercles develop and coalesce over the papilla, which may ulcerate—ulcerative form.
2. Tubercles may caseate and rupture over the renal papilla and communicate with the pelvis—ulcerocavernous form.
3. Attempt at healing produces calcification—pseudocalculi in the parenchyma of the kidney.
4. Tubercular hydronephrosis is very rare. It is due to tubercular stricture of the PUJ.
5. The opening of one of the calyces may get fibrosed leading to hydrocalyx, which may distort the rest of the calyces.
6. Cortical abscess ruptures into the perinephric space and forms a tubercular perinephric abscess. This may point at the loin and rupture to form a sinus.
7. Tubercular pyonephrosis (caseous kidney, putty kidney, cement kidney). When it gets calcified, it is called cement kidney. The entire kidney is converted into a bag of pus, which is tubercular caseous material with or without secondary infection. A complete ureteric stricture due to tuberculosis cutting off the pelvicalyceal system may result in autonephrectomy because of fibrosis.
8. Small, fibrosed, contracted, functionless kidney.
9. As a part of miliary tuberculosis—multiple small tubercles may be seen in the renal parenchyma.

Clinical Features

1. Frequency is the earliest symptom of tuberculosis. It is due to renal tubular inflammation (concentrating ability is affected, hence polyuria) and later due to tubercular cystitis.
2. Abacterial acid pyuria: The urine is opalescent, pale or yellow, and acidic in reaction. No organisms/bacteria are grown on repeated conventional culture.

Pearls of Wisdom

Sterile pyuria is seen in tuberculosis, stones, and carcinoma *in situ*.

3. Haematuria is not uncommon. Usually it is of small quantity due to ulcerocavernous variety.
4. Evening rise of temperature.
5. Loss of appetite and loss of weight.
6. Evidence of pulmonary or lymph node TB may be present.

Investigations

1. Urine for acid-fast bacilli (AFB)

- A sample of first-voided urine in the morning has to be examined to give the highest yield of AFB for 3 days.
- Ziehl-Neelsen staining and Gram staining (conventional, not in vogue).
- Lowenstein-Jensen media culture.
- Guinea pig inoculation is positive in 90% of cases.

PHOTOGRAPHS OF RENAL TUBERCULOSIS

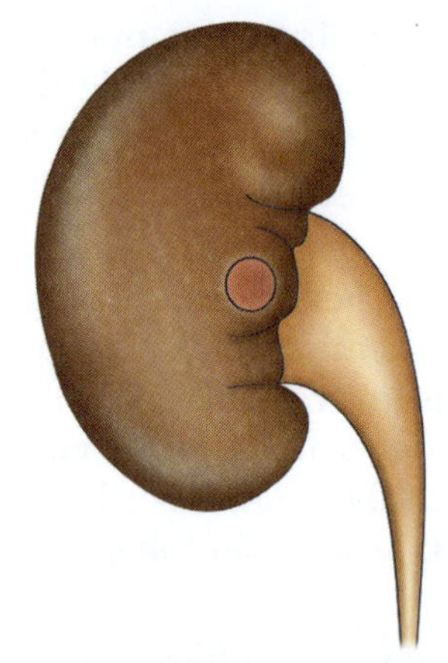

Fig. 57.25: Ulcerative form of renal tuberculosis

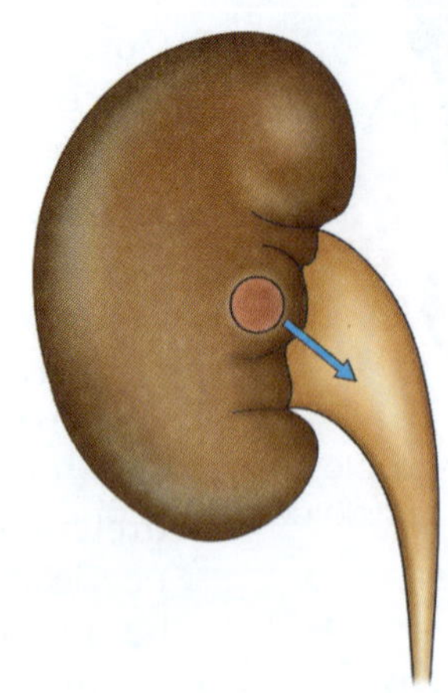

Fig. 57.26: Ulcerocavernous form of renal tuberculosis

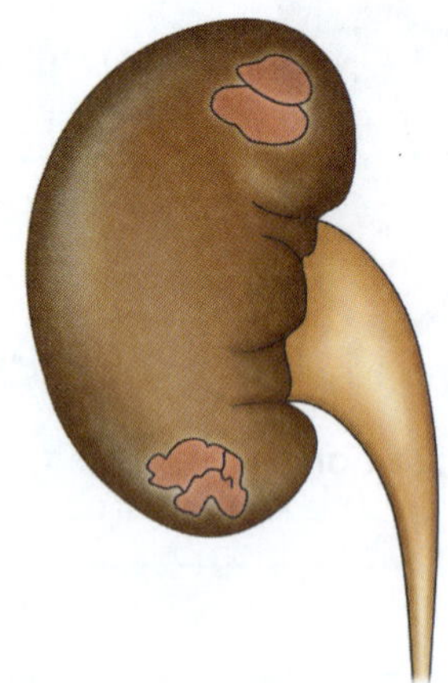

Fig. 57.27: Pseudocalculi in renal tuberculosis

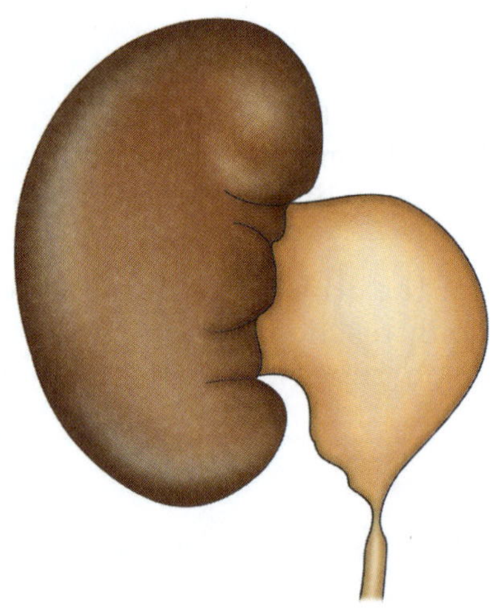

Fig. 57.28: Hydronephrosis in renal tuberculosis

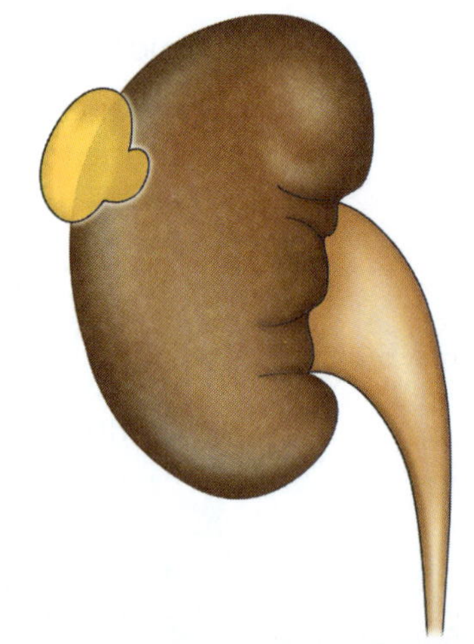

Fig. 57.29: Tuberculous perinephric abscess

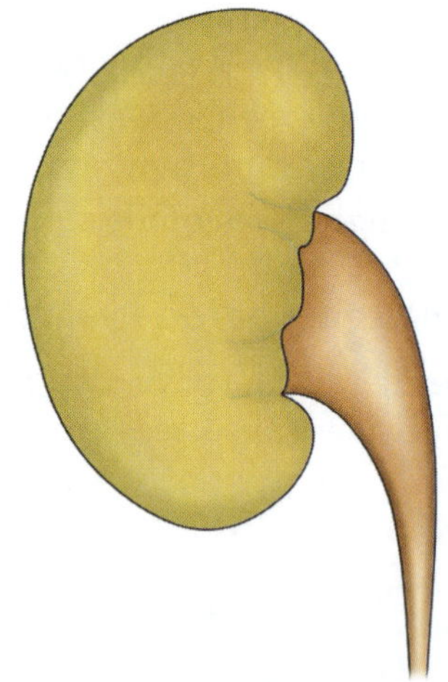

Fig. 57.30: Tuberculous pyonephrosis

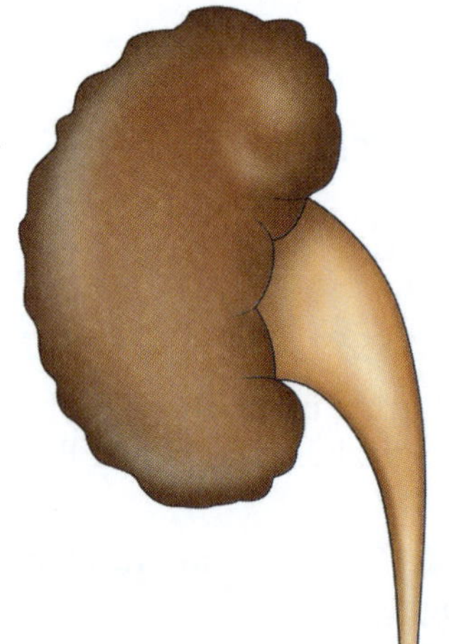

Fig. 57.31: Contracted kidney in renal tuberculosis

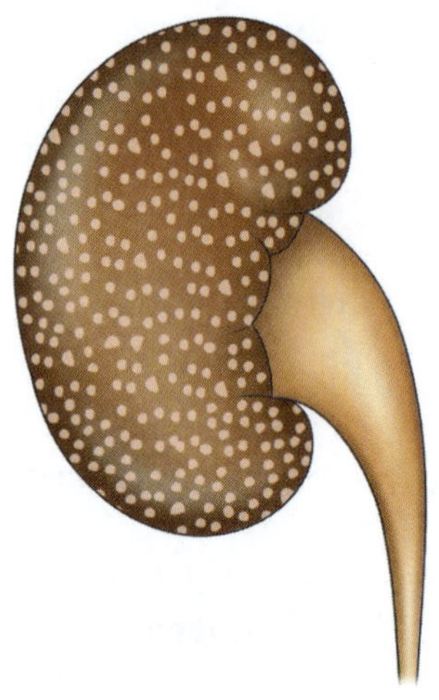

Fig. 57.32: Multiple tubercles—miliary tuberculosis

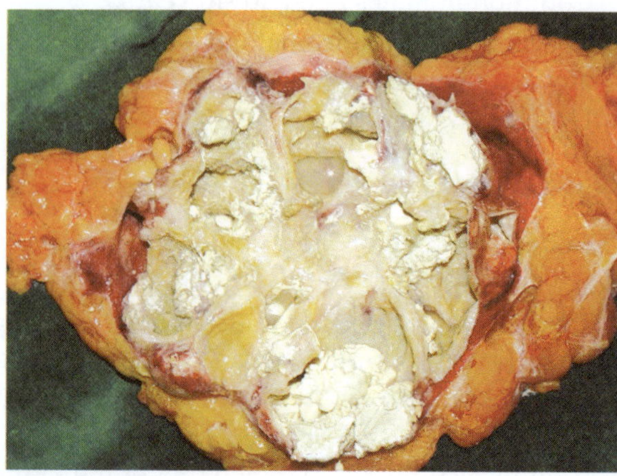

Fig. 57.33: Renal tuberculosis—entire kidney is a mass of caseous material

Pearls of Wisdom

Newer, easy methods like polymerised chain reaction (PCR) and radioisometric culture are also used. Cavitation, calcification, contraction (kidney), collecting system dilatations, and collections in the perinephric space detected by imaging studies should arouse suspicion of tuberculosis.

2. Cystoscopy

A. Earliest sign is pallor around the ureteric orifice. Initially, small ulcers are seen around the ureteric orifice. They join together and result in a larger ulcer.

- Due to extensive periureteric fibrosis, the ureter becomes thickened, shortened, and straight. The ureteric opening is lifted upwards and gapes (i.e., does not contract/ close when the bladder contracts). Such contracted, elevated, permanently opened, lower end of the ureter is called golf hole ureter (Fig. 57.34).
- As a result of this, with each bladder contraction, there is urine reflux into the kidney, which causes damage.

B. When the disease affects the urinary bladder, there will be extensive fibrosis. Soon, its capacity and compliance are reduced. At this stage, the patient suffers from strangury, which is painful ineffectual straining of urination culminating in voiding a few drops of urine. This is called "thimble bladder" or "systolic bladder".

3. IVP: Earliest sign is moth-eaten calyx. Thimble bladder and hydronephrosis may be features (Fig. 57.35).

4. CECT: It is the investigation of choice.

Treatment

1. **Conservative line of management** with antitubercular treatment is successful, provided the kidneys are functioning as in early stages (it should be pointed out that a full course of antitubercular regimen is integral, regardless of surgical treatment).
2. **Nephroureterectomy** is indicated if the kidney is nonfunctioning (Fig. 57.36).
3. **Renal cavernotomy of Henley**
   - Indicated when there is stricture of calyces resulting in hydrocalyx.
   - In this operation, the stricture is divided so that drainage improves.
4. **Treatment of thimble bladder—ileocystoplasty** (Fig. 57.37).
   - A 10–15-cm ileal loop is isolated based on the blood vessels, the fibrosed bladder dome is excised, and the intestine is split open and sutured to the urinary bladder.
   - This increases the capacity of bladder to store urine, thereby reducing frequency.
5. **Boari flap** for ureteric stricture.

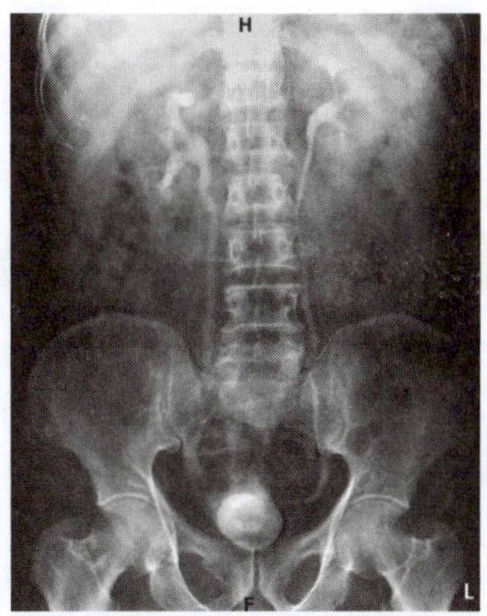

Fig. 57.35: Genitourinary tuberculosis: Left kidney is normal. Right kidney shows hydroureteronephrosis. The urinary bladder is contracted—thimble bladder

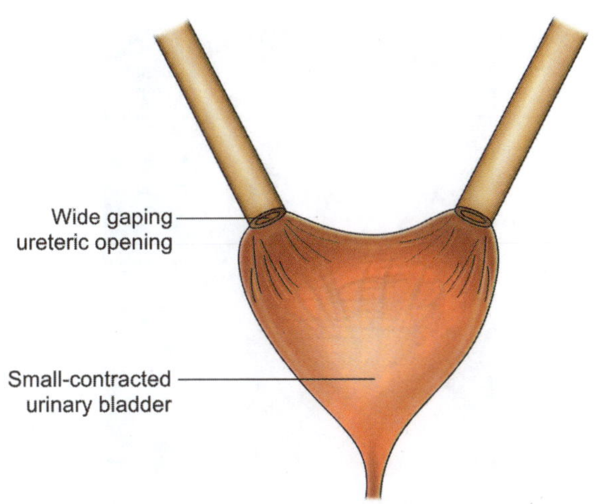

Fig. 57.34: Thimble bladder with golf hole ureter (TB)

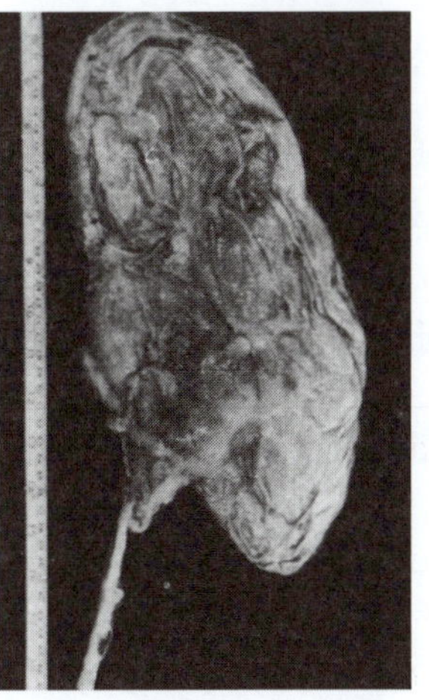

Fig. 57.36: Nephroureterectomy for renal tuberculosis (*Courtesy:* Professor Sasidharan, Manipal)

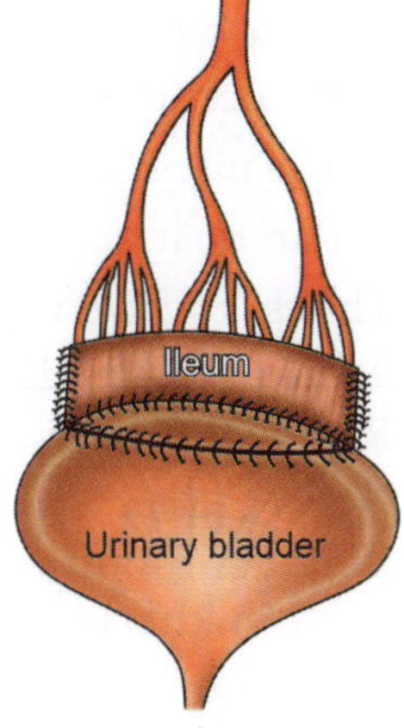

Fig. 57.37: Ileocystoplasty

Competency

SU29.6: Describe the clinical features, investigations and principles of management of renal tumours.

RENAL NEOPLASMS

Classification

- Benign: Adenoma, cortical adenoma, papilloma arising from the pelvis, haemangioma.
- Malignant: Nephroblastoma, renal cell carcinoma
- Transitional cell carcinoma (rare)
- Squamous cell carcinoma (extremely rare)

WILMS' TUMOUR (NEPHROBLASTOMA)

- This is a malignant tumour of the kidney that occurs in children.
- The tumour is composed of epithelial and mesothelial elements. It comprises blastemal, epithelial, and connective tissue (bone, cartilage, and muscle). Hence, it is called nephroblastoma (immature embryonic tissue).
- The tumour arises in one of the poles and distorts the reniform shape of the kidney. It is greyish-white or pinkish-white in colour (resembles brain tissue). At places, there may be areas of haemorrhage/necrosis.
- Microscopic features include connective tissue elements, cartilage, spindle cells, smooth striated muscle cells, and epithelial elements.
- 5% are bilateral.
- It occurs in familial and nonfamilial forms.

Clinical Features

- Both males and females are equally affected around 2–4 years of age.
  - If it occurs at < 1 year of age, it has good prognosis.
  - The upper age limit is 7 years.
  - Rarely, it may occur in adolescents.
- The child presents with abdominal distension due to a huge, nodular kidney.
- Rarely, Wilms' tumour can be bilateral.
- Haematuria is a poor prognostic symptom. It indicates rupture of the tumour into the renal pelvis. Such children usually die by 2 years of age.
- Low-grade fever may occur in rapidly growing tumours due to tumour necrosis, which releases pyrogens.
- Rapid deterioration of health is characteristic.

Investigations

1. Abdominal USG may detect a solid tumour in the kidney. Ultrasound rules out a tumour in the opposite kidney.
2. CT scan—to know the extent of lesion and spread to the adjoining structures (Fig. 57.38).
3. IVP is done to study distortion of calyces and to evaluate the function of the opposite kidney (CECT urogram has supplanted this).
4. FNAC is done to preoperatively confirm the diagnosis.

Differential Diagnosis

1. Neuroblastoma arises from adrenals. This is more common than nephroblastoma.
2. Retroperitoneal tumours
3. Adrenal tumour (Fig. 57.39)

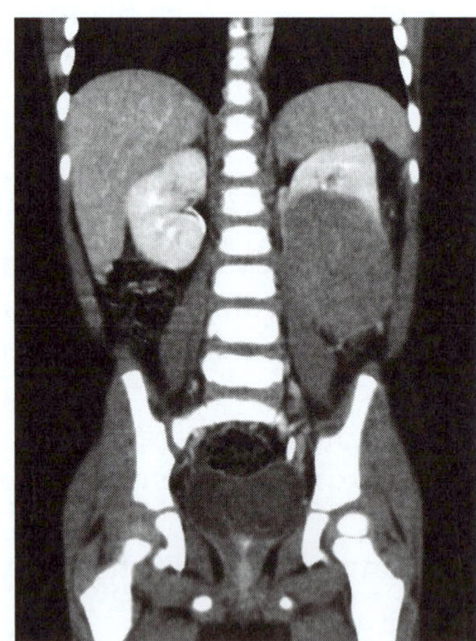

Fig. 57.38: A 3-year-old male child presented with a left loin mass. CECT abdomen and pelvis was done, which showed a large tumour in the left kidney. Left radical nephrectomy was performed, and histopathology diagnosed it as Wilms' tumour

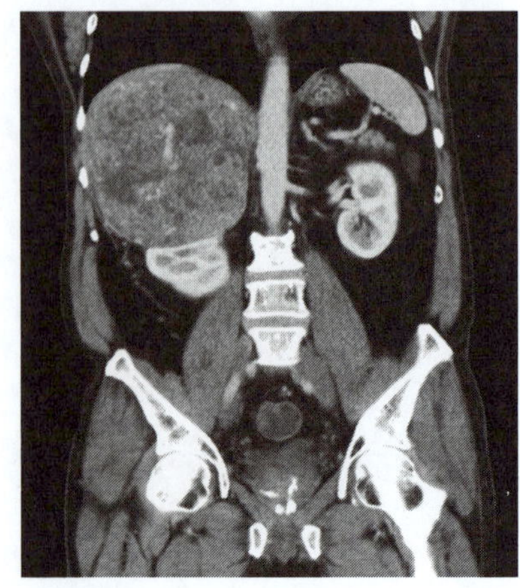

Fig. 57.39: CECT abdomen and pelvis showing a large, heterodense, right adrenal tumour

Differentiating features between Wilms' tumour and neuroblastoma (NBL)

1. **Calcification**—foci of calcification seen in NBL (85%). Less common in Wilms' (15%).
2. **Intraspinal extension**—seen in NBL
3. **Aorta and IVC** invasion by Wilms'
4. **Location**
   - Wilms'—intrarenal
   - Neuroblastoma—seen above the kidney pushing it downwards and outwards.
5. Crossing the midline—neuroblastoma
6. Urinary homovanillic acid (HVA) and vanillylmandelic acid (VMA) increase in neuroblastoma.

Spread

1. **Direct infiltration** of the capsule
2. **Lymphatic spread** occurs to the hilar, para-aortic, mediastinal, and left supraclavicular lymph nodes.
3. **Haematogenous spread** occurs to the lungs, liver, bones, brain, etc. The tumour thrombus can extend to the renal vein and inferior vena cava.

Treatment

Anaemia has to be corrected at the earliest.

1. **For tumours confined to the renal capsule** or perirenal soft tissue not infiltrating the adjacent organs, radical nephrectomy followed by chemotherapy with actinomycin D and vincristine are given for 6 months.
2. **For tumours that extend beyond the renal capsule** and perirenal soft tissue, have local infiltration to adjacent tissue, or have lymphatic metastasis, nephrectomy followed by local radiotherapy and chemotherapy are given with actinomycin D and vincristine for 15 months.
3. **If the tumour is found to be unresectable** by CT or MRI, preoperative FNAC to confirm the diagnosis is indicated, followed by preoperative radiotherapy (1000 cGy) or chemotherapy. Once the tumour regresses in size, nephrectomy should be done. Postoperative chemotherapy is given with actinomycin D, vincristine, and doxorubicin.
4. **Bilateral Wilms' tumour:** Radical nephrectomy on the side of the larger tumour and partial nephrectomy on side of the smaller tumour should be done. As much renal tissue as possible should be preserved after leaving a tumour-free margin. Postoperatively, the patient should be treated with chemotherapy. When surgery is not feasible, only radiotherapy and chemotherapy should be given. Growth disturbances and cardiac and pulmonary toxicities are complications of radiotherapy.

RENAL CELL CARCINOMA (RCC)

- It is also called hypernephroma or Grawitz tumour.
- Peak incidence at 60–70 years. Extensive use of ultrasound imaging for nonspecific abdominal symptoms has led to earlier pickup of this tumour in the fourth and fifth decades of life.
- **Male:** female ratio 2:1.
- It occurs in sporadic (common) and hereditary (rare) forms.

  Risk factors are given in Key Box 57.5.

Aetiology (Key Box 57.5)

The exact aetiology of sporadic RCC is unknown. Several environmental factors have been incriminated, such as urban dwelling, low socioeconomic status, tobacco chewing, cigarette smoking, exposure to asbestos, and analgesic abuse (phenacetin).

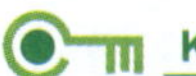 Key Box 57.5

Renal Cell Carcinoma: Aetiology

1. Chronic cystic disease
2. Chromosomal defect
3. Cadmium exposure
4. Cigarette smoking
5. Coffee drinking
6. Congenital—von Hippel-Lindau disease

Observe **6 Cs**

Comorbidities like renal failure/dialysis, obesity, hypertension, and diabetes are known to increase the risk (Key Box 57.6).

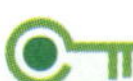 Key Box 57.6

Risk Factors for RCC

- Diabetes mellitus
- Chronic dialysis

In the hereditary or familial forms, specific oncogenes are operational. von Hippel-Lindau syndrome, in which tumorigenesis results due to loss of a tumour suppressor gene, is a well-known example of this form of RCC. A papillary variant of RCC occurs as a familial form which is characterized by trisomy 7 and 17 and is due to activation of a proto-oncogene.

Pathology

- Nearly all RCCs in adults are adenocarcinoma.
- Cell of origin: Proximal convoluted tubular epithelium.

- Starts in one of the poles (commonly in the upper pole) and usually ruptures outside the capsule, because of which the reniform shape of the kidney is maintained (Wilms' tumour grows within the capsule. Hence, the kidney shape is lost very early) (Fig. 57.40A).
- On the outer surface, it is homogenous (Wilms' tumour is pleomorphic) and yellow in colour due to lipid deposition.
- A few haemorrhagic areas are common because the tumour is very vascular (Fig. 57.40B).
- **Microscopy:** Alternate clear cells and dark cells.

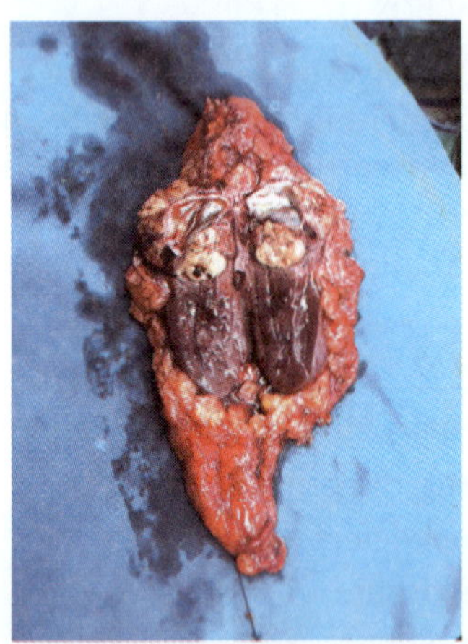

Fig. 57.40A: Renal cell carcinoma in the upper pole

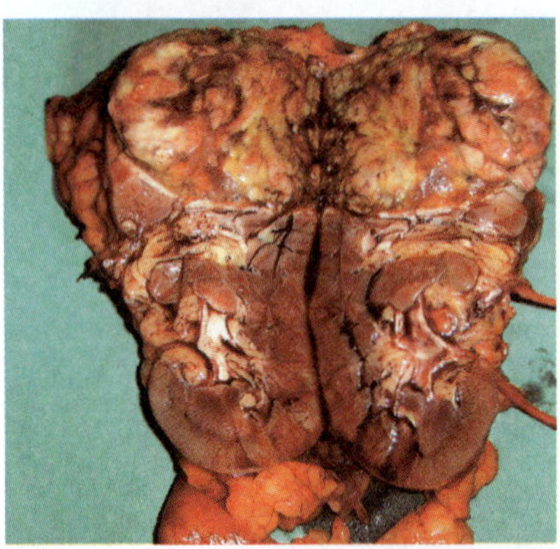

Fig. 57.40B: Upper pole RCC—observe the fleshy tumour with haemorrhage

Various Subtypes of RCC

1. **Clear cell carcinoma**
   - Most common type (70–80%)
   - It may be familial, associated with von Hippel-Lindau syndrome, or sporadic (95%).
2. **Papillary**—both familial and sporadic forms.
3. **Chromophobe**—arises from the cortical portion of the collecting duct. These tumours exhibit multiple chromosome losses and extreme hypoploidy.
4. **Renal medullary carcinoma**
   - New subtype
   - Associated with sickle-cell trait
   - Arises from calyceal epithelium.
   - Carries a poor prognosis.
5. **Collecting duct (Bellini)**—rare, occurs in young, has poor prognosis. The term "sarcomatoid" is used to describe an infiltrative and poorly differentiated variant of any of the above types.
   - Tumour cells line the blood vessels which are responsible for early blood spread from renal cell carcinoma (like follicular carcinoma of the thyroid— angioinvasion and capsular invasion).

Clinical Features (Fig. 57.41)

I. *Triad of Renal Cell Carcinoma*

Triad is seen in only 9%, but if present, it strongly indicates metastatic disease.

1. **Pain:** Dragging or intermittent colic due to blood clot blocking the ureter.
2. **Intermittent haematuria**
3. **Palpable mass:** Hard, nodular, ballotable, and bimanually palpable loin mass that moves with respiration.

II. *Other Manifestations*

1. Pathological fractures (e.g. fracture femur, humerus)—vascular, pulsatile, secondaries are common in flat

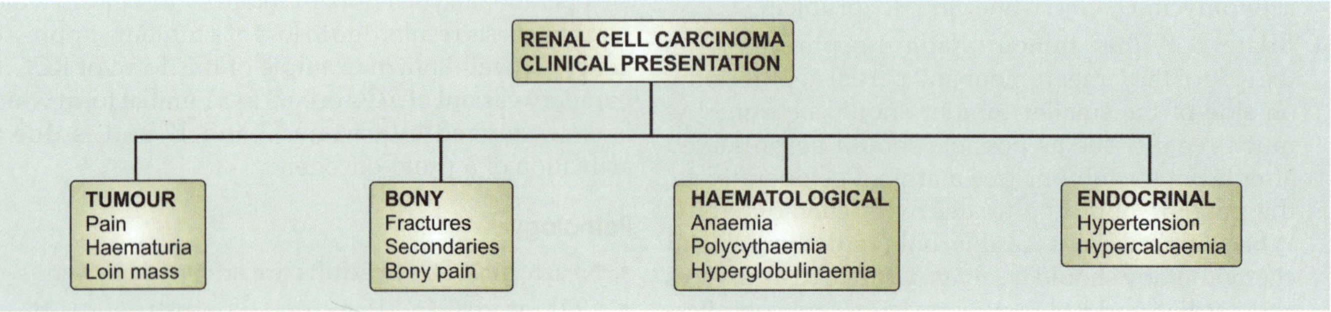

Fig. 57.41: Clinical presentation of RCC

bones (e.g., scalp, vertebra, rib, sternum) because they contain red marrow for a longer time.

2. **Anaemia** disproportionate to the amount of haematuria due to decreased production of erythropoietin.
3. Mild elevation of **temperature** due to tumour necrosis, which produces pyrogens. It can present as pyrexia of unknown origin (PUO) and is hence called internist's tumour.
4. **Nephrotic syndrome**-like features are rare.
5. Endocrinal disturbances (paraneoplastic syndromes) are rare. Increased ESR—most common paraneoplastic syndrome.
   - Renin-producing tumours are responsible for hypertension.
   - Polycythaemia is due to increased erythropoietin secretion.
   - Other hormones produced by the tumour are parathormone, adrenocorticotrophic hormone, human chorionic gonadotropin, glucagon, and prolactin.
6. **Hypertension**
7. **Liver dysfunction:** Nonmetastatic liver dysfunction (increased liver enzymes), also known as Stauffer's syndrome, improves after nephrectomy (deranged enzymatic levels normalize).

Robson's Staging of Renal Cell Carcinoma

- **Stage I:** Tumour limited to the kidney
- **Stage II:** Tumour invading the perinephric tissues or adrenal gland, but not extending beyond the Gerota's fascia.
- **Stage III:** Tumour extending into major veins or involving lymph nodes.
- **Stage IV:** Tumour invasion beyond Gerota's fascia or with distant metastasis.

Investigations

1. **Urine examination** when the patient has haematuria to look for malignant cells. In RCC, urine cytology is negative. If positive in a patient with haematuria, urothelial cancer should be suspected.
2. **Plain X-ray KUB region:** Enlarged kidney shadow can be seen (enlarged renal silhouette).
3. **IVP:** Distortion of calyces, missing calyces, or loss of the architectural pattern of the kidney.
4. **USG**
   - Enlarged kidney.
   - Locate tumour, site, and extent.
   - USG-guided FNAC can be done.
   - Can detect thrombus in the inferior vena cava (IVC).
   - In real-time examination, the IVC collapses during inspiration and opens during expiration. This is called caval kinetics. When the tumour thrombus extends into the IVC, this feature is lost in the segment housing the thrombus.

TNM STAGING **Renal cell carcinoma AJCC 8th edition**

Tx	Primary tumour cannot be assessed
T0	No tumour
T1a	<4 cm, within capsule, in greatest dimension
T1b	>4 cm but <7 cm
T2a	>7 cm but <10 cm, within capsule
T2b	>10 cm
T3a	Extracapsular but within Gerota's fascia extension
T3b	Extension into IVC below diaphragm
T3c	Extension into IVC above diaphragm
T4	Extension above diaphragm—direct invasion beyond Gerota's fascia: Ipsilateral adrenals
N0	No nodes
NX	Cannot be assessed
N1	Metastasis in regional lymph nodes
M0	No metastasis
M1	Distant metastasis present

Stage grouping

Stage I	T1 N0 M0
Stage II	T2 N0 M0
Stage III	T1 N1 M0
	T2 N1 M0
	T3 N0 M0
	T3 N1 M0
Stage IV	T4 any N, M0
	Any T, any N, M1

5. **Contrast-enhanced CT scan** is the investigation of choice for staging (Key Box 57.7 and Figs 57.42–57.46).

Pearls of Wisdom

Any renal mass which enhances after contrast on CT scan in an elderly person should be considered as RCC until proven otherwise.

Key Box 57.7

CT Scan—RCC

- Mixed density mass lesion
- Enhancement after contrast
- Secondary changes like tumour cell necrosis
- Local extent can be evaluated
- IVC thrombus and lymph node involvement can be identified.
- With CT chest, for detecting pulmonary metastases.

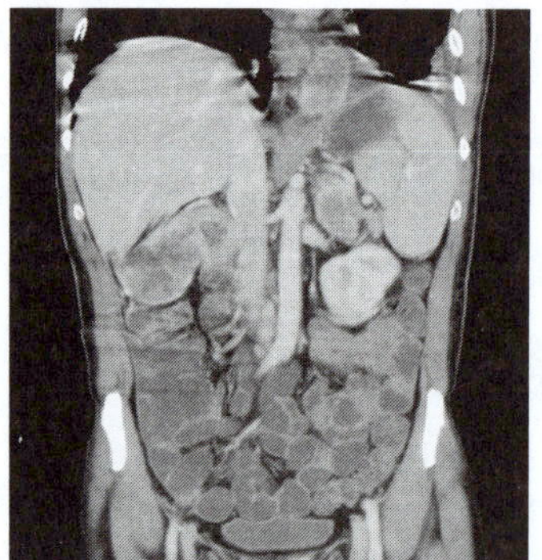

Fig. 57.42: Right RCC with left adrenal metastasis

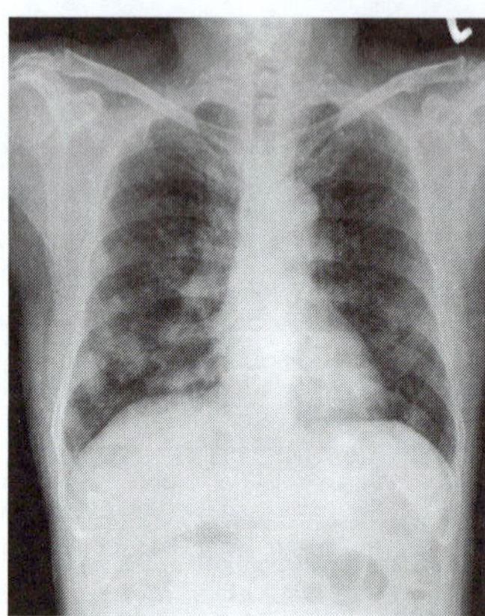

Fig. 57.43: Chest X-ray showing cannonball metastasis

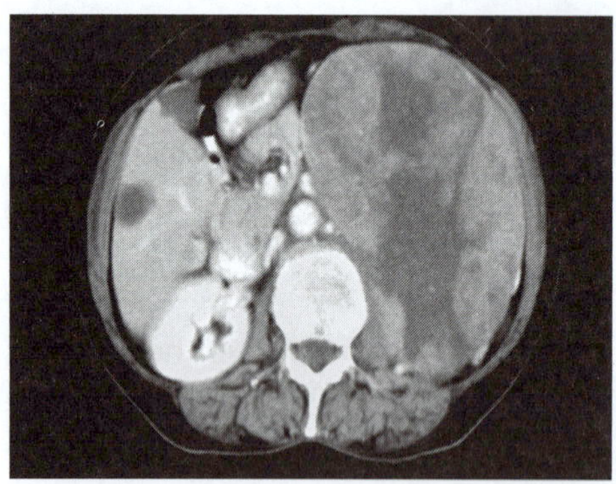

Fig. 57.44: CT scan showing left RCC

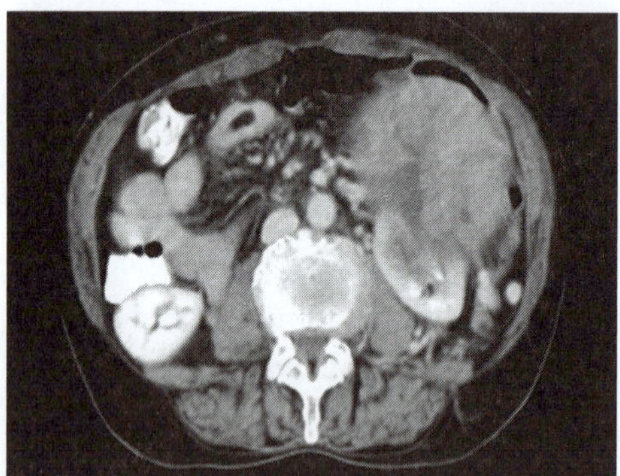

Fig. 57.45: Very extensive left RCC

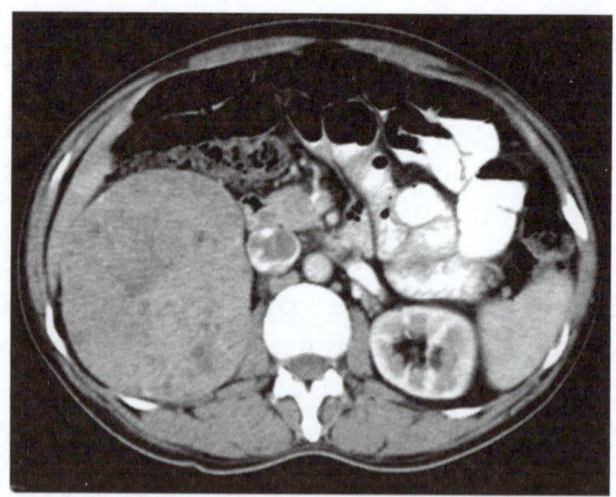

Fig. 57.46: IVC thrombus

6. **Renal angiography** is done by a retrograde transfemoral approach. Features are as follows:
   - **Neovascularisation:** Tumour blush inside the tumour.
   - Venous phase has to be observed to rule out tumour extension in the vein.
7. **MRI scan:** MRI is the investigation of choice to know the extent of IVC thrombus (better than CT).
8. **Venacavogram:** It is done to know extent of tumour in the IVC and the presence of collateral circulation.
9. **Chest X-ray**—rarely done as lung fields are surveyed during CT. Pulmonary metastases on chest X-ray are described as "cannonball lesions."

Treatment

1. **Radical nephrectomy**
   - En bloc removal of the entire Gerota's fascia with its contents (i.e. kidney, proximal ureter, adrenal gland).
   - Retroperitoneal lymph node dissection does not improve the survival rate.
   - Routine removal of the ipsilateral adrenal gland is uncommon unless the tumour involves a large portion of the upper pole of the kidney or preoperative radiologic exams suggest adrenal gland involvement.
2. **Radical nephrectomy with extraction of tumour thrombus**
   - The tumour thrombus may extend along the renal vein into the IVC and even into the right atrium (Fig. 57.47).
   - Infradiaphragmatic tumour thrombus can be removed with proximal control over the vena cava. Supradiaphragmatic IVC thrombus requires cardiopulmonary bypass (Figs 57.48 and 57.49).
   - In the absence of distant metastasis after thrombus removal, these patients survive for a long duration.
3. **Nephron-sparing surgery:** It is done in tumours <4 cm, in bilateral tumours, in those with comprised renal function, in familial RCCs, and in cases of renal cell carcinoma in solitary kidney.

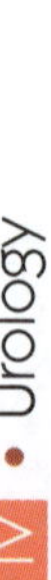

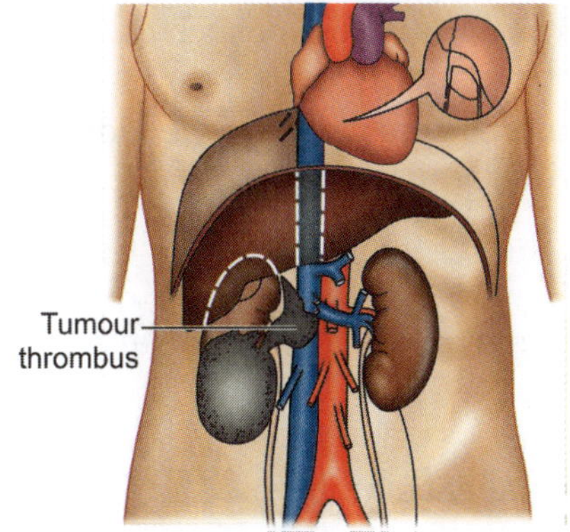

Fig. 57.47: Renal cell carcinoma with tumour thrombus in the renal vein and, inferior vena cava

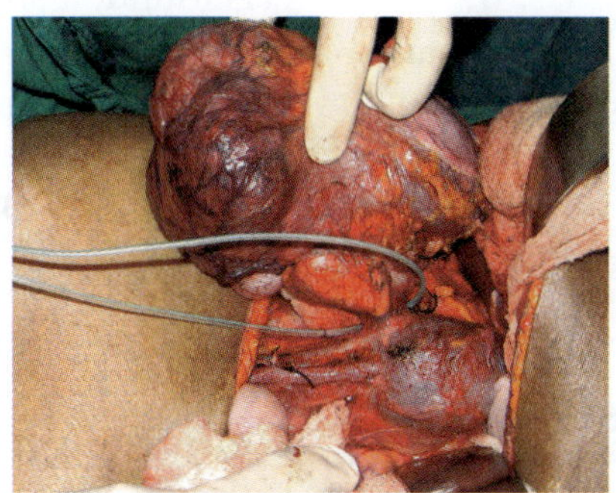

Fig. 57.48: Renal cell carcinoma with tumour thrombus removed

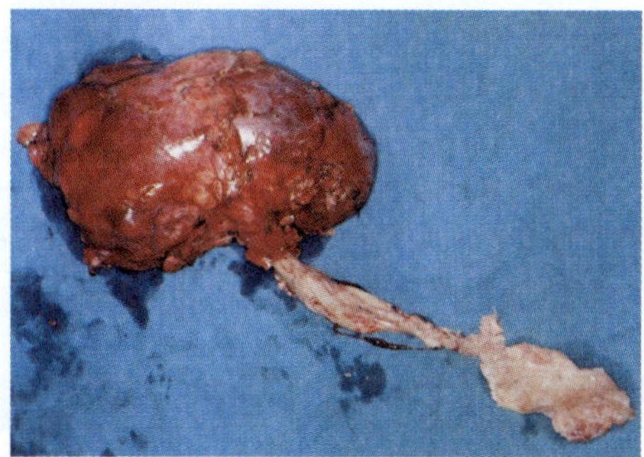

Fig. 57.49: Renal cell carcinoma—radical nephroureterectomy specimen

4. Therapeutic embolisation

- This can be used as a palliative measure in advanced carcinoma to relieve symptoms. This can also be used preoperatively to regress the size of large tumours.
- A catheter is placed in the renal artery, and substances such as gel foam, blood clot, and crushed muscle are injected.
- They block the lumen of the vessel and reduce the size of the tumour so that radical nephrectomy can be performed later.

5. Radiotherapy: Not of much use. However, it is a good form of palliation for secondaries in the lung, bone, and brain.

6. Immunotherapy: Administration of interferon or interleukin-2 has been found to improve the survival rate.

Transitional cell carcinoma of the renal pelvis is given in Key Box 57.8.

Key Box 57.8

Transitional Cell Carcinoma of the Renal Pelvis

- Uncommon tumour in the renal pelvis
- Multiple sites of urothelial mucosa are often involved
- Low-grade tumours
- Discovered late
- Haematogenous spread is common

RENAL MASS IN THE SURGICAL WARD (Table 57.2)

Clinical Features of Kidney Mass

- Moves with respiration because the fascia of Gerota encloses the kidney and fuses above the diaphragm.

Table 57.2 Renal mass in surgical ward

	Hypernephroma	*Hydronephrosis*	*Polycystic kidney*
1. Chief symptoms	Haematuria, pain in the loin, renal mass	Asymptomatic, distension, abdomen pain	Mass abdomen, hypertension, haematuria
2. Age of the patient	Over 50 years	20–30 years	30–40 years
3. Sex incidence	Common in males	Common in females	Common in females
4. Anaemia	Present	Absent	May be present
5. Features of renal failure	Absent	Can be present in bilateral cases (rare)	May be present
6. Renal mass	Unilateral, nodular, hard, may be fixed, nontender	Can be bilateral, smooth, cystic, feels firm	Bilateral, bosselated, nodular, not fixed, nontender
7. Features of kidney mass	May not have free mobility due to fixity	Not fixed, nontender	Present
8. IVU	Irregular calyces	Gross dilatation of pelvicalyceal system	Spider-leg deformity of calyces
9. CT scan	Enhancing mass	Dilated pelvicalyceal system with uniform filling of contrast	Multiple hypodense areas without enhancement
10. Treatment	Radical nephrectomy	Pyeloplasty	Symptomatic—renal transplantation

- Kidneys enlarge in the upward and downward direction.
- Bimanually palpable and ballotable. It is ballotable because of the renal pedicle and perirenal pad of fat.
- Colonic band of resonance is obliterated when the kidney enlarges, as the colon is pushed laterally.
- The upper border is not palpable because it is under the 12th rib.

ACUTE SURGICAL INFECTIONS OF THE KIDNEYS

PYONEPHROSIS

In this suppurative inflammatory condition, the entire kidney is converted into a sac containing pus or purulent urine—the renal parenchyma is almost always completely destroyed.

Causes

1. **Renal calculous disease** is the most common cause of pyonephrosis.
2. **Acute pyelonephritis** is more common in children and in females. Inadequately treated cases may develop into pyonephrosis, especially when pyelonephritis is associated with urinary tract obstruction.
3. **Infection** of a hydronephrosis.

Clinical Features

- Anaemia and fever
- Renal swelling
- Large swelling with high-grade fever with chills and rigors suggests an imminent danger of septicaemia and requires immediate drainage of pus.

Investigations

- Urine examination may be positive for coliforms and other gram-negative organisms.
- Plain X-ray KUB may reveal a stone or an enlarged renal outline.
- Ultrasound can confirm hydronephrosis.
- Intravenous urogram demonstrates poor function of the kidney on the diseased side. As a rule, the opposite kidney is normal.
- CECT is the investigation of choice.

Treatment

- Broad-spectrum antibiotics (parenteral) should be started immediately once urine and blood are sent for culture and sensitivity.
- Ultrasound-guided aspiration of pus or a percutaneous nephrostomy (preferred) and drainage of pus greatly improves the general condition of the patient.
- If any obstruction or causative agent such as a stone is found, it should be removed.
- Nephrectomy should be considered if the kidney is non-functioning with significant damage.

PERINEPHRIC ABSCESS

It refers to the collection of pus in the perirenal area.

Causes

- Infection in a perirenal haematoma
- Pyonephrosis after rupture
- Tubercular perinephric abscess
- Pus from retrocaecal appendicitis may extend into the loin and perinephric area, and may present as an abscess.

Clinical Features

- High swinging temperature
- Rigidity, tenderness, fullness in the loin
- Oedema in the loin

Investigations

- Total count: > 20,000 cells/mm3
- Urine analysis: No organisms are usually found
- X-ray spine: Scoliosis with concavity towards the abscess
- Screening chest: Diaphragm is immobile and elevated on the diseased side.

Treatment

Broad-spectrum antibiotics are started first. Ultrasound-guided pigtail insertion or percutaneous drain insertion should be attempted. If it fails, create an incision in the loin, drain the pus, and break all loculi. Closure is done with a drain. Once pus culture is available, treat accordingly.

MISCELLANEOUS

INTERESTING 'MOST COMMON' FOR RENAL CELL CARCINOMA

- Most common renal cancer in adults is adenocarcinoma.
- Most common site is the upper pole of the kidney.
- Most common presentation is mass per abdomen.
- Most common investigation of choice is CECT.
- Most common method of spread is haematogenous.
- Most common intra-abdominal malignancy that spreads within the vena cava and into the atrium.
- Most common cell of origin is the proximal renal tubular epithelium.

Dialysis and renal transplantation are discussed on page 1194.

Multiple Choice Questions

1. **Which of the following is not a feature of adult polycystic kidney disease?**
   A. It may cause renal failure
   B. Hypertension is seen in about 75% of patients
   C. It is autosomal recessive
   D. It is always bilateral

2. **Relations of right kidney include the following *except*:**
   A. Muscles posteriorly
   B. Pyloric antrum anteriorly
   C. Ascending colon laterally
   D. Adrenals medially

3. **Which of the following is a feature of horseshoe kidney?**
   A. Classically, it is the upper polar fusion of both kidneys
   B. It does not cause angulation of the ureter and hydronephrosis
   C. It may be associated with Down's syndrome
   D. Hyperextension of the spine results in pain, nausea, and vomiting

4. **Gout results in:**
   A. Calcium stones B. Cystine calculi
   C. Phosphate D. Uric acid stones

5. **Which type of stone typically causes haematuria?**
   A. Oxalate B. Phosphate
   C. Cystine D. Uric acid

6. **The following are true for calcium oxalate stones *except*:**
   A. They are called mulberry calculi
   B. They are smooth and round
   C. They are hard
   D. They are visible on X-ray

7. **The following are true about uric acid stones *except*:**
   A. They are common in those who consume red meat
   B. They are small and multiple
   C. They are also seen in gout
   D. Pure uric acid stones are radio-opaque

8. **What type of stone is staghorn calculi?**
   A. Calcium oxalate B. Phosphate
   C. Uric acid D. Cystine

9. **Which of the following is not an ideal treatment for upper ureteric stones?**
   A. ESWL
   B. Percutaneous removal
   C. Ureteroscopic removal
   D. Cystoscopic removal

10. **A patient presents with renal stones and a swelling in the neck. What is the likely diagnosis?**
    A. Medullary thyroid carcinoma
    B. Hyperparathyroidism
    C. Hyperthyroidism
    D. von Recklinghausen's disease

11. **Which of the following causes bilateral hydronephrosis?**
    A. Idiopathic retroperitoneal fibrosis
    B. Carcinoma ureter
    C. Tuberculosis of the urinary tract
    D. Aberrant artery

12. **The following are features of Dietl's crisis except:**
    A. It is called intermittent hydronephrosis
    B. It is usually seen in calculus hydronephrosis
    C. It does not produce a mass
    D. It occurs due to stone slippage

13. **Which is the investigation of choice in hydronephrosis?**
    A. Ultrasound
    B. Intravenous pyelography
    C. CT scan
    D. Isotope renography

14. **Definite indications for pyeloplasty include the following *except*:**
    A. Calculus hydronephrosis
    B. Grade III hydronephrosis
    C. Nonfunctioning kidney with cortical thickness of 0.1 cm
    D. Tuberculous hydronephrosis

15. **The following are true for renal tuberculosis *except*:**
    A. It is a primary tuberculosis
    B. Infection occurs by lymphatic spread
    C. It commonly causes hydronephrosis
    D. It causes bacterial acid pyuria

16. Which of the following is an uncommon symptom of renal tuberculosis?

A. Haematuria
B. Evening rise of temperature
C. Cystitis
D. Pyuria

17. The following are complications of renal tuberculosis *except*:

A. Thimble bladder B. Golf hole ureter
C. Putty kidney D. Hydronephrosis

18. The following are true for Wilms' tumour *except*:

A. It contains only epithelial elements
B. It commonly presents before 1 year of age
C. Its prognosis is poor if it occurs within 1 year of age
D. Haematuria indicates poor prognosis

19. The following are true about renal cell carcinoma *except*:

A. It is mainly adenocarcinoma in adults
B. Reniform shape of the kidney is maintained
C. Clear cells and dark cells are present on microscopy
D. Tumour cells do not line the blood vessels

20. Polycythaemia in renal cell carcinoma is due to the production of:

A. Renin B. Erythropoietin
C. Prolactin D. Glucagon

21. The diagnostic CT finding of renal cell carcinoma in elderly patients is:

A. Dense mass
B. Tumour necrosis
C. Lymph node enlargement
D. Enhancing mass after intravenous contrast

22. The following are true for transitional cell carcinoma *except*:

A. It is a low-grade tumour
B. Haematogenous spread is common
C. It arises from the urothelium
D. Multiple sites are usually not involved

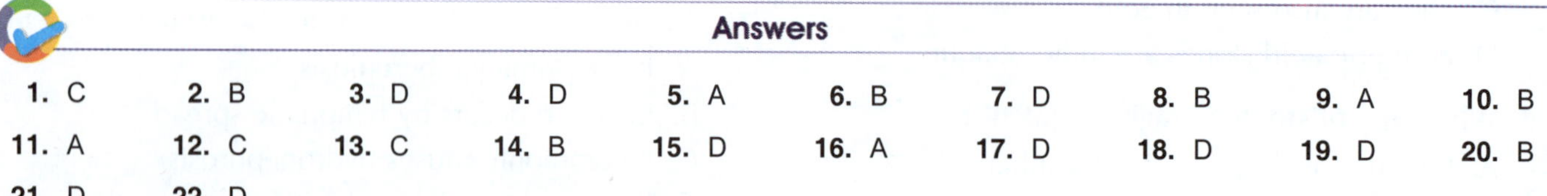

Answers

1. C	**2.** B	**3.** D	**4.** D	**5.** A	**6.** B	**7.** D	**8.** B	**9.** A	**10.** B
11. A	**12.** C	**13.** C	**14.** B	**15.** D	**16.** A	**17.** D	**18.** D	**19.** D	**20.** B
21. D	**22.** D								

CHAPTER

58

Urinary Bladder and Urethra

- Surgical anatomy
- Vesical calculus
- Carcinoma of bladder
- Ectopia vesicae
- Acute cystitis
- Diverticula
- Urinary fistulae
- Interstitial cystitis
- Schistosoma haematobium
- Urinary diversion
- Rupture bladder
- Surgical anatomy of the urethra
- Rupture urethra
- Stricture urethra
- Hypospadias
- Retention of urine
- Posterior urethral valve

SURGICAL ANATOMY OF THE BLADDER (Fig. 58.1)

Lining Epithelium

- The urinary bladder is lined by transitional epithelium (urothelium) that lies over the lamina propria (connective tissue).
- **Bladder cancers are transitional cell carcinomas.**

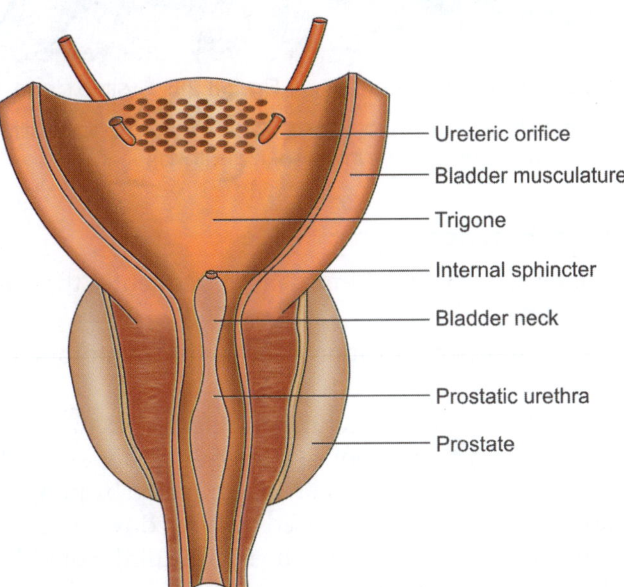

Fig. 58.1: Surgical anatomy of the urinary bladder

- However, due to metaplastic changes in the epithelium caused by chronic irritation (e.g. from a stone), other malignancies, such as squamous cell carcinoma, can occur.
- Bladder cancer can easily spread through the lamina propria into the muscle coat **(detrusor muscle)**.

Detrusor Muscle

It is a smooth muscle with intertwined fibres. Therefore, in bladder neck obstruction, it hypertrophies and leads to morphological alterations, such as trabeculations/sacculations.

Trigone

It is a triangular area that lays between the internal urethral orifice (bladder neck) inferiorly and the orifices of the ureter laterally. It is the **most sensitive part of the bladder,** and its irritation leads to increased urinary frequency and strangury.

Bladder Neck

- The internal sphincter is a smooth muscle that surrounds the bladder neck. It is innervated by α-adrenergic fibres and prevents retrograde ejaculation of urine.

- The distal urethral sphincter is a somatic striated muscle supplied by S2–S4 via the pudendal nerves.

Supports of the Bladder

- Posteriorly, the endopelvic fascia, which is continuous with the lateral ligaments of the rectum, need to be divided during radical cystectomy.
- Anteriorly, the puboprostatic ligaments need to be divided during radical cystectomy.
- **False ligaments:** The urachus and obliterated hypogastric arteries, together with the fold of peritoneum overlying these structures, are called false ligaments (medial ligaments). Peritoneal folds raised by the inferior epigastric arteries are called lateral ligaments.

Blood Supply

- **The superior and inferior vesical arteries,** which are derived from the anterior trunk of the internal iliac artery, are the main source of arterial blood supply. Minor blood supply comes from the obturator and inferior gluteal arteries and, in females, from the uterine and vaginal arteries as well.
- **Veins** form a plexus on the lateral and inferior surfaces of the bladder. Hence, during suprapubic cystostomy, these structures have to be avoided while entering the bladder.
- **The vesical** plexus, which is continuous with the prostatic plexus of veins in males, drains into the internal iliac vein.

Lymphatics

- Internal iliac nodes are the first level of lymph nodes.
- Obturator and external iliac lymph nodes get involved later.

Innervation

- **Parasympathetic** supply comes from the anterior divisions of the sacral nerves (S2, S3, S4) through the inferior hypogastric plexus. Following excision of the rectum, disturbance of micturition and sexual function may occur due to damage to the pelvic plexus.
- **Sympathetic** supply comes from T10–L2.

VESICAL CALCULUS

- **Primary:** Stones which develop in sterile urine in the absence of bladder pathology. These also include renal stones that have migrated to the bladder.
- **Secondary:** Stones develop in the presence of infection and stasis due to urinary flow obstruction. They develop secondary to bladder outlet obstruction.

Types (Figs 58.2A and 58.2B)

1. **Oxalate stone:** Moderate size, uneven surface. Mulberry stones are dark brown or black due to the presence of blood pigment. These are usually found in the kidneys.
2. **Uric acid stone:** They are the most common type of urinary bladder stones. Round to oval, smooth, pale yellow, not opaque on X-rays. They are usually formed in the bladder.
3. **Cystine:** Radiopaque due to high sulphur content.
4. **Triple phosphate:** These stones comprise ammonium, magnesium, and calcium phosphates. **They occur in urine infected with urea-splitting organisms.** Sometimes, they grow rapidly. The nucleus of the stone may contain bacteria, desquamated epithelium, or a foreign body. They are dirty white in colour.
5. **Jackstones:** Vesical calculi with jagged/spiculated surfaces.
6. In malnourished children <10 years of age, ammonium urate and calcium oxalate stones are found.

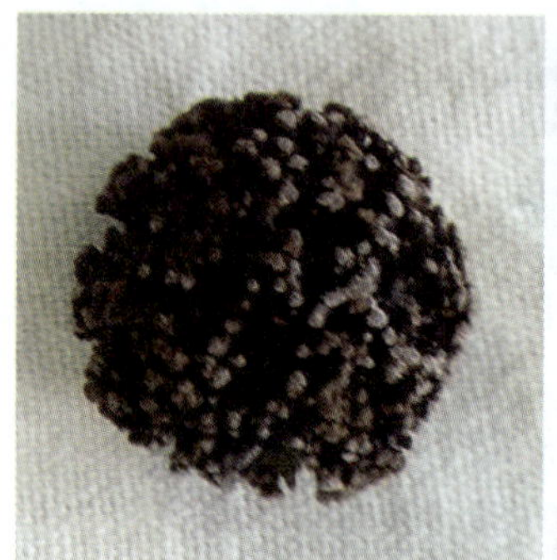

Fig. 58.2A: Oxalate stone

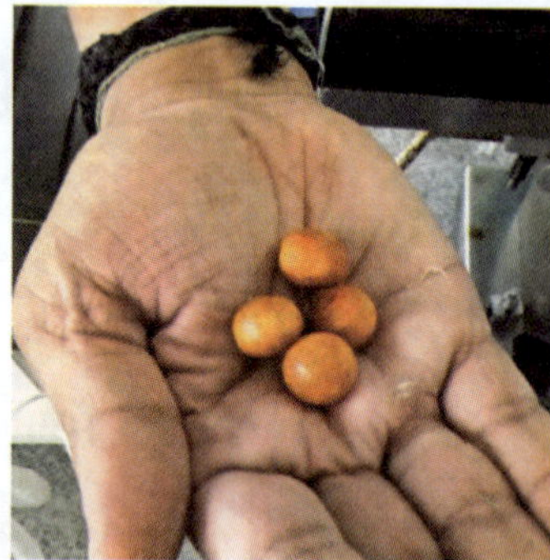

Fig. 58.2B: Cystine stone

(*Courtesy:* Dr SV Mohan, Professor of Surgery, Shivamogga Institute of Medical Sciences, Shivamogga, Karnataka)

Clinical Features

- **Males** are affected 8 times more frequently than are females.
- **Frequency** of micturition is the earliest symptom due to cystitis.
- **Pain** at the end of micturition referred to the tip of the penis in young boys suggests bladder stone. In school-going children, pain is aggravated by jumping and jolting. Pain is decreased on lying down because the stone falls away from the trigone of the bladder. Typically, oxalate stones produce pain. Painful ineffective micturition is described as strangury.

- **Haematuria** occurs if the stone causes abrasions in the bladder mucosa.
- **Acute retention of urine** is due to the calculus obstructing the internal meatus.

Investigations

- **Urine:** Red blood cells may be present—microscopic haematuria
  a. Envelope-like crystals: Oxalate stone
  b. Hexagonal plates: Cystine stone
- **Radiography:** In 90% of cases, the stone is visible (Fig. 58.3A). However, it is important to look for stones in the entire urinary tract.
- **Cystoscopy:** It is the best confirmatory investigation. The stone can be visualised.

A click can be heard when the stone comes into contact with the instrument.

Treatment

- Ultrasound lithotripsy—very safe, but only for small stones.
- Laser lithotripsy (holmium laser)—can break most large stones.
- Percutaneous suprapubic litholapaxy—using needle, guidance, and metal dilators.

I. Litholapaxy

- By introducing a cystoscopic lithotrite, the stone is firmly grasped and broken up. Small fragments of the stone are evacuated with an evacuator.

Contraindications for litholapaxy

1. **Urethra:** Obstruction such as stricture, enlarged prostate.
2. **Bladder:** Cystitis, contracted bladder, carcinoma.

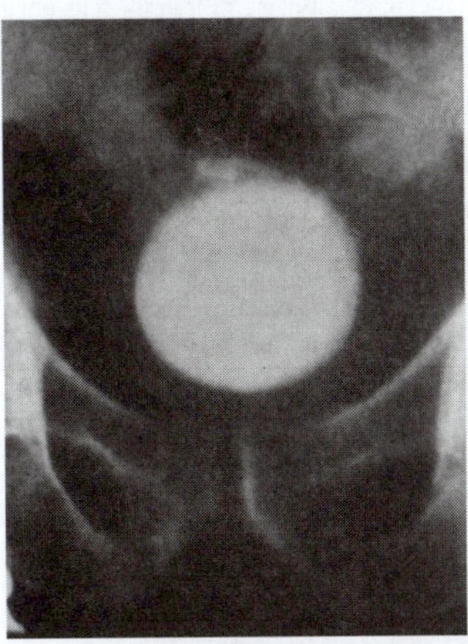

Fig. 58.3A: Bladder stone with copper-T (see clinical notes on page 1079)

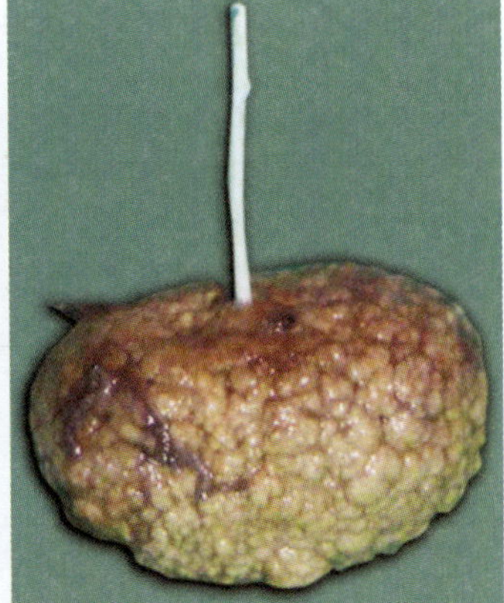

Fig. 58.3B: Bladder stone—triple phosphate stone

II. Suprapubic Cystolithotomy

- Can be done when the stone is too big (Fig. 58.3B), too hard to crush, or too soft.
  Transitional cell carcinoma—90%
  Squamous cell carcinoma—5–10%
  Adenocarcinoma—2%

Competency

SU29.8: Describe the clinical features, investigations and principles of management of bladder cancer.

CARCINOMA OF THE BLADDER

Aetiology (Key Box 58.1)

- Incidence is more in **aniline dye workers.** Products such as benzidine and 3-naphthylamine are carcinogenic.
- It is more common in men and in smokers (most common cause— >50% of cases).
- Chronic **irritation** by stones or a catheter may also produce carcinoma: 95% of tumours originate in the mucous membrane.
- **Bilharziasis or schistosomiasis** increases the risk of bladder cancer (squamous cell carcinoma).
- **Congenital anomalies** associated with an increased risk of carcinoma bladder:
  a. Patent urachus
  b. Exstrophy bladder
  c. Bladder diverticuli (can give rise to squamous cell carcinoma).

Key Box 58.1

Bladder Cancer

Aetiology	*High-risk occupations*
Bilharziasis	Aniline dye workers
Chronic irritation	Leather industry workers
Chronic smoking	Paint industry workers
Cyclophosphamide	Rubber industry workers

Pathology

1. **Malignant villous tumours:** They are transitional cell carcinomas. Multiple primaries are found in 25% of patients with bladder cancer.
   1. The villi are stunted, swollen, slow-growing, and resemble a cauliflower (verrucous).
   2. They may be sessile if high-grade.
   3. Bladder wall is more vascular.
   4. Submucous lymph nodes appear around the growth.

2. **Solid tumours are always malignant:** They are sessile and lobulated.
3. **Carcinomatous ulcer:** It arises in leukoplakia.

Histological Types

1. Transitional cell carcinoma—90% of tumours. The trigone and posterior bladder wall are affected.
2. Squamous cell carcinoma. Is seen in 5–10% of patients. The lateral wall and dome are involved.
3. Adenocarcinoma arises from urachal remnants and urethral glands--seen in 2% of patients. It occurs in conduits, pouches, etc.
4. Mixed variety
5. Undifferentiated

Clinical Features

- In 90% of cases, the initial symptom is **painless, intermittent haematuria.**
- Severe cystitis-like symptoms occur in carcinomatous ulcer.
- Later, painful, **blood-stained micturition** may occur.
- **Strangury:** Painful micturition with bleeding and incomplete emptying of the bladder.
- **Loin pain** is due to ureteric obstruction with hydronephrosis.
- **Suprapubic pain,** groin pain, and perineal pain are due to nerve infiltration. This indicates advanced nature of the growth.
- The most common site of lymph node metastasis is the pelvic (obturator) lymph nodes, and the most common site of visceral metastasis is the liver.

Investigations

1. **Urine:** Cytology of 3 freshly-voided samples.
2. **IVU:** To detect a filling defect in the bladder (Fig. 58.4).
3. **Ultrasound** to can detect bladder carcinoma (Fig. 58.5) and liver metastasis.
4. **CECT scan** is the investigation of choice, especially to know the spread of disease (Figs 58.6–58.9).
   - It is especially useful to know the infiltration of the muscle, perivesical tissue, prostate, and pelvic wall.

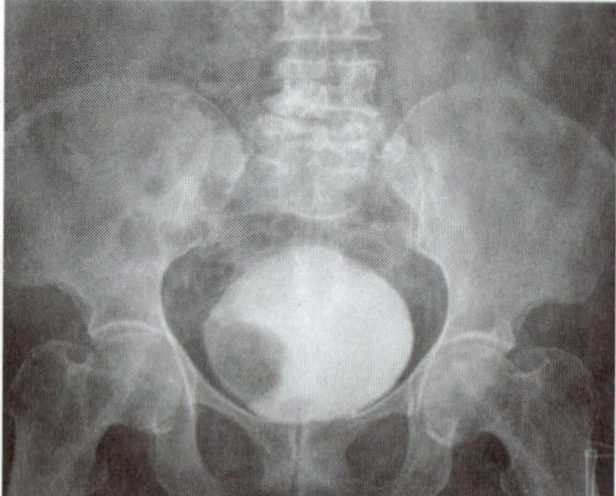

Fig. 58.4: IVU showing a filling defect

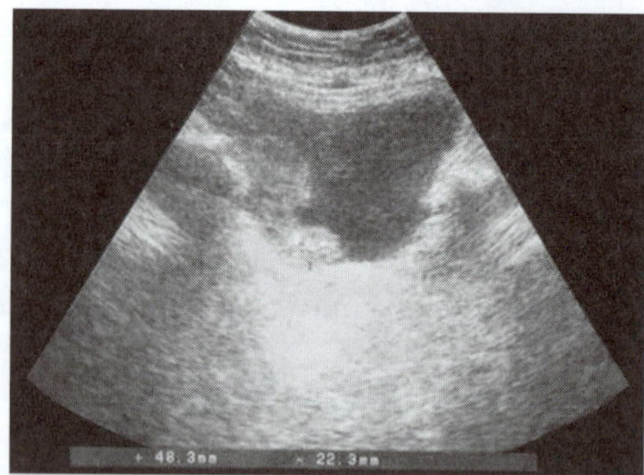

Fig. 58.5: Ultrasound suggesting carcinoma urinary bladder

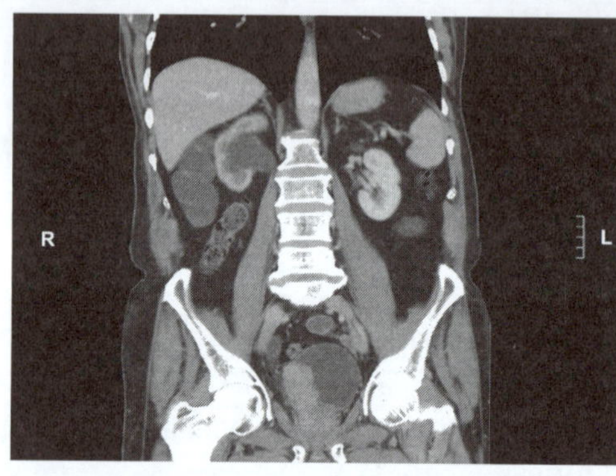

Fig. 58.6: CECT abdomen and pelvis showing a large tumour in the right lateral wall of the bladder with right hydroureteronephrosis

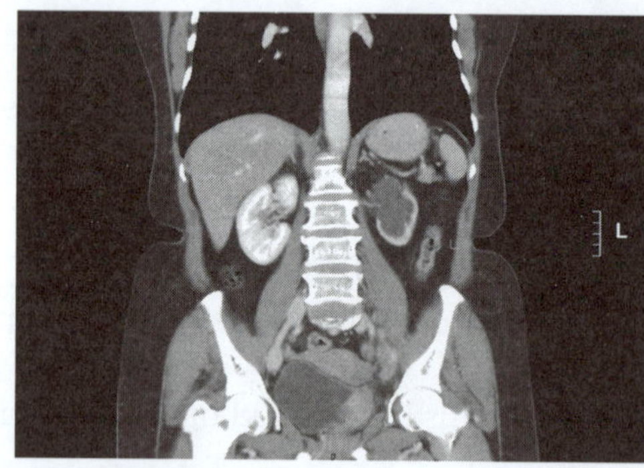

Fig. 58.7: CECT abdomen and pelvis showing a large tumour in the left lateral wall of the bladder with left hydroureteronephrosis

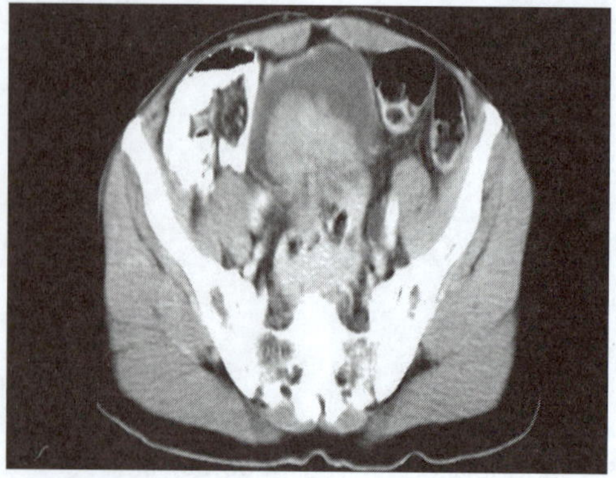

Fig. 58.8: CECT of the bladder showing a filling defect suggestive of carcinoma bladder

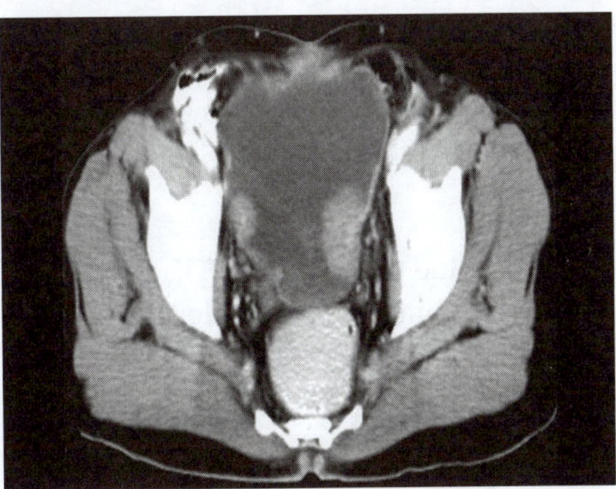

Fig. 58.9: CECT of the bladder showing filling defects in two places suggestive of carcinoma bladder

5. **Cystoscopy:** It is the gold standard investigation to locate the lesion and take a biopsy for further management (Key Box 58.2).

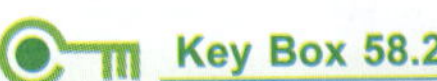

Key Box 58.2

Indications for Cystoscopy

- Haematuria with normal IVU
- Lower urinary tract symptoms
- Malignant cells on urine cytology

6. **Bimanual palpation,** rectoabdominally in males and vaginoabdominally in females, is done under general anaesthesia. Thickening of the bladder wall, mobility, fixity, and hardness can be made out.
7. **Tumour markers:** Urinary markers—BTA and NMP22.

Staging of Bladder Cancer

1. **Clinical staging:** Jewett, Strong and Marshall system
   - Clinically, the tumours are broadly classified into three groups: superficial/noninvasive, infiltrating/invasive, and carcinoma *in situ*.
2. **TNM staging**

TNM STAGING — **Transitional cell carcinoma AJCC 8th edition**

T: Primary tumour

Tx: Primary tumour cannot be detected
T0: No evidence of primary tumour
Ta: Non-invasive papillary tumour
Tis (cis): Carcinoma *in situ* (flat tumour)
T1: Involving subepithelial connective tissue
T2: Involving muscularis propria
T2a: Superficial (inner half)
T2b: Deep (outer half)
T3: Beyond muscularis propria and into perivesical fat
T3a: Microscopic
T3b: Macroscopic (macroscopic mass)
T4: Tumour involving prostate, uterus, vagina, pelvic wall, or abdominal wall
T4a: Prostate, uterus or vagina
T4b: Pelvic wall or abdominal wall

N: Regional lymph nodes

Nx: Cannot be assessed
N0: No regional nodes
N1: Metastasis in single lymph node in true pelvis (hypogastric, obturator, presacral/external iliac)
N2: Multiple lymph nodes in true pelvis
N3: Metastasis in common iliac lymph nodes

M: Metastasis

M0: No metastasis
M1: Distant metastasis
1a: Nonregional lymph nodes
1B: Distant

Treatment of Carcinoma Urinary Bladder

I. **Carcinoma not involving the muscle layer (Tis Ta, T1)**
   1. Transurethral resection of the tumour (resected base to be screened for the tumour by microscopy).
   2. Postoperative intravesical chemotherapy with thiotepa/adriamycin/mitomycin retained inside the bladder for 1 hour: 6–8 courses at weekly intervals to reduce recurrence.
   3. BCG or interferon immunotherapy is given postoperatively intravesically to prevent tumour recurrence.

II. **T2–T4 lesions: Radical cystectomy** followed by systemic chemotherapy (MVAC: Methotrexate, vinblastine, adriamycin, cisplatin).

Radical cystectomy: Removal of the bladder with pericystic fat, prostate, seminal vesicles, and urethra in men, and the bladder with pericystic fat, cervix, uterus, anterior vaginal vault, urethra, and ovaries in women. It is a major surgery with a 3–8% mortality rate.

III. **Any** T, N1, M0 or any T, N0, M1—**systemic chemotherapy (MVAC)** followed by radiation therapy or surgery should be done.

IV. **Small lesion** involving muscles in the vault of the bladder or posterolateral wall of the bladder: **Partial cystectomy** (segmental resection) of the part of the bladder containing the growth with a wide margin of 2–3 cm. This should be followed by intravesical chemotherapy.

Role of Radiotherapy

I. **Local:** If the lesion is not anaplastic and is ≤ 4 cm after open diathermy excision, radiotherapy can be given.

a. Implantation of radioactive Gold grains—^{198}Au
b. Radioactive Tantalum wire—^{192}Ta

II. Deep X-ray therapy

- Indication: Undifferentiated carcinoma
- By using Cobalt 60 or linear accelerator.

EXSTROPHY OF THE BLADDER (ECTOPIA VESICAE)

- A rare congenital anomaly seen in 1:50,000 births
- Male:Female = 4:1

Aetiopathogenesis

- This occurs due to failure of development of the lower abdominal wall and anterior wall of the urinary bladder.
- As a result, the posterior bladder wall is seen protruding out below the umbilicus. Hence, it is exstrophy of the bladder.

Types

1. **Complete:** Pubic symphysis is not formed, complete epispadias in male or bifid clitoris in female.
2. **Incomplete:** Pubic symphysis and penis/clitoris are normal.

Clinical Features (Key Box 58.3)

- More common in male children.
- **Posterior bladder wall is seen in the lower abdomen** as a pink to red mucosa and is partially inflamed.
- Umbilicus is usually absent.
- **Penis is rudimentary,** and epispadias may be present.
- Testis descends normally into a well-developed scrotum.
- **Pubic symphysis is widely separated.** It has an advantage in female patients in that it facilitates delivery.
- In **female children—umbilicus is absent,** external genitalia are poorly developed, and the clitoris is bifid.

Key Box 58.3

Ectopia Vesicae—Clinical Features

- Penis is rudimentary
- Posterior bladder wall is seen in the lower abdomen
- Pubic bone is widely separated
- Poorly developed external genitalia
- Poor health—UTI, renal failure, Ca bladder

- Constant dribbling of urine outside—therefore, patients smell of urine.
- Recurrent urinary tract infection (UTI).
- Rectal prolapse may be present.

Complications

1. Renal failure due to recurrent UTI.
2. Adenocarcinoma of the bladder at an early age (Fig. 58.10).
3. Ammoniacal dermatitis of the skin.

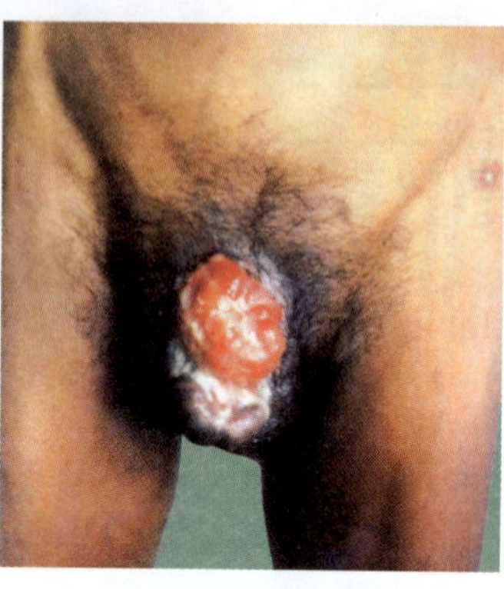

Fig. 58.10: Carcinoma bladder in a case of ectopia vesicae. (*Courtesy:* Dr PS Aralikatti, Associate Professor, BIMS, Belgaum, Karnataka)

Treatment

1. **Early presentation (neonatal or infancy):** Reconstruction of the anterior wall of the bladder with reconstruction of the bladder sphincter (enterocystoplasty).
2. **Complete:** Total cystectomy with urinary diversion by implantation of the ureters in the sigmoid colon (ureterosigmoidostomy) followed by reconstruction of the anterior abdominal wall if the patient has urinary incontinence.

ACUTE CYSTITIS—URINARY TRACT INFECTION (UTI)

Aetiology and Pathogenesis

Acute uncomplicated bacterial cystitis predominantly affects women. By definition, these infections occur in the **absence of any anatomic or functional abnormality** of the urinary tract. The ascending faecal–perineal–urethral route is the primary source of infection. Men are somewhat protected from ascending infection because of their long urethra and the antibacterial properties of prostatic secretions.

Causative Organisms

80% of bladder infections in women are caused by *E. coli* followed by other gram-negative organisms such as Klebsiella and Proteus species.

Clinical Features

Irritative voiding symptoms (frequency, urgency, dysuria) are the hallmarks of cystitis. Low backache and suprapubic pain are other complaints. Fever and other constitutional symptoms are usually present. Physical examination is frequently unremarkable, except for suprapubic tenderness.

Diagnosis

- **Urinary microscopy** is the mainstay of diagnosis. Diagnosis is strongly considered positive if microscopy shows >5 WBCs/high power field in females and 2–3 WBCs/high power field in males.
- **Urine culture** not only confirms the diagnosis but also identifies the causative organisms.
- Other tests and imaging studies are not indicated in uncomplicated infections, unless the patient presents with recurrent episodes.

Management

- Antibiotic therapy for a period of 7–10 days based on the culture and sensitivity report.
- Symptomatic treatment in the form of antipyretics, urinary analgesics, and antispasmodics may help.

DIVERTICULA OF THE BLADDER

Types

- **Congenital (situated midline anterosuperiorly):** Rare and usually asymptomatic. They represent the unobliterated vesical end of the urachus. It may require excision, if chronic infection persists.
- **Acquired:** They are pulsion diverticula and occur due to bladder outflow obstruction. Intravesical pressure is > 150 cm H_2O.

Pathology

- The diverticulum is lined by bladder mucosa.
- The opening (mouth) is situated above and to the outer side of one ureteric orifice.

Clinical Features

- Most common in males (95%) > 50 years of age.
- **Symptoms of recurrent urinary infection:** Suprapubic pain, frequency of micturition, fever with chills, etc.
- **Symptoms of lower urinary obstruction:** Frequency, urgency, hesitancy, etc.
- **Symptoms of pyelonephritis:** Backache, fever, renal angle tenderness, etc.

Pearls of Wisdom

Presence of diverticula is not an indication for surgery.

Investigations

1. **Cystoscopy:** Full bladder distension is necessary to search for diverticulum.
2. **Intravenous urography:** It can detect the site of diverticulum and hydronephrosis (Fig. 58.11).
3. **Ultrasonography**
   - It can detect residual urine.
   - It can detect diverticulum.
   - It can detect associated stone(s).

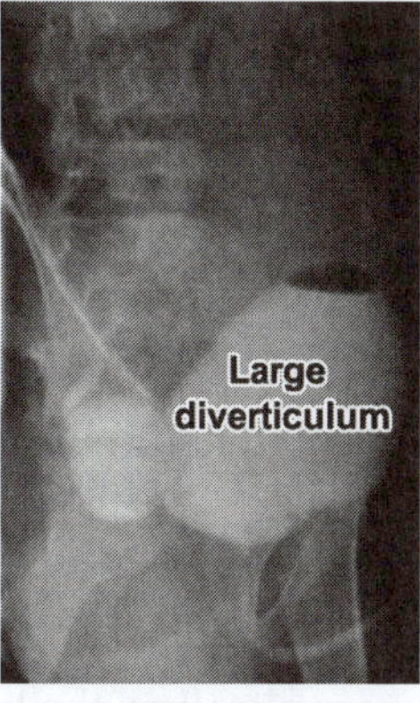

Fig. 58.11: IVU: Bladder diverticulum arising from the posterior wall. Ureter is seen entering the diverticulum

Treatment

- Combined intravesical and extravesical diverticulectomy is done if complications are present.
- Asymptomatic patients are advised to void the urine twice (double voiding).

Complications (Key Box 58.4)

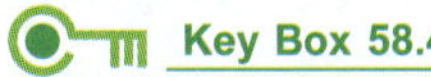 **Key Box 58.4**

Complications of Diverticula of the Bladder

- Recurrent urinary infections
- Bladder stone can occur, which may give rise to haematuria
- Hydronephrosis and hydroureter occur due to peri-diverticular inflammation and fibrosis
- Transitional cell carcinoma
- Neoplasm: Squamous metaplasia and leukoplakia

URINARY FISTULAE

Introduction

Urinary fistulae are not an uncommon problem encountered by surgeons. They are broadly classified into congenital and acquired. Congenital causes are a few (Key Box 58.5), which are discussed in more detail in their respective chapters. Acquired fistulae are more important and are discussed below. Among these, vesicovaginal fistula is discussed in more detail.

Key Box 58.5

Congenital Causes of Congenital Urinary Fistulae

- Ectopia vesicae
- Patent urachus
- Association with imperforate anus

Acquired Fistulae

1. Traumatic Urinary Fistula

Perforating wounds, penetrating wounds, or following pelvic surgery.

2. Vesicovaginal Fistula

Causes

- Protracted or neglected labour
- Gynaecological operations like total hysterectomy and anterior colporrhaphy
- Radiation causing avascular necrosis of the bladder
- Carcinoma cervix infiltrating the bladder.

Pearls of Wisdom

Leakage due to tissue necrosis usually manifests after 7 days.

Clinical features

- Leakage of urine from the vagina
- Excoriation of the vulva

Diagnosis

- Digital vaginal examination may reveal thickening on the anterior wall of the vagina.
- **Vaginal speculum examination:** Dribbling of urine into the vagina.
- **Swab test:** Methylene blue is injected into the urethra. If the vaginal swab is coloured blue, it is a vesicovaginal fistula.

Treatment

- **Low fistula:** Transvaginal repair
- **High fistula:** Suprapubic approach and repair (Modified O'Connor's repair).

3. Fistula from Renal Pelvis to Skin or Gut

- Tuberculosis causes caseation and may result in a fistula in the loin.
- Large staghorn calculi
- Pyonephrosis
- Crohn's disease of the renal pelvis.

INTERSTITIAL CYSTITIS

- It was first described by Guy Hunner (gynaecologist) in 1914 (hence, called Hunner's ulcer). It is also called as bladder pain syndrome.
- Initial symptoms are increased frequency and pain. Pain is relieved by micturition and is aggravated by overdistension of bladder.
- The characteristic linear bleeding ulcer is caused by the splitting of mucosa when the bladder is distended under anaesthesia.
- It is common in Western female patients. Many are psychiatric patients.
- There is severe fibrosis of the urinary bladder due to pancystitis, which results in a **small thimble bladder**. (In India, tuberculosis must be considered.) The capacity of such urinary bladder to store urine is about 30–60 ml.
- Frequency of micturition and pain due to decreased bladder capacity are the features. It causes sterile pyuria.
- Cystoscopy and biopsy confirm the diagnosis.
- Treatment is difficult—hydrostatic dilatation, instillation of dimethyl sulphoxide, or surgical procedures such as ileocystoplasty have been tried.

SCHISTOSOMA HAEMATOBIUM

- It is the most common cause of calcification in the bladder wall.
- It is called urinary bilharziasis.
- The disease is caused by embryos (cercariae) of schistosoma, which enter the body by penetrating the skin and reaching the bladder via the portal vein in a retrograde manner. In the bladder, ova are released and excreted back into fresh water via the urine. Fresh water snail is the intermediate host.
- Multiple pseudotubercles, nodules, granulomas, and fibrosis are the **prominent pathological** features.
- Diagnosis is suspected by painless terminal haematuria, which lasts for 5 days. Itchy skin papules are one of the early manifestations of schistosomiasis. It is known as cercarial dermatitis. Katayama fever refers to fever, itching, splenomegaly, and hepatomegaly during acute schistosomiasis.
- Cystoscopy and biopsy confirm the diagnosis.

- It is treated by long-term praziquantel, and surgery (ileocystoplasty) may be required.

Pearls of Wisdom

Urinary bilharziasis is a premalignant condition.

URINARY DIVERSION

Patients with lower urinary tract cancers or severe functional or anatomic abnormalities of the urinary bladder may require urinary diversion.

The most common method of urinary diversion incorporates various intestinal segments into the urinary tract. Virtually every segment of the intestinal tract is used.

1. **Ileal conduit:** 18–20 cm of the ileum is used as a conduit. Ureters are directly implanted into it. The end of the ileal conduit is brought through the lateral aspect of the rectus abdominis muscle, and a stoma is made. This simply acts as a conduit carrying urine from the renal pelvis or ureter to the skin, where urine is collected in an appliance attached to the skin surface. It is not a continent mechanism.
2. **Ureterosigmoidostomy** is an example of a continent urinary reservoir, wherein the ureters are anastomosed into the sigmoid colon.

Pearls of Wisdom

The most worrisome complication of this procedure is the development of adenocarcinoma at the site of ureter implantation.

- Routine sigmoidoscopy is recommended annually after 5 years of the procedure.
- Newer method of continent diversion—orthotopic bladder substitution.

3. **Nephrostomy:** It is required for drainage and decompression of the upper urinary tract and is indicated in the following situations:
   - Retrograde ureteral catheterisation is not advisable (e.g. in sepsis secondary to ureteral obstruction).
   - Retrograde ureteral catheterisation is impossible (e.g. complete ureteral obstruction by stone, tumour, or stricture).
   - It is done by a percutaneous approach.
4. **Ureteroureterostomy:** It is the anastomosis of the ureter to the ureter following resection. It can be on the same side if the resection length of the ureter is ≤4 cm or to the opposite ureter if the resection length is >4 cm.

Indications

a. Trauma to the ureter

b. Ureteric involvement by neoplastic conditions (e.g. colonic carcinoma, which requires urteric resection).
   - Mainly indicated for upper and midureteral involvement. The procedure of choice for lower ureteric involvement is reimplantation into the bladder.

RUPTURE OF THE URINARY BLADDER

Causes of Urinary Bladder Rupture

1. **Surgical (iatrogenic):** Bladder can be injured mostly during pelvic surgery (e.g. excision of the rectum) or during gynaecological procedures.
2. **Trauma:** Blunt injury to the abdomen due to road traffic accidents.
   - Kick or blow on the abdomen with a full bladder
   - Penetrating injury (extremely rare).

Types of Rupture and Clinical Features

I. Intraperitoneal Rupture

When there is surgical trauma or trauma to a distended bladder, the rupture will be intraperitoneal (Fig. 58.12A).

Clinical features

- Sudden, severe suprapubic pain, hypotension/syncope, and shock.
- Lower abdominal guarding and rigidity occur after a few hours of injury.
- Distension
- Even though the patient has not passed urine for a few hours, there is no desire to micturate.
- Shifting dullness may be elicitable.

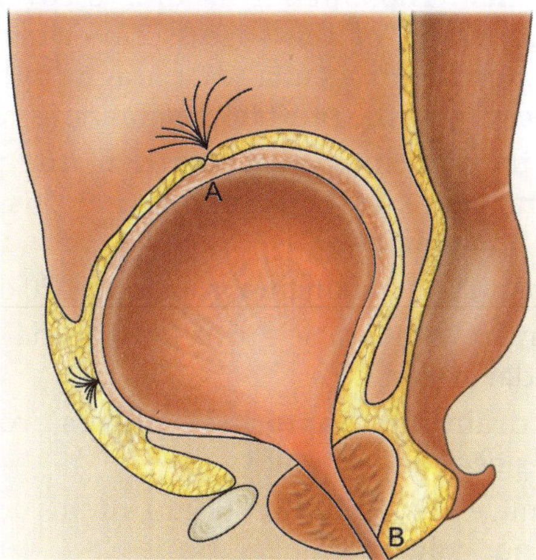

Fig. 58.12: Rupture bladder: (A) Intraperitoneal; (B) Extraperitoneal

II. Extraperitoneal Rupture (Fig. 58.12B)

- Trauma—penetrating or blunt injury with fracture of pubis gives rise to this type of injury.
- Difficult to distinguish clinically from an injury to the membranous urethra.

Investigations

1. **Plain X-ray abdomen:** Lower abdomen shows a ground glass appearance.
2. **IVP:** Extravasation of dye into the peritoneal cavity or extraperitoneally.
3. CT cystogram is the investigation of choice.

Treatment

1. **Intraperitoneal rupture:** Laparotomy and repair of the bladder in two layers with vicryl. Drain the suprapubic space with a tube drain. An indwelling urethral catheter has to be placed for 10 days to 2 weeks to keep the bladder decompressed.
2. **Extraperitoneal rupture:** Extraperitoneally expose the bladder with a suprapubic midline incision and repair the bladder. Drainage, as mentioned above, should be carried out.

Competency

SU29.11: Describe the clinical features, investigations and management of urethral strictures.

Please note: Read all about urethral injuries.

SURGICAL ANATOMY OF THE URETHRA (Fig. 58.13)

- The male urethra is divided into an anterior urethra (*bulbopenile*) and a posterior urethra (*prostatomembranous urethra*).
- The male urethra **functions as a conduit for urine and semen.** The anterior urethra is covered with erectile tissue of the corpus cavernosum and penetrates the urogenital diaphragm to enter the pelvic cavity as the prostatomembranous urethra.
- Since its margins are attached to the perineal membrane, it is **vulnerable to tear at this point in pelvic bone fracture.**
- Length of the male urethra is about 18–20 cm.
- The entire urethra is supplied by the internal pudendal artery.
- Veins drain into **Santorini's plexus** around the bladder neck and prostate.
- The female urethra is short (4 cm), drains only urine, and is not vulnerable to injuries.
- The narrowest part of the male urethra is the external meatus.

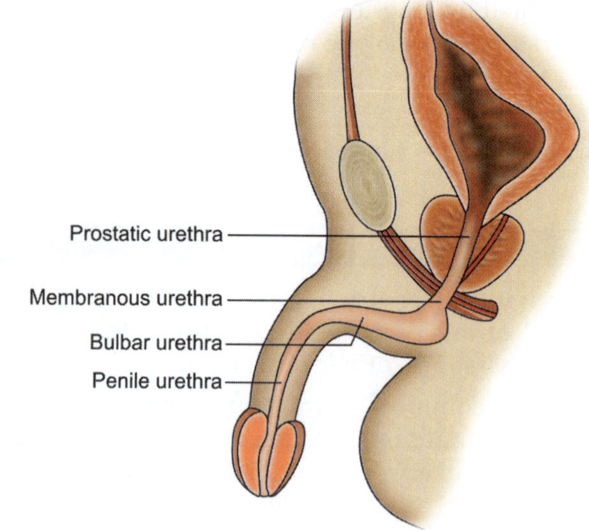

Fig. 58.13: Surgical anatomy of the urethra

- The prostatic urethra has two sphincters at each end. The internal sphincter at the bladder neck is composed of smooth muscle fibres, and **the external sphincter** is a rhabdosphincter about 2 cm long that surrounds the membranous urethra.
- Normally, urinary continence is maintained by the external sphincter. When the external sphincter is damaged (e.g. trauma, surgery) the internal sphincter maintains continence but to a lesser degree.
- Continence is not affected by ablation of the internal sphincter (e.g. post-transurethral resection of the prostate; TURP), but it **results in retrograde** ejaculation (i.e., the semen goes back into the bladder instead of exiting through the urethra).

RUPTURE URETHRA

Types

I. Rupture Bulbar Urethra

- The most common urethral injury.
- Urethra angulates in the perineum, where it gets injured.
- Superficial extravasation of urine.

Clinical triad

1. Perineal haematoma
2. **Urethral haemorrhage:** Blood at the urethral meatus
3. **Distended bladder:** Diagnosed by percussion over the suprapubic region which gives a dull note.

Treatment

- **Advise the patient to try avoiding the passage of urine.**
- Urinary antibiotics

- Shift to the operation theatre, and with aseptic precautions, gently pass a catheter. If it enters the bladder, it is kept in place **for 2 weeks, and the perineal haematoma is drained**.
- If unable to pass the catheter, **emergency suprapubic cystostomy/catheterization** is done to drain the urine, and repair of the urethra is done later.

II. Rupture Membranous Urethra

- Associated (70%) with fracture of the pelvis.
- Occurs in major road traffic accidents.
- There may be disruption of the pelvic bones and fracture symphysis pubis with avulsion of the puboprostatic ligament, leading to floating prostate.
- Deep extravasation of urine.

Types of rupture membranous urethra

1. **Complete transection** results in floating bladder. In this condition, the urethra is completely transected at the apex of the prostate. As the puboprostatic ligament is avulsed, the prostate falls back and migrates upwards. On rectal examination, the prostate is felt as though it is floating—**floating prostate (Vermooten's sign)** (Fig. 58.14).
2. **Incomplete transection**
3. **Associated with injury** to the bladder: Extraperitoneal rupture of the bladder is seen here. (Intraperitoneal rupture of bladder occurs in a distended bladder.)

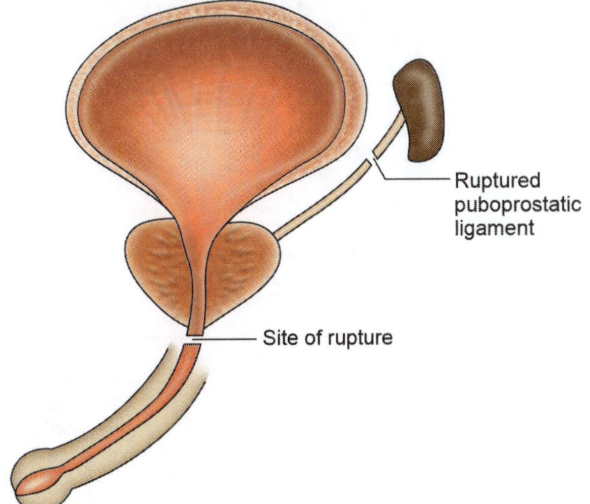

Fig. 58.14: Rupture of membranous urethra with floating prostate (Vermooten's sign). Note the ruptured puboprostatic ligaments

Clinical Features

- History of injury
- Features of shock due to significant blood loss (around 1–2 litres)
- Haematuria
- In cases of extraperitoneal rupture of the bladder, it will not be palpable due to extravasation of urine into the perineum.
- Suprapubic tenderness and dullness

Rectal examination: Floating prostate can be felt and is tender.

Investigations

1. X-ray pelvic bones may show a fracture or separation of the pubic symphysis.
2. Ascending urethrography (ASU) to confirm the rupture (Fig. 58.15).
3. Once the stricture develops, voiding cystourethrogram (VCUG) is done to know the exact location and length of the stricture.

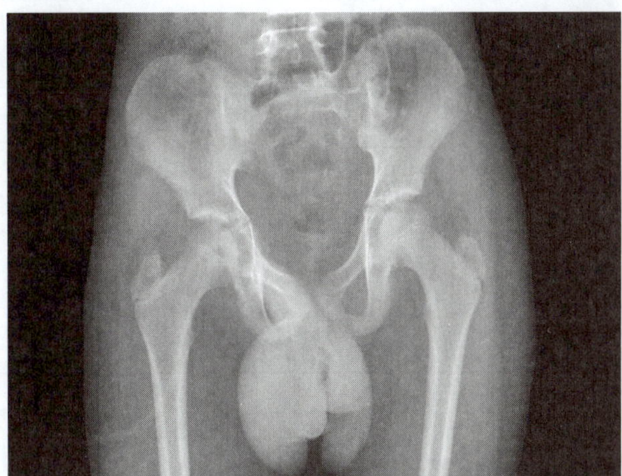

Fig. 58.15: Plain X-ray showing extravasation of dye

Treatment (Figs 58.16 and 58.17)

- Urgent blood transfusion to treat shock.
- Suprapubic cystostomy is done, and the degree of damage is assessed.
- A bougie/sound is passed from above and another similar sound is passed through the external meatus (penis). When the two meet, a click is appreciated. With both sounds in contact, the sound from the bladder is slowly withdrawn. The lower one is advanced at this stage, and a second sound appears in the bladder. A red rubber catheter is tied to it, and the sound is withdrawn through the external meatus.
- To this red rubber catheter which is seen outside, a Foley catheter is tied and is drawn into the bladder and kept in place for 15 days **(rail roading technique; progressive perineal urethroplasty)**.
- Associated injuries, such as rupture bladder, are treated by suturing.
- Antibiotics are given.

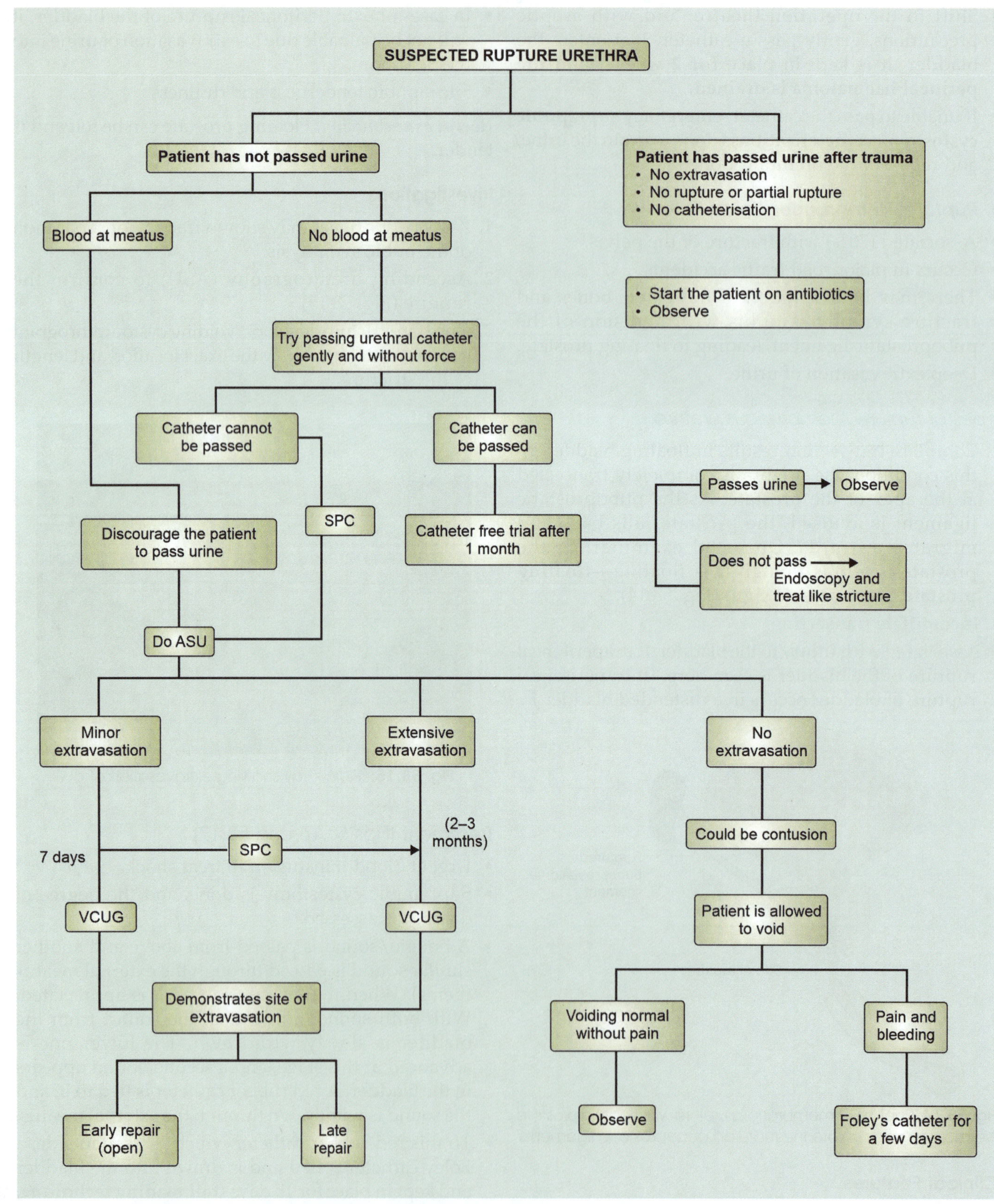

Fig. 58.16: Algorithm for managing bulbar urethral rupture (*Courtesy:* Dr Vikas Jain, Assistant Professor, Department of Surgery, KMC, Manipal, 2007–2008).

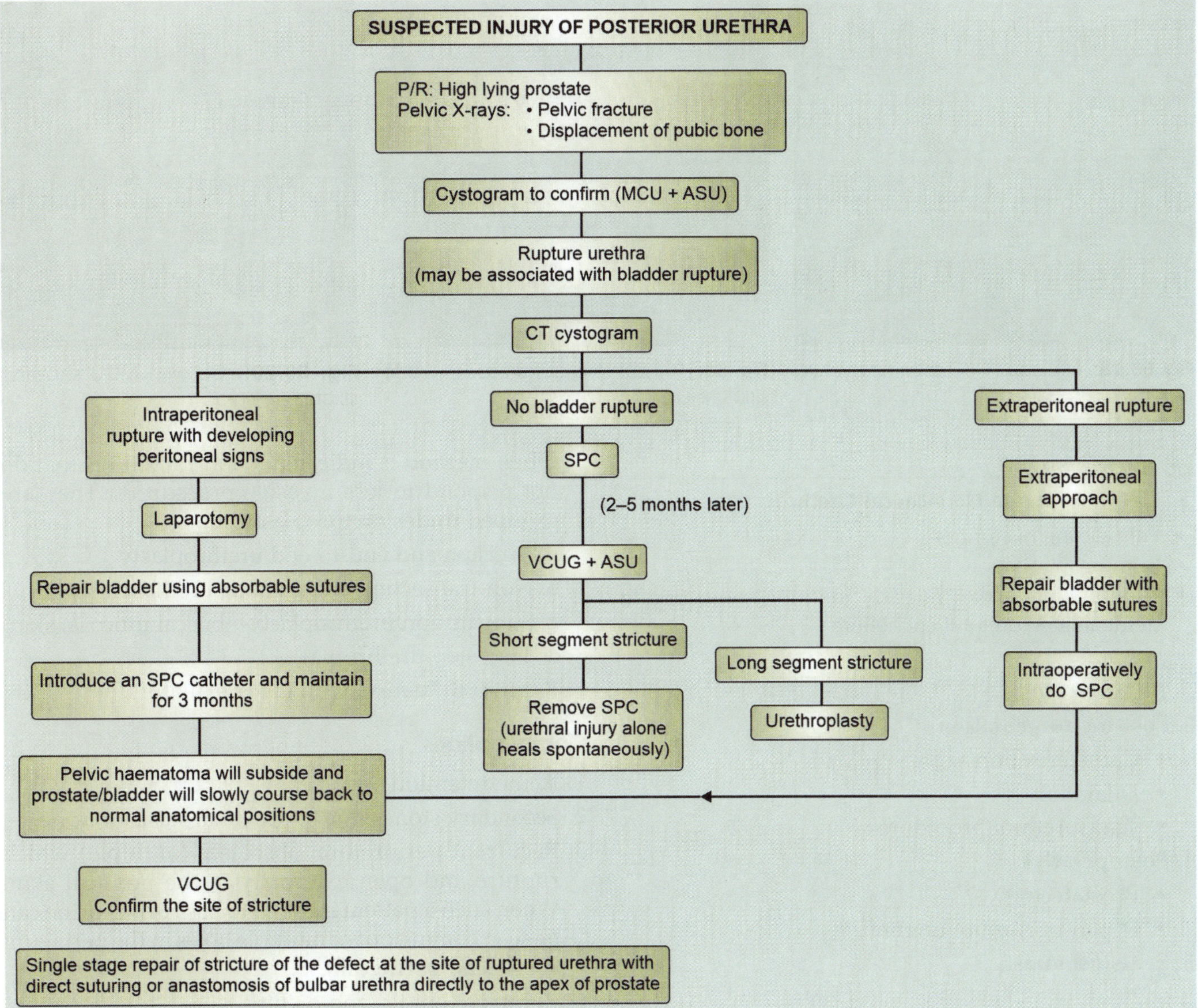

Fig. 58.17: Algorithm for managing posterior urethral rupture (*Courtesy:* Dr Vikas Jain, Assistant Professor, Department of Surgery, KMC, Manipal)

Complications of Rupture Urethra

The most dangerous complication is stricture urethra (Key Box 58.6).

Key Box 58.6

Complications of Rupture Urethra

1. Extravasation of urine into the scrotum, beneath the superficial fascia of the penis, and beneath Scarpa's fascia
2. Urethral stricture
3. Haematoma
4. Recurrent urinary tract infection

STRICTURE URETHRA

Causes (Figs 58.18–58.20)

1. **Congenital—very rare**
2. **Post-inflammatory**

A. Post-gonococcal urethritis

- Within 48 hours of exposure to the venereal disease gonorrhoea, periurethral gland involvement occurs. These are concentrated more in the bulbar urethra, so strictures are more common at this site.
- It causes periurethral fibrosis, resulting in multiple dense strictures within 1 year of infection but may not cause difficulty in micturition for 10–15 years (Key Box 58.7).

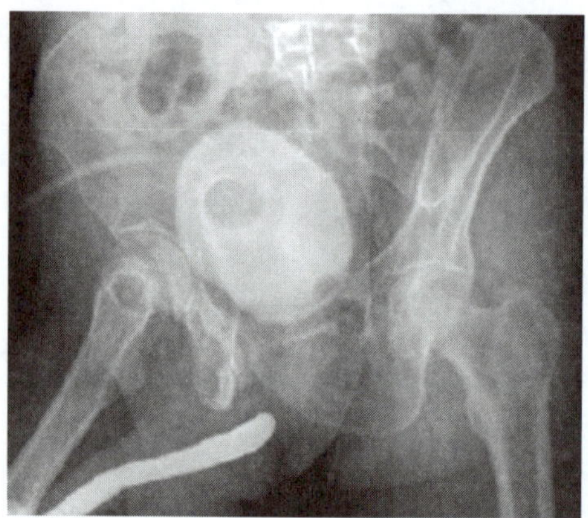
Fig. 58.18: ASU and VCUG showing stricture urethra

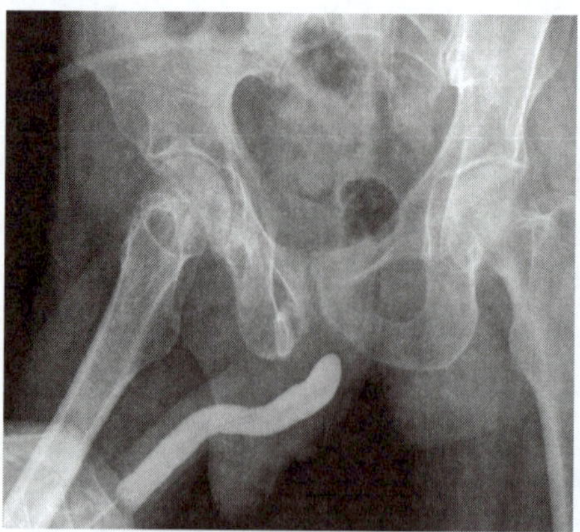
Fig. 58.19: ASU: Total cut off seen due to stricture urethra

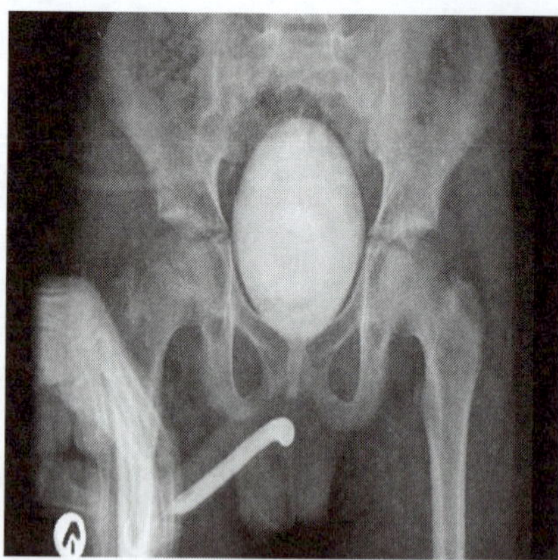
Fig. 58.20: ASU with MCU showing stricture urethra

Key Box 58.7

Acute Gonococcal Urethritis

- Pain during micturition
- Burning micturition
- Gleet: White flakes in early morning urine due to desquamated urethral epithelium

B. Tuberculosis

3. **Post-instrumentation**
   - Catheterisation
   - Dilatation
   - Transurethral procedures
4. **Postoperative**
   - Prostatectomy
   - Repair of rupture urethra
5. **Schistosomiasis**

Clinical Features

Previous history of exposure to gonorrhoea, history of instrumentation, or history of trauma to the urethra is usually present.

- Common in young age (20–40 years).
- History of straining while passing urine.
- Suprapubic pain and swelling due to distended bladder.
- Stricture urethra may be felt in the perineum as a button hole.

It should be remembered that gonococcal urethritis is not common nowadays because of effective treatment for the disease.

Treatment

Usually cut at 12 O' clock position.

1. **Visual internal urethrotomy (VIU)** by using a urethrotome.
2. **Open method** is indicated in long strictures that do not respond to less invasive procedures. They are grouped under urethroplasty.
   a. Excision and end-to-end urethroplasty
   b. Non-transecting anastomotic urethroplasty
   c. Substitution urethroplasty—buccal mucosa, skin
   d. Two-step urethroplasty
3. **Regular dilatation** with Lister's dilators.

Complications

1. Acute retention of urine.
2. Secondary stones due to proximal stasis of urine.
3. Recurrent periurethral abscesses (multiple) which rupture and open externally in the perineal skin. When such a patient is asked to pass urine, urine can be seen coming out of multiple holes in the perineum **(Watercan perineum)**.
4. Recurrent epididymo-orchitis.

HYPOSPADIAS

In this condition, some portion of the distal urethra is not developed, resulting in the external meatus being situated in the under surface of the penis. Usually, this is associated with chordee and hooded prepuce.

Types (Fig. 58.21)

1. **Glandular variety:** The external meatus is situated a few mm away from the normal site within the glans.
2. **Coronal variety**
   - It occurs due to failure of the development of the urethra that runs in the glans penis.
   - As a result of this, the urethra opens at the corona glandis—junction of the glans and shaft of the penis.

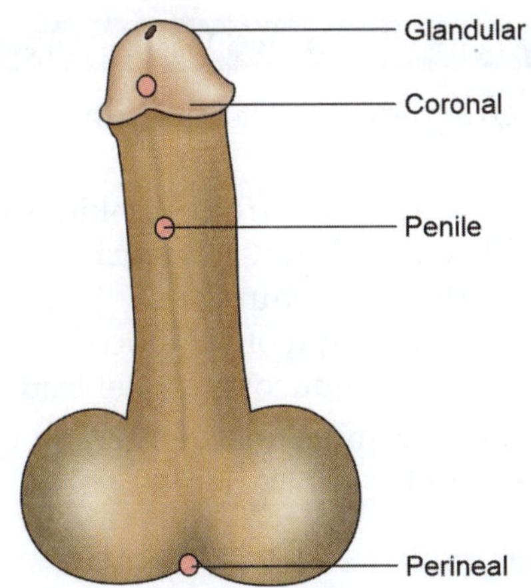

Fig. 58.21: Various types of hypospadias

- Both these varieties do not give major functional problems. It can be left alone without treatment.

3. **Penile hypospadias:** The external opening is situated somewhere in the under surface of the penis.
4. **Penoscrotal/perineal hypospadias**
   - In this condition, the entire urethra is not developed.
   - The penis is rudimentary.
   - The urethral opening is seen between two halves of the scrotum and is often split.
   - Cases may be associated with undescended testes.
   - In such cases, it is difficult to differentiate the sex of the child.

Clinical Features

- Occurs in 1:350 males.
- Micturition: Stream is good, but it wets the clothes in the third and fourth varieties.
- Chordee: Many cases are associated with bending of the penis.
- Sexual intercourse will be difficult.
- Hooded prepuce.

In severe hypospadias, the possibility of sexual differentiation disorders is settled by **karyotyping**.

Treatment

1. **One-stage urethroplasty**
   - Chordee correction: Always confirm by inducing artificial erection
   - Urethral tube formation by tubularising the urethra
   - Inner prepuceal island tube urethroplasty.
2. **Two-stage urethroplasty**
   - When the child is 6–12 months old, chordee is corrected by straightening the penis (orthoplasty).
   - When the child is 5–6 years old, reconstruction of the urethra is done using locally available skin either from the prepuce or the penile shaft (urethroplasty). Hence, circumcision should not be done in hypospadias.

Competency

SU29.7: Describe the principles of management of acute and chronic retention of urine.

DIFFERENTIAL DIAGNOSIS OF URINARY RETENTION

Causes of Urinary Retention

I. Acute Urinary Retention

A. In males

- **Benign prostatic hypertrophy (BPH):** In elderly patients > 50 years of age.
- **Stricture urethra:** In young patients.
- **Postoperative retention of urine:** Operations like haemorrhoidectomy, fistulectomy, etc., produce reflex spasm of the internal sphincter, which precipitates urinary retention. The management of such cases is given in Key Box 58.8.

Key Box 58.8

Postoperative Retention of Urine: Treatment

1. Hot water fomentation to the suprapubic region
2. Provide privacy
3. Run a tap nearby
4. Make the patient stand and pass urine
5. Catheterisation should be done as a last resort

B. In females

- Hysteria
- Retroverted gravid uterus
- Urethral stenosis

C. In children: Meatal stenosis due to meatal ulcer with a scab (due to scratching by the child).

D. In general

- Spinal anaesthesia
- Spinal injuries
- Blood clot in the bladder following prostatectomy
- Bladder stone in school-going children: Pain referred to the tip of the penis
- Acute urethritis and acute prostatitis due to bacterial infection
- Faecal impaction in the rectum
- Contracture of the bladder neck
- Urethral calculus
- Drugs: Atropine, carbachol, bethanechol.

II. Chronic Urinary Retention (Key Box 58.9)

1. Benign prostatic hypertrophy
2. Bladder neck contracture
3. Stricture urethra

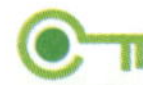 Key Box 58.9

Chronic Retention of Urine

- BPH: Most common cause
- Painless
- Suprapubic dullness
- Slow decompression is recommended

Residual urine

It is significant if > 40% of voided volume is present. Differential diagnoses include BPH, stricture urethra, and underactive bladder.

POSTERIOR URETHRAL VALVE (PUV)

- They are congenital, **symmetrical valves** in the posterior urethra.
- It is a **common cause of vesicoureteric reflux** and hydronephrosis in infants.
- The bladder wall is thickened due to obstruction and hypertrophy. The urinary bladder is palpable, hard, and felt in the suprapubic region—**cricket ball bladder.**
- Due to stasis, recurrent UTI commonly occurs.
- It is also a **common cause of renal failure** in infancy and childhood.

Investigations

- **Ultrasound:** Bilateral hydronephrosis, thickened bladder, etc.
- **Micturating cystourethrography (MCU):** Dilated proximal urethra is highly suggestive of posterior urethral valve. It is a diagnostic investigation.

Treatment

- Cystoscopic posterior urethral valve fulguration.
- In very ill patients, vesicostomy is done initially to improve renal function and stabilise the patient. Fulguration is done after 1–2 weeks.
- These patients should be monitored for renal failure by serial creatinine measurements.

Pearls of Wisdom

PUV may be associated with anorectal and vertebral malformations.

VESICOURETERIC REFLUX (VUR)

VUR is the retrograde flow of urine from the bladder to the kidneys.

Normally, urine flows from the kidneys into the bladder, and backward flow is prevented by complex anatomy at the vesicoureteric junction, most importantly a good length of submucosal tunnel of the ureter. Inadequate submucosal tunnel leads to VUR.

VUR can be of a mild to severe grade (graded I—mild to V—severe).

Clinical Features

- The child may be diagnosed with hydronephrosis antenatally, depending on the severity of reflux.
- **Recurrent UTI:** It is due to the increased amount of residual urine. When the child voids, some urine refluxes back into the kidneys, which comes back into the bladder after voiding ceases. This leads to high post-void residue (PVR) and causes recurrent infections.
- **Pyelonephritis and scarring:** Reflux of infected urine causes pyelonephritis. It can be acute or chronic. Recurrent episodes can lead to kidney scarring and decreased function, proteinuria, and hypertension. Severe scarring bilaterally may lead to chronic renal failure (CRF) and end-stage renal disease (ESRD).

Investigations

- **Urine analysis** for proteinuria and infection.
- **Complete blood picture:** Anaemia in CRF and leukocytosis in acute pyelonephritis.
- **Renal function tests:** Increased urea and creatinine in renal failure.
- **USG:** Renal size, parenchyma and hydroureteronephrosis with PVR can be assessed.
- **MCU or VCUG:** Investigation of choice for diagnosis (Figs 58.22–58.25). Procedure: Bladder is filled with contrast after catheterisation, and X-rays are taken during filling and with full bladder to look for reflux. After a full bladder, the catheter is removed, the patient is asked to void, and X-rays are taken in the voiding phase.
- **DMSA scan:** For the extent of renal scarring and function. Helps in choosing the management strategy (medical vs surgical).

Treatment

I. **Conservative management:** Low-grade reflux (grades I–III) can be managed conservatively. The aims of conservative therapy include:
   - Prophylactic/suppressive antibiotics.

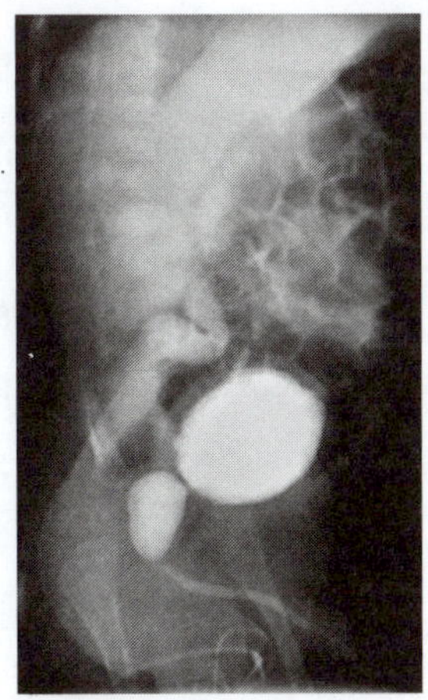

Fig. 58.22: PUV with grade IV vesicoureteric reflux

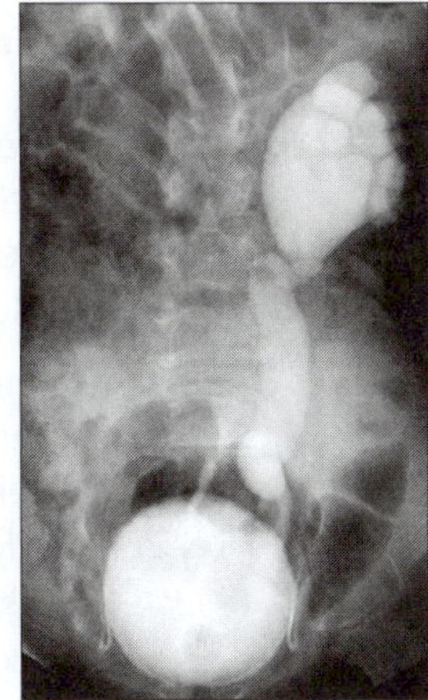

Fig. 58.23: MCU showing grade V vesicoureteric reflux

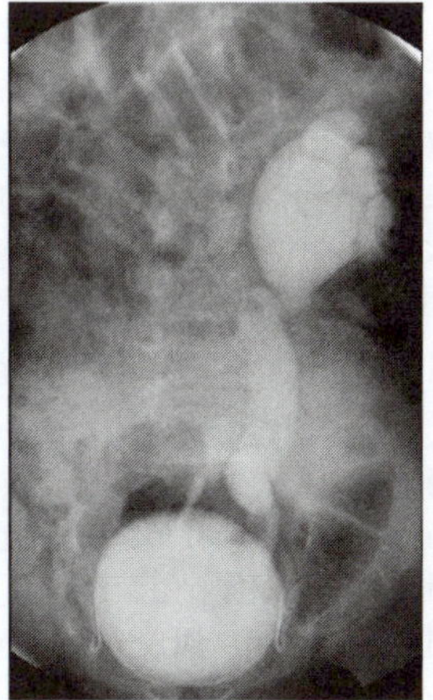

Fig. 58.24: MCU showing bilateral vesicoureteric reflux

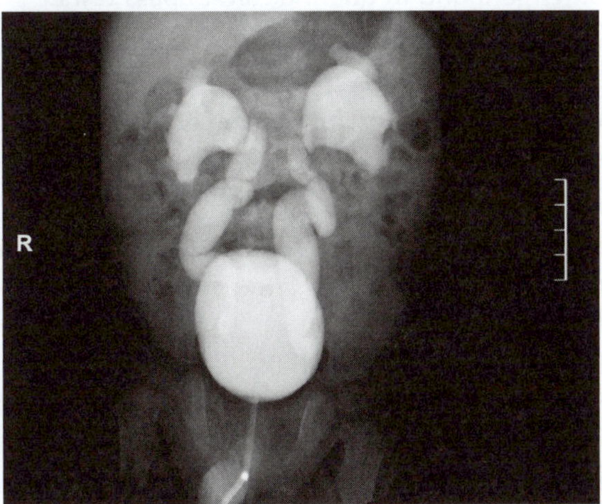

Fig. 58.25: MCU showing bilateral grade V vesicoureteric reflux

- Regular or timed voiding and double voiding to keep PVR as low as possible.
- To avoid constipation—reduces the incidence of UTI.
- With these measures, most low-grade refluxes resolve spontaneously.
- Higher-grade refluxes require endoscopic or surgical management.

II. **Endoscopic management:** Injection of a bulking agent to provide support to the VUJ helps in a few cases.

III. **Surgical management:** Ureteric reimplantation is done for high-grade reflux. The principle of surgery is to lengthen the submucosal tunnel. If one kidney is poorly functioning, nephrectomy can be done.

In some cases, bilaterally scarred, nonfunctioning kidneys may lead to ESRD. These patients require renal transplantation.

MISCELLANEOUS

INVESTIGATION OF CHOICE

- In carcinoma bladder—cystoscopy
- In rupture bladder—CT cystogram
- In rupture urethra—ASU
- In posterior urethral valve—MCU
- In vesicoureteric reflux—MCU or VCUG

Clinical Notes

A 45-year-old multiparous female was diagnosed with bladder stone. She also had pain in her genitalia for which she underwent dilatation and curettage. On dilatation, the tail of Cu-T with thread was seen in the uterus. On trying to remove the Cu-T, only the thread could be extracted. She underwent laparotomy. The uterus was found adherent to the urinary bladder. On opening the bladder, a stone of 6 × 6 cm with Cu-T impregnated in it was present. The Cu-T had perforated the anterior wall of the uterus and the posterior wall of the bladder. It was removed. (*Courtesy:* Prof Rajiv Shetty, Prof Shivaswamy, Prof Durganna, Bangalore Medical College, Bengaluru, Fig. 58.3B on page 1065)

Multiple Choice Questions

1. **The following types of malignant tumour can occur in the urinary bladder *except*:**
   A. Transitional carcinoma
   B. Adenocarcinoma
   C. Squamous cell carcinoma
   D. Leiomyosarcoma
2. **The following are true regarding the internal sphincter of the urinary bladder *except*:**
   A. It is a smooth muscle
   B. It is innervated by adrenergic fibres
   C. It prevents retrograde ejaculation
   D. It is supplied by the pudendal nerve
3. **Cystine calculi in the urinary bladder are radiopaque because of:**
   A. High calcium content
   B. High sulphur content
   C. High triple phosphate content
   D. High oxalate content
4. **The following are clinical features of urinary bladder stones *except*:**
   A. Pain referred to the testis
   B. Pain aggravated by jumping
   C. Strangury
   D. Haematuria
5. **Which of the following parasitic infestations is a strong risk factor for carcinoma urinary bladder?**
   A. Bilharziasis B. Ascariasis
   C. Leishmaniasis D. Clonorchis sinensis
6. **The following are true for carcinoma urinary bladder *except*:**
   A. Aniline dye workers are at high risk
   B. Transitional cell carcinomas are more common
   C. It presents with strangury
   D. Adenocarcinoma is due to bilharziasis
7. **The following are true in ectopia vesicae *except*:**
   A. Penis is normal
   B. Posterior wall of the urinary bladder is seen
   C. Pubic symphysis is widely separated
   D. Adenocarcinoma of the urinary bladder occurs very early
8. **The most common organism causing acute cystitis is:**
   A. *E.coli* B. Klebsiella
   C. Proteus D. Pseudomonas
9. **The following are causes for vesicovaginal fistula *except*:**
   A. Protracted labour B. Anterior colporrhaphy
   C. Radiation D. Crohn's disease
10. **The most worrying complication following ureterosigmoidostomy is:**
    A. Acidosis
    B. Adenocarcinoma
    C. Alkalosis
    D. Recurrent infection and septicaemia
11. **Which of the following is not a feature of intraperitoneal rupture of the urinary bladder?**
    A. Shock
    B. Urgent and frequent desire to pass urine
    C. Suprapubic pain
    D. Hypotension
12. **Which is the narrowest portion of the male urethra?**
    A. Penile urethra B. External meatus
    C. Perineal ureth D. Bulbar urethra
13. **Which of the following is not part of the triad of bulbar urethral rupture?**
    A. Perineal haematoma
    B. Blood at the urethral meatus
    C. Distended bladder
    D. Floating prostate
14. **What is the first advice given to patients with bulbar urethral rupture?**
    A. Blood transfusion
    B. Intravenous antibiotics
    C. Avoid passing urine
    D. Immediate catheterisation
15. **Floating prostate—Vermooten's sign is classical of:**
    A. Rupture bulbar urethra
    B. Rupture penile urethra
    C. Rupture intraperitoneal urinary bladder
    D. Rupture membranous urethra
16. **Which of the following is true for posterior urethral valves?**
    A. They are acquired
    B. Bladder is thin-walled and more prone for rupture
    C. Renal failure is uncommon
    D. They are symmetrical

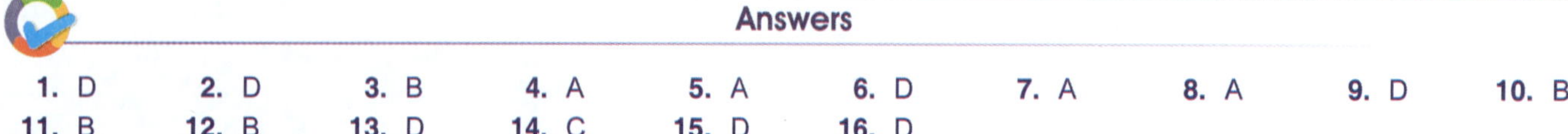

Answers

1. D **2.** D **3.** B **4.** A **5.** A **6.** D **7.** A **8.** A **9.** D **10.** B
11. B **12.** B **13.** D **14.** C **15.** D **16.** D

CHAPTER

59

Prostate and Seminal Vesicles

- Surgical anatomy
- Structural anatomy
- Benign prostatic hyperplasia (BPH)
- Carcinoma of the prostate
- Gleason score
- Prostatitis

Competency

SU29.9: Describe the clinical features, investigations and principles of management of disorders of the prostate.

SURGICAL ANATOMY

EMBRYOLOGY AND LOBES

- The prostate develops around the 12th week of intrauterine life. Primitive buds from the urethra form the glandular tissue and surrounding mesenchyme forms the fibromuscular stroma. Developmentally, the prostate has 5 lobes: Anterior, posterior, middle and 2 lateral lobes.
- **The middle lobe (median lobe)** is situated between the two ejaculatory ducts and the urethra. The enlargement of this lobe in benign prostatic hypertrophy (BPH) is responsible for urethral obstruction. This lobe enlarges upwards into the bladder (Fig. 59.1).
- In BPH, the glands of the inner adenomatous zone hypertrophy and lead to urinary outflow obstruction. **Carcinoma usually occurs in the outer non-adenomatous zone (Fig. 59.2).**
- New terminology for the BPH-arising zone is the **transitional zone** and the carcinoma-arising zone is the **peripheral zone**. Based on McNeal's zonal anatomy, in addition to the transition and peripheral zones, three more zones have been identified: The central zone, periurethral glandular tissue, and anterior fibromuscular stroma.

STRUCTURAL ANATOMY

- The prostatic urethra is surrounded by a fibroadenomatous gland.
- Urethral glands open into the prostatic urethra. These **submucosal glands are responsible for BPH.**
- When the prostate enlarges, it compresses the outer zone, resulting in a false capsule.

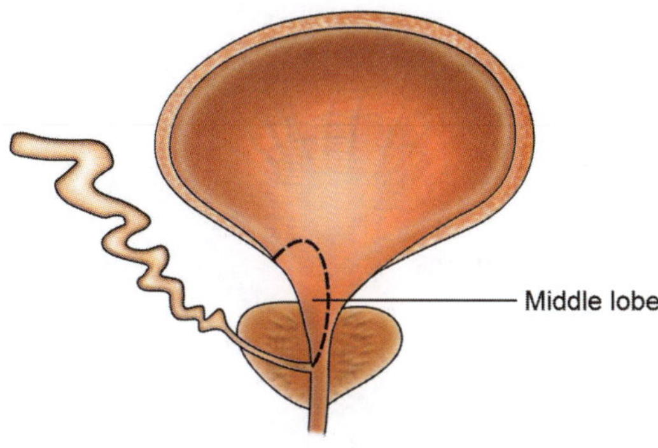

Fig. 59.1: Prostate—lobes

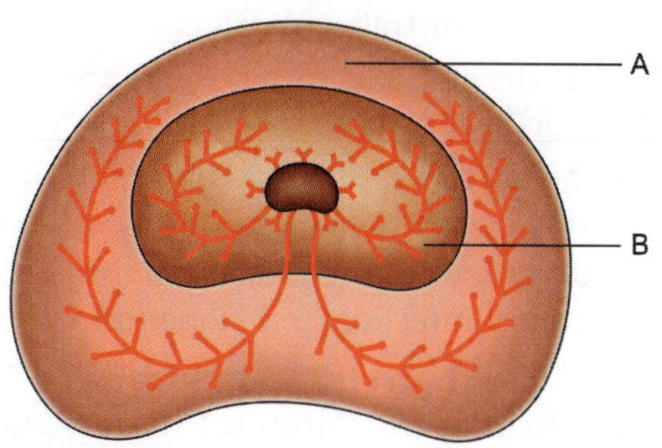

Fig. 59.2: Prostate: (A) Outer carcinomatous zone, (B) Inner adenomatous zone

- The **outermost zone** is the zone of prostatic glands proper, which is responsible for **carcinoma prostate**.
- Surrounding this, there is **fascia of Denonvilliers** which is a part of the pelvic peritoneum. This is also called the fascia that separates wind and water. (wind in the rectum and water in the bladder).
- Between the anatomical capsule and pelvic peritoneum, the prostatic venous plexus is present, which may give rise to massive haemorrhage, if injured.

BENIGN PROSTATIC HYPERPLASIA (BPH)

AETIOPATHOGENESIS

- BPH is a true hyperplastic process.

Hormonal theory: Causes of BPH are multifactorial. However, it is mainly endocrinal. The prostate maintains its ability to respond to androgens throughout life.

- It has been compared to fibroadenosis in female patients.
- As age advances, the levels of androgens come down. There is a corresponding increase in oestrogen, which stimulates the prostatic gland and produces BPH.
- There is proliferation of all elements of the prostate (fibrous, muscular, and glandular) resulting in fibromyoadenoma.
- Stromal and epitheloid elements give rise to hyperplastic nodules.

SECONDARY EFFECTS OF BPH

1. **Urethral changes**
   - Urethra gets **compressed and, elongated and gets converted into a narrow, longitudinal slit**.
   - The effect is more with median lobe enlargement due to enlargement of the subcervical glands.
   - Lateral lobes enlarge when there is involvement of the submucous glands.
2. **Changes in the bladder** (Fig. 59.3) (Key Box 59.1)
   - As a result of obstruction, the bladder musculature undergoes hypertrophy. Very prominent thick bundles of the muscle can be seen, which are called fasciculations or **trabeculations**.
   - Between the fasciculations, there are depressed areas called **sacculations**.
   - Since the sacculi are thin, as pressure increases, herniation occurs outside, resulting in diverticuli.
   - In the diverticuli, there is stasis of urine, resulting in secondary infection and stone formation.
3. **Changes in the ureter and kidney:** Bilateral hydronephrosis and bilateral hydro-ureter are the end result of BPH, which may result in renal failure.

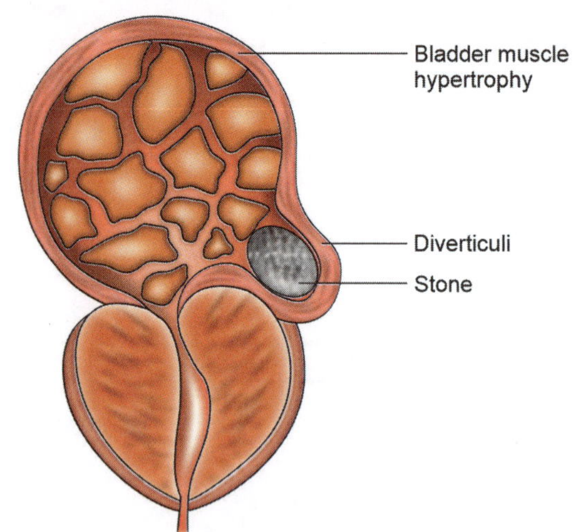

Fig. 59.3: Secondary changes in the urinary bladder due to BPH

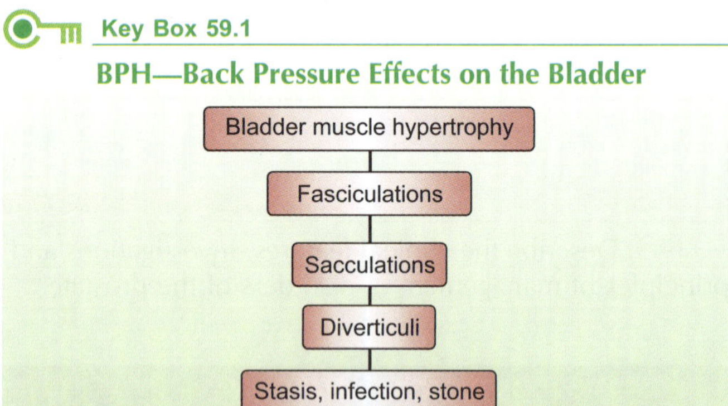

CLINICAL FEATURES OF BPH (Key Box 59.2)

- **Frequency, urgency, and hesitancy form the triad of BPH.**
  - *Frequency:* Frequency is present during the daytime followed by during the day and night (5–10 times during the night). It is due to ineffective emptying of the bladder. It results in residual urine in the bladder and precipitates cystitis.
  - *Urgency:* As the prostate enlarges, there is **vesical introversion of the sensitive mucous membrane**

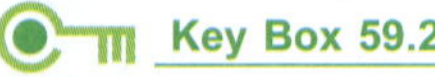

Key Box 59.2

FUN PISS

Irritative symptoms
- Frequency
- Urgency
- Nocturia

Obstructive symptoms
- Poor stream
- Intermittency
- Straining
- Sense of incomplete emptying

of the prostatic urethra within the bladder. This causes the internal sphincter to stretch and prevents contraction. Resulting in a few drops of urine trickling down the posterior urethra, causing an urgent desire to pass urine (urgency).

- *Hesitancy:* Hesitation to pass urine occurs because obstruction makes it ineffective.

- **Haematuria is rare:** It is due to congestion of the prostatic venous plexuses resulting in hyperaemia and haematuria. In a patient with haematuria and BPH, haema-turia can be due to other causes (e.g. co-existing bladder cancer). In such situations, the prostate is an innocent bystander, hence called "decoy prostate."
- **BPH with acute retention of urine:** This occurs due to postponement of micturition, following alcohol or drugs like mydriatics.
- **BPH with chronic retention of urine:** Many patients present with **chronic retention** of urine, with painless enlargement of the urinary bladder.
- **International Prostate Symptom Score (IPSS):** It can range from 0–35. Mild: 0–7, moderate: 8–19, severe: 20–35.

COMPLICATIONS

- Stones: 8 times more common
- Diverticuli
- Renal failure
- Recurrent UTI: It is the most common cause of surgical intervention.

DIAGNOSIS OF BPH

Digital rectal examination: Enlarged lateral lobes can be easily felt. Rectal mucosa is free and firm. (In an enlarged prostate, in case of carcinoma prostate, the mucosa of the rectum cannot be moved, if there infiltration into the rectum.)

Grading of prostate is as follows (Roger Barnes' grading by digital rectal examination):

I. Prostatic lobes protrude minimally into the rectal lumen by 1–2 cm, and the median sulcus is palpable.
II. Prostatic lobes protrude 2–3 cm into the rectal lumen and the median sulcus is obliterated.
III. Prostatic lobes protrude 3–4 cm into the rectal lumen.
IV. Prostatic lobes protrude >4 cm, and most of the rectal lumen is filled by the projecting prostatic lobes.

INVESTIGATIONS

1. **Blood urea and creatinine:** Raised levels indicate renal failure.
2. **Uroflowmetry:** The person is asked to void urine from their full bladder into the flowmeter. The flow rate is assessed.

   Peak flow rate
   - Normal peak flow rate: >15 ml/sec.
   - Doubtful peak obstruction: 10–15 ml/sec.
   - Definite peak obstruction: ≤10 ml/sec.
   - Thus, the degree of bladder outlet obstruction (BOO) can be secured by uroflowmetry.
3. **Ultrasonogram:** To assess the size and weight of the prostate, assess the residual urine, and look for hydroureteronephrosis and, bladder wall changes.
4. **Urodynamic studies/cystometrograms** are performed to differentiate it from neurogenic bladder.

TREATMENT

It can be classified into medical treatment and surgical treatment.

I. Medical Treatment of BPH

If the patient has mere frequency of micturition and if the residual urine is not much (<150 ml), uroflowmetry shows ≥15 ml/sec of urine flow, and there are no back pressure effects on the kidney, the patient can be reassured, and advised to avoid heavy alcohol consumption which may lead to prostatic congestion and acute urinary retention. To avoid overdistension of the bladder, patients should void urine as and when they feel the urinary sensation of micturition, (i.e. **they should not postpone micturition)**.

Drugs

a. **Finasteride acetate** 5 mg daily for 6 months. It is a 5α-reductase inhibitor. **It helps in preventing hyperplasia of the prostate. It is given for large prostates.** The other drug in this class is **dutasteride**, which is given in the dose of 0.5 mg once daily for 6–12 months.

   Side effects include decreased libido/ejaculation and, impotence.
b. **α-adrenergic blockers:** They relax the internal sphincter for better bladder drainage. They are given as monotherapy when the prostate is ≤40 g (small) as measured by ultrasound. Tamsulosin (most selective), terazosin, and alfazocin are a few examples. Silodosin (4–8 mg once nightly) is the latest drug to enter this class.

   Side effects include orthostatic hypotension and retrograde ejaculation.
c. **Combination therapy** is useful in patients with large glands.

II. Surgical Treatment of BPH

Indications for Surgery

1. **Acute urinary retention**
2. **Chronic urinary retention** with postvoid residual urine ≥200 ml.
3. If the **frequency** of micturition disturbs normal daily activities.
4. **Complications** such as haematuria (due to congestion of prostatic venous plexuses), hydroureteronephrosis, prostatic diverticulosis, vesical calculus and recurrent infections.

Surgical Methods

1. **Transurethral resection of the prostate (TURP)**
   - This is the most popular method today and is referred to as the gold standard.
   - A resectoscope is passed through the urethra, and under vision with constant irrigation with water or 1.5% glycine (best irrigation fluid), the prostate is resected into multiple pieces and removed.
   - Haemostasis is obtained with cauterization.

   Complications of TURP:
   - TURP syndrome: It manifests as nausea, confusion, vomiting and visual disturbances.
   - Incontinence (<1%)
   - Retrograde ejaculation (15%)
   - Impotence (5–10%)
   - Bladder neck contracture.
2. **Transvesical suprapubic prostatectomy (Frayer's)**
   - This method is now **restricted to glands ≥100 g in weight associated with a calculus.**
   - Ankylosis of hip/other orthopaedic conditions (difficulty in positioning).
   - Through an extraperitoneal approach, the bladder is opened, the prostate is enucleated with a finger, and bleeding is controlled by inflating the Foley bulb with 30–50 ml of air and by ligatures.
   - The bladder is drained by a Malecot's catheter, which is wider than Foley's, so that it can drain potential bleeding in the bladder.
   - During the process, the prostatic urethra is also avulsed.
   - After about 7–10 days, a tract develops along the length of the Foley catheter which heals by granulation and fibrosis, and forms the future prostatic urethra.

   Disadvantages
   - Blind resection
   - Increased risk of haemorrhage.
   - Stricture of prostatic urethra.
3. **Retropubic prostatectomy (Millin's):** It is performed by an extraperitoneal approach without opening the bladder by pushing the bladder to one side and excising the prostate.
4. **Perineal prostatectomy (Young's):** Not done nowadays.

Newer Treatments

- Holmium:YAG laser. It is the best laser for patients with ≥100 g prostate or in patients with increased bleeding.
- Intraurethral stents—in men who are grossly unfit (ASA Grade IV) for surgery.

CARCINOMA OF THE PROSTATE

- Carcinoma of the prostate is common after the age of 65 years, and its incidence increases with age.
- In Western countries, it is **the second most common type of carcinoma in males after ≥65 years** of age (first is bronchogenic carcinoma).
- Prostatectomy done for BPH does not protect against the development of prostate carcinoma because during prostatectomy the outer zone is left undisturbed (not resected).
- The most common type is adenocarcinoma.

CLINICAL FEATURES

1. **Histological surprise:** It is asymptomatic in early cases because it is in the peripheral zone. Prostatectomy is done for BPH, but histology reveals carcinoma of the prostate.
2. **Multiple bone pains**, which are often confused for rheumatism, are due to multiple metastasis.
3. **Rectal examination:** Reveals a hard nodule on the anterior wall of the rectum and obliteration of the median sulcus. The rectal mucosa cannot be moved over the prostate, but it is not ulcerated (fascia of Denonvilliers prevents the spread of carcinoma prostate into the rectum).
4. Elderly man with **bilateral sciatica** with metastasis in the thoracolumbar vertebrae.
5. **Acute retention of urine** occurs in 5–10% of cases.
6. **Difficulty** in passing urine and painful micturition (sometimes with haematuria) are due to involvement of the prostatic urethra.

SPREAD (Key Box 59.3)

1. **Haematogenous spread**
   - This is due to retrograde tumour embolisation which occurs through the prostatic venous plexus, which communicates through the emissary veins with the bone (Batson's paravertebral plexus of veins).

TNM STAGING Prostatic carcinoma (Fig. 59.4)

T: Primary tumour

Tx: Primary tumour cannot be assessed

T0: No evidence of primary tumour

T1: Clinically not palpable or not visible on imaging

T1a: Incidental histological finding ≤5% of resected tissue

T1b: Incidental finding in >5% of resected tissue

T1c: Identified on needle biopsy—(because of elevated serum PSA level)

T2: Tumour confined to prostate

T2a: Involving one half of one lobe or less

T2b: Involving more than one half of one lobe

T2c: Involving both lobes

T3: Tumour extends through prostate capsule

T3a: Unilateral or bilateral extra-prostatic carcinoma

T3b: Involving seminal vesicle/s

T4: Tumour invading adjacent structures other than seminal vesicles (bladder neck; external sphincter, rectum, pelvic floor muscles, pelvic wall)

N: Regional lymph nodes

Nx: Regional lymph node status cannot be assessed

N0: No regional lymph node metastasis

N1: Regional lymph node metastasis present

M: Distant metastases

Mx: Not assessed

M0: No metastasis

M1: Distant metastasis

M1a: Non-regional lymph node/s

M1b: Bone metastasis

M1c: Other sites

Key Box 59.3

Bones involved in Carcinoma Prostate

1. Thoracolumbar vertebrae (Fig. 59.4)
2. Pelvic bone, iliac crest
3. Femur
4. Scalp
5. Ribs

Peculiarities of secondary deposit from carcinoma prostate:

- They are multiple
- Moth-eaten appearance
- Osteoblastic (in most other secondaries, they can also be osteolytic).
- Most common site of origin for skeletal metastases.

2. **Lymphatic spread**
   - Prostatic chain of lymphatics drain into the internal iliac nodes.
   - When spread occurs along the seminal vesicle, the external iliac nodes are enlarged.
   - From this group of nodes, the para-aortic, mediastinal, left supra-clavicular nodes get involved.
3. **Local spread** (Fig. 59.4)
   - On the medial side, it can involve the prostatic urethra and cause urinary retention.
   - When it spreads upwards, the bladder can get involved, resulting in painful haematuria.
   - Superiorly, it can also involve the seminal vesicle.
   - The rectum is involved very late in carcinoma prostate because of the tough Denonvilliers' fascia.

INVESTIGATIONS

- Best screening protocol is prostate-specific antigen (PSA) and digital rectal examination (DRE).

1. **Transrectal ultrasound-guided trucut biopsy.** It is done in patients with abnormal rectal examination findings or if PSA is ≥10 ng/ml.
   Report—adenocarcinoma.
2. **X-ray of bones** (Fig. 59.5), which are likely to be involved (already mentioned).
3. **Prostatic acid phosphatase** (Key Box 59.4)
   - The enzymes which split organic phosphates are concentrated in the prostate and are responsible for acidic pH in the prostatic urethra.
   - Normally, they are drained in the urine so that they are not detectable in the serum.
   - In carcinoma prostate, it gets absorbed into the blood due to ductal blockage. Thus, high levels are reached, especially with metastasis.
   - 1 to 3 King-Armstrong units—suggestive of carcinoma of prostate.

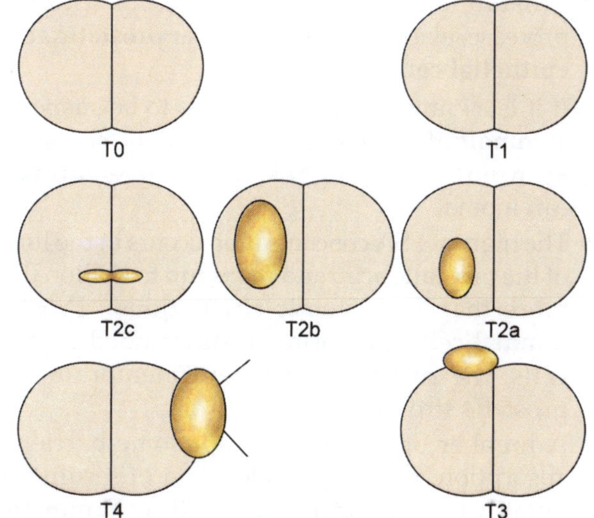

Fig. 59.4: Tumour, node, metastasis (TNM) staging for prostate cancer (*refer* to staging given in the adjacent box)

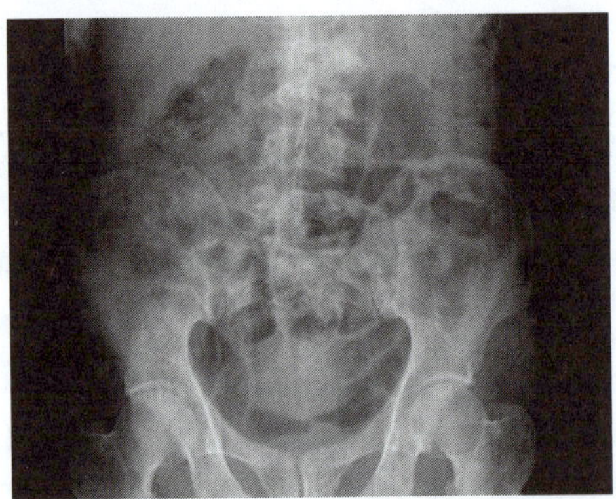

Fig. 59.5: Plain X-ray showing destruction of vertebrae

Key Box 59.4

Acid Phosphatase Increased in

1. Paget's disease of bone
2. Acute prostatitis
3. Cirrhosis of liver
4. Carcinoma prostate

Requirements before the estimation of acid phosphatase:

- Early morning blood sample
- On empty stomach
- Avoid fatty food
- Per-rectal examination should not be done before drawing the blood sample.

Significance of acid phosphatase: Levels come down with the treatment of carcinoma prostate, especially when bone metastasis disappears.

4. **Serum alkaline phosphatase:** It is increased, if there is extensive liver or bone metastasis.
5. **Prostate-specific antigen**
   - Prostate-specific antigen (PSA) is a neutral protease, elaborated by **columnar prostatic acinar epithelial cells.**
   - If it is ≥4 nmol/ml, carcinoma is to be suspected; **10 nmol/ml** is suggestive of prostatic carcinoma; **35 nmol/ml** is suggestive of: disseminated carcinoma.
   - The highest PSA concentration occurs in the lumen of the prostatic acini and ducts (up to million times more than in systemic circulations). Prostatic luminal cells are normally surrounded by basal cells, the prostatic basement membrane, and prostatic stroma.
   - A number of diseases disrupt some barriers to absorption, resulting in elevation of serum PSA, **notably prostatic cancer, prostatic inflammation, and infarction.** PSA is also transiently elevated (up to 24 hours) after ejaculation and cycling.
   - PSA measurement is the most efficient screening test for prostate cancer and it increases further, if the measurement is **combined with digital rectal examination** (DRA).
   - PSA measurement is also vital in staging prostate cancer and assessing the response to treatment.

Pearls of Wisdom

PSA is organ-specific but not cancer-specific.

6. **Abdominal and transrectal USG:** To stage the disease.
7. **Bone scan** (Fig. 59.6): It is indicated in cases of carcinoma prostate, especially in those who have bony pains, elevated alkaline phosphatase, and very high PSA levels (>20 ng/ml) (*see* clinical notes on next page).
8. **CT or MRI scan** (Fig. 59.7): These are done before proceeding to radical surgery to assess the extent of the tumour.
9. **Gallium-68 PSMA PET scan:** This is regarded as a one-stop work-up for prostatic cancer as it can provide information on both the primary tumour as well as metastases. It is a molecular imaging that targets the prostate-specific membrane antigen.

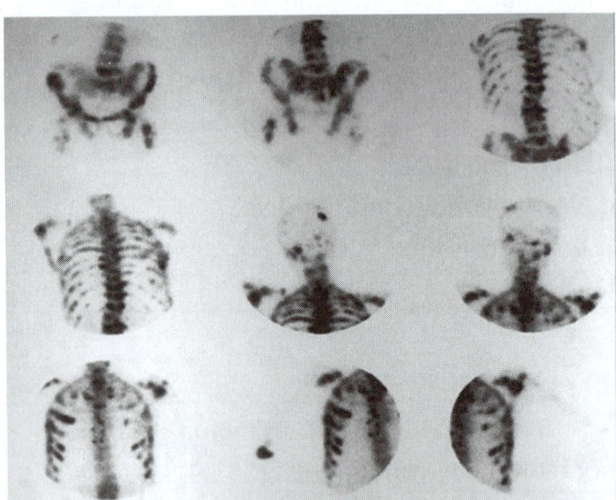

Fig. 59.6: Bone scan showing extensive metastasis

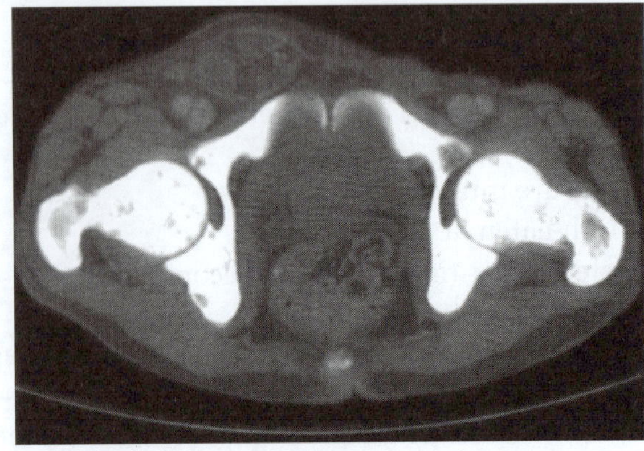

Fig. 59.7: Lytic lesions in pubic bones

Diagnosis of Carcinoma Prostate

- High index of suspicion in men >50 years of age.
- PSA >10 nmol/ml and abnormal findings on digital rectal examination.
- Proceed with TRUS guided prostatic 12 core biopsy.

Histopathological Examination

- Gleason scoring system used
- Gleason score varies from 1–5
- Two scores are used to grade the disease
  - The most common histological variant
  - The highest grade
- The final scores varies from 2–10
- Gleason score
  - >6 suggests of malignancy
  - 7 suggests—intermediate risk
  - 8–10 suggests—high-risk disease

Clinical Notes

A 75-year-old diabetic gentleman was admitted to the hospital due to giddiness and syncope. He was a diabetic. Initially, it was thought to be due to hypoglycaemia. Investigations revealed creatinine of 7.5 mg%. A diagnosis of renal failure was made. Urgent ultrasound revealed bilateral hydronephrosis due to large para-aortic nodes compressing both ureters. He underwent emergency stenting of both ureters. Rectal examination revealed a hard prostate. PSA was 20 nmol/ml suggestive of dissemination. CT scan done later showed involvement of pelvic bones, thoracolumbar vertebrae and iliac bones. It was a case of carcinoma prostate. Retrospective analysis revealed that the patient was having backache since the last 6 months.

TREATMENT OF CARCINOMA OF PROSTATE (Fig. 59.8)

It can be classified under the following headings—early malignancy and late malignancy.

I. Early Malignancy

It refers to T1 or T2, N0, M0.

A. Early prostatic malignancy with PSA levels ≤20 nmol/ml

- **Radical prostatectomy** is done for T1 and T2 and in men with a life expectancy >10 years. Metastasis should be excluded by a negative bone scan, chest radiograph, and serum PSA <20 nmol/ml. Radical prostatectomy involves pelvic lymphadenectomy and removal of the prostate and seminal vesicle including the distal the urethral sphincter followed by anastomosis of urethra to the bladder neck.
- **Most commonly injured vessel**—dorsal venous complex.
- **Radical radiotherapy** for prostate and pelvic nodes is given postoperatively.
- **Disadvantages of radical prostatectomy:** Impotence and stress incontinence may complicate the surgery.

B. Early prostatic malignancy with PSA ≥20 nmol/ml and the patient is already ≥65–70 years of age, surgery is not favoured. Radical radiotherapy is given.

II. Late Malignancy

It refer to T3 lesions, involvement of regional nodes, or the presence of metastasis.

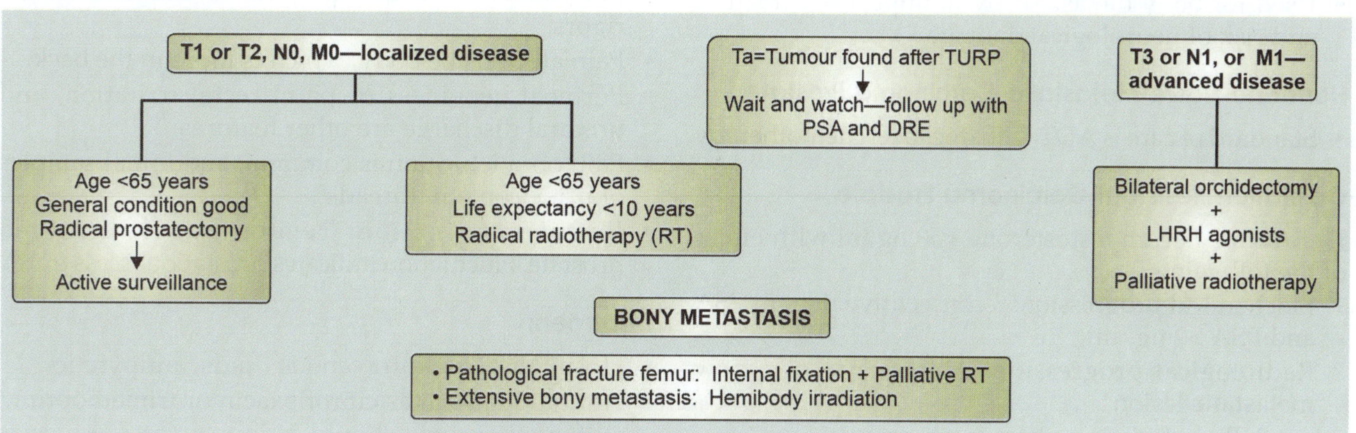

Fig. 59.8: Summary of the treatment of carcinoma prostate

Hormonal Therapy (Androgen Deprivation Therapy—ADT)

Indicated in patients with locally advanced and metastatic carcinoma prostate.

Principle: Testosterone-lowering therapy (castration).

i. *Surgical:* Bilateral orchidectomy

Advantage:
- Simple and cheap
- Quickest way to achieve castration level

Disadvantage: Irreversible

ii. *Medical*

a. **Estrogens:** Oral diethylstilbesterol (DES—not used)
- *Advantage:* Not associated with bone loss
- *Disadvantage:* Thromboembolic complications

b. **LHRH agonists:** Leuporolide

Currently, it is the main form of ADT
- Depot injections at 1, 2, 3, and 6 months and at 1 year
- It suppresses FSH and LH secretions
- *Disadvantages:* Flare-up phenomenon due to initial testosterone surge. Hence, antiandrogen therapy is given concurrently.

c. **LHRH antagonists:**
- Binds to LHRH receptors and rapidly decreases testosterone without any flare.
- *Disadvantage:* Lack of long-acting depot formulations.

iii. *Complete androgen blockade:*
- Surgical/medical + anti-androgen therapy

Chemotherapy

- **Docitaxel** is the drug of choice, 75 mg/m^2, given in 6 cycles
- **Cabazitaxel**

Radiotherapy

- Used for bony metastases with impending fracture and risk of neurological damage

Hormone Naïve Metastatic Carcinoma Prostate

- Standard of care is ADT with docitaxel chemotherapy

Castration Resistant Carcinoma Prostate

Definition: Serum testosterone <50 ng/dl with either of the following:

1. Biochemical progression: 3 consecutive rises in PSA and PSA >2 ng/ml
2. Radiological progression: Appearance of a new metastatic lesion
   a. ≥2 Bony lesions on bone scan, or
   b. New soft tissue metastasis

Treatment

1st line treatment:
- Abirateterone
- Enzulatamide
- Docetaxel
- Sipuleucel-T

2nd line treatment:
- Cabazitaxel
- Radium 223

Pearls of Wisdom

Clinically insignificant tumours—**Epstein criteria**
Tumour volume ≤0.2 ml
Gleason score <7
Organ confined cancer

PROSTATITIS

- Inflammation of the prostate can be acute or chronic.
- However, in both types, the seminal vesicles and posterior urethra are also involved.
- The diagnosis is often delayed due to varying symptoms attributed to a different cause that are being wrongly treated.
- If the treatment is in effectively given, infection persists and becomes difficult to eradicate later.

ACUTE PROSTATITIS

Aetiology

- Causative organisms are *Escherichia coli (most common), Staphylococcus aureus* and *Staphylococcus albus.*
- The infection is usually due to haematogenous spread from a distant focus or secondary to urinary tract infection.
- Instrumentation or invasive urological procedures are also factors. Catheterisation is contraindicated.

Clinical Features

- The patient is ill with high-grade fever and chills and rigors.
- Pain all over the body, which is more in the back.
- Perineal heaviness or pain, rectal irritation, and urethral discharge are other features.
- Pain on micturition is common, and initial samples of urine contain 'threads'.
- **Rectal examination:** Tender, boggy, enlarged prostate. Fluctuation indicates prostatic abscess (rare).

Treatment

- Hospitalisation, intravenous fluids, antipyretics.
- Antibiotics, such as ciprofloxacin or trimethoprim/sulfamethoxazole should be given for 4–6 weeks. Otherwise, recurrent attacks may occur.

- If **abscess is suspected,** the diagnosis can be confirmed by transrectal ultrasound and, can be drained by **transurethral unroofing of the abscess** cavity (similar technique to TURP).

CHRONIC PROSTATITIS (Key Box 59.5)

Chronic prostatitis results from inadequately treated acute prostatitis.

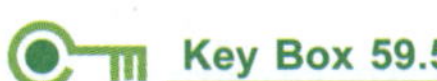
Key Box 59.5

Chronic Prostatitis

- Follows recurrent prostatitis
- Elderly men are affected
- Symptoms—misleading
- Perineal heaviness, back pain
- Postprostatic massage—threads in urine
- Pus cells and bacteria—prostatic fluid
- Prolonged antibiotics

Clinical Features

- Elderly men are affected and complain of perineal heaviness, perineal discomfort or pain on sexual intercourse.
- Intermittent fever is also a feature.
- Rectal examination may reveal a boggy and tender prostate.
- Low backache.

Diagnosis

Prostatic massage is done by a bidigital method—index finger in the rectum and the thumb in the perineum to one side. The patient is then asked to void urine. Presence of prostatic threads or mucopus in the postprostatic massage urine is diagnostic of chronic prostatitis.

Treatment

Chronic antibiotic suppression for 3–4 months—norfloxacin, trimethoprim and metronidazole are used.

MISCELLANEOUS

Prostatic calculi: They occur in middle-aged and early men. They represent calcified corpora amylacea. Consist of calcium phosphate, and lie at the periphery of the transition zone.

INTERESTING WISDOM LINES

- Do not injure the prostatic venous plexus (between the anatomical capsule and pelvic peritoneum) during prostatectomy or abdominoperineal resection (APR) done for carcinoma rectum.
- Frequency of micturition is not an indication for prostatectomy.
- Most commonly done surgery for BPH is transurethral resection.
- Prostatectomy for BPH does not protect against the development of prostatic carcinoma.
- Androgen ablation is the chief form of treatment for advanced prostatic cancers.

Multiple Choice Questions

1. **The following are true regarding the surgical anatomy of the prostate *except:***
   A. Developmentally, it has 5 lobes
   B. Median lobe enlargement causes carcinoma prostate
   C. It develops around the 12th week of intrauterine life
   D. Between the prostate and rectum, Denonvilliers' fascia is present

2. **The following are changes that occur in the urinary bladder due to BPH *except:***
   A. Fasciculations B. Sacculations
   C. Diverticuli D. Carcinoma

3. **Vesical introversion of the sensitive prostatic urethra within the urinary bladder causes:**
   A. Frequency
   B. Urgency
   C. Hesitancy
   D. Haematuria

4. **The following are complications of benign prostatic hypertrophy *except:***
   A. Stones
   B. Renal failure
   C. Recurrent urinary tract infection
   D. Carcinoma urinary bladder

5. **Which of the following drugs is used to treat benign prostatic hypertrophy?**
   A. α-adrenergic blockers
   B. β-adrenergic blockers
   C. Oral stilboestrol
   D. Oral prednisolone

6. **The following are true regarding the role of ultrasound in benign prostatic hypertrophy *except:***
   A. It can assess the size
   B. It can assess the weight
   C. It can assess residual urine
   D. It can assess the urinary flow rate

7. **The following are true regarding digital rectal examination of carcinoma prostate *except:***
   A. Hard nodule is felt
   B. Median sulcus is obliterated
   C. Rectal mucosa cannot be moved
   D. Ulcerated mucosa is present

8. **Early spread from carcinoma prostate to bones occurs through:**
   A. Batson's plexus
   B. Santorini plexus of veins
   C. Waldeyer's plexus of veins
   D. Denonvilliers' plexus of veins

9. **The following are features of bone secondaries from carcinoma prostate *except:***
   A. Thoracolumbar vertebrae are involved
   B. Moth-eaten appearance on X-ray
   C. Osteolytic lesions
   D. Multiple bones are affected

10. **Which structure is affected late in carcinoma prostate?**
   A. Prostatic urethra B. Seminal vesicles
   C. Rectum D. Urinary bladder

11. **Which of the following is not true for acid phosphatase?**
   A. It is responsible for acidic pH in prostatic urethra
   B. High values suggest carcinoma prostate
   C. It is elevated not only in carcinoma prostate but also in other conditions
   D. Early morning urine samples are best measuring this

12. **The following are true for prostate-specific antigen *except:***
   A. It is released from columnar prostatic acinar epithelial cells
   B. ≥4 nmol/ml suggests carcinoma prostate
   C. Prostatitis can also increase its levels
   D. It does not help in assessing treatment response

13. **Which of the following is not done in cases of carcinoma prostate?**
   A. Radical prostatectomy
   B. Radical radiotherapy
   C. High orchidectomy
   D. Stilboestrol therapy

14. **What is the treatment following prostatectomy for BPH if it is reported as carcinoma prostate?**
   A. Orchidectomy B. Stilboestrol
   C. Bisphosphonates D. Local radiotherapy

15. **The following are true for acute prostatitis *except:***
   A. It is usually a haematogenous infection
   B. Instrumentation can also cause this
   C. It is usually mild and self-limiting
   D. Urine samples may contain 'threads'

16. **Which of the following is true regarding posterior urethral valves?**
   A. They are acquired
   B. Bladder is thin-walled and more prone to rupture
   C. Renal failure is uncommon
   D. They are symmetrical

Answers

1. B	**2.** D	**3.** C	**4.** D	**5.** A	**6.** D	**7.** D	**8.** A	**9.** C	**10.** C
11. D	**12.** D	**13.** D	**14.** D	**15.** D	**16.** B				

CHAPTER

60

Penis, Testis and Scrotum

- Surgical anatomy of penis
- Phimosis
- Paraphimosis
- Carcinoma penis
- Peyronie's disease
- Anatomy of the testis
- Hydrocoele
- Undescended testis
- Ectopic testis
- Varicocele
- Spermatocoele
- Epididymal cyst
- Torsion testis
- Testicular tumours
- Fournier's gangrene
- Fracture of penis
- Male infertility

SURGICAL ANATOMY OF THE PENIS

- It consists of two corpora cavernosa and one corpus spongiosum (Fig. 60.1).
- **Corpora cavernosa** are vascular spaces into which **arterioles open directly**. They are corkscrew-shaped **(helicine arteries),** which allow their elongation during erection.
- **Corpus spongiosum** contains the urethra which expands distally as the glans.
- Each corpus is enclosed by a tough fibrous membrane (**tunica albuginea** of the corpus).
- The fused fibrous sheaths are attached to the under surface of the symphysis pubis by a triangular sheet of fibrous tissue **(suspensory ligament)**. This has to be divided during total amputation of the penis.

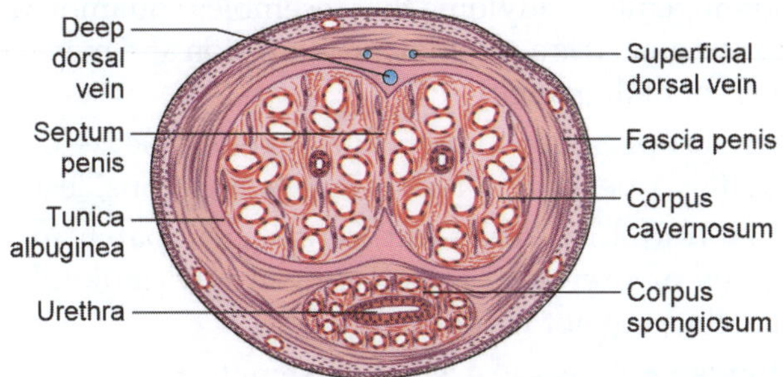

Fig. 60.1: Surgical anatomy of the penis

Blood Supply

- The artery to the bulb supplies the corpus spongiosum and the glans.
- The deep artery supplies the corpus cavernosum alone—its sole function is erection.
- The dorsal artery supplies skin, fascia and glans.
- The superficial dorsal vein drains into superficial external pudendal veins. The deep dorsal vein enters prostatic venous plexus.

Penile Urethra

- The entire penile urethra is lined with pseudostratified columnar epithelium, except for the dilated anterior part in the glans (fossa navicularis), which is lined by stratified squamous epithelium.

Lymphatic Drainage

- Medial group of superficial inguinal nodes.
- Some from the glans pass directly to the node of Cloquet

Nerve Supply

- Parasympathetic nerves—nervi erigentes: Causes erection of the external genitalia.
- Sympathetic system—hypogastric nerves: Helps in ejaculation.

Competency

SU30.1: Describe the clinical features, investigations and principles of management of phimosis, paraphimosis and carcinoma penis.

PHIMOSIS

It is the inability to retract the prepucial skin.

Causes (Key Box 60.1)

1. **Congenital:** Most common type, seen in young patients.
2. Secondary to **chronic balanoposthitis:** Balanitis means inflammation of the glans penis, and posthitis means inflammation of the prepuce. Balanoposthitis is common in diabetic patients.
3. **Chancre**
4. **Carcinoma** of the penis can present as a recent phimosis.

Clinical Features

- Inability to retract the prepuce.
- In children, ballooning of the prepuce (second bladder) can be seen, which is diagnostic.
- Balanoposthitis because of inability to clean the glans.

Complications

- Paraphimosis
- Carcinoma penis

Treatment

Circumcision: Removal of the prepuce.

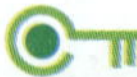

Key Box 60.1

Phimosis—Causes

- Cancer
- Chancre
- Congenital
- Chronic disease: Diabetes mellitus

PARAPHIMOSIS

In this condition, the retracted skin of the glans penis (prepuce) cannot be pulled forwards. As a result, the retracted skin acts like a tight constricting agent that compresses the corona and causes venous congestion. As venous congestion increases, the glans swells up, resulting in paraphimosis (Fig. 60.2).

Causes

1. If the retracted prepuce is not pulled forwards during catheterizations.
2. May occur after sexual intercourse.

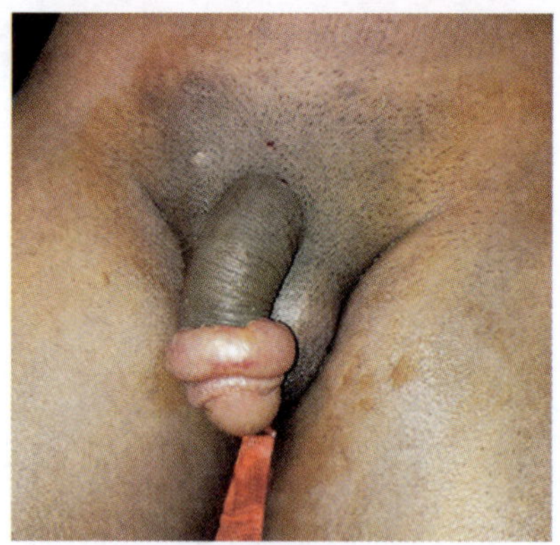

Fig. 60.2: Paraphimosis (*Courtesy:* Prof. Amith Jain, SRRM College, Bengaluru)

Clinical Features

- Severe pain in the glans penis
- Gross swelling of the retracted prepucial skin and oedema of the distal glans penis.

Treatment

1. Sedation
2. Injection hyaluronidase 250 units in 10–15 ml of saline is injected into the constriction ring (retracted prepucial skin). After 5–10 minutes, when oedema is reduced, the paraphimosis can be reduced with gentle manipulation.
3. Dorsal slit is given so that reduction can be done. Circumcision follows later.

Complications

1. Ulcers of the glans
2. Gangrene of glans (later stages).

CARCINOMA PENIS

Most common type—squamous cell carcinoma. Other varieties—melanoma, adenocarcinoma, basal cell carcinoma (BCC).

PREMALIGNANT LESIONS

1. **Genital warts: Buschke-Lowenstein** tumour is a giant penile condyloma that resembles squamous cell carcinoma. It is a cauliflower-like lesion and may have foci of malignancy.
2. **Erythroplasia of Queyrat or Paget's disease of the penis:** A persistent, red, raw, precancerous, lesion.
3. **Leukoplakia:** Persistent nonspecific patch in the glans or prepucial skin. Interestingly, leukoplakic patches are not white in the penis.
4. **Bowen's disease:** A small eczematous plaque that may develop carcinoma *in situ*.

AETIOLOGY

Phimosis

1. Extremely rare in Jews who practise circumcision immediately after birth.
2. Rare in Mohammedans who **practise** circumcision few years after birth.
3. Common in Hindus and Christians who do not practise circumcision. Due to the prepucial skin, smegma collects within, which causes chronic irritation and results in carcinoma penis.

Pearls of Wisdom

Circumcision done within 1 year confers immunity against Ca penis.

Clinical Features

1. Carcinoma penis is common in the 6th decade. The majority of patients present with a nonhealing ulcer.
2. Foul-smelling discharge is common and is occasionally blood-stained (Figs 60.3 and 60.4).
3. Recent phimosis due to growth underneath the prepuce.
4. Haematuria and pain while passing urine indicate locally advanced tumours.
5. On examination, there is often an ulcero-proliferative growth with everted edges and extensive induration (much more than the lesion). Hence, entire shaft has to be examined for evidence of induration.
6. Urethra is rarely involved in carcinoma penis because it is protected by the tough Buck's fascia, which is part of the pelvic fascia. In large fungating lesions, it may be difficult to identify the external urinary meatus. In such situations, the patient can point to the external urinary meatus.

SPREAD

1. Direct spread: Involves the glans, prepucial skin, and shaft.
2. Lymphatic spread: Inguinal nodes are enlarged. 30% of cases are due to infection. Nodes are firm and tender in infection. Hard nodes suggest metastases. Later, the internal iliac and para-aortic nodes may also get enlarged. In advanced cases, lymph nodes may show fungation (Figs 60.5 and 60.6).

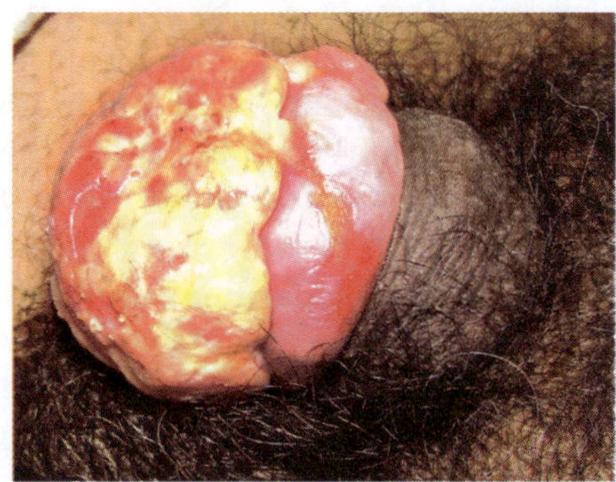

Fig. 60.3: Carcinoma penis—proliferative lesion with gross oedema due to secondary infection

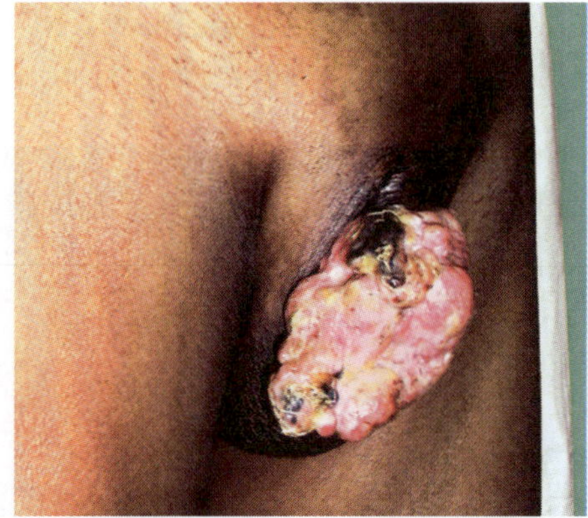

Fig. 60.4: Carcinoma penis—difficult to find penis—ask the patient from where he passes urine—he will show you the urethral opening

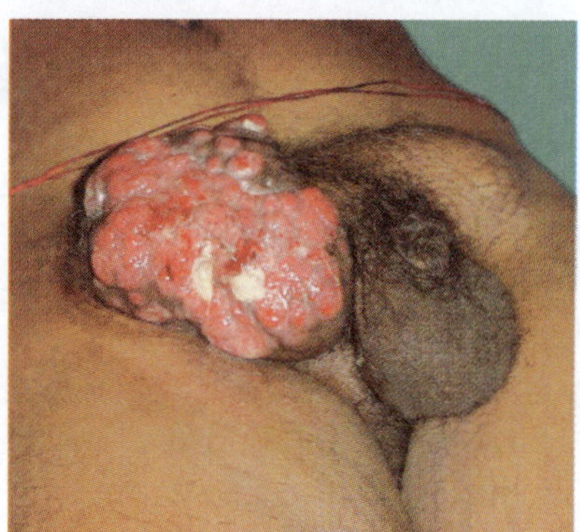

Fig. 60.5: This patient presented with fungating inguinal lymph nodes. Observe the penis—he had undergone partial amputation of the penis 2 years prior

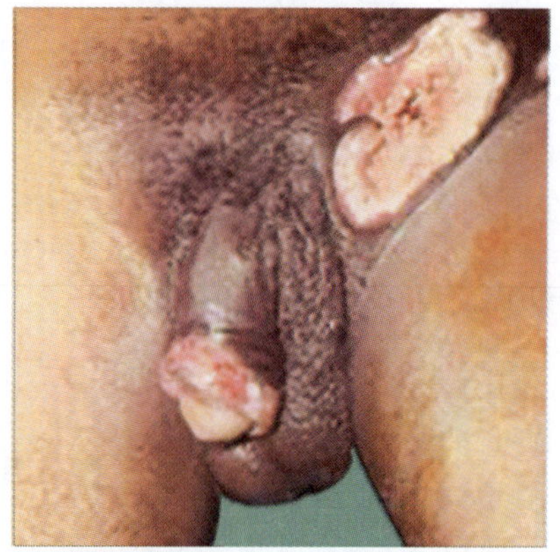

Fig. 60.6: This patient had a large foul smelling proliferative lesion in the glans penis with fungating inguinal lymph nodes. Such advanced cases have poor prognosis

Cause of Death

Death may occur due to erosion of the femoral vessels by the inguinal lymph nodes.

STAGING

I. Tumour confined to the glans or prepuce
II. Tumour involving the penile shaft or corpora cavernosa
III. Mobile regional nodal metastases, with stage I or II
IV. Tumour beyond the penile shaft, fixed regional lymph node or distant metastases.
   - Refer to TNM staging.

INVESTIGATIONS

1. Wedge biopsy from the edge of the growth, proves the diagnosis of squamous cell carcinoma nodes. Once biopsy is confirmed, metastatic work up is done.
2. Ultrasound-guided FNAC of enlarged inguinal lymph nodes.
3. MRI are helpful in lesions invading the corpora cavernosa (soft tissue details).

TNM STAGING **Carcinoma penis AJCC 8th edition**

T: Primary tumour

Tx:	Primary tumour cannot be assessed
T0:	No primary tumour
Tis:	Carcinoma *in situ*
Ta:	Non-invasive verrrucous carcinoma
T1a:	Subepithelial invasion without lymphovascular invasion and is not poorly differentiated
T1b:	With lymphovascular invasion and is poorly differentiated
T2:	Invasion of corpus spongiosum with or without urethral invasion
T3:	Invasion of cavernosum with or without urethra invasion
T4:	Invasion of adjacent structures

N: Regional lymph nodes

Nx:	Lymph node status cannot be assessed
N0:	No lymph nodal involvement
N1:	Metastasis in one inguinal node unilateral, mobile
N2:	Metastasis in multiple or bilateral superficial inguinal nodes mobile
N3:	Metastasis in deep inguinal or pelvic nodes: :Fixed, unilateral or bilateral

M: Distant metastases

Mx:	Distant metastasis cannot be assessed
M0:	No distant metastasis
M1:	Distant metastasis present

4. CT scan is useful in obese patients wherein clinical examination of inguinal nodes is difficult
5. CT-guided FNAC of pelvic nodes

DIFFERENTIAL DIAGNOSIS

1. Condyloma acuminatum
2. Buschke-Lowenstein tumour
3. Balanitis xerotica obliterans

TREATMENT

It can be divided into treatment of the primary and treatment of the secondaries.

I. Treatment of the Primary

Stage I

1. Growth confined to the prepuce—**circumcision**. Regular follow-up is necessary.
2. Growth involving the glans: **Partial amputation** with at least 2 cm margin from the palpable, indurated edge of the tumour.

Stage II

1. **Partial amputation:** After having a proximal, macroscopic tumour-free, 2 cm margin, if there is adequate length of the penile shaft (minimum 2.5 cm) to carry out sexual functions and direct the urinary stream, a partial amputation can be done (Figs 60.7 and 60.8).
2. **Total penectomy with perineal urethrostomy,** if adequate shaft cannot be retained. This is a major operation, so the patient has to be clearly instructed about the consequences and complications of it.

Complications of perineal urethrostomy

I. **Ammoniacal dermatitis** of the scrotum. To prevent this, the patient has to lift the scrotum to pass urine.
II. **Stricture of the perineal urethra,** which can be dilated by Hegar's dilators.

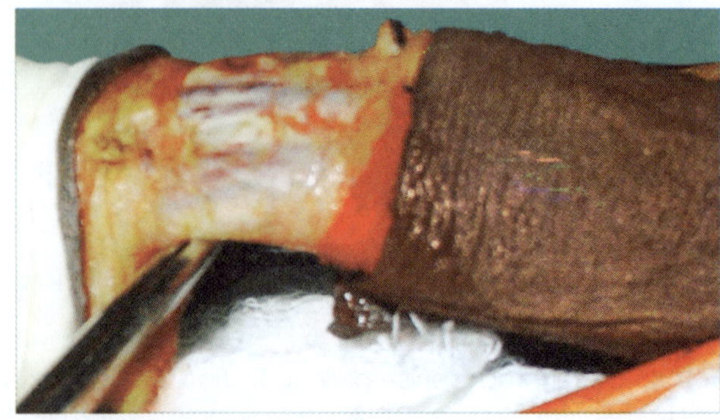

Fig. 60.7: Partial amputation in progress—veins are exposed

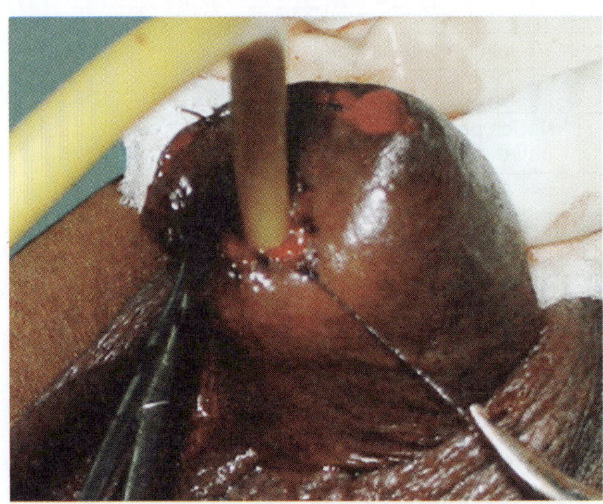

Fig. 60.8: Stump seen with catheter in place

Stage III

- Circumcision, partial amputation or total penectomy followed by ilioinguinal block dissection.

II. Treatment of Inguinal Lymph Node Secondaries

- Before discussing ilioinguinal block dissection, it is necessary to know the concept of **sentinel lymph node biopsy (SLNB)**.
- The concept of SLNB was first described by Cabana in 1977.
- He demonstrated consistent drainage of the penile lymphatics into a sentinel lymph node or groups of lymph nodes, located superomedial to the junction of the saphenous and femoral veins in the area of the superficial epigastric vein. He postulated that this SLN is the first to get involved in the penile malignancy and that if this SLN is negative for tumour, metastasis to other inguinal lymph nodes will not occur. Metastasis to this lymph node will indicate the need for complete ilioinguinal block dissection.
- **Technique:** Isosulphan blue is injected at the site of the primary tumour. After sometime, inguinal dissection is done to expose the SLN area and the lymph nodes, which take up the dye. These are removed and sent for pathological examination. Based on the report, if the node is positive for malignancy, a complete inguinal block dissection is indicated. In case of negative nodes, nothing else is required, and the patient is kept under regular follow-up.
- Only T1a patients presenting with palpable lymph nodes actually have metastasis in 50% of cases, and the remainder have lymph node enlargement secondary to inflammation. Hence, subjecting all the patients with inguinal lymphadenopathy to surgery is not recommended. Therefore, a course of antibiotics is given and a period of 4–6 weeks are waited for. If the nodes are still palpable, block dissection is carried out in T1a patients.
- However, this antibiotic policy can be followed in low-grade tumours such as *in situ* carcinoma and T1 lesions. If the lymph nodes regress, wait and watch. If the grade of the tumour is high, do not give antibiotics. FNAC is done, and it is treated accordingly.
- In addition, if the nodes are not palpable, and if the primary tumour is poorly differentiated, superficial lymph node dissection is done. If the nodes are positive, modified inguinal block dissection (Catalona) can be done.
- An algorithm to help in the management of these patients is shown in Fig. 60.9.

Pearls of Wisdom

Four weeks of antibiotics are advised after treatment of the primary to bring down the infective complications specially flap necrosis. It does not direct the future management of nodal disease.

RECENT ADVANCES IN THE TREATMENT OF CARCINOMA PENIS

Organ Preservation

Primary tumours—Tis, Ta, T1; grade 1 and grade 2 tumours—they have favourable histology.

Approaches to organ preservation

1. Topical ointments such as 5-fluorouracil or imiquimod cream in Tis only
2. Radiation therapy
3. Mohs surgery: Layer-by-layer complete excision of the penile lesion in multiple sessions with microscopic examination of the undersurface of each layer.
4. Limited excision: It can be done in selected patients who have discrete tumours, with well-differentiated carcinoma after doing an intraoperative frozen section.
5. Laser ablation: It is performed in selected patients in conjunction with frozen section biopsies. CO_2 laser has been used widely but recurrence rates are higher—about 40–50% for T1 tumours. Treatment with Nd:YAG laser has the least recurrence rates. The advantage of laser treatment is that the rate of resuming sexual activity is high.
6. **Modified radical inguinal block dissection (Catalona):** To minimise complications of inguinal block dissection, the following modifications are done.

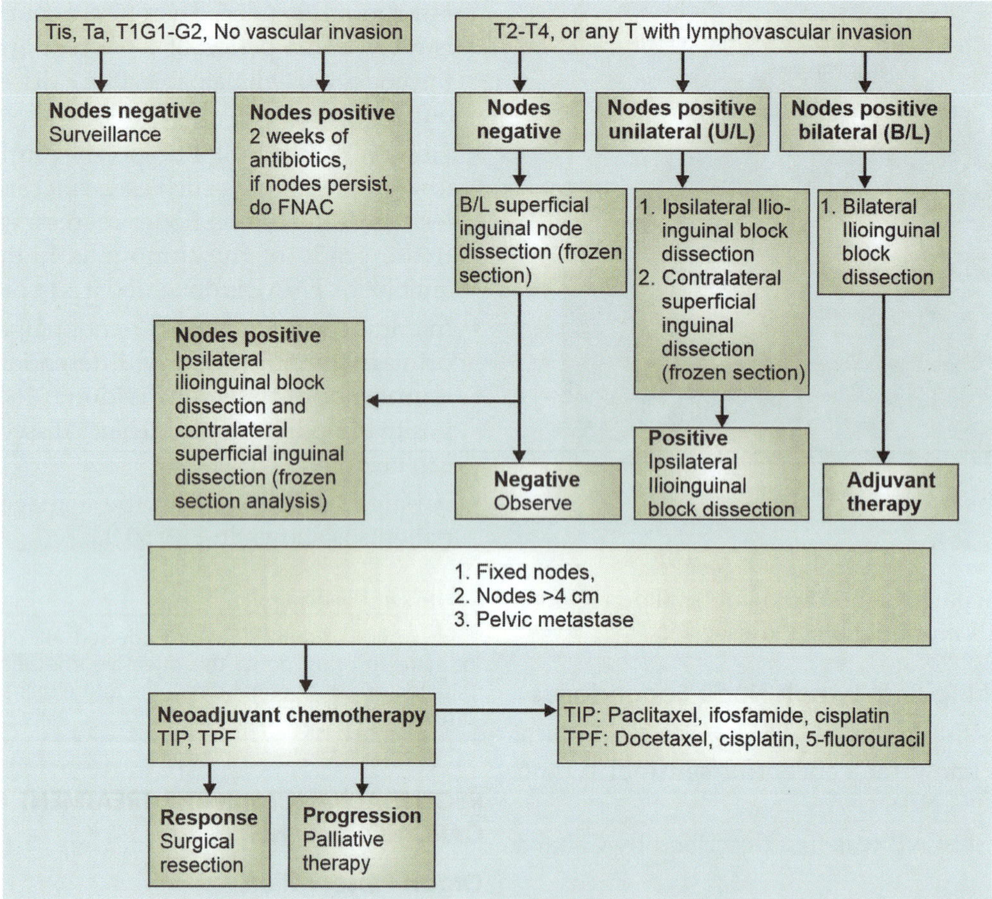

Fig. 60.9: Algorithm for managing inguinal lymph node secondaries from carcinoma penis

- Good preoperative and postoperative care
- Myocutaneous flap cover
- Preservation of the dermis
- Preservation of Scarpa's fascia
- Preservation of the saphenous vein

Stage IV

Radiotherapy + chemotherapy (cisplatin, ifosfamide and paclitaxel are the drugs used commonly).

RADIOTHERAPY (Fig. 60.10)

Indications

1. Young patients who want to have a sexual life
2. Patient refuses surgery
3. Fixed/ulcerated inguinal metastasis

Types

1. External Radiotherapy

- **Dose:** 4000–6000 cGy which may also include iliac and inguinal nodes.

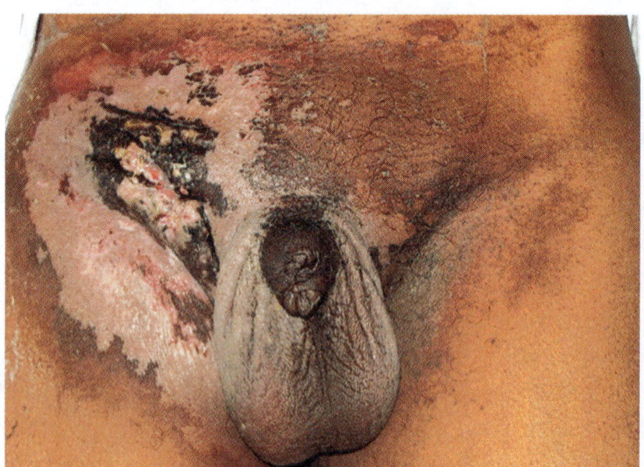

Fig. 60.10: Advanced lymph node secondaries treated with radiation

2. Interstitial Radiotherapy

Iridium wires/tantalum wires are implanted within the glans.

Complications of Radiotherapy

- Radionecrosis of the penis
  Summary of treatment (Fig. 60.11).

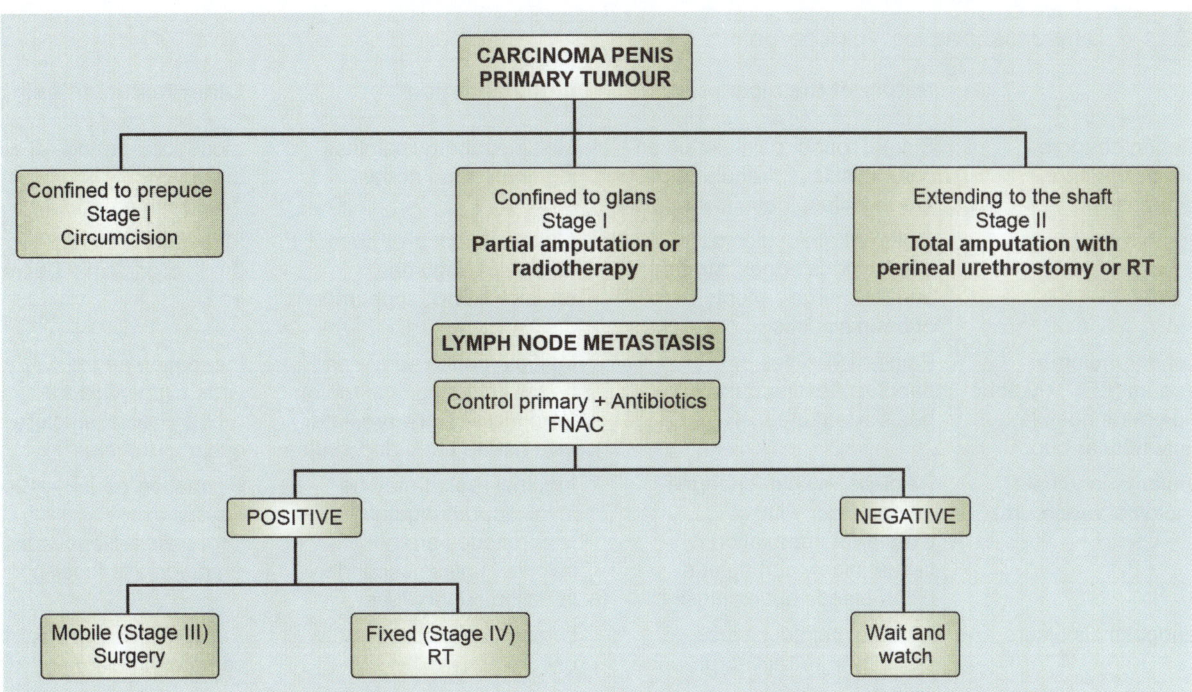

Fig. 60.11: Summary of the treatment of carcinoma penis

PEYRONIE'S DISEASE (PENILE FIBROMATOSIS)

Aetiology

- Past trauma has been considered as one of the causative factors.
- Venereal diseases have also been blamed.
- Association with Dupuytren's contracture, retroperitoneal fibrosis, and plantar fasciitis.

Clinical Features

- Hard plaques of fibrosis can be palpated along the length of the penis in the sheath of corpora cavernosa (induration–penis–plastica).
- As a result of hard plaques, erection is not proper, and the erected penis tends to bend towards the side of the plaque.

Treatment

Medical: Steroids, vitamin E, tamoxifen (poor results) colchicine therapy, intralesional verapamil. Watch and observe some cases. It may recur after a few years.

Surgical: Straightening of the penis is recommended, if the deformity is distressing.

1. **Nesbitt's operation:** Straightening the penis by placing a nonabsorabable suture in the corpora cavernosum opposite the plaque.
2. **Gelhard's operation:** Multiple incisions over the fibrous plaques with temporal fascia bridging.

DIFFERENTIAL DIAGNOSIS OF ULCER PENIS (Table 60.1)

- There are many causes of ulcer penis.
- The important ones are carcinoma and sexually transmitted diseases (Figs 60.12 to 60.14).
- The incubation period is an important clue followed by the nature of the ulcer.

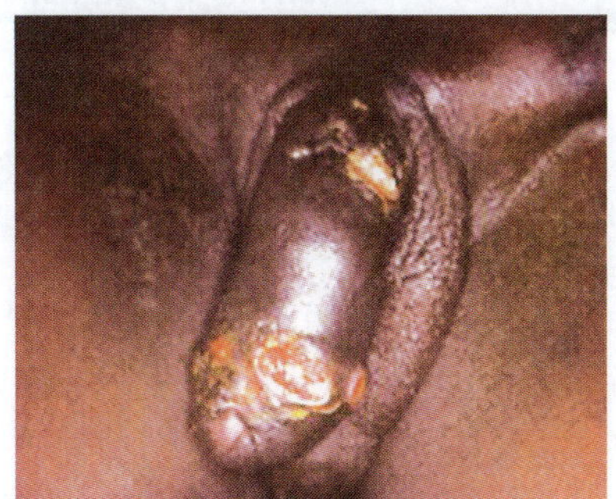

Fig. 60.12: Multiple painless ulcers due to chancroid

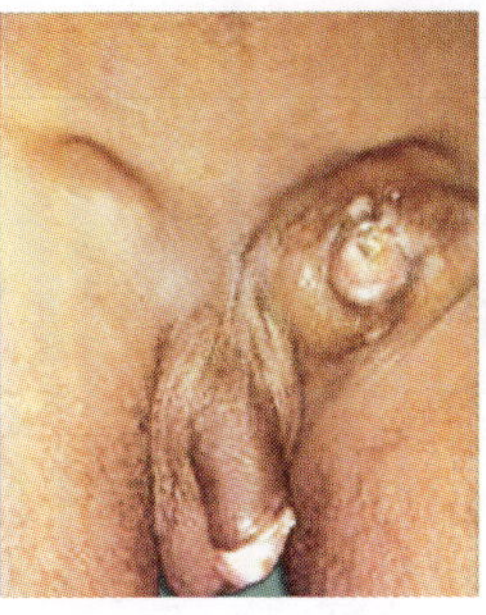

Fig. 60.13: Bubo

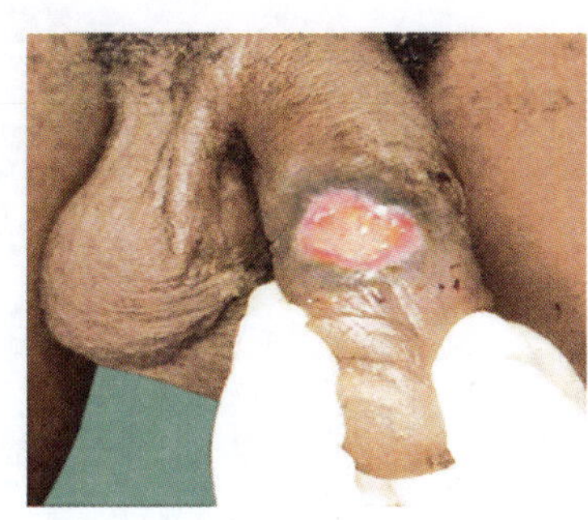

Fig. 60.14: Genital chancre

Table 60.1 Differential diagnosis of ulcer penis

	Nature of the ulcer	Inguinal region	Other features/findings
1. Hunterian chancre (syphilitic chancre, hard chancre)	Single, round, painless ulcer—coronal sulcus, frenulum, glans are the sites; base is indurated	Multiple, shotty, painless inguinal lymph nodes	Incubation period—3 weeks; organism. *Treponema pallidum*
2. Chancroid (soft sore)	Multiple painful ulcers; oedematous edges, slough and discharge—plenty of bubo-sinuses	Multiples nodes—above and below inguinal region—**bubo**; suppuration	Incubation period 3–4 days; organism—Ducrey's bacilli
3. Lymphogranuloma venereum (LGV) (lymphogranuloma inguinale, tropical tubular bubo)	Painless vesicles or papules, fleeting duration, heals spontaneously	Multiple nodes above and below in the inguinal region form **sign of groove,** later give rise to bubo and sinuses	Incubation period 1–2 weeks; virus *Chlamydia trachomatis*; rubbery rectal stricture; can occur in females
4. Granuloma inguinale (granuloma venereum)	Painless vesicle, changes into an ulcer with exuberant granulation tissue; highly contagious ulcer; bleeds but painless	Inguinal region may be involved, but inguinal lymph nodes are not involved unless secondary infection supervenes	Incubation period—10–40 days; Organism—*Donovania granulomatis* (bacilli)
5. Balanoposthitis ulcers	Multiple, painful ulcers, difficulty in retracting prepuce	Lymph node enlargement uncommon	Recurrent balanoposthitis common in diabetic patients
6. Herpes progenitalis	Vesicles and pustules on the prepuce or on the glans	Inguinal lymph nodes are not enlarged	Neuralgic pain and itching occurs before the onset of ulcer
7. Carcinomatous ulcer	Painless, indurated ulcer with everted edges; bleeds on touch	Tender nodes, hard nodes, metastasis	Phimosis is one aetiological factor

Competency

SU30.2: Describe the applied anatomy, clinical features, investigations and principles of management of undescended testis.

ANATOMY OF THE TESTIS AND EPIDIDYMIS

TESTIS (Fig. 60.15)

- **Size:** 4 × 3 × 2.5 cm, one in each scrotal sac.
- **Functional unit is a lobule:** 250 lobules filled with seminiferous tubules.
  Germ cells ⟶ Sperm production
  Leydig cells ⟶ Testosterone production
  Sertoli cells ⟶ Oestrogen production

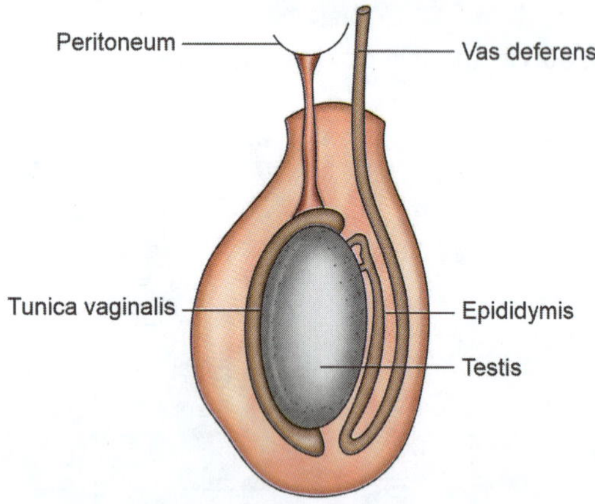

Fig. 60.15: Anatomy of the scrotum

- The seminiferous tubules converge to form a rete testis, which is connected to the epididymis through 5–7 efferent ductules.
- It is covered by thick, inseparable, fibrous tissue—**tunica albuginea**.
- The serous space in the front and lateral surface of the testis is the **tunica vaginalis**.
- **Blood supply** is by the testicular artery—a branch of the aorta. The testis gets additional blood supply from artery of the vas and the cremasteric arteries. In case of inguinal surgeries, if the testicular artery is accidentally injured, testicular vascularity is maintained by these two arteries. Veins form the pampiniform plexus in the scrotum.
- **Lymphatics:** Drain *via* the para-aortic nodes lying along the side of aorta at the level of origin of the testicular arteries (L2) just above umbilicus.

EPIDIDYMIS

- It is 6 m in length (20 feet long), highly coiled and packed, and adherent to the posterior surface of the testis.
- It has the following parts—head, body and tail. Head and body are commonly involved in tuberculosis, resulting in posterior sinus formation.
- It is lined by tall columnar epithelium.
- The head receives vasa afferentia from the rete testis and is firmly attached to the testis.

- From the tail, the vas deferens (ductus deferens), a direct continuation of the canal of the epididymis, passes up medially.
- The epididymis is supplied by a branch of the testicular artery.

Competency

SU30.5: Describe applied anatomy, clinical features, investigations and principles of management of hydrocoele.

HYDROCOELE

A collection of excessive fluid in the tunica vaginalis sac (TV sac).

I. CONGENITAL HYDROCOELE

Occurs due to a complete or partial patent processus vaginalis sac.

Types

1. **Vaginal hydrocoele** (Fig. 60.16): Occurs when the hydrocoele sac is patent only in the scrotum.
2. **Infantile hydrocoele** (Fig. 60.17): The sac from the scrotum is patent up to the deep inguinal ring.
3. **True congenital hydrocoele** (Fig. 60.18)
   - In this condition, the scrotal sac communicates with the peritoneal cavity. It is seen in infants and may be secondary to TB peritonitis. A scrotal swelling appears when the child assumes an erect posture for a long time, and it may not reduce due to the **inverted ink bottle** effect. Hence, congenital hydrocoele is not reducible. It regresses in size if the child assumes a supine position while sleeping.
4. **Encysted hydrocoele of the cord** (Figs 60.19 and 60.23–60.25)
   - In this condition, the sac is obliterated above (inguinal canal) and below (scrotum) but patent at the root of the scrotum around the spermatic cord.
   - It presents as a soft, cystic, fluctuant, transilluminant swelling separate from the testis and well above the testis.
   - Diagnosis is established by the **traction test**: The swelling has free mobility, but when gentle traction is applied, the swelling becomes fixed and moves down when the testis is pulled down. This variety of hydrocoele is treated by excision of the sac.
5. **Hydrocoele-en-bissac** (bilocular hydrocoele) (Fig. 60.20): In this condition, the scrotal sac communicates with another sac underneath the anterior abdominal wall musculature. The diagnosis is made by eliciting **cross-fluctuation**.

VARIOUS TYPES OF HYDROCOELE

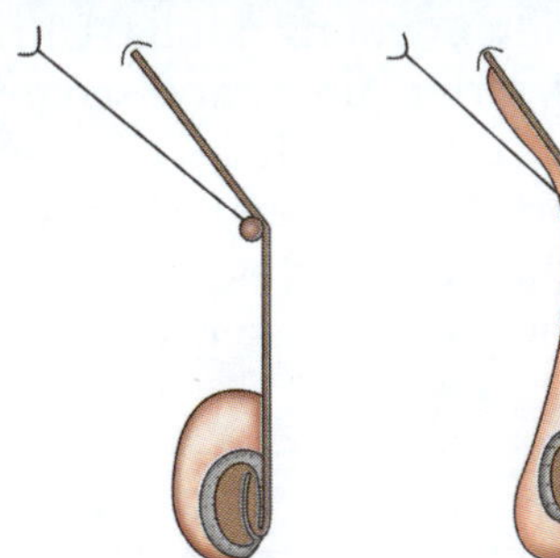
Fig. 60.16: Vaginal hydrocele

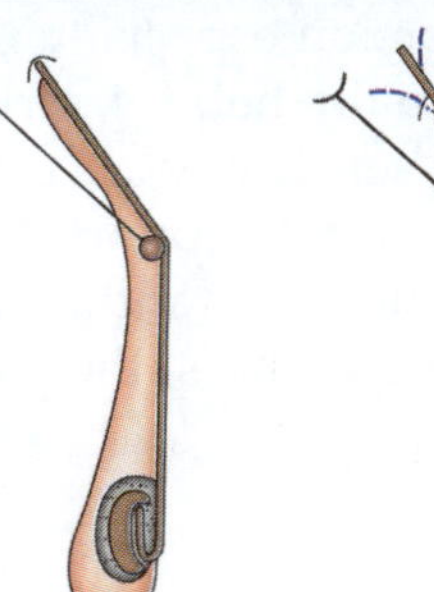
Fig. 60.17: Infantile hydrocele

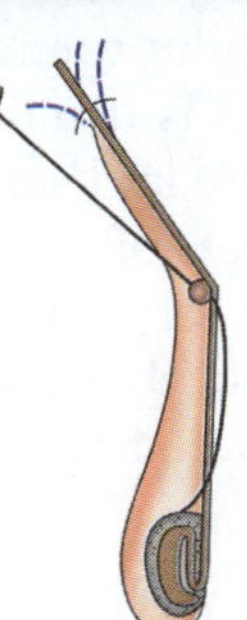
Fig. 60.18: True congenital hydrocele

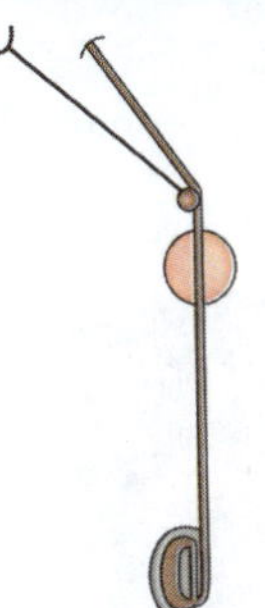
Fig. 60.19: Encysted hydrocele of the cord

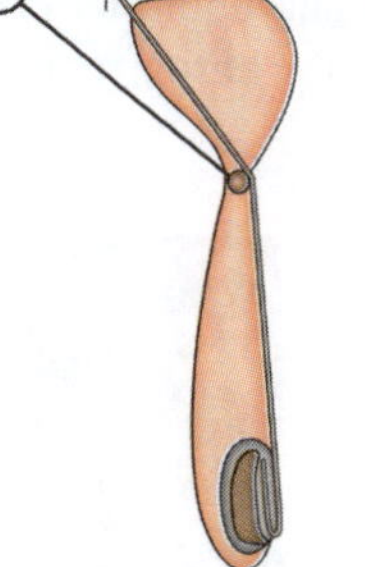
Fig. 60.20: Hydrocele en-bissac

Fig. 60.21: Hydrocele of the canal of Nuck

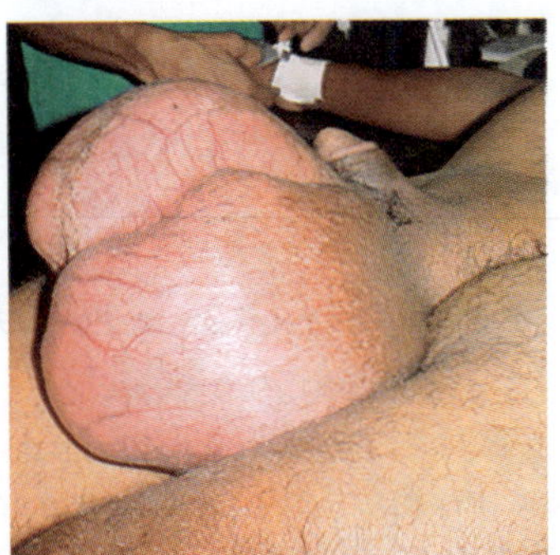
Fig. 60.22: Bilateral primary vaginal hydrocoele

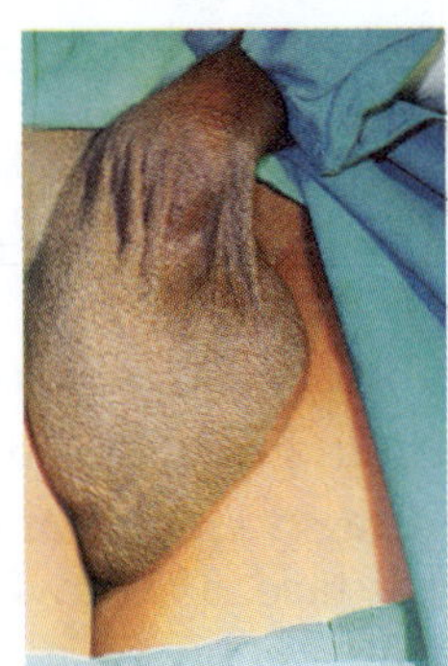
Fig. 60.23: Encysted hydrocoele

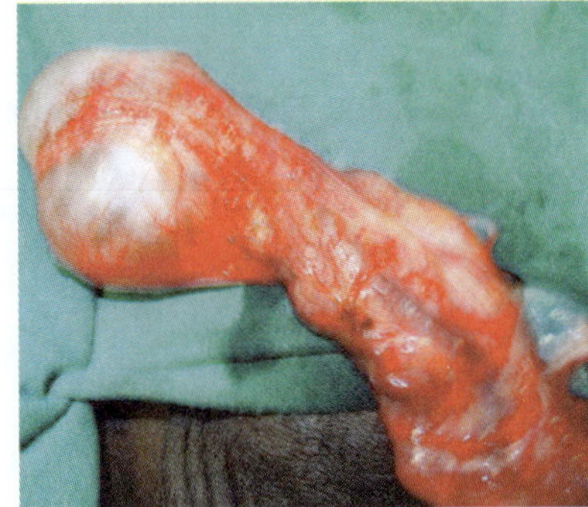
Fig. 60.24: Encysted hydrocele at surgery

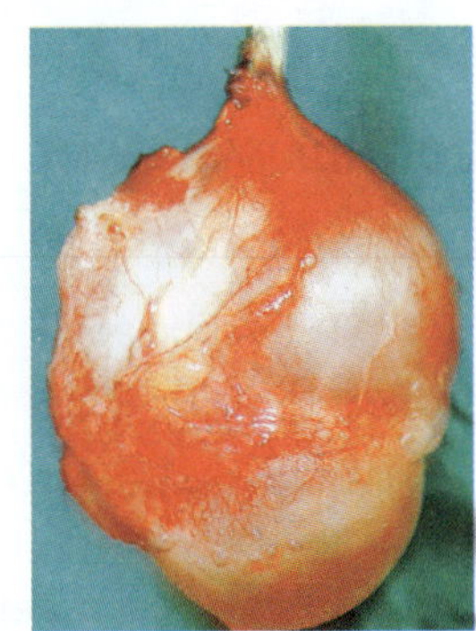
Fig. 60.25: Encysted hydrocele—excised specimen

Table 60.2 Comparison of primary hydrocoele with secondary hydrocoele

	Primary hydrocoele	Secondary hydrocoele
1. Aetiology	Defective absorption of fluid	Excessive production of fluid
2. Examples	Vaginal hydrocoele, infantile hydrocoele	Filarial hydrocoele, secondary to malignancy of the testis
3. Size	Moderate, big	Small
4. Palpation of the testis	Difficult	Easily palpable
5. Transillumination	Positive in majority of the cases	Usually negative
6. Consistency	Tensely cystic	Lax, cystic
7. Treatment	Partial excision and eversion	Treatment of the primary

6. **Hydrocoele of the canal of Nuck** (Fig. 60.21): It presents as a swelling in the inguinal region in females.

II. ACQUIRED HYDROCOELE (Table 60.2)

a. Primary or idiopathic.
b. Secondary hydrocoele.

PRIMARY VAGINAL HYDROCOELE (Fig. 60.22)

This is the most common type of hydrocoele which is seen in young adults, middle age and beyond. It is due to the following causes:

1. Defective absorption of fluid
2. Defective lymphatic drainage

Pearls of Wisdom

- Hydrocoele fluid contains albumin and fibrinogen.
- Filarial hydrocoeles contain liquid fat rich in cholesterol.
- Hydrocoele of hernia is a hernia containing hydrocoele fluid (Fig. 60.26)

Clinical Features

- Soft, cystic, fluctuant, transillumination positive swelling confined to the scrotum.
- Not reducible
- No impulse on cough
- Can get above the swelling.

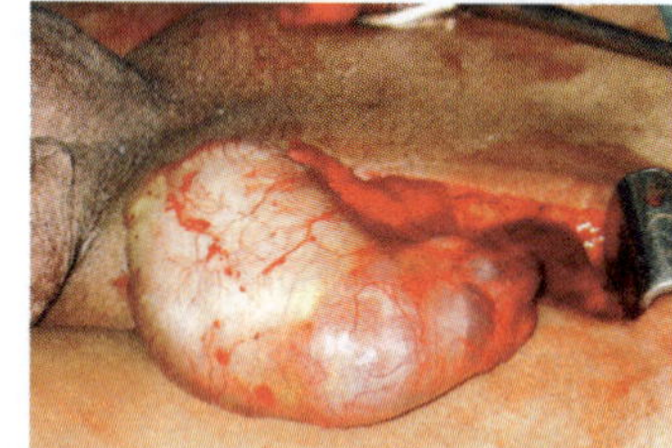

Fig. 60.26: Hydrocoele of hernia

SECONDARY HYDROCOELE

Competency

SU30.3: Describe applied anatomy, clinical features, investigations, principles of management of epididymo-orchitis.

1. **Epididymo-orchitis:** It is inflammation of epididymis and testis commonly due to infection. It is usually unilateral. **Recurrent epididymo-orchitis due to filariasis:** Fluid accumulates due to lymphatic obstruction. The fluid is milky white. Such hydrocoeles are called chylocoeles (Fig. 60.27) and often do not exhibit transillumination. (Key Box 60.2).

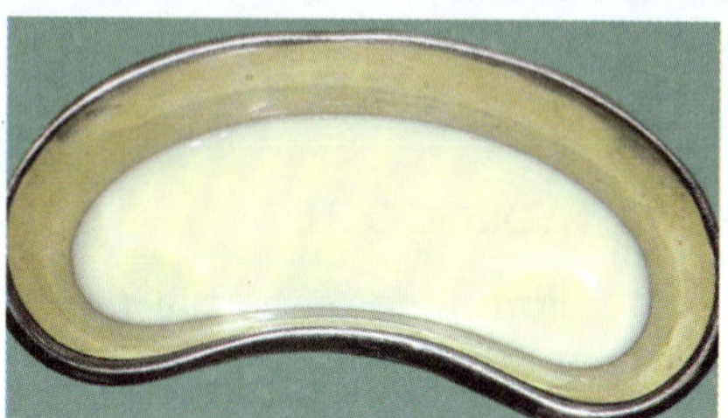

Fig. 60.27: Chylocoele fluid

Patient may present with acute scrotal pain with or without fever, dysuria or urethral discharge. Common organisms are *E. coli*, Chlamydia, *N. gonorrhoeae*, *M. tuberculosis*, etc. Mumps also causes epididymo-orchitis. It should be differentiated from testicular torsion especially in young adults. Ultrasound is usually helpful. Urine, urethral discharge culture and sensitivity are often needed. Treatment consists of scrotal support, NSAIDs and antibiotics like fluoroquinolones and/or tetracycline. In all cases of epididymo-orchitis, the partner also needs to be evaluated.

Key Box 60.2

Hydrocoele: Transillumination Negative

- Sac is very thick
- Sac is calcified
- Chylocoele (Fig. 60.27)
- Haematocoele
- Pyocoele
- Malignancy testis—blood-stained effusion

2. **Tuberculous epididymo-orchitis** (Figs 60.28 and 60.29)
   - Retrograde infection from the seminal vesicles.
   - **Craggy epididymis** refers to a rough, hard, irregular surface. This involves the epididymal head and causes fibrosis, making the epididymis feel craggy. Vas deferens feels like beads, called **beaded vas.** Secondary hydrocoele occurs in 30% of the cases.

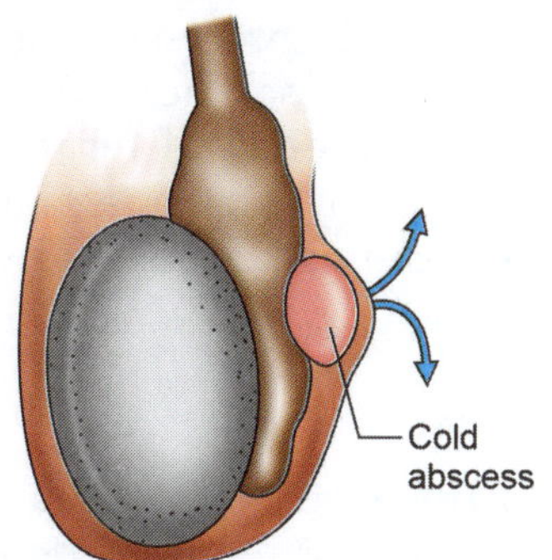

Figs 60.28 and 60.29: Tuberculous epididymo-orchitis

Eventually, it forms a **cold abscess** which ruptures and results in a **sinus posteriorly,** in the scrotum.

- It never involves the testis proper.

3. **Testicular tumours:** They can present with a swelling of the scrotum and are, often diagnosed as hydrocoele. Any young patient with a rapidly growing scrotal swelling could be having a testicular neoplasm. Fluid within the sac is haemorrhagic.
4. **Pyocoele:** Infected hydrocoele. Infection in a hydrocoele is rare because of the tunica vaginalis sac, which is relatively avascular. However, a few cases may get infected, resulting in pyocoele. These patients present with fever, chills and rigors.
5. **Haematocoele:** Trauma to the hydrocoele or spontaneous bleeding into the sac.

Treatment of Hydrocoele

(Key Box 60.3, also *see* Chapter 70)

1. **Lord's plication** is indicated in small hydrocoeles. The sac is opened, and the cut edge of the sac is plicated to tunica albuginea (the reflected portion of the processus vaginalis). As a result, the sac gets crumpled up near the testis. Testicular secretions get absorbed by subcutaneous lymphatics and the venous system.
2. **Partial excision and eversion of the sac:** Jaboulay's operation. This is indicated in large hydrocoeles. The thick, large, sac is excised and sutured behind the testis.
3. **Aspiration** is a temporary method that may introduce infection. It can be done only in high-risk patients and is a procedure to be condemned.

Key Box 60.3

Treatment of Hydrocoele

- Observe
- Lord's plication
- Jaboulay's operation

Complications of Hydrocoele

1. Haematocoele: Occurs due to minor trauma
2. Pyocoele: Infected haematocoele
3. Calcification of the hydrocoele sac
4. Rupture of the hydrocoele sac—very rare
5. **Hernia of the hydrocoele sac** occurs when there is a small tear in the sac resulting in accumulation of fluid in the subcutaneous planes (Fig. 60.30).

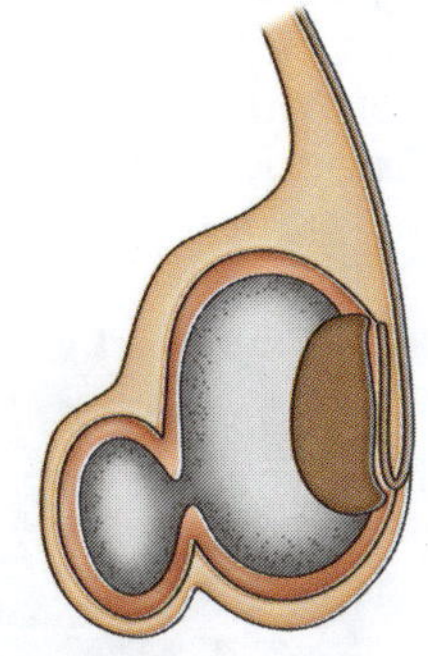

Fig. 60.30: Hernia of the hydrocoele sac

CYSTIC SWELLINGS IN THE SCROTUM

I. Hydrocoele

II. Retention cyst

1. Spermatocoele (Table 60.3 and Fig. 60.31)

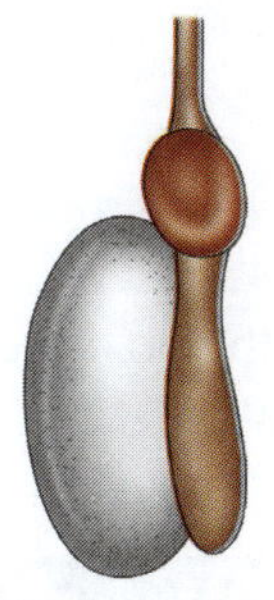

Fig. 60.31: Spermatocoele

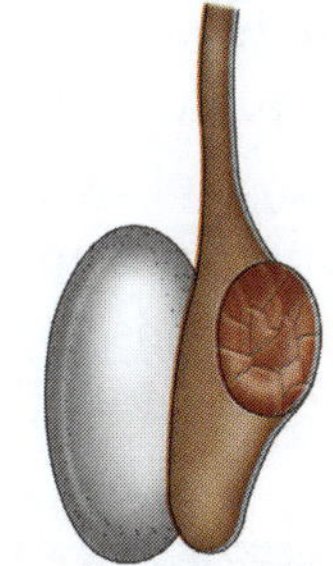

Fig. 60.32: Epididymal cyst

Table 60.3 Comparison of epididymal cyst with spermatocoele

	Epididymal cyst (Fig. 60.32)	**Spermatocoele**
1. Aetiology	Cystic degeneration of the appendages of epididymis—**congenital**	Obstruction to the sperm conducting mechanism; **acquired**—retention cyst
2. Site	Behind and above the testis in the region of epididymal head	Behind the body of the testis
3. Loculi	Multilocular	Unilocular
4. Contents	Crystal clear, watery	Barley water-like
5. Transillumination	Brilliant (Chinese lantern pattern)	Poor transillumination—very often negative
6. Aspiration	Results in recurrence as the cyst is multilocular	May cure as the cyst is unilocular
7. Excision	Excision may be necessary if the cyst is large	May be excised if aspiration is not successful

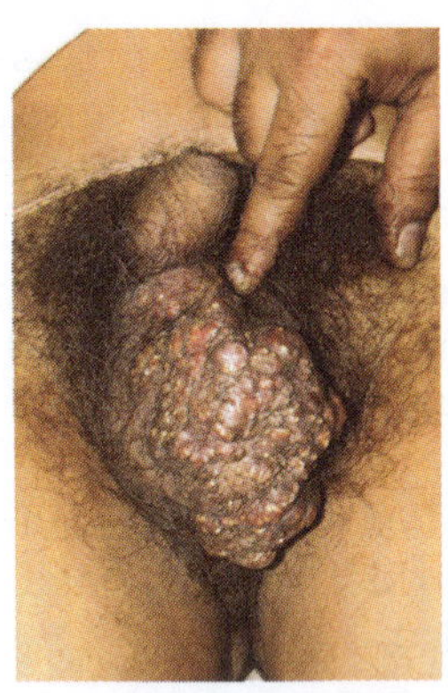

Fig. 60.33: Multiple sebaceous cysts of the scrotum (*Courtesy:* Prof Abdul Majeed, MS FRCS, Yenepoya Medical College, Mangalore)

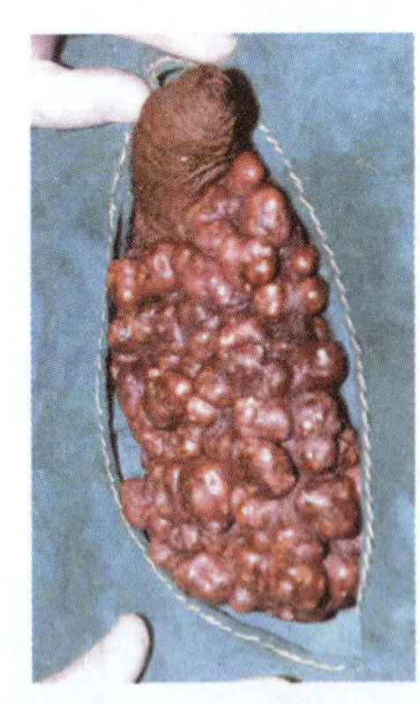

Fig. 60.34: Strawberry scrotum (*Courtesy:* Dr Umesh Bhat, General Surgeon, Kundapur, Karnataka)

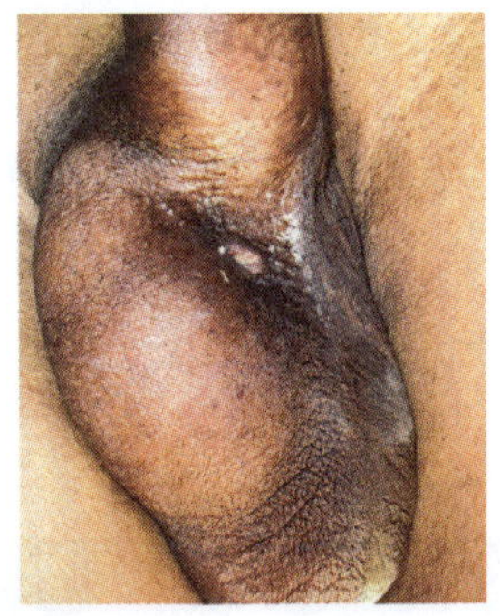

Fig. 60.35: TB sinus scrotum

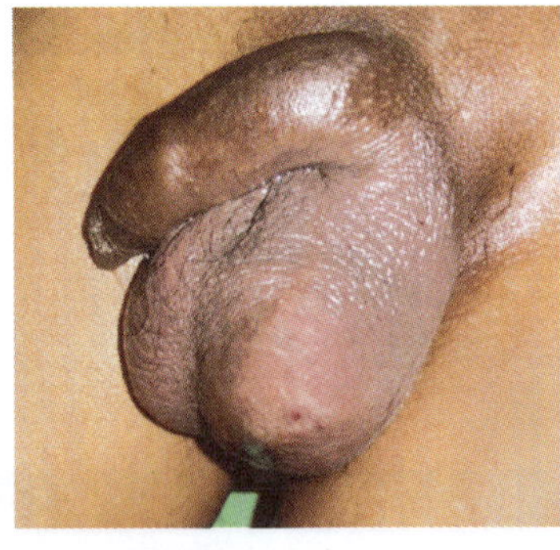

Fig. 60.36: Abscess scrotum

2. Sebaceous cyst (skin of the scrotum) (Figs 60.33 and 60.34)

III. **Congenital cyst**
1. Epididymal cyst
2. Cyst of the hydatid of Morgagni

IV. **Tubercular epididymo-orchitis**
- Cold abscess with a sinus in the posterior aspect of scrotum (Figs 60.35 and 60.36).

UNDESCENDED TESTIS

This occurs when the descent of the testis is arrested somewhere along its normal pathway to the scrotum.

Development

- The testis develops in the retroperitoneum close to the posterior abdominal wall from the genital tubercles.
- It is guided to the scrotum by the gubernaculum.
- By around the 7th month—it reaches the deep inguinal ring, by the 8th month—inguinal canal and by the 9th month—superficial inguinal pouch. In normal situations, the testis reaches the scrotum at full term.
- As it descends, it is surrounded by the processus vaginalis sac. This sac normally gets completely obliterated. A persistent processes vaginalis sac causes hernia and hydrocoele (Fig. 60.37).

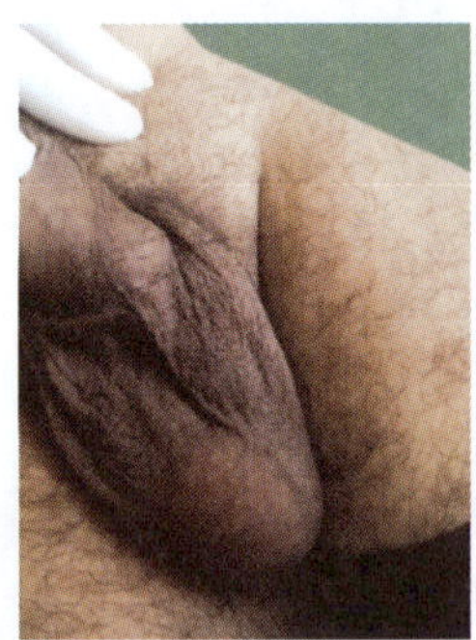

Fig. 60.37: Left testis is absent in the scrotum

Causes

1. **Muscular hypotonia:** The descent of the testis depends upon muscular contractions of the anterior abdominal wall. Hence, undescended testis is seen in children with poor muscle tone, (e.g. prune-belly syndrome and Down's syndrome).
2. **Gubernaculum dysfunction.**
3. **Maternal human chorionic gonadotrophin** (HCG) which causes development (maturation) of the testis and also helps in descent of the testis. If there is deficiency of HCG, imperfectly developed undescended testis appears.
4. **Familial**
5. Retroperitoneal adhesions.

Clinical Features

1. Right side is more often involved. Bilateral undescended testis is found in about 20% of cases.
2. **Cryptorchidism:** When both testes are impalpable as in cases of abdominal testis and inguinal testis.
3. **Retractile testis:** In this condition, the scrotum is well-developed, and the testis is palpable at the root of the scrotum and can be brought down to the scrotum. Retractile testis is harmless and spontaneously gets corrected within 1–2 years of age, without any treatment. The squatting position may help in such cases, in diagnosing the condition and in helping the testis descend to the scrotum.

Complications (can be remembered as **TESTIS**)

T Trauma produces pain

E Epididymo-orchitis will mimic an acute abdomen.

S Sterility: Histological changes start at the age of 2 years, and by the age of 12 years, irreversible damage occurs to spermatogenesis, due to testicular atrophy. Endocrine function remains normal.

T Torsion

I Indirect hernia in the majority of cases.

S Seminoma of the testis and other testicular malignancies are more common in undescended testis than in normal testis. **(Risk of seminoma in both testes, not only in undescended testis.)**

Treatment

1. **Treatment of choice is orchidopexy.**
   - It can be done by open method or laparoscopic method.
   - It can be performed as a one-stage or two-stage procedure.

   Two-stage procedure for undescended testis **(Fowler-Stephens technique).**

   Stage I—tethering spermatic blood vessels are divided.

   Stage II—testicle is placed into the scrotum after collateral blood supply to the testicle develops.

   Procedure
   - Considering functional and malignant potential of undescended testis, ideal age of surgery is between 9 months to 1 year. The inguinal canal is explored, and the testis is mobilised by dividing the adhesions, brought down into the scrotum, and fixed using nonabsorbable suture material.
   - A dartos pouch can be formed and followed later by narrowing the root of scrotum.
   - Associated hernial sac is excised.
2. **Orchidectomy** is done after the age of 14 years because of malignant potential.
3. **Ombredanne's procedure:** Testis is brought down to the opposite scrotum through the scrotal septum and kept in dartos pouch.
4. **Silber's procedure:** The testicular artery and vein can be divided and reanastomosed using microvascular techniques.

ECTOPIC TESTIS

- Testis is present in an **ectopic** site (not the route through which it descends).
- **Sites** of ectopic sites are:
  - Superficial inguinal pouch
  - Perineum
  - Root of the penis
  - Femoral triangle (thigh)
- Anatomically, the size is normal. Physiologically, it functions normally.
- **Embryology:** Testis reaches the scrotum by the scrotal tail gubernaculum. However, if this is weak, the other scrotal tail may pull it in a different direction, resulting in ectopic testis (Lockwood's theory).
- **Complication:** It is more prone to injuries.
- **Treatment:** Orchidopexy in a new scrotal pouch.

Competency

SU30.4: Describe applied anatomy, clinical features, investigations and principles of management of varicocele.

VARICOCELE

Definition

Dilated and tortuous veins of pampiniform plexus (veins draining the testis and epididymis). It lies posterior and above the testis. This can be totally missed if examination is done in the supine position. It is the most common surgically correctable cause of subfertility in males.

Anatomy

- Testicular veins, which drain the testis and epididymis, form multiple veins in the scrotum called the pampiniform plexus of veins. As they travel the inguinal canal, they are reduced to 6–8 in number. At the level of the deep ring, they are 2 in number and in the retroperitoneum, it forms the single testicular vein.
- On the right side, the testicular vein drains into the inferior vena cava directly.
- On the left side, it drains into the left renal vein at right angles where there is a valve.

Aetiology

1. Most common cause is absence/incompetent valves in internal spermatic or testicular veins.
2. Increased venous pressure in the left renal vein is also a factor. It is due to compression of the left renal vein between the aorta and superior mesenteric artery. The left renal vein can also be compressed by the sigmoid colon. Varicocele is common on the left side (because left testis is at a lower level than the right). The flow of blood from the left side is into the renal vein at an angle of 90°.
3. A recent varicocele on the right side in an elderly patient suggests renal cell carcinoma invading the renal veins. Such varicoceles are rapidly evolving and do not regress in the supine position.

Clinical Features

- Common in thin, tall patients
- Hot climates, favour the development of varicocele.
- In the **standing position**, the diseased side appears to be more swollen than the other side. It feels like a bag of worms. On asking the patient to cough, there is fluid thrill, due to regurgitation of venous blood. On the side of varicocele, the scrotum is at a lower level.

- On asking the patient to lie down, it is reducible (disappears).
- Dragging pain in the scrotum is a feature but it is nontender.
- The testis may appear small and soft with diminished testicular sensation.
- **Blow test:** On blowing, fluid thrill may be felt, and it may increase in size (Valsalva's manoeuvre).
  USG demonstrating veins ≥3.5 mm in diameter with reversal of venous flow after Valsalva manoeuvre–varicocele.

Grading of Varicocele

I (small)—palpable only with Valsalva manoeuvre, not visible

II (moderate)—palpable without Valsalva manoeuvre, not visible

III (large)—palpable and visible through scrotal skin.

Pearls of Wisdom

Subclinical varicocele: Only demonstrated by special tests or Doppler demonstrating reflux. They are neither palpable nor visible on Valsalva manoeuvre.

Effect on Spermatogenesis

Oligospermia

This occurs due to the following reasons:

A. **Venous congestion** due to the varicocele results in increased temperature in the scrotum.

B. **Reflux of blood** from the renal vein brings powerful hormones secreted from adrenal glands like corticosteroids and adrenaline.

Pearls of Wisdom

Oligospermia is a major and significant complication of varicocele. Semen quality improves in 65% of cases postoperatively.

Treatment

1. **Subinguinal microscopic (Joel Marmar's operation) varicocelectomy** for complete ligation.
2. **Inguinal approach (Ivanissevich operation):** Excision of the pampiniform plexus in the inguinal canal after ligating them. The testis still has venous drainage through the cremasteric veins.
3. **Retroperitoneal approach (Palomo's operation):** In the retroperitoneum, the testicular vein is single and separate from the vas deferens. Hence, it is ligated up in the retroperitoneum. This operation was once thought to be better than the inguinal approach since there is no danger of damaging the vas and ligation of testicular vein is easy; however, recurrence rates are high so it is not favoured nowadays.
4. **Laparoscopic varicocelectomy is popular**—retroperitoneal approach.

Complications of Varicocele Surgery

1. Hydrocele: It is because of ligation of the lymphatic channels as well. It is least after microscopic ligation.
2. Testicular atrophy is seen in ≤1% of patients.
3. Recurrence.

TORSION TESTIS (TORSION OF THE SPERMATIC CORD)

Predisposing Causes

- **Inversion of the testis** is the most common cause, where the testis lies horizontally or upside down.
- **High investment** of tunica vaginalis—bell clapper deformity.
- In cases where the body of the testis is separated from the epididymis.
- **Sudden contraction** of the spirally attached cremasteric muscle leads to rotation of the testis around its vertical axis during straining (e.g. at stools, lifting heavy weight, coitus).
- **A long, redundant spermatic cord** allows twisting of the testis on its own axis.

There are two types of testicular torsion:

- **Extravaginal torsion:** It is diagnosed in newborns and is caused by non-adherence of the tunica vaginalis to the dartos layer.
  As a result, the spermatic cord and tunica vaginalis are rotated as a unit.
- **Intravaginal torsion:** It is usually diagnosed in boys 12–18 years of age but can occur at any age.

Clinical Features

- Age: 10–25 years, sudden agonising pain in the groin and lower abdomen, may be with vomiting.
- **Scrotum is empty** and oedematous on the side of the lesion (Fig. 60.38A).
- Tender lump at the external abdominal ring—the testis is positioned high (**Deming's sign).**

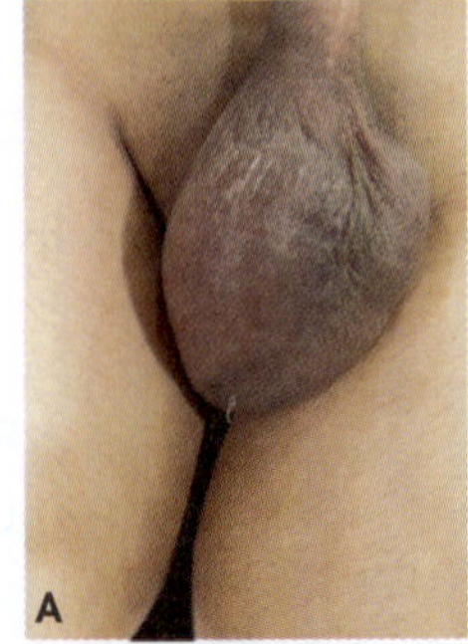

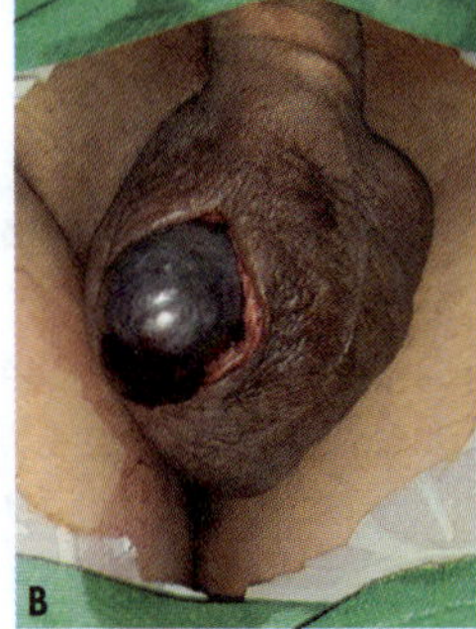

Fig. 60.38A and B: A. Torsion testis right side; B. Gangrenous testis at surgery (*Courtesy:* Prof. Amit Jain, SRRM College, Bengaluru)

- **Prehn's sign:** Elevation of the scrotum increases pain in torsion of completely descended testis (decreases pain in epididymo-orchitis).
- **Angell's sign:** The opposite testis lies horizontally because of the mesorchium.

Management

- Best results—if detorsion occurs within 4 hours of the onset of pain.
- **Scrotal Doppler** to confirm the diagnosis
  1. In the first hour, untwist the testis manually
  2. If this is not successful, urgently explore the scrotum and undo the torsion. A viable testis should be fixed to the scrotum to prevent recurrence.
  3. Gangrenous testis should be removed (Fig. 60.38B).
  4. The testis on the opposite side should be fixed at an early date to prevent torsion as it also has a high risk of undergoing torsion.

Pearls of Wisdom

Patients should be counselled and consented for orchidectomy before exploration.

Competency

SU30.6: Describe applied anatomy, clinical features, investigations and principles of management of testicular tumours.

TESTICULAR TUMOURS

They constitute 1% of all malignant tumours in males, and almost all (>90%) are malignant.

CLASSIFICATION

A. WHO Classification (Key Box 60.4)

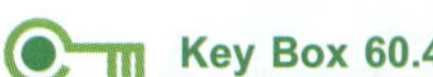

Key Box 60.4

WHO Classification Germ Cell Tumour

Seminoma	Nonseminomatous germ cell tumours
Classic (85%)	Teratoma
Spermatocytic	Embryonal cell carcinoma
Anaplastic	Choriocarcinoma
Lymphocytic	Yolk sac tumour

B. Other Classification

I. **Seminoma is the most common germ cell tumour: 50% incidence**

Types

1. Spermatocytic—good prognosis
2. Lymphocytic
3. Anaplastic

II. **Teratoma**
- Incidence: 30% (subtype will be discussed later)

III. **Combined**
- 10 to 20%

IV. **Interstitial cell tumours**
  a. Leydig cell tumour
  b. Sertoli cell tumours

V. **Lymphoma of testis:** Very rare

SEMINOMA

Aetiology

1. **Undescended testis,** undoubtedly predisposes to seminoma.
   - 1 in 20 abdominal testes, 1 in 60 testes at the level of deep ring and 1 in 80 inguinal testes are prone to testicular tumours.
   - However, it should be noted that 25% of testicular cancers in patients with crypto-orchidism occur in normal, descended testis.
2. **Klinefelter's syndrome:** These patients are prone to developing of seminoma. Other features of the disease are testicular atrophy, absence of spermatogenesis, gynaecomastia, etc.
3. **Trauma** to the testis is a coincidence. This may not precipitate a testicular tumour but draws the attention of the patient to it.

Pathology

Seminoma arises from the seminiferous tubules. As the tumour grows, it compresses the normal testicular tissue. The cut surface is smooth and homogenous (Fig. 60.39). **Microscopy: Round to oval cells** with a prominent nucleus. In a few cases, **lymphocytic infiltration** may be found.

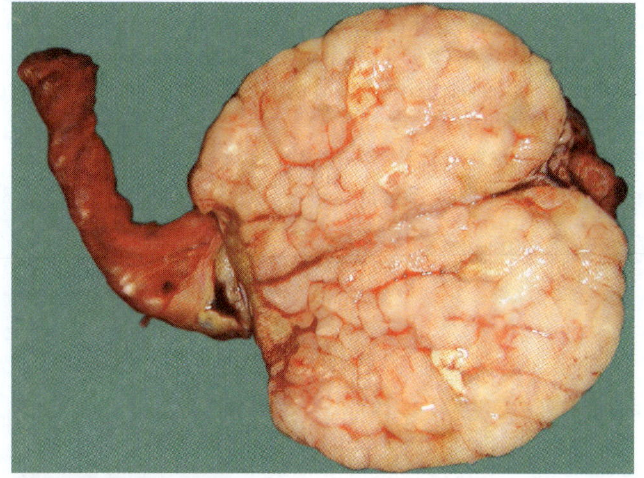

Fig. 60.39: Testicular tumour. The entire testicular parenchyma is replaced by tumour

Types of Seminoma

1. **Typical: It is the most common type of seminoma** and is also called classic variety. Syncytiotrophoblastic type produces high levels of β-HCG.
2. **Spermatocytic type:** It occurs in elderly patients. It is slow growing and rarely spreads. Hence, it has good prognosis.
3. **Anaplastic:** As the name suggests, this variety has a high mitotic index/anaplasia and thus spreads fast and carries poor prognosis.
4. **Atypical form**

TERATOMA

Teratoma arises from rete testis. The tumour contains totipotential cells, so it may have ectodermal, mesodermal and endodermal elements.

Types of Teratoma

1. **Malignant teratoma differentiated:** It is the least common variety (1%). It is almost a benign tumour—**Dermoid cyst.** Orchidectomy cures the disease.
2. **Malignant teratoma intermediate:** This is the most common variety (30%) and contains malignant and incompletely differentiated components.
3. **Malignant teratoma anaplastic:** Highly malignant tumour. Secretes alfa fetoprotein (AFP). Cells are presumed to be from the yolk sac.
4. **Malignant teratoma trophoblastic:** This is an uncommon tumour (1%) that secretes very high levels of β-human chorionic gonadotropins (β-HCG).

CLINICAL FEATURES OF TESTICULAR TUMOURS

(Key Box 60.5)

I. Typical Presentation

- **Age:** Teratoma 20–30 years, seminoma 30–40 years.
- **Testicular swelling:** More often heaviness rather than hypertrophy or if it is infiltrated with tumour but vas is never involved. This is called **sign of vas negative** (sign of vas positive in TB epididymo-orchitis where there is beading of vas).
- **Haemospermia:** Blood in the semen is rare.
- **Infertility:** Not uncommon.

Key Box 60.5

Testicular Cancer

- Irregular testis
- Indurated testis
- Nodular testis
- Nontender enlarged testis
- Young age testicular mass, small hydrocoele
- Heaviness, loss of sensation

- **Gynaecomastia** is seen in about 10% of patients.
- **Secondary hydrocoele** is not uncommon. A young adult with a small hydrocoele and enlarged testis should arouse suspicion of testicular cancer.

II. Atypical Presentation

1. Hurricane variety is the most malignant tumour. The tumour grows rapidly with pulmonary metastasis (cannonball), and death occurs within a few days.
2. Mimicking acute epididymo-orchitis: This variety presents as severe pain along with testicular swelling but does not respond to antibiotics.

III. Symptoms Mainly due to Metastases

1. **Lymphatic spread**
   - Para-aortic node mass—distension of the abdomen (Fig. 60.40).
   - Left supraclavicular node mass—swelling in the neck.
   - Iliac node mass—swelling of the leg.
2. **Blood spread:** Extensive pulmonary secondaries occur from a malignant teratoma.

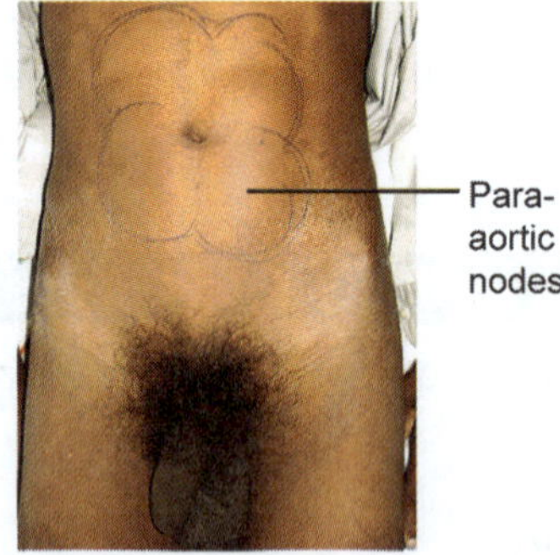

Fig. 60.40: Seminoma testis with para-aortic nodes—clinical examination of testis is very important in an upper abdominal mass

SPREAD

- Seminoma spreads lymphatically. Along the testicular vessels, it spreads to the para-aortic lymph nodes to the thoracic duct, to mediastinal nodes, and then to the left supraclavicular nodes. ***Spread does not occur to the inguinal nodes, unless the scrotum is incised.***
- Malignant teratomatous tumours spread predominantly by blood.

TNM STAGING OF TESTICULAR CANCER

- Stage I: Tumour confined to the testis only.
- Stage IIA: Tumour and lymph nodes below the diaphragm—size ≤2 cm.
- Stage IIB: Tumour and lymph nodes below the diaphragm—size ≥2 cm.

TNM STAGING	Testicular carcinoma[1]
T:	Primary tumour
Tx:	Tumour cannot be assessed
T0:	No primary tumour
Tis:	Carcinoma *in-situ*: (Intralobular germ cell neoplasia)
T1:	Tumour limited to testis and epididymis without vascular or lymphatic invasion (tumour may invade tunica albuginea but not vaginalis)
T2:	Tumour limited to testis and epididymis + vascular or lymphatic invasion or invasion of tunica vaginalis
T3:	Tumour invades spermatic cord (with or without vascular or lymphatic invasion)
T4:	Tumour invades scrotum with or without vascular or lymphatic invasion
N:	Regional lymph nodes
Nx:	Lymph node status cannot be assessed
N0:	No lymph node metastasis
N1:	Single or multiple <2 cm in greatest dimension
N2:	Nodes 2–5 cm in greatest dimension; more than 5 lymph nodes are positive but none more than 5 cm in size or no extra-nodal invasion
N3:	Nodes >5 cm in greatest dimension
M:	Distant metastasis
Mx:	Distant metastasis cannot be assessed
M0:	No distant metastasis
M1:	Distant metastasis present
M1a:	Nonregional nodal or lung metastasis
M1b:	Nonpulmonary visceral metastasis (M2)

[1]Staging also considers serum tumour markers—S-LDH, HCG, AFP

Sx: Not available/not performed

S0: Normal levels

	LDH (U/L)	HCG (mIV/mL)	AFP (ng/mL)
S1	<1.5 × N	<5000	<1000
S2	1.5–10 × N	5000–50000	1000–10000
S3	>10 × N	>50000	>10000

- Stage III: Tumour and lymph nodes above the diaphragm, mediastinal nodes, pulmonary or liver metastasis, etc. Each stage can be added letters S-means tumour markers.

Pearls of Wisdom

No biopsy should be done through the scrotal route because if the scrotal skin is involved, spread occurs to the inguinal lymph nodes opening up another lymphatic channel. Even FNAC is not recommended.

INVESTIGATIONS

1. **Ultrasound of the testis is the first investigation:** Seminoma appears as a hypoechoic lesion, and nonseminomatous tumours are non-homogenous.
2. **Chest X-ray:** To rule out cannonball secondaries, as in teratoma.
3. **Abdominal USG** to look for enlarged lymph nodes and secondaries in the liver, or to detect a tumour in an undescended testis. However, CT scan is a better investigation.
4. **MRI:** It is an excellent investigations which can diagnose testicular tumours and can also differentiate from hematoma or orchitis etc.
5. **CT scan:** Heterogenously enhancing testicular mass with retroperitoneal lymph nodes and liver metastasis can be made out (Fig. 60.41).
6. **24-hours urine sample for HCG**
   - Normal levels—≤100 IU
   - ≥1000 IU is diagnostic of chorio-carcinoma
   - Hence, it is the tumour marker of chorio-carcinoma.
7. **Human chorionic gonadotrophin: Serum HCG** (Key Box 60.6)
   - As the name suggests, it is made by chorionic elements.

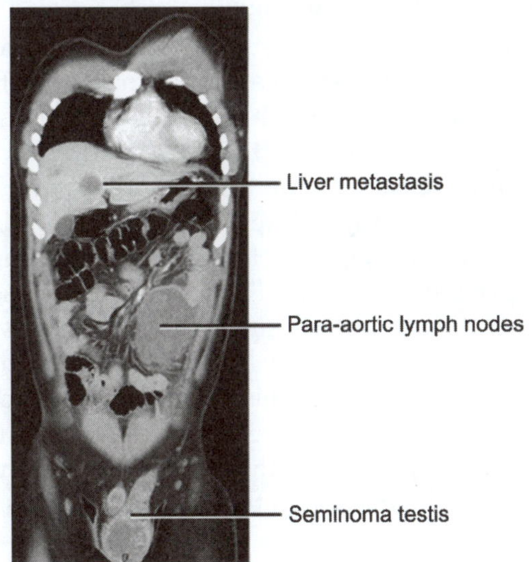

Fig. 60.41: Testicular tumour with para-aortic lymph nodes and liver metastasis

Key Box 60.6

β-HCG

- Never found in normal persons
- Secreted by syncytiotrophoblasts
- Choriocarcinoma: 100% cases
- Seminoma: 10% of cases
- Embryonal carcinoma: 65% of cases
- Increased levels after orchidectomy indicate recurrence or residual tumour
- Tumour marker of teratocarcinoma

- HCG as a whole (α- and β-HCG) may be increased in testicular neoplasm, melanoma, lymphoma, etc. It can also be raised in nonmalignant conditions, such as cirrhosis and, peptic ulcer disease.
- β-HCG is more important in diagnosing testicular neoplasms and is also useful in the postoperative period to investigate for residual or recurrent tumour.
- The blood level of **β-HCG is 0 ng/ml.**

8. **α-fetoprotein:** Increased in nonseminomatous germ cell tumours.
9. **Lactate dehydrogenase (LDH):** Increased in nonseminomatous germ cell tumours. LDH levels indicate tumour load. It is not specific for any tumour.
10. **Placental alkaline phosphatase** is increased in seminoma testis.

TREATMENT

I. Treatment of the Tumour

- **Radical inguinal orchidectomy is the treatment of choice in all testicular tumours irrespective of the histological type and stage.**

  When a patient presents with rapidly growing testicular swelling and the neoplasm is doubtful, the **testis is explored through an inguinal incision.** It is delivered out, and a **soft clamp is applied to the testicular vessels at the level of deep ring while performing the procedure so that tumour embolization does not occur.** The testis is split open and the suspicious area is biopsied and sent for frozen section. If the frozen section is positive, the cord and testicular vessels are divided at the level of the deep ring, and the testis is removed. This is called **high orchidectomy**. If frozen section is negative, the testis is sutured back and replaced in the scrotum. This type of procedure done through the inguinal route is called **Chevasu's procedure**.

II. Treatment of the Retroperitoneum and Metastasis (Key Box 60.7)

1. Seminoma

a. **Stage I-IIA (low stage):** Radiotherapy to the retroperitoneum (2500–3000 cGy) is the treatment of choice:
   - 5-year survival rate is around 95%.
   - Relapse after radiotherapy is managed by chemotherapy.

b. **Stage IIB, III, IV**
   - Radical orchidectomy + chemotherapy-PVB regimen—cisplatin, vincristine, bleomycin.
   - BEP: Bleomycin, etoposide and cisplatin.

> **Key Box 60.7**
>
> **Retroperitoneal Lymph Node Dissection (RPLND)**
>
> - It is recommended in all cases of teratoma including stage I. It is also indicated in residual disease in lymph nodes in seminomatous tumours.
> - All groups of lymph nodes draining the tumour, such as the precaval, paracaval, interaortocaval, retroaortic, para-aortic, and common iliac nodes, are removed.
> - It also involves the removal of the gonadal vein and fibrofatty tissue around the vein from its origin near the internal ring to its insertion to the renal vein on the left side and the inferior vena cava on the right side.
> - The procedure is done bilaterally.
> - Haemorrhage and injury to ureter and bowel are other complications.
> - Retrograde ejaculation is a common problem after RPLND.

c. **Treatment of residual disease in lymph nodes**
   - Stage IIB and III: If there is residual lymph nodal mass 3 cm in size even after chemotherapy, retroperitoneal lymph node dissection (RPLND) has to be done.
   - Stage IIB and III: 5 year survival rate—75%.
   - Stage IV: Poor survival.

2. Teratoma

a. **Stage I, IIA (low stage):** Radical orchidectomy ±RPLND 5-year survival–85%.

b. **Stage IIB, III:** Radical orchidectomy and chemotherapy (PVB), post-chemotherapy residual tumour in the retroperitoneum and if the tumour markers levels regress RPLND. 5-year survival rate 60%.

Comparison of seminoma with teratoma (Table 60.4)

Other tumours are given below.

INTERSTITIAL CELL TUMOURS

- Two types are clinically important: Leydig cell tumour and Sertoli cell tumour.
- They should be treated like teratoma.

a. **Leydig cell tumour**
   - A prepubertal tumour
   - Causes masculinisation due to increased androgens—infant Hercules
   - Spreads to lymph nodes and lungs
   - Good prognosis because it behaves almost like a benign lesion

Table 60.4 Comparison of seminoma with teratoma

	Seminoma	Teratoma
1. Cell of origin	Seminiferous tubules in the mediastinum of the testis	Totipotential cells in the rete testis
2. Incidence	35–40%	30%
3. Age group	30–40 years	20–30 years
4. Shape of testis	Retained	Not retained
5. Surface	Smooth	Irregular
6. Cut surface	Smooth	Variegated—nodules, cysts
7. Consistency	Firm	Firm or soft (cystic)
8. Spread	Mainly lymphatic	Predominantly blood
9. Tumour markers	—	HCG—malignant teratoma
10. Radiation response	Excellent—melts like snow	Less sensitive

b. Sertoli cell tumours

- Feminizing tumours: Gynaecomastia, loss of libido, and aspermia are other features.
- Increased oestrogen production is responsible for feminisation.
- Postpubertal tumour
- Orchidectomy is the treatment of choice.

FOURNIER'S GANGRENE (IDIOPATHIC GANGRENE OF THE SCROTAL SKIN)

Aetiopathology

Even though Fournier's gangrene is called idiopathic gangrene, certain factors precipitate.

1. Low socio-economic group patients.
2. Unhygienic conditions

It follows perianal abscesses, urogenital instrumentation or a scratch, cut or bruise in the scrotal skin (instrumentation, injury, infection—Key Box 60.8).

Causative Organisms

- Microaerophilic *Haemolytic streptococci*
- *Staphylococci*
- *E. coli*
- Anaerobes: *Clostridium welchii*

(Can be compared to **Meleney's ulcer**—synergistic gangrene—affecting the skin of the abdominal wall. Today it is grouped under necrotizing fasciitis).

Clinical Features

1. Common in young apparently healthy individuals
2. Sudden appearance of scrotal inflammation—red, swollen, very painful. Patient is toxic with fever and prostration.
3. Within 1–2 days, extensive gangrene of the scrotal skin occurs resulting in sloughing of the scrotal skin which exposes the testicles. In a few cases, the gangrene can involve the skin of the penis, the anterior abdominal wall, the medial side of thigh, and the perianal region. In such situations, it is described as **perineal phlegmon** (Figs 60.42 to 60.44).
4. Luckily, the testis does not get involved in Fournier's gangrene because of thick tunica albuginea.

Treatment

1. Broad-spectrum antibiotics are started, once pus is sent for culture and sensitivity
   - Metronidazole for anaerobes

Key Box 60.8

Fournier's Gangrene

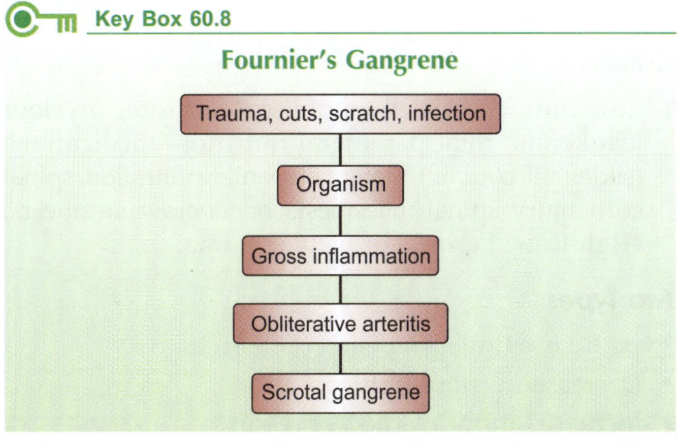

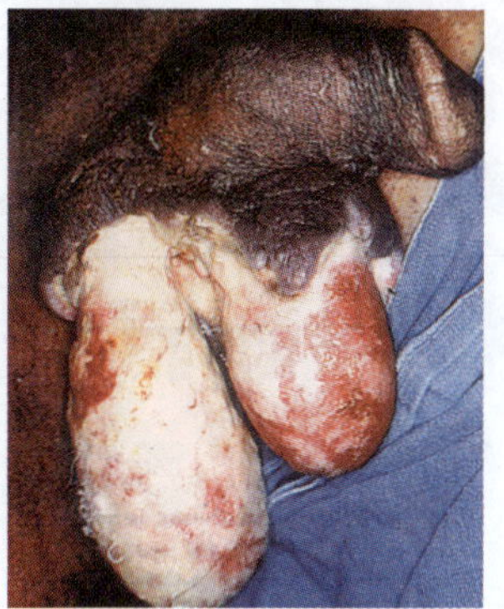

Fig. 60.42: Fournier's gangrene (*Courtesy:* Prof Santhosh Pai, Manipal)

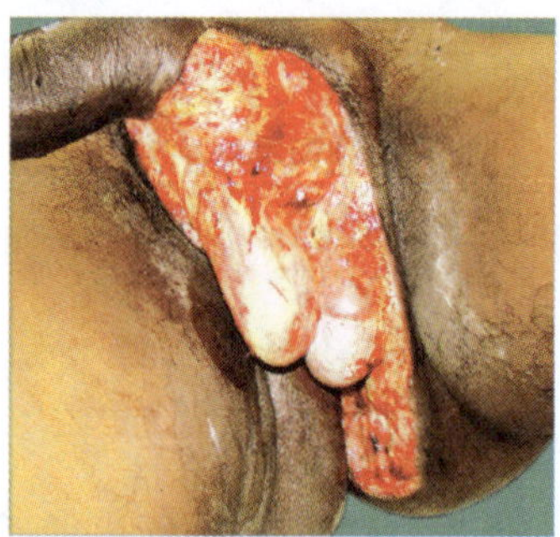

Fig. 60.43: Fournier's gangrene precipitated by a perianal abscess

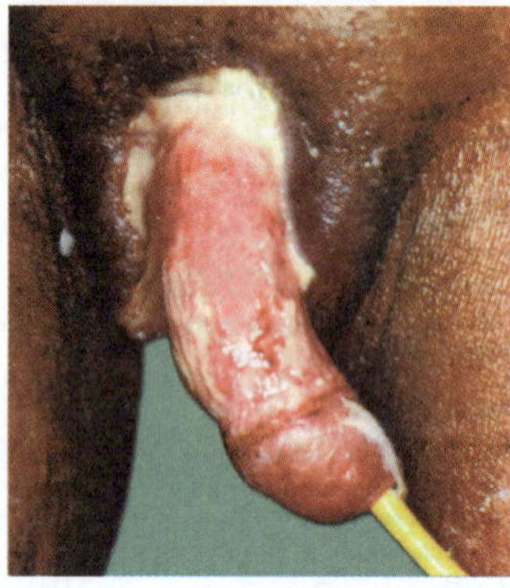

Fig. 60.44: Perineal phlegmon (*Courtesy:* Dr Ramachandra L, KMC, Manipal)

- Gentamicin for gram-negative organisms
- Ampicillin for gram-positive organisms
- Cephalosporins may have to be added if required.

2. The gangrenous portion of the scrotum has to be excised as soon as possible, which dramatically reverses the general condition of the patient from toxic to near normal.
3. If the testicles are exposed, they can be implanted in the thigh, or once inflammation subsides, skin grafting is done to cover the testicles.
4. If the penile skin is gangrenous, it is excised and covered with a split skin graft later. Surprisingly, results are better than expected! (Fig. 60.45)

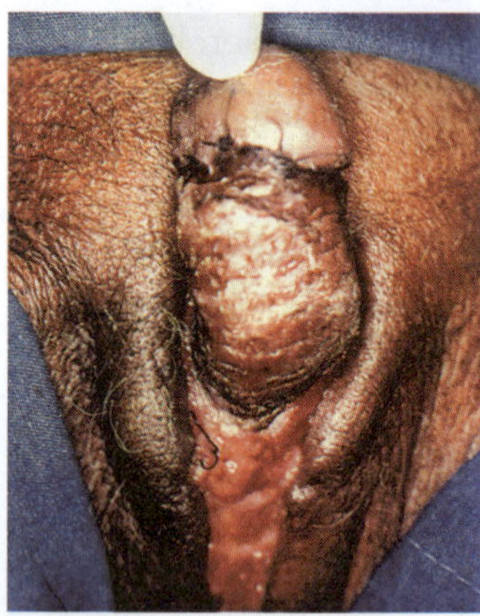

Fig. 60.45: Healing of Fournier's gangrene with skin grafting (*Courtesy:* Dr Ramachandra L, KMC, Manipal)

MISCELLANEOUS

FRACTURE OF THE PENIS

It is a misnomer.

- It is the traumatic rupture of the corpora cavernosum. It is considered a urologic emergency.
- Sudden blunt trauma or abrupt lateral bending of the penis in an erect state can break the markedly thin and stiff tunica albuginea.
- One or both corpora may be involved with concomitant urethral (38%) injury if both corpora are involved.
- **Causes:** Sexual activity, masturbation, gunshot wounds, industrial accidents, mechanical trauma.
- Diagnosed clinically.
- In equivocal cases—cavernosonography or MRI.
- Preoperative retrograde urethrography urethral injury is suspected.

Treatment

a. **Medical:** Fluids, antibiotics.
   If surgical therapy is delayed due to urethral injury, initial medical therapy consists of cold compresses, pressure dressings, anti-inflammatory medications and suprapublic cystostomy.
b. **Surgical:** Evacuate haematoma, identify site of injury, correct the defect in tunica albuginea, repair urethral injury, remove urethral catheter after 2 weeks.

Complications

Erectile dysfunction, abnormal curvature, painful erections, urethrocutaneous fistula, corpora-urethral fistula, and painful nodules.

PRIAPISM

- Priapism is a pathologic condition of a penile erection that persists beyond or is unrelated to sexual stimulation.
- It can occur in all age groups including the newborn but the peak incidence is at:
  - 5–10 years
  - 20–50 years.

Causes

1. **Low flow:** Sickle cell trait/disease, chronic myeloid leaukemia, total parenteral nutrition, medications (sildenafil, cocaine), malignant penile infiltration, spinal cord injury, spinal anaesthesia, or general anaesthesia.
2. **High flow:** Perineal or penile trauma.

Two Types

Type I: Low flow priapism (veno-occlusive)

- Decreased venous outflow
- Increased intracavernosal pressure

- Painful, fully erect penis
- Local hypoxia and acidosis
- It is the most common variety.

Type II: High flow priapism

- High inflow and high outflow
- Penis is erect but nontender
- Corporal blood gas analysis can differentiate low flow and high flow priapism.

Treatment

1. **Low flow priapism:** Corporal irrigation with normal saline and α-adrenergic intracorporal injections (epinephrine/phenylephrine/ephedrine) every 5 min till detumescence.

   In severe cases—shunts (corporoglandular, corporospongiosal or corporosaphenous) may be necessary. If patient has sickle cell disease, IV bicarbonate and blood transfusions are required.
2. **High flow priapism:** Doppler ultrasound is done to identify arterial-lacunar fistula.

   Arterial embolization or open surgical arterial ligation is done.

MALE INFERTILITY

Sperms are produced in the seminiferous tubules and are: Stored and matured in epididymis.

- The vas deferens carries the sperm from the epididymis to the prostatic urethra.
- Before opening into urethra, they are joined by the ducts of the seminal vesicles.
- The seminal vesicles and vas deferens ducts join to form the ejaculatory duct.

Semen analysis—minimal standards of adequacy:

Ejaculate volume	1.5–5.5 ml
Sperm concentration	>20 × 10^6 sperms/ml
Motility	>50%
Morphology	>30%

If abnormalities are present on semen analysis, causes may include the following:

Low ejaculate volume	Retrograde ejaculation Incomplete collection Ejaculatory duct obstruction Androgen deficiency
Oligoasthenospermia	Varicocele Drugs
Azoospermia	Non-obstructive-testicular failure (primary or secondary) Obstructive—ejaculatory duct obstruction (EjDO), congenital absence of vas deferens (CBAVD), vasectomy
Absence of fructose	Seminal vesicle agenesis/ obstruction

Evaluation of Azoospermia

Obstructive	Non-obstructive	
	Hypogonadotropic	Hypergonadotropic
• Due to obstruction	• Due to hypothalamic or pituitary failure	• Due to testicular failure
• FSH, LH, testosterone is normal	• Low FSH, LH, testosterone	• Elevated FSH
• Volume is normal	• Volume is reduced	• Volume low

FSH	LH	Testosterone	Implications
Low	Low	Low	Hypogonadotropic Hypogonadism
High	Normal	Normal	Spermatogenic failure
High	High	Low	Primary testicular failure
Normal	High	High	Androgen resistance
Normal	Normal	Normal	Non-endocrine abnormality

Sperm Retrieval Techniques for Assisted Reproductive Technology (ART)

Useful in cases where transport of sperms is not possible, (e.g. vasal agenesis).

- Pre-requisite is that production should be going on.
- Aspiration can be done from
  - **Testes:** Most recent technique—testicular sperm aspiration (TESA), testicular sperm extraction (TESE), micro-TESE.
  - **Epididymis:** Used when the vas is unavailable for aspiration—microsurgical epididymal sperm aspiration (MESA), percutaneous epididymal sperm aspiration (PESA).
  - **Vas deferens:** Most mature/fertilizable sperm present.

INTERESTING 'MOST COMMON' FOR TESTICULAR CANCER

- Most testicular tumours are malignant
- Most common cancer in young adults is testicular cancer
- Most common solid cancer in young males is seminoma
- Most common tumour is seminoma
- Most common teratoma is malignant teratoma intermediate: Teratocarcinoma

Multiple Choice Questions

1. **The following are true regarding surgical anatomy of the penis *except:***
   A. Corpora cavernosa are vascular spaces
   B. Arterioles are corkscrew-shaped
   C. Attached to symphysis pubis by suspensory ligament
   D. Deep artery supplies the corpus spongiosum alone

2. **Balanitis refers to:**
   A. Inflammation of the glans penis
   B. Inflammation of the prepuce
   C. Inflammation of glands in the fossa navicularis
   D. Inflammation of the urethral glands

3. **Dorsal slit is given for which condition?**
   A. Phimosis
   B. Paraphimosis
   C. Carcinoma penis
   D. Balanitis

4. **Following are complications of phimosis *except:***
   A. Paraphimosis
   B. Carcinoma penis
   C. Balanoposthitis
   D. Buschke-Lowenstein tumour

5. **Which of the following is a rare feature of carcinoma penis?**
   A. Foul-smelling discharge
   B. Recent phimosis
   C. Urethral involvement
   D. Extensive induration

6. **Treatment of carcinoma penis confined to the prepuce is:**
   A. Circumcision
   B. Dorsal slit and excision
   C. Partial amputation
   D. Radiotherapy

7. **The following are true for partial amputation of the penis *except:***
   A. Partial amputation is the treatment for a growth confined to the glans penis
   B. At least 2 cm proximal shaft is necessary
   C. A long ventral flap is required to cover
   D. Perineal urethrostomy may be required

8. **The following are a few important considerations in total amputation of the penis *except:***
   A. Suspensory ligaments have to be divided
   B. Perineal urethrostomy has to be done
   C. Severe excoriation of the scrotum is a complication
   D. Advantage is no stricture urethra after surgery

9. **The following are features of syphilitic chancre of the penis *except:***
   A. Single ulcer
   B. Hard chancre
   C. Firm painful lymph nodes in the axilla
   D. Contagious

10. **Testosterone is produced by:**
    A. Germ cells B. Sertoli cells
    C. Leydig cells D. Clear cells

11. **The testicular artery is a branch of the:**
    A. Aorta
    B. Common iliac artery
    C. Internal iliac artery
    D. External iliac artery

12. **The following are true for prostate specific antigen *except:***
    A. Released from columnar prostatic acinar epithelial cells
    B. More than 4 nmol/ml suggests carcinoma prostate
    C. Prostatitis can also increase its levels
    D. It does not help in assessing the response to treatment

13. **Which of the following tests differentiates encysted hydrocoele from spermatocoele?**
    A. Fluctuation
    B. Getting above the swelling
    C. Cough impulse
    D. Traction test

14. **What is the classical clinical feature of tuberculous epididymo-orchitis?**
    A. Thickened vas
    B. Atrophy of the testis
    C. Craggy epididymis
    D. Anterior sinus

15. Chinese lantern type of transillumination is classical of:

A. Spermatocoele
B. Epididymal cyst
C. Ranula
D. Cystic hygroma

16. Which of the following is true in cases of retractile testis?

A. It is premalignant
B. Testis is generally not palpable
C. Scrotum is well developed
D. Testis cannot be brought down into the scrotum

17. In torsion testis, the following are true *except:*

A. Scrotum is empty
B. Tender lump at the external abdominal ring
C. Elevation of the scrotum increases pain
D. Upper abdominal pain and vomiting are features

18. Which of the following is more prone to testicular tumour?

A. Gardner's syndrome
B. Down's syndrome
C. Klinefelter's syndrome
D. Sipple syndrome

19. Human chorionic gonadotrophin elevation is diagnostic of:

A. Choriocarcinoma
B. Seminoma
C. Leydig cell tumour
D. Sertoli cell tumour

20. Which of the following is true for seminoma?

A. It arises from rete testis
B. Undescended testis predisposes to it
C. It secretes β-HCG
D. It spreads predominantly by blood

Answers

1. D **2.** A **3.** B **4.** D **5.** C **6.** A **7.** D **8.** D **9.** C **10.** C
11. A **12.** D **13.** D **14.** C **15.** B **16.** C **17.** D **18.** C **19.** A **20.** B

CHAPTER

61

Haematuria and Urinary Tract Infections

- Causes
- History and examination
- Investigations
- Haematuria
- Urinary tract infections

Competency

SU29.1: Describe the causes, investigations and principles of management of haematuria.

CAUSES OF HAEMATURIA (Fig. 61.1 and Key Box 61.1)

I. In the Kidney

1. Infection

- Acute glomerulonephritis
- Tuberculosis

2. Infarction

- SBE with emboli causing renal infarction
- Massive haemolysis with acute renal tubular necrosis
- Mismatched blood transfusion

3. Injury

- Stab/blunt injury

4. Tumours

- Wilms' tumour: Nephroblastoma
- Hypernephroma: Renal cell carcinoma (RCC)
- Transitional cell carcinoma (TCC)

Key Box 61.1

Haematuria

Common causes

- Urolithiasis
- Tumours

Uncommon causes

- Tuberculosis
- Cystitis
- Bladder tumours
- Polycystic kidney

5. Stones

6. Polycystic kidney

II. In the Ureter

1. Stone
2. Cancer—rare

III. In the Urinary Bladder

1. Carcinoma bladder
2. Carcinoma prostate
3. Cystitis
4. Tuberculosis
5. Bilharziasis
6. Stone: Common in school-going children
7. Benign prostatic hyperplasia (BPH)

IV. Urethra

1. Stone

V. Rare Causes

1. Patients on anticoagulants
2. Sickle cell anaemia
3. Bleeding disorders

HISTORY AND EXAMINATION

1. Age and Sex

Young children	Vesical calculus
Young adults	Renal stones, TB
Elderly patients	RCC

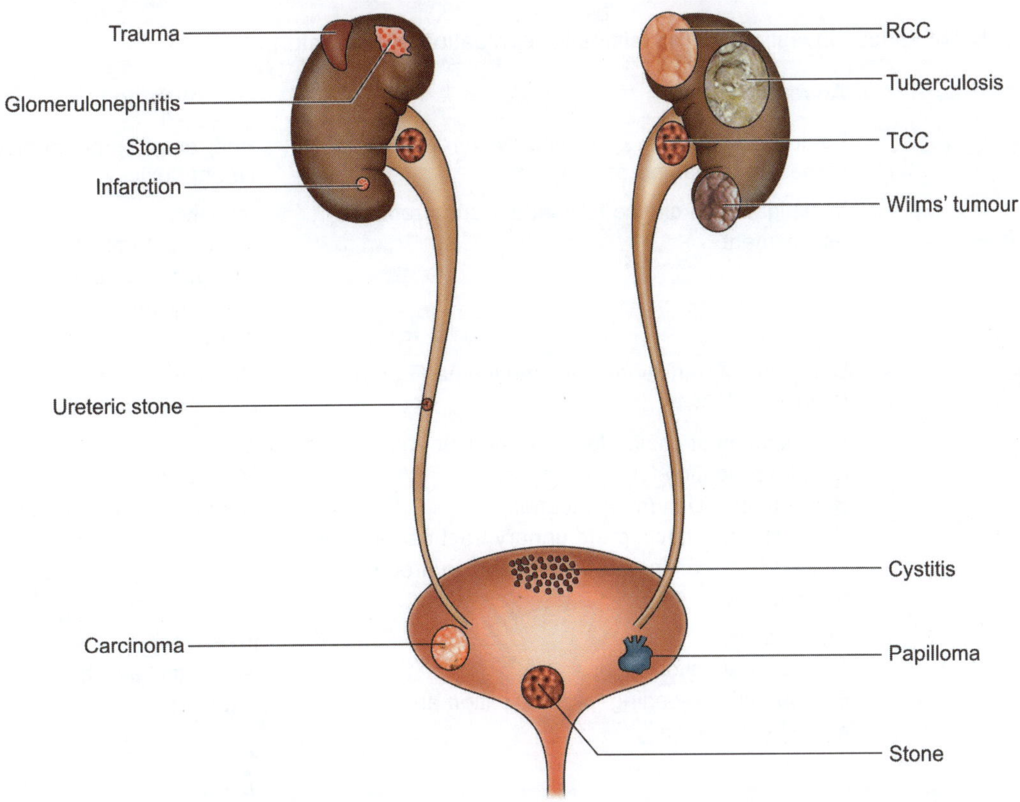

Fig. 61.1: Various causes of haematuria

2. Occupation

Aniline dye workers	Carcinoma bladder

3. Haematuria

• Bright red	• Lower urinary tract
• Altered blood	• Kidney
• Profuse	• Papilloma
• Small quantity	• Renal cell carcinoma, renal TB, stone
• Beginning of micturition	• Urethral pathology
• End of micturition	• Bladder pathology
• Mixed with urine	• Renal
• Painless haematuria	• Papilloma or carcinoma
• Painful haematuria	• Renal stone, bladder stone

4. General Physical Examination

• Gross pallor	• Significant blood loss
• Gross pallor with minimal blood loss	• RCC
• Hypertension	• Polycystic kidney
• Bony pains	• Carcinoma (prostate)

5. Abdominal Examination

• Palpable kidney	• Polycystic kidney, Wilms' tumour, RCC
• Distended bladder	• Carcinoma prostate, enlarged prostate
• Suprapubic tenderness	• Bladder stone, cystitis
• Craggy epididymis and beaded vas	• Genitourinary TB

6. Rectal Examination

• Enlarged smooth, firm prostate	• BPH
• Hard irregular prostate	• Carcinoma prostate
• Hard, thickened seminal vesicles	• Genitourinary TB
• Advanced growth	• Carcinoma rectum infiltrating urinary bladder

INVESTIGATIONS (Table 61.1 and Fig. 61.2)

1. Urine Examination

• Worm-like clots	• Growth in the ureter
• Flat disc-like	• Urethra
• Pieces of tumour	• **Papilloma** of the bladder

2. Urine Microscopy

• Pus cells	• Urinary tract infection
• Abacterial acid pyuria	• TB
• Malignant cells positive	• TCC or **papilloma** bladder

Table 61.1 Utility of various investigative modalities for evaluation of haematuria

Investigations	Advantages	Disadvantages
Intravenous urography (IVU)	Evaluation of kidney collecting system and ureter for stones, masses and obstruction	Poor assessment of bladder pathology Nephrotoxicity
Cystoscopy	Investigation of choice for bladder and urethral assessment	Invasive Significant patient discomfort Expensive equipment required Potential for complications (e.g. urethral stricture)
Urinary cytology	Diagnosis of transitional cell carcinoma (TCC) Grading of TCC	Not useful for squamous or adeno-carcinoma
CT scan	Investigation of choice for colic (noncontrast CT scan) Best investigation for renal masses Better than IVU in most situations Other organs affecting the urinary tract can also be imaged (e.g. carcinoma cervix causing ureteric obstruction)	Cost Radiation Contrast nephrotoxicity
Angiography	Aneurysms A-V fistulas/malformations Postoperative bleeding for localisation and angioembolisation	Invasive Not widely available (skilled) High cost

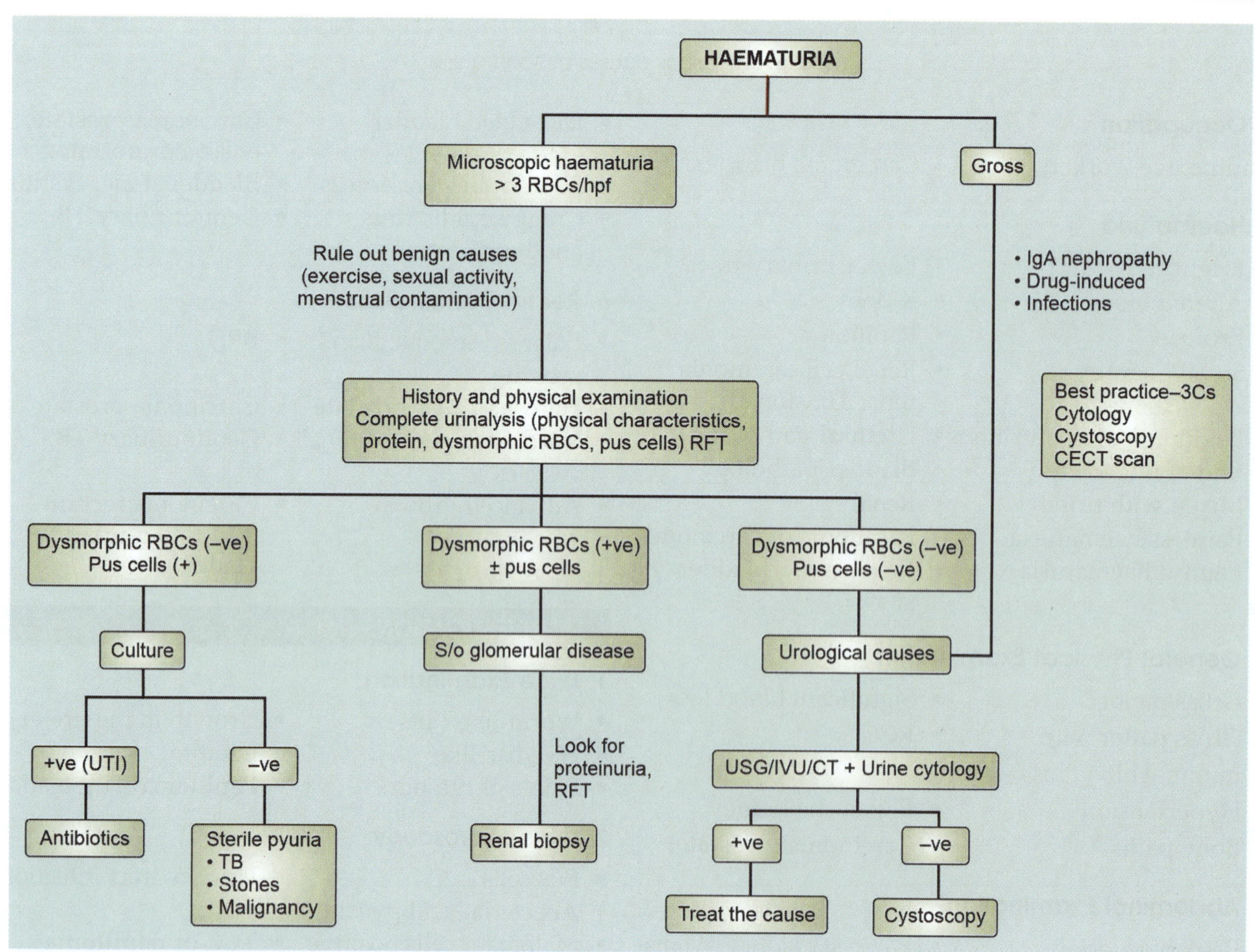

Fig. 61.2: Algorithm for investigating haematuria

3. Plain X-ray KUB

- Enlarged kidney — Polycystic kidney, RCC
- Radio-opaque shadows — Renal stones, ureteric stones, bladder stone

4. Cystoscopy

- Growth in the bladder — Papilloma bladder/TCC
- Inflammation of the bladder — Cystitis
- Ulcers, hyperaemia, golf-hole ureter — TB

5. Intravenous Urography

- Spider leg calyces — Polycystic kidney
- Irregular calyces — RCC
- Missing calyces — TB

6. Ultrasound

- Enlarged kidney — Renal cell carcinoma, polycystic kidney, Wilms' tumour, stones

Pearls of Wisdom

The differential diagnosis of haematuria is a major theory question in undergraduate examinations. I have given some ideas about how to evaluate these cases by analysing history, physical examination and investigations. This is a good exercise for students.

HAEMATURIA

Haematuria is defined as the passage of blood mixed with urine.

Classification

I. Depending upon whether the blood is seen or not:
   A. Microscopic: Not visible to the eye
   B. Macroscopic: Visible to the eye

II. Depending upon the site of origin of the blood (Table 61.2):
   A. Glomerular (renal)
   B. Non-glomerular (urological)

Macroscopic or Gross Haematuria

Urine may vary in colour from red to stale brown or chocolate coloured. It may be associated with clots. The nature of the clots may give a clue to the source or site of bleeding. Serpiginous or vermiform clots indicate bleeding from the kidneys. Amorphous clots suggest bleeding from the lower tract. Most patients with gross haematuria have some pathology in the kidneys or genitourinary tract.

It can be initial, terminal, or throughout the stream. Urethral bleeding usually manifests as the first 10–15 ml of bloodstained urine, which gradually clears. Terminal haematuria usually indicates trigonal irritation (e.g. bladder stone). It is usually associated with dysuria and strangury. Bleeding from the upper urinary tract (kidneys and ureters) is seen throughout the stream as blood mixes with the urine stored in the bladder.

Microscopic Haematuria

It is defined as the presence of ≥3 RBCs on microscopic examination. It is usually detected incidentally on urine dipstick testing and subsequent microscopic examination.

Normal RBC excretion is up to 2 million RBCs/day.

Aetiology

Evaluation: Numerous investigative modalities are available for evaluating haematuria. The choice of modality depends on clinical suspicion and important clinical signs.

Ultrasonography: It is noninvasive and less expensive

- Diagnosis of upper or lower urinary tract lesions
  a. Stones
  b. Tumours
  c. Hydronephrosis
- Renal parenchymal changes suggest a glomerular cause.
- Ultrasound examination guides towards choosing further investigations.
- Less sensitive for evaluating of ureteral causes of haematuria (Fig. 61.3).

Table 61.2 Distinguishing between glomerular and urological causes of haematuria

	Glomerular	Nonglomerular
Colour (if macroscopic)	Pale red, smoky brown or stale tea	Red or pink
Clots	Rare	More common
Proteinuria (dipstick/mg per day)	3+ or more (>500 mg/day)	<2+ (<500 mg/day)
RBC morphology	Dysmorphic RBCs	Normal
RBC casts	May be present	Absent

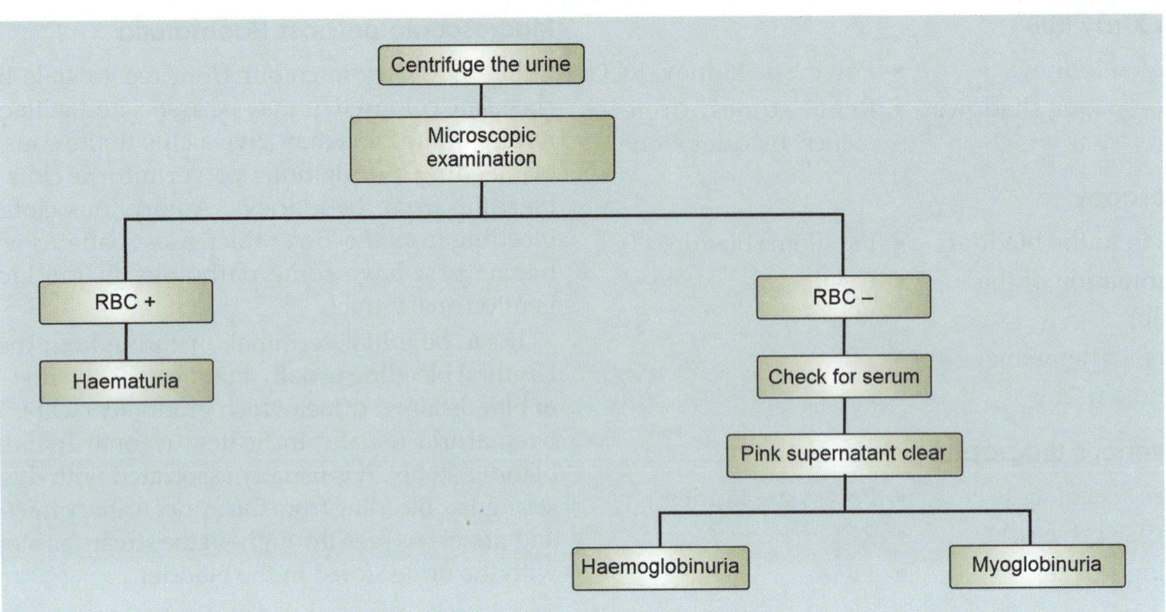

Fig. 61.3: Differentiating haematuria from haemoglobinuria and myoglobinuria

Competency

SU29.3: Describe the clinical features, investigations and principles of management of urinary tract infections.

URINARY TRACT INFECTIONS

UTI is an inflammatory response of the urothelium to bacterial invasion that is usually associated with bacteriuria and pyuria.

Bacteriuria is the presence of bacteria in the urine, which is normally free of bacteria. It can be symptomatic or asymptomatic.

Pyuria is the presence of white blood cells (WBCs) in the urine. It is generally indicative of infection and/or an inflammatory response of the urothelium to the bacterium, stones, or other indwelling foreign body.

Bacteriuria without pyuria is generally indicative of bacterial colonisation without infection of the urinary tract.

Pyuria without bacteriuria warrants evaluation for tuberculosis, stones, or cancer.

Clinical Features

Signs and Symptoms

Lower tract infections/cystitis

- Frequency, and/or urgency
- Suprapubic pain
- Haematuria is not common
- Lower tract symptoms are commonly present and usually predate the appearance of upper tract symptoms by several days.

Upper tract infections/acute pyelonephritis

- **Fever with chills**
- **Flank pain**
- Nausea and vomiting
- **Renal or perirenal abscess** may cause indolent fever and flank mass and tenderness.
- In the elderly, the symptoms may be much more subtle (e.g. epigastric or abdominal discomfort) or the patient may be asymptomatic.
- Patients with indwelling catheters often have asymptomatic bacteriuria, but fever associated with bacteremia may occur rapidly and become life threatening.

Chronic pyelonephritis describes a shrunken, scarred kidney. It is diagnosed by morphologic, radiologic, or functional evidence of renal disease that may be postinfectious but is frequently not associated with UTI.

Classification of UTI

1. **Uncomplicated UTI:** It is the infection in a healthy patient with a structurally and functionally normal urinary tract.
2. **Complicated UTI:** It is associated with factors that increase the chance of acquiring bacteria and decrease the efficacy of therapy (Key Box 61.2). Most of these patients are men.
3. **Recurrent UTI:** Recurrences of uncomplicated and/or complicated UTIs, with a frequency of at least three UTIs/year or two UTIs in the last six months.

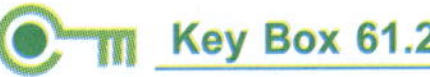
Key Box 61.2

Factors Suggesting Complicated UTI

- Functional or anatomic abnormality of urinary tract: Male gender
- Pregnancy
- Elderly patient
- Diabetes
- Immunosuppression
- Childhood urinary tract infection
- Recent antimicrobial agent use
- Indwelling urinary catheter
- Urinary tract instrumentation
- Hospital-acquired infection
- Symptoms for more than 7 days at presentation

4. **Catheter associated UTI:** CA-UTI refers to UTIs occurring in a person whose urinary tract is currently catheterised or has had a catheter in place within the past 48 hours.
5. **Urosepsis** is a life-threatening organ dysfunction caused by a dysregulated host response to infection originating from the urinary tract and/or male genital organs.

Incidence and Predisposing Factors

- Nearly 30% of women will have had a symptomatic UTI requiring antimicrobial therapy by age 24, and almost half of all women will experience a UTI during their lifetime.
- The prevalence of bacteriuria in young women is 30 times more than in men.
- The incidence of bacteriuria also increases with institutionalization or hospitalization and concurrent disease.
- Catheter-associated UTIs (CAUTIs) are the most common nosocomial infection.

Predisposing Factors

1. Pregnancy
2. Patients with spinal cord injuries
3. Diabetes
4. Multiple sclerosis
5. Human immunodeficiency virus (HIV) infection/ acquired immunodeficiency syndrome (AIDS).

Pathogenesis and Bacteriology

UTIs are a result of interactions between the uropathogen and the host. Successful infection of the urinary tract is determined in part by the virulence factors of the bacteria, the inoculum size, and the inadequacy of host defense mechanisms.

Routes of Infection

1. Ascending route
2. Haematogenous route
3. Lymphatic route

Urinary Pathogens

- Most UTIs are caused by facultative anaerobes usually originating from the bowel flora.
- Uropathogens such as *Staphylococcus epidermidis* and *Candida albicans* originate from the flora of the vagina or perineal skin.
- *E. coli* is by far **the most common cause** of UTIs, accounting for 85% of community-acquired and 50% of hospital-acquired infections.
- **Other gram-negative enterobacteriaceae,** causing community acquired UTI, are Proteus and Klebsiella
- Gram-positive *E. faecalis* and *Staphylococcus saprophyticus* are responsible for the remainder of most community-acquired infections.
- **Nosocomial infections** are caused by *E. coli,* Klebsiella, Enterobacter, Citrobacter, Serratia, *Pseudomonas aeruginosa,* Providencia, *E. faecalis,* and *S. epidermidis.*
- ***Mycobacterium tuberculosis***—do not grow under routine aerobic conditions and may be found during evaluation for sterile pyuria.
- **Less common organisms**
  - *Gardnerella vaginalis,* mycoplasma species, and *Ureaplasma urealyticum* infect patients with intermittent or indwelling catheters.
  - Anaerobic organisms are frequently found in **suppurative infections** of the genitourinary tract. The organisms found are usually *Bacteroides* species, including *B. fragilis, Fusobacterium* species, anaerobic cocci, and *Clostridium perfringens.* The growth of clostridia may be associated with Emphysematous cystitis.
  - Chlamydia

Investigations

Principle

i. Urine and the urinary tract are normally free of bacteria and inflammation.
ii. Bacteriuria and WBCs provide a presumptive diagnosis of UTI.
iii. Presence of 10^2 cfu/ml confirms a symptomatic UTI.

1. **Urine analysis and urine culture:** Sample collection
   a. Midstream urine
   b. Prostatic massage to acquire prostatic fluid during suspected prostatitis
   c. Suprapubic aspiration

2. **Imaging** is indicated in high-risk patients, including women with febrile infections and most men. Radiologic studies determine acute infectious processes that require further intervention or may find the cause of complicated infections (Key Box 61.3)

Key Box 61.3

Correctable Causes of UTI

a. Infection stones
b. Chronic bacterial prostatitis
c. Unilateral infected atrophic kidneys
d. Ureteral duplication and ectopic ureters
e. Foreign bodies
f. Urethral diverticula and infected periurethral glands
g. Unilateral medullary sponge kidneys
h. Nonrefluxing, normal-appearing, infected ureteral stumps after nephrectomy
i. Infected urachal cysts
j. Infected communicating cysts of the renal calyces, papillary necrosis
k. Perivesical abscess with fistula to bladder

a. Ultrasonography
b. Computed tomography and magnetic resonance imaging
c. Voiding cystourethrogram
d. Radionucleotide imaging

Principles of Antimicrobial Treatment

Uncomplicated cystitis	Dose	Duration
First line in woman		
Fosfomycin	3 g single dose	1 day
Nitrofurantoin	100 mg BD	5 days
Pivmecillinam	500 mg BD	3 days
Alternatives–cephalosporins		
Treatment in men		
Trimethoprim	200 mg BD	5 days
Trimethoprim/ sulphamethoxazole	160/800 mg BD	7 days

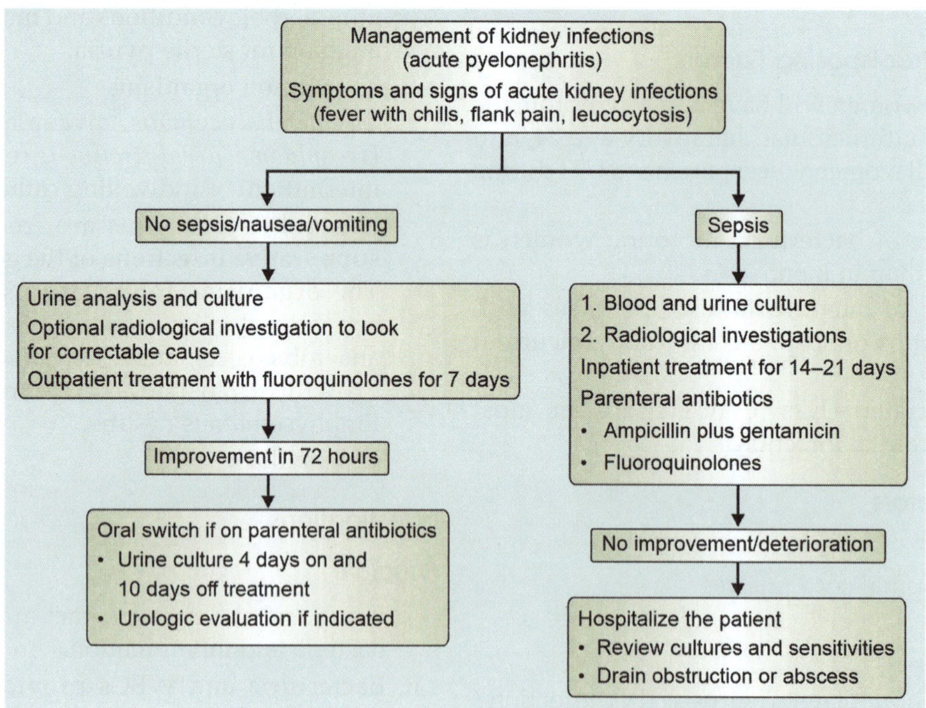

Multiple Choice Questions

1. **What causes haematuria in bacterial endocarditis?**
   A. Renal necrosis
   B. Renal sepsis
   C. Renal infarction
   D. Coagulopathy

2. **Haematuria in polycystic kidney is due to:**
   A. Hypertension
   B. Renal infarction
   C. Renal ischaemia
   D. Cyst rupture into the renal pelvis

3. **Which of the following conditions rarely gives rise to haematuria?**
   A. Renal stones
   B. Renal cell carcinoma
   C. Bilharziasis
   D. Benign prostatic hypertrophy

4. **Palpable renal masses in a 40-year-old hypertensive patient with one attack of haematuria is:**
   A. Hypernephroma B. Hydronephrosis
   C. Adenomyolipoma D. Polycystic kidney

5. **Which of the following pathologies is reflected as terminal haematuria?**
   A. Trigonal irritation
   B. Posterior urethral irritation
   C. Ureteric irritation
   D. Renal irritation

6. **In urinary tract infections due to prostatitis, which is the urinary sample asked for?**
   A. Initial sample
   B. Midstream
   C. Last sample
   D. After prostatic massage

Answers

1. A **2.** D **3.** D **4.** D **5.** A **6.** D

Section

V

Specialities

62. Chest Trauma, Cardiothoracic Surgery
63. Neurosurgery
64. Principles of Anaesthesiology
65. Organ Transplantation
66. Principles of Clinical Radiation Oncology and Chemotherapy

CHAPTER

62

Chest Trauma, Cardiothoracic Surgery

- Chest trauma
- Blunt trauma
- Pulmonary injuries
- Tracheobronchial injuries
- Myocardial contusion
- Surgical emphysema
- Mediastinal emphysema
- Mediastinal masses
- Pulmonary aspergilloma
- Congenital heart diseases
- Patent ductus arteriosus
- Coarctation of aorta
- Coronary artery bypass graft
- Off pump coronary artery bypass surgery
- Abdominal aortic aneurysms (AAA)

Competency

SU17.8: Describe the pathophysiology of chest injuries.

SU17.9: Describe clinical features and management principles of chest injuries.

CHEST TRAUMA

Introduction

In chest trauma, the mortality is very high unless promptly recognised and properly treated. The margin of safety is very slim, initial care dictates the final result. With varying degree of severity, chest injuries occur in almost 80% of road traffic accidents (Key Box 62.1).

ASSESSMENT OF INJURY

History

- Time since the injury

Key Box 62.1

Common Causes

- Automobile accidents
- Gunshot wounds
- Stab injuries
- Blast injuries
- Crush injuries

- Details of the injury from the bystander or the police
- High-speed deceleration injury (aortic and cardiac rupture to be ruled out)
- Crushing accidents (tracheobronchial and oesophageal tear)
- Sudden abdominal compression (ruptured diaphragm)
- In stab injuries, length of the knife and direction of stab.

Examination

- The clothing should be removed carefully without moving the patient.
- Palpate for clinical evidence of fracture ribs, surgical emphysema, any paradoxical movement of the ribs and auscultate for air entry in both lungs.
- Even if it is a trivial injury, the patient should be admitted and observed for a minimum of 24 hours before discharge.
- It is reasonable to do unilateral or bilateral closed tube thoracostomy (ICT) (Fig. 62.1) on suspicion of haemothorax or pneumothorax when the patient is in respiratory distress even before chest X-ray.

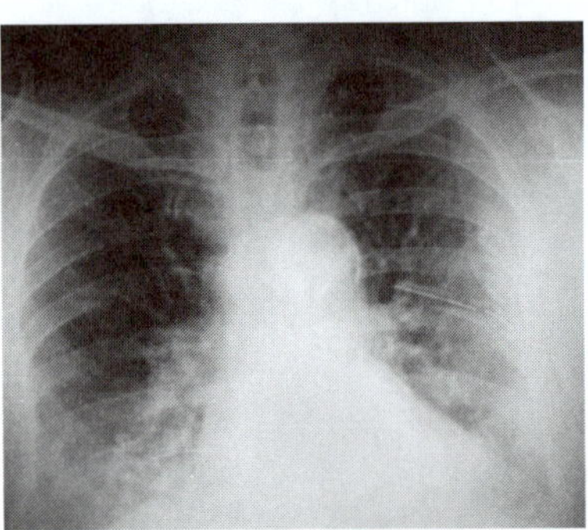

Fig. 62.1: Fracture ribs with haemothorax left side—intercostal tube has been inserted

MAIN AIMS OF RESUSCITATION

The standard method of resuscitation in all cases of polytrauma is as follows:

A. Airway

- Aspiration of blood and secretions from oral cavity, pharynx and trachea
- Introduce plastic airway
- Endotracheal intubation
- Cricothyroidotomy as necessary
- Tracheostomy as necessary

B. Breathing

- Intubation
- Intercostal chest tube (ICT)
- Closure of any open chest wounds

  These two steps (A and B) help in re-aerating the lung.

C. Circulation

- Control of major and life-threatening bleeding
- Volume infusion

D. Disability

- Neurological

E. Exposure

- All clothing to be cut open without moving the patient.

> ***Key Notes***
> - All the above steps are taken by the trauma centre team simultaneously and not one by one.
> - Relieve pain. Do not sedate.
> - All open wounds of the chest to be covered.
> - Life-threatening injuries should be identified and treated immediately.

BLUNT TRAUMA TO THE CHEST

Causes

- Road traffic accidents
- Fall from a height
- Crush injuries
- Assault with blunt object

SIMPLE RIB FRACTURE

Rib fracture can be single or multiple (Key Box 62.2).

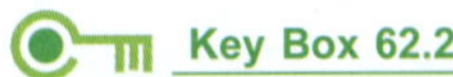

Key Box 62.2

Points to Remember

- First rib fracture is a marker of severe trauma—injury to brachial plexus, subclavian artery and vein
- Displaced fracture of 8th–10th ribs—injury to liver and spleen
- Fracture of 11th and 12th ribs—injury to kidney
- Penetrating injury to left lower chest wall—injury to heart, lung, diaphragm, stomach and spleen

Single Rib Fracture

- Often regarded as a trivial injury but should be treated with respect in elderly patients.
- Occurs due to direct injury or excessive flexion.
- The common site is at the costal angle or middle of the shaft.
- Patients will have pain on breathing, coughing and on palpation.
- They are treated with analgesics, intercostal nerve block and assurance.

Multiple Rib Fractures

- When there are multiple rib fractures without any pneumo- or **haemothorax** and no other organs are involved, intercostal nerve block and small amount of narcotics are required.
- Strapping is occasionally necessary in young adults.
- In elderly patients, consider hospitalisation for observation, pain control and pulmonary toilet.
- Chest X-ray to be repeated after 24 hours and at the time of discharge, to rule out late onset pneumothorax and haemothorax.
- Intermittent use of velcro belt rib support.
- Inform the patient of deep breathing, nebulisation, chest physiotherapy and coughing using the rib belt.
- Epidural analgesia is becoming the standard of care for pain management in patients with multiple rib fractures.

STERNAL FRACTURE

- Commonly due to steering wheel injury—blunt trauma.
- Usually occurs at the sternal angle.
- Associated with costochondral dislocations.
- Classified as **displaced and nondisplaced fractures**.
- Localised swelling, tenderness and deformity are the clinical findings.

Treatment

- Displaced fracture—requires surgical fixation with plates or steel wires.
- Nondisplaced fracture—conservative management.

FLAIL CHEST

This results from severe chest injuries with multiple rib fractures.

Here there are fracture of **three or more ribs at two places,** anteriorly and posteriorly, so that certain segments of ribs will have no attachment to the chest wall. These ribs become indrawn due to intrathoracic negative pressure as the patient inhales and is driven outwards on expiration producing instability. This is called **paradoxical respiration.** It results in hypoventilation, carbon dioxide retention and respiratory failure.

Flail chest is of three types: Anterior, posterior and lateral.

- **Anterior flail:** Fracture of the costochondral junction on both side of the sternum.
- **Posterior flail:** Fracture ribs of posterior chest wall.
- **Lateral flail:** Fracture shaft of the ribs.

Treatment

I. Commonly Done Procedures

1. **Anterior flail:** The flail segments are stabilised with metal plates and screws from costal cartilage to the sternum, introduced to stabilise the flail segments.
2. **Posterior flail:** No treatment is required as the scapula acts as a support to stabilise the flail segment.
3. **Lateral flail:** It is treated by chest wall stabilisation, by positive pressure ventilation or velcro rib belt, reduction of respiratory dead space by intercostal chest tube, removing air or blood reduction of the respiratory dead space, management of the pulmonary contusion and pain control. Epidural analgesia is recommended for pain management. Intercostal nerve blocks may also be used.

II. Other Methods

- Surgical stabilisation is rarely indicated, i.e. open reduction of rib fracture or osteofixation with metal plates and screws.
- Recent method is to intubate and stabilise the flail segments with positive pressure ventilation, which has to be done for at least one week. This is called internal pneumatic fixation.
- Physiologic stabilisation with intubation and IPPV (intermittent positive pressure ventilation) must be initiated before hypoxia develops. IPPV produces satisfactory ventilation and helps the fractured ribs to unite in the position of inspiration, thereby reducing the deformity and improving the pulmonary function.

'STOVE IN' CHEST

- Localised, severe, blunt or crush injury produces depression of a portion of the chest.
- Treatment is same as that for flail chest. Sometimes, thoracotomy may be needed if there are internal injuries.

PULMONARY INJURIES

CONTUSION OF THE LUNG

- Deceleration injuries or crush trauma often produces extensive parenchymal damage. Haemorrhage and interstitial oedema result in obliteration of alveolar spaces and consolidation of large areas of pulmonary tissue.
- Contusion of the lung can be unilateral or bilateral. The contusion can be in the form of a small area of damage with oedema and extravasation of the blood, or it may be widespread damage. Haemoptysis and excessive tracheobronchial secretions give the clue to the diagnosis (Key Box 62.3).
- Chest X-ray: Early patchy consolidation. It must be differentiated from adult respiratory distress syndrome (ARDS).
- CT scan is more specific (Fig. 62.2).

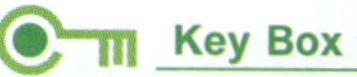

Key Box 62.3

Pulmonary Injuries

- Contusion
- Pneumothorax/haemothorax
- Laceration
- Chest wall injuries

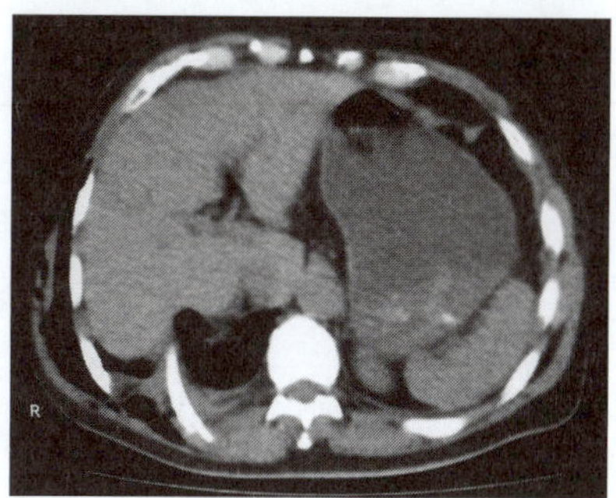

Fig. 62.2: CT scan showing rib fracture and lung injury

- Fluid restriction, pulmonary care
- Chest physiotherapy
- Steroids and rarely ventilation

  Usually self-limiting, if there are no other severe injuries.

Complications

- Pneumonia
- Atelectasis
- Respiratory failure
- ARDS

PNEUMOTHORAX

- Pneumothorax is the most common cause of respiratory insufficiency following chest trauma.
- Usually if there is a rib fracture and evidence of subcutaneous emphysema, pneumothorax is certainly present (Fig. 62.3).
- Pneumothorax can be closed (simple), open and tension.
- Small simple pneumothorax does not need any treatment.
- A repeat chest X-ray after 12–24 hours is essential to confirm that it is not progressing.
- It can be confused for a large bullae (Fig. 62.4).
- Small pneumothorax can be missed easily.

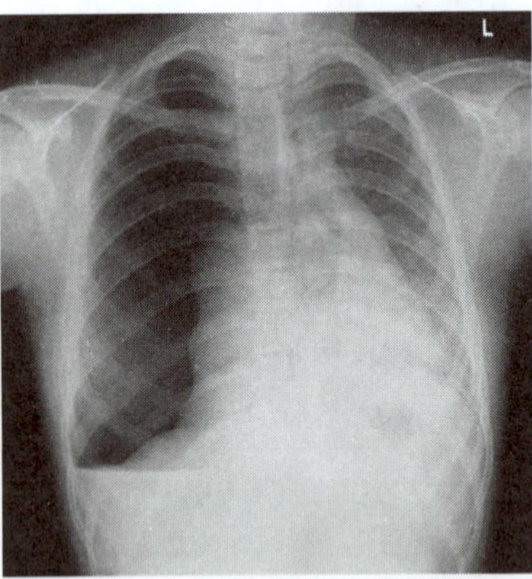

Fig. 62.3: Pneumothorax right lung

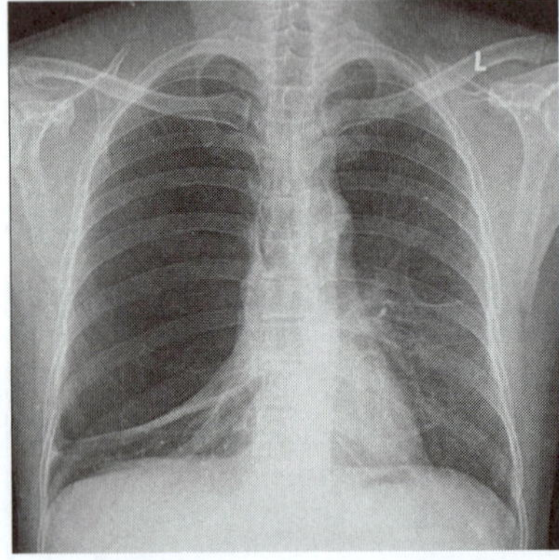

Fig. 62.4: Large bullae

- **Bilateral pneumothorax is an emergency**.
- Late pneumothorax can also occur.
- Open chest wound will produce complete collapse of lung and paradoxical shift of the mediastinum with each respiration (mediastinal flutter) causing hypoventilation and reduced cardiac output.
- Treatment is by closure of the wound, intercostal tube drainage (ICD) and surgery.

Tension Pneumothorax (Key Boxes 62.4 to 62.6)

- Injury to the lung results in continuous valvular air leak. The accumulating air collapses the lung on the same side and pushes the mediastinum to opposite side. As a result of this tension, the intrapleural pressure increases, till it is above atmospheric pressure at the time of expiration. This **reduces the venous return** to the heart as well as compromises the ventilation.
- Tension pneumothorax is **an emergency** which should be treated urgently with needle thoracocentesis in the second intercostal space in the midclavicular line to release the tension. **Thoraco-**

Key Box 62.4

Tension Pneumothorax

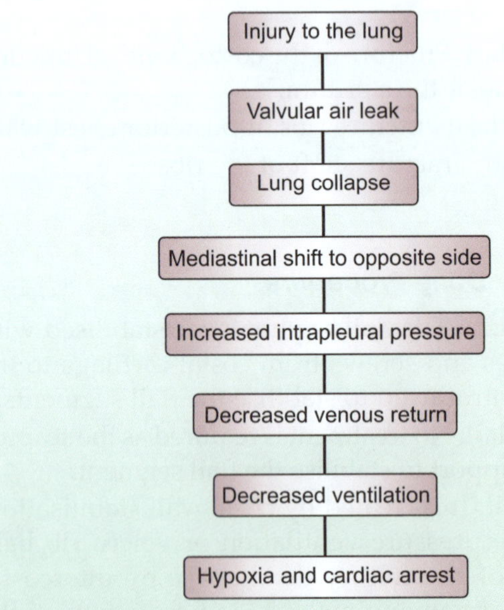

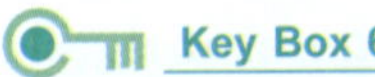

Key Box 62.5

Tension Pneumothorax: Clinical Features

Tachypnoea
Tachycardia
Tympanic note on percussion
Total absence of breath sounds
Tracheal shift *Observe* **5 Ts**

Key Box 62.6

Tension Pneumothorax

- Diagnose immediately
- Do not wait for CXR
- Thoracocentesis in 2nd intercostal space, mid-clavicular line
- Then, follow with intercostal chest tube insertion

centesis converts tension pneumothorax to simple pneumothorax.

- This should be followed by urgent ICD insertion and connected to underwater seal.
- **Do not wait for chest X-ray**.

Tension Gastrothorax

This occurs due to herniation of dilated and obstructed stomach into the mediastinum due to diaphragmatic tear resulting in haemodynamic compromise. It should be treated by reducing the hernial contents and repair of diaphragmatic tear.

HAEMOTHORAX

- May be missed in chest X-rays in the supine position.
- Results from injury to internal mammary artery, intercostal artery and vascular lung adhesions.
- **Classical signs are** reduced—chest expansion, dullness to percussion and absent breath sounds on affected side.
- Treated by intercostal chest tube insertion (Figs 62.5 and 62.6).
- If bleeding continues or features of shock develop, thoracotomy has to be considered.
- The bleeding may be delayed or may recur after several days.

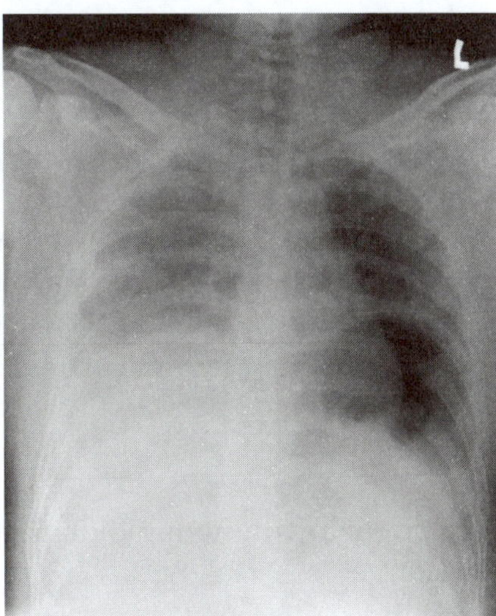

Fig. 62.5: Right haemothorax

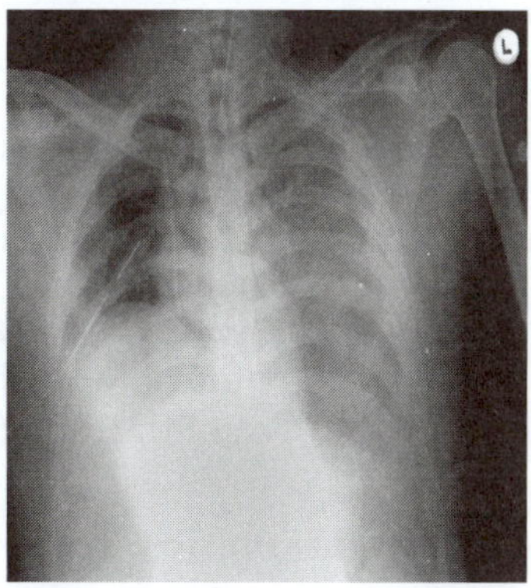

Fig. 62.6: Bilateral haemothorax—detected early and treated with ICT on the right

Indications for Thoracotomy

- Initial volume of blood loss is not as important as the amount of ongoing bleeding.
- Drainage is more than 1000 ml or 100 ml each hour for 4 hours.
- If clotted haemothorax is suspected (opacity persisting on chest X-ray even after ICD).

Complications

Failure to adequately drain a haemothorax initially results in residual clotted haemothorax and empyema or late fibrothorax.

INTERCOSTAL CHEST TUBE (ICT) INSERTION (CLOSED TUBE THORACOSTOMY) (Flowchart 62.1)

- **Second intercostal space needle thoracostomy**—anteriorly midclavicular line is ideal for pneumothorax and ICT in the fifth space in the midaxillary line for haemothorax.

Flowchart 62.1: Important steps of intercostal tube insertion

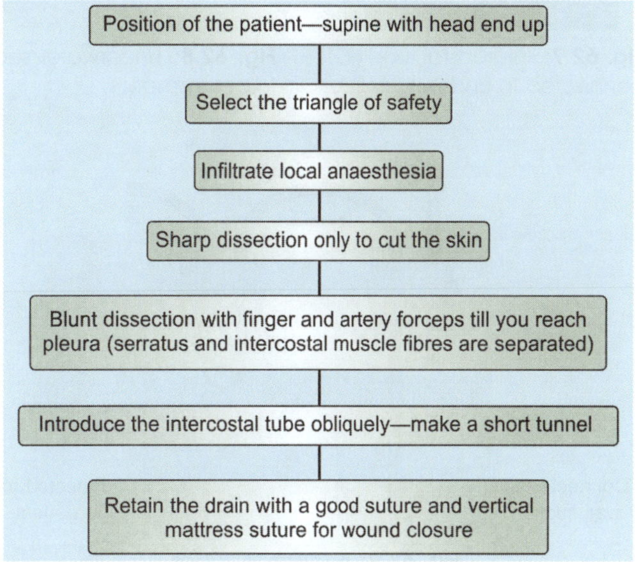

- **Triangle of safety**
  - Above the level of nipples
  - Anterior to midaxillary line
  - Below and lateral to pectoralis major muscle

- Can be introduced from fifth intercostal space mid-axillary line for pneumothorax also but the chest tube should reach the apex of the lung (Figs 62.7 and 62.8).
- **Infiltrate local anaesthetics** up to the parietal pleura.
- 2–3 cm incision parallel to the ribs—deepened, suture taken.
- Insert the chest tube with trocar into the pleural cavity. Push the tube pointing towards the shoulder and not the mediastinum.
- Then the trocar is removed and the chest tube is connected to underwater seal. The ICT is fixed.
- Intercostal drainage (ICD) can also be done by connecting to 2 bottles (Fig. 62.9). When low thoracic suction is not available, the ICT is connected to wall suction.

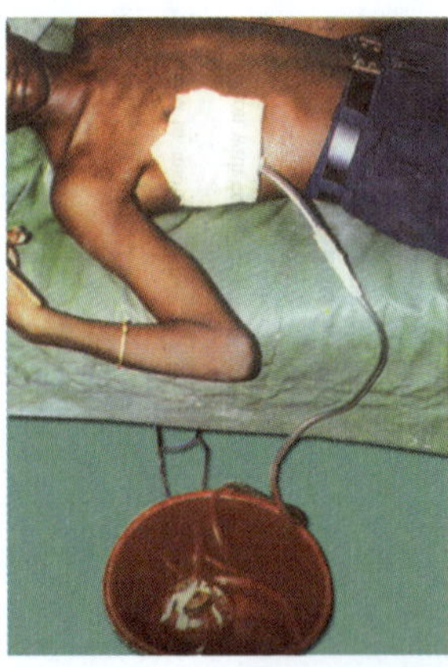

Fig. 62.7: Intercostal tube (ICT) connected to underwater seal

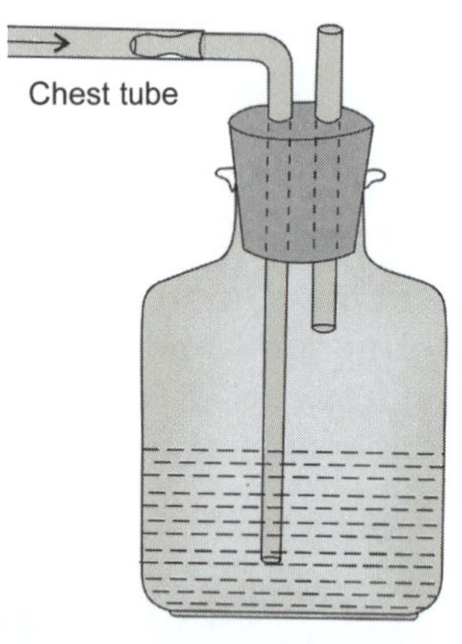

Fig. 62.8: Underwater seal (diagrammatic)

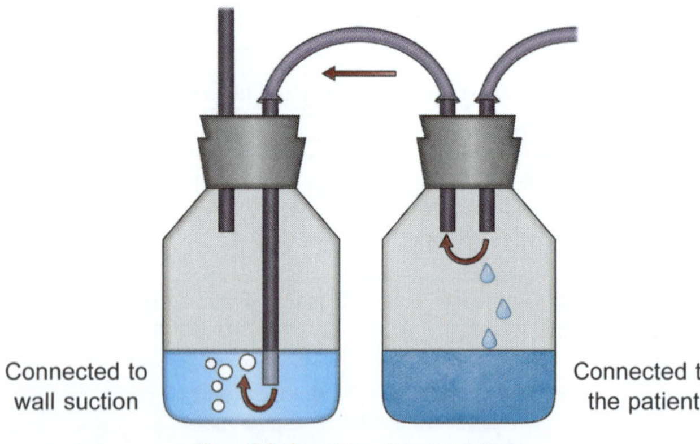

Fig. 62.9: ICD with 2 bottles

Removal of ICT (Key Box 62.7)

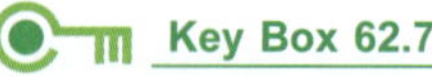

ICT—Removal

- Chest X-ray—lung fully expanded and drainage should be less than 100 ml for two days and no air leak. Patient should not be on a ventilator
- Clamp the tube for 24 hours
- Removal after 24 hours of clamping, provided the patient is comfortable and lung remains fully expanded

TEN COMMANDMENTS OF PRECAUTIONS WHILE USING ICT–ICD

1. Should select triangle of safety
2. Should direct the tube towards apex in cases of haemothorax and pneumothorax
3. Should direct the tube towards base in empyema
4. Should confirm that all the holes are inside
5. Should be connected to under water seal
6. Should observe for movement of the fluid column with respiration
7. Should take an X-ray after the insertion of the tube
8. Should avoid kinking of the tube
9. Should not clamp the ICD, if there is air leak
10. Should be always lower than patient level in the supine position. Otherwise, contents of the bottle will enter the pleural space

LUNG LACERATION

- **Minor laceration:** Haemopneumothorax. Usually intercostal chest tube is enough.
- **Major laceration:** Haemopneumothorax
  i. Introduce intercostal chest tube
  ii. Continuous air leak or bleeding through ICT and lung not expanding. Requires thoracotomy and repair or resection of lobe.

SHOCK LUNG

Definition

- Alveolar collapse due to shock as a result of oedema, impaired perfusion, and reduction in alveolar space resulting in respiratory failure is called shock lung.
- It is also called **A**cute **R**espiratory **D**istress **S**yndrome (**ARDS**).

Causes

- Major chest trauma with multiple rib fractures and lung contusion
- Septic shock and septicaemia
- Disseminated intravascular coagulation

- Massive blood transfusion
- Major burns
- Cardiopulmonary bypass (also called 'Pump lung')
- Acute pancreatitis
- Aspiration of gastric contents

Pathogenesis

- Diffuse inflammation of the lung
- Extensive intravascular coagulation due to microthromboembolism
- Focal disorders of the circulation, primarily because of sluggish microcirculation due to leukostasis, sludge, leading to extensive hyaline thromboses
- Increased capillary permeability due to damaged capillaries
- Diffuse alveolar damage, decreased production of surfactant by type II pneumocytes leading to bilateral extensive fine atelectasis
- Net result is pulmonary consolidation, decrease in the lung compliance, poor gas exchange leading to stiff lung.

Investigations

- Arterial blood gas analysis
- Chest X-ray
- CT scan

Treatment

- Ventilatory support (intermittent positive pressure ventilation)
- Antibiotics—broad spectrum
- Low to moderate doses of steroids may help in early ARDS, in patients requiring high doses of vasopressors to maintain blood pressure.

- Intensive care—supportive therapy can be remembered as **FASTHUG**
  F—Feeding (usually enteral)
  A—Analgesia
  S—Sedation once a day and check neurological status
  T—Thromboembolism prophylaxis
  H—Head-end elevation (20–30°)
  U—Ulcer (gastric) prophylaxis, and
  G—Glucose (blood) control.

INJURY TO TRACHEA AND MAJOR BRONCHI

TRACHEAL INJURIES

Injuries occur as a result of trauma sustained due to crush injuries. Common in cervical trachea.

Symptoms

- Acute airway obstruction
- Subcutaneous emphysema—mediastinal and cervical
- Pneumothorax
- Voice impairment

Treatment

Intubation, tracheostomy, surgery and repair.

MAJOR BRONCHIAL INJURIES

- Blunt trauma produces stereotype injury to main bronchus of either side. Lobar bronchi are less commonly injured (Table 62.1).
- Lesion is often a circumferential laceration with complete separation or a partial tear.

Symptoms

- Pneumothorax, uncontrolled air leak
- Haemoptysis
- Surgical emphysema
- Bronchoscopy for confirmation

Surgery

- Endobronchial intubation
- Bronchoplasty, injury to the lobar bronchus—resection of the lobe of the lung.

INJURY TO THE DIAPHRAGM

Features

- Due to crush injury
- Industrial—due to fall of heavy weights over the abdomen.
- Commonly, left diaphragm tear occurs.
- Missed in chest X-ray in the supine position.

Table 62.1 Summary of blunt chest injury

Rib fractures	Pulmonary injuries	Tracheobronchial	Diaphragm
Flail chest	Contusion	Mediastinal emphysema	Breathlessness
Stove-in chest	Pneumothorax	Shock	Coils of bowel within thorax
Subclavian injury	Haemothorax	Airway obstruction	
Surgical emphysema	Laceration	Death	

- Diagnosed by CECT of the abdomen or chest X-ray reveals the Ryle's tube in the chest or coils of bowel (gas shadow) in the chest and elevated fundic air bubble (Figs 62.10 to 62.12). Diagnostic laparoscopy is also a good investigation in cases of rupture diaphragm.
- When in doubt, do diagnostic laparotomy.

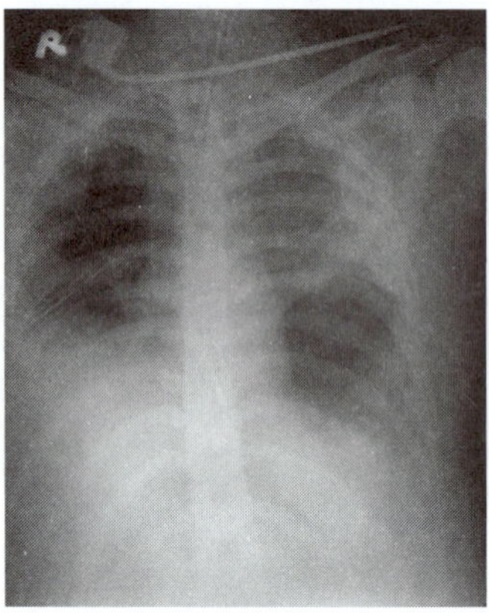

Fig. 62.10: Chest X-ray left haemothorax with elevated fundic air bubble

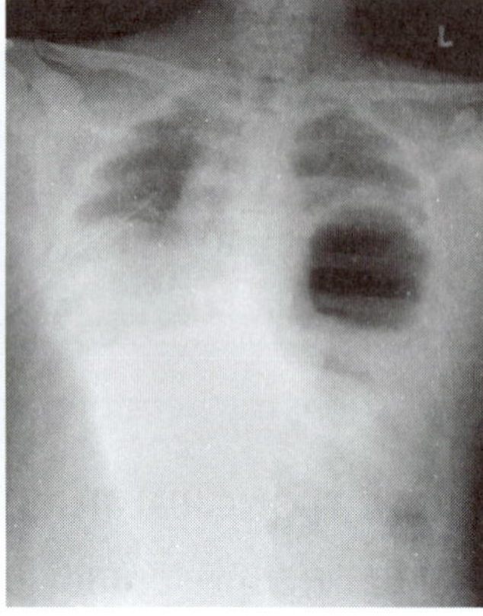

Fig. 62.11: Fundic air bubble in the thorax

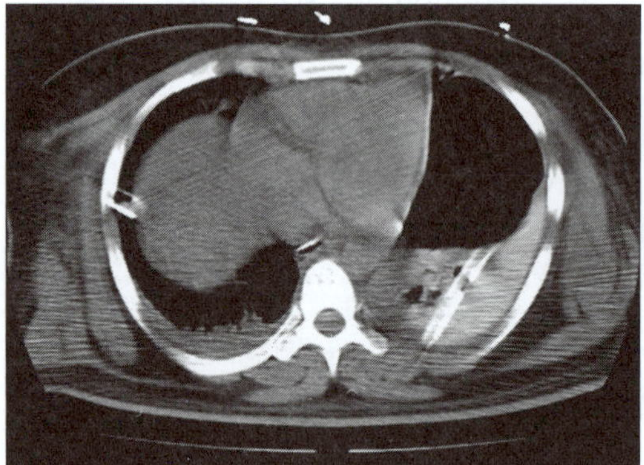

Fig. 62.12: ICT in the stomach

INJURY TO THE AORTA (RUPTURE OF THE AORTA)

- Deceleration injuries
- Gets avulsed at the region of ligamentum arteriosus
- Complete rupture—immediate death
- Incomplete rupture—shock, widening of mediastinum, unequal pulses.

Surgery

- Repair is done using cardiopulmonary bypass.

MYOCARDIAL CONTUSION

- Deceleration injuries
- Anterior chest impact
- Clinical features include arrhythmias, reduced cardiac output, cardiac tamponade.

SURGICAL EMPHYSEMA

Types

1. Localised
2. Extensive from the eyelids to the scrotum, quite alarming in appearance. Indicates lung injury (Fig. 62.13).

Pearls of Wisdom

Palpable crepitus is diagnostic of surgical emphysema.

X-ray chest may show pneumothorax or air in the subcutaneous plane (Fig. 62.14).

Treatment

- **Localised:** Not extending, no pneumothorax—observation.
- Pneumothorax—ICT.
- **Extensive:** ICT to be introduced on the side where it is maximum.
- ICT may be required on both sides.

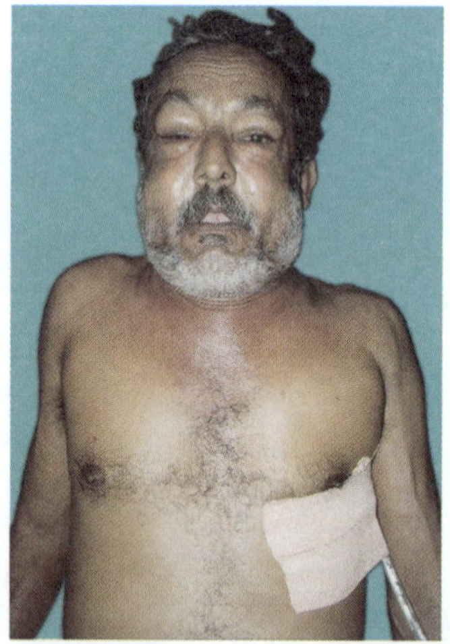

Fig. 62.13: Surgical emphysema

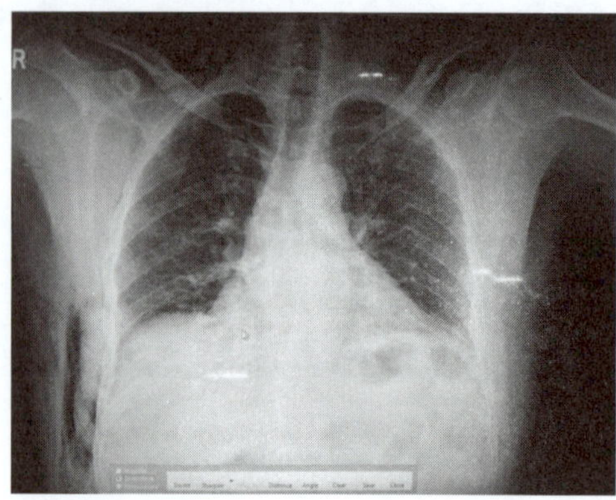

Fig. 62.14: Chest X-ray showing 10th rib fracture with surgical emphysema on the right side

Key Box 62.8

Surgical Emphysema

- Air in the subcutaneous tissue
- Palpable crepitus
- Sometimes, can be gross
- Disfigurement is more than symptoms and signs
- Rib stabbing the lung
- Rupture of bronchus—mediastinal emphysema

- Two ICT, one apical and the other basal, may need to be introduced if there is continuous air leak.
- The emphysema usually subsides within a week. Multiple incisions and expelling the air from the subcutaneous space manually are not required but may be carried out for cosmetic purposes or if patient has respiratory distress (Key Box 62.8).

PENETRATING THORACIC WOUNDS

Stab Wounds

They depend on type of weapon, length and direction of the stab (Key Box 62.9).

Projectile Wounds

- Relatively low velocity revolver bullets may perforate one or two lobes of the lung with a little damage and only drainage of the pleural space is required. There will be entry and exit wounds.
- High velocity perforating wounds cause more damage to the tissue, adjacent to the tract. If the damage is extensive, lobectomy or pneumonectomy has to be considered.
- Bomb fragments, because of irregular shape, commonly carry with them pieces of ribs and are associated not only with **severe haemorrhage** and air leak from the torn pulmonary vessels and bronchus but also with haemorrhage from irregular entry and exit wounds. Urgent thoracotomy is necessary.

Treatment

Emergency thoracotomy is a life-saving procedure in the trauma centre. Thoracotomy for polytrauma has a poor prognosis than for isolated thoracic injuries.

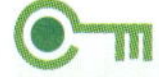
Key Box 62.9

Penetrating Wounds

- Represents mainly stab and gunshot wounds
- Immediately pack the wound
- Intercostal chest tube
- Thoracotomy mandatory

Indications

- Decompression of cardiac tamponade
- Control of bleeding, allow for internal cardiac massage
- Clamping of descending thoracic aorta for exsanguinous bleeding in the abdomen.

Surgery

Anterolateral thoracotomy through 5th intercostal space, entered in 1–2 minutes.

MEDIASTINAL EMPHYSEMA

- The emphysema is mainly **suprasternal.**
- On auscultation, **pericardial crunching sounds** synchronous with the heart beat, are heard.
- If there is haemodynamic instability, bilateral intrapleural ICT has to be introduced as a precaution against tension pneumothorax.
- Rule out oesophageal and tracheal injury.

Principles of Managing Chest Injuries

1. **Pulmonary physiotherapy:** Most important in all chest injury patients.
2. **Aspiration of secretions:** Tracheal aspiration, nasotracheal suction, aspiration of oral cavity and pharynx.
3. **Relieving pain:** Oral narcotics, parenteral narcotics, thoracic epidural analgesia, intercostal nerve block.
4. **Physiotherapy assistance**
   - Encourage coughing
   - Chest percussion and vibration
   - Deep inspiratory efforts
   - Humidification of air, nebulisation
   - Early mobilisation
5. **Treatment of pneumothorax or haemothorax:** Insertion of intercostal chest tube.
6. **Treatment of shock:** First of all, the causes of shock in chest injuries has to be determined by thorough assessment of the patient. Once the cause is found out, depending upon the nature of the problem, the patient is treated in an intensive care unit (Key Box 62.10).

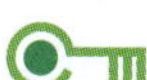
Key Box 62.10

Causes of Shock

- Tension pneumothorax
- Massive haemothorax
- Cardiac tamponade
- Myocardial contusion
- Air embolism
- Ruptured diaphragm
- Injury to the great vessels

7. **FAST (Focussed Abdominal Sonography in Trauma):** Focussed assessment with ultrasonography for trauma and rapid assessment for ruling out fluid collection in the abdomen, chest and pericardium.
8. **Surgery:** Depending upon the severity and location, surgery is done.
9. **Treatment of complications** (Key Box 62.11)
   - Thromboembolism
   - Tracheostomy complications
   - Prolonged ICU complications.

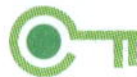 **Key Box 62.11**

Complications

- Empyema
- Bronchopleural fistula
- Bronchial stenosis
- Chylothorax
- Clotted haemothorax
- ARDS
- Atelectasis

Nontraumatic Rib Fractures (Key Box 62.12)

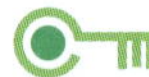 **Key Box 62.12**

Nontraumatic Rib Fractures

- Stress fractures
- Metastatic disease
- Metabolic disease such as hyperparathyroidism
- Osteogenesis imperfecta
- Consider child abuse, 'shaken baby' syndrome
- Older patients after violent coughing

EMPYEMA

Definition

Collection of the pus in the pleural space is called empyema.

Aetiopathogenesis

- It is the end stage result of pleural effusion and infection. A few examples are—following haemothorax, lung abscess, pneumonia. In India, tuberculosis is an important cause of empyema (Figs 62.15 and 62.16).
- Oesophageal perforations—iatrogenic or spontaneous also result in empyema.
- Rupture of subphrenic abscess, rupture of hydatid cyst, rupture of amoebic liver abscess also can result in empyema.
- The classical events which follow empyema following pneumonia are exudative phase with pleural effusion, followed by thickening of fluid—fibropurulent stage and when the lung is covered by thick cortex, it is called organising phase.

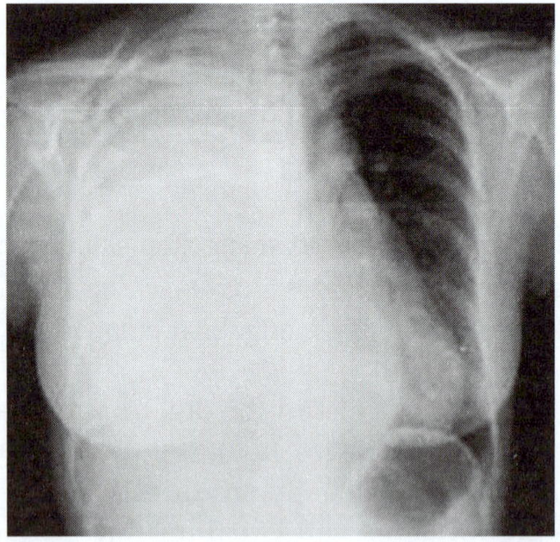

Fig. 62.15: Effusion

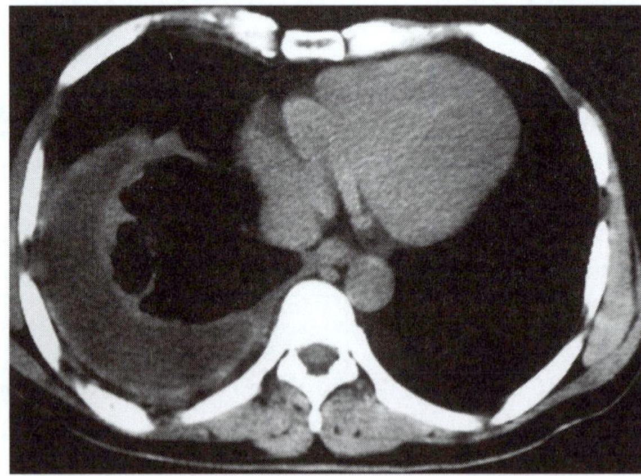

Fig. 62.16: Right empyema split pleura sign

Diagnosis

- History of fever diagnosed as pneumonia or tuberculosis
- Pain in the chest, difficulty in breathing
- Tenderness over the chest
- Toxic features in acute empyema specially in children
- Presence of thick pus with thick cortex of fibrin and coagulum over the lung.

Investigations

- Chest X-ray may show collapse of the lung, tracheal deviation, evidence of pneumonia or tuberculosis.
- Aspiration of pleural fluid and analysis—exudative in cases of pneumonia. Send for bacterial culture.
- CT scan may show split pleura sign. Tuberculous spine can be diagnosed as a cause of empyema (Fig. 62.17).

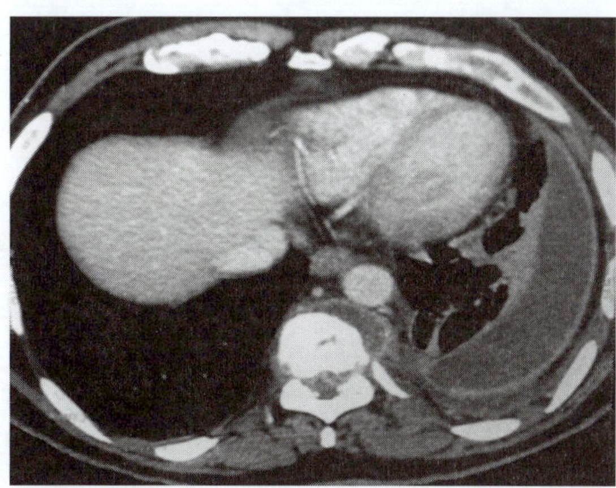

Fig. 62.17: Empyema left with Koch's spine—split pleura sign (*Courtesy:* Figs 62.15 to 62.18 are contributed by Dr CS Rajan, Senior Consultant and Head, Department of Thoracic Surgery, St. Martha's Hospital, Bengaluru)

Surgical Management of Pleural Effusions and Empyema

- **V**ideo-**A**ssisted **T**horacoscopic **S**urgery (**VATS**): With 3–4 ports, video-assisted procedures have become very popular. Minimal incision, less pain and recovery is fast. Drainage, pleural biopsy, talc pleurodesis, debridement of empyema, intercostal tube drainage (ICD) all can be done.
- Rib resections, and drainage through a window—Eloesser's method.
  - Modified Eloesser drainage surgery soon after completion of surgery.
  - This surgery is a palliative operation for chronic empyema collapsed lung and bronchopleural fistula. In these patients, any major lung resection is fraught with high risk of sepsis and stump blow-out.
  - An inverted U-shaped incision is taken on the lower rib and the flap is stitched to the diaphragm for clearing of the purulent secretions.
  - The Eloesser flap is a surgical method devised by "Dr Leo Eloesser in 1935." It was originally planned for tuberculous empyema (Fig. 62.18A and 62.18B).
- **Decortication:** More radical procedure involves thoracotomy, debridement, excision of thick cortex or the covering of the lung, so that lung will expand. This is done by posterolateral thoracotomy.

Complications

- Toxicity, septic shock, multiorgan failure in untreated cases
- Damage to the lungs—lobectomy, pneumonectomy

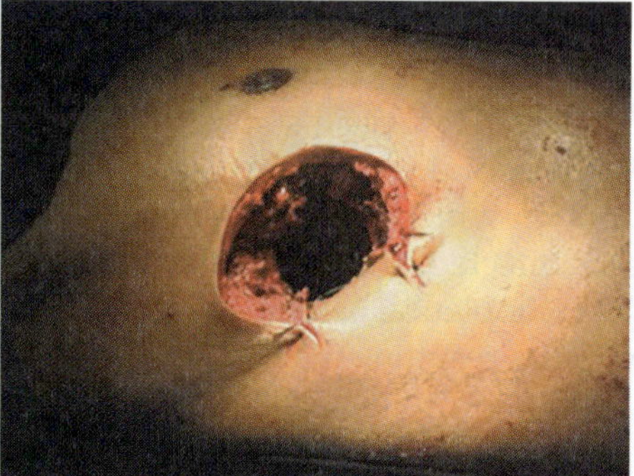

Fig. 62.18A: Initial picture of Eloesser drainage of empyema

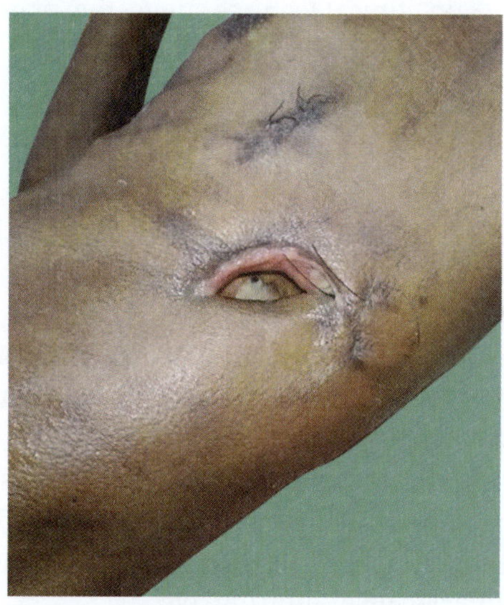

Fig. 62.18B: Same patient after six months of Eloesser drainage

Empyema necessitans: It is a type of empyema which presents as a swelling in the subcutaneous plane with communication to the pleural space/cavity. It is a tense, tender, fluctuant swelling with local rise of temperature. Intercostal bulge is also seen. On asking the patient to cough, expansile impulse is felt. Otherwise, management is similar to that of empyema such as drainage, treating the cause, ATT in tuberculosis and antibiotics in pyogenic infections.

BRONCHOPLEURAL FISTULA

Definition

It is fistulous communication between the main stem, lobar and segmental bronchus to the pleural space.

Causes

- Following lobectomy or pneumonectomy or bacterial/tuberculous infection.
- It may occur when large airways are in communication with the pleural space.

Pathogenesis

- There will be a large empty space left behind following pneumonectomy. This space will be filled with air. Over a period of time, air is absorbed and fluid gets filled up which gets fibrosed slowly. When this fluid gets infected, the stump may break down and cause bronchopleural fistula. The gaping of bronchial stump occurs resulting in bronchopleural fistula.
- Invariably the fluid which accumulates later will be infected.

Clinical Features

- History and clinical features suggestive of empyema
- History of lung surgery
- Persistent air leak in the intercostal drain
- Pus in the ICD

Chest X-ray

- Lung does not fully expand.

Treatment

- Treatment is extremely difficult and disappointing.
- Propped up/sitting position and turn to the diseased side so as to get a dependent drainage
- Intercostal drain connected to underwater seal
- Pleurocutaneous window drainage can be done
- Specific treatment includes control of infection, treat the primary cause, suturing, etc.

Competency

SU26.3: Describe the clinical features of mediastinal diseases and the principles of management.

SURGICAL ANATOMY OF MEDIASTINUM AND MEDIASTINAL MASSES

The **mediastinum** is a broad central partition that separates the two laterally placed pleural cavities. It extends from the sternum to the bodies of the vertebrae; and from the superior thoracic aperture to the diaphragm.

Contents: The thymus gland, pericardial sac, heart, trachea and major arteries and veins. It also serves as a passageway for structures such as the oesophagus, thoracic duct and various components of the nervous system as they traverse the thorax on their way to the abdomen.

Division of Mediastinum (Fig. 62.19)

- A transverse plane extending from the sternal angle (the junction between manubrium and the body of the sternum) to the intervertebral disc between 4th and 5th thoracic vertebrae separates the mediastinum into the **superior mediastinum** and **inferior mediastinum**.

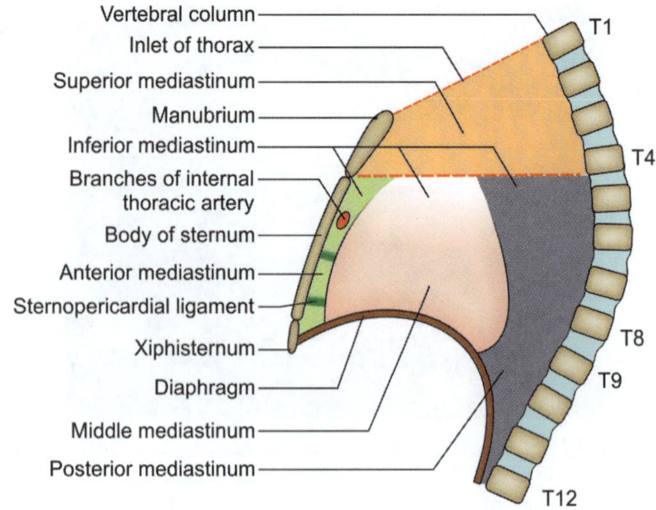

Fig. 62.19: Subdivisions of the mediastinum

- **Inferior mediastinum** is further partitioned into the **anterior, middle, and posterior mediastinum** by the pericardial sac.
- **Anterior mediastinum:** It lies between the back of the sternum and the anterior aspect of the great vessels and pericardium. It contains the thymus, internal mammary arteries, lymph nodes, connective tissue and fat.
- **Middle mediastinum:** It extends from the pericardium anteriorly to the ventral surface of the thoracic spine posteriorly. It contains the pericardium, heart, great vessels, airway and oesophagus.
- **Posterior mediastinum:** It is made up of the spine and includes the costovertebral sulci. The posterior compartment contains the proximal intercostal neurovascular bundles, the spinal ganglia, the sympathetic chain, lymphatic tissue, and connective tissue.

  Differential diagnosis of mediastinal masses is shown in Table 62.2.

ANTERIOR MEDIASTINAL MASSES

"Terrible Ts": Thymic tumours, Teratoma/germ cell tumour, (Terrible) lymphoma, and Thyroid.

1. Thymoma

- Most common anterior mediastinal primary tumour; 20% of adult mediastinal neoplasms.
- Presentation between ages 30 and 50 (most patients are >40 years old).
- 50% are asymptomatic but others have symptoms secondary to compression: Chest pain, cough, dyspnoea, compression of the superior vena cava resulting in head and neck venous congestion, facial oedema.

Table 62.2 Differential diagnosis of mediastinal masses

Anterior mediastinum	Middle mediastinum	Posterior mediastinum
Thymus • Thymoma • Thymic cyst • Thymic hyperplasia • Thymic carcinoma	Bronchogenic cyst	**Neurogenic tumours** • Neurofibroma • Neurilemmoma • Neurosarcoma • Ganglioneuroma • Ganglioneuroblastoma • Neuroblastoma • Chemodectoma • Phaeochromocytoma
Lymphoma **Germ cell tumour** • Teratoma/dermoid cyst • Seminoma • Nonseminoma – Yolk sac tumour – Embryonal carcinoma – Choriocarcinoma	Pericardial cyst Lymphadenopathy • Lymphoma • Sarcoid • Metastatic lung cancer	Meningocoeles Thoracic spine lesion (e.g. Pott's disease)
Intrathoracic thyroid • Substernal goitre • Ectopic thyroid tissue Parathyroid adenoma Haemangioma Lipoma Liposarcoma Fibroma Fibrosarcoma Foramen of Morgagni hernia	Enteric cyst Oesophageal tumours Vascular masses and enlargement	

- **Myasthenia gravis:** Seen in 30–50% of thymoma patients; others can have hypogammaglobulinemia (10%), endocrine disorders, connective tissue disorders.

Staging (Table 62.3)

Investigations

- Chest X-ray may show a mediastinal mass.
- Contrast CT scan of the thorax is the investigation of choice which will detect a mass lesion and its relationship to the adjacent structures (Fig. 62.20).

Table 62.3 Masaoka's clinical stage

Stage I:	Macroscopically completely encapsulated and microscopically no capsular invasion
Stage II:	Macroscopic invasion into surrounding fatty tissue or mediastinal pleura, or microscopic invasion into capsule
Stage III:	Macroscopic invasion into neighbouring organ, i.e. pericardium, great vessels, or lung
Stage IVa:	Pleural or pericardial dissemination
Stage IVb:	Lymphogenous or haematogenous metastasis

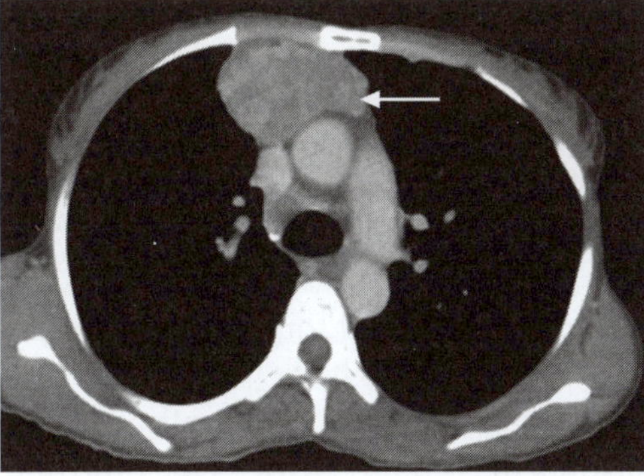

Fig. 62.20: Thymoma

- MRI can also be done.
- Preoperative biopsy is not necessary (Key Box 62.13).

Surgery

- Surgery is the main modality of the treatment—a complete resection of the thymus. Median sternotomy is done to remove the tumour.
- A minimally invasive (thoracoscopic or robotic) approach is another option.

Key Box 62.13

Preoperative Biopsy is not Necessary for the Resection of Following Tumours

1. Thymoma
2. Pleomorphic adenoma
3. Testicular tumours
4. Renal cell carcinoma
5. Hepatocellular carcinoma

2. Germ Cell Tumours (GCT)

- The mediastinum is the most common location for extragonadal germ cell tumours in adults.
- They are classified as benign (teratomas, dermoid cysts) or malignant (seminomas, nonseminomatous GCTs).
- Seminomas are more common than nonseminomatous GCTs.
- Occur in the second decade—late teens
- 20% are malignant
- Cystic teratomas are dermoid cysts, less malignant compared to solid teratomas which have more chances of malignancy.
- Diagnosis is by tumour markers: Alfa fetoproteins (AFP) and beta-hCG. AFP is normal in teratoma and "pure" seminomas. Ninety percent of nonseminomatous germ cell tumours have elevated AFP and/or beta-hCG.
- They are highly radiosensitive (Key Box 62.14).

3. Lymphomas

- The most common are nodular sclerosing Hodgkin's lymphoma and primary mediastinal B-cell lymphoma.
- May present with systemic symptoms such as fevers, weight loss or night sweats but can also present with symptoms such as chest pain, dyspnoea, wheezing, stridor, hoarseness, dysphagia, or **superior vena cava syndrome** due to compression of mediastinal structures.
- **Core biopsy** is required for the diagnosis. Immunohistochemistry studies have to be done.
- **CT scan will help in ruling out other diseases**.
- Mediastinal mass ratio (MMR)—the ratio of the mass to the chest diameter is calculated (*see* page 222 of Chapter 29).
- **Chemotherapy** is the treatment of choice.

Key Box 62.14

Tumours which are Highly Radiosensitive

1. Germ cell tumours
2. Seminoma
3. Lymphoma
4. Squamous cell carcinoma

4. Thyroid Masses

- Intrathoracic thyroid tissue—**ectopic or substernal**, typically causes symptoms of shortness of breath or dysphagia. Sometimes they produce dangerous airway obstruction, deviation of the trachea or narrowing.
- The intrathoracic mass is usually continuous with the thyroid gland in the neck; only 2% of cases are separate from the cervical thyroid and are truly intrathoracic.
- Diagnosis is by CT scan and technetium scan.
- Majority can be managed with cervical incision—a few may require sternotomy.
- Less commonly, intrathoracic mobilisation *via* **VATS** is done.
- Possibility of collapse of trachea should be kept in mind after thyroidectomy—one should be ready with re-intubation/tracheostomy.

MIDDLE MEDIASTINAL MASSES

- Lymphadenopathy is the most common lesion presenting as a mass in the middle compartment of the mediastinum.
- The most common causes include lymphoma, sarcoid and metastatic lung cancer.
- Mediastinoscopy is a very useful technique to biopsy lymphadenopathy in this region.
- Cystic masses comprise approximately 20% of middle mediastinal masses.

1. Bronchogenic Cysts

- Bronchogenic cysts are the most common cystic lesion.
- Secondary to abnormal lung budding during development.
- Bronchogenic cysts are more common in men, in the right paratracheal region and in the subcarinal location.
- Often presents with substernal pain, cough, recurrent infection symptoms or dyspnoea.

2. Enteric Cysts

- They are the third most common benign oesophageal masses after leiomyomas and polyps, and are usually asymptomatic.
- **Three criteria** are required to establish their diagnosis:
  a. Oesophageal attachment
  b. The presence of two layers of muscularis propria
  c. Epithelium characteristic of the gastrointestinal tract.

3. Pericardial Cysts

- Seventy percent arise in the right cardiophrenic angle.
- Symptoms can include shortness of breath, right heart failure secondary to compression, infection and bleeding.

Management

- Bronchogenic and enteric cysts need surgical resection to establish a definitive diagnosis and to decrease the risk of infection or malignant degeneration.
- Pericardial cysts can be typically observed, if asymptomatic, but resection can be utilised, if there are symptoms or if the diagnosis is not completely established by imaging.
- Simple drainage is generally not recommended because *these cysts typically* recur without complete resection.

POSTERIOR MEDIASTINAL MASSES

Neurogenic tumours represent more than 60% of posterior mediastinal masses. These lesions are classified based upon their neural cell of origin. 95% of posterior mediastinal masses arise in the intercostal nerve rami or the sympathetic chain region.

1. Schwannomas and Neurofibromas

- These are benign lesions that arise from the intercostal nerve sheath and make up 90% of adult neurogenic tumours.
- Neurilemmomas or schwannomas constitute 75% of this group of masses. These tumours are firm, encapsulated masses consisting of Schwann cells.
- Neurofibromas are nonencapsulated, soft, friable and are associated with von Recklinghausen neurofibromatosis.
- The surgery of choice for removal of these tumours is by thorocoscopy or thoracotomy.
- Postoperative complications include Horner's syndrome, partial sympathectomy, recurrent laryngeal nerve damage and paraplegia.

2. Malignant Tumours of Nerve Sheath Origin

- Malignant nerve sheath tumours are spindle cell sarcomas of the posterior mediastinum and include malignant neurofibromas, malignant schwannomas and neurogenic fibrosarcomas.
- They affect men and women equally in the third to fifth decades of life and are closely associated with neurofibromatosis, with a 5% risk of sarcomatous degeneration.
- Pain and nerve deficits are common.
- Complete surgical resection is the optimal treatment but in patients with unresectable tumours, adjuvant chemotherapy and radiation are options.

3. Autonomic Ganglionic Tumours

- Neuroblastomas and ganglioneuroblastomas are malignant tumours that occur most commonly in children and originate from the sympathetic ganglia.
- Ganglioneuromas are benign lesions that arise from the sympathetic ganglia, and are most common in young adults. Lesions that arise from paraganglionic cells include phaeochromocytomas and paragangliomas.
- Some neurogenic tumours are "dumb-bell shaped" and arise near intervertebral foramen, and have a posterior mediastinal and intraspinal component.
- Resection usually requires a combined approach with neurosurgery and thoracic surgery.

PULMONARY ASPERGILLOMA

- Pulmonary **aspergilloma**, is a **mycetoma** or **fungus ball**, caused by fungus of *Aspergillus* species.
- The most common place affected by aspergillomas is the lung.
- Tuberculosis of the lungs and immunocompromised conditions are risk factors.
- The fungus settles in a cavity and grows to a big ball—called fungal ball.
- Majority of the cases are asymptomatic.
- Cough, chest pain, haemoptysis, abscess formation are the features.
- Diagnosis is by chest X-ray and CT scan (Fig. 62.21), majority of the cases do not require any treatment.
- In symptomatic cases—recurrent hemoptysis (rarely), removal of the lesion, lobectomy may be required (Fig. 62.22).

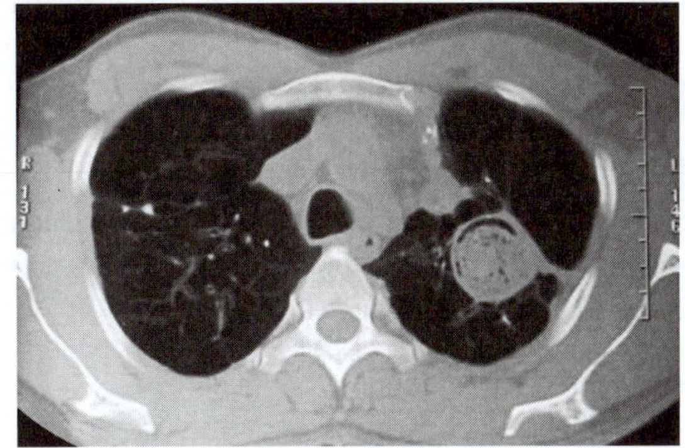

Fig. 62.21: CT chest showing crescent sign—pulmonary aspergilloma

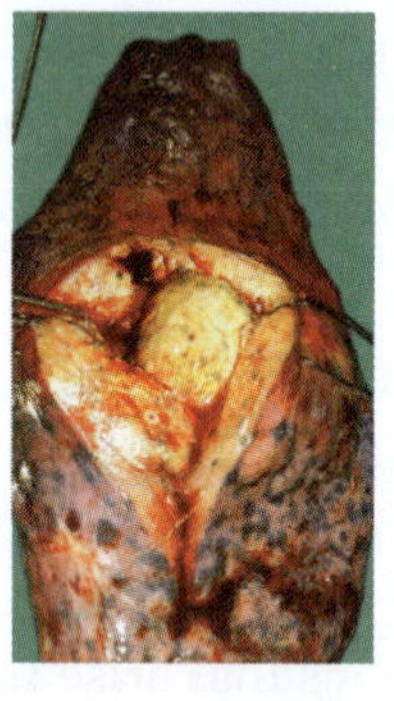

Fig. 62.22: Pulmonary aspergilloma—cut open specimen (*Courtesy:* Figs 62.21 and 62.22, Dr CS Rajan, Senior Consultant and Head, Dept of Thoracic Surgery, St. Martha's Hospital, Bangalore)

Competency

SU26.4: Describe the etiology, pathogenesis, clinical features of tumours of lung and the principles of management.

BRONCHOGENIC CARCINOMA

Introduction

Bronchogenic cancer is the most frequent cause of cancer death in men and women and accounts for 14.5% of all cancer diagnoses and 27.6% of all cancer deaths in the United States. Cigarette smoking is unequivocally the most important risk factor in the development of lung cancer. In India, bronchogenic carcinoma has become number one cancer in men overtaking other cancers. The diagnosis is often delayed. Many patients present as metastasis in bones. Surgical resection alone cannot be curative in many cases because of late presentation of the cases. Prognosis is poor in spite of the treatment.

Risk Factors

- **Cigarette smoking:** It is described as pack years—a pack containing 20 cigarettes. It is calculated by number of packs of cigarette smoked per day by the number of years he has smoked, e.g. one pack year is equal to smoking 20 cigarettes per day for one year.
- **Industrial carcinogens:** Asbestos, arsenic, chromium or nickel, organic chemicals, radon.
- **Radon** is the second leading cause of lung cancer. Radon is a natural radioactive gas released from the normal decay of uranium in the soil.

Pathology—Types

1. **Adenocarcinoma** (ADA) of the lung is the most frequent histologic type and accounts for approximately 45% of all lung cancers. Women smokers have more incidence of adenocarcinoma. Adenocarcinoma of the lung develops from the mucus-producing cells of the bronchial epithelium. Cells are cuboidal to columnar cells. Most of these tumours (75%) are peripherally located. Adenocarcinoma of the lung tends to metastasise earlier than squamous cell carcinoma of the lung and more frequently to the central nervous system (CNS)—cases can present as weakness of the limbs, hemiparesis, etc.
2. **Bronchioloalveolar carcinoma** is an adenocarcinoma. Sometimes it can be a more indolent disease. It is well differentiated and spreads along alveolar walls without invasion of stroma, blood vessels or pleura.
3. **Squamous cell carcinoma** (SCCA) of the lung occurs in approximately 30% of patients with lung cancer. Approximately 75% of these tumours are centrally located and tend to expand against the bronchus, causing extrinsic compression. These tumours are prone to undergo central necrosis and cavitation. **Squamous cell carcinoma** tends to metastasise later than adenocarcinoma. Microscopically, keratinisation, stratification and intercellular bridge formation are exhibited. SCCA may be more readily detected on sputum cytology than ADA.
4. **Large cell undifferentiated carcinoma** may be made in approximately 10% of all lung tumours. These tumours tend to occur peripherally and may metastasise relatively early. Small cell lung cancer represents approximately 20% of all lung cancers; approximately 80% are centrally located. The disease is characterised by an aggressive tendency to metastasise. It often spreads early to mediastinal lymph nodes and distant sites, especially bone marrow and brain.
5. **Small cell lung cancer** appears to arise in cells derived from the embryologic neural crest. Microscopically, these cells appear as **sheets or clusters of small dense cells**, with dark nuclei and little cytoplasm. This oat-like appearance under the microscope gives the term oat cell carcinoma to this disease. These tumours are often advanced at presentation, with an aggressive tendency to metastasise both by lymphatics and by blood. Chemoradiotherapy is generally used for treatment. However, the 5-year survival rate is only 5%.

Table 62.4 shows differences between adenocarcinoma and squamous cell carcinoma.

Table 62.4 Clinical comparison of extrahepatic with intrahepatic portal hypertension

Factors	Adenocarcinoma	Squamous cell carcinoma
1. Incidence	Most common—45%	30%
2. Metastasis	Early	Later
3. Locations	Peripheral	Central
4. Metastasis to brain	More frequent	Less frequent

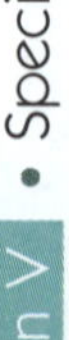

Clinical Features

- Cough and haemoptysis: It is a nonspecific symptom in many patients and diagnosis is delayed because it is often thought to be a smoker's cough.
- Dyspnoea is due to pleural effusion or due to restrictive pulmonary disease.
- Bloody effusion, clubbing of the fingers, localised chest pain are other features.
- Hoarseness due to recurrent laryngeal nerve paralysis, back ache due to metastasis in vertebrae, or neurological features due to metastasis in brain are also presenting features in many cases.
- Myopathy similar to myasthenia gravis can occur in small cell carcinoma.

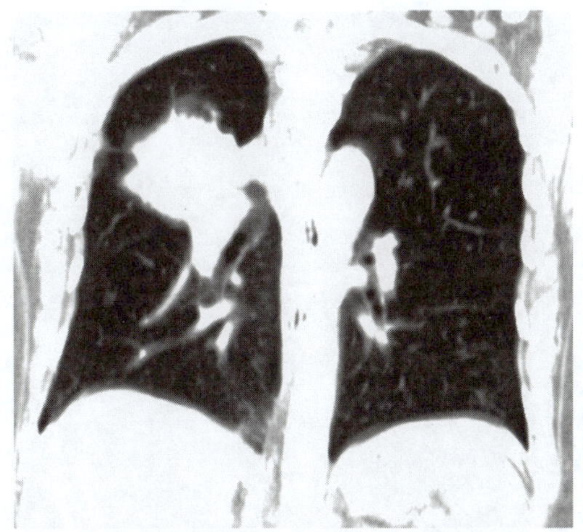

Fig. 62.23: CT of lungs showing bronchogenic carcinoma

Diagnosis and Spread

- In addition to chest X-ray, CT scan, sputum for malignant cells, diagnosis can also be made with bronchoscopic biopsy and CT-guided biopsy. Spread is common PET scan: 18F-fluorodeoxyglucose positron emission tomography (FDG-PET) is the investigation of choice to detect the distant lesions (Figs 62.23 to 62.25).
- Brain CT or magnetic resonance imaging (MRI) (Fig. 62.26).
- Mediastinoscopy.
- CT of the chest, abdomen, MRI brain: Mediastinal lymph node masses, metastases to the adrenal glands, brain, lung and bone are common.
- Bone metastases are osteolytic. Whole body bone scan is needed.

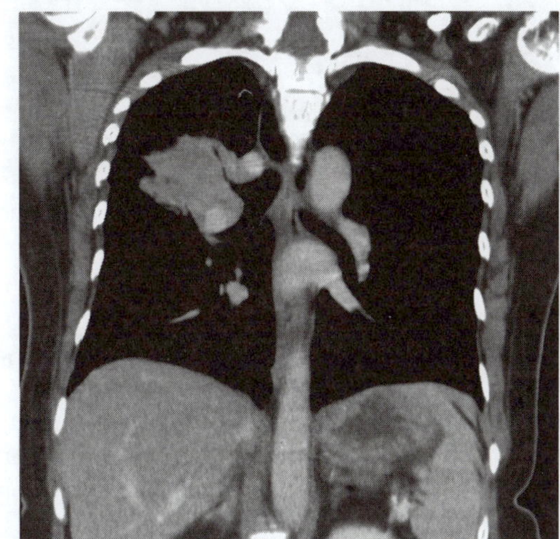

Fig. 62.24: Sagittal section of the CT showing bronchogenic carcinoma right lung

Treatment

Can be grouped into three major categories:

1. *Stages I and II tumours* are contained within the lung and may be completely resected with surgery.
2. *Resectable stages IIIA and IIIB tumours* are locally advanced tumours with metastasis to the ipsilateral mediastinal (N2) lymph nodes (stage IIIA) or involving mediastinal structures (T4N0M0). These tumours, by their advanced nature, may be mechanically removed with surgery followed by systemic chemotherapy. Radiotherapy can also be given to locally advanced disease.
3. *Stage IV disease* includes metastatic disease and is not typically treated by surgery, except for patients requiring surgical palliation. Systemic therapies—chemotherapy for metastatic disease are common.

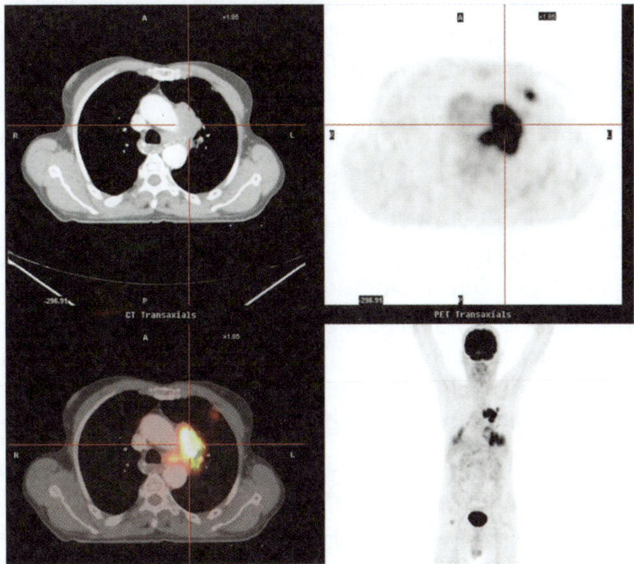

PET-CT of a patient who was diagnosed to have carcinoma lung on bronchoscopy. PET-CT shows a hilar mass with a nodule anteriorly on left side of pleura. It also shows pneumonic patch on lower zone of left lung which is FDG avid

Fig. 62.25: PET scan of lung showing bronchogenic carcinoma

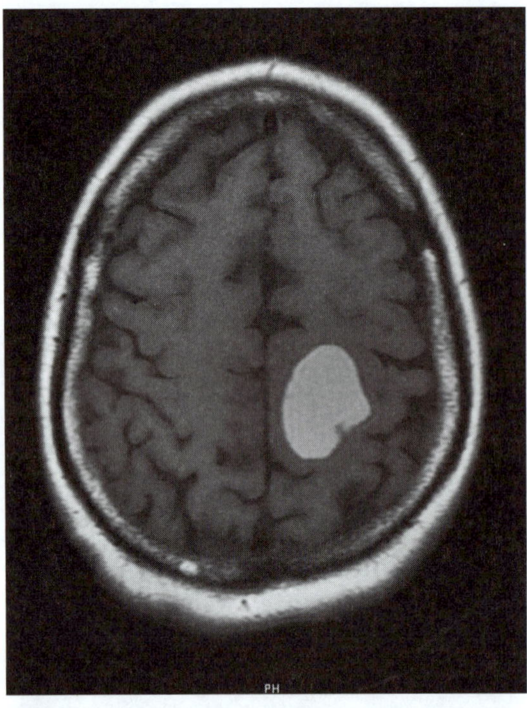

Fig. 62.26: MRI brain showing metastasis from bronchogenic carcinoma

TNM STAGING

Stage	T	N	M
Occult cancer	TX	N0	M0
0	Tis	N0	M0
IA	T1a/b	N0	M0
IB	T2a	N0	M0
IIA	T2b	N0	M0
	T1a/b; T2a	N1	M0
IIB	T2b	N1	M0
	T3	N0	M0
IIIA	Any T1; T2	N2	M0
	T3	N1/N2	M0
	T4	N0/N1	M0
IIIB	T4	N2	M0
	Any T	N2	M0
	Any T	N5	M0
IV	Any T	Any N	M1a/b

TNM STAGING The international tumour–node–metastasis staging

T (Primary tumour)

TX: Primary tumour cannot be assessed, or tumour proven by the presence of malignant cells in sputum or bronchial washings but not visualised by imaging or bronchoscopy

T0: No evidence of primary tumour

Tis: Carcinoma *in situ*

T1: Tumour ≤3 cm in greatest dimension, surrounded by lung or visceral pleura, without bronchoscopic evidence of invasion, more proximal than the lobar bronchus (i.e. not in the main bronchus)

- T1a tumour ≤2 cm in greatest dimension
- T1b tumour >2 cm but ≤3 cm in greatest dimension

T2 tumour >3 cm but ≤7 cm or tumour with any of the following features:

- Involves main bronchus ≥2 cm distal to the carina
- Invades visceral pleura associated with atelectasis or obstructive pneumonitis that extends to the hilar region but does not involve the entire lung
- T2a tumour >3 cm but ≤5 cm in greatest dimension
- T2b tumour >5 cm but ≤7 cm in greatest dimension

T3 tumour >7 cm or one that directly invades any of the following: Chest wall (including superior sulcus tumours), diaphragm, phrenic nerve, mediastinal pleura, parietal pericardium; or tumour in the main bronchus <2 cm distal to the carina but without involvement of the carina or associated atelectasis/obstructive pneumonitis of the entire lung or separate tumour nodule(s) in the same lobe

T4 tumour of any size that invades any of the following: Mediastinum, heart, great vessels, trachea, recurrent laryngeal nerve, oesophagus, vertebral body, carina; or separate tumour nodule(s) in a different ipsilateral lobe

N (Regional lymph nodes)

NX: Regional lymph nodes cannot be assessed

N0: No regional lymph node metastasis

N1: Metastasis in ipsilateral peribronchial and/or ipsilateral hilar lymph nodes and intrapulmonary nodes including involvement by direct extension

N2: Metastasis in ipsilateral mediastinal and/or subcarinal lymph node(s)

N3: Metastasis in contralateral mediastinal, contralateral hilar, ipsilateral or contralateral scalene or supraclavicular lymph node(s)

M (Distant metastasis)

MX: Distant metastasis cannot be assessed

M0: No distant metastasis

M1: Distant metastasis

- M1a separate tumour nodule(s) in a contralateral lobe; tumour with pleural nodules or malignant pleural (or pericardial) effusion
- M1b: Distant metastasis

Competency

SU26.1: Outline the role of surgery in the management of coronary heart disease, valvular heart diseases and congenital heart diseases.

CONGENITAL HEART DISEASES

Introduction

- Abnormal heart structures since birth.
- It develops between 3rd and 8th week of foetal life.
- 1st operation for congenital heart disease was ligation of PDA by Gross in 1938.
- With new advances in neonatal cardiopulmonary bypass (CPB), outcomes have improved.

Development

- At 12 weeks, primitive vascular tube is fully developed.
- Foetal circulation differs from adult in that right and left ventricles pump blood in parallel rather than in series to receive increasingly oxygenated blood.
- **3 important structures are ductus venosus, foramen ovale and ductus arteriosus.**

Changes at Birth

- Pulmonary vascular resistance falls (breathing).
- Pulmonary vasodilation and ductus arteriosus constricts within 30 minutes of delivery (due to increased oxygen levels).
- Reversal of pulmonary and systemic pressure gradient. Termination of blood flow from pulmonary artery into aorta.
- Taping/cutting umbilical cord.
- Venous return from placenta stops.
- IVC and right atrial pressure decrease and left right atrial pressure increases (due to increased systemic vascular resistance).
- Foramen ovale closes.

Abnormalities

- Persistence of normal channels (patent ductus arteriosus—PDA, patent foramen ovale).
- Failure of septation (atrial septal defect—ASD, ventricular septal defect—VSD, tetralogy of Fallot—TOF).
- Stenosis (intracardiac—supravalvular, valvular, infravalvular, coarctation of aorta).
- Atresia/abnormal connections (transposition of great arteries—TGA, total anomalous pulmonary venous connections—TAPVC).

Incidence

Eight cases per 1000 live births in UK.

Aetiology

Unclear: Infection/envirotoxins/genetics.

Diagnosis

In utero foetal ECHO.

Classification

- Cyanotic (1/3rd) and acyanotic (2/3rd)
- Right to left shunts (similar to TOF)
- Left to right shunts (similar to ASD, VSD, PDA)
- Parallel systemic and pulmonary flow (similar to TGV)
- Aortic stenosis, coarctation of aorta
- Mixing of systemic and pulmonary flow (similar to TAPVC): Heart failure in infancy.

CYANOTIC CONGENITAL HEART DISEASE

1. Tetralogy of Fallot (TOF)

Most common cyanotic congenital heart disease

Child adopts squatting posture during hypoxic spells which increases systemic vascular resistance and venous return to heart. This directs the blood into pulmonary circulation and oxygenation improves. Chest X-ray shows boot-shaped heart. Treatment—single or two-stage surgery (Key Box 62.15).

2. Transposition of Great Vessels (TGA)

- **Most common cause of cyanosis in newborn.**

Features

- Aorta arises from right ventricle and pulmonary artery from left ventricle.
- Incompatible with life unless associated with ASD or VSD.
- **Chest X-ray—'Egg on side' appearance.**

Treatment

- Rashkind percutaneous balloon atrial septoplasty.
- Definitive repair—arterial switch (2 stages).
- Mustard or Senning surgery.

3. Total Anomalous Pulmonary Venous Drainage

- Pulmonary venous drain disconnected from left atrium and drains to right side, e.g. inferior vena cava (IVC) or superior vena cava (SVC).

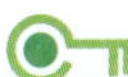

Key Box 62.15

Components

1. VSD
2. Overriding aorta
3. Pulmonary stenosis
4. Right ventricular hypertrophy

- Presents with failure to thrive.
- Treatment—surgery.

4. Eisenmenger's Syndrome

- It occurs following reversal of a previous left to right shunt as with ASD or VSD.
- Similar to pulmonary hypertension.
- Closure of shunt contraindicated.

ACYANOTIC CONGENITAL HEART DISEASE

1. Patent Ductus Arteriosus

Definition

Persistence of the foetal ductus arteriosus in the postnatal period.

Embryology

- Derived from the 6th aortic arch
- Essential for the foetal circulation
- Blood ejected by right ventricle flows exclusively through the ductus to the lower extremity and placenta bypassing the high resistance pulmonary circulation in the foetus.

At Birth

- Physiological closure occurs in 1–6 days
- Anatomical closure occurs in 2–3 weeks

Mode of Closure

Smooth muscle constriction in response to rising arterial oxygen tension.

Pathophysiology

Shunt occurs across the ductus both in systole and diastole resulting in left ventricle overload and pulmonary plethora.

- Shunt depends on the size of the ductus and pulmonary and systemic vascular resistance. Continuous murmur is due to shunt during both systole and diastole.

Clinical Features

- Incidence: M : F = 1:2
- It depends on the size of the ductus, pulmonary vascular resistance, age at presentation and associated anomalies.
  a. **Small ductus: Asymptomatic**
  b. **Infants:** Congestive heart failure
  c. **Children:** Dyspnoea on exertion, repeated respiratory tract infection (Key Box 62.16).

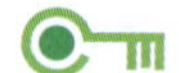 **Key Box 62.16**

Diagnosis

- Hyperdynamic precordium and bounding peripheral pulses in large shunt
- Machinery or **continuous murmur (Gibson's murmur)** in the left second intercostal space, radiating to the left infraclavicular area
- ECG: Left ventricular hypertrophy
- Chest X-ray: Cardiomegaly
- Pulmonary congestion in large ductus and hilar dance on fluoroscopy
- Two-dimensional echo is diagnostic—in suprasternal view, the PDA is seen

Pearls of Wisdom

Occurs 1 in 5000 live births. 50% in premature babies

Complications

- Reversal of shunt
- Infective endocarditis
- Congestive heart failure

Treatment

It can be divided into surgical and nonsurgical methods.

I. Surgical methods

- Presence of PDA is sufficient indication for surgery even without symptoms.
- **In infants:** Large PDA with congestive cardiac failure not responding to antifailure measures, surgery is indicated.

Surgery

- Triple ligation
- Division and suturing
- Right lateral position and posterolateral thoracotomy
- Thorax entered through 4th intercostal space
- **It can also be done by thoracoscopy** and video-assisted thoracoscopic surgery (VATS) and clipping of PDA.

Care during surgery

Left recurrent laryngeal nerve must be carefully preserved.

Complications during surgery

- Haemorrhage, left recurrent laryngeal nerve palsy
- Chylothorax

II. Nonsurgical methods

- **Pharmacological closure:** In preterm infants—indomethacin
- **Transcatheter closure:** Interventional cardiology
- Double umbrella device—Rashkind
- Gianturco coils
- Lock Clamshell occluder.

2. Coarctation of Aorta

Definition

Congenital narrowing of the descending thoracic aorta usually occurring just distal to the left subclavian artery origin, adjacent to the site of insertion of the ductus arteriosus.

Incidence

- 0.2–0.6 per 1000 live births
- 5–8% of all cases of congenital heart diseases.

Aetiology

Flow theory: Reduced flow in the aorta due to multiple abnormalities in the heart during the foetal period.

Ductal sling theory: When there is isolated coarctation, this theory is applicable. Abnormal extension of contractile ductal tissue into the adjacent aorta which results in coarctation.

Types

Infantile—preductal and adult—juxtaductal.

Classification

- Group I: Isolated coarctation
- Group II: Coarctation with VSD
- Group III: Coarctation with complex intracardiac anomalies (Key Box 62.17).

Clinical Features

Depend on: Age and symptoms at presentation, location of the coarctation, severity of the coarctation, associated anomalies.

Symptoms

- Visual disturbances, exertional dyspnoea

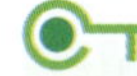 **Key Box 62.17**

Associated Congenital Anomalies

- Ventricular septal defect
- Bicuspid aortic valve
- Patent ductus arteriosus
- Mitral valve abnormalities

- Upper extremity hypertension
- Headache, epistaxis
- Claudication of the lower limbs

Signs

- Systolic murmur heard over the precordium and posteriorly between the scapula.
- **Feeble femoral pulses.**
- Enlarged collateral vessels are seen (Suzman's sign) and palpable between scapula and bruit can be heard here.
- Systolic gradient between arm and leg blood pressure.

Collaterals

- Subclavian artery and its branches
- Internal mammary artery
- Intercostal artery
- Scapular, cervical, vertebral, epigastric and spinal arteries.

Investigations

- **ECG:** LVH with LV strain
- **CXR:** Notching of the ribs **(Dock's sign)** from third rib onwards, above four years of age.

Diagnosis

- Two-dimensional echocardiogram, cardiac catheterisation
- Transoesophageal echocardiogram (TEE)
- Angiogram

Pearls of Wisdom

Classic 'three' sign: Formed by dilated left subclavian artery, narrowing of the coarctation and the poststenotic dilatation of aorta.

Complications (Key Box 62.18)

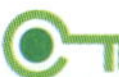 **Key Box 62.18**

Complications

- Circle of Willis aneurysm rupture
- Aortic dissection
- Early coronary atherosclerosis
- Bacterial endocarditis
- Congestive heart failure
- Spontaneous rupture of aorta

Treatment

A. Nonsurgical (infants): Balloon dilation and stenting.

B. Surgery

- Left posterolateral thoracotomy
- Thorax entered through fourth intercostal space
- Arterial line in the right upper limb
- Preserve the vagus and recurrent laryngeal nerves
- Arterial line in the lower limb
- Lower limb pressure during cross-clamping of aorta, to be kept above 45 mmHg
- If the pressure is low, then create a shunt from the aortic arch to the descending thoracic aorta with the help of a cannula.
- Patch aortoplasty.

Complications of surgery

- Haemorrhage, RLN injury, phrenic nerve injury
- Horner's syndrome, chylothorax
- Paradoxical hypertension, paraplegia, stroke.

Late complications

- Recoarctation, aneurysm and left arm ischaemia (when subclavian flap aortoplasty is done).

Pseudocoarctation: Rare condition which results from congenital elongation of the aortic arch which leads to redundancy and kinking of the aorta and may appear similar to coarctation but there is no obstruction to blood flow.

3. Atrial Septal Defect

Defect in septum between left and right atrium leading to left to right shunt.

Types

ASD is of three types:

- **Ostium secundum:** Defect in floor of fossa ovalis. Presents late in life.
- **Ostium primum:** Endocardial cushion defect associated with mitral valve defects (mitral regurgitation) and trisomy 21. Presents earlier in life.
- **Sinus venosus:** Defect near junction of SVC and atrium.

Treatment

Open heart surgery with CPB and closure of defect directly with sutures or with pericardial or synthetic patch.

4. Ventricular Septal Defect

VSD is of four types:

- Perimembranous defect (in membranous septum): 70–80%
- Muscular defect (multiple): 10%
- Atrioventricular defect: 5%
- Subarterial defect: 5–10%

O/E: Pansystolic murmur

Treatment

Surgical repair: Open heart surgery with patch.

CORONARY ARTERY BYPASS SURGERY

Introduction

Often simply called bypass surgery, it is the **most commonly performed open heart surgery all over the world.** The incidence of coronary artery disease is rapidly rising in the developing countries. A **vein graft** from the lower limb or an **arterial graft** (internal mammary artery or the radial artery) is used to bypass the obstructed coronary artery. The bypass is done from the root of the aorta to the distal coronary artery.

- The obstruction or the block is not touched.

Risk Factors for Coronary Artery Disease

(Key Box 62.19)

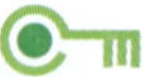
Key Box 62.19

Risk Factors

I. Nonmodifiable
- Age, sex, family history

II. Modifiable, controlled or treated by medicines:
- Smoking, uncontrolled diabetes
- Uncontrolled hypertension
- Obesity, overweight, lack of physical exercise
- Individual response to stress
- High blood cholesterol or lipid abnormalities

Incidence

Least in Japan and highest in Finland.

Indications for Surgery

1. Usually indicated in symptomatic or for prognostic reasons (i.e. balance between expectant benefit and risk faced by patient).
   a. >50% stenosis of left main stem artery
   b. >70% stenosis of proximal left anterior interventricular artery
   c. Triple vessel disease
   d. Poor ventricular function associated with CAD.
2. Chronic stable angina
3. Acute coronary syndrome

4. Surgery for complications of MI such as ventricular septal rupture, etc.

Pearls of Wisdom

With interventional cardiology progressing rapidly the indications for surgery are getting blurred.

Investigations

- ECG/cardiac enzymes—Trop T and Trop I
- 2D echocardiogram—new stress ECHO
- Holter monitoring, thallium scan-201 or ^{99m}Tc
- Stress test (exercise tolerance test)
- Coronary angiogram
- Radionucleotide studies and cardiac MRI
- CT (multislice high resolution)

Contraindications of CABG

- Small, diffusely diseased arteries
- Diffuse disease and heart failure
- Acute myocardial infarction over 6 hours old
- Moribund patients after resuscitation

Surgery

- Bypass surgery with vein or artery graft
- Endarterectomy
- Venous patch

Bypass Surgery

1. Techniques of bypass
    - **Cold cardioplegia** with moderate hypothermia and cardiopulmonary bypass.
    - Ischaemic cross-clamp with moderate hypothermia with cardiopulmonary bypass.
    - **Empty beating heart**, normothermic with cardiopulmonary bypass.
    - **Beating heart surgery,** no heart lung machine.
2. Grafts
    - Veins—lower limbs (long saphenous vein)
    - Upper limb (cephalic vein) rarely used
    - Arteries—radial (Key Box 62.20)
    - Internal mammary artery both right and left
    - Gastroepiploic
    - Inferior epigastric
    - Inferior mesenteric
3. Nonautogenic conduits
    - Cryopreserved human saphenous vein allograft
    - Processed bovine sacral artery
    - Polytetrafluoroethylene graft (Gore-Tex)

Key Box 62.20

Advantages of Arterial Graft

- It is artery to artery anastomosis
- Compatible size
- Flow adaptation
- IMA advantages: No vasa vasorum
- Dense nonfenestrated intact internal elastic lamina that inhibits cellular migration and subsequent initiation of hyperplasia
- Thin medial layer with a few smooth muscle cells which provide a little vasoreactivity
- Produces more prostacyclin which is a vasodilator and platelet inhibitor

Standard Surgical Procedure

- Median sternotomy
- Internal mammary artery dissection done
- Pericardium opened
- Systemic heparinisation 3 mg/kg
- Aortic and venous cannulation.
- Cardiopulmonary bypass started
- Aorta cross-clamped and cold K^+ rich solution given in the aortic root
- Heart arrested in diastole to achieve immobile surgical field
- Distal anastomosis completed
- Proximal anastomosis done with the heart beating
- Weaned off CPB
- Protamine given and decannulation carried out
- Sternum closed, extubation 6–8 hours later.

Complications of Surgery

1. Perioperative MI (2–3%)
2. Stroke
3. Arrhythmias (30%)
4. Sinus tachycardia
5. Atrial fibrillation
6. Reinfarct
7. Wound infection
8. Bleeding
9. General weakness
10. Mortality (2–3%)
11. Persistent poor cardiac output requiring inotropes or mechanical support

Mechanical support to low cardiac output patients post-CABG: Intra-aortic balloon pump (IABP)

- Inserted percutaneously in common femoral artery, threaded into aorta till its tip lies in distal arch vessels.

- Balloon is triggered by the ECG, deflating during ventricular systole (decreasing afterload) and inflating during diastole (increasing diastolic pressure and blood flow to coronaries).

Prognosis

- Ability to return to normal lifestyle
- Improvement in ventricular function
- Work capacity better than preoperative
- Risk of arrhythmias unchanged
- Minimal medications
- Complete and dramatic relief of chest pain.

Patency

Year	Artery	Vein
1	97	90
5	95	60
10	90	40

Recent Advances

- Age limitation changed (CABG done in 80 years old also)
- Improved myocardial preservation
- Composite arterial grafts
- Sutureless anastomosis
- Endoscopic vein harvesting
- Intracoronary injections of vascular endothelial growth factor (VEGF)

Composite Arterial Grafts

- Arterial grafts have long-term patency.
- Patients with total arterial grafts may not require future surgery.
- Arterial grafts are used in the shape of T or Y.
- It can revascularise almost all blocked major vessels.

Endoscopic Vein Harvesting

- Only two small incisions
- With help of a subcutaneous tunnel, the vein is dissected
- Requires expensive equipment
- Major branches are tied and smaller ones are controlled by pressure
- Cosmetic advantage
- Takes longer time

OFF PUMP CORONARY ARTERY BYPASS SURGERY

Procedure

- Beating heart surgery, no heart lung machine
- Sternotomy, stabilisation devices used
- Short-acting beta-blockers to reduce the heart rate.
- Proper positioning of the heart with mechanical stabilisation device for proper visual presentation
- CPB standby, all vessels can be bypassed by proper position of heart, quick recovery, early extubation
- No CPB, less trauma, reduced risk of bleeding and kidney failure, reduced hospital stay.

Advantages

- Avoids physiological stress associated with CPB.
- Aortic manipulation leading to neurological complications avoided. Whole body inflammatory response that occurs due to CPB is decreased.
- Incidence of postoperative renal failure due to CPB is decreased.

Future Developments/Recent Advances

1. Bypass graft coupling devices to facilitate anastomosis (clips, stents).
2. Normalising left ventricular geometry with intracardiac devices.
3. Myocardial protection during CPB (ventricular assist devices). Ischaemic preconditioning pharmacologically preoperatively.
4. **Vascular intimal hyperplasia:** Important cause of graft occlusion. Gene-based therapies to prevent this before grafting the veins.
5. Minimally invasive direct coronary artery bypass **(MIDCAB)** surgery: Anterior submammary incision. LIMA dissected down with the aid of a thoracoscope and grafted to the LAD.

ABDOMINAL AORTIC ANEURYSMS (AAA)

- Aneurysms are defined as a focal dilatation of at least 50% larger than the expected normal arterial diameter.
- For AAA—transverse diameter 3 cm or greater.

Pearls of Wisdom

Most common type of true aneurysm with high propensity to rupture and it is the 15th overall leading cause of death.

Risk Factors for AAA (Key Box 62.21)

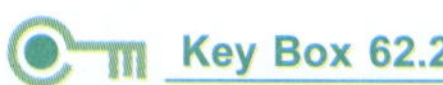

Key Box 62.21

Most Important Risk Factors of AAA

1. Age: Peak incidence at 80 to 85 years
2. Male: Female ratio—4 : 1
3. Genetic: First-degree relatives: 11-fold increase in relative risk
4. Tobacco use: 8 : 1 preponderance of aneurysms in smokers
5. Other factors: 55% demonstrate *C. pneumoniae* by immunohistochemistry

Site

95%—infrarenal aorta, 5%—suprarenal aorta.

Salient Features

Fates of aneurysm

- Infection, rupture (free/contained), thrombosis, embolism.

Growth Rates

<5 cm diameter—0.3 cm/year >5 cm diameter—0.5 cm/year.

Clinical Features

Incidental finding

- Pulsatile abdominal mass on palpation, detected during evaluation for another abdominal pathology or detected at surgery for unrelated abdominal or pelvic operation.

Classical triad

1. Sudden-onset midabdominal or flank pain
2. Shock
3. Presence of a pulsatile abdominal mass (expansile pulsation).

Palpation findings

Firm mass, expansile pulsation over the mass and if upper border is palpable, then the origin is probably infrarenal.

Diagnosis

1. **Chest X-ray** (Fig. 62.27)—round opacity, eggshell pattern of calcification
2. **Abdominal ultrasound**
   a. Detail of the vessel wall
   b. Presence of plaques
   c. Size
3. **CT—most precise**
   a. Proximal and distal extent can be made out.
   b. Amount and location of mural thrombus (Fig. 62.28)

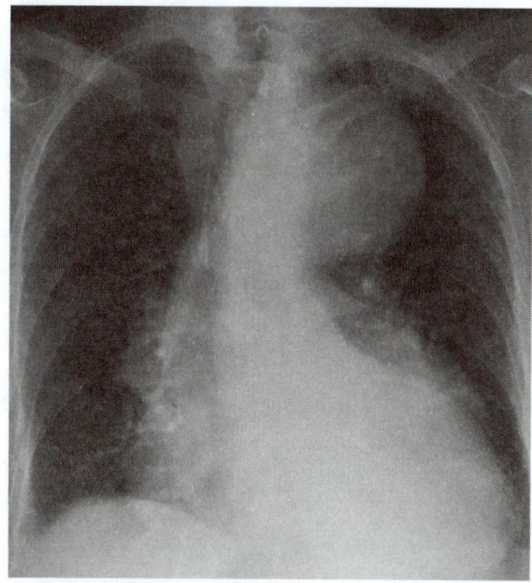

Fig. 62.27: Large arotic aneurysm

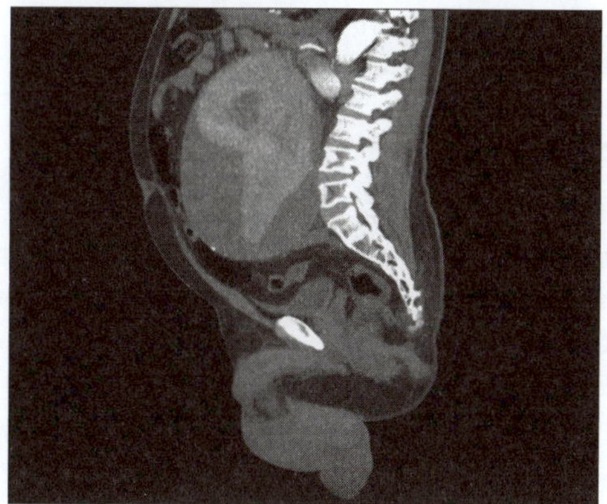

Fig. 62.28: Ruptured aneurysm of aorta with thrombus

   c. Calcifications
   d. Adjacent structures
4. **MRI/MRA**
   a. Less frequently used
   b. Used if patient has renal failure
5. **Contrast arteriography**
   Less frequently used

Complications (Key Box 62.22)

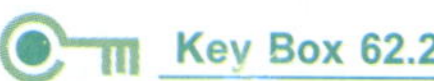

Key Box 62.22

Complications

1. Most frequent—nonfatal MI and renal failure
2. Bleeding
3. Most serious GI complication—ischaemia of the left colon and rectum
4. Lower extremity ischaemia
5. Ischaemic injury to the spinal cord or lumbosacral plexus
6. Postoperative sexual dysfunction
7. Deep vein thrombosis (DVT)

Management

Low-risk AAAs

- Followed with serial size measurements. Reduce expansion rate and rupture risk by conservative treatment such as:
  1. Smoking cessation
  2. Blood pressure control
  3. Reduction of cholesterol
  4. Risk factor modifications
  5. Drugs used: α-blockers, NSAIDs—inhibit elastase
- MMP inhibitors—doxycycline
- Repair is indicated when it is symptomatic or >1 cm/year growth.

High-risk patients

- Delay in repair until larger diameter
- Endovascular aneurysmal repair (EVAR) can be tried.

Techniques of Open Repair

1. **Transperitoneal approach**
2. **Retroperitoneal approach** is indicated in cases of hostile abdomen, suprarenal aneurysm, horseshoe kidney, peritoneal dialysis, inflammatory aneurysm and in ascites.
3. **Minimal incision aortic surgery:** 12 to 15 cm incision, 9 cm proximal to the umbilicus.

Endovascular Aortic Aneurysm Repair

Stent-graft is introduced into the aneurysm through the femoral arteries and fixed in place to the nonaneurysmal aortic neck and iliac arteries with self-expanding or balloon-expandable stents (Palmaz stents), or with barbs, pins or hooks.

Special Considerations

1. Inflammatory aneurysm

- Incidence is about 5%
- Adherent to: Duodenum, IVC, left renal vein, ureters—the reason being lymphatic obstruction during aneurysm expansion and secondary fibrosis and infection from chronic contained rupture
- Rupture is uncommon (as it is often symptomatic and treated before rupture)
- Retroperitoneal approach is preferred.

2. Aortocaval fistula

a. Continuous abdominal bruit +
b. High-output cardiac failure
c. 'Steal' phenomenon—ischaemia to the lower limbs.

Treatment: Fistula closure followed by AAA repair.

3. Horseshoe kidney

a. Kidney usually fused anterior to the aorta
b. Left retroperitoneal approach
c. Endovascular repair is not possible.

RUPTURED ABDOMINAL AORTIC ANEURYSM

Types of Rupture

Anteriorly—into peritoneal cavity.

Posteriorly—into retroperitoneum.

Clinical Features

Back and abdominal pain, pallor, diaphoresis and syncope. If untreated, it is fatal in all cases.

Treatment

- Immediate surgical repair.
- If patient is unstable + previously diagnosed or a pulsatile mass, he is transferred immediately to OT.
- If stable + questionable diagnosis, a CT and open surgical repair, control the haemorrhage + resuscitation + aneurysm repair. Early postoperative mortality rate is 45%.

Differential Diagnosis of Ruptured AAA

- Angina pectoris, perforated peptic ulcer
- Acute pancreatitis, acute cholecystitis
- Acute diverticulitis, mesenteric vascular occlusion
- Prolapsed lumbar intervertebral disc, sciatica

INTERESTING 'MOST COMMON' FOR INTESTINES

- The most common cause of respiratory insufficiency following chest trauma is pneumothorax.
- Most common cyanotic congenital heart disease is tetralogy of Fallot.
- Most common cause of cyanosis in newborn is transposition of great vessels.
- Most commonly performed open heart surgery all over the world is CABG.
- Most common type of true aneurysm with high propensity to rupture is abdominal aortic aneurysm.
- Most common type of AAA is infrarenal.
- Most commonly done investigation for AAA is CT scan.
- Most common noncardiac complication after repair of AAA is renal failure.

Multiple Choice Questions

1. Fracture of the following rib is a marker of severe trauma:
A. First B. Fourth
C. Eighth D. Tenth

2. Treatment of posterior flail segment is:
A. Strapping
B. Open reduction and fixation
C. No treatment is required
D. External fixator application

3. Posterior flail segment does not require treatment because:
A. Scapula supports the flail segment
B. It does not cause complications
C. It heals by itself
D. It has no physiological implications

4. 'Internal pneumatic fixation' for flail chest is the term used for:
A. Insertion of a balloon into the chest
B. Internal fixation with screws
C. Endotracheal intubation and positive pressure ventilation
D. Valsalva manoeuvre

5. Tension pneumothorax should immediately be treated with:
A. Intercostal tube insertion
B. Needle thoracostomy
C. Thoracotomy
D. Thoracoscopic drainage

6. Features of tension pneumothorax include all of the following *except*:
A. Tachypnoea
B. Hypotension
C. Dull note on percussion
D. Tachycardia

7. Indications for thoracotomy in haemothorax include all of the following *except*:
A. Drainage more than 1000 ml
B. Drainage of more than 100 ml/hour for 4 hours
C. If clotted, haemothorax is suspected
D. Coagulation abnormalities

8. The intercostal drain can be removed in all of the following situations *except*:
A. Lung is fully expanded
B. Drainage < 100 ml
C. No air leak
D. The patient is on a ventilator

9. The following is diagnostic of surgical emphysema:
A. The lungs are emphysematous
B. Always follows surgery
C. Palpable crepitus
D. Infiltrates on chest X-ray

10. The following is true about mediastinal emphysema *except*:
A. The emphysema is mainly suprasternal
B. Mediastinal drain needs to be inserted
C. Pericardial crunching sounds can be heard on auscultation
D. Oesophageal and tracheal injury need to be ruled out

11. Nontraumatic rib fractures may be seen in all of the following *except*:
A. Hypoparathyroidism
B. Metastatic disease
C. Older patients after violent coughing
D. Osteogenesis imperfecta

12. The classic 'three' sign of coarctation of aorta is formed by all of the following *except*:
A. Dilated left subclavian artery
B. Narrowing of coarctation
C. Post-stenotic dilatation of aorta
D. Dilated pulmonary artery

13. Most common type of aneurysm with a propensity to rupture:
A. Abdominal aortic aneurysm
B. Carotid artery aneurysm
C. Radial artery aneurysm
D. Cerebral artery aneurysm

14. The most common cause of noncardiac complication after abdominal aortic aneurysm repair is:
A. Pulmonary insufficiency
B. Cerebral insufficiency
C. Renal insufficiency
D. Hepatic insufficiency

15. The most common cause of respiratory insufficiency following chest trauma is:
A. Pulmonary contusion B. Pneumothorax
C. Flail chest D. Haemothorax

Answers

1. A	**2.** C	**3.** A	**4.** C	**5.** B	**6.** C	**7.** D	**8.** D	**9.** C	**10.** B
11. A	**12.** D	**13.** A	**14.** C	**15.** B					

CHAPTER

63

Neurosurgery

- Head injuries
  - Classification
  - Primary lesions
  - Secondary lesions
- Extradural/epidural haematoma
- Chronic subdural haematoma
- Raised intracranial pressure
- Fracture skull
- CSF rhinorrhoea
- Pott's puffy tumour
- Hydrocephalus
- Brain tumours
- Trigeminal neuralgia
- Brainstem death

Introduction

Head injuries derive their importance because of the fact that many patients who die or who are disabled belong to the younger age groups. Head injuries account for 1% of all deaths, one-fourth of deaths due to trauma and they are responsible for **half of all deaths** from road traffic accidents. Majority of the patients are young, adult males.

PATHOPHYSIOLOGY AND MECHANISM OF HEAD INJURIES

Competency

SU17.4: Describe pathophysiology, mechanism of head injuries.

Classification

I. Based on clinical type

1. Open
2. Closed

II. Based on type of injury

1. Blunt injury—acceleration, deceleration
2. Missile injuries

- The term **open head injury** is used to denote a type of injury in which there is a **fracture of the skull associated with tear of the dura and arachnoid,** resulting in cerebrospinal fluid leak either to the external environment or into one of the **potentially infective areas in the base of the skull, e.g. CSF rhinorrhoea or otorrhoea.**
- **A closed head injury** is one where there is **no such leakage.** The advantage of this classification is that it helps the treating physician to recognise a group of patients who are likely to develop an infective complication following the head injury and he can initiate measures to prevent it.
- **Blunt injuries,** depending on the severity of impact, can result in an open or closed head injury. Missile injuries tend to result in an open head injury most often.
- The brain is protected by a bony box which has a **vault** and **base of the skull.** The **base** of skull in contrast to the vault is a **rough terrain** due to the various **bony prominences, ridges** and **foramina**.
- This factor is important in causing extensive brain damage to the brain in acceleration/deceleration type of injuries. In addition to the linear acceleration/deceleration, **rotational acceleration** is also capable of producing damage to the brain as the **brain swirls about** inside the skull. Such injuries result in maximal damage at interfaces between structures of different densities such as **grey matter–white matter junctions.**

Pathology

The pathological changes due to trauma to the brain can be classified into primary and secondary.

I. Primary lesions

- Diffuse axonal injury
- Shearing lesions
- Contusions and burst lobe

II. Secondary lesions

- Swelling, haemorrhage
- Extradural haematoma
- Subdural, intracerebral haematoma
- Infection, SAH

I. Primary Lesions (Key Box 63.1)

A few important primary lesions are discussed below.

- **Diffuse neuronal damage is the most constant** feature of blunt injuries. Immediately after an injury, no changes may be seen but changes begin **after 14 hours of injury and maximum effects** may last up to **one week. Prolonged unconsciousness** may follow injuries which produce only diffuse neuronal damage without any obvious macroscopic changes. Shearing lesions of the nerve fibres account for some severe injuries without any conspicuous changes to naked eye examination of the brain.
- **Cerebral concussion:** Alteration in consciousness without structural damage as a result of non-penetrating traumatic brain injury. There might be loss of consciousness, confusion and amnesia. These are the features. Widespread degeneration of white matter occurs without much changes in the nervous system cortex or brainstem. These patients have spasticity in all four limbs after injury and **when they regain consciousness**, they are found to be severely demented (Key Box 63.2).

Key Box 63.1

Primary Lesions

- Diffuse neuronal damage
- Cerebral contusion
- Cerebral laceration

Key Box 63.2

Cerebral Concussion

- Temporary physiological paralysis of the nervous system
- Loss of consciousness
- Post-traumatic amnesia
- Recovery may be complete
- Some can develop complications

- **Contusion and burst lobe** are the obvious naked eye changes seen after injuries and were thought to be the main injuries before diffuse neuronal damage and shearing lesions were described. Contusions are seen on the summit of the gyri which get injured against the bone. **The overlying pia is torn and the blood seeps into the subarachnoid space.** A bleeding cortical vessel may result in the formation of the **acute subdural haematoma or intracerebral haemorrhage. Brain oedema** which develops surrounding the contusion and lacerations is the one that determines the outcome. Most often contusions are seen at the **poles of the frontal and temporal lobes, under surface of frontal and temporal lobes, over corpus callosum, superior and anterior surfaces of cerebellum and anterior surface of brainstem.**

II. Secondary Lesions (Key Box 63.3)

- **Brain swelling:** This is a vague term applied to increase in brain bulk due to both oedema and venous congestion. It is aggravated by hypoxia or respiratory insufficiency which may be due to associated lung injury or obstruction to upper respiratory passages.

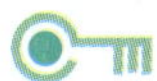
Key Box 63.3

Secondary Lesions

1. Brain swelling
   - Oedema
   - Venous congestion
   - Hypoxia
2. Intracranial haemorrhage
   - Extradural
   - Subdural SAH
3. Infections
   - A. Open head injury
     - Generalised meningitis/fulminant meningitis
     - Subdural empyema
   - B. Closed head injury
     - Pott's puffy tumour

Sometimes such a swelling can lead to severe brain compression which is difficult to relieve, since there is no single mass lesion.

Pearls of Wisdom

Malignant cerebral oedema has close to 100% mortality. This is more common in children.

- **Intracranial haemorrhage:** Extradural or subdural haemorrhages may develop as a clean cut secondary event, even though bleeding may have started at the time of injury. These cause compression of brain, secondary rise in intracranial pressure and can cause death, if not detected and treated early.

- **Infections:** All open head injuries are liable to result in intracranial infection either as generalised meningitis or focal infection such as **subdural empyema or brain abscess, osteomyelitis of skull**. After closed head injuries, infection of a sub-pericranial blood clot may result in **Pott's puffy tumour.** When infection supervenes on an already injured brain, it may retard the recovery or may even lead to death. Hence, it becomes mandatory to treat all infections vigorously.

Cause of Death in Head Injuries

- It is instructive to consider the pathological findings in fatal cases and to speculate the **deaths** which might have been prevented. For example, earlier many deaths which had occurred as a result of aggravation of brain swelling **due to hypoxia** could have been prevented by **ventilation** and **anti-oedema measures**. It should be emphasised that the role of the treating physician is to anticipate and take appropriate measures to prevent the patient from succumbing to the secondary injuries (damages—seizures, hypoxia). **In extensive primary damage to the brain, apart from supportive treatment, one may have to wait and hope.**
- Extensive injury to vital areas such as diencephalon, or patients with **diffuse damage** are **not likely to survive**. These are patients who are unconscious from the time of injury with bilateral, dilated, fixed pupils, flaccidity in all 4 limbs and autonomic disturbances.
- Sometimes a head injury associated with extensive injuries to chest, abdomen or the limbs by their sheer severity can cause death.
- Intracranial complications such as haematomas, brain swelling, infection, and extracranial complications such as chest injury/metabolic abnormalities, if recognised and treated early, can go a long way in saving the life of the patients.

INTRACRANIAL HAEMATOMA

- Most of the head injuries are mild or minor and irrespective of how they are managed, the patient recovers on his own. All those who are unconscious, even if briefly, run the risk of respiratory obstruction. Some of the so-called trivially injured run the risk of developing an intracranial haematoma. Hence, all head injuries must be taken seriously. A **complicated head injury** is one where anyone of the **secondary pathological changes** may occur and threaten the life of the patient. **Uncomplicated** head injury is one where no **such events** occur. However, it could be a severe one where the unconsciousness is prolonged.
- These haematomas could develop in any one of the planes intracranially. Extradural (epidural), subdural, intracerebral haematoma, or a haemorrhagic contusion.
- The clinical presentations of these haematomas are due to either increase in the intracranial pressure or due to signs of cerebral compression. In the case of acute subdural haematoma or intracerebral haematoma, the clinical picture and the outcome of treatment is also dependent on associated brain damage, age of the patient, time of presentation and GCS at presentation.

EXTRADURAL/EPIDURAL HAEMATOMA (Fig. 63.1)

- The clot collects between the dura and the inner table of skull. A majority of them occur in the **middle cranial fossa,** since injury to **middle meningeal vessels (vein and artery) is the commonest cause.** However, about 20–25% of the extradural haematomas can occur in the frontal, parietal regions, at the vertex or in the posterior fossa. Injuries to the dural venous sinuses or a large diploic venous channel are the other causes for the formation of a haematoma. Depending upon the source of bleeding, the haematoma could collect rapidly (hyperacute type) or slowly over a period of a few hours to a few days and present as a **chronic calcified lesion**. 60–80% of these patients have an associated fracture of the skull bone and only a few of them may present with classical symptoms with **lucid interval**. In the remaining patients, the initial picture can vary from an unconscious state to a fully conscious person with or without a history of post-traumatic amnesia. With the widespread availability and use of CT scan, the diagnosis has become much simpler nowadays. However, a few clinical features are worth mentioning.

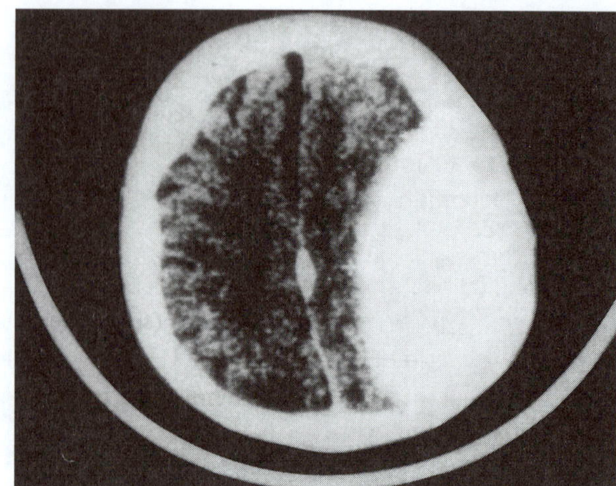

Fig. 63.1: CT scan showing extradural haematoma

Competency

SU17.5: Describe clinical features for neurological assessment and GCS in head injuries.

Neurological assessment by Glasgow Coma Scale

1. Eyes open
   - Spontaneously 4
   - To speech 3
   - To pain 2
   - None 1
2. Best verbal response
   - Oriented 5
   - Confused 4
   - Inappropriate words 3
   - Incomprehensible sounds 2
   - None 1
3. Best motor response
   - Obeys commands 6
   - Localises the pain 5
   - Withdrawal to pain 4
   - Flexion to pain 3
   - Extension to pain 2 (severe damage with increase of ICP)
   - None 1

- Total score is 15; minimum score is 3. Any patient who has a coma score of 8 or less than 8 is said to be in coma.

1. Deteriorating Consciousness Level

- This is one of the hallmarks for the diagnosis of intracranial haematoma. The term **'lucid interval'** is used when a patient recovers from an initial period of unconscious state. Though in earlier days, this was said to be associated with intracranial haematomas, it can occur in other conditions such as brain oedema, multiple contusions. To assess the consciousness level properly, instead of using vaguely defined terms such as semiconscious, obtunded, etc. the **'Glasgow Coma Score'** is widely used, to avoid observer errors in the observation of such patients.
- **Restlessness** in a previously quiet patient indicates **increasing intracranial pressure**, which again needs to be investigated. At the earliest appearance of focal neuronal deficit, the patient has to be taken up for exploratory burr holes.
- Progressive neurological deficit indicates cerebral compression and the manifestation may depend on the area of the brain affected.

2. Pupillary Abnormalities

These are to be considered as a late manifestation. It is due to pressure by the **herniating** uncus of the **temporal lobe on the ipsilateral third nerve at the tentorial hiatus**. In the **early stages** due to irritation of the nerve, there is a sluggish response to the light source. This is called early third nerve and is associated with neurological obtundation, bradycardia and constriction. Since it is a transient phenomenon, the early constriction goes unnoticed most of time. The patients are often detected in the **next stage**, i.e. **pupillary dilatation,** caused by **paralysis of pupilloconstrictor fibres in the third nerve**. However, if the cerebral compression is unrelieved, this may go onto bilateral. Pupillary dilatation is due to **ischaemia of third nerve nucleus** at the midbrain which is caused by pressure on the posterior cerebral artery. These series of pupillary changes have been termed **Hutchinsonian pupils.** The dilated pupil has a definite localising value in that if an exploratory burr hole has been decided upon, it should be done on the side of the initially dilated pupil.

3. Autonomic Disturbances

Bradycardia, though said to be a definite sign, is a late and not an early sign. Initially, there may be a rise in the pulse rate (tachycardia) which may progress to bradycardia, when the systolic blood pressure increases. At times there may be a rise in the diastolic pressure also. These **changes occur due to changes in the cerebral blood flow as a consequence of increased intracranial pressure.** Respirations become deep and slow rate (bradypnoea) and later patients may develop Cheyne-Stokes ventilation due to brainstem ischaemia.

4. Non-Localising Signs

Kernonhan's notch—contralateral pupillary dilatation 6th nerve and 8th nerve palsy in posterior fossa lesions and CVJ anomalies.

Pearls of Wisdom

Cushing's triad of increased intracranial pressure (ICP)
- Bradycardia
- Hypertension
- Irregular respiration

- Local scalp swelling is seen in more than half of the cases. Thus, examination of the head for any such swelling becomes important.
- Some of these patients may have a stiff neck either due to increased intracranial pressure or due to associated injury to neck muscles. Mild fever may, at times, occur and this sometimes confuses the observer. In such a case, the patients must be investigated with a definitive investigation like CT scan. If much time is not available, one should not hesitate to proceed to exploratory burr holes or a 'trauma craniotomy flap' has to be employed to rule out a haematoma.

- Though in adults, 'shock' is a rare complication of head injury, in children with intracranial haematoma and associated cephalohaematomas, due to volume depletion 'shock' may be encountered. Even in adults, if there is a large scalp injury which is not sutured immediately, shock can occur.
- Posterior fossa haematomas in any plane are dangerous because of the lesser space available for the haematomas. As a result of this, rapid brainstem compression can occur which may prove fatal. The availability of CT scan has made detection of these so-called 'unusual haematomas' more frequent. In a suspected case, even if **facilities are not available,** the treating physician should **explore the posterior fossa**, if the clinical features suggest haematoma, or if the skull X-rays show a fracture line extending across the occipital bone towards the foramen magnum.

Investigations (Key Box 63.4)

Competency

SU17.6: Choose appropriate investigations and discuss the principles of management of head injuries.

As has been pointed out earlier, the advent of CT scan of the head has made the diagnosis easier and more specific. However, it should be emphasised that **in the absence of CT scan,** if adequate clinical features point out to the **possibility of an intracranial haematoma**, the patient must be taken up immediately for an exploratory surgery rather than wait and allow him to develop irreversible brainstem damage. Since 60–80% of patients with an intracranial haematoma have a skull bone fracture, irrespective of his consciousness level has to be observed for at least 24–48 hours. Occasionally, one may have to resort to old investigations such as angiography not only to establish the haematoma but also to rule out associated vascular anomalies.

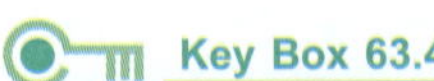
Key Box 63.4

Indications for Skull Radiology

- Loss of consciousness
- Obvious depression on the skull
- Compound fracture
- Laceration or contusion of the scalp
- Focal neurological signs

TREATMENT OF HEAD INJURIES IN GENERAL

I. Resuscitation and Support

1. Admission is indicated when

a. Definite history of unconsciousness
b. Fracture temporal bone
c. Person who cannot be attended by the doctors immediately, i.e. no medical facilities nearby.
d. Post-traumatic seizures—patient should be admitted.

2. Casualty reception

a. Airway
- Mouth gag—to prevent tongue falling backwards.
- Endotracheal intubation with positive pressure ventilation. Hypoxia is an important cause of cerebral oedema which worsens the level of consciousness.

b. General assessment of patient
- To rule out abdominal injuries such as splenic rupture.
- Haemothorax—may need an intercostal tube.
- Long bone fractures

c. General assessment of the degree of shock by pulse, blood pressure monitoring and treatment.

d. Neurological assessment by Glasgow Coma Scale
- Total score is 15; minimum score is 3. Any patient who has a coma score of 8 or less than 8 is said to be in coma.

II. Care of the Unconscious

a. Ryle's tube aspiration or feeding (in the absence of skull base fractures)
b. Care of the eyes—padding
c. Catheter for drainage of urine
d. Change of position to avoid bedsores.
e. Intubation for elective ventilation/airway protection

III. Surgical Treatment for Extradural Haematoma

Immediate surgery for removal of haematoma and relief of cerebral compression is a must. Extradural haematoma, in particular, is a neurosurgical emergency and patient survival will depend upon the speed with which the compression is relieved. It is not an exaggeration to state that even if decompression has to be done with unsterile instruments, at the bedside it may be worth the effort. In every neurosurgeon's career, at least one such situation might have occurred and a live patient may justify the means employed. Once consciousness is lost, pupils are dilated and decerebrate rigidity and periodic breathing develop, it may be only a few minutes that may be available to save the life of the patient and one should not wait and waste time. In the case of extradural haematoma, the **outcome is dependent on the size of the haematoma and the stage in which** the patient was taken up for surgery. In the case of acute subdural and intracerebral haematoma, it depends on associated brain damage. If the associated brain damage is very severe, patients succumbs to the brain damage (Key Box 63.5 and Fig. 63.2).

Acute Subdural Haematoma

Impact damage is more as compared to epidural haematoma. There is associated underlying brain injury.

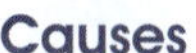 Key Box 63.5

Extradural Haematoma

- 3 cm vertical incision immediately above the midpoint of zygoma
- Strip the pericranium
- Burr hole with Hudson's brace
- Evacuate 'black-currant jelly' clot
- Extend the burr hole and control bleeding middle-meningeal artery by bipolar diathermy
- Dural hitch sutures to prevent stripping of dura

Symptoms are due to compression of underlying brain with midline shift, in addition to parenchymal brain injury.

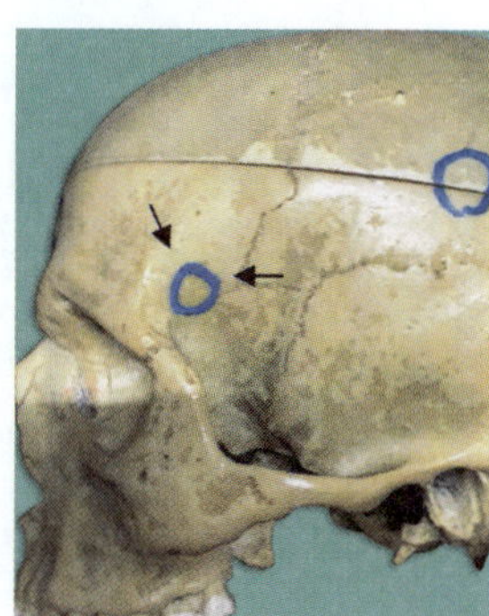

Fig. 63.2: Burr hole site

Causes

- Parenchymal laceration bleed
- Torn cortical bridging vessel

May occur in people who are on anticoagulant therapy.

Mortality—50–90%

Outcome is better, if surgery is done within 4 hours.

CHRONIC SUBDURAL HAEMATOMA

- Common in old people.
- In the elderly, the distance between the dura and the brain increases because of the shrinkage of the brain. Even a minor trauma can tear the cortical veins resulting in collection of blood.
- Bleeding is never progressive and the blood in the subdural space slowly forms membranes and the inflammatory cytokines cause seepage of fluid into this potential space causing increase in ICP and symptoms compress the brain causing features of raised intracranial pressure (ICP).

Clinical Features

- Elderly patients with history of minor trauma
- Bilateral headache, mental apathy
- Slowness, confusion—later alteration in the level of consciousness may progress to unconsciousness
- Waxing and waning of the level of consciousness is seen in some patients. If such a history is elicited, one should always suspect chronic subdural haematoma.
- Unilateral weakness (contralateral), alterations in speech, seizures.

Diagnosis

CT scan or, if feasible, MRI scan are the ideal investigations (cerebral angiography had been used and is still being used in some centres where access to the latest imaging facilities are not available).

Treatment

- Burr hole and drainage of the haematoma usually under local anaesthesia or occasionally under general anaesthesia is often the practised mode of treatment.
- At times, the patient may need two or more burr holes to ensure adequate evacuation.
- If the brain fails to expand and obliterate the cavity, especially in older people or in persons with a very thick inner membrane, a large craniotomy and wide excision of the subdural membrane has to be carried out to remove the constricting effect.
- Adequate bedrest and plenty of fluid administration are also important postoperative measures.
- Ideally, 2 burr holes and a posterior wick drain is placed for 24 hours, with 3 days of bed rest and adequate hydration.

RAISED INTRACRANIAL PRESSURE

Normal ICP is 8–12 mmHg.

Measures to Reduce the Raised ICP

Aim is to keep ICP 20 mmHg

- Head and elevation up to 30°
- Hyperventilation
- Sedation—with or without muscle relaxant
- Use of diuretics—furosemide, mannitol
- Thermoregulation
- Use of barbiturates—thiopentone—reduces brain metabolic rate
- Maintaining fluid and electrolyte balance
- Seizure control
- Steroids in severe head injury are associated with increased mortality and should not be used. (On the contrary, they are used for reducing vasogenic oedema secondary to tumours).

FRACTURE SKULL

Anterior Fossa Fracture

1. Fracture cribriform plate can result in CSF rhinorrhoea.

2. Fracture may extend to the orbit—subconjunctival haemorrhage.
3. Olfactory nerve involvement—partial anosmia.
4. Optic nerve may be contused or fracture may involve the optic foramen resulting in partial or total loss of vision.
5. Rarely, 3rd nerve palsy gives rise to dilated pupil. Traumatic mydriasis
6. Raccoon eyes

Middle Cranial Fossa Fracture

1. Epistaxis due to fracture venous/sphenoid sinuses.
2. CSF from the ear: Blood mixes with CSF and so, does not clot.
3. 7th nerve palsy.
4. Rarely 6th and 8th nerves are also involved.
5. Battle sign: Discolouration of skin and haemosinus within the mastoid air cells.

Posterior Cranial Fossa Fracture

1. Extravasation of blood in the suboccipital region causing boggy swelling in the nape of the neck.
2. 9th, 10th, and 11th cranial nerves may be involved.
3. **Battle sign:** Discolouration of skin and collection of blood occur in the region of mastoid process.

CSF RHINORRHOEA

- There should be a communication between the intradural cavity (subarachnoid space) and the nose.
- It indicates tear of the dura mainly in the basal region and a fracture involving paranasal sinuses—frontal, ethmoidal or sphenoidal.
- There is always an injury to a small portion of the brain. It (the portion of brain) plugs the tear, preventing the dura from healing. Thus, the rhinorrhoea persists for many days.
- This leads to complication, i.e. infection and meningitis.
- **Two types**
  1. **Traumatic:** It can be iatrogenic following surgery or can be post-traumatic (62 to 80%).
  2. **Nontraumatic spontaneous:** It can be due to high pressure (hydrocephalus) or congenital.
- Confirmation of CSF rhinorrhoea is on the bedside by following clinical signs.
  1. **Ring sign:** Onto linen, ring of blood with 1 layer ring of clear fluid. Halo or target sign.
  2. **Reservoir sign:** Gush of CSF in certain position of the head.
- β_2 transferrin is the most accurate method.
- CSF may be collected and fluid glucose can be assessed to differentiate from nasal discharge.

Treatment

- Acetazolamide 250 mg three times a day.
- Lumbar drainage can be done in the absence of raised ICP.
- Prophylactic antibiotics.
- If the rhinorrhoea persists, repair of the dural defect alone, (or) at times with a shunt procedure will be needed.
- Conservative management may be tried for up to 2 weeks before resorting to anterior cranial fossa floor repair.

POTT'S PUFFY TUMOUR

- This is **subperiosteal infection** usually caused by osteomyelitis of the underlying skull.
- It is common in the frontal region and the **frontal bone is commonly involved.**
- The cause of infection is through frontal sinusitis.
- Another common cause of infection of a subpericranial haematoma following needle aspiration.
- It can also follow **chronic suppurative otitis media.**
- Pus collects in the subpericranial space and extradural plane, which communicate with each other (dumb-bell type abscess).
- It causes a **boggy swelling in the frontal region** and tenderness over the scalp.
- Pitting oedema over the scalp is conclusively called **Pott's puffy tumour**.
- Severe headache, vomiting and blurring of vision should clinch the diagnosis.

Treatment

1. CT scan to confirm the diagnosis.
2. A burr hole and aspiration of pus can be done followed by 6–8 weeks of antibiotics.
3. In chronic cases, the wall of the abscess may have to be removed. The associated osteomyelitic skull bone requires a radical removal under cover of antibiotics.

HYDROCEPHALUS

Definition

This is a condition that occurs due to disturbances of CSF flow and imbalance between CSF production and absorption resulting in the accumulation of CSF and dilatation of ventricles.

CSF Production

CSF is mainly produced by the choroid plexus of lateral ventricles by an active autoregulated process.

Daily production: 450 ml—total volume is 150 ml.

CSF Circulation (Fig. 63.3)

Lateral ventricle

↓ *via* foramen of Monro

3rd ventricle

↓ *via* aqueduct of Sylvius

4th ventricle

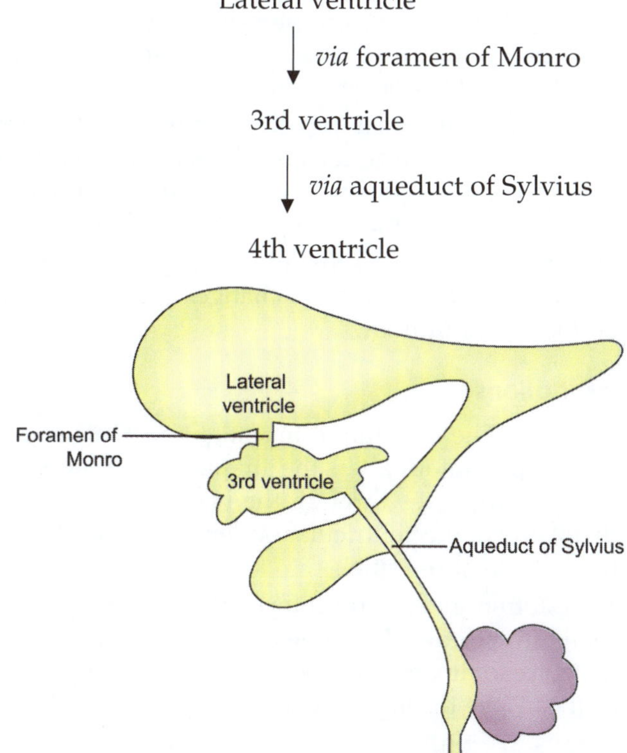

Fig. 63.3: Ventricular system

CSF leaves the 4th ventricle by foramen of Luschka and Magendie to circulate over the convexity where it is finally absorbed over arachnoid granulations.

Aetiopathology

Hydrocephalus occurs due to **two reasons:**

- If there is overproduction of CSF, or CSF circulation.
- If there is decreased absorption.

A. **Overproduction:** True overproduction is rare and occurs in cases of **choroid plexus papilloma.**

B. **Decreased absorption:** Failure of CSF absorption is much more common due to infection and haemorrhage. Other causes being: Structural abnormality occurring in CSF pathway—tumour, congenital malformation such as aqueduct stenosis.

Types

1. **Communicating:** Due to obstruction in sub-arachnoid space.
2. **Noncommunicating:** Due to obstruction in ventricular system. Obstructive hydrocephalus.

Clinical Features

I. Infantile Hydrocephalus

- Difficulty in delivery of large head (Key Box 63.6)
- Craniofacial disproportion

Key Box 63.6

Differential Diagnosis of Large Head

1. Megalencephaly	Intracranial pressure is normal
2. Chronic subdural haematoma	Enlargement of parietal region
3. Cerebral atrophy	May cause ventricular enlargement
4. Cerebral tumours	

External hydrocephalus

Primary–idiopathic–hydrocephalus–obstructive hydrocephalus–secondary to aqueductal stenosis or intraventricular tumors

Megalencephaly

- Increase in head circumference more than 2 cm/ month
- Scalp is thin, shiny and prominent veins
- Fontanelles: Bulging and tense especially on crying
- Sutures: Open, excessive irritability.
- **Macewen's sign**—cracked pot sound on percussing over dilated ventricles.
- Inability to retain feeds, mental retardation, delayed milestones, hypothalamic disturbances.
- **Sun-set sign:** Weakness of upward gaze palsy.

II. Childhood/Adult Hydrocephalus

- By this time, fontanelles have closed.
- Features of increased intracranial pressure: Headache, nausea, vomiting.
- Irritability, indifference, apathy, drowsiness.
- Blurring of vision is not the sign of papilloedema.
- Blindness is due to ophthalmoplegia.
- Bradycardia, systemic hypertension, altered respiratory rate is due to distortion of brainstem. Untreated cases also develop unilateral or bilateral abducens palsy or upward gaze palsy.

Treatment

Aim

1. **To decrease CSF production** by using pharmacological agents:
   - Acetazolamide
   - Furosemide
   - Isosorbide
   - Glycerol
2. **Direct removal** of cause of obstruction.
3. **Diversion** of CSF to another viscus for reabsorption by means of various shunt procedures.

SHUNTS

Ventriculoperitoneal shunt and ventriculoatrial shunt (Figs 63.4 and 63.5).

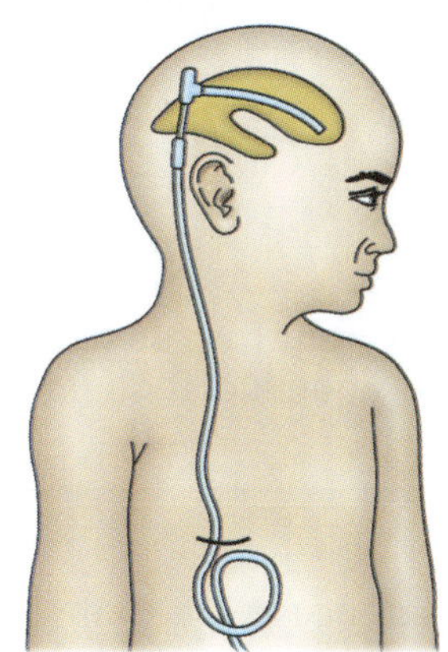

Fig. 63.4: Ventriculoperitoneal shunt

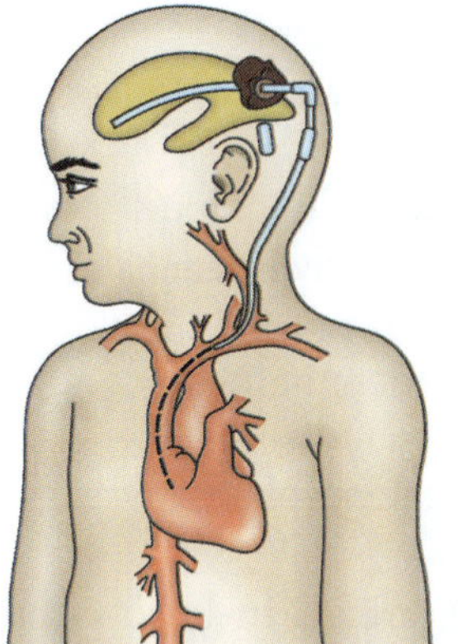

Fig. 63.5: Ventriculoatrial shunt

Complications of Shunts (Key Box 63.7)

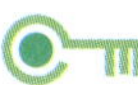

Key Box 63.7

Complications of Shunts

1. Shunt obstruction
2. Shunt infection
3. Seizures
4. Extracerebral fluid collection
5. Subdural haematoma
6. Spontaneous pneumocephalus
7. Ascites/pseudocyst
8. Distal end herniation/perforation into large bowel/ dislodgement of ventricular end

TUMOURS

Eight percent of all primary cancers arises in the CNS. In adults, it constitutes the sixth largest group of cancers and in children the CNS is the commonest site for solid tumours.

Pearls of Wisdom

Most adult brain tumours are supratentorial but 60% of tumours in children are infratentorial and arise in the posterior fossa.

Presenting Feature

1. **Progressive neurological deficit:** In up to two-thirds of the patients, a focal motor weakness is the most common presentation. This deficit arises from the direct neuronal damage or are due to compression on brain or cranial nerves by the tumour. Sudden change may be due to haemorrhage into a pre-existing tumour.
2. **Headache:** It occurs in over 50% of patients caused by raised intracranial pressure (ICP). Only 10% patients have the classic presentation of headache with early morning worsening, associated with nausea and a temporary relief by vomiting.
3. **Generalised or focal seizures** occur in 25%. Focal seizures may help to localise the site of tumour. A high index of suspicion is required for patients past the second decade with recent onset epilepsy.
4. **Other presentations** include visual disturbances, visual field defects, mental changes, etc. depending on the site of tumour.

Investigations

1. **CT scan:** The best initial investigation. This shows where the tumour alters the attenuation of the X-ray beam as it passes through the brain. It also shows distortion of the ventricular system or obliteration of the pattern of the sulci.
2. **MRI:** Often gives extra information and may eventually supersede CT completely. It is the investigation of choice for imaging the posterior fossa and the spine as it can 'see through' bone.
3. **X-rays** are only of anecdotal interest picking up incidental calcifications or erosion of parts of the skull. Newer imaging modalities including SPECT and PET scans are increasingly being used in higher centres.
4. **DSA/CT angio/MR angio** when indicated to assess and visualize the vascularity of the tumour or to plan interventional procedures.

SPECIFIC TYPES OF BRAIN TUMOURS

Gliomas

- Astrocytoma
- Oligodendroglioma
- Mixed tumours

Astrocytoma: WHO Classification

Grade 1 : Pilocytic
Grade 2 : Diffuse
Grade 3 : Anaplastic
Grade 4 : Glioblastoma multiforme

- This is the **most common primary brain tumour** arising from the supporting glial cells and diffusely infiltrates brain tissue early on.
- **Two grading systems** are available: WHO and St Anne/Mayo. Grade 1 and Grade 2 (low grade) tumours are slow growing and compatible with good quality survival. Grades 3 and 4 are rapidly growing. Grade 4 tumours are also called glioblastoma multi-

forme are highly radio and chemoresistant with median survival of only 12 months even with optimal treatment. Even low grade astrocytomas may evolve over time into secondary glioblastomas.

Glioblastoma Multiforme

- Most common in 5th and 6th decades.
- Treatment includes surgery to confirm the diagnosis and achieve a macroscopic excision, followed by a high dose (60 gy) of irradiation.
- Chemotherapy wafers impregnated with carmustine must be inserted GLIADIL wafers.

Oligodendroglioma

- This type of glioma is usually a **slow-growing tumour** and over half arise in the frontal lobes.
- There may be a **history of epilepsy** or even focal neurological signs of many years' duration.
- They may show **calcification,** both microscopically and macroscopically.

Ependymoma

- These glial tumours arise from cells that line the ventricles of the brain and the central canal of the spinal cord.
- They are **most common in the fourth ventricle** in children and young adults where they block CSF flow and often present with hydrocephalus. In adults, they are considered as a differential for intramedullary lower spinal cord lesion.

Embryonal Tumours

- Primitive neuroectodermal tumours (PNETs) are a group of **highly malignant tumours** of which the cerebellar PNET or medulloblastoma is the archetype.
- Commonest in children and young adults. It may originate from primitive cell nests which have undergone malignant transformation. Medulloblastoma is the most common brain tumour in children.
- The patient presents with truncal ataxia, headache, vomiting and sometimes diplopia. All PNETs are prone to spread within the CNS producing **'sugarcoating metastasis'** which are best seen on MRI of the spine.

Schwannoma (Neurilemmoma)

- Peripheral neurons get their myelin sheaths from Schwann cells. Occasionally, these form slow growing benign tumours on cranial or spinal nerves.
- The cranial nerve most affected is the **vestibular division of the 8th cranial nerve** and the tumour is then usually called **acoustic neuroma**. Newer terminology is **vestibular schwannoma.**

Pearls of Wisdom

Even though it does not arise from the acoustic division and is not a neuroma, it is still called an acoustic neuroma.

- It causes progressive deafness, hydrocephalus and ataxia. It is slow growing. Less often it may involve the trigeminal or the vagus nerve.
- Often associated with NF2, especially in bilateral acoustic tumours and multiple meningiomas.
- Commonest presentation: Unilateral or bilateral progressive deafness (sensorineural hearing loss—SNHL) with tinnitus and vertigo.

Meningioma

- Eighty percent are supratentorial.
- These tumours arise from the arachnoid layer of the meninges and the arachnoid villi. They are commonest over the falx and the convexity of the skull but rarely may also arise from the skull base (especially from the sphenoid wing and olfactory groove) or inside the lateral ventricle.
- Commonest in middle-aged women and may occur at the site of a previous radiation field. Most are benign and slowly growing. Signs occur based on the site of tumour (Key Box 63.8).
- They tend to provoke endosteal hypertrophy or exostosis of the overlying skull and is still occasionally detected on an incidental skull film or even by palpation of the skull. Patient with neurofibromatosis type 2 often have multiple meningiomas. Rarely, they are malignant.
- Paediatric meningiomas tend to be atypical in location.
- Recurrence depends on the extent of resection (SIMPSON's grading of excision).

Pituitary Tumours

- 10–15% of all intracranial tumours
- Majority are benign adenoma
- Prolactinoma—30%
- Nonfunctioning adenoma—20%
- GH secreting adenoma—15%

Key Box 63.8

Sites of Meningioma

Site		%
❍ Convexity of skull	:	20%
❍ Parafalcine arc	:	20%
❍ Sphenoid ridge	:	10%
❍ Tuberculum sella	:	10%
❍ Olfactory groove	:	10%
❍ Ventricle	:	2–5%

- ACTH secreting adenoma—10%.
- May produce **mass effect**—bitemporal hemianopia or cranial nerve dysfunction.
- **Endocrine dysfunction** such as galactorrhoea, primary/secondary amenorrhoea, Cushing's syndrome, acromegaly.
- **Pituitary apoplexy—**results in sudden onset of headache, visual loss, ophthalmoplegia and altered conscious level.
  Caused by haemorrhagic infarction of a pituitary tumour.

Other Tumours

They are pineal region tumours, pituitary adenomas, craniopharyngiomas, choroid plexus tumours, etc.

Metastases

One-fourth of all cancer patients have intracerebral metastases at the time of death. Common primary sites include the bronchus (50%), breast (15%), and melanoma (10%).

Treatment

They can be divided into medical and surgical line of treatment.

I. **Medical**
   - Acutely raised intracranial pressure (ICP) is treated with **IV mannitol 0.5–1 g/kg body weight**.
   - Hydrocephalus can be relieved using a **CSF diversion** system (closed external ventricular drainage or a **ventriculoperitoneal shunt**).
   - Seizures are treated with **lorazepam and phenytoin** commonly and maintained on phenytoin.
   - **Corticosteroids**, especially dexamethasone 4 mg qid is given to reduce symptoms of raised ICP, which may make surgery easier.

II. **Surgery**
   - This is the **mainstay of treatment**. The aim of surgery is to obtain a complete tumour excision without producing a neurological deficit.
   - This is not always possible due to the site of the tumour, in which case compromises must be made and a **debulking procedure** is done.
   - Any residual tissue may be observed or treated with adjuvant radiotherapy.
   - **Stereotactic guided surgery** is now a well-established concept in brain surgery allowing more targeted treatment of the lesion with minimal surrounding damage.

III. **Radiotherapy:** Intracranial tumours are relatively **radioresistant**, and radiotherapy is primarily a palliative treatment.

IV. **Chemotherapy:** No definite benefit of chemotherapy for the treatment of brain tumours. **Temozolomide** is a promising new drug for the treatment of brain tumours.

Outcome

Surgery offers good prospects for the treatment of benign brain tumours such as meningioma or pituitary adenoma, but outcome of treatment of malignant tumours is still poor.

TRIGEMINAL NEURALGIA

- Superior cerebellar artery or multiple sclerosis plaque can cause this condition.
- Severe episodic lancinating facial pain occurring in the distribution of V cranial nerve.
- Vascular compression of the nerve near the root entry zone, multiple sclerosis may be causative factors.
- Investigation—MRI.

Treatment

- Carbamazepine or gabapentin.
- 75% will not respond to medical treatment.
- Surgery: Refractory cases
  1. Percutaneous glycerol injection, radiofrequency ablation, thermocoagulation, balloon compression, local nerve block.
  2. Microvascular decompression *via* craniotomy.
  3. Stereotactic radiosurgery.

BRAINSTEM DEATH

Irreversible loss of consciousness, loss of brainstem reflexes and apnoea.

Diagnosis of brainstem death is done in three stages:

1. Identification of the cause of irreversible coma.
2. Exclusion of reversible causes of coma.
3. Clinical demonstration of absence of brainstem reflexes.

Brainstem Reflexes

- Pupillary reaction to light, corneal reflexes, vestibular ocular reflex, cough reflex, gag reflex, motor response to pain.
- Apnoea test—apnoea despite a CO_2 increase to >6.65 kPa or 50 mmHg.
- All reflexes must be absent and are tested independently twice by 2 doctors.

CT SCANS OF HEAD INJURIES (Figs 63.6 to 63.14)

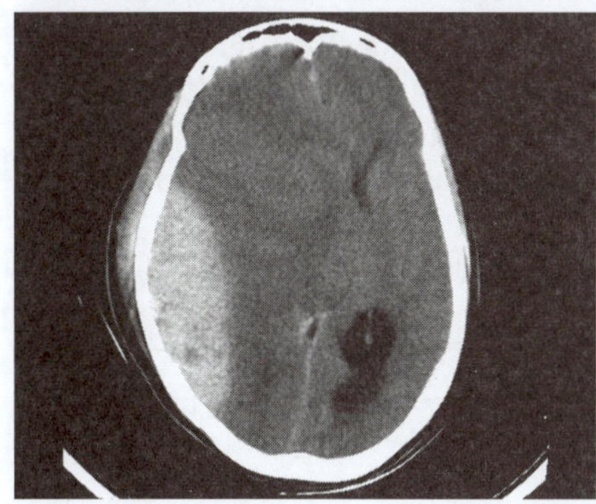

Fig. 63.6: Right temporoparietal extradural haematoma (EDH) showing mass effect with midline shift with subfalcine herniation

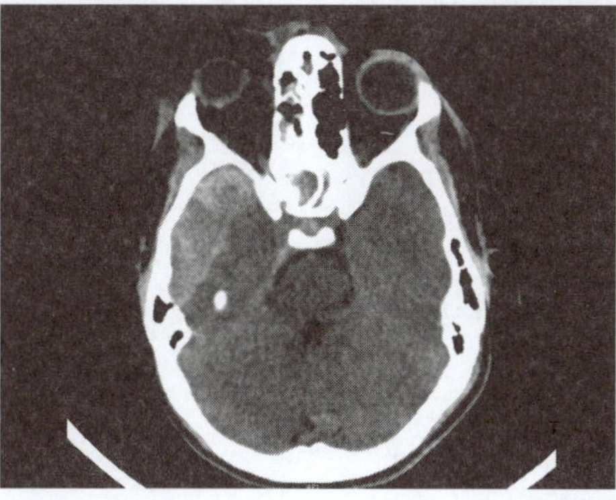

Fig. 63.7: Right temporal extradural haematoma

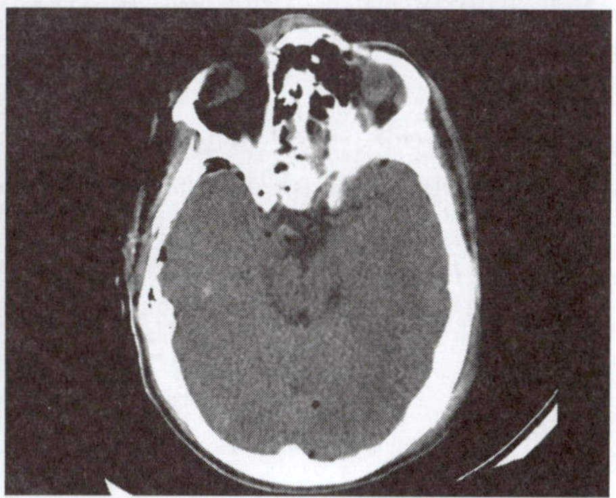

Fig. 63.8: Postoperative scan—no EDH. Post right temporal craniotomy with pneumocephalous

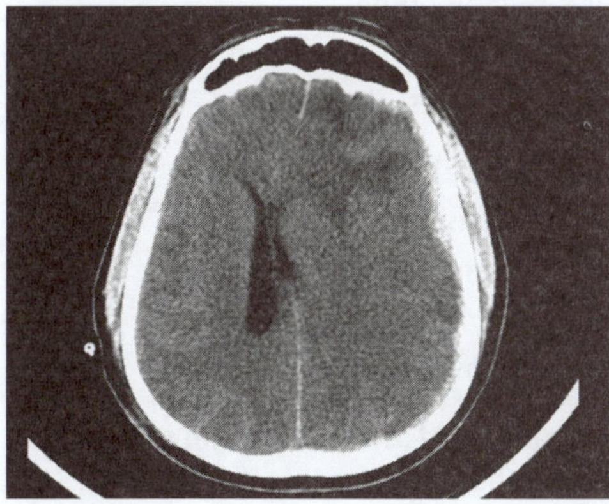

Fig. 63.9: Left frontoparietal acute subdural haematoma. Left frontal and temporal nonhaemorrhagic contusion with subfalcine herniation with midline shift

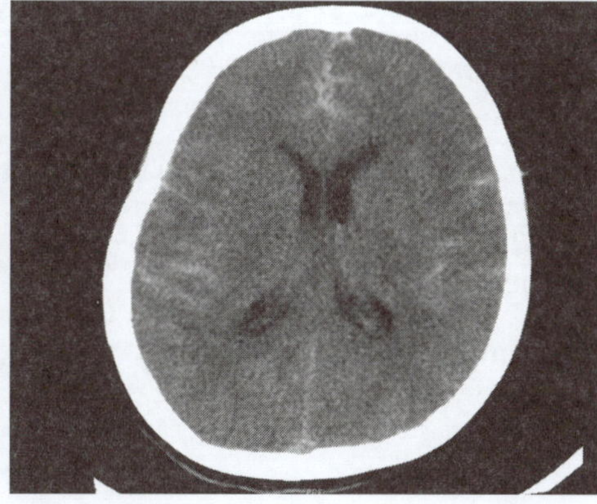

Fig. 63.10: Traumatic right more than left frontoparietal and anterior interhemispheric subarachnoid haemorrhage

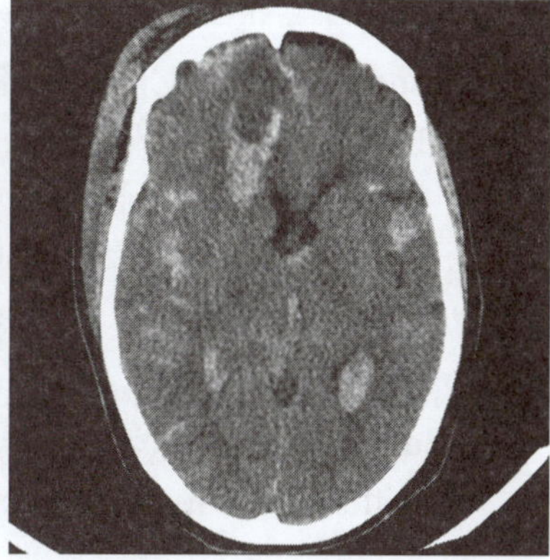

Fig. 63.11: Diffuse axonal injury—right frontal, left temporal contusion, right frontoparietal region—subarachnoid haemorrhage and intraventricular haemorrhage

Contributed by Dr Sunil Upadhyay—Assistant Professor, Department of Neurosurgery, KMC, Manipal

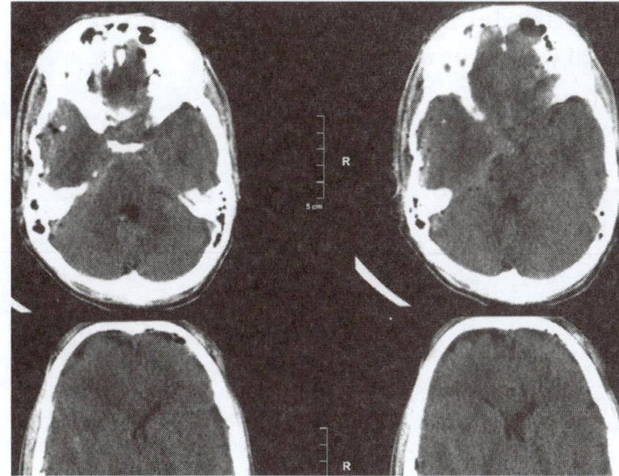

Fig. 63.12: Right temporal depressed fracture with temporal EDH with pneumocephalous

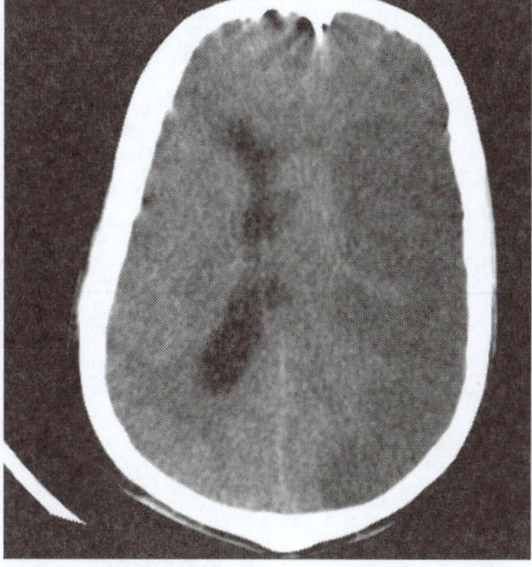

Fig. 63.13: Left frontoparietal hypodence area suggestive of left middle cerebral artery stem infarct

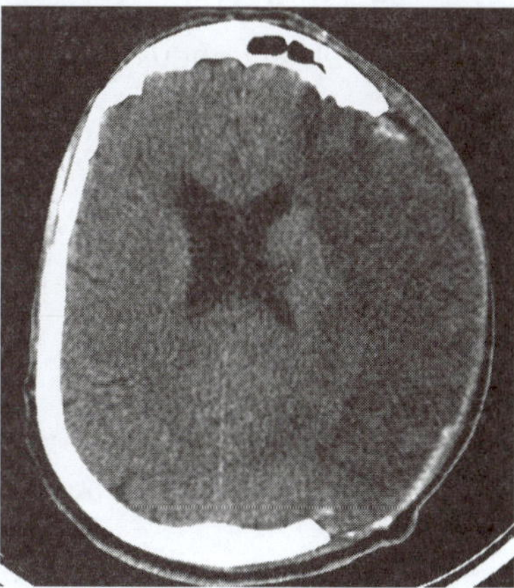

Fig. 63.14: Left FTP decompressive craniectomy brain herniation outside the skull

VERY IMPORTANT WISDOM LINES IN HEAD INJURY

- If an exploratory burr hole has been decided upon, it should be done on the side of the initially dilated pupil.
- Bradycardia is due to raised intracranial pressure.
- If hypotension responds to volume replacement in trauma centre in a comatose patient, the coma is most likely not due to head injury.
- Admit the patient, if there is fracture temporal bone.
- Hypoxia is an important cause of cerebral oedema which worsens the level of consciousness.
- Steroids in severe head injury are associated with increased mortality and should not be used.
- CSF rhinorrhoea indicates tear of the dura mainly in the basal region and a fracture involving paranasal sinuses.
- Glasgow Coma Score of less than 8 means patient is in coma.

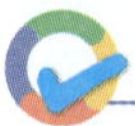

Multiple Choice Questions

1. Following is not the feature of Glasgow Coma Scale:
A. Eyes opening B. Motor response
C. Verbal response D. Sensory response

2. Closed head injury include following *except:*
A. Head injury with fracture skull
B. Head injury with black eye
C. Head injury with facial nerve palsy
D. Head injury with CSF rhinorrhoea

3. Which of the following is included under secondary lesions following head injury?
A. Diffuse neuronal damage
B. Contusions
C. Lacerations
D. Swelling

4. Post-traumatic amnesia is a feature of:
A. Raised intracranial tension
B. Fall from a height
C. Fracture skull
D. Cerebral concussion

5. Which is an important cause of brain swelling following head injury?
A. Infection B. Oedema
C. Acidosis D. Bleeding

6. The cause of extradural haematoma is bleeding from:
A. Venous sinuses
B. Cavernous sinus bleeding
C. Basal veins bleeding
D. Middle meningeal vessels bleeding

7. Lucid interval is typically seen in:
A. Extradural haematoma
B. Acute subdural haematoma
C. Chronic subdural haematoma
D. Pontine haematoma

8. Which nerve is paralysed after herniation of temporal lobe in extradural haematoma?
A. Oculomotor nerve B. Ophthalmic nerve
C. Trigeminal nerve D. Facial nerve

9. Pupillary dilatation following head injury is due to ischaemia of the third nerve caused by:
A. Middle cerebral artery B. Posterior cerebral artery
C. Inferior cerebral artery D. Anterior cerebral artery

10. Following are definite indications for admission in a head injury patient *except:*
A. Fracture skull
B. CSF rhinorrhoea
C. History of unconsciousness
D. Scalp bleeding

Answers

1. D **2.** D **3.** D **4.** D **5.** B **6.** D **7.** A **8.** B **9.** B **10.** D

CHAPTER

64

Principles of Anaesthesiology

- Preoperative assessment and premedication
- Regional anaesthesia
- Endotracheal intubation
- Monitoring in anaesthesia
- Local anaesthetics
- Complications of anaesthesia
- General anaesthetic agents
- Muscle relaxants

Introduction

Surgery has been practised for ages. However, the advent of modern techniques of anaesthesia has allowed surgery to develop by leaps and bounds. If there is a well-informed, vigilant and safe anaesthesiologist taking care of the patient, the surgeon is able to concentrate on the surgical procedure unhindered. An anaesthesiologist is also a perioperative physician. An anaesthesiologist's understanding of anatomy, physiology and pharmacology, and his expertise of management of critical illness and pain give him a wider scope of practice including intensive care, pain and palliative care.

A good understanding of the physiology and pharmacology, complemented by continuous and vigilant monitoring, has made the practice of anaesthesia safer. Safe practice of anaesthesia comprises the following steps: A good rapport with the patient, a thorough preoperative preparation and premedication, monitoring and perioperative care.

TYPES OF ANAESTHESIA

The choice of anaesthesia depends on several factors: The site and duration of surgery, general condition of the patient, expertise of the anaesthesiologist and preference of the patient.

Anaesthesia can be classified into two main categories: General anaesthesia and regional anaesthesia.

Competency

SU11.2.1: Enumerate the indications of general anaesthesia.

General Anaesthesia (GA)

In this type of anaesthesia, the patient is rendered unconscious by the administration of anaesthetic agents. These agents produce a generalised and reversible depression of the central nervous system. The components of general anaesthesia include anaesthesia (unconscious with no sensation), analgesia (no pain), amnesia (no recall) and muscle relaxation.

Indications for General Anaesthesia

- When the surgical procedure involves areas that cannot be easily performed under regional anaesthesia such as head and neck procedures
- Prolonged surgical procedures that make it uncomfortable for patients to lie in the same position for a long period of time
- Extensive surgical procedures involving body cavities (thorax, abdomen)
- Surgeries involving multiple parts of the body
- Haemodynamically unstable patients
- Patients with coagulation disorders
- Patient request

Contraindications

The only absolute contraindication to general anaesthesia is patient refusal. However, if the patient's general condition is poor and is at risk of deterioration with the administration of general anaesthesia, one may attempt to avoid general anaesthesia by adopting regional anaesthesia, if possible or defer surgery till the patient is optimized to tolerate it.

Competency

SU11.2.2: Describe the various techniques of general anaesthesia.

Techniques of General Anaesthesia

General anaesthesia (GA) has three important phases: Induction, maintenance and emergence. GA may be provided using administration of either inhalational anaesthetic agents, intravenous anaesthetics or a combination.

Preoperative assessment, preparation and premedication: Induction of general anaesthesia alters the physiology of the patient in many ways and it is important to do a preoperative assessment *(described in detail later)* to know the baseline condition. The patient is then prepared for surgery if he has any condition that needs to be optimized before surgery. For example, asthma. The patient is given preoperative instructions regarding fasting before surgery. Certain medications may be prescribed as premedication (to reduce anxiety, pain. etc).

Induction and airway management: In the operation theatre, an intravenous access is secured (called 'lifeline' of the patient) and monitoring commenced. Once the anaesthetist is satisfied that the patient's vitals are within acceptable limits, he/she proceeds to induce general anaesthesia by either intravenous or inhalation anaesthesia. The patient becomes unconscious and as a consequence, the tongue and the epiglottis fall back into the pharynx and the airway gets obstructed. To overcome this, the anaesthetist maintains a patent airway using an endotracheal tube or a supraglottic airway such as laryngeal mask airway or I-gel after the induction of general anaesthesia *(described in detail later)*.

Maintenance: The induction agents are short acting and hence, maintenance of anaesthesia must be done with continued administration of inhalation anaesthetic agents or infusion of intravenous anaesthetic agents. Muscle relaxants may be given to facilitate surgery, especially for intracavitory surgeries. The patient is monitored throughout surgery and interventions made as required.

Emergence: Once surgery is complete, the patient is allowed to wake up, after adequate reversal of neuromuscular blockade and the circulation anaesthetics. The artificial airway is removed after full return of consciousness and airway reflexes. The patient is shifted to the postoperative care unit where the patients will be cared for till discharge.

PREOPERATIVE ASSESSMENT AND PREMEDICATION

Every patient is anxious when he comes into the operating room. The causes of anxiety can be varied: Fear of the disease condition, surgery, anaesthetic and the anticipated pain. A good rapport developed between the patient and the anaesthesiologist can build up his confidence and help allay many of these fears.

Anaesthesia is associated with changes in the internal homeostasis. Normally, these are well tolerated by the different systems. However, if the patient has a preexisting derangement, his capacity to withstand changes in his internal milieu may be limited. It is thus very important to assess preoperatively the baseline condition of the patient, irrespective of the scheduled surgery and anaesthesia. This will be detailed in an elective case and a more directed assessment in an emergency.

History

A detailed history of the patient with symptoms pertaining to the presenting complaint must be elicited. The patient should be questioned about symptoms pertaining to the presence of any comorbidities such as hypertension, diabetes, ischaemic heart disease, respiratory illness, neurological illness, renal and hepatic dysfunction. History of previous surgery, exposure to anaesthetics, medication history, allergies, smoking, alcohol, recent respiratory infections and his current effort tolerance should also be elicited.

Physical Examination

A detailed physical examination is done and the relevant history specially borne in mind. General physical examination includes:

Vital signs: Blood pressure, heart rate, respiratory rate, temperature and oxygen saturation.

PICCLE: Pallor, icterus, cyanosis, clubbing, lymphadenopathy, oedema and raised jugular venous pulse.

Spine: To rule out infection over the skin covering the spine, tenderness, stiffness or fractures of spine, to check spaces.

Veins: Ease of obtaining venous access is also assessed.

Assessment of Airway

Whenever a person becomes unconscious, the tongue and epiglottis fall back onto the pharynx and obstruct the airway. Since the patient may need sedation or may be made unconscious during a general anaesthetic, the anaesthetist must ensure ability to secure the patient's airway. Hence, preoperative assessment of the airway becomes important.

The assessment is done as follows:

The 1–2–3 Test

- When a person opens his mouth, one should be able to insinuate one finger in the temporomandibular joint.
- There should be at least two finger breadths' distance between his incisors.
- There should be at least three finger breadths' distance between the chin and the thyroid cartilage (thyromental distance) of the patient.

Mallampati Test

The patient is made to sit upright, open his mouth wide and protrude his tongue. The structures visualised are classified as given in Fig. 64.1. These classes roughly correlate with the following grades of laryngoscopic views (Fig. 64.2). Difficult airway may be anticipated in Mallampati Class III and IV and the anaesthesiologist must be prepared to secure airway in such patients.

Neck Movements

Restriction of neck movements, especially extension makes endotracheal intubation more difficult.

Systemic Examination

A detailed examination of the various systems is then carried out and relevant findings noted.

Investigations

There is no place for routine investigations to be ordered before any surgery. Investigations that are required to assess the baseline status of the patient and have a bearing on the perioperative course must be done. Thus, they should be tailored to the individual patient. The common investigations ordered are as follows:

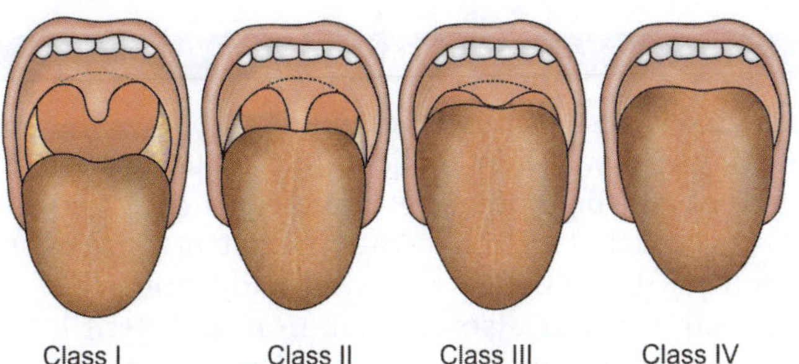

Fig. 64.1: Mallampati classification of the airway

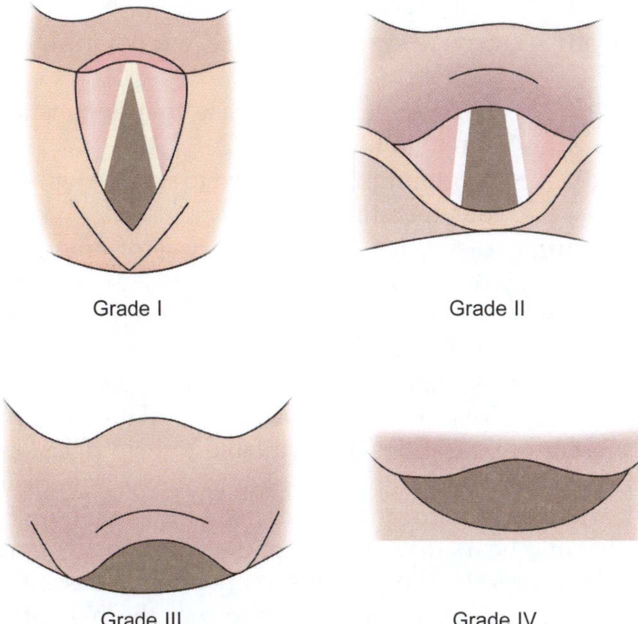

Fig. 64.2: Modified Cormack-Lehane grading of laryngoscopic view

Haemoglobin estimation: All patients.

Electrocardiogram, blood sugar estimation, blood urea, serum creatinine and electrolytes: Male patients >40 years, smokers and female patients above 50 years.

Total and differential white cell count: If infection is suspected.

Platelet count and coagulation profile: If any abnormality is suspected or bleeding is anticipated.

Chest X-ray is ordered if a major abdominal or thoracic surgery is planned, postoperative ventilation is expected or cardiorespiratory disease is suspected.

Stress test, echocardiogram, pulmonary function test or a blood gas analysis are obtained as necessary.

Blood grouping and cross-matching are requested if the surgery may be associated with major blood loss.

ASA Physical Status Classification

The patient's preoperative physical status can be classified into five different categories. The American Society of Anaesthesiologists classification of Physical Status is as follows:

ASA I : Healthy patient, no medical problems

ASA II : Mild systemic disease
ASA III : Severe systemic disease, but not incapacitating
ASA IV : Severe systemic disease that is constant threat to life
ASA V : Moribund, not expected to survive without the operation

A suffix E is added if the surgery is of emergent nature. A sixth category called ASA VI is given to the patient who is declared brain dead, whose organs are being removed for donor purposes.

The risks associated with anaesthesia in a patient with concurrent diseases must be assessed. Algorithms by different organisations are available to help decision-making in individual patients: For example, American Heart Association recommendations for evaluation of ischaemic heart disease in a patient posted for non-cardiac surgery. The goal of preoperative assessment and preparation is thus to ensure that the patient is optimised and is in the best possible condition prior to surgery and anaesthesia.

Informed Consent

The patient is explained about the planned anaesthetic, the problems anticipated and the risks involved in his own language and a **written and informed consent** is obtained.

Preoperative Instructions

The patient is permitted to take solids and milk up to 6–8 hours and clear fluids up to 3 hours prior to surgery. This may be relaxed for neonates and infants where a four-hour fast for breast milk is sufficient. Formula feeds and milk from any other source are treated as solids. If the last food intake contained a considerable amount of fat, gastric emptying time may be delayed.

Premedication

This term refers to administration of certain medications prior to anaesthesia. The drugs used and their objectives are as follows:

1. **To allay anxiety:** Certain degree of anxiety is felt by most patients before surgery. A good rapport developed between the patient and the anaesthesiologist helps relieve this anxiety. Any of the following medications may be used to reduce anxiety.

   Adults (night before and morning of surgery)

   Tab Alprazolam 0.25–0.5 mg

   Tab Lorazepam 2–4 mg orally

   Children: To enable easy separation from parents.

   Midazolam 0.5 mg/kg (maximum 10 mg) mixed with 5 ml of paracetamol syrup is given orally 15–20 minutes prior to the procedure.

   Triclofos syrup, 75–100 mg/kg, one hour prior to surgery.
2. **To relieve pain:** If the patient has any painful condition that could get aggravated on movement, a narcotic in appropriate doses can be added to reduce the pain during shifting from the ward, e.g. fractures. Care must be taken to avoid excessive sedation and respiratory depression.
3. **To dry secretions:** An anticholinergic such as **glycopyrrolate** (0.2 mg) is added if a fibreoptic intubation is planned so that oral secretions do not hinder vision. Local anaesthetic agents produce better local anaesthesia of the upper airway when the mucosa is dry. It may be given intravenously just prior to surgery in ENT surgeries and oral surgeries.
4. **To help anaesthesia induction:** Premedication with a narcotic provides analgesia and helps induce anaesthesia more smoothly.
5. **To blunt baroreceptor reflexes:** A small dose of β-blockers or clonidine may be given in certain patients to blunt baroreceptor reflexes during intubation.
6. **To reduce gastric volume and acidity:** Some patients are at risk of regurgitation of gastric contents and aspiration. They may be premedicated with a prokinetic such as **metoclopramide** (10 mg) and a H_2 blocker such as **ranitidine** (150 mg orally). **Pantoprazole** 40 mg may be given instead of ranitidine. The consequences of aspiration of gastric contents depend on its quantity and acidity. Particulate matter, if aspirated, can cause mechanical blockage of the airways. Metoclopramide reduces residual gastric content by hastening gastric emptying and ranitidine reduces the acidity. Sometimes, a nonparticulate antacid such as sodium citrate may be given to neutralise existing gastric acid. Multiple factors during anaesthesia and surgery increase the chances of nausea and vomiting. Since anaesthesia involves blunting of airway reflexes, patients are at risk of aspiration. This is why patients are kept fasting before elective surgery. This may not be possible for patients who are posted for emergency surgery. It is assumed that these patients are 'full-stomach' and appropriate precautions are taken.

AIRWAY MANAGEMENT

General anaesthesia involves induction of unconsciousness during which the patient's ability to maintain his airway and breathing are impaired. It thus becomes necessary that the anaesthesiologist maintains and protects the patient's airway. In addition, not only anaesthesia but also oxygenation and ventilation are maintained well only if the airway is patent and secured.

Management of airway is one of the basic skills acquired by an anaesthesiologist. This is relatively easy in most individuals. Difficult airway is the term given when there is difficulty with mask ventilation, endotracheal intubation, or both.

BAG-MASK VENTILATION

When a person becomes unconscious, the tongue and the epiglottis fall back and obstruct the airway. Since they are attached to the mandible, lifting up of the mandible also lifts these two structures and opens airway. This is usually done by head-tilt and chin-lift method as during cardiopulmonary resuscitation. Jaw thrust is more popular with anaesthesiologists. The patient may be ventilated using a 'bag' (either a self-inflating bag or anaesthetic circuit) and a facemask (Fig. 64.3). The mask is triangular in shape, the narrow portion of which is placed at the bridge of the nose and the base placed in the depression between the lower lip and chin. The mask is held in place by an E-C technique (Fig. 64.4).

ENDOTRACHEAL INTUBATION

Endotracheal intubation is the most definitive way of maintaining airway in patients who require muscle paralysis and require intermittent positive pressure ventilation. It involves introduction of a tube into the trachea for maintaining the patency and protecting the airway as well as to ensure adequate oxygenation and ventilation. Whenever general anaesthesia is induced and needs to be maintained for long periods, endotracheal intubation is done.

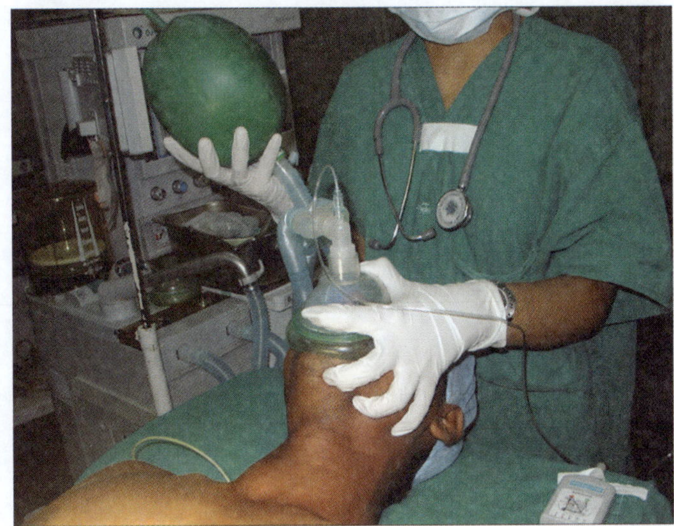

Fig. 64.3: Maintenance of airway and ventilation using bag (anaesthetic circuit) and mask

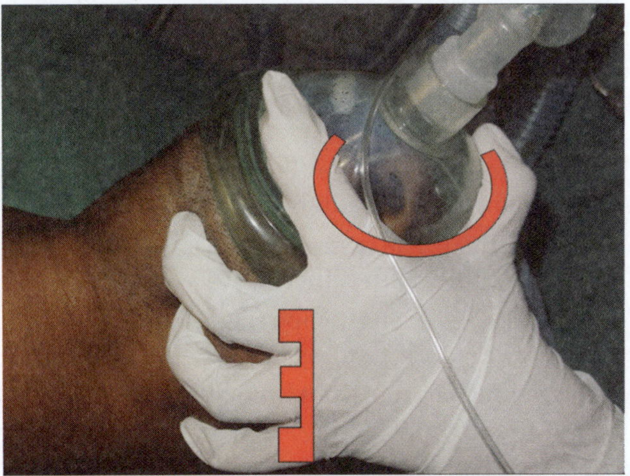

Fig. 64.4: The E-C technique of holding a face mask to get airway seal. The thumb and index fingers form a 'C' at the top of the mask holding it firmly down on the face. The middle, and ring fingers lift up the mandible as well as provide head tilt. The little finger aids in providing jaw thrust. Note that the finger pressure should be given on the bony part and not on the soft tissues under the chin

Indications

- To administer general anaesthesia for long (>1–2 h) periods.
- To maintain patency of the airway in unconscious patients.
- To protect lungs from aspiration of regurgitated gastric contents.
- To ensure delivery of adequate tidal volumes to the lungs.
- To clear excessive and retained secretions from the lungs.

Contraindications

Endotracheal intubation may be extremely difficult or even impossible and a tracheostomy may be better in certain situations:

- When the upper airway integrity is lost as in extensive maxillofacial injury with bilateral fractures of mandible and maxillae.
- Injuries to the neck with laryngeal rupture
- Large tumours of the upper airway.

Equipment

Laryngoscopes

These consist of a handle and a blade:

- The handle contains batteries. The blade has a flange to push the tongue towards the left side. This ensures more room for visualisation of the glottis. A bulb nearer the tip of the blade lights up when the handle and blade are at right angles to each other and electrical contact is made.

- There are several types of laryngoscopes to aid in different situations.
  - **Macintosh type blade** (Fig. 64.5) **is curved** and is popular for use in adults
  - **The Miller blade is straight** and is used in children and in adults with difficult airway
  - **The McCoy laryngoscope** (Fig. 64.6) has a **tiltable tip**.
  - Fibreoptic laryngoscopes are flexible.

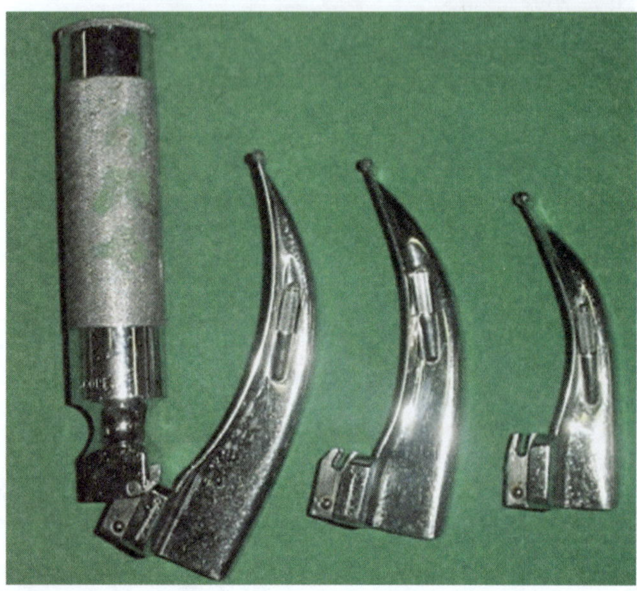

Fig. 64.5: Macintosh laryngoscope. Note the curved blade. Sizes 1, 2 and 3 are displayed

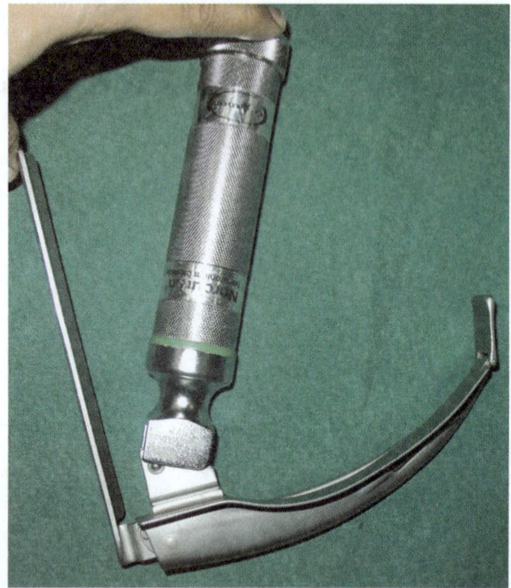

Fig. 64.6: McCoy laryngoscope. Note the retractable tip of the laryngoscope blade

  - **Videolaryngoscopes** have a small camera on the blade a little proximal to the tip and provide a better view of 'difficult to see' larynx.
  - **Short-handled laryngoscopes** are available for use in difficult airways, e.g. pregnant women, obese patients.

Endotracheal Tubes (Fig. 64.7)

It is a C-shaped tube and is commonly made of polyvinyl chloride (PVC). The machine end has a standard 15 mm diameter connector. The patient end is bevelled and has an opening on the side just proximal to the tip called the Murphy's eye. This ensures patency of the tube even if the bevelled tip is against the tracheal wall.

Endotracheal tube size

Endotracheal tubes are available in different sizes. Their size is indicated as the internal diameter in millimetre (Key Box 64.1). However, the correct size will depend on the growth of the child.

Depth of insertion

- The distance of several points on the tube from the patient end is marked in centimetre along the tube. The tube is fixed at 22 or 23 cm in adult men and at 20 or 21 cm in adult women.
- In children, the following formula is used: Age/2 + 12 cm.

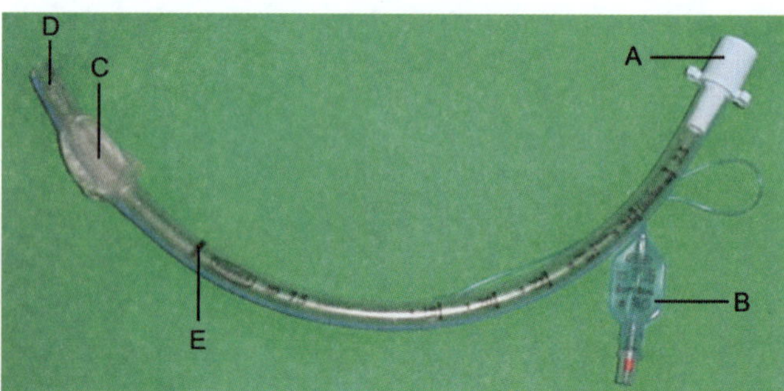

Fig. 64.7: Endotracheal tube. (A) Standard 15 mm connector, (B) pilot balloon, (C) inflatable cuff, (D) beveled patient-end, (E) black line to indicate optimum positioning of the tube. This line is usually placed just above the glottis

Key Box 64.1

Endotracheal Tube Size

Adult male	8 or 8.5 mm ID
Adult female	7 or 7.5 mm ID
Children <6 years	Age/3 + 3.5 mm ID
Children >6 years	Age/4 + 4.5 mm ID

The tube should be positioned such that its tip must lie above the carina but well below the glottis. Air entry should be heard bilaterally on auscultation of the chest.

Position

A pillow (7–10 cm) under the patient's head enables mild flexion at the cervical spine. The head is then extended at the atlanto-occipital joint. This is called the intubating position or "sniffing position".

Route

Endotracheal intubation can be done either orally or nasally (Figs 64.8 and 64.9). It can be done either under direct vision or indirectly using a fibreoptic scope. It may need to be done blindly when visualisation of the glottis by direct means is not possible and a fibreoptic scope is not available.

In such cases, if the regular antegrade technique (mouth or nose to larynx) is not possible, retrograde intubation (larynx to mouth) may be tried. In the retrograde technique, a guidewire is passed from the cricothyroid membrane upward into the mouth or nose and the endotracheal tube is guided over it towards the larynx.

Procedure (Key Box 64.2)

The patient's head is placed in the sniffing position. The mouth is opened and the laryngoscope blade is introduced through the right angle of mouth along the tongue into the pharynx. Once the epiglottis is seen, the tip of the laryngoscope blade is pressed into the vallecula. This lifts up the epiglottis to reveal the glottis. The glottis is identified by the two pearly white vocal cords. Once the cords are seen, the endotracheal tube is inserted between them into the trachea.

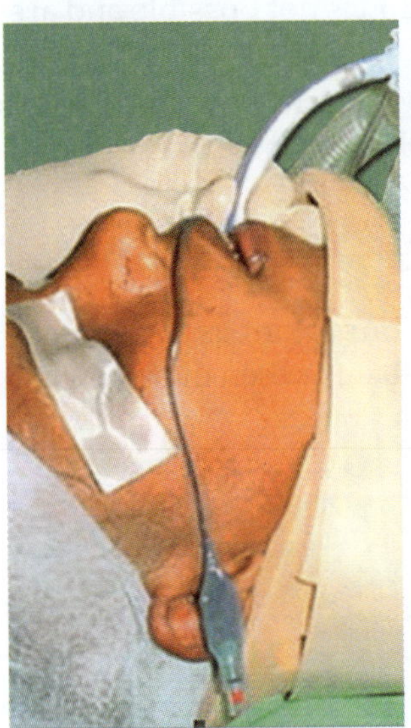

Fig. 64.8: Oral endotracheal intubation

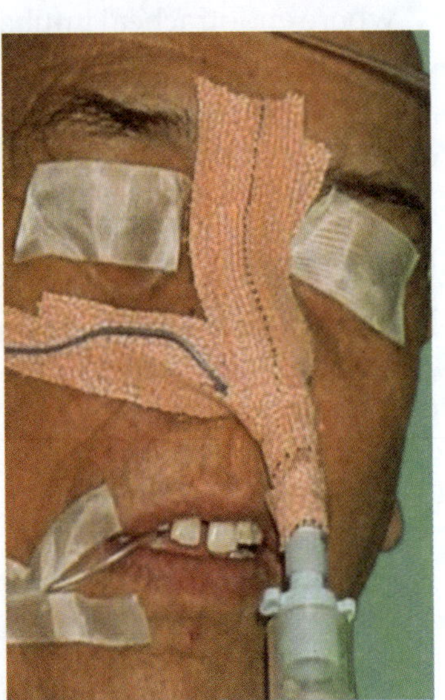

Fig. 64.9: Nasal endotracheal intubation

Key Box 64.2

Endotracheal Intubation

- Orotracheal or nasotracheal
- Direct or indirect (using fibreoptic laryngoscope)
- Under vision or blind
- Anaesthetised or awake
- Antegrade or retrograde

It may also be done with the patient awake after administering local anaesthesia to the upper airway when a difficult intubation is anticipated.

Many airway adjuncts are available for use when a difficult airway is encountered, especially when it is unanticipated. These include oropharyngeal airway, nasopharyngeal airway, laryngeal mask airway and Combitube®.

Confirmation of Correct Placement of Endotracheal Tube

Correct position of the endotracheal tube may be confirmed by the following:

- Endotracheal intubation under vision
- Bilateral visible chest rise
- Bilateral equal air entry in the lungs
- Absent breath sounds in the epigastrium
- A square wave normal capnogram—gold standard
- Prompt inflation of the deflated bulb of oesophageal detector device.

Complications

The complications of endotracheal intubation may be classified as follows:

Immediate

- Trauma to teeth, lips, tongue, pharynx or larynx
- Haemodynamic changes—tachycardia, hypertension, myocardial ischaemia
- Misplaced tube—accidental extubation, oesophageal intubation.

Delayed

Laryngeal granuloma, laryngeal or subglottic stenosis.

Oropharyngeal Airway (Figs 64.10 and 64.11)

- It is available in various sizes. The correct size is chosen such that when it is placed along the side of the patient's face, it should extend from **the angle of mouth up to the tragus.** This is inserted along the tongue and reaches up to the posterior pharyngeal wall.

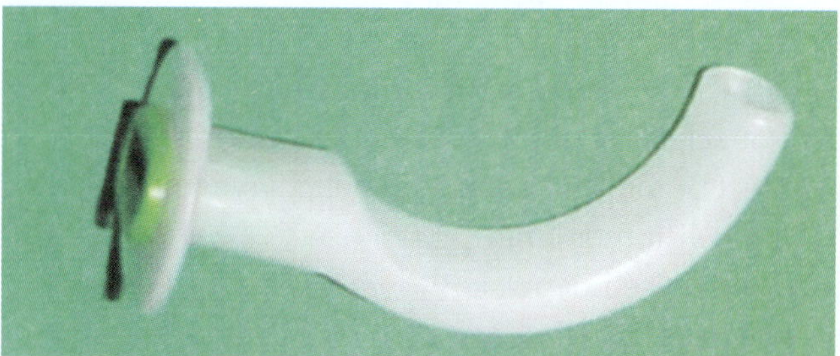

Fig. 64.10: Oropharyngeal airway

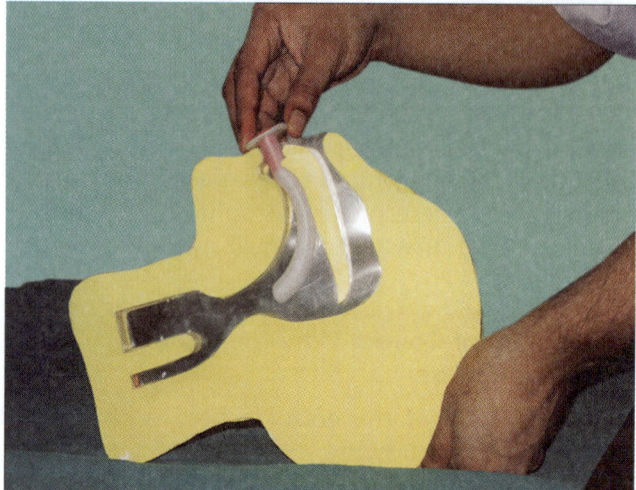

Fig. 64.11: Insertion of oropharyngeal airway. Take care not to push the tongue backwards

- Care should be taken not to push the tongue backwards with the airway itself.
- To avoid that, the airway is inserted with its concavity towards the palate and then turned once 50% of it is inserted and passed further.
- Please note that an oropharyngeal airway is excellent in patients who are completely unconscious. Patients who are conscious do not tolerate it. In patients who are semiconscious, it may initiate a gag reflex and induce vomiting. In such patients, a nasopharyngeal airway is a better choice.

Nasopharyngeal Airway (Figs 64.12 and 64.13)

- It is a soft tube made of latex or silicon. It is available in various sizes. The correct size is the same size as an endotracheal tube for that patient.

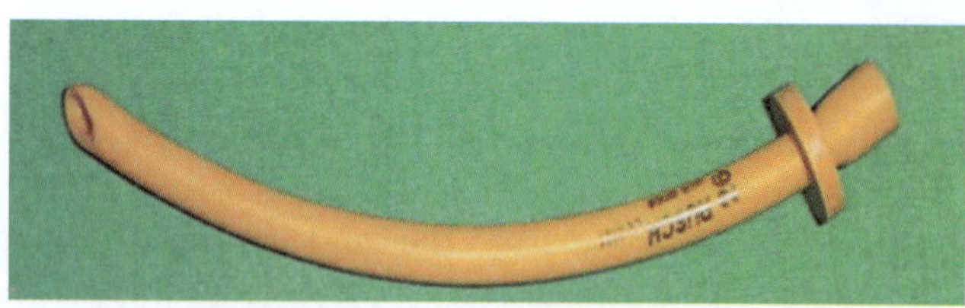

Fig. 64.12: Nasopharyngeal airway

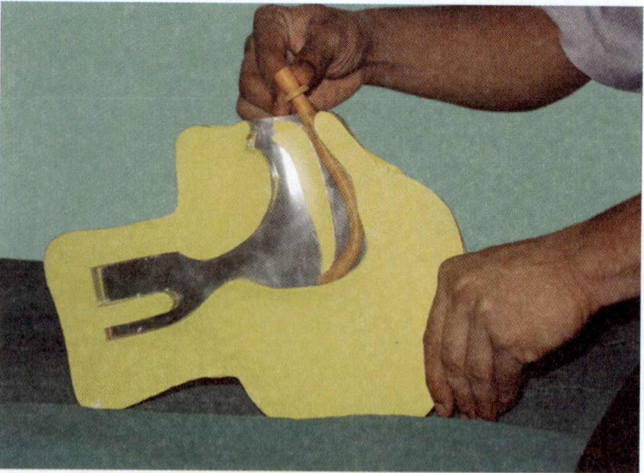

Fig. 64.13: Insertion of nasopharyngeal airway

The correct length is chosen such that when it is placed along the side of the patient's face, it should extend from the **nostril up to the tragus**. This is inserted along the nose and reaches up to the posterior pharyngeal wall.

Laryngeal Mask Airway (Fig. 64.14)

This is a supraglottic airway that has revolutionised airway management during anaesthesia. It has a tube or a shaft with a standard 15 mm connector at the proximal end to connect to the anaesthetic circuit. The patient end has an oval-shaped inflatable cuff which when inserted rests just above the larynx and creates an airtight seal.

Uses

- To administer anaesthesia
- To maintain airway in patients with difficult airway where endotracheal intubation is not possible and are at risk of hypoxia
- It may also be used as a conduit for passage of endotracheal tube, either blindly or with the use of fibreoptic bronchoscope.

Endotracheal Extubation

Endotracheal extubation is as important as intubation. A patient's trachea may be extubated when the following criteria are met

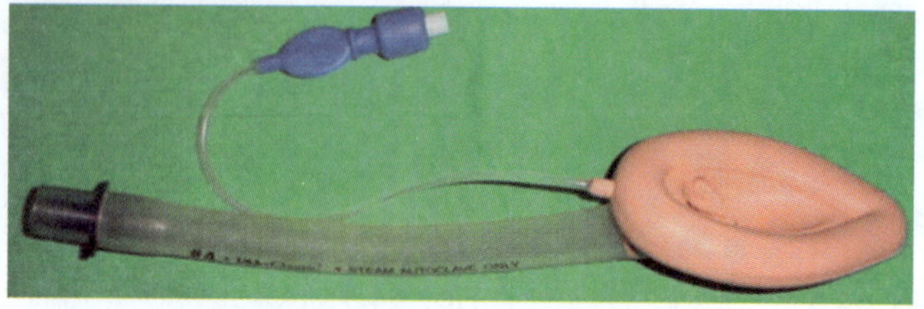

Fig. 64.14: Laryngeal mask airway

- Oxygenation and ventilation are satisfactory
- Patient is haemodynamically stable
- Patient is fully conscious
- Able to maintain his airway patency
- Airway reflexes are intact
- Able to cough and clear airway.

Equipment for reintubation and personnel skilled in intubation should be readily available. After a good oropharyngeal suction to clear the secretions, the cuff is deflated and the tube removed. Oxygen should be administered by face mask and the patient monitored till he is stable and ready to go to the ward.

MONITORING IN ANAESTHESIA

The administration of anaesthesia is associated with changes in the internal homeostasis of the patient, especially the cardiac and respiratory systems. Constant monitoring of the various body systems is necessary to ensure the well-being of the patient and prompt recovery from anaesthesia at the end of surgery. Identification and prompt treatment of any untoward changes should alleviate complications due to anaesthesia.

- Monitoring used in anaesthesia may be classified into: **Noninvasive and invasive monitoring.** The extent of monitoring depends on the patient's preoperative condition, the extent of surgery, the type of anaesthesia and the facilities available.
- Most patients are noninvasively monitored. Basic noninvasive monitoring includes **clinical observation of the patient** and monitoring of the patient's haemodynamic parameters. **Adequate cardiac output is associated with good urine output, warm and well-perfused peripheries and good capillary refill.** Heart rate may be monitored with a finger on the pulse. Blood pressure may be measured using a standard sphygmomanometer. More conveniently and accurately, heart rate and rhythm are continuously monitored using the electrocardiogram and blood pressure using automated noninvasive blood pressure monitoring systems.
- Invasive monitoring becomes necessary when considerable haemodynamic instability exists or is expected to occur perioperatively. This may include invasive arterial pressure, central venous pressure and several others as required.
- **Minimum monitoring standards** (according to guidelines from Indian Society of Anaesthesiologists) for a patient undergoing any type of anaesthesia are:
  - Noninvasive blood pressure (NIBP)
  - Electrocardiogram (ECG)
  - Pulse oximetry
- Monitoring capnography, although not mandatory in India, is an important monitor in patients undergoing anaesthesia. In addition, monitoring of body temperature, anaesthetic gases and neuromuscular blockade is desirable.

Competency

SU11.2.3: Describe advantages and complications of regional anaesthesia.

SU11.2.4: Enumerate the types of regional anaesthesia.

SU11.2.5: Enumerate the indications of regional anaesthesia.

REGIONAL ANAESTHESIA

This involves injection of local anaesthetic agents in close proximity to the nerves, nerve plexuses or spinal cord segments supplying the site of surgery. There are three types of regional anaesthesia: Central neuraxial block, peripheral nerve block and local anaesthesia.

Central Neuraxial Block

Regional anaesthesia induced by injecting the local anaesthetic agents around the spinal cord is called central neuraxial block. It includes spinal, epidural and caudal anaesthesia/analgesia. If the drug is injected into the cerebrospinal fluid (subarachnoid space), it is called subarachnoid block or spinal anaesthesia. If the drug is injected into the epidural space, it is called epidural anaesthesia. The drug can also be injected into the sacral epidural space accessed through the sacral hiatus. This is called caudal epidural block.

Peripheral Nerve Block

When regional anaesthesia is induced by injecting the local anaesthetic agents around nerve plexuses (plexus block) or individual nerves, it is called peripheral nerve block.

Indications

Surgeries that can be done by blocking nerve supply to the surgical area. For example: Surgeries on the lower limbs or below umbilicus can be done under spinal or epidural anaesthesia. Surgeries on the upper limb can be done under brachial plexus block.

Contraindications

- Patient refusal
- Infection at the site of injection
- Coagulation abnormalities

Advantages of Regional Anaesthesia

- Only the part that needs to be operated upon is anaesthetized.

- The patient will be able to resume oral fluid intake early after surgery.
- There is minimum cardiorespiratory depression, especially after peripheral nerve blocks.
- Systemic effects of anaesthetics can be avoided.

Disadvantages

It is difficult for a patient to lie immobile for long periods of time.

- The patient can get restless and irritable.
- Occasionally, neurological injury and other complications (as described below) can occur.
- Regional anaesthesia has a small failure rate and certain surgeries may outlast the duration of block provided by the regional block, in which case general anaesthesia may need to be given. Thus, even though the primary anaesthetic contemplated is regional anaesthesia, it must be ensured that the patients are also fit for general anaesthesia before taking up for surgery.

Competency

SU11.2.6: Describe indications, advantages, complications of local anaesthesia.

LOCAL ANAESTHETICS

Local anaesthetics are drugs when injected around the nerves block impulse conduction distal to the site of injection and produce analgesia and anaesthesia in that area.

Classification

Local anaesthetics consist of a hydrophilic tertiary amine group linked to a lipophilic aromatic group. They are classified into two main categories based on this linking group: The aminoamides and the aminoesters.

- **Aminoesters:** Procaine, chloroprocaine, tetracaine.
- **Aminoamides:** Lignocaine, bupivacaine, ropivacaine.

Mechanism of Action

A nerve impulse is transmitted by progressive opening of sodium channels across the membrane and sudden influx of sodium into the intracellular fluid. Local anaesthetics produce **sodium channel blockade.** They block the fast sodium channels and the sodium influx, thus blocking all impulse transmission across the membrane.

Local anaesthetic exists in two forms: Ionised and nonionised. The nonionised form is lipophilic and crosses the phospholipid membrane more easily. The ionised form is hydrophilic, blocks the channel in the open state and blocks nerve transmission (use-dependent blockade). The drug blocks the channel from the intracellular direction.

Factors Influencing Activity

Lipid solubility

Higher the lipid solubility, higher is its ability to penetrate the lipoprotein membrane and hence greater is its potency.

pKa

The pKa of a drug is the pH at which the ionised and nonionised portions of the drug are equal. The lower the pKa, lower is the degree of ionisation for any given pH. The nonionised portion is lipophilic and crosses the cell membrane more easily hastening the onset of nerve blockade. For example, lignocaine has a pKa of 7.9 and acts faster than bupivacaine with a pKa of 8.1.

pH

Acidosis decreases the proportion of the nonionised drug and reduces the amount of drug able to cross the membrane. That is why local anaesthetics do not work optimally when injected into an infected tissue (pH is acidic in these tissues).

Protein binding

The greater the degree of protein (membrane proteins) binding, longer is the duration of action.

Choice of Local Anaesthetic Agents

- **Lignocaine:** Skin infiltration—0.5–1% Minor nerve block—1% Epidural—1.5–2%

  Spinal anaesthesia—5% hyperbaric (heavy)

  Two topical preparations—2% lignocaine jelly and 4% lignocaine spray for the mucosal surfaces of the body. ***Note:*** 1% means each ml contains 10 mg of the drug, 2% to 20 mg/ml, and so on.
- **Bupivacaine:** Skin infiltration, epidural—0.25%, 0.5% Spinal anaesthesia—0.5%, hyperbaric (heavy).
- **Levobupivacaine:** Bupivacaine is a racemic mixture containing levo and dextrorotatory forms. The dextrorotatory form is cardiotoxic. The levorotatory form of bupivacaine is now available as levobupivacaine (0.25 and 0.5%) and is much safer.
- **Ropivacaine:** Available as 0.2% for providing post-operative analgesia, labour analgesia and as 0.75% for spinal and epidural anaesthesia and nerve blocks.
- **Chloroprocaine:** This is a short-acting ester local anaesthetic now reintroduced for clinical use. There were a few cases of cauda equina syndrome in the

1980s when it was used for subarachnoid block and its use was abandoned. The cause of the neurological injury was then traced to the metabisulfite added to the solution as a preservative. It has now been reintroduced in a concentration of 1% for intrathecal use in a preservative-free form. It is approved for use in the US and Europe. Its advantages are its short duration of action (40 min approximately) and is suitable for procedures of short duration.

Maximum Recommended Doses of Local Anaesthetics for Infiltration and Blocks

- Lignocaine—3 mg/kg
- Lignocaine with adrenaline—7 mg/kg
- Bupivacaine—2 mg/kg
- Ropivacaine—2.5 mg/kg, not to exceed 200 mg for minor nerve blocks.

Clinical Effects

Local effects

Local anaesthetics block the sodium channels in the neuronal membrane and thus the propagation of impulses across it.

Systemic effects

These drugs can produce systemic effects when high plasma levels of the drug are achieved. This may also be deliberate as and when lignocaine is used as an antiarrhythmic agent. It is classified as Class Ia drug (sodium channel blockers) in the Vaughan Williams classification of antiarrhythmic agents.

When high plasma concentrations of local anaesthetics are achieved, either due to accidental intravenous injection of the drug or due to intravascular absorption of large amount of drug infiltrated in a region, systemic toxicity can occur.

Pearls of Wisdom

Adrenaline containing preparations should not be used for nerve blocks of fingers, toes and penis as it can cause ischaemia.

Toxicity of Local Anaesthetics

Systemic toxicity

If significant amount of local anaesthetics reach the tissues of heart and brain, they exert the same membrane stabilising effect as on peripheral nerve, resulting in progressive depression of function. The toxicity of local anaesthetics is dose-dependent. These drugs always produce central nervous system (CNS) toxicity first. As the plasma level rises, cardiovascular toxicity and collapse occur.

The plasma levels of lignocaine required to produce cardiovascular collapse (CVS toxicity) is seven times that required to produce convulsions (CNS toxicity). Bupivacaine requires only three times the plasma level to produce cardiac toxicity as for CNS toxicity. Thus, bupivacaine has a greater potential for cardiotoxicity.

Pearls of Wisdom

With all local anaesthetics, central nervous system toxicity always comes first. This is followed by cardiac toxicity.

Clinical features of local anaesthetic toxicity are related to the plasma level of the local anaesthetic. The clinical effects and their relation to plasma level of lignocaine are given in Table 64.1.

The likelihood of toxicity of local anaesthetics depends on several factors:

1. Amount of drug injected
2. Site of injection—vascularity
3. Addition of vasoconstrictors
4. Rapidity of injection
5. Nature of drug given
6. Presence of associated conditions such as low cardiac output or renal failure.

Amount and nature of drug injected

Lignocaine is mostly used to produce peripheral neural conduction blockade. It can be used in doses not exceeding 5 mg/kg body weight for plexus blocks or

Table 64.1 The clinical effects and their relation to plasma level of lignocaine

Plasma	CNS toxicity	CVS toxicity
Concentration (μg/ml)		
5	Tingling, numbness, tinnitus, light-headedness	
5–10	Slurred speech, muscle twitching	
10	Loss of consciousness	
10–15	Convulsions	
15	Coma	Myocardial depression
20	Respiratory arrest	Cardiac arrhythmias
25		Ventricular arrest

infiltration. When combined with vasopressors such as adrenaline (1:200,000 = 5 μm/ml), the dose can be increased up to 7 mg/kg. The intravenous dose of lignocaine is 1–1.5 mg/kg when used as an anti-arrhythmic. However, even a small dose such as 20 mg in an adult when injected accidentally into the carotid artery may be sufficient to produce convulsions.

Bupivacaine is used only for nerve blocks or infiltration. It is not an antiarrhythmic drug. Bupivacaine is cardiotoxic and care should be taken not to exceed the prescribed doses. Circulatory collapse and cardiac arrest due to large doses of bupivacaine can be very resistant to resuscitation. It can be used in a dose of up to 2.5 mg/kg body weight.

Ropivacaine is a newer amide local anaesthetic agent which is similar to bupivacaine but with less cardiotoxicity. A levo isomer of bupivacaine, called levobupivacaine is also less cardiotoxic and has been put into clinical use recently.

Site of injection

Certain sites are very vascular as compared to others. A higher plasma level of local anaesthetic is reached when the same amount of local anaesthetic is used for multiple intercostal nerve blocks as compared to brachial plexus block.

Prevention of toxicity

- Do not exceed recommended doses.
- Aspirate to rule out presence of the needle tip in a vessel before injecting the drug.
- Avoid injecting large boluses at once. Small boluses, given slowly to achieve the desired effect, are safer.

Treatment of local anaesthetic toxicity

The toxicity of local anaesthetics manifests as CNS depression and convulsions. Maintenance of airway, breathing and circulation must be a priority. These convulsions generally last for a short period of time.

- Patency of the airway must be maintained.
- Oxygen by face mask.
- Ventilation, if apnoea occurs.
- Convulsions are treated with intravenous diazepam or thiopentone in incremental doses.
- Cardiovascular collapse with ephedrine, inotropes and vasoconstrictors, and CPR as needed.
- Arrhythmias must be treated appropriately.
- Intralipid 20%: This is now recommended for use in local anaesthetic toxicity with cardiovascular collapse. Intralipid molecules act like a sink to mop up local anaesthetic molecules. When LA toxicity with cardiovascular collapse occurs, it is advised to give intralipid in a dose of 1.5 ml/kg over 2–3 min followed by 0.25 ml/kg/min for 15–20 min. If the patient is still unstable, can repeat the bolus once or twice at the same dose and the infusion rate can be doubled. The maximum dose of intralipid is 12 ml/kg.

SPINAL AND EPIDURAL ANAESTHESIA

- Injection of local anaesthetics around the spinal cord to produce a reversible blockade of impulses that pass through it, is called **central neuraxial blockade**.
- When the local anaesthetic is injected into the cerebrospinal fluid bathing the spinal cord, it is called **spinal anaesthesia** (subarachnoid block).
- When the local anaesthetics are injected into the epidural space to block the nerves that emerge from the spinal cord, it is called **epidural anaesthesia**.

SPINAL ANAESTHESIA

Physiological Effects

Nervous system

The local anaesthetics spread from the site of injection by mixing with the cerebrospinal fluid (CSF). They reach the nerve fibres in the spinal cord and block transmission of impulses below the highest level of spread. The concentration of the drug is higher in the caudal regions and reduces with increasing distance cranially. A lower concentration of the drug is sufficient to block smaller fibres (C and Aδ), whereas the thick motor fibres (Aα) require a larger concentration to get blocked. Thus, **a differential blockade** is seen after a spinal anaesthetic and is as follows:

- Motor block up to a certain level (depends on the dose of drug injected).
- Sensory level of block 2 segments higher than motor block.
- Sympathetic block about two to four segments above the level of sensory block.

Cardiovascular system

- **Hypotension:** Due to the blockade of sympathetic nerves below the level of spinal block, there is profound vasodilatation in the affected areas. A relative hypovolaemia occurs and hypotension is usually seen. The extent of hypovolaemia depends on the preoperative volume status, level of block and ability to compensate for the vasodilatation. The vessels in the upper limbs constrict to compensate for vasodilatation in the lower limbs. This is described as **pink trousers, blue jacket** phenomenon.
- **Bradycardia:** Heart rate is maintained in low blocks, but in higher blocks (high thoracic), sympathetic

nerve block of the cardioaccelerator nerves can occur causing unopposed action of the parasympathetic system and bradycardia.

- **Cardiac output also reduces** in high spinal anaesthetics.

Respiratory system

- No changes in respiratory function are seen in spinal anaesthetics below T10 level.
- When the level of spinal anaesthesia ascends, the intercostal nerves are gradually blocked.
- The diaphragm is not easily paralysed as the phrenic nerve is a thick and strong nerve and arises from cervical nerve roots (C3, C4, C5).
- In high spinals, the alveolar ventilation reduces and may lead to hypoxia and hypercarbia.

Gastrointestinal system

- Unopposed parasympathetic activity leads to constriction of gut with increased peristaltic activity.
- Nausea, retching or vomiting may occur and may be the symptom of impending hypotension. These symptoms disappear when the hypotension is corrected. Occasionally, it may need administration of an anticholinergic or an antiemetic agent.
- However, since the bowel is contracted and small and the skeletal muscle relaxation produced is greater, the surgeons find it easier to operate on such a gut.

Indications

- Lower abdominal surgery
- Lower limb surgery
- Caesarean section
- Prostate surgery

Contraindications

Absolute

- Patient refusal
- Infection at the site of injection
- Bleeding tendencies

Relative

- Hypovolaemia
- Severe stenotic valvular heart disease

Limitation

Limited duration of block.

Preprocedure Check

A preprocedure check of the anaesthesia equipment, resuscitation equipment and drugs is made. An intravenous line is placed and monitoring commenced. The patient is then positioned for spinal anaesthesia.

Position

The spinal anaesthetic may be administered with the patient in lateral or sitting position.

Lateral: The patient lies either in the left or right lateral position. The back should be parallel to the edge of the operating table and perpendicular to the ground. The legs should be flexed at the hips as much as possible.

Sitting position: The patient sits on the table, with the back bent forward. He is allowed to rest his arms on pillows. The back is cleaned with spirit and betadine and draped. Under aseptic precautions, the vertebral spines are identified in the lumbar region. The highest point of the iliac crest corresponds to L3–4 space. The L2–3, L3–4, L4–5 intervertebral spaces can also be used. A space higher than this is not used as the spinal cord ends at L1 in adults. This point is lower in children and should be borne in mind in paediatric spinals.

Approach

The subarachnoid space may be approached either from the midline or by a paramedian technique. A subcutaneous wheal of local anaesthetic is raised in the chosen intervertebral space.

Midline approach: The lumbar puncture needle is inserted in the midline, midway between the spines and perpendicular to the skin. The spinal needle passes through the following structures to reach the subarachnoid space:

1. Skin
2. Subcutaneous tissue
3. Supraspinous ligaments
4. Interspinous ligaments
5. Ligamentum flavum
6. Dura and arachnoid

Paramedian approach: The needle is inserted a fingerbreadth lateral to the spine and advanced in a slightly cephalad direction towards the midline. If the needle touches the lamina, it should be redirected medially. The correct position of the needle is identified by obtaining a free flow of CSF. This approach helps access the subarachnoid space in those patients whose interspinous and supraspinous ligaments are calcified or in patients unable to bend enough to open the interspaces well. The local anaesthetic is now injected into the CSF, taking care not to displace the needle.

Complications

These may be classified into **Minor** and **Major based on the reversibility and seriousness of the complication.**

Minor

Hypotension

This is treated with intravenous fluids to compensate for the vasodilatation. If necessary, incremental doses of a vasoconstrictor may also be used.

Bradycardia

If the cardioaccelerator nerves (T1–T4) are blocked. This is usually easily treated with an anticholinergic such as atropine or glycopyrrolate. If profound, a small dose of adrenaline may be required (very rare).

Postdural puncture headache (PDPH)

The incidence of PDPH depends on the size of the needle used, number of punctures made, fluid status and ambulation. With finer needles (25 or 26 G) and good hydration of the patient, PDPH is uncommon. This may be treated with rest, increased fluid intake, plenty of coffee and NSAIDs. Rarely, an epidural blood patch *(vide infra)* may be required.

Respiratory depression

If the level of spinal anaesthesia is high and all intercostal muscles are paralysed, respiratory depression may occur. However, diaphragm, the principal muscle of respiration is supplied by the thick phrenic nerve which does not get blocked easily. Any respiratory depression seen during spinal anaesthesia is more due to hypoperfusion of the respiratory centre (due to hypotension). This can be treated with respiratory support as required and stabilisation of blood pressure.

Retention of urine

Backache: This is not a problem of spinal anaesthesia *per se* but may be due to faulty positioning during surgery.

Major

1. **Infection:** Arachnoiditis, meningitis.
2. **Nerve injury:** Cauda equina syndrome.

EPIDURAL ANAESTHESIA (Table 64.2)

In this type of central neuraxial blockade, local anaesthetic is injected in the space around the dura (epidural space). The local anaesthetic blocks the nerves as they emerge through the intervertebral foramen. Some of it diffuses through the meninges into the spinal cord and acts on the spinal cord.

Preprocedure Check

A preprocedure check of the anaesthesia equipment, resuscitation equipment and drugs is made. An intravenous line is placed and monitoring of heart rate, electrocardiogram, blood pressure and oxygen saturation is established and the baseline noted.

Table 64.2 Comparison of spinal and epidural anaesthesia

Spinal anaesthesia	Epidural anaesthesia
1. Done in the lumbar region only	Can be done in the lumbar, sacral (caudal), thoracic or cervical regions
2. Confirmation of correct placement of needle by ensuring free flow of CSF	Placement confirmed by using loss of resistance to injection of air, saline or both
3. A small amount of local anaesthetic is used	Larger mass of local anaesthetic is injected
4. 23–29 G lumbar puncture (LP) needles used	Larger needles (16–20 G) are required
5. Test doses not required	Use of test doses advisable
6. Onset of neural blockade is fast. So, also side-effects	Onset slow as drugs have to penetrate the dura. So, less hypotension
7. All the nerves are blocked below the level of anaesthesia	The local anaesthetic spreads both caudad and cephalad. Segmental block can be achieved
8. Limited duration. Continuous spinals are not routinely used	Epidural catheters are routinely introduced and hence duration of anaesthesia can be prolonged with repeated boluses or continuous infusion through catheters
9. Postdural puncture headache possible	PDPH not seen, unless dura is inadvertently punctured
10. No such problem	Inadvertent intrathecal or intravascular injection of large amount of drugs possible, with consequent complications such as total spinal blockade and local anaesthetic toxicity respectively

Position

The epidural puncture can be done with the patient in sitting position or in the lateral decubitus position.

Technique

The patient's back is cleaned with an antiseptic and then draped. Under aseptic precautions, epidural puncture is done using a 16 or 18# Tuohy needle. This needle has a **blunt tip** to reduce the risk of dural puncture. The needle is inserted either in the **midline** or by a **paramedian** approach. It passes through the same tissues as in lumbar puncture except the subarachnoid space. The needle is inserted along with its stylet and always advanced slowly from skin onwards. Once the subcutaneous tissue is entered, the stylet is removed. A 2 ml or 5 ml syringe with a freely moving plunger and containing either air, saline or both is then connected to the needle hub. A gentle attempt at injection of this air or saline is made as the needle advances through the tissues. The entry of the needle into the epidural space is heralded when it penetrates the ligamentum flavum and there is a **loss of resistance to injection of air or saline**. This is taken as the end-point. An epidural catheter is passed through this needle and advanced to about 3–4 cm into the space. The needle is removed and the catheter taped and fixed to the back. A bacterial filter is attached to the injection port of the catheter (Figs 64.15A to C).

The epidural needle or catheter may accidentally enter an epidural vein or the subarachnoid space. To avoid injecting a large dose of local anaesthetic into either of these spaces, a test-dose containing a small amount of local anaesthetic (3 ml of 2% = 60 mg lignocaine) and 15 µg of adrenaline is injected. Any sensory or motor block following this dose would suggest an accidental dural puncture resulting in spinal anaesthesia. An accidental intravascular injection is identified by an increase in the heart rate and blood pressure within a minute of the injection. In either situation, the epidural catheter may need to be withdrawn or replaced. If neither response is seen, an epidural placement is assumed and the full dose of local anaesthetic is injected in divided doses. The patient should be continuously monitored till the block wears off.

Complications

1. Postdural puncture headache (PDPH)

The epidural needles are large and dural puncture results in a larger leak of cerebrospinal fluid (CSF). This results in low CSF pressures. Whenever the patient sits up or becomes ambulatory, a drag occurs on the brain and the meninges due to gravity and loss of CSF. This results in a typical postural headache referred to the occipital region. The pain disappears when he lies down supine. This is more common in obstetric patients. It may occur up to 2 to 7 days after lumbar puncture and may persist for up to 6 weeks.

Treatment: Plenty of oral fluids may increase CSF production. Rest, plenty of coffee and NSAIDs may also help. Rarely, an epidural blood patch may be required.

Epidural blood patch: If the headache is very severe, an epidural blood patch may be given. 15–20 ml of patient's own blood is drawn under aseptic precautions. Simultaneously, epidural puncture is made in the same space as the previous epidural puncture. The freshly drawn blood is injected into the epidural space which clots and seals the puncture hole. This is nearly 100% effective in relieving the headache.

2. Total spinal block

When a large dose of local anaesthetic is injected intrathecally inadvertently, all spinal nerves are blocked, causing profound hypotension, bradycardia and collapse. If the patient is continuously monitored and treated promptly, this is completely reversible.

Treatment

1. Volume infusion and vasopressors
2. Endotracheal intubation and ventilation as necessary

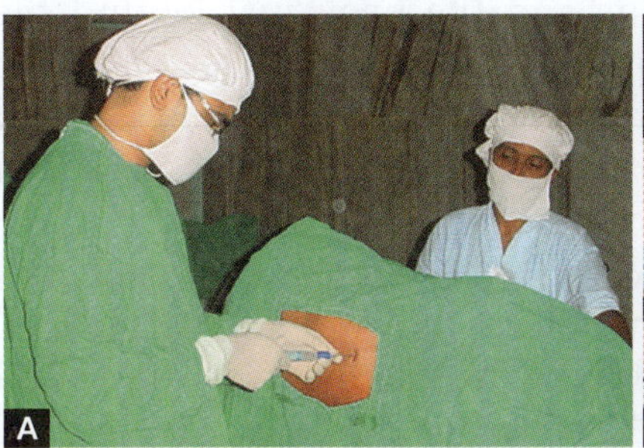
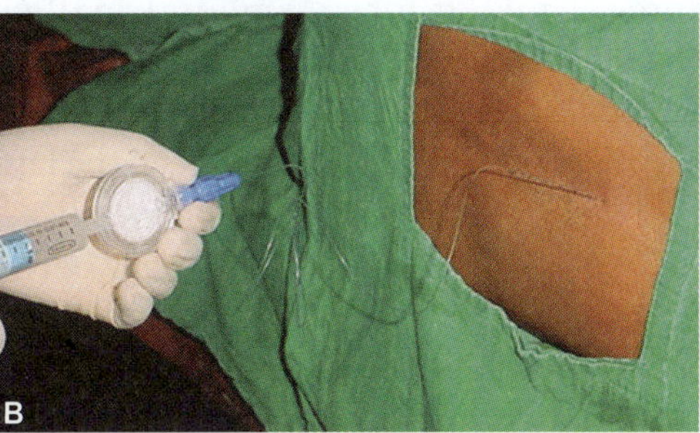
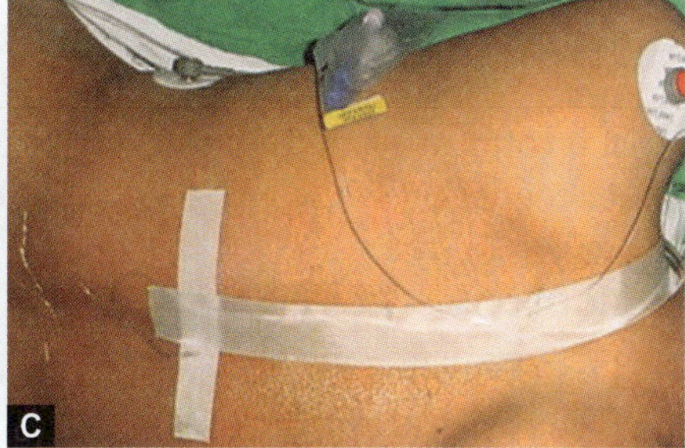

Figs 64.15A to C: Epidural anaesthesia. (A) Eliciting loss of resistance to air; (B) Epidural catheter attached to bacterial filter; (C) Epidural catheter taped to the back

3. Urinary retention
4. **Meningitis,** if aseptic precautions are not followed.
5. Cauda equina syndrome, adhesive arachnoiditis: Extremely rare.

OTHER REGIONAL TECHNIQUES

CAUDAL ANALGESIA

This is a very popular technique in providing post-operative analgesia in children. It involves injection of local anaesthetics with or without opioids in the caudal epidural space.

Procedure

Position

The patient is positioned in lateral position with the knees flexed and the back perpendicular to the ground. It can also be given with the patient in prone position. The area over the sacrum and the gluteal region is cleaned and draped.

Needles

A 22 or 23 G hypodermic needle or a scalp vein set is used to administer the block.

Technique

The needle is inserted at the apex of the sacral hiatus at a 60° angle to the skin. A distinct 'pop' or a 'give way' is felt as the needle punctures the sacrococcygeal membrane. The angle of the needle is then changed to about 15° to 20° to the skin and advanced a little further into the sacral epidural space. The latter step is optional and has to be done with caution as the dural sac may end relatively low in infants. After careful aspiration to rule out blood or CSF, a small dose of local anaesthetic is injected. There should be no resistance to injection. A subcutaneous injection should also be ruled out.

Drugs

0.25% bupivacaine in a dose of 0.5 ml/kg is sufficient for perineal and low sacral procedures, 1 ml/kg for lumbosacral procedures and 1.5 ml/kg for lower abdominal procedures. However, a total volume of 20 ml and a total dose of 2.5 mg/kg of bupivacaine may not be exceeded.

Indications

- Postoperative pain relief in children for perineal and lumbosacral procedures.
- It is also used to supplement general anaesthesia for perianal procedures in adults.

Contraindications

- Absence of consent from parents/patients
- Local infection
- Bleeding tendencies.

Complications

- Intrathecal injection is possible, especially in smaller infants who have extension of dural sac down to S3.
- Intravascular injection of large dose of local anaesthetics.

BRACHIAL PLEXUS BLOCK

Injection of local anaesthetics injected around the brachial plexus produces analgesia and even surgical anaesthesia in the upper limb. The brachial plexus can be blocked by four different approaches: Interscalene, supraclavicular, infraclavicular and the axillary. Peripheral nerve blocks are most often given under direct visualization using ultrasound. Other methods include use of a peripheral nerve stimulator or landmark-guided techniques.

ANKLE BLOCK

This is a popular technique in providing intra- and post-operative analgesia in adults undergoing procedures on the foot.

Position

The patient is positioned supine. The foot is raised by an assistant and the area around the ankle is cleaned and draped.

Needles

A 22 G hypodermic needle is used to administer the block.

Technique

Ankle block involves blocking of **5 nerves**.

1. The **posterior tibial nerve** is blocked with 3–5 ml of local anaesthetic at a point midway between the medial malleolus and the heel, just behind the posterior tibial arterial pulsations.
2. The **sural nerve** may be blocked at a point midway between the lateral malleolus and the heel, just lateral to the Achilles tendon.
3. The **deep peroneal nerve** is blocked at a point midway between the lateral and the medial malleoli lateral to the tendon of extensor hallucis longus and anterior tibial artery.
4. The **saphenous nerve** and the **superficial peroneal nerves** are easily blocked by raising a subcutaneous

wheal of local anaesthetic between the malleoli anteriorly.

Drugs

Lignocaine plain not exceeding 5 mg/kg or bupivacaine not exceeding 2.5 mg/kg may be used.

Indications

Postoperative pain relief in adults for procedures on the foot.

Contraindications

Absence of consent from patients, local infection, bleeding tendencies.

COMPLICATIONS OF ANAESTHESIA

The practice of anaesthesia has become very safe due to better preoperative evaluation and preparation, careful choice of patients, better monitoring, availability of safer drugs and safer anaesthetic techniques. The incidence of complications has come down drastically. However, complications can still occur. The perioperative (pre-, intra-, and postoperative periods) complications can be classified as follows.

Respiratory

- Airway obstruction
- Bronchospasm
- Respiratory failure

Cardiovascular

- Hypertension
- Hypotension
- Arrhythmias
- Shock

Central Nervous System

- Postoperative drowsiness
- Postoperative nausea and vomiting
- Neurologic complications of regional blockade.

Renal and Hepatic Failure

Impairment of urea, creatinine and liver enzymes can occur.

RESPIRATORY COMPLICATIONS

Airway Obstruction

Airway obstruction may occur during the induction of general anaesthesia. When a person becomes unconscious, the tongue and the epiglottis fall back and can obstruct the airway. The patency of the airway is usually maintained fairly easily by the anaesthesiologist by using chin lift or jaw thrust manoeuvres. A definitive airway such as an endotracheal tube may then be inserted into the trachea.

Occasionally, the chin lift or jaw thrust manoeuvres are inadequate to maintain a patent airway as in patients with abnormal airways. Insertion of an endotracheal tube may also prove to be difficult in certain individuals. An oral or nasopharyngeal airway may be inserted to overcome this obstruction and maintenance of the airway for a short duration. If there is difficulty in inserting the endotracheal tube due to supraglottic causes and oral or nasopharyngeal airways are not sufficient to relieve the obstruction, insertion of a laryngeal mask airway or a Combitube® may be attempted. If the problem is at the glottis or subglottis and the airway is obstructed, an emergency cricothyrotomy or a tracheostomy may be required.

Perioperative airway obstruction may also be due to any of the following causes:

- Trauma—maxillofacial, head injury
- Foreign body aspiration
- Laryngospasm
- Infection—Ludwig's angina, retropharyngeal abscess
- Oedema—laryngeal/pharyngeal oedema
- Neurological—recurrent laryngeal nerve injury
- Endocrine—thyroid enlargement
- Tumour—malignancy of the airway (tongue, cheek, larynx or the pharynx)

A thorough assessment of the airway must be done preoperatively and a management plan A formulated. Plan B and Plan C also should be considered in the eventuality of failure of Plan A. Generally loss of life occurs not because of inability to intubate but due to an inability to oxygenate and ventilate the patient. This situation, also called, 'cannot intubate—cannot ventilate' (CVCI) is one of the most dreaded situations faced by an anaesthesiologist.

Bronchospasm

Bronchospasm may occur in a patient under anaesthesia. The possible causes are as follows:

- Irritable airways as in a known asthmatic, chronic obstructive airways disease, i.e. exacerbation of preexisting bronchospastic disease.
- Endobronchial intubation and carinal stimulation
- As part of allergic reaction to anaesthetic drugs, antibiotics
- Aspiration of regurgitated gastric contents
- Pneumothorax
- Upper airway obstruction and laryngospasm can reflexly stimulate bronchospasm.

Treatment involves treatment of the precipitating cause and bronchodilators.

Respiratory Failure

A patient is said to be in respiratory failure if he is unable to maintain adequate oxygenation and ventilation, i.e. arterial blood gas tension of O_2 less than 60 mmHg (when patient is breathing 60% O_2) and CO_2 more than 50 mmHg. This could be acute or acute exacerbation of chronic respiratory failure.

Causes

Central

- Head injury
- Depressant drugs—anaesthetics, opioids
- Hypoxic encephalopathy
- Metabolic causes such as hyponatraemia, hypoglycaemia, hypokalaemia, hyperglycaemia.

Peripheral

- Lung parenchymal disorders such as pneumonia, atelectasis, aspiration, pneumothorax, pulmonary embolism.
- Inadequate respiratory excursion due to pain or thoracic cage abnormalities such as kyphoscoliosis.
- Weakness of muscles, e.g. prolonged effect of muscle relaxants, myasthenia gravis.

Treatment

- Treat the cause
- Intermittent positive pressure ventilation and ventilatory support till the patient improves.

CARDIOVASCULAR COMPLICATIONS

Hypertension, hypotension and arrhythmias occur perioperatively due to various reasons such as inadequate preoperative treatment, surgical stress, inadequate anaesthesia, metabolic or endocrine causes or even drug interactions. Brief periods of haemodynamic instability, although common are well-tolerated by healthy individuals. Continuous and appropriate monitoring and prompt treatment should avoid long-term complications.

Hypotension may be due to decreased preload, reduced contractility or decreased afterload to the left ventricle. If not identified or treated in time, it may progress to shock and cardiac arrest. Hypovolaemic shock is the commonest type of shock encountered during surgery. However, cardiogenic shock due to perioperative myocardial infarction, anaphylactic shock due to allergic reaction to anaesthetics or neurogenic shock due to vasovagal attack, high spinals may also occur in susceptible individuals.

Perioperative myocardial infarction (MI) is a complication that occurs in susceptible individuals. It may be caused due to extreme and sustained variations in haemodynamics such as hypotension, hypertension or tachycardia. It may also be caused due to thrombosis as the patient is in a hypercoagulable state due to stress of surgery. The highest incidence of perioperative MI is seen not on the day of surgery (when the patient is under the vigilant care of the anaesthesiologist) but on the second or the third day when the attention given to him is less in terms of pain relief or haemodynamic changes.

CENTRAL NERVOUS SYSTEM COMPLICATIONS

Awareness

Rarely, a patient under general anaesthesia (GA) might recall events that occurred during the procedure. This is termed awareness during anaesthesia and is one of the most dreaded complications by both anaesthesiologist and the patient. This is more likely to occur if the patient's haemodynamics are very unstable (as in postpartum haemorrhage, trauma) and the anaesthesiologist fears further cardiac depression may occur with the use of inhalation agents. The use of opioids and nitrous oxide may provide analgesia but not the amnesia and anaesthesia required. With increased awareness of this complication among anaesthesiologists coupled with the use of benzodiazepines and modern anaesthetic agents which are more cardiostable, the incidence of this is reduced. A 'depth of anaesthesia' monitor is called BIS index monitor provides some information of the conscious state of the patient but is not widely available yet.

Postoperative Drowsiness

A patient may be slow to awaken after anaesthesia due to persistent effect of the anaesthetic agents or opioids administered during the anaesthesia. However, it may be due to metabolic causes such as hypoxia, hypothermia, hypo- or hypernatraemia, hypo- or hyperglycaemia. If all these causes are ruled out, a neurological consultation is obtained to rule out any space-occupying lesions in the central nervous system, stroke or hypoxic encephalopathy.

Postoperative Nausea and Vomiting (PONV)

PONV is a frequent complication of anaesthesia. It is common in women, after laparoscopic surgeries, squint surgeries and is associated with the use of nitrous oxide and opioids or even early oral intake postoperatively. It may be treated with IV metoclopramide (10 mg), ondansetron (4–8 mg) or dexamethasone (4–8 mg) in an average adult.

Nerve Injuries

Nerve injuries may arise as a complication of regional blockade. Complications such as adhesive arachnoiditis, cauda equina syndrome or paraplegia have been reported after spinal and epidural anaesthesia but are extremely rare. The use of tourniquet, if prolonged or if very high pressures are used, can also cause nerve injuries.

Peripheral nerve injuries may occur perioperatively due to improper positioning under regional or general anaesthesia. The common peroneal nerve and the sciatic nerve can be injured during lithotomy position. The ulnar and the radial nerves may be affected in the arm or at the elbow due to inadequate attention to positioning. Brachial plexus stretch injury can occur if the arms are allowed to be abducted more than ninety degrees. Injury to optic nerves or the retina may occur in prone position due to compression of the eyeball. Corneal injury may occur due to exposure in an unconscious patient.

RENAL FAILURE

Renal failure, usually prerenal is associated with large fluid shifts or major haemodynamic instability. Direct injury to the kidneys (acute tubular necrosis) may occur if adequate attention is not given to prerenal failure. Methoxyflurane, an inhalation anaesthetic agent can cause renal failure but is no longer in clinical use. Renal failure can also occur as part of hepatorenal syndrome or after a mismatched blood transfusion.

HEPATIC FAILURE

A patient with compromised hepatic function may proceed to hepatic failure perioperatively, e.g. cirrhosis of liver, obstructive jaundice. Hepatic failure may also occur due to infective complications such as hepatitis or sepsis. Massive hepatic necrosis has been reported after repeated use of halothane. The incidence of this is very rare and must be a diagnosis of exclusion.

> Competency
>
> **SU11.2.7:** Describe the drugs used in general, regional and local anaesthesia.

GENERAL ANAESTHETIC AGENTS

General anaesthetic agents are of two main types: Inhalational anaesthetic agents or Intravenous anaesthetic agents.

INHALATIONAL ANAESTHETIC AGENTS

- **Volatile anaesthetics:** The volatile anaesthetic agents need a vaporiser to calibrate and deliver the vapour accurately in measured doses, e.g. isoflurane.
- **Nonvolatile anaesthetics:** For example, nitrous oxide.

Classification

I. Agents of mainly historical interest

1. Ethyl chloride
2. Chloroform
3. Trichloroethylene
4. Cyclopropane
5. Methoxyflurane
6. Enflurane
7. Diethyl ether
8. Halothane

II. Agents in clinical use

1. Isoflurane
2. Sevoflurane
3. Desflurane
4. Nitrous oxide

III. Agent undergoing clinical trials—Xenon

A comparison of clinical effects of common inhalational anaesthetic agents in use is given in Table 64.3. Only important effects have been mentioned for the benefit of students.

HALOTHANE

This was a very popular anaesthetic agent till recently but is largely replaced by isoflurane. Reasons for dwindling popularity are:

- Myocardial depression
- Arrhythmogenicity
- Remote possibility of halothane hepatitis
- Easier availability of isoflurane (a safer agent).

Halothane Hepatotoxicity

Two types of halothane induced hepatic dysfunction are recognised:

Type I: It is mild, self-limiting and more common. It is associated with mild increases in liver enzymes but not jaundice. It is caused by reductive metabolism of halothane.

Type II: On extremely rare occasions (widely quoted incidence 1:35,000), the administration of halothane may be associated with the production of hepatitis. This entity, known as halothane hepatitis, is largely a diagnosis of exclusion. It is fulminant with a high

Table 64.3 Comparison of different inhalation anaesthetics

Parameter	Halothane	Isoflurane	Sevoflurane	Desflurane
Smell	Pleasant	Pungent	Pleasant	
Parameter	Halothane	Isoflurane	Sevoflurane	Desflurane
Smell	Pleasant	Pungent	Pleasant	Pungent
Inhalation induction	Suitable	Not suitable	Suitable	Not suitable
Effect on CNS				
CNS depression	Rapid, progressive	Rapid, progressive	Rapid, progressive	Rapid, progressive
Induction and recovery	Fast	Faster	Fastest	Fastest
Effect on RS				
Minute ventilation	Depressed	Depressed	Depressed	Depressed
Bronchodilatation	+++	++	++	Cough
Effect on CVS				
Myocardial contractility	↓↓↓	↓↓	↔	↔
Heart rate	↓↓	↑↑	↔	↑↑
Blood pressure	↓↓	↓↓↓	↓	↓
Arrhythmias	+++	↔	↔	↔
Effect on uterine muscle tone	↓↓	↓	↓	↓
Effect on skeletal muscle	Relaxes	Relaxes	Relaxes	Relaxes

mortality rate (up to 50%). It is associated with fever, jaundice and grossly elevated liver enzymes. The toxic metabolite, trifluoroacetic acid reacts with liver proteins and triggers immune-mediated reaction in genetically susceptible individuals. Risk factors for development of halothane hepatitis are female gender, obesity, prior history of postanaesthetic jaundice, genetic susceptibility, repeated administration and enzyme-inducing drugs such as phenobarbitone.

Halothane is metabolised up to 20%, and sevoflurane (2%) and isoflurane (0.2%). Thus, hepatic dysfunction, although reported with sevoflurane and isoflurane, is extremely rare.

ISOFLURANE

- It is a halogenated ether.
- It is not expensive.
- It causes **less cerebral vasodilatation** than halothane.
- It is associated with only a remote risk of hepatitis
- Isoflurane is now **routinely used** for all cases because it produces less arrhythmias and myocardial depression.
- It has a **pungent** smell and hence cannot be used for inhalation induction.

SEVOFLURANE

- It is a newer general anaesthetic agent and has a sweet smell.
- **Useful for** inhalation induction, especially in children.
- Induction and recovery are faster than with halothane.
- It produces minimal myocardial depression.
- It is also a useful agent for induction of anaesthesia in patients with **difficult airways.**
- It is expensive but more affordable than previously. Thus, it is being increasingly used for neurosurgery, cardiac surgery and in patients who can afford it, because of better haemodynamic stability and faster recovery.

DESFLURANE

- It is another new volatile anaesthetic agent.
- It causes vasodilatation and increase in heart rate.
- Induction and recovery are **very fast.**
- However, it is **irritant to the respiratory tract** and hence is not suitable for inhalational induction.
- It also requires a specially constructed **heated vaporiser** because of its high volatility.
- Desflurane has a very low blood-gas solubility coefficient. Hence, emergence from desflurane anaesthesia is very fast and thus it is an ideal agent to use in obese patients. It is very expensive.
- Desflurane is a greenhouse gas and can contribute to air pollution. Hence its use has reduced and many hospitals across the world have stopped its use.

NITROUS OXIDE

- It is an anaesthetic gas which is compressed and supplied as a **liquid in blue cylinders.**

- It is sweet smelling and nonirritant.
- It provides **analgesia** but is insufficient to produce an adequate depth of anaesthesia when used alone.
- It **enhances induction** of anaesthesia with the volatile anaesthetics and reduces their requirement.
- It does not produce significant depression of the cardiovascular system.

Uses

- It is used along with volatile anaesthetic agents as part of balanced anaesthesia.
- A combination of 50% nitrous oxide and 50% oxygen is available as Entonox. It can be used to provide labour analgesia.
- It may also be used to provide analgesia for small procedures in dentistry.

Side Effects

- It can **diffuse into closed gas spaces** such as pneumothorax, obstructed intestines, sinuses and middle ear, and can cause barotrauma. The volume of a cavity can increase 3 to 4 times within 1–2 hours. Hence, nitrous oxide is best avoided in patients in whom such expansion may be anticipated.
- Its use is associated with increased incidence of **post-operative nausea and vomiting.**
- In prolonged administrations, it can affect vitamin B_{12} synthesis causing megaloblastic anaemia.
- **Teratogenicity:** This has been observed in pregnant rats exposed to nitrous oxide for prolonged periods but not proved in human beings. Nitrous oxide is best avoided in early pregnancy.
- Like desflurane, nitrous oxide is also a greenhouse gas and its clinical use has reduced considerably.

INTRAVENOUS ANAESTHETIC AGENTS

Intravenously administered anaesthetic agents are more popular for induction of anaesthesia because it is more rapid and smooth than that associated with inhalational agents. They can also be used for maintenance of anaesthesia, sedation during regional anaesthesia, sedation in the ICU and treatment of status epilepticus.

They can be classified into **rapidly-acting** (acting within one arm-brain circulation time) and **slower-acting** (those that take longer than one arm-brain circulation time).

INTRAVENOUS ANAESTHETICS

- Rapidly-acting: Thiopentone, propofol, etomidate.
- Slower-acting: Ketamine, high dose opioids, benzodiazepines.

THIOPENTONE SODIUM

It is an ultra-short acting barbiturate, available as a yellowish powder. It is used as a 2.5% solution (25 mg/ml). It is used in a dose of 4–5 mg/kg intravenously.

Clinical Effects

CNS

- Generalised depression of the CNS is observed within 15 to 20 seconds of IV injection of thiopentone. **Loss of eyelash reflex is used as an end-point.**
- It is a potent anticonvulsant.
- It is not an analgesic. To the contrary, it increases pain sensation **(antanalgesic)**. Consciousness is regained within 5 to 10 minutes.

CVS

- It produces myocardial depression, peripheral vasodilatation and hypotension especially when large doses are administered rapidly.
- Profound hypotension may occur, especially in a patient with hypovolaemia or cardiac disease. It may induce tachycardia.

RS

- It reduces respiratory drive. A short period of apnoea is common.
- It can precipitate asthma following airway obstruction in susceptible individuals.

Skeletal muscle

There is poor muscle relaxation with thiopentone.

Uterus and placenta

- There is a little effect on resting uterine tone.
- It crosses placenta rapidly, although foetal blood concentration is far less than that observed in the mother.

Eye

- It reduces intraocular pressure.
- The corneal, eyelash and eyelid reflexes are abolished.

Side Effects

- Hypotension, tachycardia
- Respiratory depression
- Irritant to veins and can cause thrombophlebitis. If it extravasates, can cause tissue necrosis.
- Intra-arterial injection: Accidental intra-arterial injection of thiopentone results in severe arterial

spasm and pain. This may be treated with vasodilators and heparin.
- Allergic reactions: Very rare.

Contraindications

Absolute	*Relative*
1. Airway obstruction	1. Hypovolaemia
2. Acute intermittent porphyria	2. Asthma
3. Previous hypersensitivity reaction	

PROPOFOL

This drug became commercially available in 1986. It is comparable to thiopentone but is five times more expensive. It is highly lipid soluble and is formulated in a white, aqueous emulsion containing soya bean oil and egg phosphatide. It is used in a dose of 2–2.5 mg/kg intravenously. The dose should be reduced in the elderly and in haemodynamically unstable patients.

Clinical Effects

CNS

- Propofol depresses the central nervous system within 20 to 40 seconds of injection. Loss of verbal contact is used as an end-point.
- Recovery is rapid and there is a minimal "hang-over" effect even in the immediate post-anaesthetic period.

CVS

- The arterial pressure decreases more than with thiopentone. This is due to peripheral vasodilatation. The degree of hypotension can be reduced by slowing the rate of administration.
- Heart rate increases slightly.

RS

- After induction, apnoea occurs commonly and for a longer duration than with thiopentone.
- It causes ventilatory depression, particularly with opioids.
- It may prevent development of bronchospasm because it blunts airway reflexes.

GIT, uterus and placenta: Propofol has no significant effect on GI motility but causes mild transient decrease in or hepatorenal function.

Uses (Table 64.4)

- As an **induction agent**
- As an infusion, can be used to provide **total intravenous anaesthesia**
- To provide **conscious sedation**
- As continuous infusion to **sedate patients in the ICU**, since its half-life is very short.

Adverse Effects

- Cardiovascular depression
- Respiratory depression
- Pain on injection
- Allergic reactions.

Table 64.4 Comparison of different intravenous anaesthetics

Parameter	Thiopentone	Propofol	Ketamine
Onset	Rapid	Rapid	Slow
Effect on CNS			
CNS depression	↓↓↓	↓↓↓	Dissociative anaesthesia
Cerebral blood flow	↓↓	↓↓	↑↑
Pain sensation	Antanalgesia	No change	Profound analgesia
Hallucinations	None	None	Present
Effect on RS			
Minute ventilation	↓	↓↓	↔
Bronchodilatation	Can precipitate bronchospasm	No effect	Bronchodilator
Airway reflexes	Not blunted	Blunted	Maintained
Effect on CVS			
Myocardial contractility	↓	↓	↑↑
Heart rate	↑	↑	↑↑
Blood pressure	↓	↓↓	↑↑
Arrhythmias	↔	↔	↔
Muscle tone	↓	↓	↑
Intraocular pressure	↓	↓	↑

ETOMIDATE

- Etomidate is a rapidly acting intravenous anaesthetic agent with a short duration of action of 3–5 minutes.
- It is a **very cardiostable** agent and is used to induce anaesthesia in cardiac patients and in haemodynamically unstable patients.
- However, continuous infusions are not advisable as it is known to depress synthesis of cortisol by the adrenal gland and impair response to ACTH.
- It is used in a dose of 0.2–0.3 mg/kg IV.

Adverse Effects

1. Adrenocortical suppression when used as infusion
2. Excitatory phenomena: Involuntary movements, cough
3. Pain on injection and venous thrombosis
4. Nausea and vomiting

KETAMINE HYDROCHLORIDE

Ketamine differs from other intravenous anaesthetic agents in many respects and produces dissociative anaesthesia, rather than generalised depression of the central nervous system. It is used in a dose of 1–2 mg/ kg IV or 4–5 mg/kg IM.

Clinical Effects

CNS

- It induces anaesthesia within 30–60 seconds of intravenous injection and lasts for 10–20 minutes. It is effective within 3–4 minutes of intramuscular injection and lasts for 15–25 minutes.
- It produces anaesthesia by dissociating the cerebral cortex from the limbic system.
- It is a potent analgesic.
- It increases cerebral blood flow and intracranial pressure.

CVS

The heart rate, blood pressure and cardiac output increase.

RS

- Respiration is usually well-maintained with ketamine although transient apnoea may occur occasionally.
- Ketamine is a good **bronchodilator**.

Skeletal muscle

There is increased muscle tone. Some spontaneous and involuntary movements may occur.

GIT

Increased salivation can occur and can be prevented by using anticholinergic agents.

Eye

Intraocular pressure increases.

Uterus and placenta

It readily crosses the placental barrier and hence should be given in lower doses in pregnant patients.

Adverse Effects

- Emergence delirium
- Hypertension and tachycardia
- Increased intracranial pressure
- Vivid and unpleasant hallucinations are known with ketamine and can be prevented by prior injections of benzodiazepines.

Uses

- Patients in severe hypotension, shock
- Paediatric anaesthesia
- Analgesia and sedation
- Bronchial asthma
- **Difficult locations:** Accident sites, war casualties.

PHYSIOLOGY OF NEUROMUSCULAR JUNCTION

When a nerve impulse arrives at the neuromuscular junction through the motor neuron, acetylcholine (ACh) molecules are liberated from the nerve endings into the junctional cleft. Acetylcholine molecules act as neurotransmitters by interacting with the **nicotinic ACh receptors** on the postjunctional muscle membrane at the motor end plates. This induces the opening of ionic channel of the receptor to allow ionic (sodium, calcium) flux into the muscle. The sudden influx of sodium results in depolarisation and muscle contraction.

Acetylcholine Receptor

The acetylcholine receptor is flower-shaped with five petal-like structures. These five subunits are named $\alpha(2)$, $\beta(1)$, $\varepsilon(1)$ and $\delta(1)$. Each alpha subunit must be occupied by an acetylcholine molecule to open the channel. This acetylcholine receptor at the neuromuscular junction is nicotinic in nature and thus different from those in the rest of the body.

MUSCLE RELAXANTS

These are drugs that interfere with the combination of acetylcholine molecules with their receptors. These block neuromuscular transmission and cause relaxation of the muscle resulting in muscle paralysis.

Neuromuscular blockers are of two types: **Depolarising** and **nondepolarising muscle relaxants**.

DEPOLARISING MUSCLE RELAXANTS (SUCCINYLCHOLINE)

It is the only depolarising muscle relaxant in clinical use. It has a molecular structure similar to acetylcholine. It combines with the alpha subunit of the ACh receptor and produces muscle contraction. However, unlike acetylcholine, it has a prolonged action. Continued depolarisation of a muscle results in **accommodation blockade** and the muscle relaxes.

Dose: 1–1.5 mg/kg intravenously.

Onset of action: Within 60 seconds.

Duration of action: 3–5 minutes.

Metabolism: By plasma cholinesterase.

Uses

Succinylcholine is the only muscle relaxant which has the **shortest time to onset of action** (60 seconds) **and shortest duration of action** (3–5 minutes). It is used:

- To facilitate endotracheal intubation in 'full-stomach' patients.
- It is useful in patients with difficult airway because it gives very good relaxation to facilitate intubation but if intubation fails, the patient is likely to resume spontaneous breathing early and hypoxic brain injury may be avoided.
- To maintain paralysis for short procedures.

Adverse Effects

- **Muscle pains:** The initial depolarisation that occurs due to succinylcholine causes uncoordinated contraction (fasciculations) of different groups of muscle fibres. This can cause severe muscle pain postoperatively.
- **Bradycardia,** especially if a second dose of succinylcholine is given. It is easily avoided by pretreatment with atropine.
- **Hyperkalaemia** in patients with renal failure, burns, massive crush injury, etc.
- **Increase in intracranial pressure**
- **Increase in intraocular pressure**
- **Prolonged action** in patients deficient in pseudocholinesterase (plasma cholinesterase). This occurs as a genetic problem in a small number of patients but may be an acquired problem as in severe liver disease.
- **Malignant hyperthermia** is a disorder that is unique and life-threatening precipitated by exposure to **inhalation anaesthetics and succinylcholine** in susceptible patients. In malignant hyperthermia, the metabolic rate of muscle cells is increased tremendously due to a defective **ryanodine** receptor which is necessary for **reuptake of calcium** after a depolarisation.

Those with a family history of anaesthetic mishaps, neuromuscular diseases such as muscular dystrophy may be susceptible to this disorder and succinylcholine is best avoided in these patients. It is not always possible to identify latent muscular dystrophies in infants and children. Administration of succinylcholine in these patients can be disastrous. Hence, the use of succinylcholine should be avoided in children less than 2 years unless an indication such as a full stomach exists. Even then, rocuronium may be considered as an alternative.

NONDEPOLARISING MUSCLE RELAXANTS

Pancuronium, vecuronium, rocuronium, atracurium and cisatracurium are drugs belonging to this group in clinical use. The nondepolarising muscle relaxants combine with the ACh receptors but do not have any intrinsic effect on the muscle. They cause muscle paralysis by preventing the ACh molecules that are released from the nerve terminal from combining with the ACh receptors on the postsynaptic membrane and producing their action (competitive inhibition). Even if one alpha subunit is combined with a molecule of nondepolarising muscle relaxant, the muscle cannot contract in response to a nerve impulse and gets paralysed. The muscle regains its power when the muscle relaxant gets metabolised.

The nondepolarising muscle relaxants can be classified according to their duration of action as follows:

- **Short-acting (10–20 min):** Mivacurium
- **Intermediate-acting (20–30 min):** Atracurium, vecuronium and rocuronium
- **Long-acting (>45 min):** d-Tubocurarine and pancuronium.

Uses

1. To facilitate endotracheal intubation
2. To maintain paralysis during anaesthesia and in the ICU.

REVERSAL OF NEUROMUSCULAR BLOCKADE

At the end of anaesthesia, the muscle relaxation produced by the nondepolarising muscle relaxant is usually reversed. This is to ensure good recovery of muscle power to maintain airway and respiration.

ACh molecules are broken down by cholinesterases. Anticholinesterases such as neostigmine block the action of cholinesterase, thus allowing ACh molecules to accumulate in the neuromuscular junction. The block produced by the nondepolarising muscle relaxants is competitive. When ACh molecules increase in number due to the action of the anticholinesterase, and non-depolarising muscle relaxant molecules decrease in number due to metabolism, muscle power returns. **Neostigmine** is the only anticholinesterase in clinical use. Its dose is 0.05 mg/kg body weight. Neostigmine increases the amount of ACh not only at the neuromuscular junction but also in the entire body. It can cause the muscarinic effects of ACh such as bradycardia, bronchoconstriction, etc. Hence, neostigmine is always combined with atropine (0.025 mg/kg) or glycopyrrolate (0.01 mg/kg) to counter the muscarinic effects.

Recovery from Neuromuscular Blockade

Clinical indicators

- Opening of eyes without furrowing of forehead
- Good handgrip
- Raising arms against gravity
- Good cough
- Ability to lift head against gravity (sustained head-lift) for at least five seconds.
- Good cough and sustained head-lift are reliable indicators of adequate recovery, whereas simple opening of eyes and handgrip may still be associated with incomplete recovery.

Objective criteria

The amount of neuromuscular blockade can be checked using a peripheral nerve stimulator. The ulnar nerve is stimulated and the response of the adductor pollicis muscle is checked. If good muscle contractions are seen in response to the nerve stimulation, the muscle power is said to have returned. Similarly, posterior tibial nerve and facial nerve may also be used to monitor neuromuscular junction.

The patient is allowed to breathe spontaneously and his trachea extubated only when there is clinical evidence of complete recovery from neuromuscular blockade. If there is inadequate recovery of muscle power, the patient may need to be ventilated artificially till muscle power is normal.

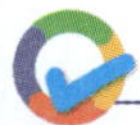

Multiple Choice Questions

1. With the mouth wide open and tongue protruded in a patient in sitting position, if only soft and hard palate are seen, his airway is classified as Mallampati class:

A. I B. II
C. III D. IV

2. The following period is adequate fasting before administration of anaesthesia after taking a glass of cow's milk:

A. 2 hours
B. 4 hours
C. 6 hours
D. 8 hours

3. American Society of anaesthesiologists physical status (ASA–PS) 6 would be appropriate to describe the following patient:

A. Patient with moderately controlled diabetes mellitus on insulin
B. Patient posted for surgery for 6 times before
C. Patient in severe hypovolaemic shock undergoing fluid resuscitation
D. Brain dead patient for organ donation

4. The following is an ideal anaesthetic agent for inhalation induction:

A. Isoflurane
B. Sevoflurane
C. Desflurane
D. Diethyl ether

5. Succinylcholine is contraindicated in all of the following *except*:

A. Full stomach
B. Raised intracranial pressure
C. Open eye injury
D. Crush injury

6. The following inhalation anaesthetic requires a heated vaporiser:

A. Isoflurane B. Sevoflurane
C. Desflurane D. Diethyl ether

7. The following anaesthetic can be given by nasal, intramuscular and intravenous routes for induction of anaesthesia:

A. Thiopentone B. Ketamine
C. Etomidate D. Propofol

8. The following intravenous anaesthetic is useful in status asthmaticus for its bronchodilatory effect:

A. Thiopentone
B. Ketamine
C. Etomidate
D. Propofol

9. The following intravenous anaesthetic produces dissociative anaesthesia:

A. Thiopentone B. Ketamine
C. Etomidate D. Propofol

10. The following local anaesthetic is also Class 1b antiarrhythmic agent:

A. Lignocaine B. Bupivacaine
C. Prilocaine D. Cocaine

11. The following local anaesthetic is very cardio-toxic:

A. Lignocaine B. Bupivacaine
C. Prilocaine D. Ropivacaine

12. The following anaesthetic is described as an antanalgesic:

A. Thiopentone B. Ketamine
C. Etomidate D. Propofol

13. The following drug is absolutely contraindicated in acute intermittent porphyria:

A. Thiopentone B. Ketamine
C. Etomidate D. Propofol

14. The following muscle relaxant produces 'accommodation blockade':

A. Succinylcholine B. Atracurium
C. Vecuronium D. Tubocurarine

15. The gold standard for confirmation of endotracheal tube position is:

A. Presence of bilateral air entry
B. Absent breath sounds in the epigastrium
C. A square wave capnogram
D. Bilateral visible chest rise

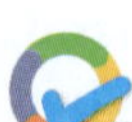

Answers

1. C	2. C	3. D	4. A	5. A	6. C	7. B	8. B	9. B	10. A
11. B	12. A	13. A	14. A	15. C					

CHAPTER

65

Organ Transplantation

- **Principles of Transplantation**
  - Pathophysiology
  - Major histocompatibility complex
  - Graft rejection
- **Liver Transplantation**
  - Indications
  - Contraindications
  - Donor criteria
  - MELD score
  - Types
  - Procedures
- **Renal Transplantation**
  - Donor
  - Procedures
  - Postoperative management
  - Complications
- **Small Bowel Transplant**
  - Indications
  - Contraindications
  - Recipient evaluation
  - Procedures
  - Complications
- **Islet Cell Transplantation**
  - Indications
  - Contraindications
  - Islet cell preparation
  - Technique
  - Complications
- **Drugs used for Immunosuppression**

PRINCIPLES OF TRANSPLANTATION

Introduction

For end stage renal or liver disease, transplantation is the best answer as of today. Over 25,000 transplantations are performed annually for different conditions and more than 100,000 patients are awaiting an organ for kidney, liver or other organs. The acceptance of an organ depends often on the beliefs and decisions related to the country, race and religion. In certain countries, living donor transplantation, even though risky, is the only realistic organ donation method, greatly limiting the potential for transplantation of organs from cadaver. Surgical advances have permitted successful transplantation of lung, pancreas and intestine from living donors. Because of the limited supply, use of living donors may be the only means to achieve timely kidney or liver transplantation as it is happening in India. First let us study the principles and pathophysiology of organ transplant.

Competency

SU13.1: Describe the immunological basis of organ transplantation.

Pathophysiology of Organ Transplant

Generally the word "immunity" is used in the context of infections. "Immunity" implies defense against infections. Immunity is of two types, namely:

1. Innate immunity
2. Adaptive or acquired immunity

Innate immunity: Important components of innate immunity are:

- Phagocytic neutrophils
- Natural killer cells (NK cells)
- Circulating plasma proteins mainly complements.

Adaptive immunity: Adaptive immunity is normally quiescent but is pressed into action by the presence of suitable stimulus such as microbes. Components of adaptive immunity are lymphocytes and their products. Adaptive immunity may be

- Humoral immunity—mediated by antibodies which are synthesised by B-lymphocytes (B cells). They offer protection against extracellular microbes.
- Cell mediated immunity—mediated by T-lymphocytes (T cells). T cells may be CD4 T cells which indirectly facilitate killing of microbes by macrophages or CD8 T cells which directly kill microbes. CD8 T cells are also called cytotoxic T cells.

Major Histocompatibility Complex (MHC)

The MHC complex is also known as human leucocyte antigen (HLA) complex. It consists of a cluster of genes located on chromosome 6. MHC gene products are displayed on the cell surface to the notice of circulating T cells. Such MHC gene products fall into two categories.

1. Class 1 MHC molecules—which display peptides synthesised within the cytoplasm of the respective cell. Class 1 MHC molecules are present in all cells.
2. Class 2 MHC molecules—which display antigens synthesised outside the cell. Class 2 MHC molecules are mainly expressed in antigen processing cells (APCs) or dendritic cells.

Role of MHC in Organ Transplant

Following an allograft, the host cells recognise the foreign nature of the graft by two mechanisms.

1. Direct recognition—the T cells recognise the foreign class 1 MHC because of immunologic cross reaction. Subsequently cytotoxic T cells are activated which kill the graft cells.
2. Indirect recognition—the host APCs present the antigens in the graft (transplant) in class 2 MHC. This activates T cells which secrete cytokines, induce inflammation and damage the graft.

Towards Improving Graft Survival

- ABO blood group antigens are expressed in all cells and are not just by RBCs. ABO incompatibility results in hyperacute rejection of graft. Hence, it is recommended to ensure ABO compatibility.
- Better HLA matching improves transplant outcomes. This is particularly relevant in live donor kidney transplant. However, HLA matching is not done in heart, lung and liver transplants as the urgency of transplant requirement overweighs the benefits of HLA matching. Also in these situations other factors such as size of the graft assume more practical significance.

Graft Rejection

Based on the timing and mediators of rejection, graft rejection may be classified as follows:

1. **Hyperacute rejection**
   - Occurs within minutes to days following transplant
   - Mediated by preformed antibodies
   - Untreatable but preventable
   - Cross-matching prevents hyperacute rejection
   - Methods of cross-matching include—lymphocytotoxic assay, flow cytometric technique, bead-based screening assays, panel-reactive antibody assay.
2. **Acute rejection**
   - Occurs in weeks to months following transplant
   - Mediated by T cells to a great extent and B cells to a lesser extent.
   - Accordingly they are termed T cell-mediated rejection (TCMR) or antibody mediated rejection (ABMR).
   - Immune suppression helps to overcome acute rejection
3. **Chronic rejection**
   - Most common cause of long-term allograft loss
   - Occurs over months to years following transplant
   - Involves both T cells and B cells
   - Examples for chronic graft rejection—interstitial fibrosis, tubular atrophy and chronic allograft nephropathy in renal transplant, vanishing bile duct syndrome in liver transplant and bronchiolitis obliterans in lung transplant.

LIVER TRANSPLANTATION

Introduction

Liver transplantation is a lifesaving procedure for patients who have chronic end-stage liver disease and acute liver failure (ALF) when there are no alternative treatment options. In 1963, Dr Thomas Starzl performed the first three human liver transplantations at the University of Colorado but patient suffered from biliary atresia, had coagulopathy and did not survive surgery. Introduction to cyclosporine for immunosuppression in solid organ transplantation revolutionised the liver transplantation surgery.

Indications for Liver Transplant

1. **Fulminant hepatic failure:** It is acute onset of liver failure in the absence of pre-existing liver disease. Here coagulopathy sets in within 8 weeks of onset of jaundice. Causes are acetaminophen overdose and hepatitis B infection in Asia. If left untreated, patients most often succumb to coma due to cerebral oedema.
2. **Hepatitis C**: Chronic hepatitis C is the commonest indication for liver transplant in the West. However, hepatitis C recurs even after liver transplantation because the virus persists in the extrahepatic tissues. Pre-transplant and post-transplant treatment with interferon and ribavirin can potentially improve the outcome in these patients.
3. Hepatitis B

4. Primary biliary cirrhosis
5. Primary sclerosing cholangitis
6. Alcoholic liver disease (Figs 65.1 and 65.2)
7. Nonalcoholic steatohepatitis (NASH)
8. Biliary atresia—it is the commonest indication for liver transplant in the paediatric age group.
9. **Hepatocellular carcinoma:** Theoretically liver transplant should offer the best chance of cure in HCC but there is always the risk of recurrence of HCC following transplant. Many transplant centres follow "Milan criteria" to decide the feasibility of liver transplant in HCC, which says that liver transplant can be considered in HCC when there is a single nodule of <5 cm or there are fewer than 3 nodules, the largest of which is measuring <3 cm. Those who follow the "**Milan criteria**" believe that the recurrence of HCC is very low if the criteria are strictly adhered to.

Contraindications for Liver Transplant

1. Systemic infections other than liver infections
2. Pulmonary manifestations of chronic liver disease
3. Inability to abstain from alcohol when liver transplantation is being contemplated for alcoholic liver disease.
4. Lack of commitment to immunosuppressive drugs
5. Metastatic HCC

Following are **not contraindications** for liver transplantation:

- Failure of other organs in addition to liver, e.g. amyloidosis—here combined liver and kidney transplants can be undertaken.
- HIV infection
- Portal vein thrombosis

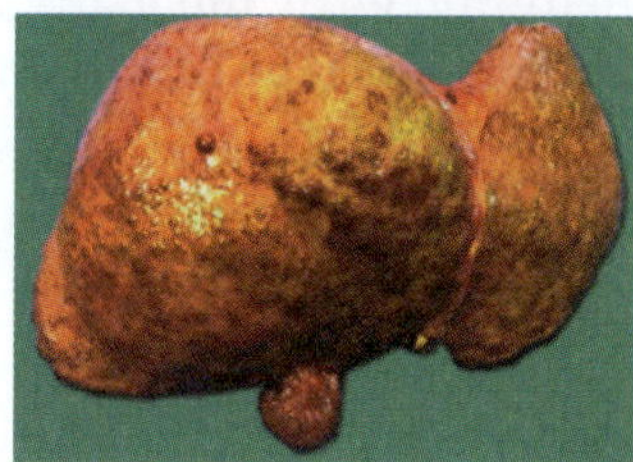

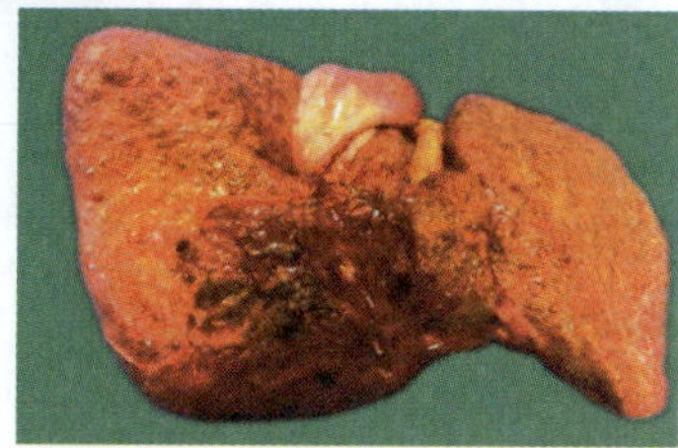

Figs 65.1 and 65.2: Cirrhotic liver which was removed (*Courtesy:* Dr Sachidananda N, hepatobiliary and liver transplant surgeon, Prof of Surgery, Akash Institute of Medical Sciences and Research, Devanahalli, Bangalore)

Donor Criteria for Liver Transplantation

Donors for liver transplant can be deceased donors or live donors. The outcomes are better with deceased donors, but the limitation is shortage of such donors. The ideal donor should be young and otherwise healthy. The donor factors associated with increased risk are older age, a fatty infiltration and use of split liver from these donors. Two categories of donors who are increasingly considered although not ideal are:

- **Older donors:** If liver from older donors are used for hepatitis C recipients, there is an increased risk of development of cirrhosis in the transplanted liver.
- **Donor after cardiac death:** These are donors who do not meet brain death criteria but become donors once life support is taken off. Liver from such donors can be considered for transplant with cut off time of 30 minutes.

Model for End-stage Liver Disease (MELD Score)

Candidates needing liver transplant far outnumber the available donors. Therefore, candidates needing liver transplant are listed in the transplant register in organ transplant programmes. The order in which candidates are placed in the waiting list for liver transplant is determined by MELD formula. MELD formula incorporates three components, namely—creatinine, bilirubin and INR. These components provide an objective assessment of severity of liver disease.

MELD score =

[0.957 × Ln creatinine (mg/dl)] +
[0.378 × Ln bilirubin (mg/dl)] +
[1.120 × Ln INR]

In the waiting list, candidates with higher MELD score come first. MELD score is nowadays preferred to Child-Pugh's score for being more objective.

Competency

SU13.2.2: Enumerate indications, describe surgical principles, management of organ transplantation.

Types of Liver Transplantation

1. **Conventional liver transplant:** This is performed to replace the diseased liver with a healthy liver from a deceased donor.
2. **Expanded criteria donor (ECD):** A diseased donor over the age of 60 with mild liver abnormalities. The term "expanded" is used because an expansion of the donor pool is considered to increase transplantation. With an ECD liver, the waiting time may be shorter—not done in India.
3. **Living donor liver transplantation (LDLT):** A procedure in which a healthy, living person donates

a portion of his or her liver to another person. Finding a living donor match shortens waiting time, increases long-term transplant success and gives the flexibility of scheduling the date of surgery.

4. **Split liver transplant:** A deceased donor liver is split into two functioning units, which are used for transplantation to a child (left lobe) and an adult (right lobe).
5. **Combined organ transplant:** A person may receive more than one organ during the same transplant procedure such as liver and kidney or liver and heart. This may be recommended for patients who are experiencing multiple organ failure.

Technical Aspects of Liver Transplantation

More often the donor in liver transplant is deceased. However, with severe shortage of donors, live donor liver transplants are becoming common. The donor liver transplant is placed in its native position in the abdomen of recipient after removing the diseased liver. Hence, the term "Orthotopic liver transplant" is used. (This may be compared with kidney transplant where the transplanted kidney is placed in the iliac fossa, thereby deriving the term heterotopic transplant.) Sometimes, the donor liver is split and the left liver is used for a paediatric recipient and the right liver is used for an adult recipient. Such a liver transplant is termed "split liver transplant". A few operative steps in the back table where the donor live is prepared for transplantation is given in Key Box 65.1.

Key Box 65.1

Key Points in the Back Table Surgery

1. Dissection and removal of extra tissue such as diaphragm, adrenal gland, pancreatic, tissue, etc.
2. Preparation of cuffs of the suprahepatic and infrahepatic vena cava, cleaning of the portal vein and artery, and inspection of the bile duct.
3. Verification of secure ligatures on small retrohepatic caval, portal vein and hepatic arterial branches.
4. Confirm the continuity and integrity of all major structures that must be anastomosed to the companion recipient structures.

Competency

SU13.2.1: Describe the principles of immunosuppresive therapy.

Immunosuppression after Liver Transplantation

Chronic rejection is uncommon following liver transplantation. The need for immunosuppression decreases over time. Combination of calcineurin inhibitors (tacrolimus, cyclosporin), steroids (methylprednisolone) and antiproliferative agents (mycophenolate mofetil) are used. In the context of liver transplantation sirolimus deserves a special mention:

- It has antineoplastic activity, hence, is an attractive option in HCC.
- It delays wound healing.
- It is associated with hepatic artery thrombosis.

Complications of Liver Transplantation

1. Primary non-function—these patients need retransplant.
2. Hepatic artery thrombosis—these patients need early thrombectomy or retransplant.
3. Portal vein thrombosis
4. Bile duct leak and stricture
5. Other complications—bleeding, coagulopathy

Future Trends

Hepatocyte transplantation: In chronic liver diseases due to specific enzyme deficiencies like Crigler-Najjar syndrome, hepatocytes or stem cell transplant seems logical. With only a few cells needed to restore functioning of liver, this concept makes sense as it avoids the morbidity and mortality of a major surgical procedure.

RENAL TRANSPLANTATION

Preparation for Transplantation

Recipient is prepared by haemodialysis. It also enhances the chances of success of a transplant.

Donors: Two Sources

A. Cadaver kidney is obtained from 'brain dead' patients who are still living with mechanical ventilatory support. Consent should be taken from patient's relatives.

B. Living

Living related

Living non-related

Criteria of an Ideal Donor

1. Less than 60 years of age
2. No previous renal disease
3. No diabetes
4. No hypertension
5. Adequate renal perfusion 50 ml/hour urine output is necessary.
6. No systemic infections such as hepatitis B, C, HIV infection.
7. No malignancy

Living Related Donors

- An identical twin is ideal
- Father or mother
- Son or daughter
- Brother or sister

Tests Done before Transplantation

- Blood group ABO compatibility
- Biochemical investigations
- Complete blood picture
- Renal function tests
- Rule out: Diabetes, hypertension, hepatitis B infection, hepatitis C infection, HIV.
- Bilateral renal angiography to study vascular pattern. Tissue typing.

Pearls of Wisdom

Recipient contraindication to renal transplantation is if the recipient is suffering from diseases such as heart disease or malignancy (advanced), which compromises his survival.

Competency

SU13.2.2: Enumerate indications, describe surgical principles, management of organ transplantation.

Operation Technique

Donor Operation

1. **Living related donor:** Donor nephrectomy with preservation of as much length of the artery, vein and ureter.
2. **Cadaver donor:** The donor kidney is perfused with icy perfusion fluid and removed along with vena cava and aorta, and packed in plastic bags surrounded by ice in an insulated box. It can be stored like this for 72 hours.

Perfusion fluid: It has high concentration of potassium (80 mmol/l) and high osmolarity (400 mOsm/kg). This is used during transplant anastomosis.

Recipient operation: Kidney is transplanted in the right iliac fossa by anastomosing renal artery to internal iliac artery and renal vein to external iliac vein. Ureter is implanted in the bladder (Figs 65.3 to 65.5).

Postoperative Management

1. **Immunosuppression:** Cyclosporin A is given alone or in combination with low doses of azathioprine and steroids.
2. **Fluid balance:** Aim to maintain urinary output at the rate of 20 ml/hour. Even an anephric patient needs 500 ml of fluid/day to replace insensible loss. CVP is ideal for management of fluids in the postoperative period.
3. **Postoperative oliguria:** Monitoring of renal function—serum creatinine should drop by 50% in 48 hours post-transplant period.

Causes

a. **Acute tubular necrosis (ATN):** Minimal ATN is common due to short ischaemic time. Hence, oliguria phase may be a few hours.

b. **Rejection:** More likely on the 5th day. Twice weekly DTPA (diethyl triamine penta-acetic acid) isotope renography and gamma camera scan of the kidney confirms perfusion of the kidney when oliguria is present. Percutaneous needle biopsy can confirm the rejection.

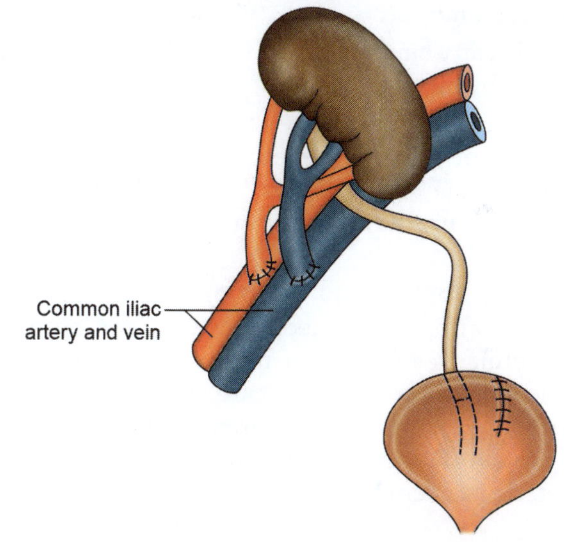

Fig. 65.3: Diagrammatic representation of renal transplantation

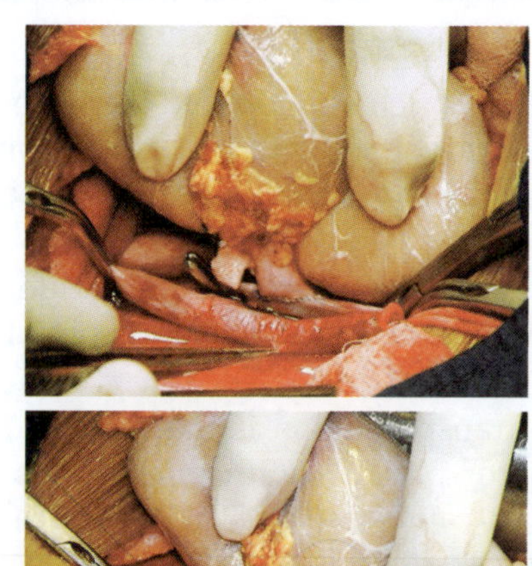

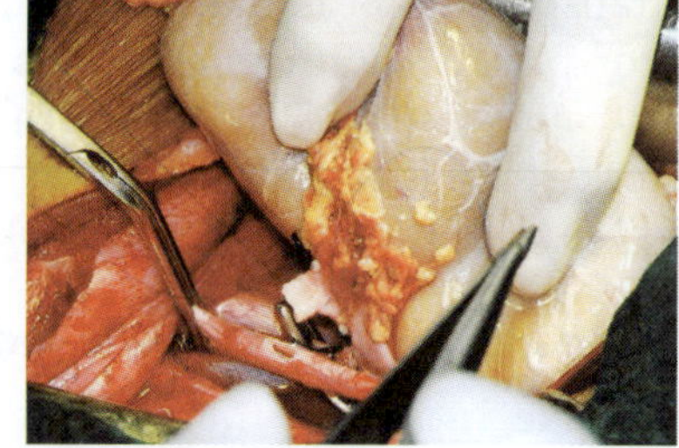

Figs 65.4 and 65.5: Renal artery and renal vein are ready to be sutured to common iliac artery and vein during renal transplantation (*Courtesy:* Dr Arun Chawla, Head Department of Urology, KMC Manipal)

Treatment of Rejection

1. **Acute rejection:** Within 3 months, this responds to high doses of intravenous steroids. 90 mg methylprednisolone IV/day × 3 days.
2. **Chronic rejection** involves the vascular element. It does not respond to steroids.

Surgical Complications

1. **Haemorrhage** manifests as oliguria, hypotension. Wound should be re-explored and bleeding vessels should be ligated.
2. **Renal artery thrombosis** results in nonfunctioning of the transplanted kidney. It can be diagnosed by ultrasonogram and isotope studies. This is treated by nephrectomy.
3. **Renal artery stenosis** can develop later. It should be treated by an angioplasty.
4. **Lymphocoele** can develop due to perivascular dissection and increased flow of lymph. Such lymphocoele can lead to ureteric obstruction. Small collection needs to be observed, large ones need drainage.
5. **Ureteric obstruction** or urinary leakage due to disruption of ureteroneocystostomy can be due to ischaemia or necrosis of the distal ureter. During donor nephrocystostomy, care should be taken not to remove too much of periureteric tissues and avoid too much dissection in the renal hilum to prevent ureteric ischaemia.

SMALL BOWEL TRANSPLANT

Introduction

- Small bowel is rich in lymphoid tissue and the large mucosal surface area with major histocompatibility antigens. This definitely evokes a fight between graft and host.
- Small bowel is colonised by a multitude of bacteria and other micro-organisms. This is one of the reasons for failure.
- Intestinal transplantation is an established treatment modality for patients with intestinal failure. Any patient who cannot meet >50% of their calorie needs via the enteric route is considered to have intestinal failure and they require intestinal transplantation.

Common Causes for Intestinal Failure: Indications

- **Common cause in adults:** Massive resection of intestine for SMA/SMV thrombosis, Crohn's disease, radiation injury or trauma. After massive small intestine resection, one has to do intestinal transplantation within fifteen days and if it is not possible for any reason, then wait for at least four to six weeks, allow for the infection/inflammation to settle before performing intestinal transplantation.
- **Common cause in children:** Necrotizing enterocolitis, long segment intestinal atresia, midgut volvulus.
- **Uncommon causes in children:** Gastroschisis, motility disorders, microvillous inclusion disease, tufting enteropathy. Even though these children have full length of intestine, it is not functional and will not allow them to eat normal food and grow.

Contraindications

Lack of central venous access, presence of active infection, aggressive malignancy, multisystem organ failure, cerebral oedema, and HIV are contraindications for intestinal transplantation.

Managing Patients with Intestinal Failure

- It is ideal to maintain continuity of the intestine, use the remaining length to its maximum capacity. If the colon along with ileocecal valve is intact, one may attempt at rehabilitating the intestine, allow it to adapt. Successful intestinal rehabilitation is more often successful in children compared to adults.
- Most of these patients need total parenteral nutrition to survive and meet their calorie requirement.

Managing Total Parenteral Nutrition (TPN)

- **Placing of lines:** Tunneled lines (Hickman's line) placed in the neck or upper extremity are preferred for long-term TPN. These lines carry less risk of infection and it can be used for home TPN.
- **The calorie requirements** are calculated based on standard formula. For weight reduction, 20 to 25 cal/kg/day for weight maintenance 25 to 30 kcal/kg/day and for weight gaining 30 to 35 kcal/kg/day. Of these calories 60% must be met with carbohydrates, 30% with fat and 10% with proteins. Limiting lipids to less than 2 gm/kg/day, and will help protect liver from cholestasis. Giving lipids three days a week will also help achieve this goal. For long-term TPN one has to pay attention to micro-nutrients as well and have replace vitamins and selenium, manganese, chromium, iodine on regular basis. Iron stores are most often enough for a few months and iron injections will be needed only when TPN is continued for more than six months.
- Giving these calories in limited volume is a challenge in children, but in adults it is usually not a problem. Long-term TPN must be managed by dedicated physician along with dietician. Giving dextrose, amino acids and lipids separately will not give rise to acid–base balance problems in the short term, but

in the long run patients will develop acidosis and other deficiencies. It is best to custom prepare the TPN for those who need long-term TPN.

Managing Central Line Infections

- When there is suspected central line related infection, tendency is to remove the line and give appropriate antibiotics.
- In patients with short gut and those who are dependent on TPN the central venous accesses are precious and one has to make attempts to save them. Repeated access to these central access will lead to stenosis/ thrombosis of the veins and we loose those venous accesses. Hence we usually treat them for the infection while we retain the lines.
- Remove them only when it is absolutely necessary or when they have repeated fungal infections.

Pretransplant Evaluation of the Recipient

The team includes transplant surgeon, gastroenterologist, social worker, nutritionist, psychologist and financial co-ordinator, infectious disease specialist, cardiologist and pulmonologist.

Investigations

- Ultrasound of liver and central veins
- Serology tests: CMV, EBV, HIV, HBsAg, anti-HCV
- Blood group, HLA typing
- Hypercoagulable status and liver biopsy—if indicated
- Cardiopulmonary evaluation

Donor Selection

- Haemodynamically stable, heart beating brain dead donor with no intestinal pathology is preferred.
- CMV positive donors are accepted for CMV positive recipients.

The Donor Procurement

- It is similar to procurement of the liver. A long midline incision from suprasternal notch to pubic-symphysis is made and the concerned teams assess their concerned organs. Intestine is assessed for any injury. The contents are milked either into the stomach or large intestine without creating any serosal tears. SMA and portal veins are dissected and looped at their origin using vessel loops.
- Organs are preserved in university of Wisconsin solution or HTK (custodial) solution. Cold ischaemia time is kept to minimum by co-ordinating timing of the donor operation with the recipient's surgery team. Acceptable cold ischaemia time for small intestine is less than 12 hours.

Types and Operative Procedure

Three primary procedures

1. Isolated transplantation of the small intestine (with or without the portion of the right colon with the ileocaecal valve).
2. Combined transplantation of the intestine and liver as separate grafts.
3. Multivisceral transplantation (MVT), which is the simultaneous transplantation of a composite graft including the liver, stomach, duodenum, pancreas, and small intestine.

Details (Figs 65.6 to 65.13)

1. **Isolated intestinal transplantation** is performed for patients with isolated intestinal failure. If they have liver failure also then they would require multivisceral transplant (combined liver, intestine along with pancreas in one cluster).
   - The incision is carefully planned keeping in mind the previous surgery, stoma and the need to create new stoma. The arterial flow is usually provided from infra-renal aorta (via a conduit) and venous outflow to the portal vein.
   - In patients with mesenteric vein thrombus, it is provided to inferior vena cava. The portal outflow is preferred because it provides growth factors to liver for optimal hepatocyte function.
   - Intestine continuity is maintained by enteroenterostomy performed in side to side fashion (there may be size discrepancy) in four layers.
   - Ileostomy, feeding jejunostomy and venting gastrostomy may also be performed if needed. Stoma (ileostomy) is used to perform biopsy in the early postoperative period to monitor for possible rejection.
   - The abdominal wall closure may be difficult in some patients due to multiple past surgeries, recurrent infection, scar tissue formation and contracted abdominal cavity. In some cases, temporary mesh may be used. In some cases, plastic surgery procedures like flaps may be needed to obtain closure. Some surgeons have used abdominal wall transplantation (from same cad donor) based on inferior epigastric vessels (donor) connected to (rec) femoral or iliac vessels.

Living donor small intestinal transplantation

- It is a way of increasing the donor pool where there is very long waiting time for recipients. A segment of terminal ileum (200 cm for adults and 150 cm for children) is harvested about 20 to 30 cm proximal to ileocaecal valve.
- The donor is left with >60% of the intestine.

PHOTOS OF SMALL BOWEL TRANSPLANTATION

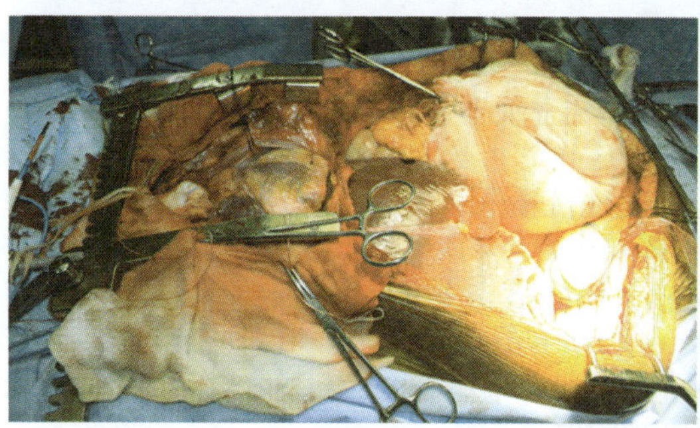

Fig. 65.6: Incision from sternal notch to pubic symphysis, with chest open exposing the thoracic and abdominal organs. Intestine is wrapped in a towel

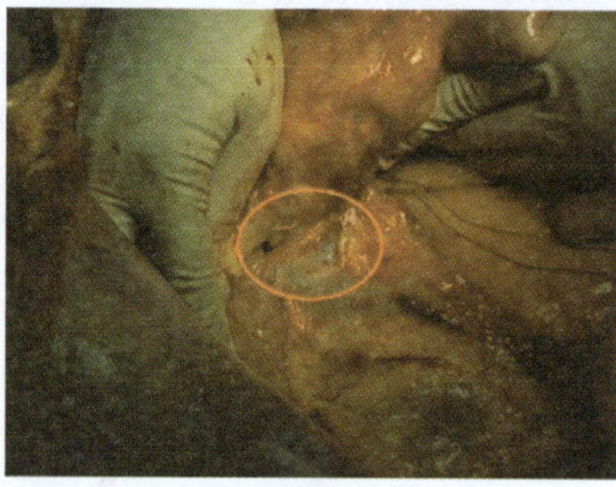

Fig. 65.7: Ascending colon and duodenum are mobilized and moved to left side till left renal vein is identified (red oval). Silk is seen around the IMV. SMA can be felt superior to the left renal vein

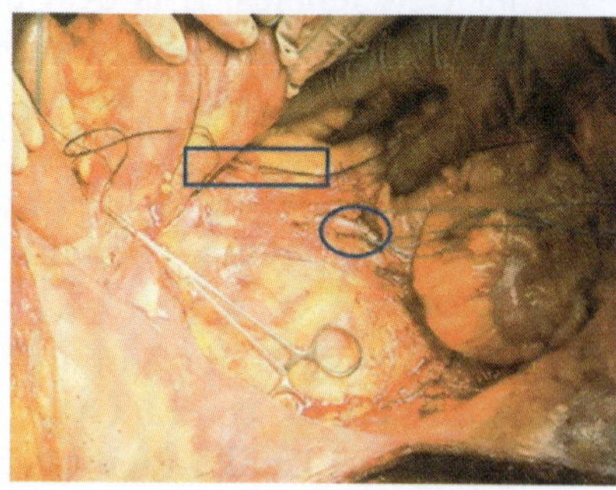

Fig. 65.8: Green suture (ethibond) seen around the infra-renal aorta. Silk sutures are seen around the IMV

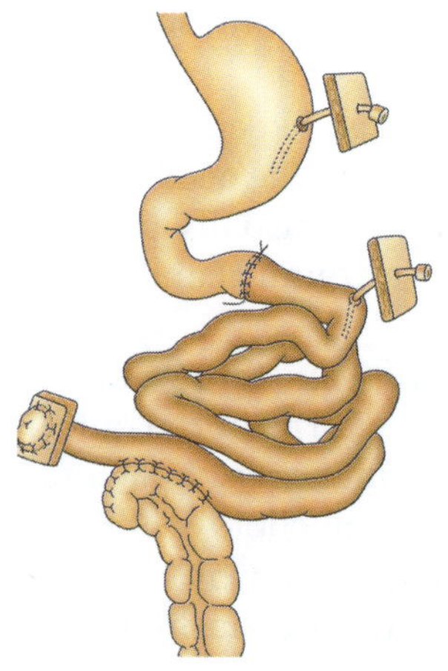

Fig. 65.9: Showing how to maintain intestinal continuity and how the stoma is created to monitor for rejection. Organ drawn in pink is transplanted organ, rest are patients own native organs

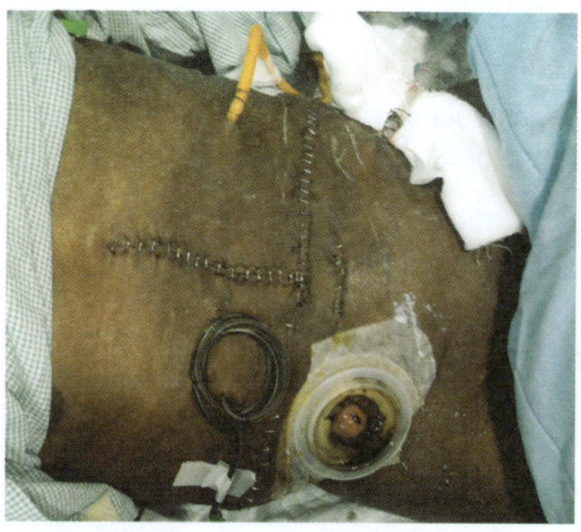

Fig. 65.10: Recipient's abdomen after intestine transplant. Foley is used as venting gastrostomy. Ryles tube is used as feeding jejunostomy. Terminal ileum is brought out as stoma

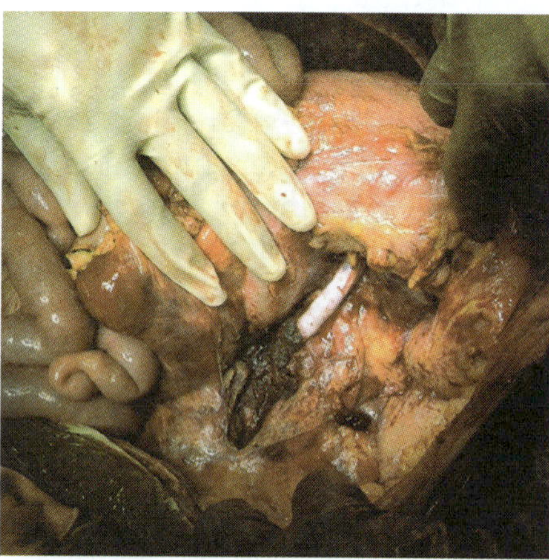

Fig. 65.11: Showing aortic conduit created to provide arterial inflow to intestine

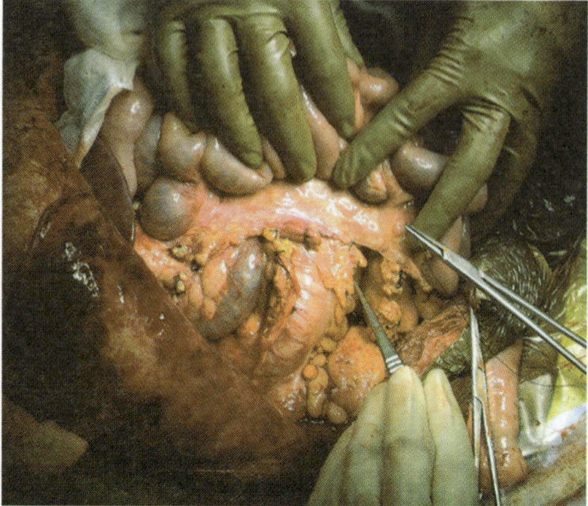

Fig. 65.12: After implanting small intestine, fixing the mesentery to retroperitoneum to avoid volvulus

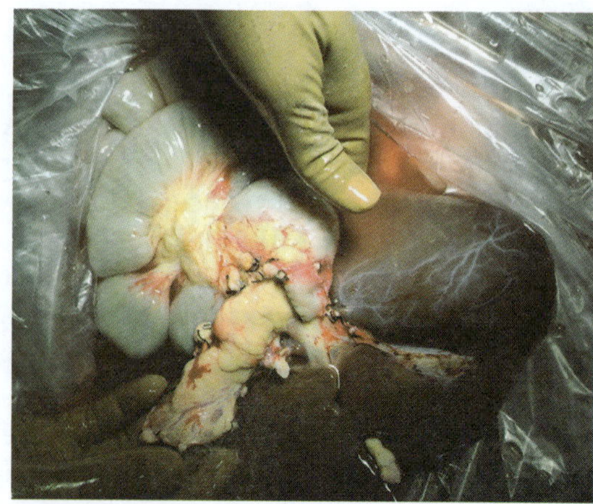

Fig. 65.13: Showing multivisceral organs ready to be implanted

(*Courtesy:* Dr Mahesh Gopa Setty, Consultant Transplant Surgeon,Bengaluru, Karnataka)

2. **Combined transplantation of the intestine and liver**
   - It is indicated when patients have cholestatic jaundice also secondary to TPN and require combined liver and small bowel transplantation.
   - When combined liver and small bowel transplantation is carried out, the two grafts are transplanted *en bloc*.
   - The donor aorta is fashioned into a conduit including the superior mesenteric and coeliac arteries and anastomosed to the recipient aorta.
   - The portal vein anastomosis is similar to that in liver transplantation.
3. **Multivisceral transplantation (MVT)**
   - Multivisceral, also called 'cluster' transplants may be necessary in the case of large desmoid tumours.

Immunosuppression

- Intestinal transplantation is more successful now because of better immunosuppression available.
- Most centers use induction with steroids, antithymocyte globulin or OKT3. Long-term maintenance is achieved with tacrolimus, mycofenolate with or without steroids.

Postoperative Care

Intestine output is monitored carefully. Excessive stoma output may be associated with rejection or CMV infection. They are monitored with intestinal biopsy and blood test respectively. While intestinal motility comes to normal and the anastomosis heal, the patients are given TPN. It may take a few weeks to couple of months for the intestinal function to come back to normal.

Complications

A. **Technical complications:** Encountered are bleeding, thrombosis and anastomotic leaks. These require re-exploration. They are sources of morbidity and mortality. Bleeding is easy to control. If there is thrombosis (incidence <10%) of the graft vessel, it is difficult to salvage it and we may have to take out the transplanted organ.

B. **Rejection**

1. **Acute cellular rejection:** Acute cellular rejection usually occurs within the first year post-transplantation but can occur at any time. Clinically, it can present as diarrhoea, unexplained fever, abdominal pain and/or cramping.
2. **Chronic rejection:** Clinically, these patients may have chronic diarrhoea despite adequate treatment. Patients have an obliterative arteriopathy.

C. **Infection**

1. **Bacterial:** Bacterial infections can manifest as intra-abdominal infection, opportunistic infections, surgical site infections, pneumonia. Pathogenic organisms are: *Escherichia coli, Klebsiella, Enterobacter, Enterococci,* and commonly, polymicrobial infections.
2. **Viral:** Cytomegalovirus (CMV) is a common pathogen post-intestinal transplantation, which often affects the allograft. Treatment with ganciclovir and/or CMV immunoglobulin and rarely, reduction in immunosuppression are methods that are used to minimise graft loss.
3. **EBV (Epstein-Barr virus)** also presents a unique challenge to intestinal transplant recipients because of the higher rates of post-transplantation lymphoproliferative disorder (PTLD) when compared with other solid organ transplant recipients.

D. **GVHD:** Graft-versus-host disease (GVHD) occurs when donor lymphoid cells begin to target recipient tissues, most notably the epithelial cells in the skin and intestine. It is relatively uncommon.

E. **Other complications:** Postoperative haemorrhage, biliary (if liver is also used) thrombosis of vessels resulting in graft loss, bowel anastomosis leak and wound infections.

ISLET CELL TRANSPLANTATION

Introduction

- Type 1 diabetes mellitus, also known as juvenile-onset or insulin-dependent diabetes, is a chronic polygenic autoimmune disorder that has a strong hereditary basis in the human leucocyte antigen system. It results from destruction of pancreatic beta cells in the islets of Langerhans. Beta cells constitute 28–75% of pancreatic islets.
- Percutaneous islet cell transplantation is a minimally invasive cellular replacement therapy. It avoids risk of hypoglycaemia which is one of the major problems of exogenous insulin.

Indications

- Type 1 diabetes mellitus (DM) with disease presence for at least 5 years, absence of endogenous C-peptide secretion.
- Islet cell transplantation may be performed alone, in combination with renal transplantation, or following kidney transplantation. Example: Diabetic patients with imminent or established end-stage renal disease.

Contraindications

- Age less than 18 years or greater than 70 years
- DM duration less than 5 years
- Residual C-peptide secretion (i.e. stimulated C-peptide level: 0.5 ng/dL).
- Proliferative diabetic retinopathy, portal hypertension.
- Active infection (including hepatitis C, hepatitis B, HIV and tuberculosis).

Islet Cell Preparation (Flowchart 65.1)

- After cold perfusion of the abdominal organs, the pancreas, spleen and duodenum is removed *en bloc*. The portal vein is transected at the duodenal border and the common bile duct is transected close to the pancreatic border.
- The organ is packed in a triple-barrier bag with cold preservation solution and stored at 4°C for transportation. The maximum cold ischaemia time is 12 hours.
- The most commonly used preservation solution is University of Wisconsin solution.
- **Obtaining islet cells:** The initial step is infusion of collagenase through the main pancreatic duct; the collagenase is delivered with pressure monitoring aimed at duct distension with minimum leakage of the enzyme. Collagenase cannot digest thick interlobar fibrous tissue. This is achieved by the **Ricordi chamber**. The chamber includes five or six stainless steel balls, which provide mechanical fracture of the fibrous tissue. Thus, it provides effective digestion, dilution and collection of the digested tissue. The purity of the final cell suspension is analysed and the cells are washed and placed in culture media for 12–72 hours in an incubator at 22°–37°C. The isolated islets are then transplanted.

Flowchart 65.1: Islet cell preparation

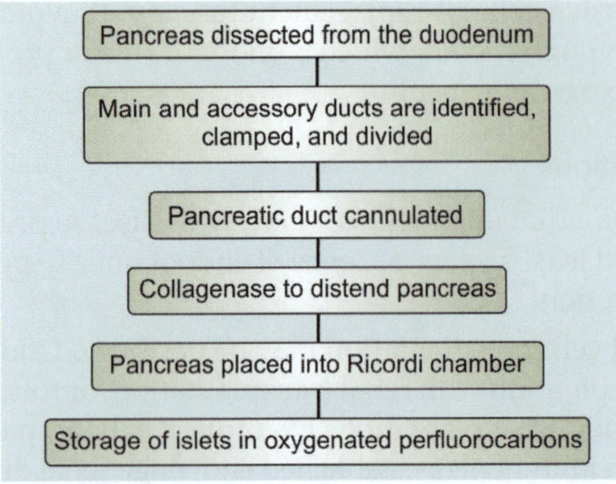

Technique of Transplantation

- The portal venous system is used for islet cell transplantation (Fig. 65.14).
- With ultrasound (US) and/or fluoroscopic guidance, a branch of portal vein is punctured with a 20–22-gauge needle *via* a percutaneous transhepatic approach.
- The percutaneous access is dilated to accept a 5–6 F catheter or vascular sheath, which is advanced into the main portal vein.
- Confirm the catheter placement using ultrasound.
- Systemic anticoagulation with heparin should be initiated—5000 units is routinely administered.

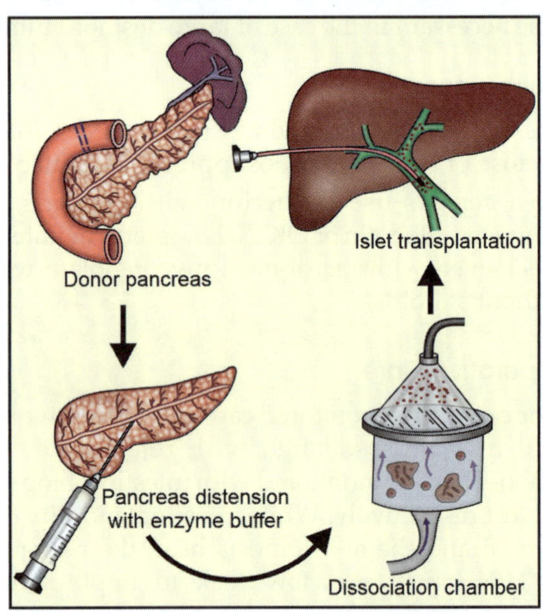

Fig. 65.14: Islet cells transplantation

Islet Cell Infusion

- At least 10,000 islet equivalents per kilogram of body weight.
- An islet equivalent refers to an islet measuring at least 150 µm in diameter. In general, harvested islet cells are infused by using gravity flow or direct syringe injection.
- Other sites of injecting islet cells (Key Box 65.2)

Key Box 65.2

Other Sites of Injecting Islet Cells

- Intrahepatic
- Renal subcapsular
- Intrasplenic
- Intraperitoneal
- Subcutaneous

Competency

SU13.2.1: Describe the principles of immunosuppresive therapy.

Peri- and Post-procedural Imaging, DM Management and Immunosuppression

It includes a combination of a T cell-depleting agent and interleukin-2 monoclonal antibody receptor blocker (daclizumab) for induction and maintenance with a combination of a calcineurin inhibitor (tacrolimus) and a mammalian target of rapamycin inhibitor (sirolimus).

Complications of Islet Cell Transplantation

- Bleeding—either intraperitoneal or liver subcapsular is the most common procedure-related complication. Fortunately, effective hepatic parenchymal tract embolisation significantly reduces bleeding.
- Partial portal vein thrombosis is another complication. It is because of activation of coagulation system by transplanted cells.
- Other complications of islet cell transplantation include transient liver enzyme elevation, abdominal pain, focal hepatic steatosis and severe hypoglycaemia.

Drugs used for Maintenance Therapy after Transplantation

Steroids: Prednisolone is commonly used. Side effects are hypertension, Cushing's syndrome, diabetes, cataract, muscle wasting.

Antiproliferating agents: Azathioprine is the drug used. It inhibits both humoral and cell mediated immunity. Bone marrow suppression and toxic hepatitis are side effects.

T cell directed immunosuppressants: Cyclosporine, Tacrolimus and Sirolimus are a few drugs. Cyclosporine inhibits formation of mature CD4 and CD8 T cells in the thymus. It does not cause myelosuppression. Side effects are nephrotoxicity, hypertension, hyperkalaemia, hirsutism, etc. It is used in a dose of 4 mg/kg in 500 ml saline, IV and later oral therapy with 12 mg/kg daily. After a few weeks tapered to 5 mg/kg/day.

Tacrolimus: Used in liver transplant and in acute rejection of the kidney. Effects are similar to cyclosporine. Side effects are also similar to cyclosporin but without hirsutism and gingival hypertrophy.

Competency

SU13.3: Discuss legal and ethical issues concerning organ donation.

MEDICOLEGAL ASPECTS OF ORGAN DONATION

Transplantation of Human Organs Act (THOA) 1994: It regulates the removal, storage, and transplantation of human organs for therapeutic purposes and prevents the commercial trade of human organs. The organs that can be donated as per the act are the kidneys, cornea, liver, heart, lungs, pancreas, ear drum, and ear bones. There are three types of live organ donations as per the act: (1) Relatives by blood, (2) spouse, and (3) out of affection. Applications of unrelated transplants are scrutinized by state authorization committees. Registration of hospitals conducting transplantation should be done with these committees.

Cadaver organ donation: Organs can be donated if brainstem death has occurred, which is certified twice by a panel of doctors over a period of at least 6 hours. The panel should include:

1. Registered medical practitioner in-charge of the hospital in which the brainstem death has occurred.
2. Registered medical practitioner nominated from the panel of names approved by the appropriate authority.
3. Neurologist/neurosurgeon nominated from the panel of names approved by the appropriate authority.
4. Registered medical practitioner treating the deceased person.

Beating heart donor: This method is used for cadaveric organ transplantation. After the declaration of death, the person is connected to artificial life-sustaining methods. This will better preserve the organs, which can then be successfully transplanted to the recipient.

Punishments for commercial dealings involving human organs:

10 years of imprisonment and a fine of 20 lakh rupees.

Doctor: 3 years suspension (temporary erasure) from medical register by regulatory body (NMC) with permanent erasure for subsequent offence.

Multiple Choice Questions

1. **Which of the following is not a component of innate immunity?**
   A. Phagocytic neutrophils
   B. Natural killer cells
   C. Complements
   D. Mast cells
2. **Which of the following is a cytotoxic T cell?**
   A. CD8
   B. CD4
   C. CD6
   D. CD2
3. **Which of the following are included under MELD score in liver transplantation?**
   A. Creatinine, bilirubin, albumin
   B. Creatinine, bilirubin, INR
   C. Creatinine, bilirubin, bleeding time
   D. Creatinine, bilirubin, ammonia
4. **Tacrolimus is a:**
   A. Calcineurin inhibitor
   B. Steroids
   C. Antiproliferative agents
   D. Antibacterial agent
5. **Following intestinal transplantation, which is the common intestinal pathogen causing infection?**
   A. Shigella
   B. Cytomegalovirus
   C. Streptococci
   D. Meningococci

Answers

1. C **2.** A **3.** B **4.** A **5.** B

CHAPTER

66

Principles of Clinical Radiation Oncology and Chemotherapy

- Radiation
- Dose fractionation
- Sources and methods
- Measurement
- Clinical use
- Curative treatment
- Palliative treatment
- Radiotherapy reactions
- Advances in radiation therapy
- Oncology: Concise concepts of chemotherapy
- Early detection of cancer and multidisciplinary approach

Introduction

Radiation oncology is that discipline of human medicine concerned with the generation, conservation, and dissemination of knowledge concerning the causes, prevention, and treatment of cancer and other diseases involving special expertise in the therapeutic applications of ionising radiation.

Leopold Freund was the first to report in 1897, the use of ionising radiation to "cure" a large nevus pigmentosus on the back of a young girl. With time, ionising radiation became more precise; high-energy photons, electrons, protons, neutrons, and carbon ions became available; and treatment planning and delivery became more accurate and reproducible. Advances in computer and electronic technology fostered the development of more sophisticated treatment-planning and delivery techniques, leading to the development and eventually broad implementation of three-dimensional conformal radiation therapy (3DCRT) and intensity-modulated radiation therapy (IMRT), stereotactic body radiation therapy (SBRT), etc.

RADIATION

The term radiation applies to the emission and propagation of **energy** through space and material medium. Radiation travels with the speed of light in a vacuum, and interacts with living or nonliving matter resulting in varying degrees of energy transfer to the biological medium. This process of deposition of energy within the cells is brought about by **ionisation** (removal of an orbital electron) of atoms and molecules. Ionising radiations are off very high frequency (3×10^{21} hertz) and short wavelength (10^{13} m) electromagnetic waves. Ionisation can occur within the nuclear DNA molecule of a cell (**directly acting**) or interaction with other molecules, mainly water (H_2O) to produce **free radicals (indirectly)**, which in turn can damage DNA and result in cell death or mutagenesis.

By damaging DNA, radiation interferes with cell division and can result in **reproductive** death of a cell. This process in a malignant tumour could mean the loss of its ability for uncontrolled cell division or proliferation. This process is unselective; it occurs both in cells of normal tissues and in those of tumours. Therapeutic usefulness of radiotherapy, therefore, depends on the differential sensitivity of tissues (normal *vs* tumour cell), on careful treatment planning and dose prescription to minimise normal tissue damage and the patient's tolerance to radiation.

DOSE FRACTIONATION

The **5 Rs** of radiobiology provide the basis for fractional radiotherapy (Key Box 66.1). In clinical practice dividing a dose into a number of fractions has the following advantages:

1. The **acute effects** of single doses of radiation can be decreased with fractionation. The patient's symptomatic tolerance improves with **fractional radiation.**

Key Box 66.1

Basis of Fractional Radiotherapy

- **R**epair
- **R**edistribution
- **R**eoxygenation
- **R**epopulation/recovery
- **R**adiosensitivity

2. Fractionation exploits the difference in **recovery rate** between normal tissues and tumours. Effects on normal tissues are less because of repair of sublethal damage between dose fractions and normal cellular **repopulation.**
3. Radiation-induced **redistribution** of cells within the cell cycle tends to sensitise the rapidly proliferating cells, which is seen more in tumours.
4. **Radiosensitivity** of cells depends markedly on the phase of the cell cycle at which they receive the radiation. Cells in **mitosis and G2 phase are the most sensitive** and cells in early Gl, and late S phases are the most resistant.
5. Reduction in the number of hypoxic cells is brought about through cell kill and **reoxygenation**. Also blood vessels compressed by a growing cancer are decompressed as the cancer shrinks, permitting better oxygenation.

Oxygen Effect

The biologic effects of ionising radiations are greatly influenced by the presence of normal oxygen concentration within the cells. The absence or low oxygen content conveys a resistance to radiation requiring about three times the dose to produce the same biologic effects. Certain solid tumours and large tumours are likely to contain 10–15% of hypoxic cells.

For routine practice the "Conventional or Standard" dose fractionation schedule is followed. This consists of 180–200 cGy fraction per day, and 5 fractions per week over 4–6 weeks (depending on the total dose). The choice of optimal dose/time/fractionation schedules for various tumours should be individualised according to the cell kinetic characteristics and clinical observations.

Radiocurability refers to the eradication of tumour at the primary or regional site and reflects the direct effect of irradiation, which may or may not parallel the patient's ultimate outcome.

PROBABILITY OF TUMOUR CONTROL (Fig. 66.1)

It is axiomatic in radiation therapy that higher doses of radiation produce better tumour control, and numerous

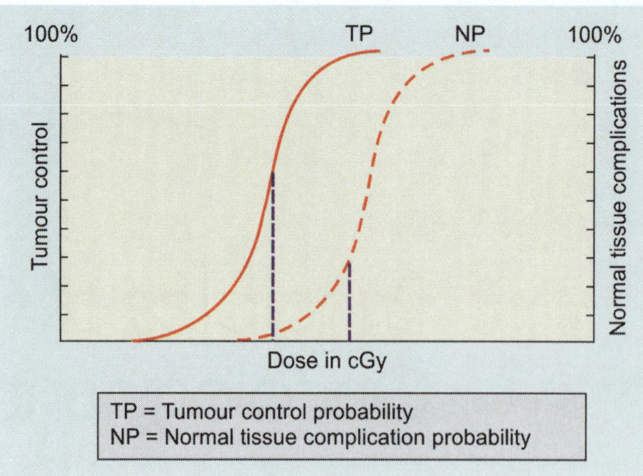

Fig. 66.1: The graph showing tumour probability control

dose–response curves (sigmoid in shape) in a variety of tumours have been published.

For every increment of dose a certain fraction of cells will be killed. Therefore, the total number of surviving cells will be proportional to the initial number present and the fraction killed with each dose. Thus, it is apparent that **various levels of irradiation yield a different probability of tumour control**, depending on the extent of lesion or number of clonogenic cells present.

For **subclinical disease** (10^{3-4} cells) in squamous cell carcinoma of the upper respiratory tract or for adenocarcinoma of the breast, doses of 4500–5000 cGy result in control of disease in over 90% of patients.

For **microscopic residual disease** or cell aggregates greater than $10^6/10^9$ are required for the pathologist to detect them. Therefore, these volumes must receive higher doses of radiation in the range of 6000–6500 cGy in 6–7 weeks for epithelial tumours.

For **clinically palpable tumours (gross disease)**, doses of 6000 cGy (for T1) to 7500 cGy to 8000 cGy (for T4 tumours) are required (200 cGy/day/5 fractions weekly). This dose range and probability of tumour control have been documented for various tumours.

RADIOTHERAPY—SOURCES AND METHODS OF DELIVERY

Radiotherapy is the therapeutic use of high-energy ionising radiation in the treatment/management of malignant disease.

These are either electromagnetic waves, X-rays, gamma rays or corpuscular (subatomic particles) electrons, protons, neutrons, alpha particles, or heavy ion nuclei. Ionising radiation penetrates tissues to different depths according to its type of energy and physical nature. Radiotherapy treatment planning is an important part of the radiation oncologist's work.

SOURCE OF RADIATION (Fig. 66.2)

Gamma and beta rays from radioactive isotopes (cobalt 60, caesium 137, indium 197) and X-rays and electrons from a high energy X-ray machine (linear accelerator). Protons, neutrons and heavy ion nuclei from cyclotrons.

X-rays and gamma rays are identical in properties but are produced by different sources. Ionising radiations can be classified according to their density of ionisations per unit length of the distance in the absorbing media as low and high LET (linear energy transfer) radiation.

IONISING RADIATION

- Low LET—X-rays, gamma rays and electron.
- High LET—neutrons, protons, α-particles and negative ions.
- High LET radiation has a mass heavier than electrons. Hence, they cause dense ionisation and are biologically more effective (damaging) than low LET radiation. They are also less dependent on repair of sublethal damage, cell cycle phases and oxygen content of the cells for radio-sensitivity.
- High LET radiation is available in limited cancer centres around the world, require expensive equipment to produce and are undergoing clinical trials.

METHODS OF DELIVERY

Ionising radiations may be delivered clinically in three ways:

I. External Beam Irradiation

From sources at a distance (usually 80–100 cm) from the body surface. This includes ^{60}Co Teletherapy Units and X-ray sources, such as linear accelerators (Fig. 66.3).

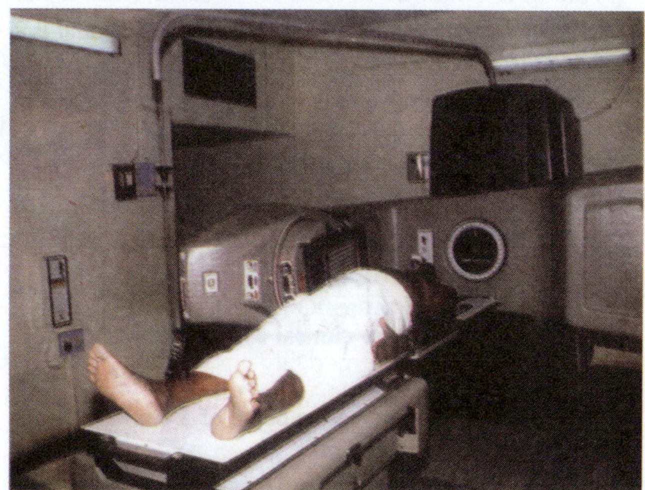

Fig. 66.2: Cobalt teletherapy unit

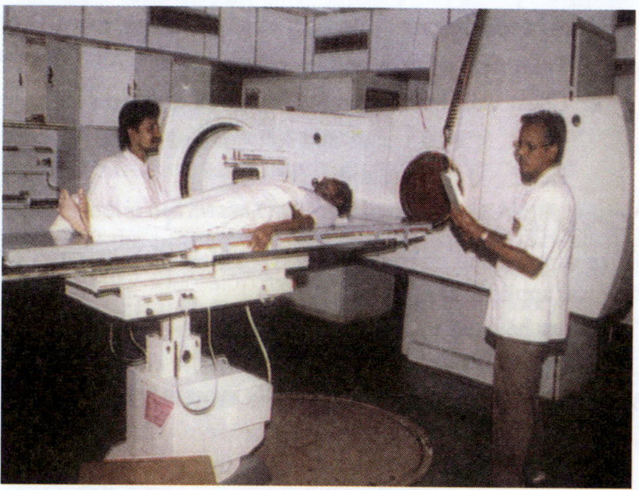

Fig. 66.3: Linear accelerator

Advantages of Megavoltage Beam RT

1. Deeper penetration
2. Sharp beam edges
3. Skin sparing
4. Equal absorption in bone and soft tissues
5. Improved dose distribution within tissue.

II. Brachytherapy (Key Box 66.2)

Brachytherapy refers to use of radiation sources in or close to the tumour.

Use of sealed (closed containers) radioactive sources for radiation treatment from a short distance.

Types of Brachytherapy

1. **Intracavitary** (within a cavity), e.g. uterine cavity, vaginal cavity, oesophageal and bronchial lumen.
2. **Interstitial** when radioactive needles and wires are inserted into and around a tumour.
3. **Surface moulds or plaques** as radioactive surface applicators, e.g. skin cancer, eye cancers.

With this mode of therapy a high dose can be delivered locally to the tumour with rapid dose fall off in the surrounding normal tissue. In the past,

Key Box 66.2

Advantages of Brachytherapy

1. High localised dose to limited volume
2. Minimal dose to adjacent tissues
3. Spares deeper normal tissues
4. Continuous RT in a single course
5. Short overall time (high dose rate)
6. Alone: Rarely (early stage)
   Combined: Often (as boost)

brachytherapy was carried out mostly with radium or radon sources. Currently, use of artificially produced radionuclides such as ^{137}Cs (caesium 137), ^{192}Ir (iridium 192), ^{198}Au (gold 198), and ^{125}I (iodine 125) is rapidly increasing.

New technical developments have stimulated increased interest in brachytherapy. Examples

1. Introduction of improved artificial isotopes
2. Manual afterloading devices to reduce personnel exposure
3. Remote afterloading, high dose rate (HDR) machines, have increased accuracy, improved dosimetry, reduced (short) treatment time, treatment on outpatient basis and have improved patient compliance.

Brachytherapy is used very often. **Combined** with **external beam treatment** and **rarely alone** (early stage). The rationale behind combining the two is to treat the primary site and regional spread (very often subclinical disease) with external RT and to deliver a higher dose (boost) to the primary (gross disease) with brachytherapy. Aim is not to exceed the normal tissue tolerance and at the same time the tumour should receive adequate curative dose. Brachytherapy can also be used as palliative therapy, e.g. bronchial and oesophageal obstruction.

III. Internal or Systemic Irradiation

From unsealed radioactive sources (i.e. ^{131}I, ^{32}P, ^{89}Sr) administered enterally, intracavitarily or intravenously, for diagnostic (nuclear medicine) and therapeutic purposes, e.g. carcinoma thyroid, bone tumours and thyrotoxicosis.

MEASUREMENT OF IONISING RADIATION

1. The **Roentgen** is a unit of exposure. It is a measure of ionisations produced per unit volume of air by X-rays and gamma rays and cannot be used for photon energies above 3 Mev.
   - The SI unit for exposure is Coulomb per kilogram (C/kg).
   - 1 R = 2.58 × 10^4 C/kg air.
2. **Radiation absorbed dose (RAD)**
   - Absorbed dose is a measure of the biologically significant effects produced by ionising radiation. Absorbed dose = De/dm, De is the mean energy imparted by the ionising radiation to material of mass dm. The old unit of dose is rad and represents the absorption of 100 ergs of energy per gram of absorbing material.
   - 1 rad == 100 ergs/g = 10^2 J/kg
   - The SI unit of absorbed dose is gray (Gy) and is defined as:

     1 Gy = 1 J/kg

Thus the relationship between rad and gray is 1 Gy = 100 rad or 1 cGy = 1 rad.

ELECTRON BEAM THERAPY

Source

Mainly linear accelerators.

Energy

Most useful range for clinical use is 6 to 20 Mev.

Use

1. Superficial tumours up to a depth of 5 cm
2. Local boost

Advantages

1. Characteristic sharp dose fall off beyond the tumour
2. Dose uniformity within the target volume

Principal Applications

1. Treatment of skin and lip cancers
2. Chest wall irradiation for breast cancer
3. Boost dose to nodes and tumour bed
4. Head and neck cancers.

Clinical Use of Radiotherapy (Key Box 66.3)

Like surgery and chemotherapy, radiation therapy (RT) has definite indications and contraindications for its application.

It can be used alone to cure or, in combination with other methods, as an adjuvant. Currently 50–60% of all patients with cancer receive RT during the course of their illness. If properly used, 50% of these patients could get cured. For the other half, incurable by any current method, palliation of specific symptoms and signs can improve quality of life (Table 66.1).

Key Box 66.3

Radiotherapy Use in Four Settings

1. As a primary **curative** modality
2. As an **adjuvant** for curative therapy (combined modality)
3. As **prophylactic radiation**
4. As **palliative** treatment

Table 66.1 Differences between radical and palliative radiotherapy

Radical radiotherapy	Palliative radiotherapy
• Treatment is intended to eradicate all clonogenic malignant cells. • High dose curative courses of RT needed and considerable normal tissue morbidity (acute) may be associated. • Late side-effects of adjacent normal tissues may be dose limiting. • Patient often needs high doses and long courses of treatment.	• Treatment is intended to control symptoms to improve quality of life. • Minimum doses of RT to achieve maximum control with minimal side-effects. • Short patient survival times, less concern with long-term limiting, morbidity. • Patient prefers a few hospital visits, so short courses of treatment used.

Before treating a patient with radiotherapy, the radiotherapist must be satisfied that the working diagnosis is correct, pretreatment investigations and staging have to be complete. Then the radiation oncologist must address two questions:

1. Is the treatment intent ***curative*** or ***palliative***?
2. What is the best approach to achieve this goal?

The first question is vital, for there are important differences between radical and palliative radiotherapy.

The second question recognises that cancer can be treated by surgery, radiotherapy and drugs. In many instances, radiotherapy is the best approach. In view of the increasing complexity of curative cancer management for many tumours, with different combinations of surgery, radiotherapy and chemotherapy for different stages of the disease, require a co-ordinated **multi-disciplinary** approach. The correct initial choice gives the best prospect for cure or good palliation.

AS A PRIMARY CURATIVE MODALITY (Key Box 66.4)

A. **RT frequently may be the sole agent used with curative intent** for anatomically limited tumours of the retina, optic nerve, brain (craniopharyngioma, medulloblastoma, ependymoma), spinal cord (low-grade glioma), skin, oral cavity, pharynx, larynx, oesophagus, uterine cervix, vagina, prostate and reticuloendothelial system (Hodgkin's disease, stages I, II and IIIA).

B. **When no other potentially curative treatment exists.** Some cancers remain localised for all or much of their natural history. These cancers might also be unresectable by virtue of their anatomical location or because of local infiltration into surrounding normal/vital structures, which would mean that surgery will severely affect physiological function, e.g. locally advanced head and neck cancer, cervical cancers stage IIb-III, medulloblastoma (alternative to surgery for inaccessible and inoperable malignancies).

Key Box 66.4

Indications for Curative RT

Stages I and II

Testis	Seminoma
Ovary	Dysgerminoma
Skin	Basal cell and squamous cell carcinoma
Lymphatic	Hodgkin's lymphoma
Cervix	Cervix, uterus, vagina
Bladder	Transitional cell Ca
Prostate	Adenocarcinoma
Anal canal	Carcinoma
Head and neck	Cancers
Oesophagus	Cancer
Lung	Non-small cell cancer
Brain	Medulloblastoma

C. **Where alternative therapy is considered more "toxic".** Carcinoma of the larynx, anal canal, breast can all be managed by ablative surgery and in each case the anatomy and physiology of the respective organ is lost. Each of these cancers can be managed by irradiation with preservation of anatomy and function.

Preservation of organ and its function (larynx, breast, anal canal, limbs, cervix, tongue, bladder).

ADJUVANT FOR CURATIVE THERAPY (COMBINED MODALITY) (Key Box 66.5)

RT is combined with surgery for advanced cancers of the head and neck, cancers of the lung, uterus, breast, urinary bladder, testis (seminoma), rectum, soft tissue sarcomas and primary bone tumours.

RT is an adjuvant to chemotherapy for some patients with lymphomas, lung cancers and cancer in children (rhabdomyosarcoma, Wilms' tumour, neuroblastoma).

In some clinical situations the combined benefits of surgery, RT and chemotherapy might be exploited. It has been most useful in the management of breast cancer, bone sarcoma and Wilms' tumour.

Key Box 66.5

Adjuvant RT (SURG+RT+/–CT)

- Head and neck cancer locally advanced
- Brain tumours
- Breast cancer
- Rectal cancer
- Soft tissue sarcoma
- Bone sarcoma
- Endometrial Ca
- Paediatric solid tumours (Wilms', rhabdomyosarcoma, neuroblastoma)

COMBINED TREATMENT
(SURGERY AND RADIATION THERAPY)

In many situations radiation therapy alone is inadequate for achieving maximum cure levels. This can be because the number of tumour stem cells is too large, some or all of the cancer cells are radioresistant, or tolerance of the contiguous normal tissues is too low. The rationale for combining surgery and radiation therapy is the differing mechanisms of the two disciplines. Radiation therapy fails at the centre of the tumour where the concentrations of the tumour cells is the largest and the conditions may be hypoxic (less sensitive to RT).

Surgical resection fails because the tumour extends further than the margins of excision, infesting contiguous tissues with undetectable microscopic foci. Radiation therapy is efficient in the sterilisation of these tumour cell numbers that are well vascularised, and the surgical resection is efficient in removing the gross necrotic tumour masses.

Radiation can be combined with surgery either preoperatively or postoperatively.

Aims and Advantages of Preoperative RT

1. Unresectable cancer to resectable cancer
2. Prevent iatrogenic metastases
3. Reduction of size and vascularity
4. Destroys microscopic foci beyond surgical margin

Disadvantages

1. Delay in surgical (primary) treatment
2. Delay in wound healing
3. Pathologic downstaging to influence other adjuvant treatment
4. Alters anatomical staging (precise pathological extent)
5. Inability to tailor RT to high risk areas.

POSTOPERATIVE RT (Key Box 66.6)

Clinical situations may indicate different sequences but such combinations of surgery and radiation therapy improve the local tumour control rate for many advanced cancers. Combined therapy may also improve the cure rate, at the same time reducing the morbidity associated with more aggressive single modality treatment.

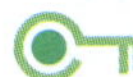
Key Box 66.6

Aim and Advantages

1. Exact disease extent known so as to tailor the treatment individually.
2. Operative margins are well-defined—gross or microscopic.
3. Less postoperative complications—wound healing intact.
4. GI anastomoses and ileal conduits can be done in a non-irradiated field.
5. Potential for unnecessary irradiation in some patients is reduced.

Disadvantages

1. Delay in RT due to postoperative complications—delay wound healing.
2. Decreased radiosensitivity of the tumour due to rich oxygen in vascular tumour.
3. Postoperative adhesions of organs/structures increase RT complication rate.
4. No effect on dissemination during surgery.
5. Volume of normal tissue to be irradiated is more. Usually all tissue planes are potentially contaminated by surgery.

COMBINATION OF RADIOTHERAPY WITH CHEMOTHERAPY

In general, chemotherapy is used in an adjuvant way to control subclinical disease elsewhere in the body or in an additive way to enhance the local effects of the radiation to achieve higher rate of local control. Many other agents will act in both ways.

Agents of choice are those whose toxic effects are in organs not included in the radiation target volume. An example is the combination of the cisplatin compounds with radiation therapy for head and neck cancers. Here, the toxicity of chemotherapy is primarily haematogenous and renal. The toxicity of RT is on the oral mucosa.

Chemotherapy could be combined with RT in three main ways

1. Neoadjuvant: 1–3 courses before definitive RT.
2. Adjuvant: After completion of definitive RT.
3. Concurrent: During a course of radiotherapy.
4. Combinations of the above.

PROPHYLACTIC CRANIAL RADIATION

Certain cancers have a high incidence of developing brain (CNS) metastases even after their primary disease is controlled, because of the blood–brain barrier which can act as a sanctuary site for relapse. Among such patients, it is possible to reduce their local CNS relapse rate and improve survival by treating the CNS by prophylactic cranial RT ± intrathecal chemotherapy. The total dose needed is low (18–24 Gy) and has minimal side effects, e.g. acute lymphoblastic leukaemia/high grade lymphomas (Key Box 66.7).

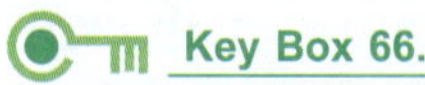 Key Box 66.7

Palliative Treatment

Objectives of palliative irradiation include:

- Relief of pain, usually from metastases to bone.
- Relief of headache and neurological dysfunction from intracranial metastases.
- Relief of obstruction, such as tumours involving ureter, oesophagus, bronchus, lymphatic and blood vessels.
- Promotion of healing of surface wounds by local tumour control.
- Haemostatic for cervical/bladder cancers.

MANAGEMENT: RADIOTHERAPY REACTIONS (Table 66.2)

The incidence of systemic symptoms from radiotherapy is variable. In broad terms, the larger the treatment yield, the fraction size and the total given dose, the greater will be the chance of the patient developing problems. The dose of radiation that can be delivered is limited by acute reactions and by late irreversible organ/tissue damage. Each organ has a known tolerance which should not be exceeded.

However, in order to achieve a given level of tumour control probability certain amount of normal tissue sequelae are unavoidable.

During a course of radiotherapy mild to moderate grade acute reactions occur frequently and can be usually conservatively managed and might require a short break in the treatment, whereas chronic reactions are usually the dose limiting complications. Severe grade reactions should be avoided using proper time dose fractionation regimens, accurate treatment planning and execution.

Some of the important acute reactions following RT, their threshold doses and management are shown in Table 66.2.

Table 66.2 Complications and management of RT

Organ toxicity		Approx. dose threshold Gy	Specific management points
Skin	Erythema	10–12	No specific treatment required
Skin	Dry desquamation	40–50	Proflavine and emollients may produce symptomatic relief
Shin	Moist desquamation	45–55	Keep the affected area dry. Gentian violet may be helpful in drying the affected area
Mucous	Mucositis	30–40	Topical benzydamine hydrochloride mouth rinse or spray. Stop smoking. Mucaine for oesophageal mucositis. Always exclude candidiasis
Hair	Alopecia	30–40	Warm patient prior to starting treatment. Advise a wig fitting
Lung	Pneumonitis with cough, dyspnoea	20	Consider systemic corticosteroids
GI tract	Nausea, vomiting	Any dose	Regular antiemetics may be required
GI tract	Diarrhoea	30–40	Advise low fibre diet when starting treatment. Antidiarrhoeal preparations may be required for symptomatic relief
Bladder	Urinary frequency and dysuria	40–50	Exclude urinary tract infection and consider antimuscarinic drugs
Bone marrow	Suppression especially of white blood cells and platelets during wide-field radiotherapy	10–20	Check full blood count regularly

ADVANCES IN RADIATION THERAPY

Current research in radiation oncology is of such significance that it promises a new standard of care for patients with cancer. Recent advances in radiation therapy include efforts to improve the effectiveness of radiation and to improve the quality of life of treated patients. Innovations in radiobiology, imaging technology, computer technology and treatment machine technology has resulted in marked changes in the way radiotherapy is practised at present. The newer methods aim at increasing the accuracy of treatment, planning and dose delivery using the highly sophisticated features offered by the modern day equipment (Key Box 66.8).

1. **3-D conformal radiotherapy** (three-dimensional treatment planning and conformal dose delivery). In 3-D CRT, patient immobilisation, image-guided treatment planning and computer-controlled treatment delivery can create a radiation dose distribution that conforms to the shape of the tumour volume (Key Box 66.9). The tumour volume containing the cancer and areas of potential cancer is much more accurately outlined as are normal tissues to be avoided. The target radiation dose can be increased when necessary without increased toxicity to normal tissue. This is accomplished using volumetric CT data in a 3-D treatment planning computer.

Key Box 66.8

Advances in Radiation Therapy

1. 3D conformal radiotherapy (3-dimensional)
2. IMRT (intensity modulated radiation therapy)
3. SRS/SRT (stereotactic radiosurgery and radiotherapy)
4. IGRT (image-guided radiation therapy)
5. SBRT (stereotactic body radiation therapy)
6. Proton therapy
7. Intravascular brachytherapy
8. CyberKnife

Key Box 66.9

Cancers Being Treated with IMRT

- Prostate cancer, pancreatic tumours, lung cancer
- Metastatic brain tumours, primary brain tumours (glioblastomas, gliomas, etc.)
- Liver tumours (metastases, hepatocellular carcinoma)
- Head and neck cancer (larynx, tongue, sinus, base of skull, mouth, etc.)
- Radiosurgery (single fraction) and stereotactic radiation therapy (fractionated)

2. **IMRT:** IMRT is an advanced form of 3-DCRT. It is one of the technologically most advanced treatment methods available in external beam radiation therapy. IMRT allows very precise external beam radiotherapy treatments. Rather than having a single large radiation beam pass through the body, with IMRT the radiation is effectively broken up into thousands of tiny pencil-thin radiation beams of varying intensity with millimetre accuracy. These beams enter the body from many angles and intersect on the cancer. This results in a high dosage to the tumour and a lower dose to the surrounding healthy tissues.
   - **Intensity modulation radiotherapy** can allow us to treat tumours to a higher dose, retreat cancers that have previously been irradiated, and safely treat tumours that are located very close to delicate organs like the eye, spinal cord, or rectum. Simply put, this can translate into a higher cancer control rate and a lower rate of side effects.
3. **SRS/SRT (stereotactic radiosurgery and radiotherapy):** High-dose highly focused radiation therapy for small (SRS = Single fraction, SRT = Multiple fractions) target lesions (<2–4 cm) can be accomplished by either gamma knife (multiple, fixed, precisely aimed cobalt teletherapy beams) or stereotactic radiation therapy (multiple rotational arcs of photon beams from a linear accelerator). Both techniques are similar in their use of standard energy photon beams for treatment and rely on meticulous patient immobilisation to deliver treatment to a precisely localised target within a co-ordinate mapping system. These techniques have been widely used and well described for the treatment of intracranial neoplasms (meningiomas, acoustic neuromas and metastatic tumours) and for the ablation of arteriovenous malformations and ocular melanomas. [Equipment used: 1. Gamma knife (Multiple ^{60}Co sources) or 2. X- knife (modified linear accelerator)].
4. **IGRT**
   - Image-guided radiation therapy (IGRT), is one of the most cutting-edge innovations in cancer technology available. Tumors can move, because of breathing and other movement in the body. Real-time imaging of the treatment target and normal organs during each treatment allows for minimisation of reduction of irradiated volumes, as well decreases the chance of missing a target, helping to limit radiation exposure to healthy tissue and reduce common radiation side effects.
   - In IGRT, the linear accelerators are equipped with imaging technology that take pictures of the tumour immediately before or even during the time radiation is delivered.

There are numerous types of imaging modalities that can be incorporated into an IGRT system. Examples include: Ultrasound images, low-energy (kV) CT scan images, high-energy (MV) CT scan images, etc.

5. **SBRT:** Stereotactic body radiation therapy (SBRT) is a technique that utilises precisely targeted radiation to a tumour while minimising radiation to adjacent normal tissue (Fig. 66.4). This targeting allows treatment of small or moderate sized tumours in either a single or limited number of dose fractions. SBRT has been used in hepatocellular carcinoma, lung cancer, prostate cancer, pancreatic cancer. As with any form of radiation therapy, careful attention to matters of patient selection and technical quality assurance is essential for the effective and safe implementation of SBRT.
6. **Proton therapy**
   - **Proton beam:** Proton radiation reduces the dose to normal tissues by allowing for more precise dose delivery because of the unique physical properties of heavy particles. Protons penetrate tissue to a variable depth, depending upon their energy, and then deposit that energy in the tissue in a sharp peak, known as a Bragg peak. This rapid dose fall off at a depth that can be controlled by the initial energy of the protons allows for decreased radiation to adjoining normal tissue by a factor of 2 to 3.
   - Protons are used for uveal melanoma (ocular tumours), skull base and paraspinal tumors (chondrosarcoma and chordoma), and unresectable sarcomas, pediatric neoplasms (such as medulloblastoma) and prostate cancer.
7. **Intravascular brachytherapy:** Arterial renarrowing after angioplasty or restenosis occurs in 30 to 40% of patients and results from neointimal proliferation and constrictive remodelling of the angio-injured artery. Coronary stenting has led to a 30 to 50% decrease in the rate of restenosis primarily by preventing the constrictive remodeling of the artery but at the cost of an increase in neointimal proliferation. The system used for intra-arterial beta-radiation therapy has Yttrium-90 beta ray emitting source (half-life, 64 hours; maximal energy, 2.284 MeV), a centering balloon and an automated delivery device. An 18-Gy dose not only prevents the renarrowing of the lumen typically observed after successful balloon angioplasty but actually induces luminal enlargement.

   Drawback (all techniques)
   - High cost of treatment (expensive equipment + time and labour-intensive)
   - Lack of long-term data (survival/late morbidity).
8. **CyberKnife: CyberKnife radiosurgery** is the non-invasive alternative to surgery for the precise treatment and effective removal of **cancerous tumours** (Fig. 66.5) from the body.
   - The system has a miniaturised linear accelerator mounted on a robotic arm with 6 different points of axis where it can bend, turn, tilt or swivel with submillimetre accuracy.
   - Destroys tumours with highly precise beams of radiation, tumours virtually anywhere in the body, quickly, painlessly and without downtime or hospital stay in one to five sessions (hypofractionation).
   - Thus offers new hope to patients who have inoperable or surgically complex tumours and for those who may be looking for an alternative to more invasive surgery.

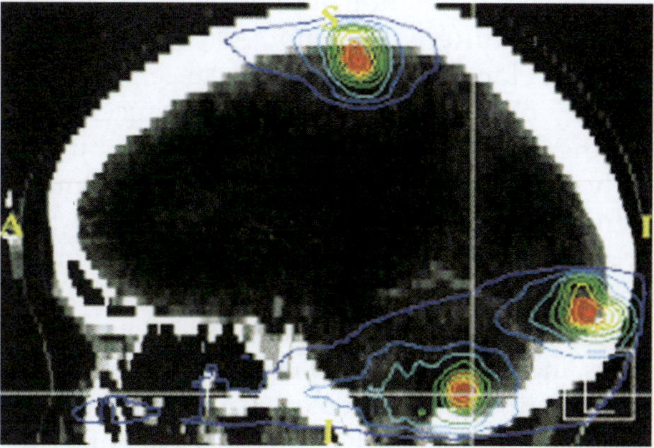

Fig. 66.4: Stereotactic radiosurgery brain (metastasis)

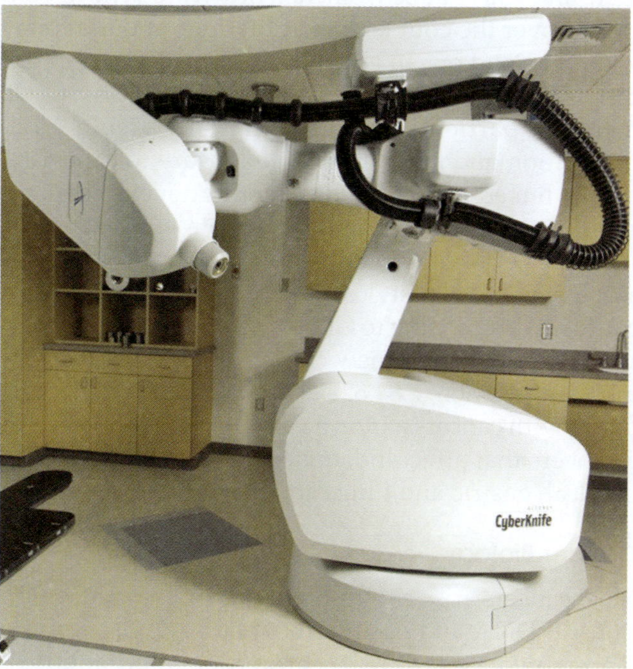

Fig. 66.5: CyberKnife

ONCOLOGY: CONCISE CONCEPTS OF CHEMOTHERAPY

INTRODUCTION

Cancer (also called malignancy) is a term used for diseases in which abnormal cells divide without control and can invade and spread to nearby and distant tissues and organs through the blood and lymph systems. There are different types of cancers depending on the tissue of origin. Carcinoma is a cancer that develops in the skin, mucosa or in tissues that line or cover internal organs. Sarcoma is a cancer that originates in the bone, cartilage, or other connective or supportive tissue. Leukemia is a cancer of the blood and bone marrow. Lymphoma and multiple myeloma are cancers that begin in the cells of the immune system like lymph nodes, spleen or bone marrow.

Oncology is a branch of medicine that specializes in the diagnosis and treatment of cancer. It includes:

- Medical oncology—the branch that deals with the use of chemotherapy or drugs to treat cancer.
- Radiation oncology—the branch that deals with use of radiation therapy to treat cancer.
- Surgical oncology—the branch that deals with use of surgery to treat cancer.

Epidemiology of Cancer

The new global cancer data suggests that the global cancer burden has risen to 18.1 million cases and 9.6 million cancer deaths. The International Agency for Research on Cancer (IARC) estimates that one in five men and one in six women worldwide will develop cancer over the course of their lifetime, and that one in eight men and one in eleven women will die from their disease. A number of factors appear to be driving this increase, particularly a growing and ageing global population and an increase in exposure to cancer risk factors linked to social and economic development. For rapidly growing economies, the data suggests a shift from poverty or infection related cancers to those associated with lifestyles more typical in industrialized countries. According to GLOBOCAN 2018 data, in 2018 there were 11,57,294 new cancer cases in India in both men and women, 7,84,821 deaths and 22,58,208 people living with cancer (within 5 years of diagnosis). The top 5 cancers that affect Indian population are breast, oral, cervical, gastric and lung cancers.

Cancer Biology

Most cancers arise as a result of multiple somatic mutations to DNA and occur only after a cell has acquired many mutations to create chromosomal instability. As a cell acquires mutations, it undergoes a variety of changes. There is a continuum from a perfectly normal cell to a cancer cell. Along this continuum, cells often change their appearance and behaviour, a phenomenon known as dysplasia, before they become malignant. While mutations in DNA are a fundamental cause of cancer, other causes exist as well. Epigenetic changes affect both DNA and associated chromatin, without affecting the nucleotide sequence, and contribute to carcinogenesis by influencing gene expression.

Genes

1. **Oncogenes:** Proto-oncogenes are essential to growth and mitosis in a normal cell. However, mutations in proto-oncogenes give rise to oncogenes, which contribute to the formation of cancer cells.
2. **Tumour suppressor genes:** Tumour suppressor genes represent another common class of genes frequently altered in cancers. Tumour suppressor genes encode proteins which downregulate cell proliferation and control cell cycle checkpoints necessary for cell growth. Tumour cells commonly exhibit mutations in tumour suppressor genes such as Rb and p53.
3. **DNA repair genes:** DNA mutations can occur with remarkable frequency in the life of a cell through errors introduced during replication. A variety of DNA repair enzymes exist to remove and fix these mutations. Loss of DNA repair enzymes leads to an increased risk of permanent DNA damage with consequences including progression to cancer.

It is thought that cancers possess a population of stem cells sufficient to propagate a tumour. These cancer stem cells need not arise from a pool of normal stem cells. Rather, somatic mutations may result in a differentiated cell reverting to a stem cell phenotype. If this hypothesis is correct, true eradication of cancers would require therapy targeting the stem cell population.

Cancer cells are prone to acquire additional mutations. It is therefore common for cancers to have multiple sub-clones of the original malignant cell. These new clones possess different metastatic abilities or develop resistance to different chemotherapeutic drugs. The presence of clonal variation within cancers explains the frequently observed phenomenon of cancers initially shrinking in response to chemotherapy, but subsequently growing back. Metastases are the hallmark of a malignant tumour. They represent spread of tumour cells away from the primary tumour. Normal cells typically adhere to their neighboring cells and the surrounding extracellular matrix. A variety of protein families, including integrins, cadhedrins, selectins, and other cell adhesion molecules (CAMs) anchor cells to one another. Mutations in CAMs are frequently present in cancer cells. These mutations make it easier for cancer cells to disaggregate from one another in order to spread out beyond the normal cell's usual anatomic boundary. In order to metastasize, a cell or group of cells must detach from the primary tumour, digest and move through the intercellular matrix and penetrate the vascular basement membrane. Enzymes, like matrix metalloproteinases, are upregulated in cancer cells to facilitate this process. As soon as cancer cells have moved to a new location, their growth will be limited unless they can establish a blood supply. Diffusion of oxygen and nutrients into a collection of cells only permits growth of spherical colonies smaller than a few hundred microns. Larger growth requires the formation of new tumoral blood vessels. Successful cancers can elaborate growth factors such as vascular endothelial growth factor to stimulate angiogenesis (new blood vessel growth).

Cell Cycle Regulation and Anti-Cancer Drugs

Normal cells have regulated cell cycles composed of the following phases: Quiescent phase [G0], growth phase [G1, S, G2] and mitotic phase [M] with checkpoints and a regulated process of programmed cell death (apoptosis). The G1/S checkpoint is involved in most malignancies. This point is referred to as the restriction point and is a point of irreversible progression towards cell division. Cells will normally continue proliferation in early-midG1, unless inhibited by inhibitory signals or growth factor deprivation. There tinoblastoma protein (RB) is a key regulator for irreversible initiation of cell division. Inactivation of the RB by phosphorylation allows the cell to continue to the S phase. In the event of DNA damage, the ATM (ataxia telangiectasia mutated) signal transduction pathway may act to arrest replication (G1 or G2 phases) or prolong replication (G1, S, G2 phases) for repair of the DNA damage. The ATM pathway phosphorylates MDM2 bound to p53. The dissociated p53 is now able to stop cell cycle progression, synthesize repair enzymes and initiate apoptosis. Apoptosis is the process of programmed cell death during cell development or after cellular injury. Apoptosis can be readily identified on histologic sections by the following features—cell shrinkage, chromatin condensation, formation of cytoplasmic blebs, and phagocytizing macrophages. Cells with irreparable DNA damage are flagged for apoptosis, thereby limiting the potential for uncontrolled cell proliferation. However, in most cancers there is one or more genetic alteration in this G1 checkpoint.

Most antineoplastic agents are classified according to their structure or cell cycle activity—either cell cycle phase specific or cell cycle phase non-specific:

- Cell cycle phase specific agents act on the cells in a specific phase. They are most effective against tumours that have a large proportion of cells actively moving through the cell cycle and cycling at a fast rate. Rapid cycling ensures that the cell passes through the phase in which it is vulnerable to the drugs' effects.
- Cell cycle phase non-specific agents are not dependent on the cell being in a particular phase of the cell cycle for them to work—they affect cells in all phases of the cell cycle. Resting cells (phase G0) are as vulnerable as dividing cells to the cytotoxic effects of these agents. As a result, phase non-specific agents have been found to be some of the most effective drugs against slow-growing tumours (Fig. 66.6).

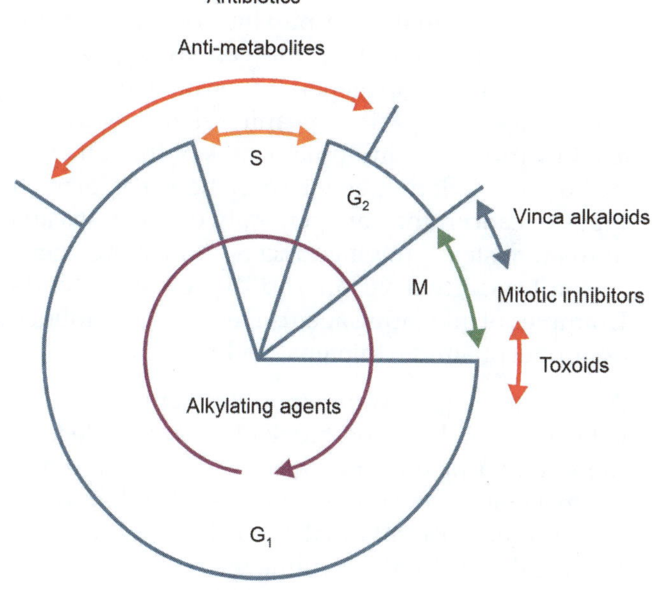

Fig. 66.6: Cell cycle

Cancer Treatment Drugs

Depending on the type of cancer and the kind of drug used, chemotherapy drugs may be administered differently. They can be administered orally (oral chemotherapy), or injected into a muscle (intramuscular injection), injected under the skin (subcutaneous injection), or into a vein (intravenous chemotherapy). In special cases, chemotherapy drugs may be injected into the fluid around the spine (intrathecal chemotherapy). Two or more methods of administration may be used at the same time under certain circumstances. No matter what method is used, chemotherapy drugs are absorbed into the blood and carried around the body. Of all the methods of chemotherapy drug administration mentioned above, intravenous injection is most commonly used. It is the most efficient way to get the medication into the bloodstream. Oral chemotherapy is more convenient and does not require any specialized equipment. In chemotherapy, cancer patients may be given one or several drugs from the available anti-cancer drugs. Since different chemical agents damage cancer cells in different ways and at different phases in the cell cycle, a combination of drugs is often employed to increase the cancerous cell-killing effectiveness. This is called combination chemotherapy.

The different types of chemotherapeutic drugs used are (Fig. 66.7):

a. The Cytotoxics

1. **Alkylating agents:** Alkylating agents were among the first anti-cancer drugs and are the most commonly used drugs in chemotherapy today. Alkylating agents act directly on DNA, causing cross-linking of DNA strands, abnormal base pairing, or DNA strand breaks, thus preventing the cell from dividing. Alkylating agents are generally considered to be cell cycle phase nonspecific, meaning that they kill the cell in various and multiple phases of the cell cycle. Although alkylating agents may be used for most types of cancer, they are generally of greatest value in treating slow-growing cancers. Alkylating agents are not as effective on rapidly growing cells. Examples of alkylating agents include chlorambucil, cyclophosphamide, thiotepa, and busulfan.
2. **Antimetabolites:** Antimetabolites replace natural substances as building blocks in DNA molecules, thereby altering the function of enzymes required for cell metabolism and protein synthesis. In other words, they mimic nutrients that the cell needs to grow, tricking the cell into consuming them, so it eventually starves to death. Antimetabolites are cell cycle specific. Antimetabolites are most effective during the S-phase of cell division because they primarily act upon cells undergoing synthesis of new DNA for formation of new cells. The toxicities associated with these drugs are seen in cells that are growing and dividing quickly. Examples of antimetabolites include purine antagonists, pyrimidine antagonists, and folate antagonists.
3. **Plant alkaloids:** Plant alkaloids are antitumor agents derived from plants. These drugs act specifically by blocking the ability of a cancer cell to divide and become two cells. Although they act throughout the cell cycle, some are more effective during the S- and M-phases, making these drugs cell cycle specific. Examples of plant alkaloids used in chemotherapy are actinomycin D, doxorubicin, and mitomycin.
4. **Antitumor antibiotic:** Antitumor antibiotics are cell cycle nonspecific. They act by binding with DNA and preventing RNA (ribonucleic acid) synthesis, a key step in the creation of proteins, which are necessary for cell survival. They are not the same as antibiotics used to treat bacterial infections. Rather, these drugs cause the strands of genetic material that make up DNA to uncoil, thereby preventing the cell from reproducing. Doxorubicin, mitoxantrone, and bleomycin are some examples of antitumour antibiotics.

b. Targeted Therapies

Targeted therapy implies drug treatment directed at a particular tumour cell biologic characteristic. Examples include expression of the estrogen receptor or over-expression of the HER2 gene in breast cancer, driver mutations in lung cancer, Philadelphia chromosome positivity in chronic myeloid leukemia and acute lymphoblastic leukemia, CD20 positivity in non-Hodgkin lymphomas.

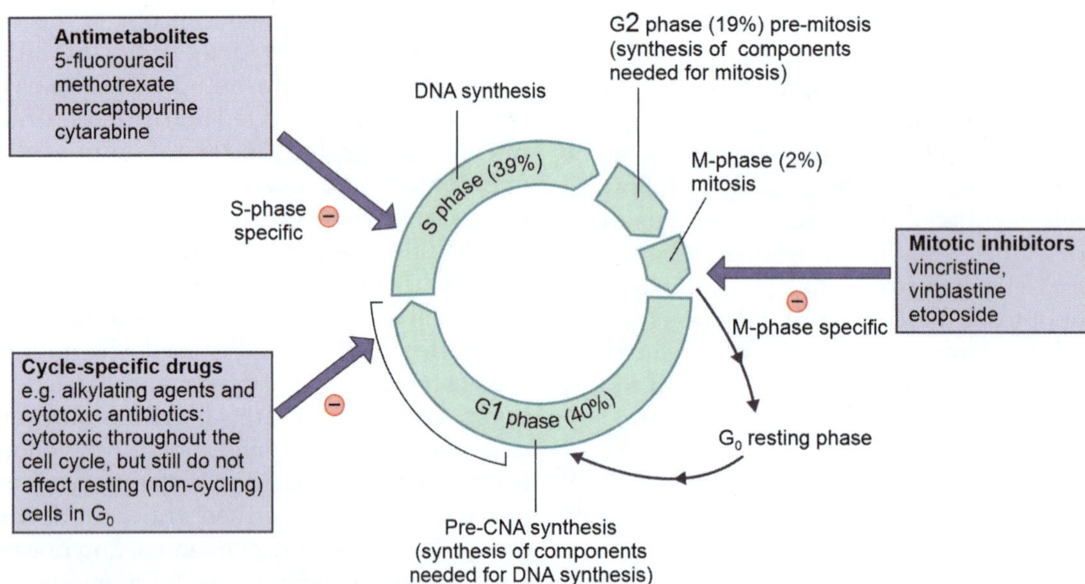

Fig. 66.7: Chemotherapeutic drugs and their action

c. Immunotherapy

There have been many attempts to develop vaccines, cytokines, and antibodies to treat cancer immunologically. The concept of using the immune system to treat cancer is the basis of immunotherapy. The human body clearly can generate an immune response to cancers. A biopsy of a cancerous tissue will frequently show a large number of tumor infiltrating lymphocytes (TIL) within the tumor. Some studies have correlated the presence of TIL with better outcomes in some cancers (melanoma, breast). However, despite the presence of an immune response, most cancers evade immune surveillance. One mechanism by which this is accomplished is using checkpoints on regulatory T cells to shutdown the immune response. Antibodies have been developed that inhibit these checkpoints and have been successfully used in the treatment of cancers like melanoma, lung cancer, head and neck cancers, lymphomas, etc.

Role of Medical Oncology

Medical oncology is the branch of internal medicine that specializes in the treatment of cancer in adult patients and are the physicians who prescribe chemotherapy. Anti-cancer drugs can work by mobilizing the immune system (e.g. interleukin-2, ipilumumab), blocking hormones (e.g. tamoxifen), interrupting intracellular pathways (e.g. temsirolimus), or mutating DNA (e.g. nitrogen mustard) to list a few of the actions. The side effects from these anti-neoplastic agents can range from life-threatening bone marrow suppression to emotionally distressing alopecia. And hence it should be appreciated that there are different indications, mechanisms, and toxicities for each agent.

The common indications for chemotherapy are:

1. Neoadjuvant chemotherapy—chemotherapy administered before the definitive treatment. *For example*, chemotherapy given before surgery (in breast cancer, ovarian cancer) or radiation therapy (head and neck cancer).
2. Adjuvant chemotherapy—chemotherapy administered after the definitive treatment. *For example*, chemotherapy given after surgery (after colonic carcinoma resection or gastric carcinoma resection).
3. Definitive chemotherapy—chemotherapy administered as the primary modality of treatment. *For example*, chemotherapy given in lymphomas, leukemia.
4. Concurrent chemotherapy—chemotherapy administered along with radiation therapy (concurrent chemoradiotherapy in cervical or head and neck cancer).
5. Palliative chemotherapy—chemotherapy administered for palliation. *For example*, chemotherapy given in advanced lung cancer or advanced breast cancer.
6. Metronomic chemotherapy—chemotherapy administered in small doses given at regular intervals to avoid toxicities. *For example*, oral chemotherapy given in head and neck cancers.
7. Targeted chemotherapy—chemotherapy administered against a specific target. *For example*, anti-Her2/neu chemotherapy in breast cancer, Rituximab in lymphomas.

Competency

SU9.2: Biological basis for early detection of cancer and multidisciplinary approach in management of cancer.

SU9.2.1: Describe the basis for early detection of cancer with colorectal tumorogenesis as an example.

SU9.2.2: Define the "screening".

SU9.2.3: Enumerate the cancers which are amenable for screening.

SU9.2.4: Classify the criteria for screening.

SU9.2.5: List the advantages and disadvantages of screening.

SU9.2.6: Describe the need for a multidisciplinary team in management of cancer.

SU9.2.7: List the composition of the multidisciplinary team.

SU9.2.8: Enumerate the advantages and disadvantages of a multidisciplinary team.

EARLY DETECTION OF CANCER AND MULTIDISCIPLINARY APPROACH IN MANAGEMENT OF CANCER

Multidisciplinary Approach in Management of Cancer

Cancer is to a large extent avoidable. Many cancers can be prevented and others can be detected early in their development, treated and cured. Even with late stage cancer, the pain can be reduced, the progression of the cancer slowed, and patients and their families can be helped to cope. A comprehensive cancer management approach is to implement the four basic components of cancer care—prevention, early detection, diagnosis and treatment, and palliative care.

Multidisciplinary cancer care has an established position internationally and has been recommended by cancer organizations, governments, and learned societies as best practice in cancer care. Multidisciplinary team (MDT) focuses on patient-centered, specialized, and integrated multidisciplinary care, which involves professionals with expertise in all of the major treatment modalities and those skilled in providing appropriate support. All of the professions and disciplines involved in cancer care are included in this concept, including the doctors, cancer nurses, and the many professions that are allied to the provision of cancer management. In an effective MDT, everyone works together to manage individual patients and thus serve as a key resource for the development of strategies for cancer services locally, regionally, and nationally.

Concept of Best Cancer Practice

Effective prevention (lifestyle, vaccination, public health, etc.)

Well-managed screening programs (cervix, breast, colorectal cancer [CRC]).

Prompt diagnosis and rapid referral.

Prompt access to best care.

Patient—centered, specialized, and integrated multidisciplinary care in:

- Surgery
- Radiotherapy
- Chemotherapy
- Biologic therapy
- Psychosocial and survivorship care
- Palliative care at all stages

Access promoted to good care for socially disadvantaged groups.

Research and innovation as a core part of the work of the cancer care team.

Practical Applications

- MDTs caring for patients with cancer can improve patient outcomes by reviewing their organization, processes, and the quality of their decisions regularly and seeking to continuously improve their practice.
- MDTs caring for patients with cancer can improve patient outcomes by recruiting patients into a clinical trials portfolio.
- MDTs caring for patients with cancer can improve patient outcomes by updating their required inputs from molecular pathology each year.
- MDTs caring for patients with cancer can improve patient outcomes by having a policy for patient engagement in individual care and in policy development for the team.
- MDTs caring for patients with cancer can improve patient outcomes by exploring, initially in pilot form, the use of PROM data to assist in patient evaluation and monitoring.

Cancer Screening

Diagnosing symptomatic cancer earlier is a feasible and cost-effective strategy, that can contribute to better clinical outcomes and improve patient experience. Effective asymptomatic detection (screening) is currently only available for a few cancers, and even in countries with established population-based screening programs, the majority of patients with cancer are diagnosed following symptomatic presentation. In low-resource settings where screening programs are not available or feasible, early diagnosis (also known as clinical downstaging) strategies can support their introduction by improving clinical pathways and building diagnostic capacity.

Early diagnosis programs consist of supporting prompt help-seeking among symptomatic individuals and/or enabling timely access to diagnosis and treatment. Public education campaigns aiming to raise awareness of cancer and its symptoms and signs among the general population have been conducted in many countries. The timeliness of cancer diagnosis and treatment in symptomatic patients has been conceptualized as a series of intervals starting from symptom onset. Local or contextualized epidemiological knowledge about the incidence, mortality, and survival associated with different cancers in a given setting can inform the prioritization of cancer types when designing an early diagnosis program.

The early diagnosis program framework comprises four components:

- Conduct of a need assessment (based on cancer site–specific statistics) to identify the cancers that may benefit most from early diagnosis in the target population.
- Consideration of symptom epidemiology to inform prioritization within an intervention.
- Identification of factors influencing prompt help-seeking at individual and system level to support the design and evaluation of interventions.
- Appraisal of factors influencing the health systems' capacity to promptly assess patients.

Prevention of cancer especially when integrated with the prevention of chronic diseases and other related problems (such as reproductive health, hepatitis B immunization, HIV/AIDS, occupational and environmental health), offers the greatest public health potential and the most cost-effective long-term method of cancer control. There is sufficient knowledge now to prevent around 40% of all cancers. Most cancers are linked to tobacco use, unhealthy diet, or infectious agents. Early detection detects (or diagnoses) the disease at an early stage, when it has a high potential for cure (e.g. cervical or breast cancer). Interventions are available which permit the early detection and effective treatment of around one-third of cases.

There are two strategies for early detection:

- Early diagnosis, often involving the patient's awareness of early signs and symptoms, leading to a consultation with a health provider—who then promptly refers the patient for confirmation of diagnosis and treatment.
- National or regional screening of asymptomatic and apparently healthy individuals to detect precancerous lesions or an early stage of cancer, and to arrange referral for diagnosis and treatment.

Screening

Certain tests help find specific types of cancer before signs or symptoms appear. This is called screening. The main goals of cancer screening are to:

- Reduce the number of people who die from cancer
- Reduce the number of people who develop the disease

In general, the benefit of cancer screening derives from detecting cancer in earlier and more treatable stages, and thereby, reducing mortality from cancer. In addition, for some cancer types and screening modalities, such as endoscopic screening for colorectal cancer and Papanicolaou (Pap) smears for cervical cancer, screening can also prevent the occurrence of cancer by identifying and removing cancer precursors. Screening may also reduce cancer morbidity when the treatment for earlier-stage cancer is associated with fewer side effects than the treatment for advanced cancers.

Each type of cancer has its own screening tests. Some types of cancer currently do not have an effective screening method. Developing new cancer screening tests is an area of active research.

Performance characteristics	Definition
Sensitivity	Proportion of subjects with cancer who test positive
Specificity	Proportion of subjects without cancer who test negative
Receiver-operating characteristic (ROC) curve	Curve of sensitivity at varying levels of 1-specificity
Area under the ROC curve (AUC)	Area below the ROC curve; 1 = perfect prediction, 0.5 = no predictive ability
Positive predictive value (PPV)	Proportion of subjects who test positive that have cancer
Negative predictive value (NPV)	Proportion of subjects who test negative that do not have cancer

The RCT is the gold standard for assessing the effectiveness of a cancer screening modality. In a randomized controlled trial (RCT) of cancer screening, the primary outcome is typically cancer-specific mortality, defined as the rate of death from the cancer of interest. Overall mortality is not used as the primary endpoint in cancer screening trials because, since deaths from the cancer of interest will be a small fraction of all deaths, there is too much "noise" from non-relevant deaths and the trial would require enormous sample size to be adequately statistically powered. The reduction in mortality that is attributable to screening is often difficult to assess unless there is a dramatic effect, such as with cervical cancer, where the screening modality reduced incidence and very sharply reduced mortality. Colorectal cancer screening also reduces cancer incidence, although the effects to date have not been as dramatic as for cervical cancer screening.

Researchers must often rely on observational or population-level studies to help assess screening benefit. Two common related biases in non-randomized studies of screening are lead time bias and over-diagnosis bias. Early detection through screening implies an advancement in the time of diagnosis of the cancer from what would have otherwise occurred in the absence of screening. The concept of "lead time" refers to the length of this period of time advancement. Since diagnosis is advanced and before any symptoms, it is possible that, in the absence of screening, clinical diagnosis would never have occurred, either due to the inherent indolence of the cancer or due to competing causes of death. This phenomenon of screening detecting a cancer that never would have otherwise become clinically apparent is known as over-diagnosis. Both over-diagnosis and lead-time are theoretical concepts, in that they can generally not be observed in a given individual but can be estimated statistically in populations. Lead time and over-diagnosis can lead to scenarios in observational studies where screening appears to be beneficial even though the modality may actually have no effectiveness in reducing mortality from the cancer.

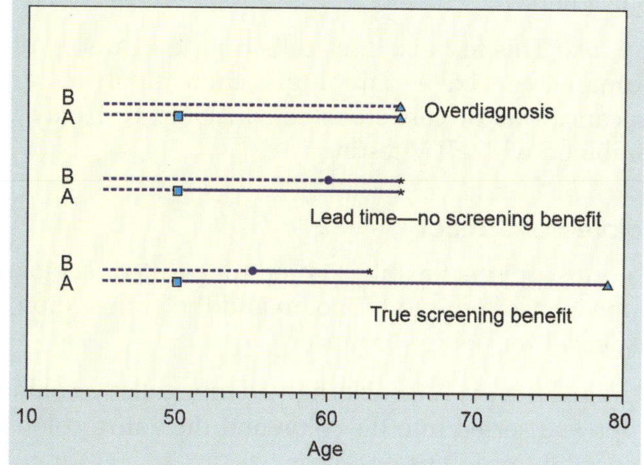

Another bias in evaluating the effect of screening is selection bias. This issue arises when one examines the (cancer-specific) mortality rate among a group undergoing screening to that in a group not undergoing screening or to population-wide statistics. Since those who choose to be screened may be different with respect to the incidence of and survival from the cancer of interest, these underlying factors, and not the screening itself, may be contributing to any observed differences in mortality rates between the screened and non-screened (or population-wide) group.

Breast Cancer

Mammography: Mammography is a type of X-ray specifically designed to view the breast. The images produced by mammography (mammograms) can show tumors or irregularities in the breast.

Clinical breast examination: A medical professional looks and feels for any changes in the breast's size or shape. The examiner also looks for changes in the skin of the breasts and nipples.

Breast self-examination: During this exam, a woman looks and feels for changes in her own breasts. If she notices any changes, she should see a doctor.

Magnetic resonance imaging (MRI): An MRI is not regularly used to screen for breast cancer. But it may be helpful for women with a higher risk of breast cancer, young age (<40 years), those with dense breasts.

Cervical Cancer

Human papillomavirus (HPV) testing: Cells are scraped from the outside of a woman's cervix. These cells are tested for specific strains of HPV. Some strains of HPV are more strongly linked to an increased risk of cervical cancer. This test may be done alone or combined with a Pap test. An HPV test may also be done on a sample of cells from a woman's vagina that she can collect herself.

Pap test: This test also uses cells from the outside of a woman's cervix. A pathologist then identifies any precancerous or cancerous cells. A Pap test may be combined with HPV testing.

Colorectal Cancer

Colonoscopy: A flexible, lighted tube called a colonoscope is inserted into the colon and the entire colon is inspected for polyps or cancer.

Sigmoidoscopy: A flexible, lighted tube called a colonoscope is inserted into the colon and the entire colon is inspected for polyps or cancer.

Fecal occult blood test (FOBT): Test finds blood in the feces, or stool, which can be a sign of polyps or cancer. There are two types FOBT: Guaiac and immunochemical.

Double contrast barium enema: This is an X-ray of the colon and rectum. The barium enema helps the outline of the colon and rectum stand out on the X-rays. This test is used to screen people who cannot have a colonoscopy.

Stool (Fecal) DNA tests: This test analyzes DNA from a person's stool sample to look for cancer. It uses DNA changes found in polyps and cancers.

Head and Neck Cancers

General health screening exam. The doctor looks in the nose, mouth, and throat for abnormalities and feels for lumps in the neck. Regular dental check-ups are also important to screen for head and neck cancers.

Lung Cancer

Low-dose helical or spiral computed tomography (CT or CAT) scan: A CT scan takes X-rays of the inside of the body from different angles. A computer then combines these images into a detailed, 3-dimensional image that shows any abnormalities or tumors.

Prostate Cancer

Digital rectal examination (DRE): A DRE is a test in which the doctor inserts a gloved lubricated finger into a man's rectum and feels the surface of the prostate for any irregularities.

Prostate-specific antigen (PSA) test: This blood test measures the level of a substance called PSA. PSA is usually found at higher-than-normal levels in men with prostate cancer. But a high PSA level may also be a sign of conditions that are not cancerous like urinary tract infection, etc.

Skin Cancer

Complete skin exam: A doctor checks the skin for signs of skin cancer.

Skin self-examination: People examine their entire body in a mirror for signs of skin cancer. It often helps to have another person check the scalp and back of the neck.

Dermoscopy: A handheld device to evaluate the size, shape, and pigmentation patterns of skin lesions. Dermoscopy is usually used for the early detection of melanoma.

Advantages of Screening

Risks of screening:

There are documented harms from screening as follows:

- The possibility of serious test-related complications, which may be immediate (e.g. perforation with colonoscopy) or delayed (e.g. potential carcinogenesis from radiation exposure).
- A false-positive screening test result, which may cause anxiety and lead to additional invasive diagnostic procedures.
- Over-diagnosis, which occurs when screening procedures detect cancers that would never become clinically apparent in the absence of screening.
- Increased testing with additional tests that a person may not need because of over-diagnosis and false positives. These tests can be physically invasive, costly, and can cause unnecessary stress and worry.

Key Points

- Early detection of cancer screening can reduce cancer mortality; detection of precancerous lesions, achievable currently with colorectal and cervical cancer screening, reduces cancer incidence as well.
- Sensitivity and specificity are critical metrics for researchers assessing the predictive ability of a screening modality; positive predictive value (probability of cancer given a positive test) is more relevant for clinicians.
- The gold standard for evaluating cancers screening tests is the randomized controlled trial (RCT). Caution must be taken when using observational data, and especially survival statistics, to assess cancer screening.
- Harms from screening include false positive tests and their downstream sequellae, inclufing invasive diagnostic tests and complications thereof, as well as overdiagnosed and overtreated cancers.
- Targeting screening to high risk subjects is a strategy to make screening more efficient, in terms of optimizing the benefits to harms tradeoff and the cost-effectiveness of screening.

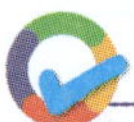

Multiple Choice Questions

1. **The following statements about radiation are correct *except*:**
   A. Fractional radiation reduces the acute effects of single dose of radiation on normal tissues
   B. Cells in mitosis and G2 phase are most sensitive to radiation
   C. Oxygen concentration within cells is directly proportional to the radiation dose required to kill them
   D. Standard dose of radiation is 180–200 cGy per day and 5 per week over 4–6 cycles

2. **A dose-response curve for radiation is of which shape?**
   A. Sigmoidal B. Linear-rising
   C. Bell-shaped D. Irregular

3. **The following are the principles of brachytherapy *except*:**
   A. It is a type of method of delivery of ionising radiation from sources inside or close to the tumour
   B. External RT is used to deliver a higher dose (boost) to treat the primary site while brachytherapy treats the regional spread
   C. It is highly localised, specific to a given tumour volume
   D. It has a high dose rate, given as continuous RT in a single course

4. **1 cGy is:**
   A. 1 rad B. 10 rad
   C. 100 rad D. 1000 rad

5. **The most commonly used chemotherapeutic agent with radiation for head and neck cancers is:**
   A. Vincristine
   B. Doxorubicin
   C. Cisplatin
   D. Etoposide

6. **Which of the following statements regarding chemotherapy adjuvant to radiotherapy is false?**
   A. Agent of choice will have minimum toxic effects on the organs included in the radiation target volume
   B. Neoadjuvant chemotherapy refers to 1–3 courses of CT after definitive RT
   C. Adjuvant CT refers to a course after completion on definitive RT
   D. Intrathecal CT is a prophylactic measure to prevent CNS metastasis in cancers like ALL or high grade lymphomas

7. **IMRT refers to:**
   A. Intensity modified radiation therapy
   B. Intensity modulated radiation therapy
   C. Intensive method of radiation therapy
   D. Intravascular method of radiation therapy

8. **Intra-arterial brachytherapy uses which of the following?**
   A. Technetium-99 B. Yttrium-90
   C. Iodine-123 D. Cobalt-60

9. **The following is true about electron beam therapy *except*:**
   A. The source is mainly a linear accelerator
   B. Most useful range is 6–20 Mev
   C. Deeply situated tumours at a depth of >5 cm are treated with this
   D. Provides dose uniformity within the target volume

10. **The following is true about postoperative RT:**
    A. Exact disease extent is known and treatment can be individualised
    B. Postoperative complications, especially wound healing is affected
    C. Operative margins are ill-defined
    D. Potential for unnecessary radiation increases

Answers

1. C 2. A 3. B 4. A 5. C 6. B 7. B 8. B 9. C 10. A

Section

VI

VIVA VOCE EXAMINATION

67. Principles of Radiology, Imaging, *Viva Voce* Examination
68. Instruments
69. Specimens
70. Operative Surgery, Laparoscopic Surgery and Accessories

CHAPTER

67

Principles of Radiology, Imaging, *Viva Voce* Examination

- Plain X-rays
- Barium swallow
- Barium meal
- Enteroclysis
- Barium enema
- Angiography
- Ultrasonography
- Computed tomography
- Virtual colonoscopy
- Cholangiogram/ERCP/MRCP
- Magnetic resonance imaging
- PET scan
- Interventional radiology

Introduction

One of the sessions in the undergraduate and post-graduate examinations is questions on plain X-rays and images. More and more images such as ultrasound, CT scan, MRI, PET scan, etc. have been used in the evaluation of the patients. These investigations are done to achieve evidence based science and surgery. Several CT images have been included in the book. Students are requested to study the principles behind these investigations so as to understand the investigations properly. This is only an exercise for you to perform better in the final examination.

PLAIN X-RAYS

- When a plain X-ray is projected look carefully and identify the side—right or left. To give an example, if fundic air bubble is seen and cardiac shadow is seen it is on the left side. Similarly, because of the liver, diaphragm on the right side is usually elevated compared to the left side.
- Look at the bony cage—clavicle, ribs, sternum, vertebrae.
- Chest X-ray is taken always PA view so as to avoid sternal shadow.
- Then look at the soft tissue shadows—in the lungs, oesophageal shadow, cardiac shadow for any cardiomegaly and aortic shadow for any prominence.
- A Few examples are given below which are commonly asked questions.

I. PLAIN X-RAY CHEST PA VIEW SHOWING COLLECTION OF FREE GAS UNDER THE RIGHT DOME OF THE DIAPHRAGM

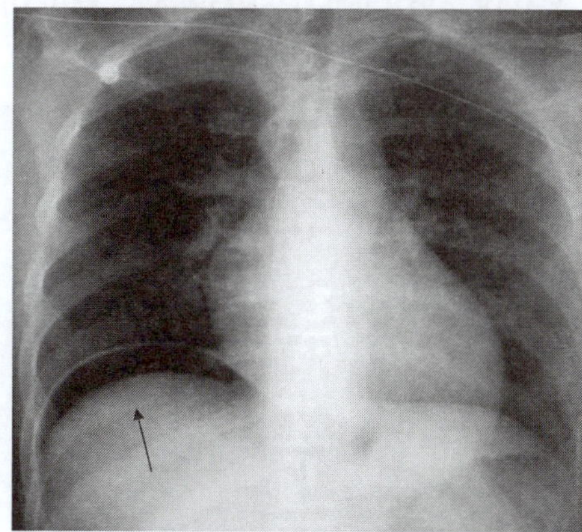

Fig. 67.1: X-ray chest PA view showing free gas under the right dome of the diaphragm

Normally, fundic air bubble is present on the left side. Hence, importance is given to the gas on the right side.

1. **What are the causes of free gas under the right dome of the diaphragm?**
   - Perforation of hollow viscus. *Examples:* Duodenal ulcer, gastric ulcer, enteric ulcer, Meckel's diverticulum, Malignant ulcers—colonic, gastric, perforation of the tuberculous ulcer—ileum

- Abdominal stab injury, laparotomy
- Tubal insufflation test done for tubal patency—not done nowadays

2. Is there any other finding in the X-ray?

- Ground glass appearance indicates significant fluid in the peritoneal cavity.

3. How do you manage a case of perforated duodenal ulcer?

- With antibiotic coverage, Ryle's tube aspiration and early resuscitation with intravenous fluids, exploratory laparotomy is done. The site of perforation is identified which is in the first part of the duodenum. The perforation is closed by using nonabsorbable sutures. Omentum can be used to reinforce the suture line. This is called **Roscoe Graham operation.** Tube drain is used to drain peritoneal cavity.

4. Will you do elective surgery such as GJ and vagotomy or HSV at this stage?

- Since the general condition of the patient will be very poor at this acute stage because of hypovolaemic and septic shock, elective surgery is not done.

5. What are the stages of duodenal ulcer perforation?

- Stage of chemical peritonitis
- Stage of illusion or delusion
- Stage of bacterial peritonitis

II. PLAIN X-RAY ABDOMEN SHOWING MULTIPLE GAS AND FLUID LEVELS

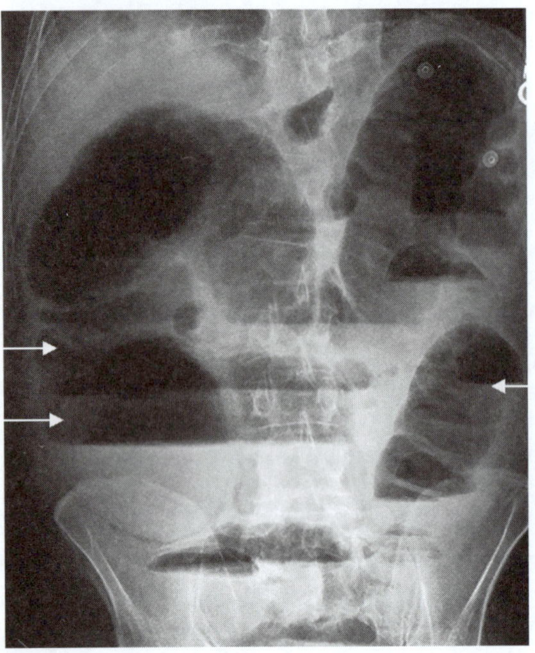

Fig. 67.2: Plain X-ray abdomen showing multiple gas and fluid levels with prominent valvulae conniventes

1. What is the diagnosis?

- Since jejunal loops are prominently seen and loops are centrally located, it is probably terminal ileal obstruction.

2. What are the common causes of terminal ileal obstruction?

- Tuberculous stricture
- Bands—congenital
- Adhesions
- 'Worm ball' in children
- Obstructed hernia

3. How do you identify jejunum, ileum and colon in a plain X-ray?

- Jejunum—valvulae conniventes—regularly placed mucosal folds placed opposite to each other.
- Ileum—no character—**characterless loop of Wangensteen**.
- Colon—**haustrations**—a large incomplete mucosal folds **not placed** opposite to each other.

4. How do you treat tuberculous strictures?

- Resection and end-to-end anastomosis.

5. Can any other surgical procedure be done?

- Stricturoplasty (like pyloroplasty), if there is a single stricture.

III. PLAIN X-RAY ABDOMEN SHOWING RADIO-OPAQUE SHADOW IN THE RIGHT UPPER ABDOMEN

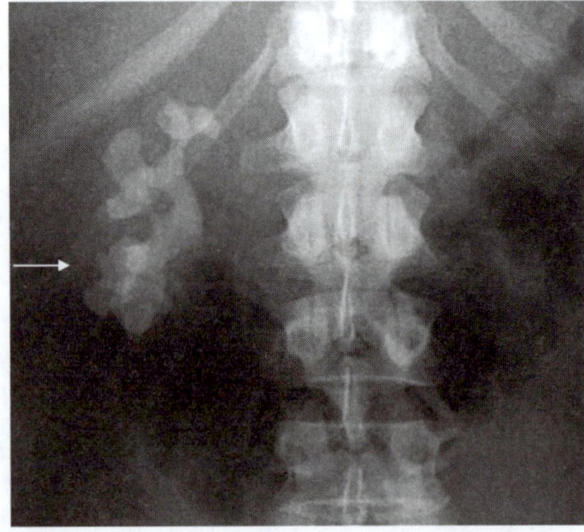

Fig. 67.3: Plain X-ray abdomen showing staghorn calculi right kidney region

1. What is the diagnosis?

- Probably renal stone

2. Why is it not a gallstone?

- The location of the stone is at lower level when compared to gallstone.
- The shape of the stone suggests that it is a stone in the pelvis growing within calyces.

3. What do you call such a stone?
- Staghorn calculus

4. What type of X-ray is ideal to distinguish renal stone from gallbladder stone?
- Lateral view

5. What will be the findings in case of renal stones in a lateral picture?
- Renal stones are found superimposed on vertebral bodies. On the other hand, gallstones are found anterior to it.

IV. PLAIN X-RAY ABDOMEN SHOWING RADIO-OPAQUE SHADOW IN THE REGION OF GALLBLADDER

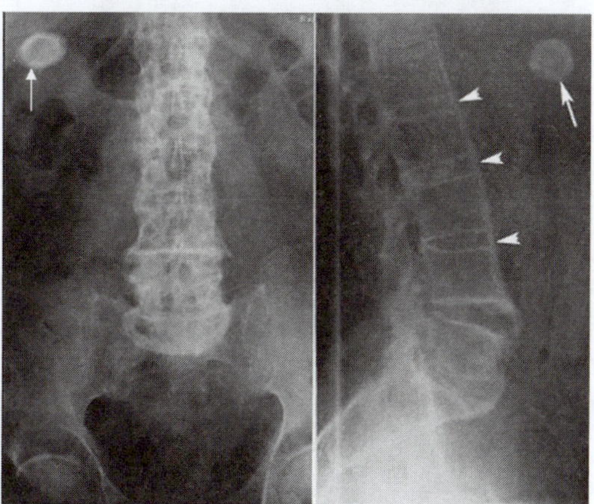

Fig. 67.4: Plain X-ray abdomen AP and lateral view, showing gallstone

1. What is the diagnosis?
- It is gallstone because in the lateral picture it is in front of vertebral column

2. What percentage of gallstones are visible in a plain X-ray?
- Only 10%

3. What is the reason for that?
- The calcium content in gallstones is very less.

4. What are the causes of radio-opaque shadow in the abdomen?
- Gallstones
- Renal stones
- Pancreatic stones
- Renal tuberculosis
- 'Chip' fracture of the transverse process of the vertebrae
- Calcified lymph nodes—tuberculosis
- Faecoliths
- Phleboliths

5. What is the treatment of symptomatic gallstones?
- Cholecystectomy

V. X-RAY CHEST PA VIEW SHOWING MULTIPLE ROUND SHADOW IN BOTH LUNG FIELDS

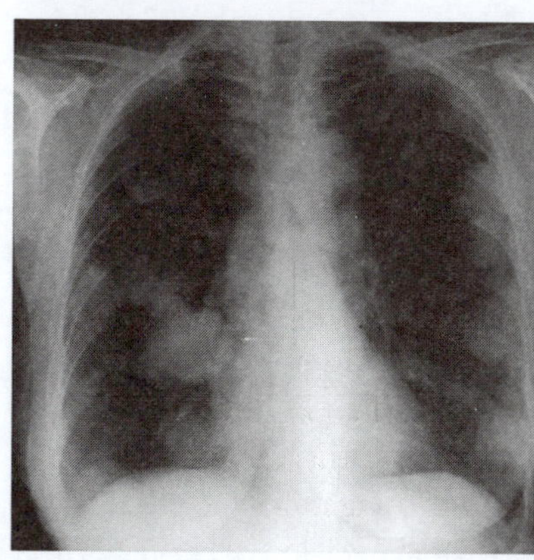

Fig. 67.5: Chest X-ray PA view showing cannonball secondaries

1. What is the diagnosis?
- Bilateral chest secondaries

2. What are they called?
- Cannonball secondaries

3. Why are secondaries in the lung round?
- Lung is an elastic tissue, it has resilience. Hence, during the act of inspiration and expiration, equal amount of pressure is exerted on secondaries, which are growing. Hence, they tend to become round.

4. What are the common causes of chest secondaries?
- Carcinoma breast
- Carcinoma testis
- Malignant melanoma
- Hepatoma
- Renal cell carcinoma
- Sarcoma

5. Is there any other differential diagnosis?
- Miliary tuberculosis: The shadows will be very small and numerous.

VI. X-RAY CERVICAL VERTEBRAE WITH UPPER RIBS SHOWING BILATERAL CERVICAL RIBS

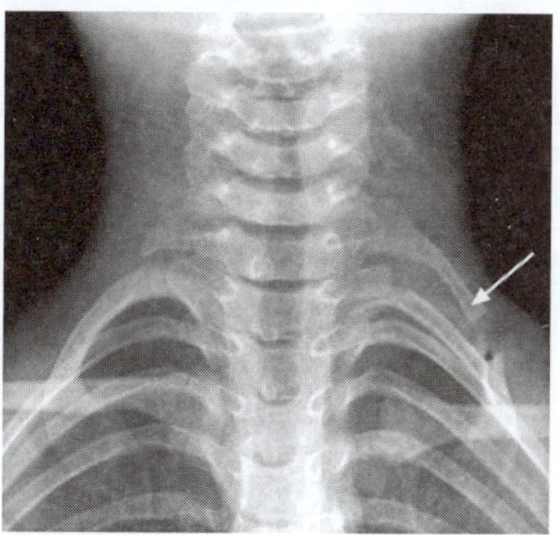

Fig. 67.6: X-ray cervical vertebrae with upper ribs showing bilateral cervical ribs

1. **What is a cervical rib?**
   - It is an extra rib arising from 7th cervical vertebra.
2. **What are 4 types of cervical rib?**
   - Incomplete bony
   - Complete bony with anterior expanded bony end.
   - Partly fibrous, partly bony
   - Complete fibrous band
3. **What variety gives rise to vascular symptoms?**
   - The fibrous band variety
4. **What is your finding here?**
   - On the right side, it is complete variety and on the left side, it is incomplete.
5. **If cervical rib is symptomatic, what is the treatment?**
   - Extraperiosteal excision of cervical rib which means removal of the rib along with the periosteum. Some surgeons also do cervical sympathectomy to decrease vasomotor tone of vessels.

VII. X-RAY LATERAL VIEW OF THE SKULL SHOWING A LARGE SWELLING WITH EROSION IN THE PERICRANIUM

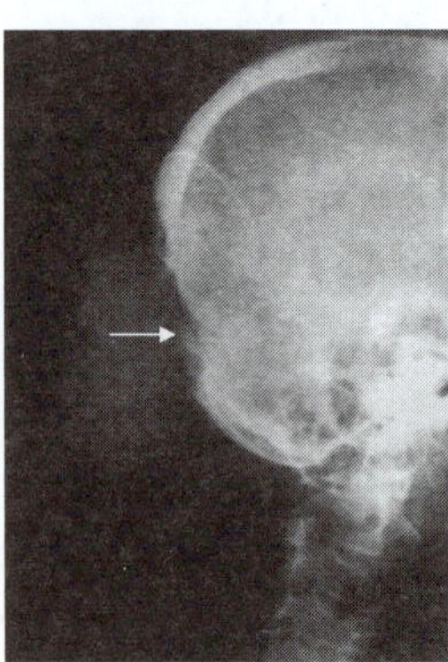

Fig. 67.7: X-ray lateral view of the skull showing a large swelling with erosion in the pericranium

1. **What is the diagnosis?**
   - Secondary deposit in the skull
2. **Why is it not a lipoma or neurofibroma?**
   - Erosion of the bone is seen in malignancy, not in benign tumours.
3. **If this patient is a female aged 40 years, what are the causes?**
   - Follicular carcinoma thyroid
   - Carcinoma of the breast
   - Renal cell carcinoma
4. **What is the treatment if this is follicular carcinoma thyroid?**
   - Near total/total thyroidectomy followed by radio-iodine therapy and external radiotherapy for metastasis in bones.
5. **How do you diagnose follicular carcinoma thyroid histologically?**
   - Angioinvasion and capsular invasion (lobectomy–total thyroidectomy).

VIII. PLAIN X-RAY ABDOMEN SHOWING EXTENSIVE CALCIFICATION IN THE REGION OF PANCREAS

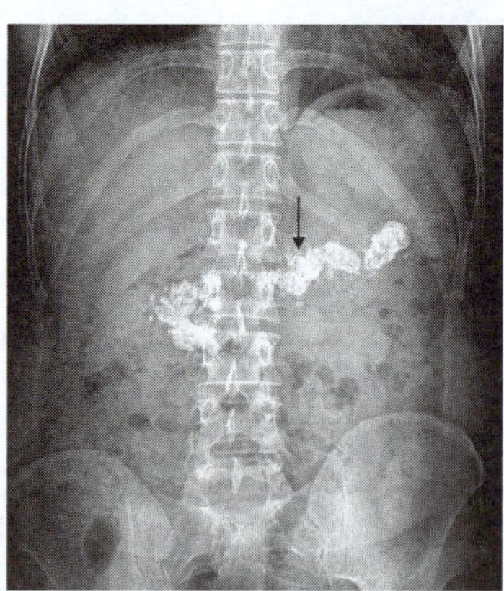

Fig. 67.8: Plain X-ray abdomen showing extensive calcification in the center of the abdomen

1. **What is the diagnosis?**
   - Chronic pancreatitis
2. **Why do you say so?**
   - Extensive calcification involving head, body and tail of pancreas.
3. **What other investigation can be done here, which is used for therapeutic purpose?**
   - ERCP-stent can be placed-one of the methods of treatment of chronic pancreatitis.
4. **What are the manifestations of chronic pancreatitis?**
   - Severe abdominal pain, diabetes, steatorrhoea, multiple strictures.
5. **If pancreatic duct is dilated more than 8 mm in a patient with severe abdominal pain with chronic pancreatitis, what is the treatment?**
   - Longitudinal pancreaticojejunostomy—Puestow's operation. In this operation, pancreatic duct is laid open, strictures are divided, and the duct is anastomosed to jejunum.

BARIUM STUDIES

This is the study of the gastrointestinal tract by instillation/ingestion of barium suspension made up of/made from pure **barium sulphate**.

BARIUM SWALLOW

It is the contrast study from the oral cavity up to the fundus of the stomach.

Indications

Dysphagia and obstruction, odynophagia, assessment of mediastinal masses, motility disorders of oesophagus—achalasia, scleroderma.

Relative Contraindications

- Tracheo-oesophageal fistula, perforation.

Procedure

One mouthful of contrast media is given and the act of deglutition is observed fluoroscopically. After a mouthful of barium, films are exposed to the region of interest.

Interpretation of Study

1. Malignant obstructions are seen as annular constrictions, shouldering cranial and caudal to the lesion, mucosal destruction, ulceration and fistulae formation.
2. Benign strictures are long segment narrowings with no mucosal abnormalities.
3. Achalasia cardia is evident as 'rat tail' appearance of the lower end of the oesophagus, with gross dilatation of the oesophagus proximally and thin streaks of contrast entering the stomach.
4. Scleroderma shows dilatation, atonicity, poor or absent peristalsis and free gastro-oesophageal reflux.

A few examples of barium swallow X-rays

1. BARIUM SWALLOW SHOWING INTRINSIC, IRREGULAR, AND PERSISTENT FILLING DEFECT IN THE LOWER OESOPHAGUS

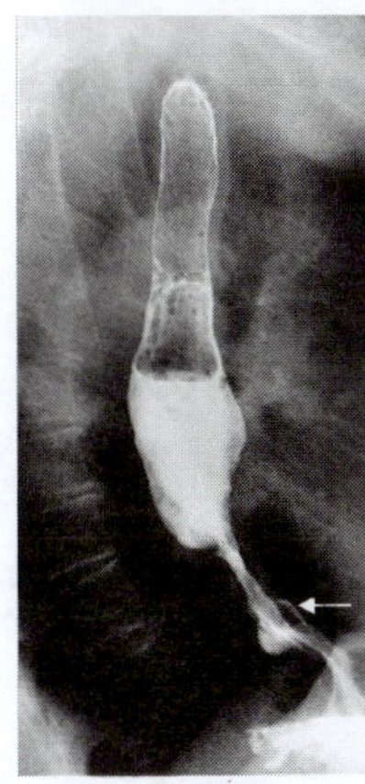

Fig. 67.9: Barium swallow showing filling defect in the lower oesophagus

1. **What is the diagnosis?**
   - Carcinoma lower one-third of oesophagus.
2. **What are the other findings?**
   - Proximal shouldering is very characteristic of malignancy.
3. **How do you confirm the diagnosis?**
   - Oesophagoscopy and biopsy
4. **If biopsy report is adenocarcinoma, what is the treatment?**
   - Operable—oesophagogastrectomy
   - Inoperable—to relieve **D**ysphagia, **S**elf **E**xpandable **M**etallic stents **(SEMS)** can be introduced. Thus, surgery can be avoided.
5. **What are the premalignant conditions?**
   - Achalasia cardia
   - Reflux oesophagitis
   - Corrosive stricture
   - Plummer-Vinson syndrome

2. BARIUM SWALLOW SHOWING EXTENSIVE AND IRREGULAR FILLING DEFECT INVOLVING MIDDLE ONE-THIRD OF OESOPHAGUS

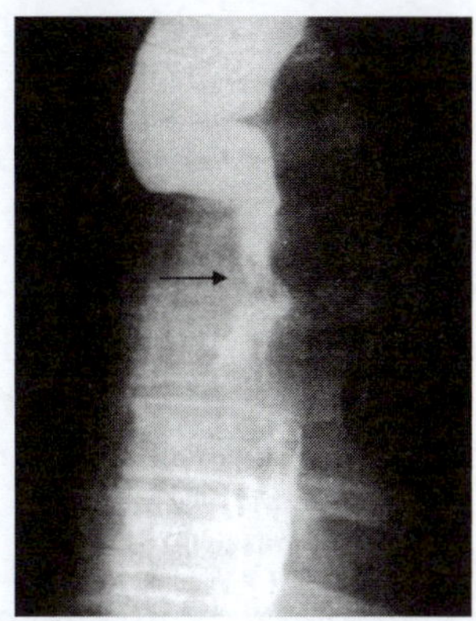

Fig. 67.10: Barium swallow showing extensive and irregular filling defect involving middle one-third of oesophagus

1. **What is the diagnosis?**
   - Carcinoma middle one-third of oesophagus
2. **How do you confirm the diagnosis?**
   - Oesophagoscopy and biopsy
3. **What will be the biopsy report?**
   - Squamous cell carcinoma
4. **What other investigations are necessary in such case?**
   - Bronchoscopy, CT scan of the chest and endosonography are important investigations.
5. **Looking at this advanced lesion, what is probably the best treatment for this patient?**
   - Chemotherapy and radiotherapy followed by dilatation of the oesophagus, since chances of fibrosis and narrowing of the lumen following radiotherapy are high.

BARIUM MEAL

This is the radiological study of oesophagus, stomach, duodenum and proximal jejunum.

Indications

- Symptoms of vomiting, epigastric pain, heart burn, dyspepsia
- Upper abdominal mass
- Gastrointestinal haemorrhage
- Gastric or duodenal obstruction
- Malignancies

Contraindications

- Suspected perforation
- Suspicion of aspiration
- Large bowel obstruction

Procedure

An undiluted barium suspension is given and deglutition is seen under fluoroscopy. Once barium reaches the stomach, the patient is rotated so as to coat the entire stomach and filming is done. More barium is given to distend the stomach wall. Filming is done as contrast enters the duodenum and opacifies proximal jejunum.

Interpretation of Study

1. **Hiatus hernia** is evident as presence of the stomach above the oesophageal hiatus. In addition, gastro-esophageal reflux will be evident. Mucosal ulceration and strictures may be demonstrable in long-standing cases.
2. **Gastric and duodenal ulcers** appear as projections from the normal contour with pooling of contrast. Benign **ulcers** usually **project out** and have the mucosal folds radiating up to the edge of the ulcer. Deformity of the stomach and duodenal cap are seen in chronic stages.
3. **Bezoars of stomach** are seen as radiolucent masses in the stomach and the barium fills the crevices between the particles forming a characteristic appearance.
4. **Infantile hypertrophic pyloric stenosis:** Thin **streak** of barium is seen extending across pylorus—indentation of barium-filled antrum is seen.
5. **Persistent, irregular filling defect** is seen in carcinoma of the stomach.

Few examples of barium meal X-rays

1. BARIUM MEAL: CONTRAST OPACIFIED STOMACH DEMONSTRATING A PROJECTION FROM LESSER CURVATURE

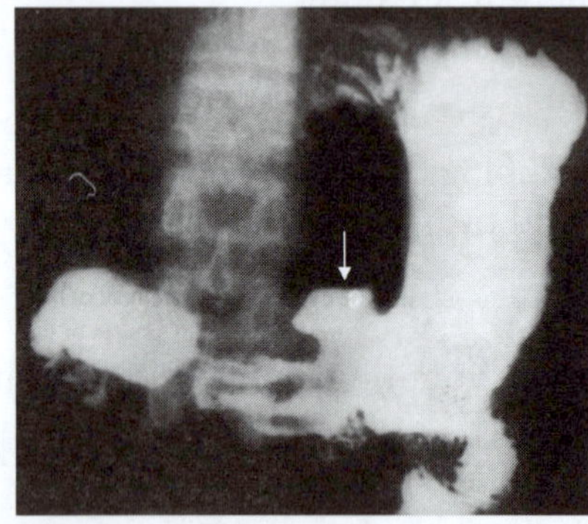

Fig. 67.11: Barium meal: Contrast opacified stomach demonstrating a projection from lesser curvature due to a benign gastric ulcer (niche)

1. **What is the diagnosis?**
   - Benign gastric ulcer
2. **What is the finding called?**
   - Niche
3. **Will you do a biopsy?**
   - Yes because 1–2% of gastric ulcers can turn into malignancy
4. **What is the treatment of benign gastric ulcer?**
   - Avoid irritants such as smoking, spicy food, alcohol and drugs such as non-steroidal anti-inflammatory drugs.
5. **Mention complications of gastric ulcer.**
   - Bleeding, tea pot deformity, hour glass contracture, perforation and carcinoma.

2. BARIUM MEAL SHOWING INTRINSIC, IRREGULAR, AND PERSISTENT FILLING DEFECT INVOLVING PYLORIC ANTRUM

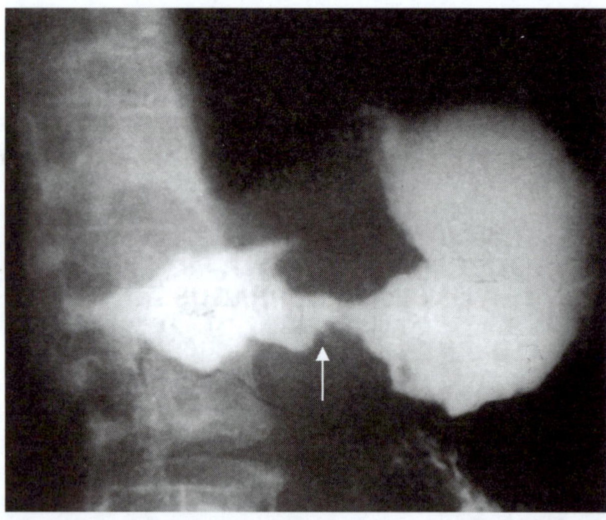

Fig. 67.12: Barium meal showing intrinsic, irregular and persistent filling defect involving pyloric antrum

1. **What is the diagnosis?**
   - Carcinoma pyloric antrum
2. **How do you confirm diagnosis?**
   - Gastroscopic biopsy
3. **What will be the biopsy report?**
   - Adenocarcinoma
4. **What is the treatment, if it is operable?**
   - Subtotal gastrectomy
5. **What structures are removed in the operation?**
   - Growth along with 60–70% of distal stomach, omentum, removal of primary of group of lymph nodes along the lesser and greater curvature, and in the vicinity of major blood vessels followed by gastrojejunal anastomosis—D2 gastrectomy.

3. BARIUM MEAL X-RAY SHOWING ENORMOUS DILATATION OF THE STOMACH AND FAILURE OF BARIUM TO FILL INTO THE DISTAL INTESTINE

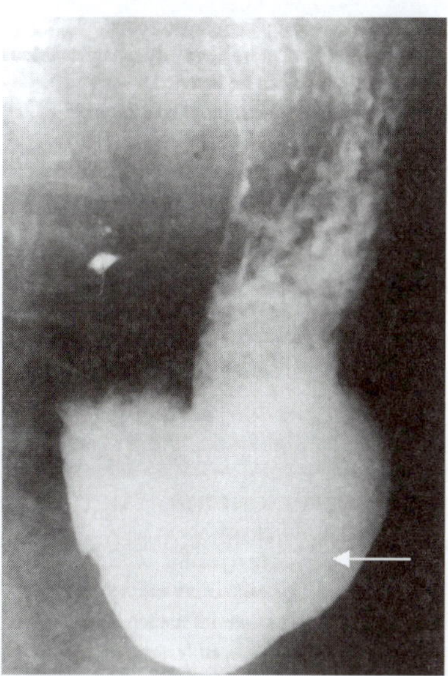

Fig. 67.13: Barium meal X-ray showing enormous dilatation of the stomach and failure of barium to fill into the distal intestine

1. **What is the diagnosis?**
   - Gastric outlet obstruction due to chronic cicatrized duodenal ulcer (pyloric stenosis is an old terminology).
2. **Why is it not due to carcinoma pyloric antrum?**
   - There is no filling defect in the pyloric antrum.
3. **How do you treat this case?**
   - With a preoperative stomach wash, adequate intravenous fluids, total truncal vagotomy with GJ is the treatment of choice.
4. **Why GJ and vagotomy?**
   - After vagotomy, motility of the stomach is lost and in pyloric stenosis, there is already obstruction at the pyloric antrum. Hence, gastrojejunostomy is the drainage procedure of choice.
5. **Why not pyloroplasty or highly selective vagotomy?**
   - Pylorus is scarred and deformed. Hence, it is not safe to do pyloroplasty. HSV is contraindicated in the presence of pyloric obstruction.

SMALL BOWEL ENEMA OR ENTEROCLYSIS

This is the radiological study of the small bowel (from jejunum to the ileocecal junction) by intubation of the jejunum and instillation of contrast media through the tube. This investigation has replaced barium meal follow through. Refer to Key Boxes 67.1 and 67.2.

Key Box 67.1

Indications

- Mechanical obstruction
- GIT bleeding
- Tumours of small intestine
- Unexplained abdominal pain
- Diarrhoea

Key Box 67.2

Contraindications

- Complete obstruction
- Suspected perforation
- Massive dilatation of small bowel
- Duodenal obstruction
- Gastrojejunostomy

Procedure

- Bilbao Dotter tube is inserted with the guide wire through one of the nostrils and advanced caudally with the swallowing action till the tip reaches the stomach. The tube is then advanced through the antrum of the stomach to the pyloric canal. Then it is advanced under fluoroscopic guidance to about 4–5 cm distal to the Treitz ligament (duodenojejunal junction).
- 200 ml barium suspension is injected at a rate of 75 ml/min followed by 5% of methylcellulose at a rate of 100 ml/min. The head of the barium column is followed with intermittent fluoroscopy and films exposed wherever necessary.
- Ileocaecal spot films are taken when the junction is opacified and distended.

Interpretation of Study

1. Normal small bowel shows a decrease in calibre from jejunum to ileum and the change of prominent valvulae conniventes to featureless ileum is evident.
2. Malignancies and lymphomas show evidence of strictures, proximal dilatations and mucosal abnormality. Large mesenteric nodal masses displace the bowel loops.
3. Strictures and ulceration of terminal ileum: Dilatation of the segment proximal to the narrowed segment and conical shrunken caecum are seen in ileocaecal tuberculosis. In later stages, ileal strictures, fistulae, etc. may be seen.

Complications

Perforation, inspissation of barium, transient bacteraemia.

One example of small bowel enteroclysis or small bowel enema

1. SMALL BOWEL ENEMA SHOWING STRICTURE TERMINAL ILEUM

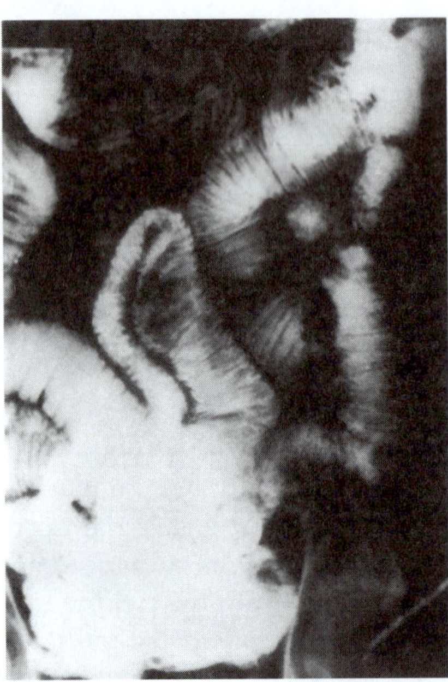

Fig. 67.14: Small bowel enema showing stricture terminal ileum

1. **What is the diagnosis?**
   - Most probably intestinal tuberculosis.
2. **What are the nature of the strictures in tuberculosis?**
   - Transverse
3. **How do you confirm the diagnosis?**
   - CT enterography can be done. Later balloon enteroscopy is done and biopsy can be taken.
4. **What is the treatment?**
   - Single stricture can be treated by stricturoplasty and multiple strictures are treated by resection anastomosis.
5. **What are the complications of tubercular stricture?**
   - Intestinal obstruction, perforation peritonitis.

BARIUM ENEMA

This is the radiographic study of the large bowel by administration of contrast media through the rectum.

Types

Single contrast barium enema and double contrast barium enema.

Indications

Change in bowel habit, melaena, mass suspected to be arising from colon.

Contraindications

Toxic megacolon, pseudomembranous colitis, rectal biopsy done recently (procedure withheld for 7 days).

Procedure

- Bowel is prepared with low residue diet, purgation and cleansing water enema. High density barium suspension is allowed to flow up to the ileocaecal junction and reflux into the terminal ileum. Single contrast filming is done. The patient is asked to evacuate the barium and a post-evacuation film is taken. Once barium is evacuated properly, air insufflation is carried out so as to distend colon up to the ileocaecal junction.
- Filming is done to demonstrate the double contrast of large bowel with additional spots of hepatic, splenic flexures and rectosigmoid junction in oblique positions so as to open up these regions.

Interpretation of Study

A few examples are:

1. **Ulcerative colitis**
   - Loss of haustral pattern, fine granularity of mucosa
   - Strictures, pipe stem colon, increase in presacral space
2. **Malignant lesions**
   - Circumferential/eccentric growth narrowing the lumen
   - Hold up of barium proximal to the lesion, mucosal abnormality—ulcerations
3. **Tuberculosis:** Ileocaecal region is the commonest site. Deformed, elevated caecum, stricture and ulceration involving ascending colon and ileum.
4. **Crohn's disease:** Multiple ulcerations, thickening and distortion of valvulae conniventes, short or long strictures, cobblestone pattern and separation of bowel loops are the features.
5. **Malabsorption:** Dilution of barium, segmentation of the column of barium, 'Moulage sign' (barium in a featureless tube) and jejunal dilatation are the findings.

A few examples of barium enema studies

1. BARIUM ENEMA SHOWING THE LEFT COLON, TRANSVERSE COLON AND A PART OF ASCENDING COLON

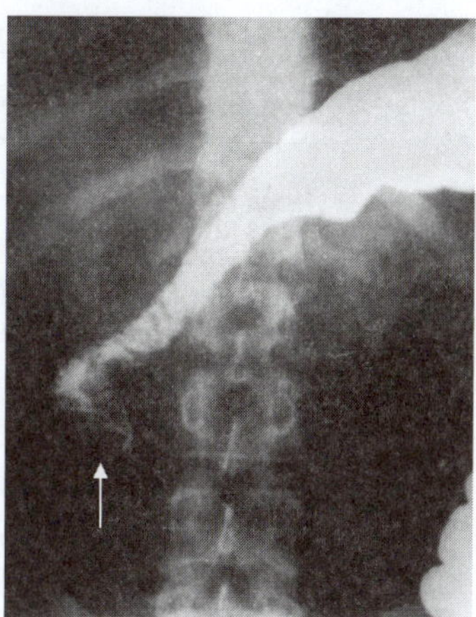

Fig. 67.15: Barium enema showing the left colon, transverse colon and a part of ascending colon with pincer ending

1. **What is the diagnosis?**
   - Ileocolic intussusception
2. **Why do you say so?**
   - The 'claw' like ending or pincer ending is typical of intussusception.
3. **What are the causes of intussusception in adults?**
   - Submucous lipoma, or polyps
   - Meckel's diverticulum
   - Growth in the caecum
   - Leiomyoma of the ileum
4. **In a child, what are the causes?**
   - Weaning of the diet or viral infection.
5. **What is the treatment of adult intussusception?**
   - Resection because there is a precipitating cause.

2. BARIUM ENEMA SHOWING INTRINSIC, IRREGULAR AND PERSISTENT FILLING DEFECT IN THE ASCENDING COLON

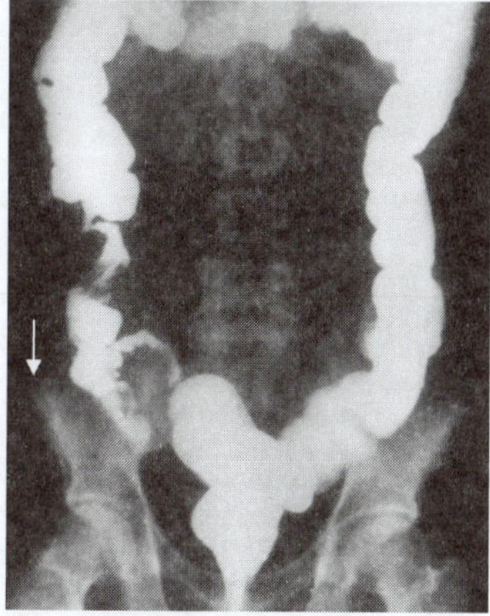

Fig. 67.16: Barium enema showing intrinsic, irregular and persistent filling defect in the ascending colon

1. **What is the diagnosis?**
   - Carcinoma ascending colon
2. **What is the confirmatory investigation?**
   - Colonoscopy and biopsy
3. **What is the report, if it is carcinoma?**
   - Adenocarcinoma
4. **What is the treatment?**
   - Right radical hemicolectomy, if it is operable. Structures removed in this operation include terminal ileum (6–8 cm), caecum including appendix, ascending colon and 1/3rd of right transverse colon. If it is inoperable, part of ileum is anastomosed to the transverse colon to prevent or relieve intestinal obstruction (side to side). One need not remove two feet of ileum.
5. **What is the differential diagnosis?**
   - Ileocaecal tuberculosis: In this condition:
     A. Irregular filling defect is not seen.
     B. Caecum is usually pulled up and then ileocaecal angle becomes obtuse.

3. BARIUM ENEMA SHOWING LOSS OF HAUSTRATIONS IN THE LEFT COLON, SMALL AND MULTIPLE, REGULAR FILLING DEFECTS DUE TO PSEUDOPOLYPOSIS

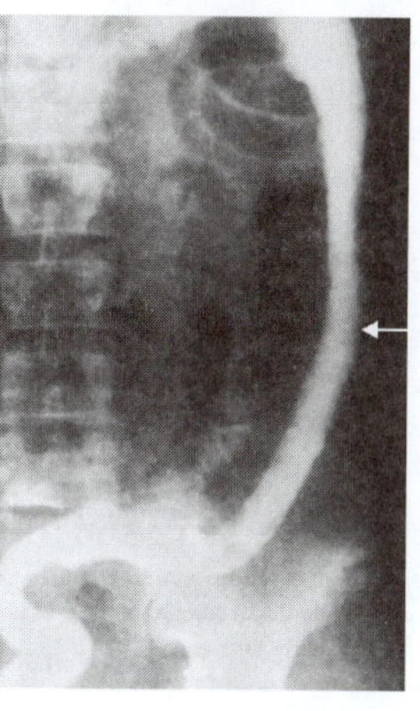

Fig. 67.17: Barium enema showing loss of haustrations in the left colon, small and multiple, and regular filling defects due to pseudopolyposis

1. **What is the diagnosis?**
   - Ulcerative colitis.
2. **What is pseudopolyposis?**
   - An attempt at healing in between the ulcers produces granulation tissues which have the appearance of polyps. Hence, pseudopolyposis.
3. **What are the dangerous complications of ulcerative colitis?**
   - Haemorrhage, toxic megacolon, perforation and malignancy.
4. **What are the drugs used in the treatment of ulcerative colitis?**
   - Salazopyrines and corticosteroids

5. **What are the surgical treatments?**
   - Total colectomy with permanent ileostomy. OR
   - Total colectomy, creation of a pouch with anastomosis of the pouch to the anal canal.

4. BARIUM ENEMA SHOWING PULLED UP CAECUM

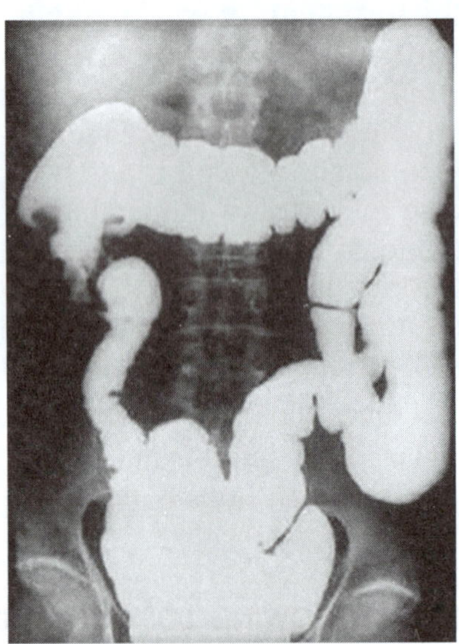

Fig. 67.18: Barium enema showing pulled up caecum—an increase in the ileocaecal angle from acute to obtuse

1. **What is the diagnosis?**
   - Ileocaecal tuberculosis
2. **Why caecum is pulled up?**
   - Involved caecum and ascending colon are contracted and fibrosed resulting in caecum in a higher position.
3. **What are the other signs you will look for in this case?**
   - Narrowing of terminal ileum (Fleischner's sign), fibrotic terminal ileum opening into the contracted caecum (Stierlin's sign).
4. **What about ileocaecal angle?**
   - Normal angle is acute. In this case, it becomes obtuse.
5. **What are the surgical treatments?**
   - If obstruction is present, better to do limited colectomy followed by anti-tuberculous treatment.

ANGIOGRAPHY

Definition

This is the study of blood vessels by injection of a contrast medium containing iodine into the vessel. For lower limbs, femoral artery is selected because it is superficial and easily palpable. It is punctured under local anaesthesia. Today majority of the cases undergo CT angiogram. In CT angiogram, iodine-based contrast is injected through the intravenous line, thus avoiding a direct puncture of artery, thus avoiding complications such as pseudoaneurysm formation, bleeding, etc. Investigation is designed to increase the absorption of X-ray photons and thereby enhancing the image contrast of blood vessels and well-perfused tissues.

Indications

1. Primary vascular diseases such as vaso-occlusive disease, aneurysm, arteriovenous malformation (AVM).
2. Vascularity assessment of a tumour.
3. Congenital vascular conditions such as coarctation.
4. Percutaneous interventional vascular procedures.

Contraindications

1. Bleeding tendencies
2. Skin infections at site of entry
3. Cardiovascular disease such as recent myocardial infarction, overt congestive cardiac failure
4. Hepatic failure

Procedure

- Local anaesthesia at site of puncture is preferred except in children or restless patients, wherein general anaesthesia is preferred. Using a Seldinger needle the artery is punctured.
- The catheter of appropriate dimension is placed into the artery and negotiated into the desired vessel to be studied. Contrast is injected and filming is done (Figs 67.19 and 67.20).

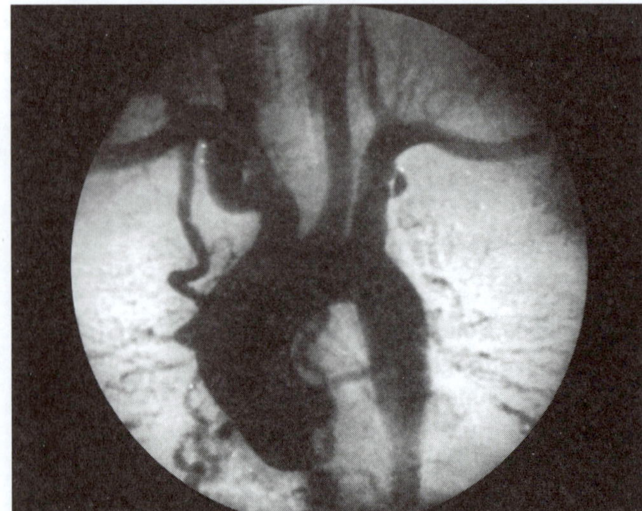

Fig. 67.19: Arch aortogram: Contrast in the arch of aorta demonstrating the major vessels arising from it

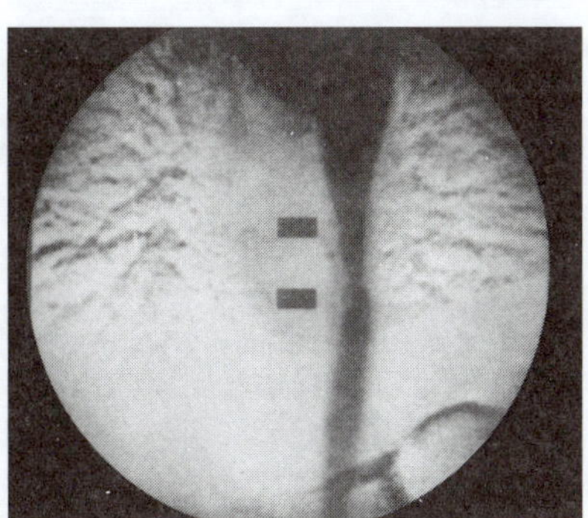

Fig. 67.20: Aortogram: Contrast in the thoracic aorta showing narrowing

Puncture Sites

Femoral artery, axillary artery and brachial artery.

Interpretation of Study

1. Aneurysms are seen as focal dilatations of vessel or projecting from the main vessel through a neck.
2. Tumour vessels show abnormal branching pattern, vascular encasement, displacement, arteriovenous shunting and pooling of contrast in the lesion.
3. AVM shows evidence of a dilated feeding artery/ abnormal blush and early draining vein.
4. Vascular occlusions are seen as abrupt or gradual tapering of vessel with collateral supply distally.

Complications

- Damage to arterial walls at the site of puncture
- Severe hypotensive reactions
- Thrombosis of arteries, catheter clot embolus, haematoma at puncture site
- Vagal inhibition
- Allergic reactions to contrast
- Damage to nerves and to organs

A few examples:

1. RETROGRADE ANGIOGRAPHY SHOWING OCCLUSION OF FEMORAL ARTERY ON THE LEFT SIDE

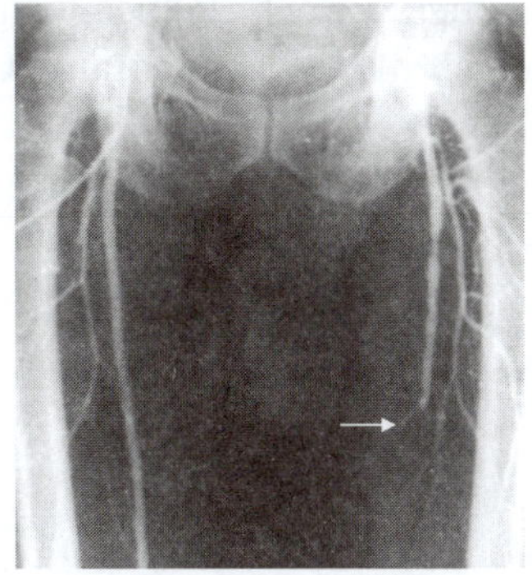

Fig. 67.21: Retrograde angiography showing occlusion of femoral artery on the left side

1. **What is the technique employed in this angiography?**
   - Seldinger's technique—percutaneous, transfemoral, retrograde.
2. **What is the probable cause in our country?**
   - Buerger's disease (thromboangiitis obliterans).
3. **Why do you say so?**
   - Buerger's disease affects medium-sized vessels and narrowing of femoral artery is segmental in this radiograph.
4. **What is the surgical treatment for Buerger's disease?**
   - Lumbar sympathectomy
5. **How does lumbar sympathectomy help these patients?**
   - By reducing the sympathetic tone of the lower limb, arterioles and capillaries get dilated allowing cutaneous ulcers to heal.
6. **If patient is 65 years old, what diagnosis you would have considered? What is the treatment in such cases?**
   - Atherosclerosis. Femoropopliteal bypass.

2. CT ANGIOGRAM SHOWING FEMORAL ARTERY AND ITS BRANCHES

1. **What is the technique employed in this angiography?**
   - It is CT angiogram.
2. **What is the indication?**
   - Patient with severe claudication with or without ulcers as in atherosclerotic disease.
3. **What are the findings?**
   - In the first film (Fig. 67.22A), superficial femoral artery is narrowed and in the second picture (Fig. 67.22B), you can see dye flowing freely after dilatation—angioplasty. It is done by a balloon

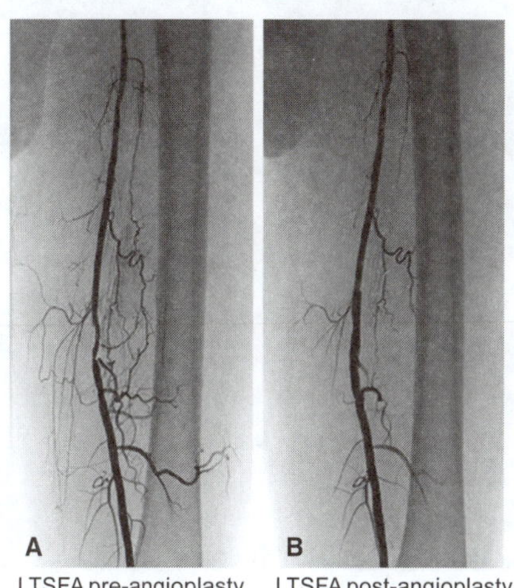

Fig. 67.22: A. CT angiogram showing narrowing of superficial femoral artery; B. Balloon angioplasty is done

Key Box 67.3

Nitinol Stents

1. These are combination of nickel-titanium alloys
2. Self-expanding stents
3. Good memory and good elasticity of these stents
4. Resistant to corrosion
5. Biocompatible

dilatation using 6 or 7 mm and stent of the same size is used. Stents used are nitinol stents (Key Box 67.3).

4. How angioplasty is done?

- Under local anaesthesia, thin catheter is advanced into the femoral artery and with help of balloon it is dilated followed by a small stent is placed.

5. What is the usual site of obstruction of femoral artery?

- It is in the hiatus of adductor magnus—Hunterian canal.

ULTRASONOGRAPHY (Figs 67.23 and 67.24)

Principle

This imaging modality is based on the **piezoelectric effect** which is the property of certain substances to convert **electrical energy to sound energy.** These are the active portions of the ultrasonic transducers. **The commonly used substance in the transducer is lead zirconate titanate (PZT).**

Applications (Key Box 67.4)

- Ultrasonic beam of **high frequency** gives excellent resolution images of only superficial structures. This is used for study of musculoskeletal system, joints, thyroid, scrotum, etc. For imaging **deeper structures of abdomen, a low frequency** probe with greater **penetrancy** is used.

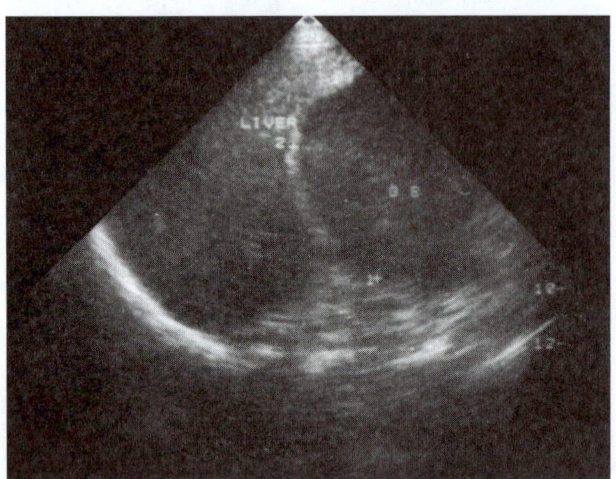

Fig. 67.23: Ultrasound of liver and gallbladder demonstrating an isoechoic mass lesion occupying the lumen of gallbladder which was due to malignancy

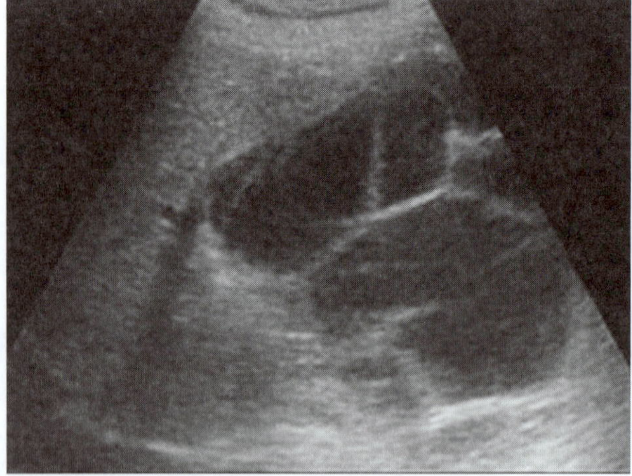

Fig. 67.24: Ultrasound of liver shows hydatid cyst which is anechoic with multiple daughter cysts

Key Box 67.4

Frequency of Various Ultrasound Beam

- **2.5 to 3.5 MHz:** Deep abdomen, obstetric and gynaecological imaging
- **5.0 MHz:** Vascular, breast, pelvic imaging
- **7.5 MHz:** Breast, thyroid
- **10.0 MHz:** Breast, thyroid, superficial veins, superficial masses such as parotid swelling, musculoskeletal imaging
- **15.0 MHz:** Superficial structures such as lipoma, musculoskeletal imaging including soft tissue sarcoma

Interpretation of Images

- Images are dependent on the **intensity of echoes** received back by the transducer.
- Structures which reflect all the sound waves back are depicted as **bright echoes** and **termed hyperechoic.**
- Structures which reflect **moderate** level of sound waves appear as uniform grains and are **termed isoechoic.**
- Fluid-filled structures which transmit all the sound waves, **do not reflect any echoes and are termed hypoechoic.**
- The reflection of sound waves in the form of echoes depends on the density of the organ and the transmission of sound through the same.

Advantages of Ultrasonography

1. It is a cost-effective investigation.
2. It is widely available.
3. Noninvasive.
4. Owing to the relatively small size of the apparatus, it is fairly portable, and can thus be brought to the bedside of the moribund patient.
5. It does not involve the use of ionising radiation, and can, therefore, be safely used in a pregnant patient and can be repeatedly used as a follow-up modality.

Limitations of Ultrasonography

1. Its use is limited in thorax.
2. Limited use in the abdomen when there is gaseous distension.
3. Operator expertise is all important.
4. It cannot image bone.

COMPUTED TOMOGRAPHY (CT)

This is an imaging procedure where detailed information is obtained from thin sections in collimated X-rays.

Indications

- Structural evaluation of intracranial lesions (Fig. 67.25)
- Detailed evaluation of lung, mediastinal pathologies

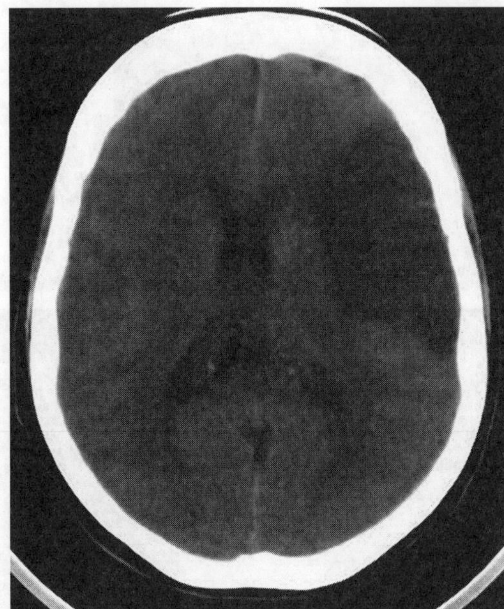

Fig. 67.25: Cranial CT: Hypodensity of the left (L) frontoparietal cerebral parenchyma suggestive of a (L) middle cerebral artery territory infarct

- Intra-abdominal and pelvic masses where exact site of origin and relation to adjacent structures can be evaluated.
- Extra-osseous and soft tissue extension of bone tumours.
- Vascularity of the normal organ and the abnormal tissue can be evaluated and compared.

Contraindications (Relative)

- Pregnancy
- Restless patients

Interpretation of Images

- Structures imaged appear densely white to densely black depending on the absorption of X-rays and the emerging resultant X-rays which are detected. **The composite picture is actually a collection of Hounsfield numbers.** Each Hounsfield number being assigned a specific shade of grey, thus producing a picture that might be easily understood. Some of the common densities to be encountered in practice are as follows (Hounsfield units = HU):

Air	–1000 HU
Fat	–50 to –100 HU
Water	0 HU
CSF	0 to +3 HU
White matter	+22 to +32 HU
Grey matter	+36 to +46 HU
Clotted blood	+60 to +80 HU
Calcification bone	+80 to +1000 HU

- In order to increase the contrast that may exist between the structures in the body, **intravenous contrast (iodine containing) is administered.** Certain tissues show enhancement of their density and various pathologies also show fairly characteristic contrast uptake patterns (Figs 67.26 to 67.29).
- In abdominal scanning, **oral contrast** is administered to the patient before the procedure, to enable the operator to accurately separate the bowel loops from the other intra-abdominal structures.
- The advantages of CT over conventional radiology are that it can visualise extremely small pathology, not evident on conventional films, is cost-effective as multiple X-ray films and procedures can be avoided. It is noninvasive and the radiation levels applied to the patient are extremely low.

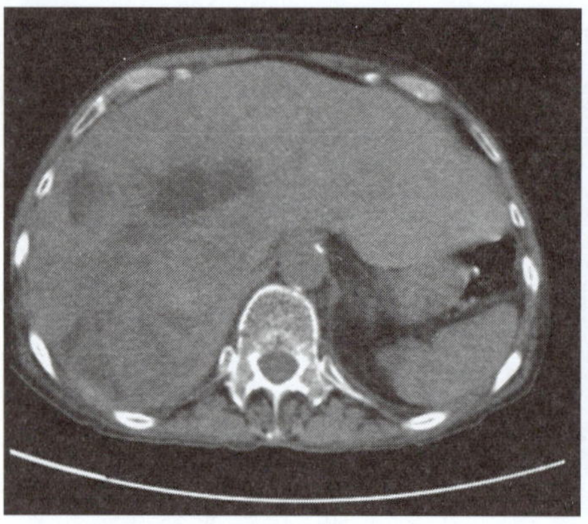
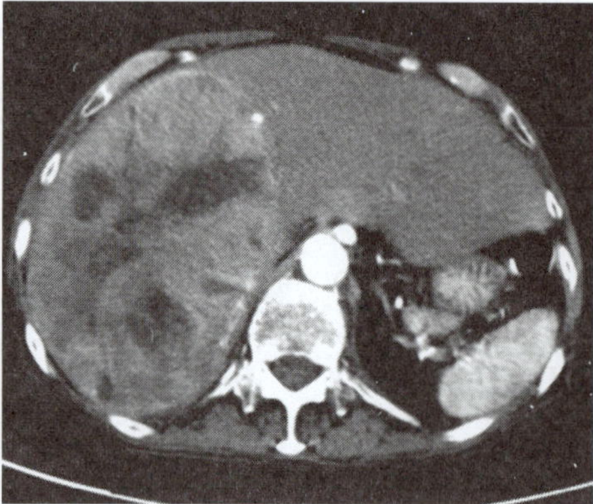
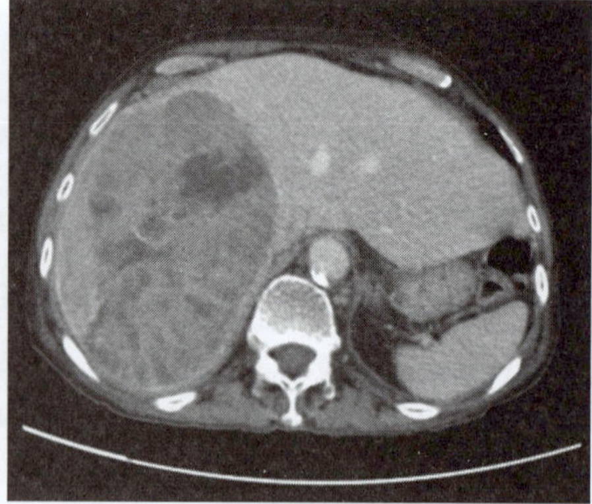

Figs 67.26 to 67.28: CT scan axial section through liver shows large mass in plain scan. Brightly enhancing in arterial phase of contrast study. Finally wash-out of contrast in portovenous phase which is a classical feature of hepatocellular carcinoma in multiphase contrast CT scan

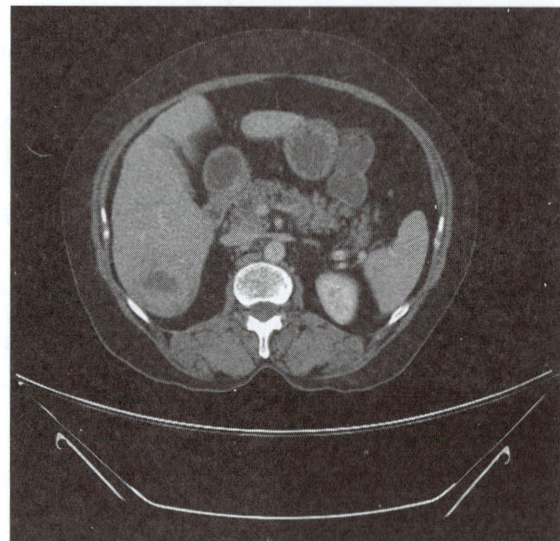

Fig. 67.29: CT scan of abdomen: Contrast-enhanced scan demonstrating a hypodense lesion in right lobe of liver posteriorly due to an abscess

VIRTUAL COLONOSCOPY

- It is a recently developed technique that uses a CT scanner and computer virtual reality software to look inside the body without having to insert a long tube (conventional colonoscopy) into the colon or without having to fill the colon with liquid barium (barium enema).
- More formally known as three-dimensional CT colonography, the virtual procedure allows radiologists to obtain 3D images from different angles, providing a sort of movie of the colon's interior without having to insert an endoscope into the bowel.

Advantages

- Noninvasive procedure, well-tolerated by patient
- Requires no sedation, less time-consuming
- Useful in elderly who are frail and infirm
- Useful when a tumour is large enough to block passage of scope (Figs 67.30 and 67.31).

Disadvantages

- Exposure to radiation, less detail of inner lining of colon
- Small polyps are located more reliably by colonoscopy
- Strictly a diagnostic procedure (unlike colonoscopy).

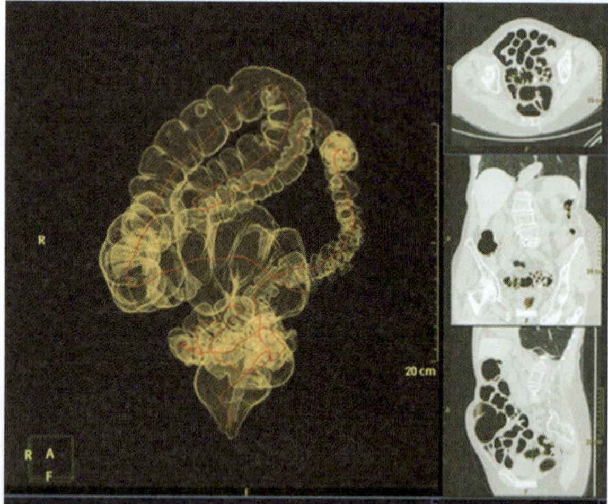

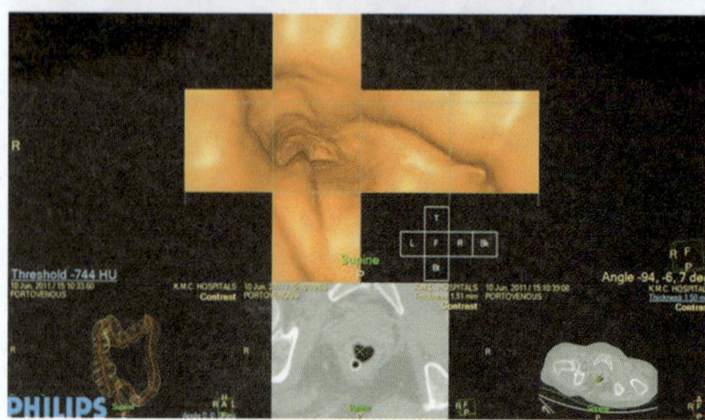

Figs 67.30 and 67.31: Virtual colonoscopy shows opened-up view to look for small mass or polyp

A few examples are given below.

1. CONTRAST ENHANCED (CE) CT ABDOMEN SHOWING MASS IN THE RIGHT ILIAC FOSSA

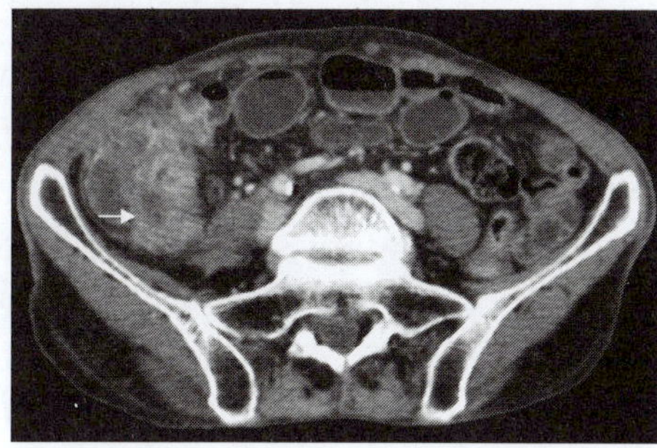

Fig. 67.32: A hypodense mass in the right iliac fossa involving caecum

1. **What is this investigation?**
   - Contrast enhanced CT scan
2. **How to interpret the CT scan?**
   - Structures imaged appear as densely white or black.
3. **What is the name used to the picture in terms of number of units?**
   - Hounsfield units
4. **Why do you give contrast?**
   - This is to increase the density between various structures. *Example:* Aorta appears bright with contrast.
5. **What are the precautions?**
   - Pregnancy is a contraindication. Iodine containing contrast can give rise to nephropathy. Allergy to contrast can happen. Hence, dehydration should be corrected. Serum creatinine should be checked before contrast.
6. **When do you use oral contrast?**
   - While studying abdominal viscera, e.g. if leak is suspected.
7. **What is the finding here?**
   - It is showing a hypodense lesion in the right iliac fossa.
8. **What is the diagnosis?**
   - Mostly carcinoma caecum
9. **Why do you say so?**
   - Anatomically it is a lesion occupying the right iliac fossa involving caecum.
10. **How do you describe this?**
    - It is a hypodense mass with solid and cystic areas. Cystic areas represent tumour degeneration.
11. **What else is seen in this picture?**
    - Fat planes between the mass and the abdominal wall is obliterated.
12. **What is the importance of that?**
    - Probably it is infiltrating the abdominal wall.
13. **Why do you want to know this information?**
    - At surgery, the involved portion of the abdominal wall has to be removed.
14. **How do you confirm the diagnosis?**
    - Colonoscopy and biopsy
15. **What will be the report expected?**
    - In majority of the cases it is adenocarcinoma
16. **What is the treatment, if it is operable?**
    - Right radical hemicolectomy
17. **If it is inoperable, what is the treatment?**
    - Palliative ileo-transverse anastomosis

2. CECT SHOWING HYPODENSE LESION WITH AIR POCKETS IN THE LEFT SUBPHRAENIC SPACE

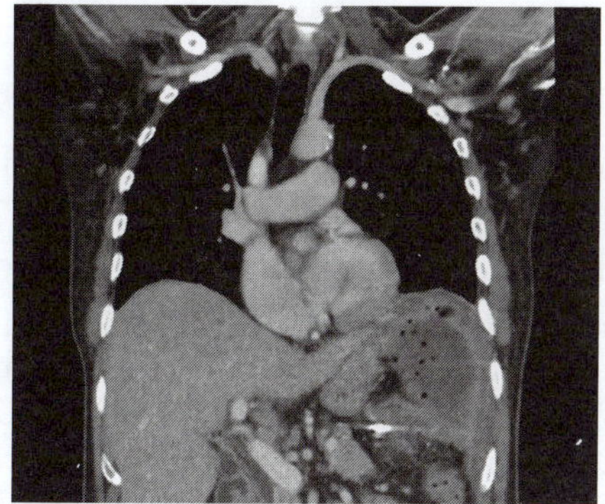

Fig. 67.33: CECT showing left subphrenic abscess

1. **What are the findings in this film?**
   - About 5 cm sized hypodense lesion with air-filled lesion.
2. **What is the most likely diagnosis?**
   - Abscess
3. **What are causes of abscess in that location?**
   - Pancreatic necrosis, posterior gastric perforations, ruptures liver abscess
4. **Left posterior subphrenic space is called as what?**
   - Lesser sac
5. **What is the treatment?**
   - Ultrasound-guided per cutaneous aspiration of pus.

CHOLANGIOGRAM/ERCP/MRCP

Introduction: These are used in the evaluation of biliary tract and pancreas. Details have been given in the gallbladder and pancreas chapter. T-tube cholangiogram is used following open choledochotomy. ERCP is preferred for evaluation of lower biliary obstructions, classical example being stones in the CBD. MRCP is used in the evaluation of high bile duct strictures or obstructions. A few examples are given below.

1. T-TUBE CHOLANGIOGRAPHY SHOWING A FILLING DEFECT IN THE LOWER END OF THE COMMON BILE DUCT (CBD)

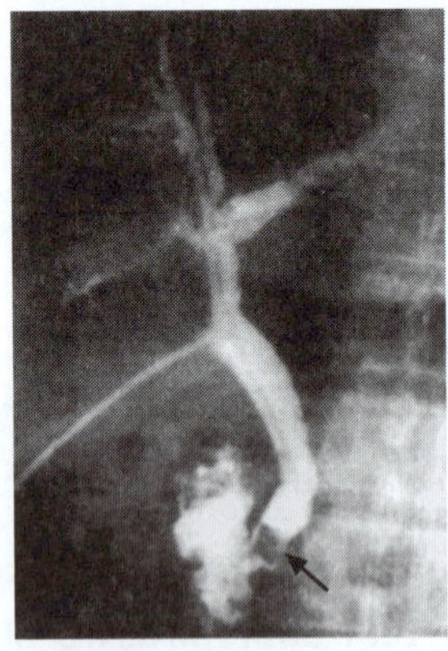

Fig. 67.34: T-tube cholangiography showing a filling defect in the lower end of the common bile duct (CBD)

1. **What is the diagnosis?**
   - Postcholecystectomy—residual stone in the CBD
2. **What is the surgery done for this patient?**
   - Cholecystectomy and choledocholithotomy
3. **Why do you insert a T-tube after CBD exploration?**
   - In case of distal obstruction by a residual stone, the bile starts leaking from the suture line on the CBD and may result in biliary peritonitis. In such situations, T-tube helps in drainage of the bile.
4. **What material is T-tube made of?**
   - Latex
5. **How do you treat this patient in order to extract the stone?**
   - Endoscopic sphincterotomy and extraction of the stone.

2. ERCP SHOWING FILLING OF THE DYE IN THE DUODENUM LOWER CBD AND PARTIAL FILLING OF INTRAHEPATIC BILE DUCT RADICALS. ALSO 3 CLIPS ARE VISIBLE ALONG THE LENGTH OF COMMON HEPATIC DUCT. GALLBLADDER IS NOT VISUALIZED

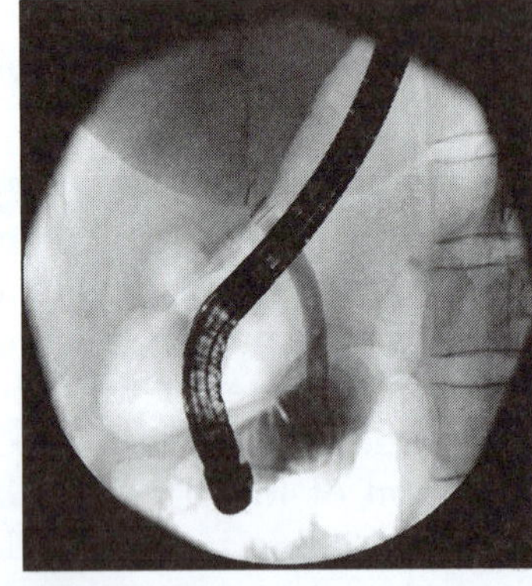

Fig. 67.35: ERCP showing partial obstruction of CBD/CHD caused by clips. Gallbladder is not seen.

1. **What is the diagnosis?**
   - Postcholecystectomy—stricture common hepatic duct/common hepatic duct.
2. **What is the type of injury is this?**
   - Strasberg D—probably a lateral injury due to partial clips.
3. **What is the next investigation?**
   - CET is done to know any significant bile collection/ biloma—if present and if sepsis is present, better to explore.
4. **How do you treat this patient in order to eliminate sepsis?**
   - Explore, drain the bile, remove clips, if possible insert T-tube drain, Morrison's pouch and come out
5. **In cases of complete transections, how do you treat?**
   - If detected on table, do primary repair—hepatico-jejunostomy. If detected later, assess for sepsis—treat it, improve nutrition and surgery can be done 4 to 6 weeks later.

MAGNETIC RESONANCE IMAGING (MRI)

Principle

Certain atomic nuclei, which possess unpaired protons or neutrons, have an inherent spin. The nucleus is positively charged and therefore creates a small magnetic field around itself, when it spins. The human body contains in abundance such spinning nuclei in the atoms of hydrogen which is found in water and lipids (Figs 67.36 to 67.40).

When the tissues containing these nuclei are within a strong magnetic field, the nuclei tend to align themselves along the lines of the force. The spinning protons now tend to precess, i.e. wobble about the axis of the main magnetic field. Now a radiofrequency (RF) is applied, being of the same frequency as the processing but at right angles to the main magnetic field. This excites the protons at low energy states into higher energy states. Thus, an absorption of energy takes place, which is used, as the excited protons 'relax' back to their original energy level when the radiofrequency is switched off. The relaxation of protons back to equilibrium and lower energy state is termed **spin-lattice relaxation** or **longitudinal relaxation**. It is exponential and referred to by the time **constant** T1. When the RF pulse is applied the protons process together in synchronism or in phase with each other. During relaxation, however, they go quickly out of

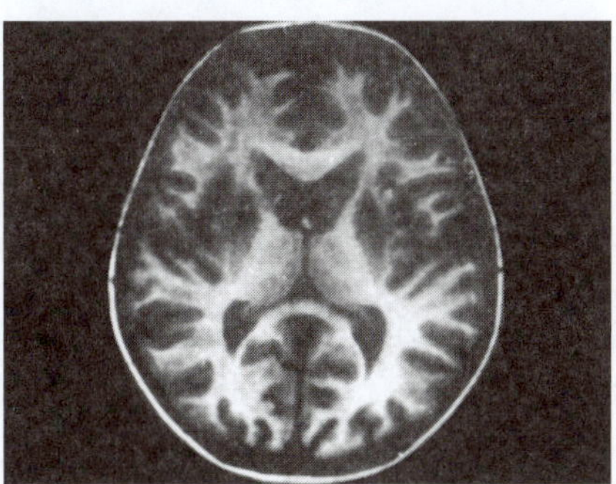

Fig. 67.36: MRI: T1 and T2 weighted axial and coronal scans of normal brain

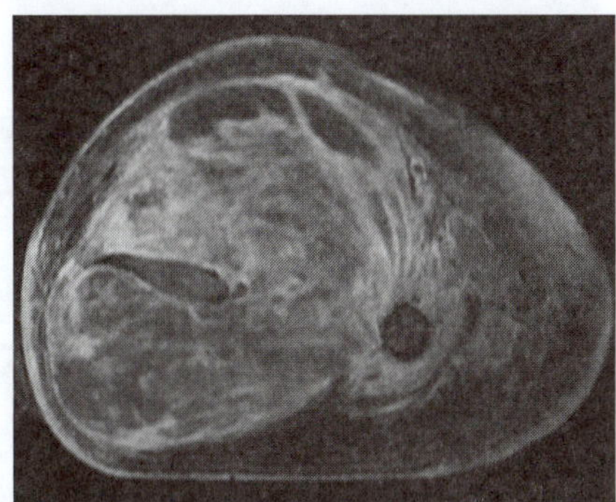

Fig. 67.37: Soft tissue sarcoma involving the muscle of thigh. The lesion is hyperintense in appearance

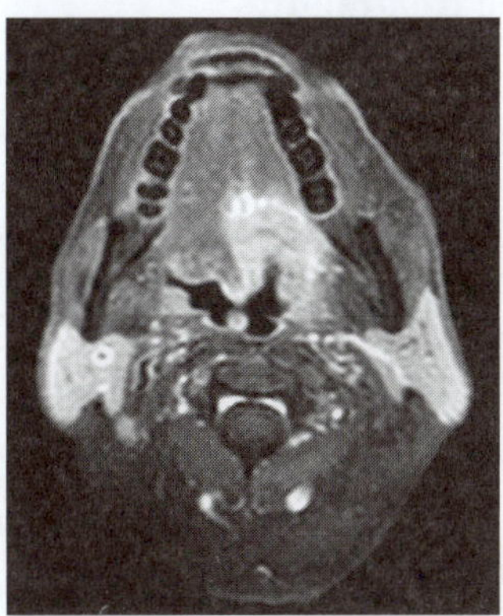

Fig. 67.38: Carcinoma tongue. MRI image shows hyperintense lesion is involving the posterior and base of the tongue on the left side. The other bright structures seen bilaterally are parotid glands

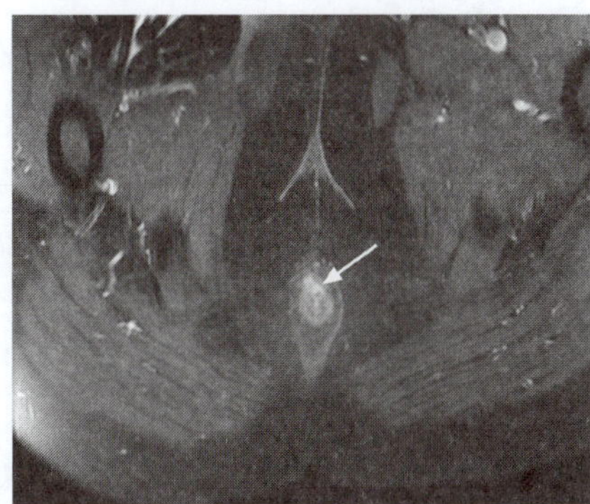

Fig. 67.39: Intersphincteric fistula—axial section of MRI pelvis showing hyperintense fistula (arrow)

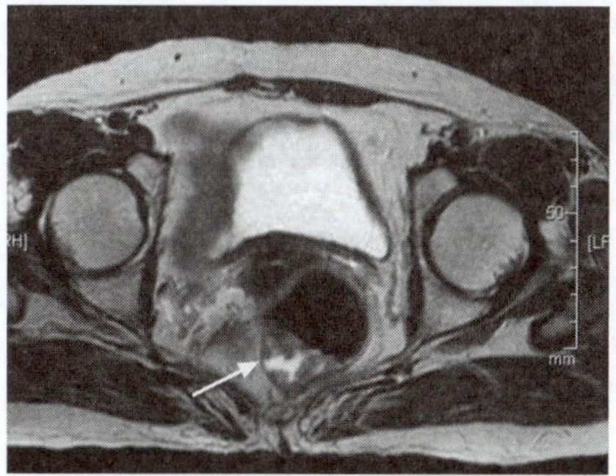

Fig. 67.40: Axial section of pelvis shows wall thickening of the rectal wall (arrow)

phase due to small variations in local magnetic fields. This loss of phase is termed **spin-spin relaxation** or **transverse relaxation**. It is also an exponential and referred to by the time constant T2. Depending on the type of tissue under study, the T1 and T2 relaxation times will differ, thus giving rise to differences in the image.

The MRI image depends upon four main factors:

1. The T1 relaxation time
2. The T2 relaxation time
3. The proton density
4. The blood flow

Depending on the characteristics of the above four parameters, the signal intensity of the image will vary, thus deciding the appearance that any given tissue will finally cast.

Advantages of MRI

1. It is noninvasive.
2. It does not involve the use of ionising radiation. Hence, it is safe in that respect.
3. It gives high intrinsic contrast.
4. Direct transverse, sagittal and normal imaging possible.
5. No bone/air artefact.
6. It has no known biological hazard.

Disadvantages of MRI

1. The imaging time is long. Hence, movement of the patients may produce artefacts.
2. Due to variety of protocol options during scanning, the final image is highly operator-dependent and this requires expert technical staff.
3. Expensive
4. Poor bone and calcium detail
5. **Patients with pacemakers, metallic implants and critically ill patients cannot be scanned.**

A few examples are given below.

1. MRI SHOWING STONES IN THE CBD

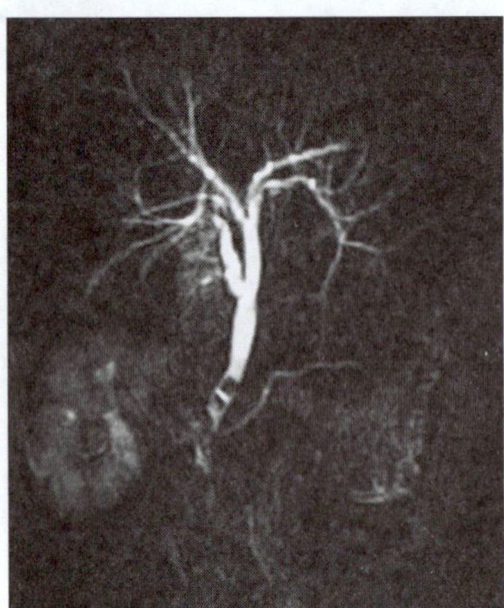

Fig. 67.41

1. **What structures are seen here?**
   - Intrahepatic radicles, common bile duct and duodenum.
2. **What are the findings?**
   - Filling defects are seen as dark shadows in the CBD.
3. **What is the final diagnosis?**
   - Choledocholithiasis
4. **What are the advantages of MRI?**
   - It is non-ionizing and no contrast is used.
5. **How do you treat this condition?**
   - ERCP, basketting of stones followed by laparoscopic cholecystectomy.

2. MRI OF THE THIGH

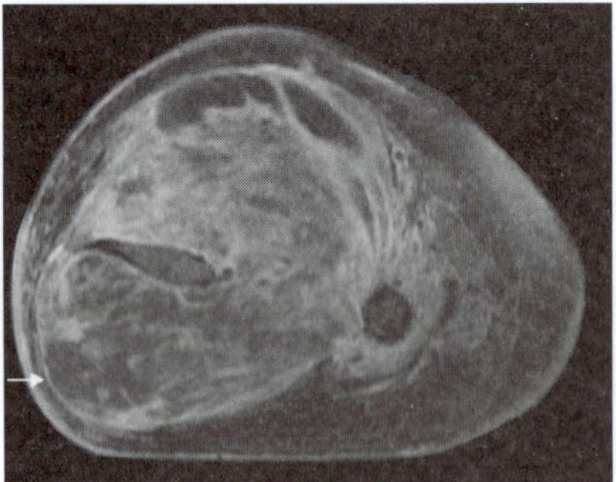

Fig. 67.42: MRI of the thigh

1. **Name this investigation.**
   - Magnetic resonance imaging
2. **What are the principles of MRI?**
   - Certain atomic nuclei, which possess unpaired protons or neutrons, possess an inherent spin. The nucleus is positively charged and, therefore, creates a small magnetic field around itself, when it spins. The human body contains in abundance such spinning nuclei in the atoms of hydrogen, which is found in water and lipids.
3. **What are the chief advantages of MRI over CT scan?**
   - It is noninvasive and does not involve the use of ionising radiation. Hence, it is safe.
4. **What are the disadvantages of MRI?**
   - The imaging time is long. Hence, movement of the patients may produce artefacts.
   - Expensive
   - Patients with pacemakers, metallic implant and critically ill patients cannot be scanned.
   - Claustrophobia
5. **What does this picture show?**
   - A hyperintense mass occupying the thigh region.
6. **What is the diagnosis?**
   - Soft tissue sarcoma
7. **How do you confirm the diagnosis?**
   - Trucut biopsy
8. **Why not FNAC?**
   - FNAC cannot diagnose the type of sarcoma
9. **What are common tumours in this location?**
   - Malignant fibrous histiocytoma (MFH) and liposarcoma.
10. **What is the treatment?**
    - Wide excision with 2–3 cm margin.

Few MRI images:

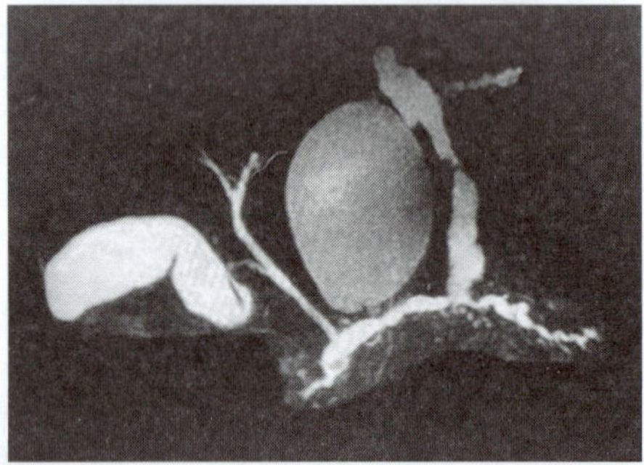

Fig. 67.43: MRI showing pancreaticopleural fistula

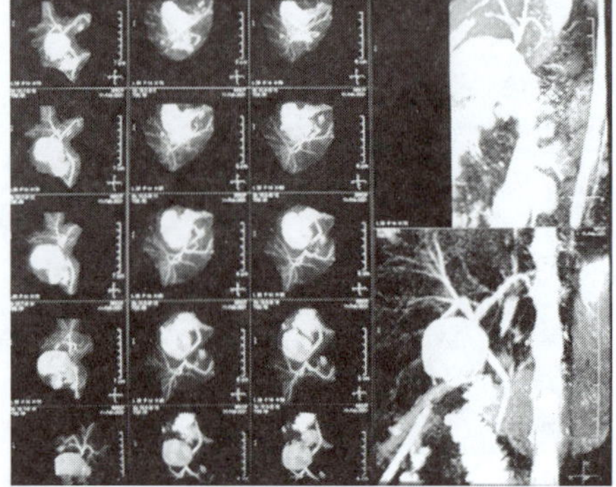

Fig. 67.44: MRI showing leak from bile duct after cholecystectomy

POSITRON EMISSION TOMOGRAPHY (PET SCAN)

- PET scan is a medical imaging technique that combines computed tomography (CT) and nuclear scanning. It is used to determine the metabolic or biochemical activity in the brain, heart and other organs by tracking the movement and concentration of a radioactive tracer injected into the blood stream.
- A camera records the tracer's signal as it travels through the body and collects information about the organs. A computer then converts the signals into 3D images of the examined organ, which provide a clear view of an abnormality.
- One of the main differences between PET scan and other imaging tests like CT or MRI is that the PET scan reveals the cellular level metabolic changes occurring in an organ and functional changes at cellular level. A PET scan often detects these changes very early, whereas CT or MRI detect changes a little later as the disease begins to cause structural changes in organs or tissues.
- Positron emission tomography (PET-CT) constitutes major progress in management of cancer patients for the initial diagnosis, staging and follow-up of various malignancies. PET-CT is also useful in the follow-up of patients following chemotherapy or surgical resection of tumour, since, most of them have a confusing appearance at CT or MR imaging due to postoperative changes or scar tissue (Figs 67.45 to 67.50).

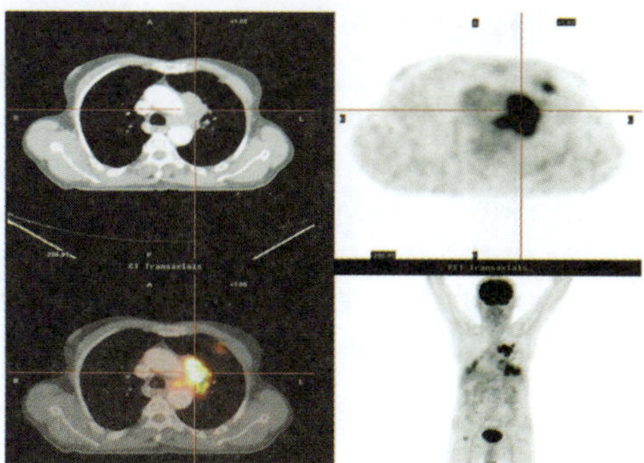

Fig. 67.45: Carcinoma breast with metastasis

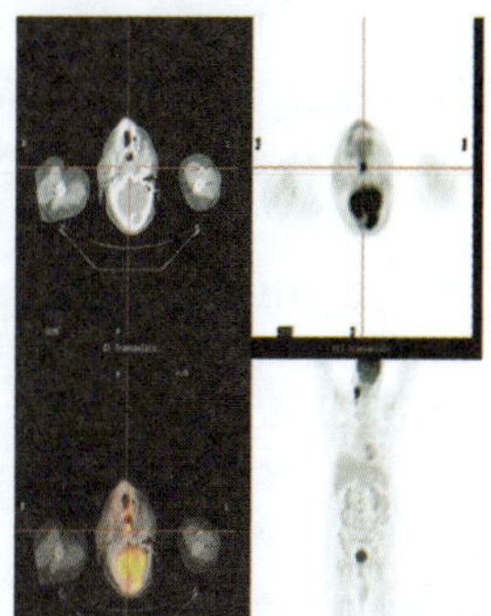

Fig. 67.46: Carcinoma oesophagus

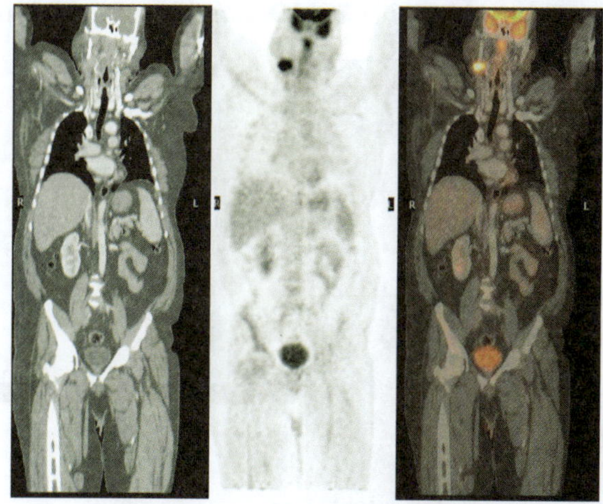

Fig. 67.47: Carcinoma lung—PET-CT scan

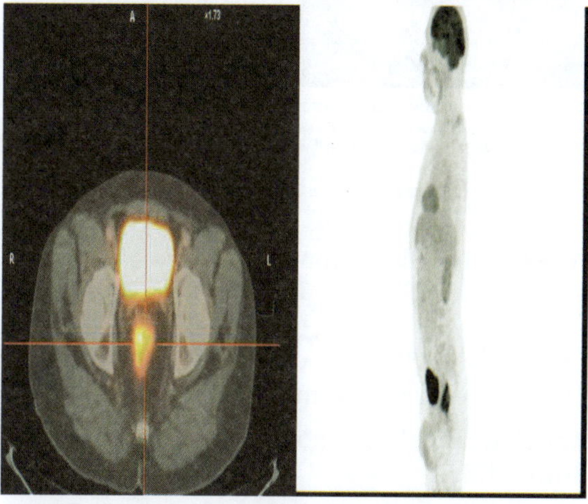

Fig. 67.48: Carcinoma nasopharynx—PET-CT scan

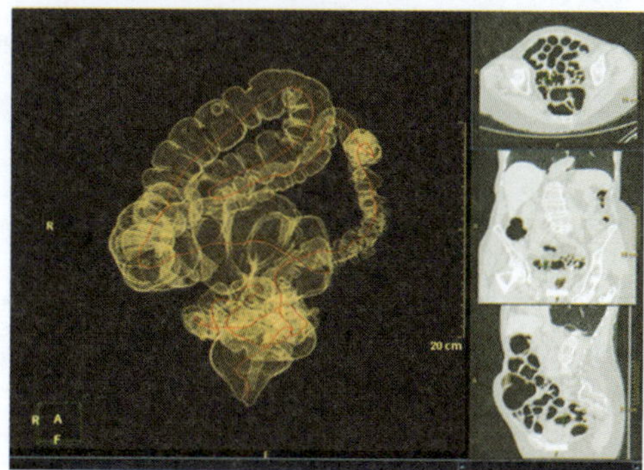

Fig. 67.49: Another case of carcinoma nasopharynx

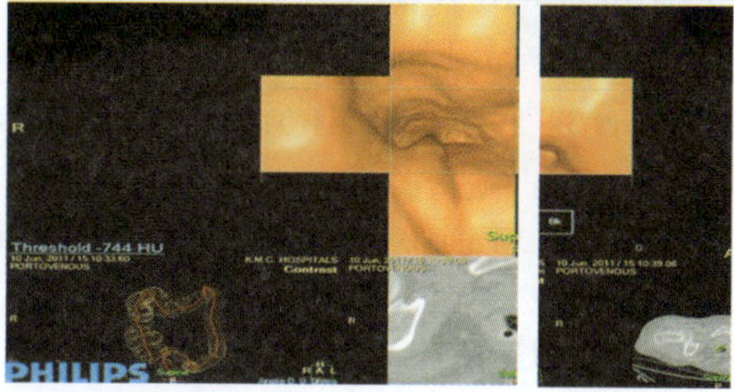

Fig. 67.50: Carcinoma rectum—PET-CT scan

1. POSITRON EMISSION TOMOGRAPHY (PET) SCAN

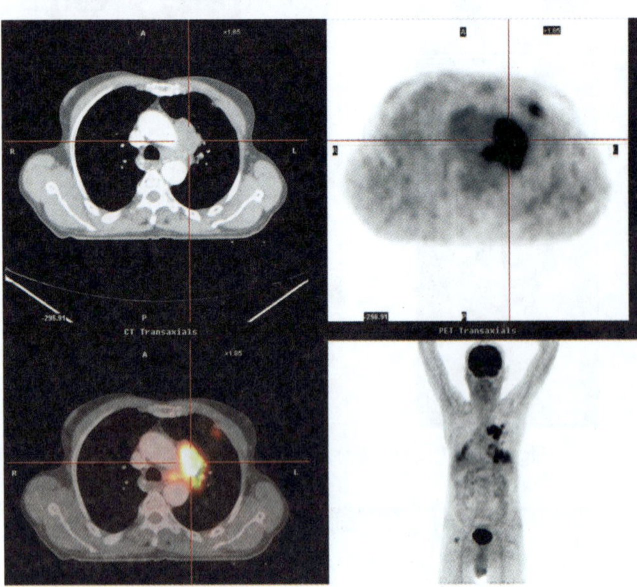

PET-CT of a patient who was diagnosed to have carcinoma lung on bronchoscopy.
PET-CT shows a hilar mass with a nodule anteriorly on left side of pleura.
It also shows pneumonic patch on lower zone of left lung which is FDG avid

Fig. 67.51: CT and PET of lung

1. **Name this investigation.**
   - PET-CT scan
2. **What is PET scan?**
   - Positron emission tomography
3. **What is the most commonly used positron emitting radionuclide?**
   - Fluoro-deoxyglucose (FDG)
4. **What are the chief uses of PET scan?**
   - For myocardial perfusion and viability, detection of metastasis from cancer—carcinoma lung, colon, nasopharynx, etc.
5. **What are the disadvantages?**
   - Very expensive and limited availability
6. **What does this picture show?**
   - Hilar mass with a nodule anteriorly on the left side of pleura
7. **What may be the diagnosis?**
   - Carcinoma lung
8. **How do you confirm the diagnosis?**
   - Bronchoscopy and biopsy
9. **If the report is adenocarcinoma lung, what is the next step?**
   - To stage the disease by whole body bone scan, PET scan, and CT scan.
10. **If confined to lung, what is the treatment?**
    - Lobectomy/pneumonectomy.

INTERVENTIONAL RADIOLOGY

The role of radiology was limited as only a diagnostic art until mid 1970s. However, now radiology has taken on an exciting new aspect and has entered the field of interventional radiology. Two main types of interventional procedures: Vascular and nonvascular.

Vascular

1. **Angioplasty:** This is performed by the use of intraluminal balloon catheters and may be performed for almost any diseased vessel in the body. The more commonly treated vessels are the coronaries, renal arteries, peripheral limb vessels, etc.
2. **Embolisation:** This procedure is performed either preoperatively to reduce the vascularity of certain tumours, or as a curative treatment for vascular malformations, aneurysms, GI bleeding, etc. Temporary embolisation may be achieved by using gel foam or autologous clots and permanent embolisation by using balloons, steel coils, ethanol, etc. Inferior vena cava (IVC) umbrella placement, IVC membranotomy are also done.
3. **Intravascular ultrasound:** The use of ultrasound inside a blood vessel to visualise the interior of the vessel in order to detect problems inside the blood vessel.
4. **Stent placement:** A tiny, expandable coil, called a stent, is placed inside a blood vessel at the site of a blockage. The stent is expanded to open up the blockage.
   - **Important types of stents and stent selection: Self-expanding stents** are compressed within a catheter device and released by removing a constraining sheath or membrane. The final diameter of the stent is a function of the outward elastic load of the stent and the inward recoil of the elastic wall.
   - **Balloon expandable stents** are mounted on angioplasty balloons in a compressed state and then deployed by balloon inflation. These stents retain the diameter imposed by angioplasty balloon unless externally compressed.
5. **Foreign body extraction:** The use of a catheter inserted into a blood vessel to retrieve a foreign body in the vessel.
6. **Needle biopsy:** A small needle is inserted into the abnormal area in almost any part of the body, guided by imaging techniques, to obtain a tissue biopsy. This type of biopsy can provide a diagnosis without surgical intervention.
7. **Blood clot filters:** A small filter is inserted into a blood clot to catch and break up blood clots.

8. **Injection of clot-lysing agents:** Clot-lysing agents, such as tissue plasminogen activator (tPA) are injected into the body to dissolve blood clots, thereby increasing blood flow to the heart or brain.
9. **Catheter insertions:** A catheter is inserted into large veins for giving chemotherapy drugs, nutritional support, and haemodialysis. A catheter may also be inserted prior to bone marrow transplantation.
10. **Cancer treatment:** Administering cancer medications directly to the tumour site.

Nonvascular

1. **Hepatobiliary:** Percutaneous transhepatic biliary drainage (PTBD) is widely accepted in cases of biliary obstruction, along with percutaneous biliary calculus removal. Biliary stent placement across a malignant lesion is widely being done in inoperable cases as a palliative procedure.
2. **Urinary:** Percutaneous nephrostomy, percutaneous stenting and percutaneous nephrolithotomy are being performed.
3. **Guided biopsy:** Fluoroscopy, ultrasound or CT-guided biopsy of various lesions are now part of routine technique.
4. **Other interventional procedures:** Percutaneous gastrostomy, catheter drainage of abscesses, pseudocysts, ultrasound-guided intrauterine foetal surgeries, etc.

Advantages of Interventional Procedures

1. Patient compliance is high as surgery is avoided.
2. Cost-effectiveness is high.
3. Infection rates are low.
4. Can be repeated as it is relatively noninvasive.
5. Certain untreatable conditions are treated palliatively with interventional procedures.

> ***Please Note:*** X-rays discussed here are the common X-rays which are asked in the MBBS examination. However, modern investigations such as mammogram, ultrasound, CT scan and MRI also may be asked. You are requested to read the chapters on radiology and breast for more details about these investigations.

Multiple Choice Questions

1. Niche and a notch mark is an absolute contra-indication for myelography

A. Chronic duodenal ulcer
B. Chronic gastric ulcer
C. Carcinoma stomach
D. Stromal tumour

2. Trifoliate/clover deformity is diagnostic of:

A. Chronic duodenal ulcer
B. Chronic gastric ulcer
C. Carcinoma stomach
D. Stromal tumour

3. The substance used in barium studies is:

A. Barium chloride
B. Barium sulphate
C. Barium carbonate
D. Barium sulphide

4. Barium follow through extends up to:

A. Proximal duodenum
B. Fundus of the stomach
C. Ileocaecal junction
D. Proximal jejunum

5. Which of the following is a contraindication for barium study?

A. Dysphagia and odynophagia
B. Motility disorders of the GIT
C. Perforation of gastric mucosa
D. Assessing mediastinal masses

6. Achalasia cardia shows the following findings on barium swallow *except*:

A. Shouldering effect cranial and caudal to the lesion
B. Rat tail appearance of lower end of the oesophagus
C. Gross dilatation of the proximal oesophagus
D. Thin streaks of contrast entering the stomach

7. 'Moulage' sign (barium in a featureless tube) is a feature of:

A. Crohn's disease B. Intestinal TB
C. Ulcerative colitis D. Malabsorption

8. Which of the following statements is false?

A. Angiographic studies use ^{123}I as contrast substance
B. Enteroclysis is done for mechanical obstruction of the intestine
C. Peripheral venography done for deep vein thrombosis uses ^{125}I
D. Papilloedema is an absolute contraindication for myelography

9. Which of the following statements is false?

A. Ultrasound is based on the principle of piezo-electric effect, the most common substance used in ultrasonic transducers being lead zirconate titanate (PZT)

B. MRI uses ionising radiation, hence it is unsafe

C. Patients with pacemakers and critically ill patients cannot be scanned using MRI

D. CT scan gives good bone and calcium detail

10. The most common side effect of peripheral venography is:

A. Complications due to contrast

B. Tissue necrosis

C. Thrombophlebitis

D. Pulmonary embolism due to dislodged clot

11. Which of the following statements is false about PET scan?

A. PET scan uses protons for radiological examination

B. It combines CT and nuclear scanning

C. It detects changes at the cellular level

D. It helps in early detection of changes in various pathologies.

12. BI-RADS score of 5 indicates which of the following?

A. Normal mammogram, no evidence of cancer

B. Mammogram normal, some evidence of cancer present

C. Suspicious findings on mammogram, 20–35% chance of cancer

D. Mammogram findings highly suspicious, 95% chance of cancer

13. The following statements about virtual colonoscopy are true *except*:

A. It is also called CT pneumocolon, purely diagnostic

B. It is invasive, requires sedation and contraindicated in elderly

C. It involves exposure to radiation

D. It cannot identify polyps measuring between 2 and 10 mm

14. Which of the following in future may be a gold standard test for screening of colorectal cancer?

A. PET scan

B. Sigmoidoscopy and colonoscopy

C. MRI

D. Virtual colonoscopy

15. The following is true about MRI *except*:

A. It is noninvasive

B. Gives high intrinsic contrast

C. Imaging possible in transverse, sagittal and normal views

D. Bone/air artefact can be a problem

Answers

1. B **2.** A **3.** B **4.** C **5.** C **6.** A **7.** D **8.** A **9.** B **10.** A
11. A **12.** D **13.** B **14.** D **15.** D

CHAPTER

68

Instruments

- Forceps
- Retractors
- Occlusion clamps
- Dilators
- Tracheostomy tube
- Rubber tubes
- Catheters
- Sengstaken tube
- Needles

ARTERY FORCEPS (HAEMOSTAT)

- It is also called **Spencer Well's artery forceps**. It has a ratchet and two blades with uniform serrations.
- It is used to control bleeding, not only from arteries but also from veins and capillaries. Once the bleeding points are caught, they are coagulated or ligature is applied.
- The curved artery is commonly used (Fig. 68.1B).
- The smaller version of this is called mosquito forceps (Fig. 68.1A). This is extremely useful in repair of harelip, cleft palate or other plastic surgery operations.
- It is also available as straight artery which is used to hold the stay sutures (Fig. 68.1C).

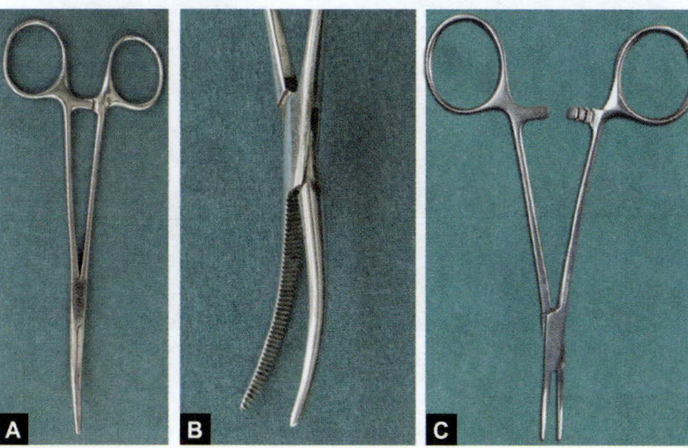

Figs 68.1A to C: (A) Mosquito forceps; (B) Curved artery forceps; (C) Straight artery forceps

ALLIS TISSUE HOLDING FORCEPS (Fig. 68.2)

- It has a ratchet and triangular expansion at the tip, where serrations are present.
- It can be used to **hold tough structures** such as fascia, aponeurosis, etc.
- Even though it can cause trauma, because of its better grip, it can be used to hold the duodenum for duodenal closure during gastrectomy.

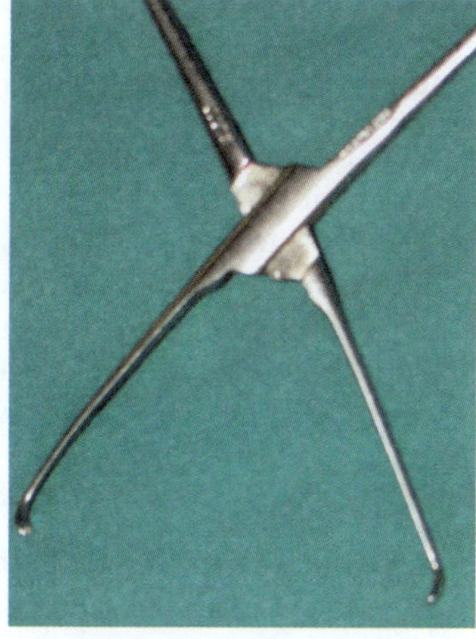

Fig. 68.2: Allis forceps

KOCHER'S FORCEPS

(Fig. 68.3 and Key Box 68.1)

- This is similar to an artery forceps with serrations. It is available as curved and straight.
- There is a sharp tooth at the tip of the instrument. Hence, it has a better grip.
- Kocher's forceps can be used to **hold tough structures** like **aponeurosis, fascia**, etc.
- During thyroidectomy, it can be used to hold the strap muscles for dividing them.
- Theodor Kocher, a Swiss surgeon, got the Nobel prize for his contribution to thyroid surgery.

Key Box 68.1

Remember

- Kocher's forceps
- Kocher's test
- Kocher's collar incision for thyroidectomy
- Kocher's sign—eyelid phenomenon in hyperthyroidism-staring and frightened look
- Kocher's thyroid dissector
- Kocher's vein
- Kocher's subcostal incision
- Kocher's gland holding forceps

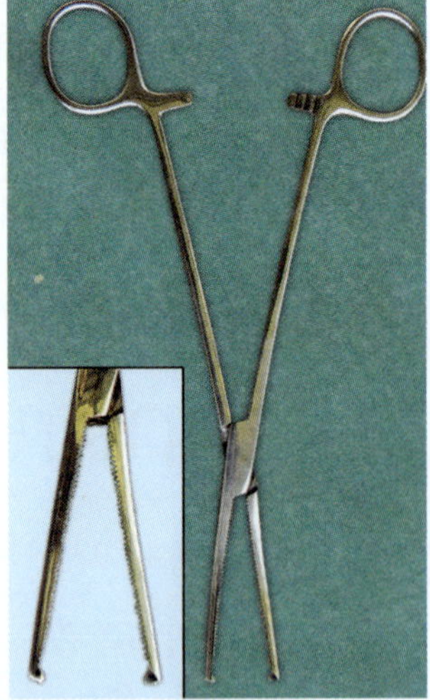

Fig. 68.3: Kocher's forceps

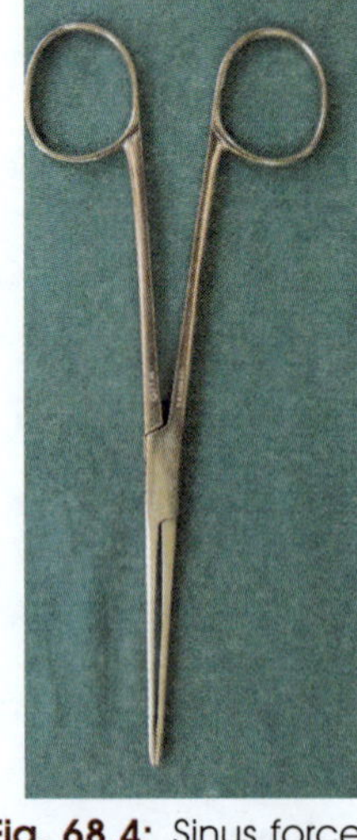

Fig. 68.4: Sinus forceps

SINUS FORCEPS (Fig. 68.4)

- This is like an artery forceps which has **No ratchet**.
- Serrations are confined to the tip so as to hold the wall of an abscess cavity, for biopsy.
- In ***Hilton's method*** of drainage of an abscess, once the incision is made, the sinus forceps is thrust into the abscess cavity and by opening the blades in all directions, the loculi are broken. To facilitate free opening of the blades, sinus forceps has no ratchet.

SWAB HOLDING FORCEPS (Fig. 68.5)

- This has a ratchet and two long blades
- Operating end is rounded with serrations
- It is used to hold the swab (gauze pieces) to prepare the parts with antiseptic agents at the time of surgery.
- This instrument can also be used as a blunt 'dissector' with the swab, while dissecting at a depth, e.g. lumbar sympathectomy, vagotomy.

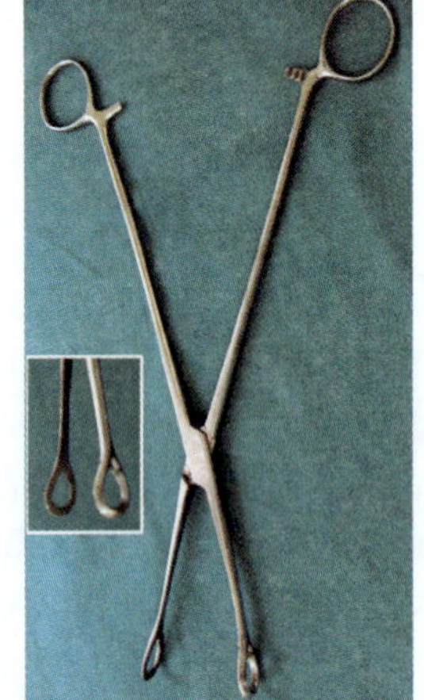

Fig. 68.5: Swab holding forceps

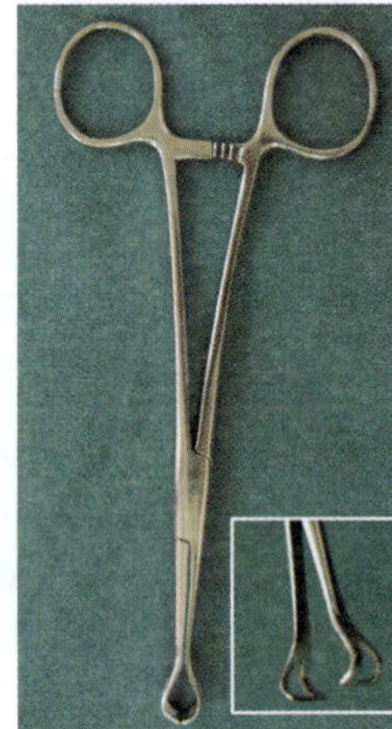

Fig. 68.6: Babcock's forceps

BABCOCK'S FORCEPS (Fig. 68.6)

- An instrument with a ratchet and a triangular expansion with fenestrations at the operating end. It does not have any teeth. Thus, it is used to hold intestines during anastomosis or resection.
- This instrument can also be used to hold many other structures such as thyroid gland, mesoappendix, uterine tubes, etc.

LANE'S FORCEPS (Fig. 68.7)

- This is similar to Babcock's forceps but the tip is more broad, expanded with a bigger opening.
- It is used to hold the appendix
- However, it does not seem to have any additional advantage when compared to Babcock's forceps.

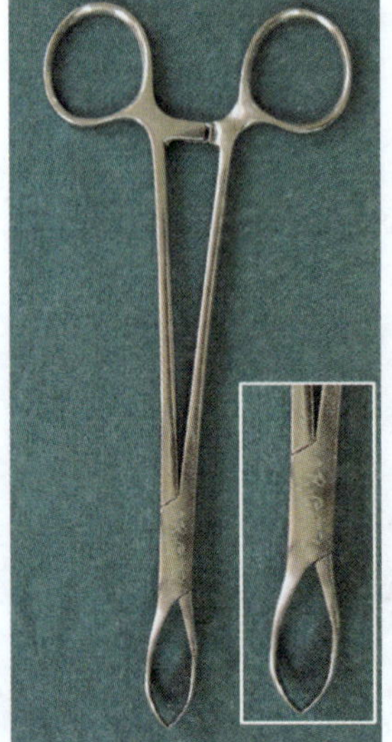

Fig. 68.7: Lane's forceps

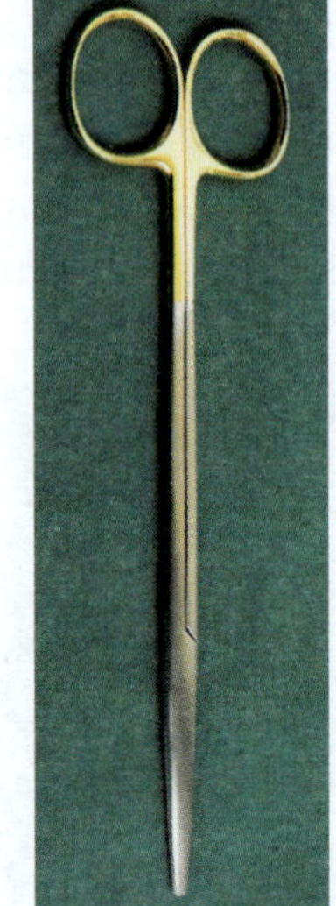

Fig. 68.8: Mayo's scissors

DISSECTING SCISSORS

- This is also called **Mayo's scissors** (Fig. 68.8 and Key Box 68.2).
- It does not have ratchet and operating end is sharp
- This is used to dissect tissue planes during surgical operations and to cut or divide important structures.
- It is popularly called **tissue scissors**.

Key Box 68.2

Remember

- Mayo's scissors
- Mayo's herniorrhaphy
- Mayo's posterior GJ
- Mayo's vein
- Mayo's needle (used for hernia repair)

STRAIGHT SCISSORS (Fig. 68.9)

It is used to cut the sutures or knots. Hence, called suture-cutting scissors.

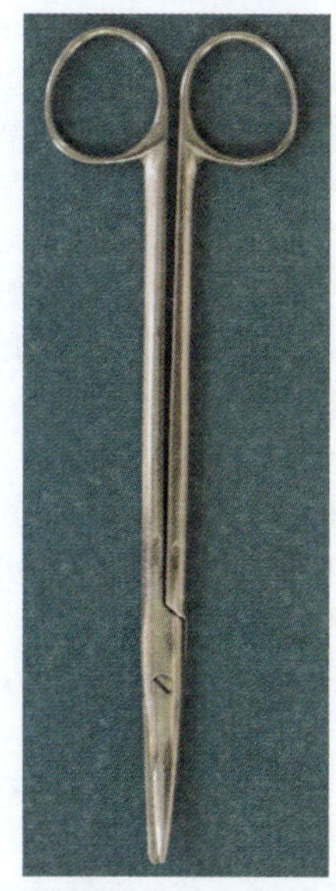

Fig. 68.9: Straight scissors

DISSECTING FORCEPS (Fig. 68.10)

- This is a toothed forceps. It is also available as non-toothed forceps.
- Dissecting forceps with dissecting scissors makes good 'tool' for a surgeon to develop a tissue plane in majority of surgeries.
- The forceps is very useful to 'pick' individual layers such as serosa, seromuscular layers, mucosa, etc. during anastomosis.

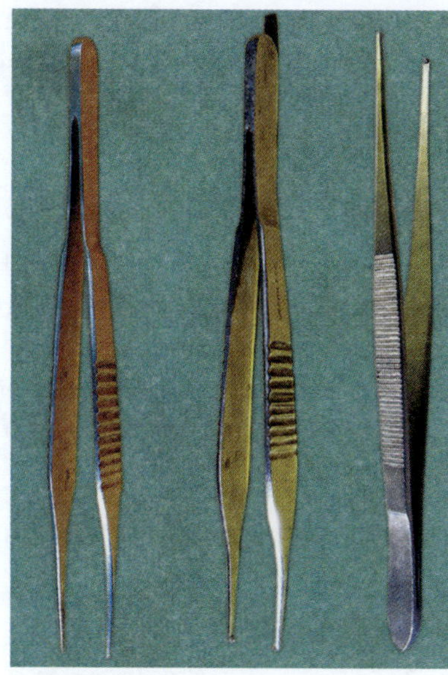

Fig. 68.10: Dissecting forceps

NEEDLE HOLDER (Fig. 68.11)

- This is a long instrument with a ratchet at non-operating end.
- The operating end has two small blades with serrations.
- The instrument is used to **hold the curved needles** which are used to suture the parts.
- A firm grip is essential to apply proper sutures.

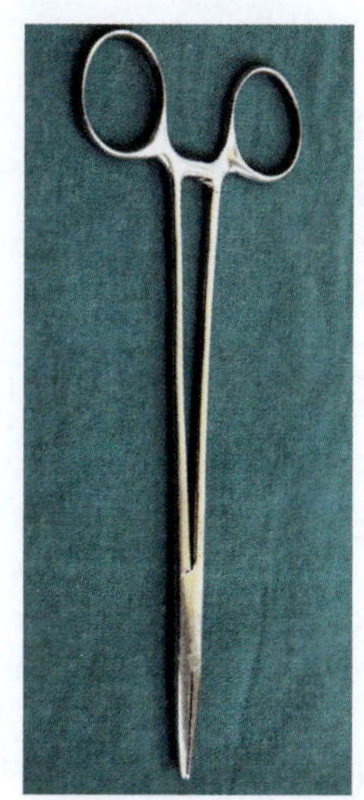

Fig. 68.11: Needle holder

SCALPEL WITH BLADE (Fig. 68.12)

- This is popularly called **surgeon's knife.**
- This is used to incise the skin and subcutaneous tissue.
- Due to the sharp nature, it can be used to divide a major vascular pedicle once ligatures are applied.

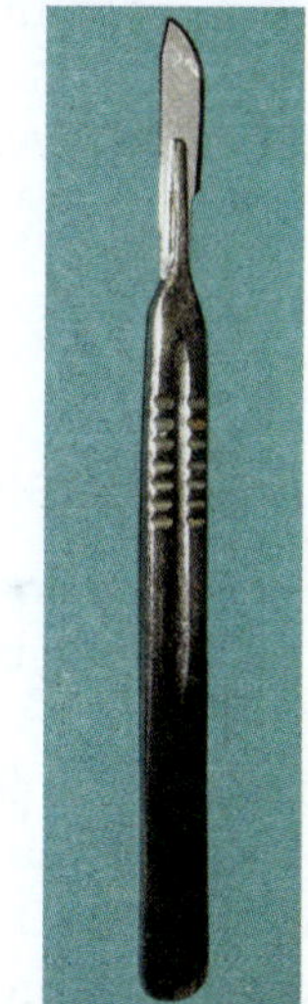

Fig. 68.12: Scalpel with blade

CHEATLES FORCEPS (Fig. 68.13)

- It is a long instrument having a curved shaft
- The **handle has no lock**
- It is kept dipped in antiseptic solutions
- This instrument is used to pick up sterilised articles such as sponges, gauze pieces or other instruments and to transfer to the instrument trolley.

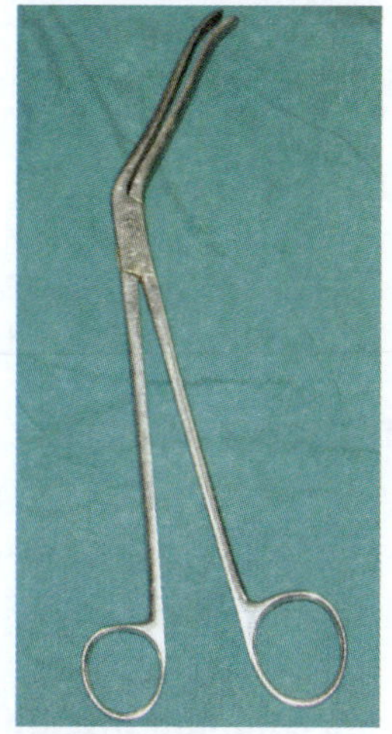

Fig. 68.13: Cheatles forceps

DEAVER RETRACTOR (Fig. 68.14)

- This is popularly called **Deaver liver retractor**
- It has a long blade and operating end is curved
- It can be used to retract the liver during vagotomy, cholecystectomy or gastrectomy, etc.

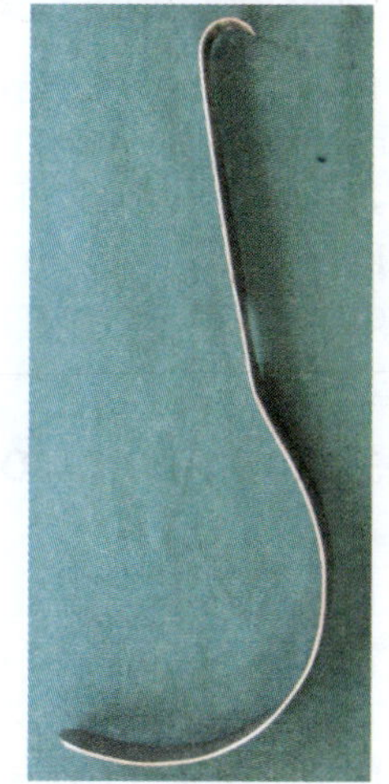

Fig. 68.14: Deaver retractor

- Since it has long blades, it can be used to retract the kidney upwards, during lumbar sympathectomy or to retract the urinary bladder during surgery on the rectum.

MORRIS RETRACTOR (Fig. 68.15)

- This is a long instrument with broad operating end.
- This is used t**o retract the abdominal wall**, once the peritoneum is opened.
- However, if a self-retaining retractor is used to widen the laparotomy wound, the use of Morris retractor gets limited.

CZERNY RETRACTOR (Fig. 68.16)

- This is a double-hooked retractor on one side and a single blade on the other side.
- This is a **superficial retractor**, can be used to retract layers of the abdominal wall, muscles, etc. Thus, during appendicectomy, herniorrhaphy or thyroidectomy, this instrument is very useful.

LANGENBECK RETRACTOR (Fig. 68.17)

- This instrument has only **one blade**
- The uses of this are similar to that of Czerny's retractor.

MOYNIHAN'S STRAIGHT OCCLUSION CLAMP (Fig. 68.18)

- This is a long instrument with a ratchet. The operating end has two long blades with serrations in the line of blades.
- This instrument is used to **occlude the intestinal lumen** to prevent spillage of intestinal contents during intestinal resection or intestinal anastomosis.
- This does not interfere with the vascularity of the intestine.

PAYR'S CRUSHING CLAMP (Fig. 68.19)

- This is a heavy instrument with **double lever system**, because of which it has a better grip
- The two short blades have uniform serrations
- During gastrectomy, when portion of the stomach is excised, this instrument is applied on the stomach side so that the stomach with this instrument is excised.

DESJARDIN'S CHOLEDOCHOLITHOTOMY FORCEPS (Fig. 68.20)

- This is a long curved instrument with no **ratchet**
- The operating end is expanded with fenestrations
- The tip is blunt
- It is used to **extract stones from common bile duct**. It can also be used to extract stones from the ureter.

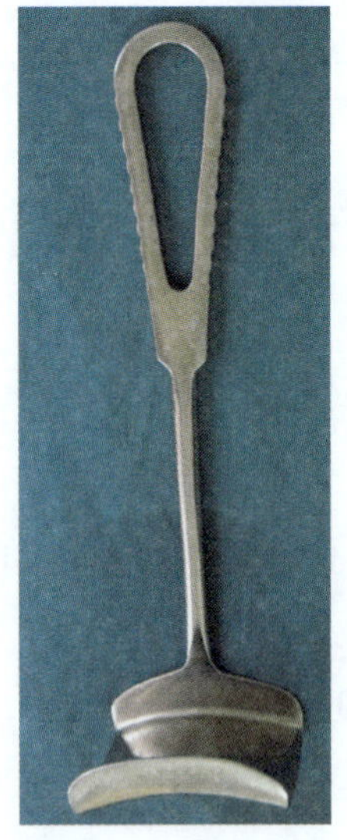

Fig. 68.15: Morris retractor

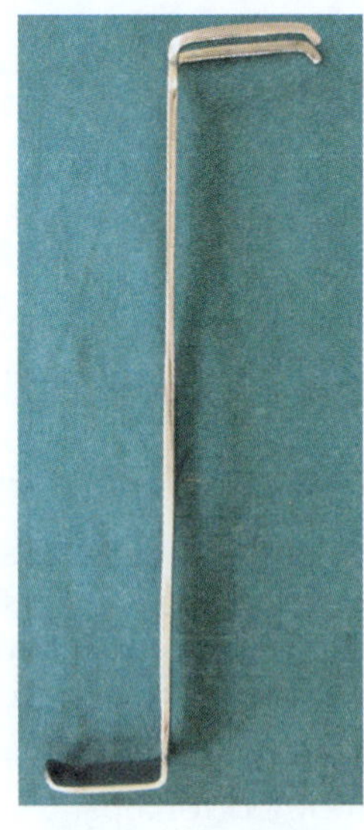

Fig. 68.16: Czerny retractor

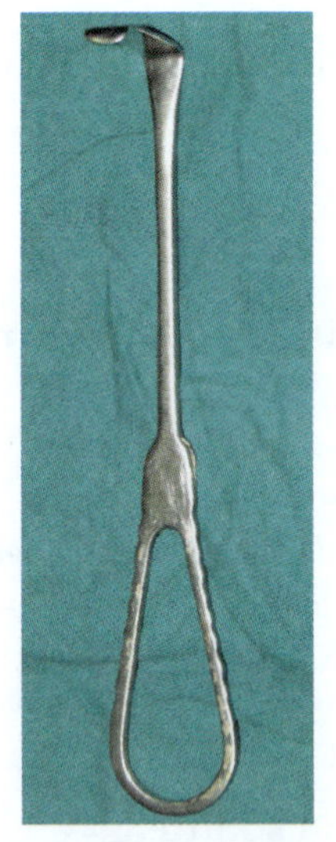

Fig. 68.17: Langenbeck retractor

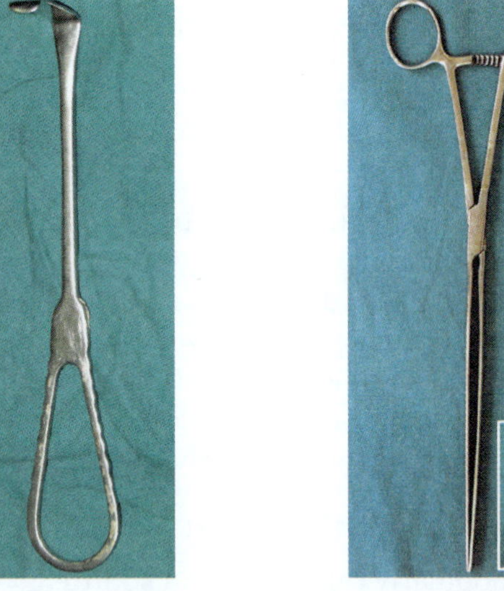

Fig. 68.18: Moynihan's occlusion clamp

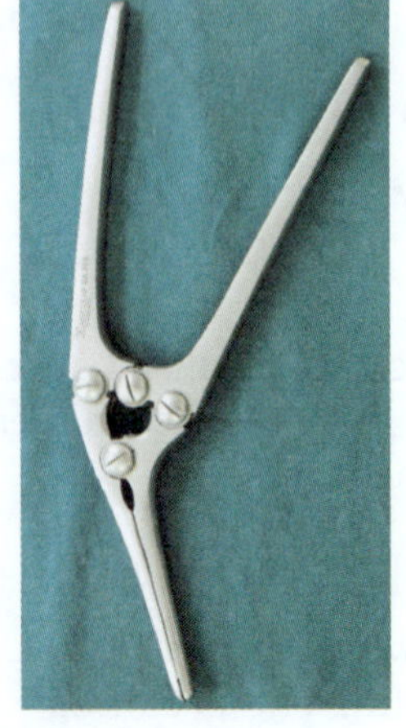

Fig. 68.19: Payr's crushing clamp

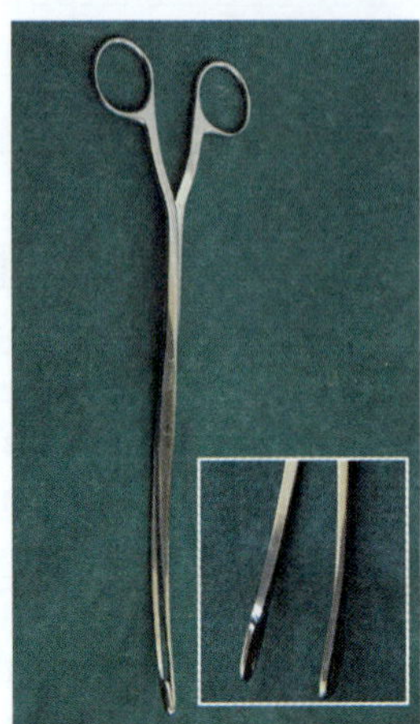

Fig. 68.20: Desjardin's forceps

- Since there is no ratchet, free opening is possible, and the stones do not get crushed.

BAKE'S DILATOR (Fig. 68.21)

- This is a long malleable instrument available in various diameters.
- It has a handle, long body and the tip is blunt.
- Once common bile duct exploration is completed, this dilator is passed, to assess for any distal obstruction.
- The free passage of Bake's dilators of different sizes indicate that there is no distal obstruction (however, to be confirmed by cholangiogram).

KOCHER'S THYROID DISSECTOR (Fig. 68.22)

- This has a long handle and the operating end is small and blunt with an opening.
- A few longitudinal serrations are present at the tip.
- This was used to dissect the upper pole of thyroid gland.
- This instrument can also be used to dissect the isthmus of the thyroid gland from the trachea.
- **Silk thread can be fed** into the opening so as to ligate the vascular pedicle or isthmus.
- With the availability of the right-angled forceps, this instrument is not in routine use nowadays.

ANEURYSM NEEDLE (Fig. 68.23)

- It is a long instrument with an *eye* at the operating end.
- It is called aneurysm needle because it was used to ligate the feeding artery in an aneurysm. However today, this instrument is of limited use.
- During **venesection or cut down**, the silk suture can be threaded within the *eye*, passed round the vein and it is tied.

TROCAR AND CANNULA (Fig. 68.24)

- This has two parts. The inner sharp part is the trocar and outer blunt part is cannula.
- It is used to drain hydrocoele fluid.
- Once hydrocoele sac is delivered, it is punctured with trocar and cannula, the trocar removed and the fluid drained.
- Make sure that trocar and cannula should match, otherwise injury to the deeper structures (testis) can occur.

HUMBY'S KNIFE (Fig. 68.25)

- This instrument has a handle and a long sheath.
- When in use, a disposable blade can be attached to it.
- The instrument is used to take skin graft. Hence, it is also called skin grafting knife.
- To facilitate the exact thickness of the skin to be removed, there is a screw at the operating end, with which, prior adjustment should be done.

MYER'S METAL STRIPPER (Fig. 68.26)

- This is a long metallic chain or a stripper used in varicose vein surgery.
- It has a handle which is T-shaped and the 'advancing' end which enters the vein. This is blunt. Once this end comes out of the cut end of the vein, a medium-sized head is connected to it.
- With gentle force (traction) exerted on the handle, the varicose vein can be stripped.
- Hence, it is also called vein stripper

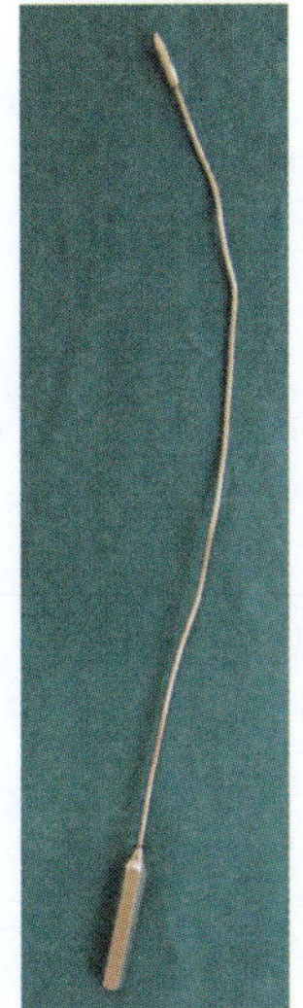
Fig. 68.21: Bake's dilator

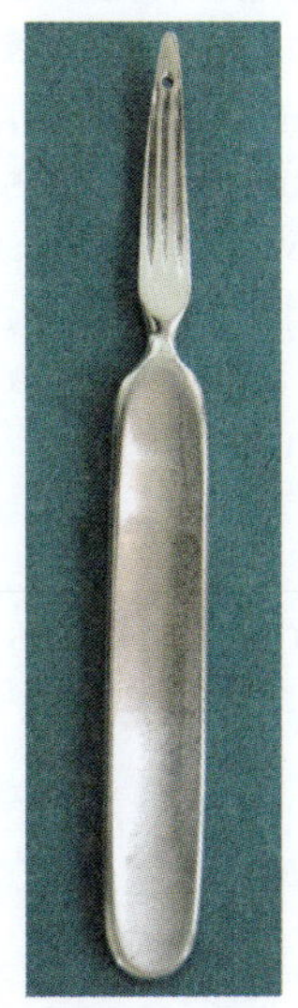
Fig. 68.22: Kocher's thyroid dissector

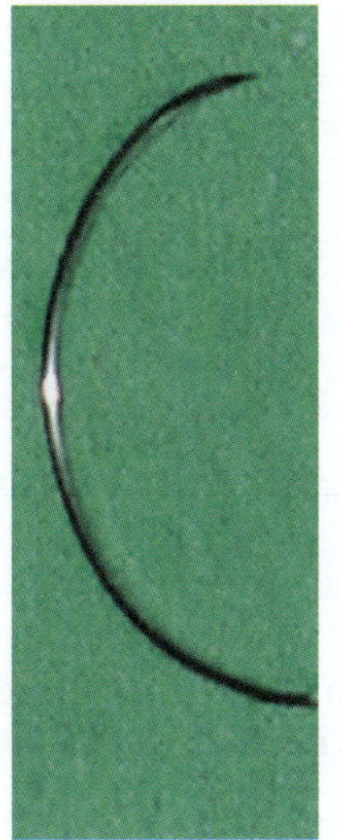
Fig. 68.23: Aneurysm needle

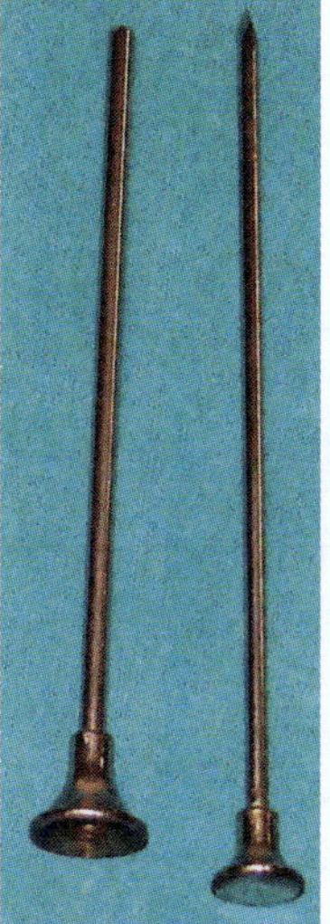
Fig. 68.24: Trocar and cannula

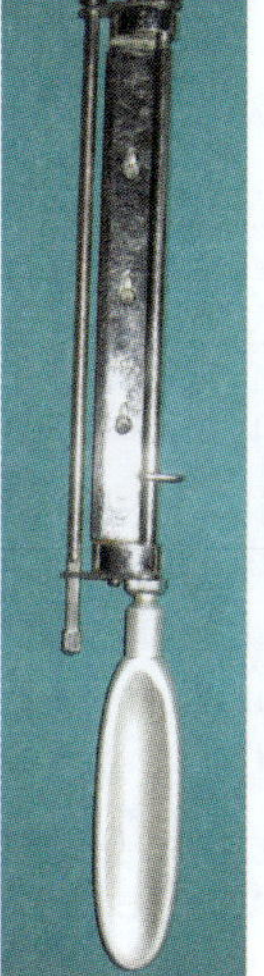
Fig. 68.25: Humby's knife

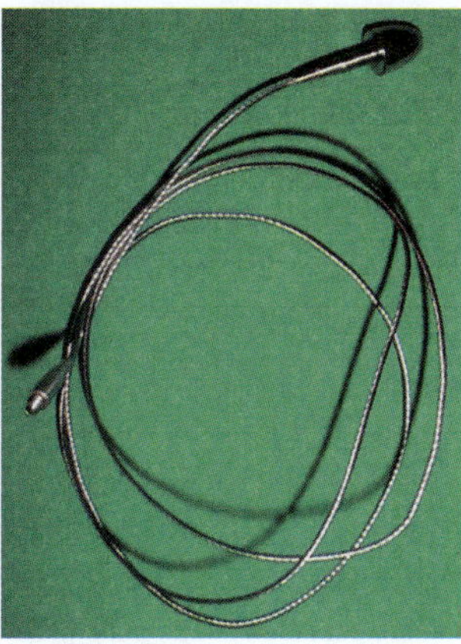
Fig. 68.26: Myer's metal stripper

SELF-RETAINING RETRACTOR (Fig. 68.27)

- It is a strong, heavy instrument, with two blades.
- This is used to spread the laparotomy wound. Hence, it is called self-retaining retractor.

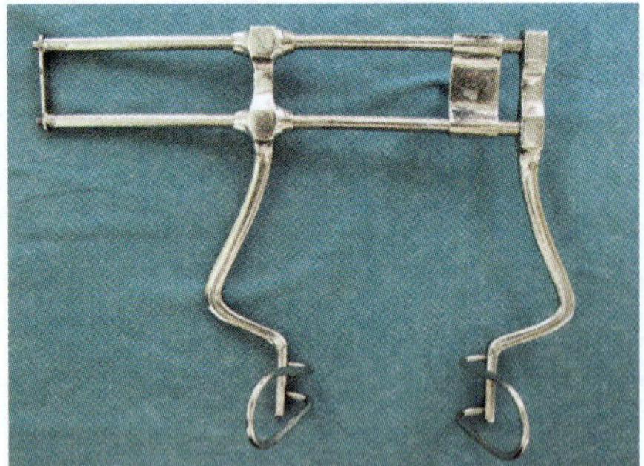

Fig. 68.27: Self-retaining retractor

RIB SPREADER (Fig. 68.28)

- This is also a strong heavy instrument with two long blades.
- Once an incision is deepened through the intercostal spaces and the pleura is opened, the rib spreader is used and by rotating the latch handle, the ribs are spread apart.

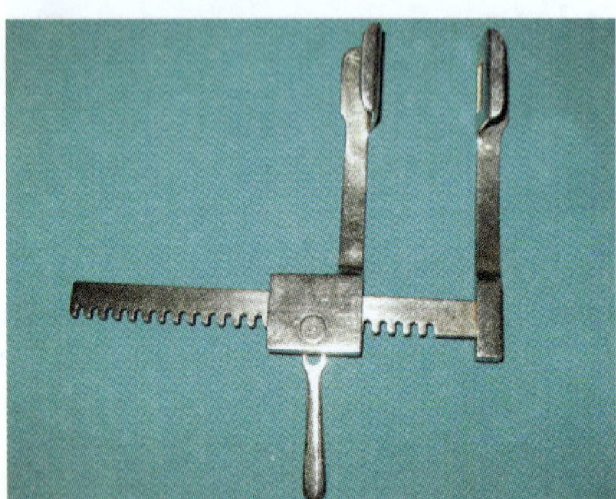

Fig. 68.28: Rib spreader

PROCTOSCOPE (Fig. 68.29)

- This is an instrument used to visualise the rectum and the anal canal.
- It has an outer sheath with the handle (A).
- An inner blunt part is called obturator (B).
- Before introducing the proctoscope one must make sure that obturator and the outer sheath must match. Lubricate the instrument well before introducing.
- In painful conditions such as fissure *in ano*, proctoscopy is contraindicated.
- Once rectal examination is done, proctoscope is held firmly with the left hand (buttocks separated), the obturator is supported by the right hand. The instrument is slowly introduced inside. The obturator is removed and rectum is visualised using light source.

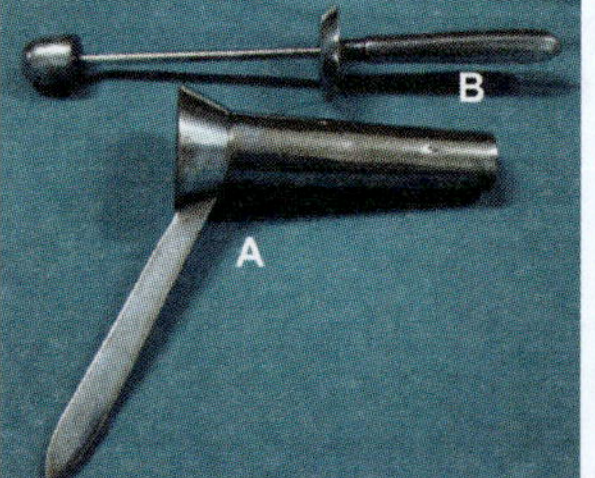

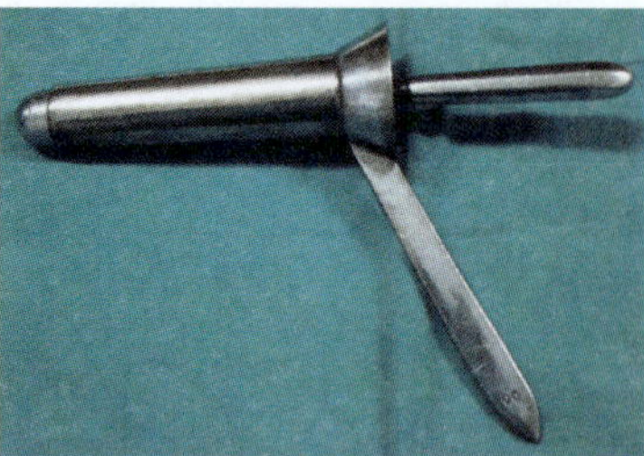

Fig. 68.29: Proctoscope

- Proctoscope is used to diagnose haemorrhoids, carcinoma rectum or rectal ulcers, etc. Biopsy can be taken with a biopsy forceps in nonhealing ulcers of the rectum. Haemorrhoids can be injected and pelvic abscess can be drained into the rectum with the help of a proctoscope.

LISTER'S METAL DILATOR (LISTER'S BOUGIE)

- This is a long instrument curved at the tip. Its diameter is written near the handle. It is available in various diameters. The difference between the two numbers is 3. The maximum size of the Lister's dilator is 9/12 (Fig. 68.30).
- The tip is olive-pointed and the end of the handle is round. The minimum and maximum diameter of the instrument is written on the handle. The other type of bougie is Glutton's bougie with a plain tip and the end of the handle is trapezoid. The maximum size of Glutton's bougie is 24/28 and difference between the two numbers is 4.

MALE METALLIC CATHETER (Fig. 68.31A)

- These catheters are used to drain urine in cases of retention of urine when rubber catheter fails.
- It is a long instrument which is curved because the male urethra is long and curved.
- It has two eyes at the distal end which are situated laterally and at different levels so that the instrument does not become weak at that spot.
- Once the urine is drained, the catheter can be left in place by passing a thread through the two rings present at the proximal end and fixing them to patient's thigh.
- Due to the fear of false passage, injury to the urethra and introducing infection, this catheter is not used nowadays. It is replaced by trocar suprapubic cystostomy.

FEMALE METALLIC CATHETER (Fig. 68.31B)

- Used to drain urine in females
- This is a short and straight instrument because the urethra is short and straight in females.

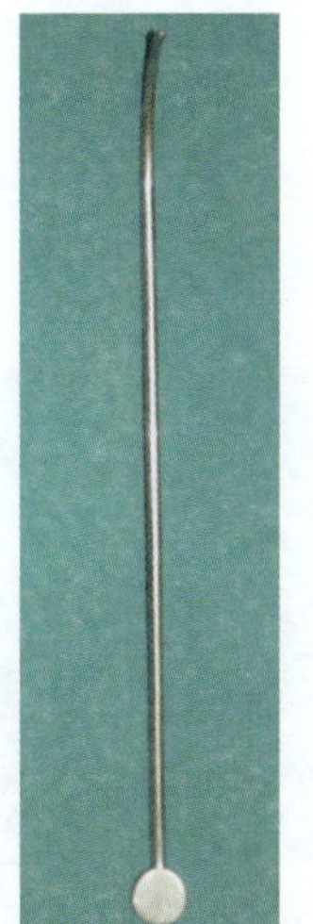

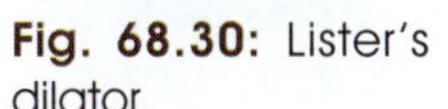

Fig. 68.30: Lister's dilator

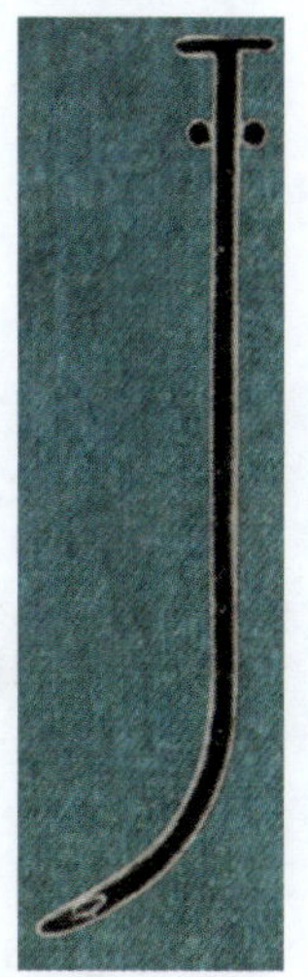

Fig. 68.31A: Male metallic catheter

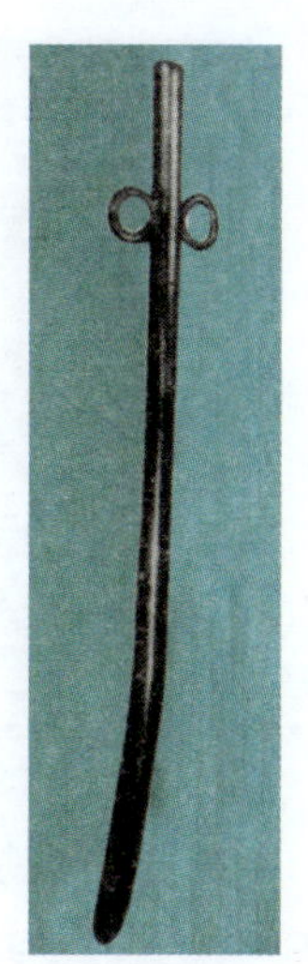

Fig. 68.31B: Female metallic catheter

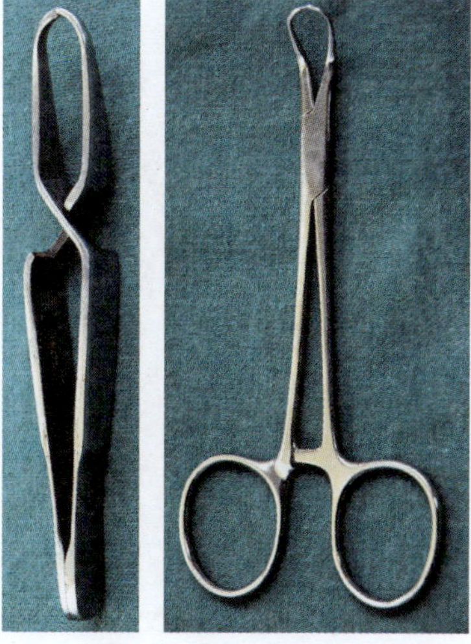

Fig. 68.32: Towel clip

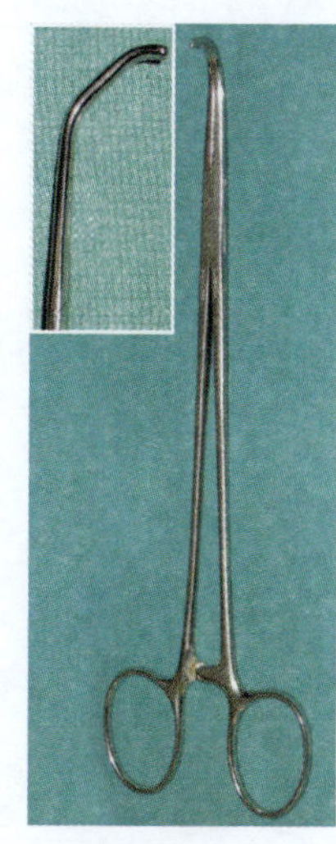

Fig. 68.33: Right-angled forceps

- It has multiple holes at the tip
- Indications for usage of this catheter are very rare because acute retention of urine is rare in females and even if it occurs, a red rubber catheter can be passed.
- It is used to empty bladder before vaginal hysterectomy and other gynaecologic surgeries.
- Emptying the bladder is mandatory before any gynaecological examination of a patient.

TOWEL CLIP (Fig. 68.32)

- This instrument has a ratchet and the operating end is sharp.
- This is available in different sizes.
- Once the part is cleaned and draped the clips are used to hold the towels in place.

RIGHT-ANGLED FORCEPS: LAHEY'S FORCEPS

- This is a long instrument with right angle at the operating end (Fig. 68.33).
- This instrument is extremely useful in **ligating the major vascular pedicles**, e.g. superior thyroid pedicle—thyroidectomy.
- Cystic artery: Cholecystectomy
- Lumbar veins: Lumbar sympathectomy

HUDSON'S BRACE AND THE BURR (Fig. 68.34)

- This is a heavy instrument with a brace and the burr (drill).
- This is used to create **openings into the cranium** so as to get an access to the structures within.
- Thus once a 'burr' is made, drainage of blood, fluid or pus can be done.

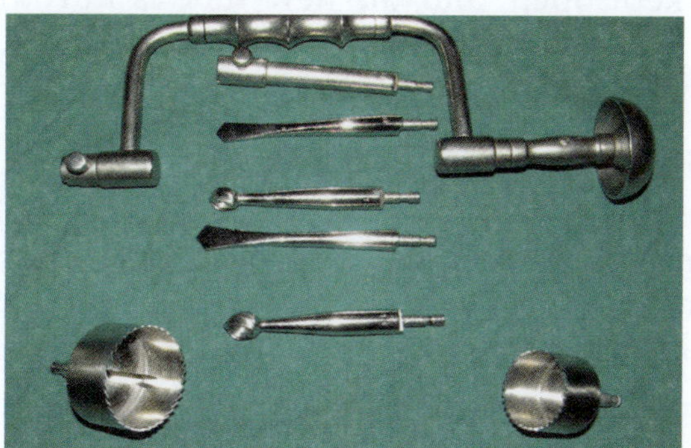

Fig. 68.34: Hudson's brace and the burr

CRICOID HOOK (Fig. 68.35)

- This has a broad handle and a thin shaft with a hook at the operating end.
- This is used to stabilise the trachea by hooking the cricoid cartilage 'up'.
- This step is essential in children wherein veins are very superficial and can get injured easily when child moves the head and neck. By stabilising the trachea, it is easy to incise the trachea, without injuring the vessels.

TRACHEAL DILATOR (Fig. 68.36)

- This is an instrument with **no ratchet at** the non-operating end.
- The operating end is blunt and curved.
- The peculiarity of this instrument is that **when the handle is opened, operating end is closed** and **when the handle is closed, operating end is opened**.
- Tracheal dilator is used in the **post-tracheostomy period**, when the tube has to be changed due to blockage. In such situations, once the tube is removed,

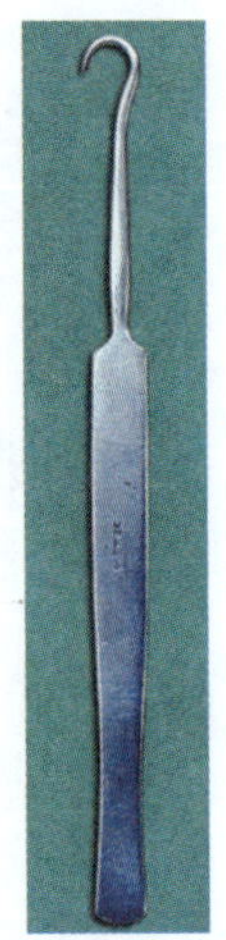
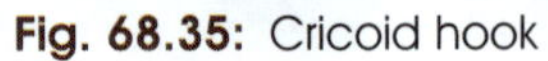

Fig. 68.35: Cricoid hook

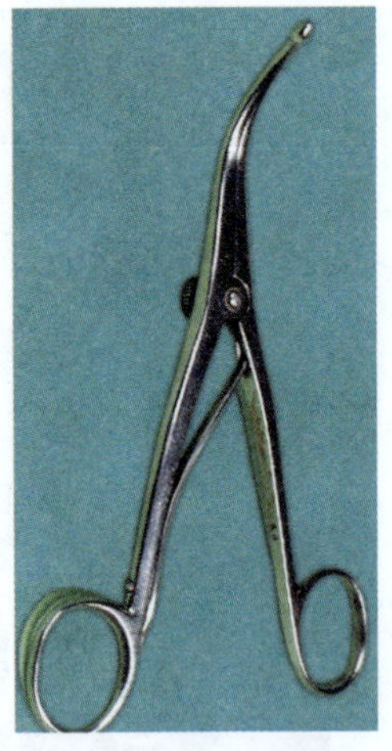

Fig. 68.36: Tracheal dilator

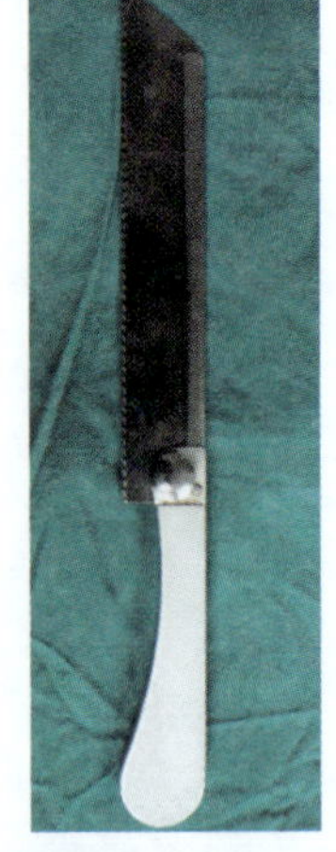

Fig. 68.37: Fergusson's amputation saw

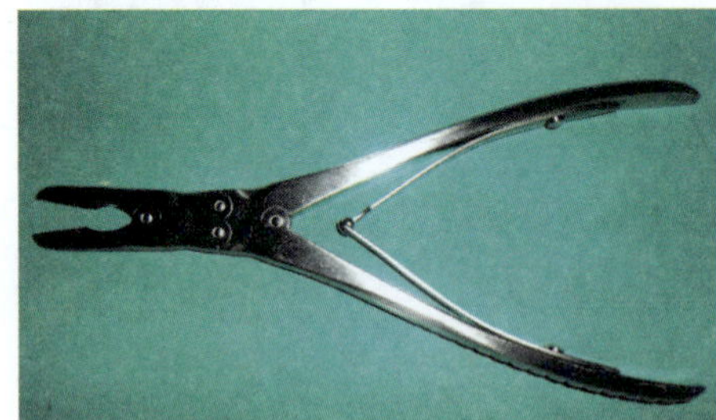

Fig. 68.38: Bone nibbler

tracheal dilator is introduced, the opening in trachea is kept open, and the new tube is introduced. However, once the track is formed, tracheal dilator need not be used.

FERGUSSON'S AMPUTATION SAW (Fig. 68.37)

Amputation saw has teeth on its cutting edge to facilitate cutting through the bone and is of different sizes. They are manufactured with one- or two-sided cutting edge for limb amputations.

Uses: In lower limb, amputations commonly—above knee (AK) amputation and below knee (BK) amputation.

BONE NIBBLER (Fig. 68.38)

It is also called double action bone nibbler, identified by long handle and small jaws, top jaw is used for cutting and lower jaw is used to hold the tissue firmly.

Uses: To make cut end of the bone smooth after amputation rib cutting and to enlarge burr hole.

BONE FILE/RASPATORY (Fig. 68.39)

One side of the raspatory is used to hold as a handle, while its other side has sharp projections with both fine and coarse teeth on both sides with a flat blade.

Uses: Blunt separation of the periosteum and connective tissue from the surface of the bone, smoothening of sharp bony edges after amputation and before fixing fractures.

VOLKMANN CURETTE (Fig. 68.40)

The edges of the distal spoon-shaped part of this instrument are sharp which make it possible to remove the tissues.

Uses: Scoop the granulation tissue, to clean the base of the infected wound, and to remove the infected bone in the case of osteomyelitis.

DEBAKEY FORCEPS (BAYONET STYLE) (Fig. 68.41)

They are typically large—some examples are upwards of 12 inches (36 cm) long, and have a distinct coarsely ribbed grip panel, as opposed to the finer ribbing on most other tissue forceps, a type of atraumatic tissue forceps.

Uses: In vascular procedures to avoid tissue damage during manipulation. Less traumatic manipulation of tissue and used during suturing.

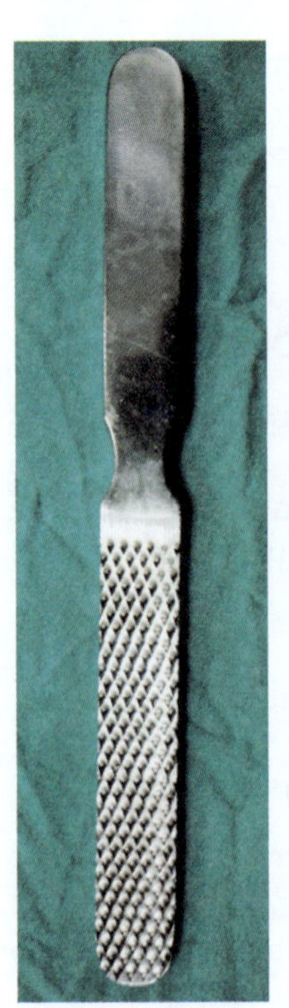

Fig. 68.39: Bone file

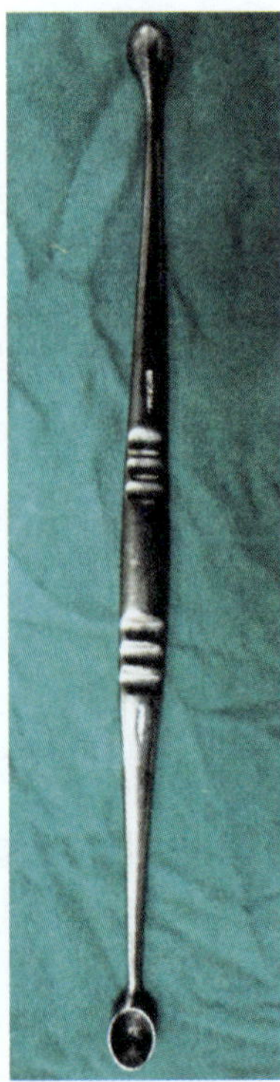

Fig. 68.40: Volkmann Curette

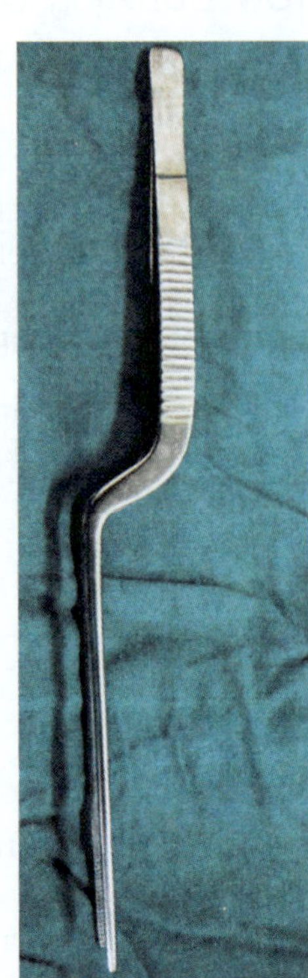

Fig. 68.41: Debakey forceps

BECKMAN-ADSON LAMINECTOMY RETRACTOR (Fig. 68.42)

It has hinged blades with 4 × 4 prongs, an adjustable swivel arms and a ratchet to hold tissue apart.

Uses: Retraction in procedures involving deep tissues like in laminectomy for spinal surgeries.

RIBBON MALLEABLE RETRACTOR (Fig. 68.43)

A malleable or ribbon retractor (manual) may be bent to various shapes.

Uses: It is used at the end of the case to keep the viscera away during the fascial closure and is also used to retract deep wounds.

THE HARMONIC SCALPEL (Fig. 68.44)

The harmonic scalpel is a new device that has been introduced to surgery during the last decade. It is a device that uses high-frequency mechanical energy to cut and coagulate tissues at the same time.

It uses ultrasound technology to cut tissues while simultaneously sealing the edges of the cut. (More details on page 1310).

Active tips of the harmonic scalpel employ a rigid active lower blade through which the vibrating energy is transmitted. The movable upper jaw is used to compress the vessel against the lower blade, thus allowing transfer of the vibrational energy.

The instrument is similar to an electrosurgery instrument and can be used in all open and laparoscopic surgeries, but superior in that it can cut through thicker tissue, creates less toxic surgical smoke and may offer greater precision especially during a laparoscopic surgery.

BIPOLAR CAUTERY (Fig. 68.45)

When the electric current is passing between the two parts of the instrument, we call it the bipolar diathermy/ cautery (e.g. bipolar forceps).

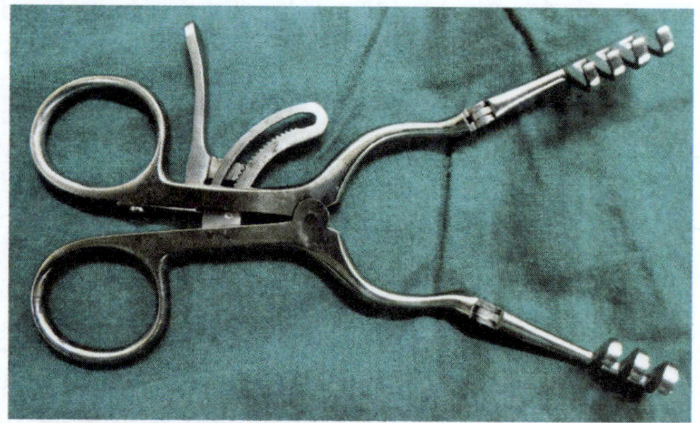

Fig. 68.42: Beckman-Adson laminectomy retractor

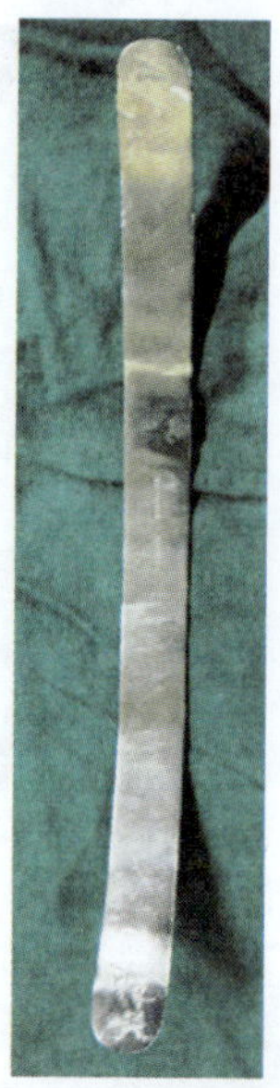

Fig. 68.43: Malleable retractor

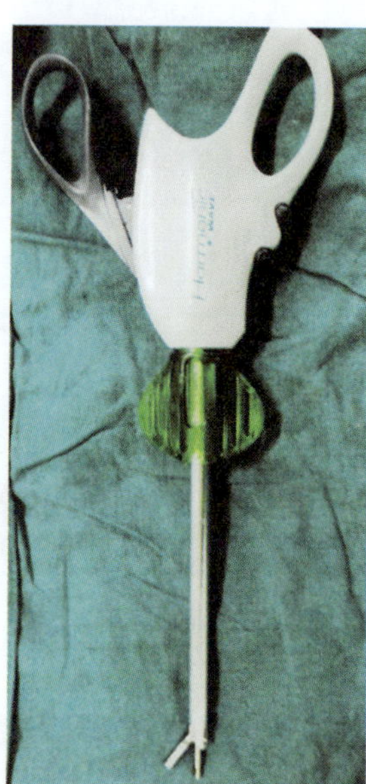

Fig. 68.44: Harmonic scalpel

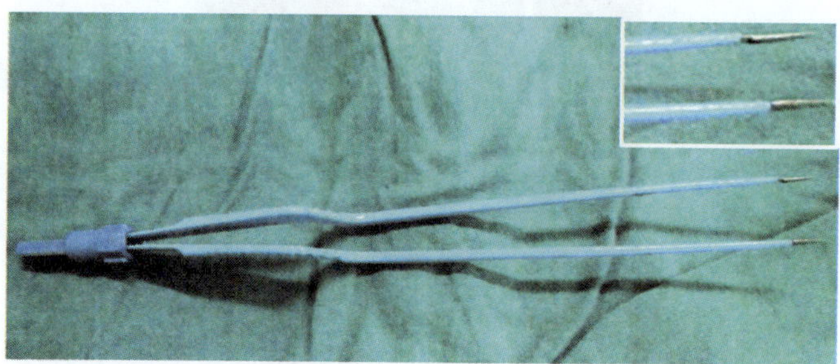

Fig. 68.45: Bipolar cautery

It makes possible to perform a more precise work and the size of the burned area is small and is more useful when haemostasis is required close to the nerves.

Uses: Thyroid surgery when close to RLN (recurrent laryngeal nerve) neurosurgery or spinal surgeries.

ALLISON'S LUNG RETRACTOR (Fig. 68.46)

It is retractor with a special type of blade, made of wires, in the form of a net over one end and a handle at the other end.

Uses: For retraction of the lung in thoracotomy. It does not damage the lungs and the lungs can expand in between the wires.

GIGLI SAW (Fig. 68.47)

Composed of a wire as a blade and two handles to hold the wire on either side.

Uses: For bone cutting in amputation surgeries similar to amputation saw such as below knee and above knee amputations commonly.

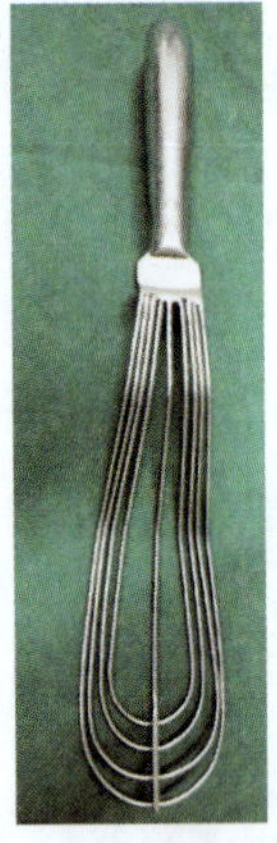

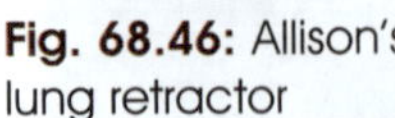

Fig. 68.46: Allison's lung retractor

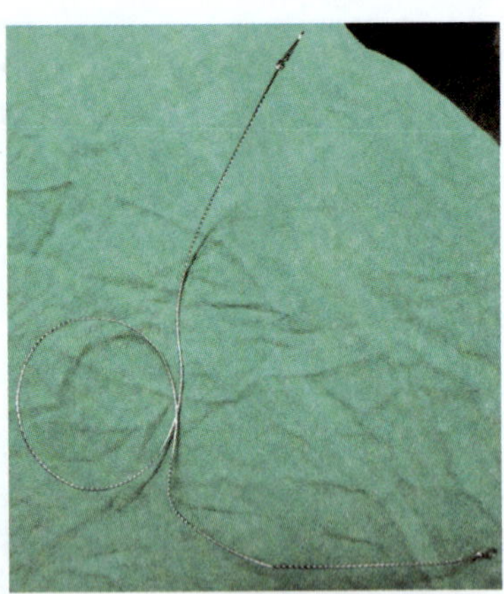

Fig. 68.47: Gigli saw

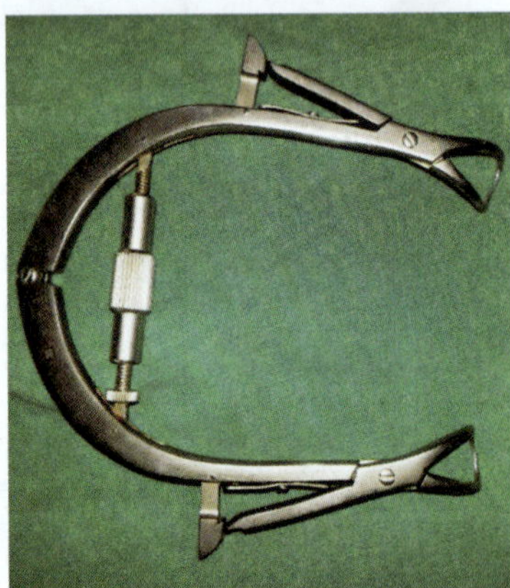

Fig. 68.48: Joll's retractor

JOLL'S THYROID RETRACTOR (Fig. 68.48)

It is a self-retaining retractor, which is held by the two towel clip like forceps on both sides to hold the flaps and can be adjusted using a screw in between.

Uses: To retract skin flaps during thyroid surgery.

METAL TRACHEOSTOMY TUBE (Fig. 68.49)

- This has **two tubes**, the inner long and the outer short tube.
- This has no **cuff**.
- Once the tube is introduced, the tape is passed around the neck, passed through the opening and tied so as to keep the tube in place.
- If the tube is blocked, the inner tube can be removed, cleaned and reintroduced.
- Metal tracheostomy tubes are useful as permanent tracheostomy tube.

CUFFED TRACHEOSTOMY TUBE (Fig. 68.50)

- This is made of polyvinyl chloride. It is a **single tube**.
- Once the tube is introduced within the trachea, the cuff is inflated by using 3–5 ml of air.

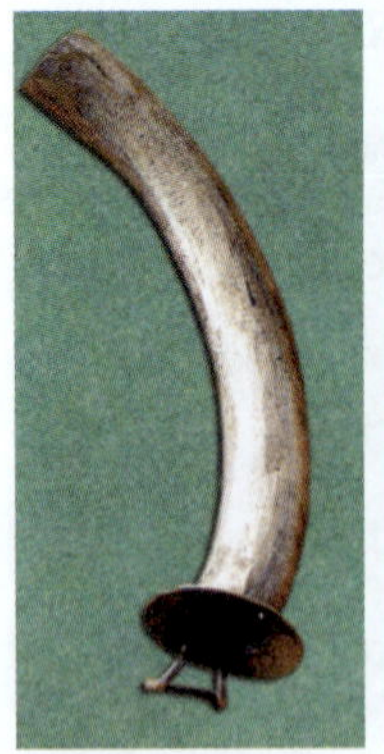

Fig. 68.49: Metal tracheostomy tube

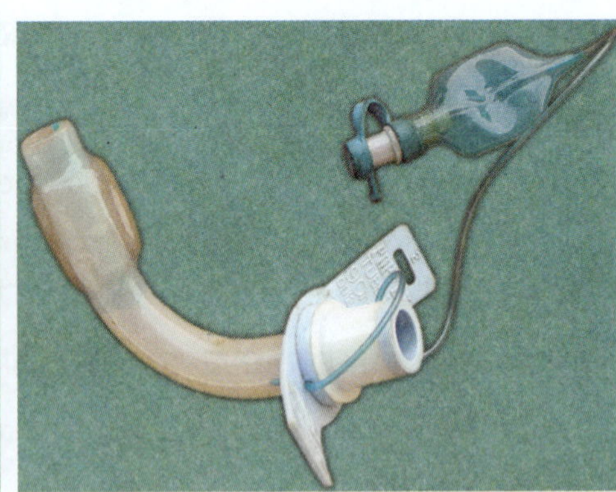

Fig. 68.50: Cuffed tracheostomy

- The cuff prevents leakage of air and prevents **acid aspiration syndrome (Mendelson's syndrome)**.
- If this tube is blocked, it is an emergency. In such cases, the tube has to be cleaned and mucus plugs have to be removed. Otherwise, the tube is removed, the tracheal opening is kept open with the help of tracheal dilator and a new tube is introduced. Alternatively, endotracheal intubation may need to be done to ensure patency of the airway.

CORRUGATED RED RUBBER DRAIN (Fig. 68.51)

- It is made of red rubber. It has corrugations on both sides. Whenever a major surgery is done, some amount of blood loss or anastomotic leakage is expected. This drain is used so that **fluid can escape freely outside**.
- Thus, it is used after thyroidectomy, gastrectomy, cholecystectomy, etc. The drain is removed after it stops draining. Usually it takes about 3–5 days.
- After laparotomy for peritonitis, these drains are used to prevent residual abscess in the postoperative period.

MALECOT'S CATHETER (Fig. 68.52)

This is made of red rubber. It has flower-shaped end and has a wide diameter. It is used to drain amoebic liver abscess. It is straightened with the help of an introducer and left in cavity and brought outside. It is a self-retaining catheter. This is used to drain urinary bladder after transvesical prostatectomy or can be used as feeding gastrostomy tube. It can also be used to drain empyema thoracis.

MOUSSEAU BARBIN'S TUBE (Fig. 68.53)

- This is also called MB tube. It is a funnel-shaped tube with Ryle's tube like attachment. It is used in inoperable cases of carcinoma oesophagus to palliate

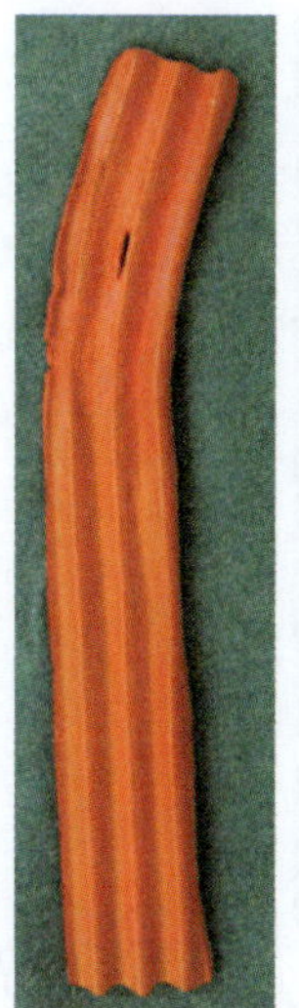
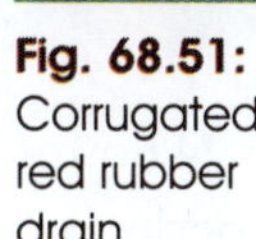

Fig. 68.51: Corrugated red rubber drain

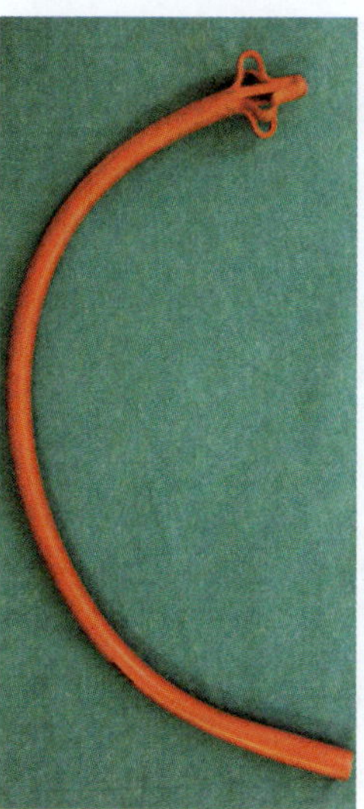

Fig. 68.52: Malecot's catheter

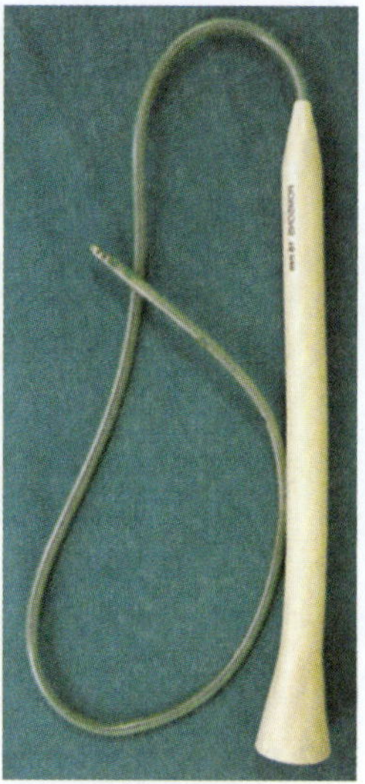

Fig. 68.53: Mousseau Barbin's tube

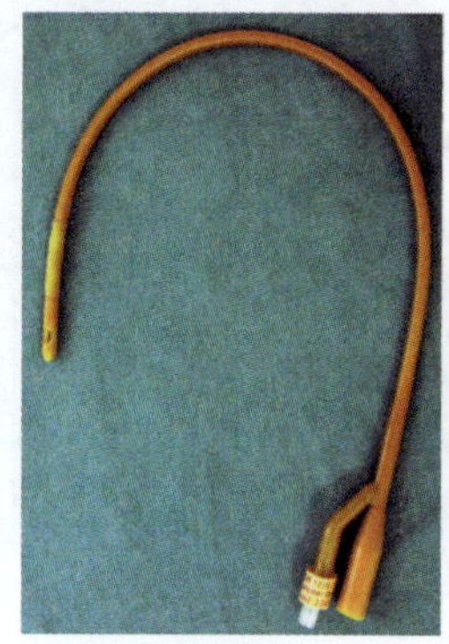

Fig. 68.54A: Foley catheter

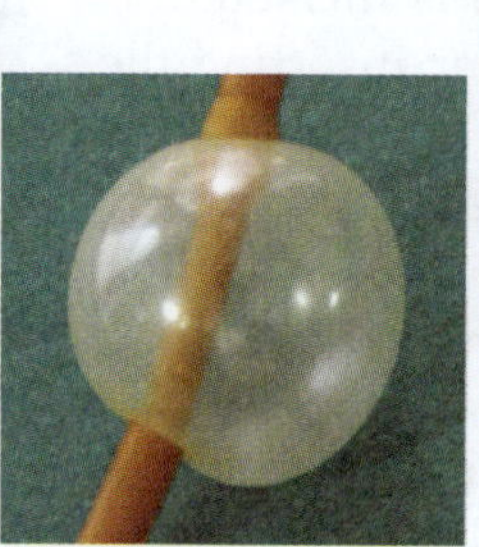

Fig. 68.54B: Distended bulb

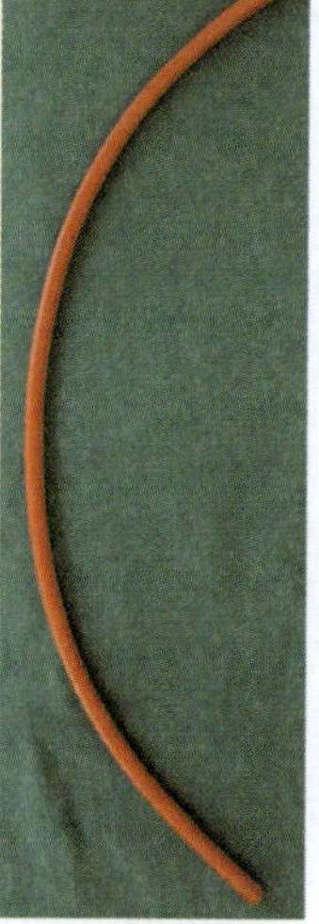

Fig. 68.55: Red rubber catheter

dysphagia. It is stitched to the Ryle's tube which is brought out through the mouth and it is slowly drawn in by pulling the other end of Ryle's tube which is in the stomach, after doing a gastrostomy.

- Once the tube is below the level of growth, it is cut at a sufficient distance and is stitched to the stomach wall.
- With the availability of laser coagulation of the growth, and considering discomfort caused by the tube including its migration, the MB tube is not popular and not preferred.

FOLEY'S SELF-RETAINING URINARY CATHETER
(Figs 68.54A and B)

- This is made of **latex with silicon coating**. At the tip, there is a bulb, capacity of which is written at the other end.
- Before inflating the bulb, one must make sure that **catheter is in the urinary bladder, not in the urethra**. This is assessed by free flow of urine.
- After introducing the catheter, the bulb is inflated using saline. Thus, it becomes self-retaining. After the usage, it is removed by deflating the bulb. It can also be used to drain peritoneal cavity as in biliary peritonitis. Inflated bulb compresses the prostatic bed and controls bleeding after prostatectomy.

RED RUBBER CATHETER (Fig. 68.55)

This is used to drain urine temporarily. It causes urethritis if it is left long in the urinary bladder. Once the urine is emptied, it is removed. It is not a self-retaining catheter. Not routinely used nowadays because of availability of Foley's catheter. It is more stiff than Foley catheter. Hence, **in cases of stricture urethra,** where **Foley's catheter cannot be passed, red rubber catheter may be used.**

NASOGASTRIC TUBE/RYLE'S TUBE (Fig. 68.56)

- This is also called **nasogastric tube.** At the end of this tube there are **lead shots.** After introducing within the stomach, its position is confirmed by pushing 5–10 ml of air and auscultating in the epigastrium or aspirating gastric juice. It is a long tube having 3 marks. When the tube is passed up to the 1st mark, it enters the stomach. Usually it is passed up to 2nd mark. Life-saving use of **Ryle's tube** is in **acute gastric dilatation.**

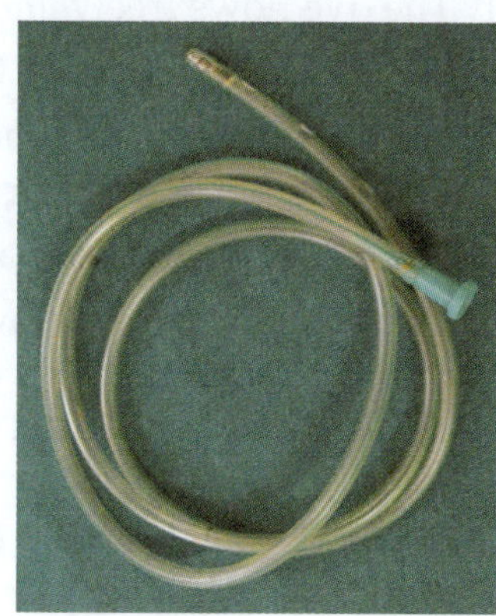

Fig. 68.56: Ryle's tube

- **In volvulus of the stomach, it is impossible to pass a Ryle's tube.**
- Ryle's tube is used to decompress the stomach as in intestinal obstruction or pyloric stenosis.
- It is used in the diagnosis of GI haemorrhage.
- It is also used to provide enteral nutrition to comatose patients or critically ill patients.

T-TUBE (KEHR'S)

- This is a flexible tube made of latex with a long vertical limb and a short horizontal limb.
- Whenever the **common bile duct (CBD) is incised**, it is sutured after inserting the T-tube. The short horizontal limb is placed vertically within the common bile duct after making 2–3 holes within. Some surgeons slit open the entire length of the short limb.

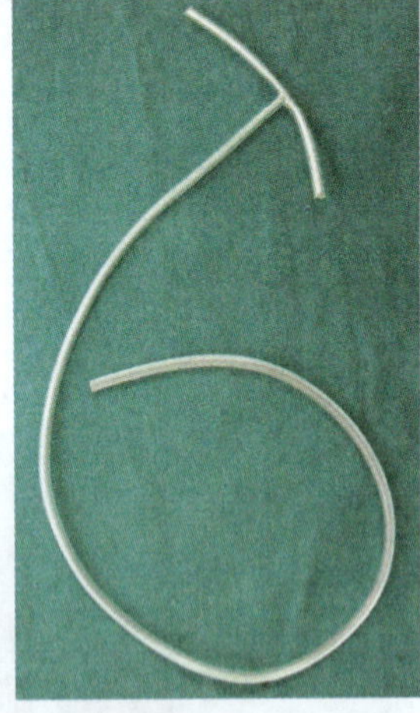

Fig. 68.57: T-tube (Kehr's)

- The long limb is brought to the exterior from the most dependent part of the common bile duct and connected to a sterile container.
- Presence of the T-tube may prevent peritonitis due to biliary leakage in cases of residual stones blocking the lower end of the CBD.

REMOVAL OF THE TUBE

About 7–10 days later, a T-tube cholangiography is done and the T-tube is removed with a gentle pull, provided following criteria are fulfilled.

1. The dye flows freely into the duodenum.
2. No filling defects in the CBD.
3. After clamping the tube for 24 hours, there is no abdominal pain or fever.
4. Patient is passing normal coloured stools.

Once the tube is withdrawn, some amount of biliary leak may persist for 2–3 days and it stops by itself provided there is no distal obstruction.

SENGSTAKEN-BLAKEMORE DOUBLE BALLOON TRIPLE LUMEN TUBE (Fig. 68.58)

- It is used in controlling bleeding **oesophageal varices.** It has 3 lumens and 2 balloons, a gastric balloon and an oesophageal balloon.
- **Gastric balloon is inflated** with about **200–250 ml** of air and oesophageal balloon is inflated with about **40–60 ml of air**. It is pulled upwards so as to snugly fit at the oesophagogastric junction and thus it acts by internal tamponade.
- Sengstaken tube should not be kept in place for more than 48 hours because it can cause pressure necrosis of oesophagus.

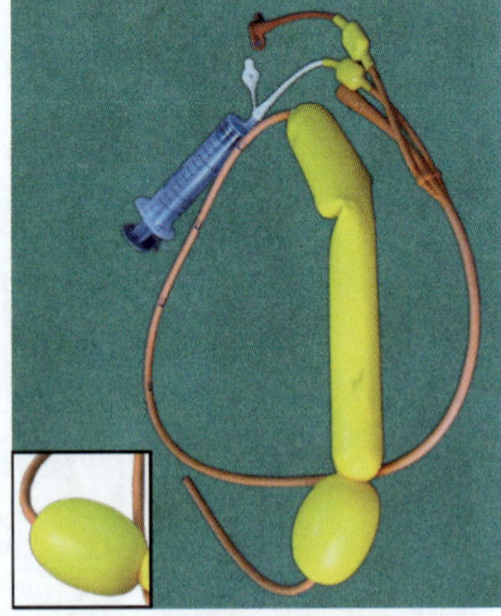

Fig. 68.58: Sengstaken-Blakemore double balloon triple lumen tube

- It should be deflated for a few minutes after 24 hours.
- Sengstaken tube should be used by an experienced physician. Oesophageal secretions and saliva cannot be aspirated while using this tube, and if gastric balloon is deflated suddenly, it slides up and causes choking. The oesophageal balloon should be immediately deflated in such situations.
- **Modification of Sengstaken tube is called Minnesota tube or 4 lumen tube.** It has 4 lumens. The 1st to inflate oesophageal balloon, the 2nd to inflate gastric balloon, the 3rd to aspirate like a Ryle's tube, and the 4th lumen is used to aspirate oesophageal secretions. If there is any difficulty in breathing while using Sengstaken tube or Minnesota tube, bulb should be deflated or tube should be cut.

SUTURING NEEDLES (Fig. 68.59)

Traumatic

- Round body needle is an eyed needle. These are used to suture soft tissues, muscles, tendons, vessels, intestines, etc.

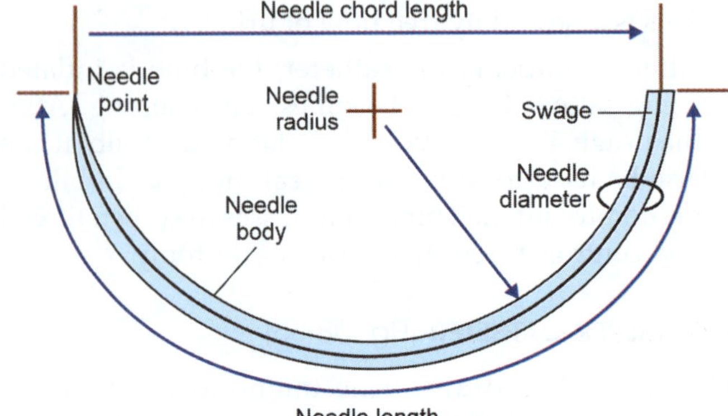

Fig. 68.59: Needle and parts

- Cutting needles are used to suture slim and some tough structures. The cutting tip is limited to the point of the needle which tapers out to merge smoothly into a round cross-section. These are used in vascular anastomosis/surgery.
- Reverse cutting needle is used to suture mucoperiosteum: It is triangular in cross-section. It's effects of the cutting edge is on the outer surface of the needle curvature. Advantage of reverse cutting is strength and increases the resistance to bending.

These needles have an eye. The eye is wider than body of the needle, so tissue trauma is more.

Atraumatic Needle

- These needles have no eye. **Suture** is attached to the needle by a process called **swaging**. Tissue trauma is less, and hence is used in suturing vessels or to repair a small tear in the bowl, etc. **This was first devices by George Merson of England, hence most of these sutures are called Mersutures.** These are disposable needles hence sharpness is not affected.
- **Needles:** They are the essential tools of a surgeon for suturing the defects of skin/fascia/intestinal anastomosis, vascular anastomosis.

  Parts of the needle: Needle has three main parts—shank, body, point. The body of the needle is either round, triangular or flattened.
- They are made of stainless steel.
- **Traumatic :** Needles with eye, suture material loaded into the eye. Needle holes in tissues are larger that suture material.

Types

Round bodied, cutting, reverse cutting, taper cut, blunt.

- Round-bodied needles: Uniformly round, gradually taper to a point designed to separate tissue fibres rather than cut through them soft tissue; intestinal and cardiovascular surgery. Cutting needles are used for suturing tough or dense tissue, e.g. skin, fascia.
- Reverse cutting in which the cutting edge is on the outside of the needle curvature.

Taper cut needle: It is a combination of round body needle (minimal trace) and penetration like a cutting needle.

Parts of the needle:

Eye/eyeless: Here you thread the suture material.

Junction of eye and body: Weakest

Body: Straight/curved

Needle length: Circumferential

Tip: Pointed

Needle chord length: Linear distance between tip and end of needle (eye).

Round body needle	Cutting needle
• Uniformly round needle	• No uniform shape
• Tip is tapered	• Sharp end has a triangular shape on cross-section.
• They separate the tissue.	• They cut, penetrate, fibres and tough structures.
• Used to suture tissue fibres muscles, intestines, vessels.	• Used to suture fascia aponeurosis, linea alba and skin

SUTURE MATERIALS (Key Box 68.3)

ABSORBABLE

1. Plain catgut (7-day catgut)

- The word catgut is derived from kit-gut, which means the violin strings. It is the oldest suture material known.
- Catgut is derived from the submucosa of the sheep intestines.
- The plain catgut lasts for **7–10 days**. Hence, its uses are minimal.
- It can be used to put 'fat stitches' (subcutaneous fat).
- It is biological, absorbable and monofilament.
- Sheep's submucosa has a rich content of elastic tissue.

2. Chromic catgut (21-day catgut)

- When plain catgut is mixed with chromic salts, chromic catgut is obtained.
- The strength of the chromic catgut is about 15–25 days.
- Chromic catgut is widely used in intestinal anastomosis, closure of urinary bladder, closure of common bile duct, gastrojejunostomy, etc.

Key Box 68.3

Colour	Suture Material
Yellow	Plain catgut
Brown	Chromic catgut
Violet	Vicryl
Creamy yellow	Dexon
Creamy	PDS
Blue	Prolene
Black	Silk
White	Cotton

- Catgut is biological, absorbable, monofilament suture material.
- Chromic catgut is packed along with round body needle.
- The number 2–0 refers to the thickness of the suture.
- Knotting property is good.
- The catgut is preserved in 70% alcohol and is kept soft due to 5% glycerine.

3. **Vicryl (polyglactin)**
   - This is a copolymer of glycolide and lactide.
   - It is a synthetic and absorbable suture.
   - Unlike catgut, this is absorbed by hydrolysis.
   - **Since the strength and reliability is more than catgut, vicryl is being used more and more for small intestinal and colonic anastomosis. It has replaced catgut in suturing bile duct also.**
   - Being synthetic, tissue reaction is less than that of chromic catgut.
   - This has also replaced catgut while suturing common bile duct.
   - Knotting property is good
   - Vicryl can be used in the presence of infection.
4. **Dexon (polyglycolic acid)**
   - Synthetic absorbable
   - Braided
   - Used like vicryl
5. **PDS (polydioxanone suture)**
   - Like vicryl
   - Costly
   - Creamy in colour

NONABSORBABLE

1. **Prolene**
   - This is polypropylene and nonabsorbable.
   - It is monofilament, artificial and uncoated. Does not harbour micro-organism. Hence, the chances of infection are less.
   - Since it is nonabsorbable, prolene can be used for abdominal closure, repair of hernias, repair of incisional hernia, etc.
   - It has high memory (recoiling tendency after removal from the pocket) and hence multiple knots are required.
2. **Sutupack**
   - It is a monofilament or multifilament polyamide.
   - Black in colour
   - It is braided, uncoated and nonabsorbable.
   - Uses of sutupack are similar to prolene.
   - Knotting property is not very good. Hence, it is mandatory to put 4–5 knots.
3. **Mersilk**
   - This is nonabsorbable, braided silk, black in colour.
   - It has been provided with a round body. This can be used in ligating bleeding points or anastomosis, etc.
4. **Black silk**
   - This is a nonabsorbable suture material.
   - It is biological and derived from the **cocoon of the silkworm larva**.
   - It is braided, coated with wax to reduce capillary action. Tissue reaction is much more with black silk because it is a foreign protein.
   - In spite of this, it is widely used because of its easy availability and is cheap.
   - Knotting property is excellent.
5. **Cotton**
   - White in colour
   - Multifilament—infection rate is high
   - Nonabsorbable, cheap

Note to students: For more details about the instruments, you may refer to *Manipal Manual of Instruments*.

CHAPTER

69

Specimens

- TB lymphadenitis
- Hodgkin's lymphoma
- Carcinoma tongue
- Chronic gastric ulcer
- Linitis plastica
- Intussusception
- Carcinoma rectum
- Gangrenous appendicitis
- Carcinoma colon
- Meckel's diverticulum
- Polycystic kidney
- Renal cell carcinoma
- Hydronephrosis
- Carcinoma penis
- Seminoma testis
- Cholecystectomy
- Hydatid cyst
- Carcinoma stomach
- Lipoma
- Malignant melanoma
- Thyroidectomy
- Wide excision of skin
- Whipple's pancreaticoduodenectomy
- Splenectomy

I. TUBERCULOUS (TB) LYMPHADENITIS

1. What is this specimen?

- Specimen of lymph nodes which are matted. Cut surface shows caseation. Hence, it is tuberculous lymphadenitis.

2. What is the microscopic picture?

- Central caseation surrounded by epithelioid cells, Langhans' type of giant cells.

3. What are the stages of TB lymphadenitis?

- Stage of lymphadenitis
- Stage of matting
- Stage of cold abscess
- Stage of collar stud abscess
- Stage of sinus formation

4. Why is matting seen in TB lymphadenitis?

- It is because of periadenitis

5. What is the treatment of cold abscess?

- Nondependent aspiration by using wide bore needle, to avoid sinus formation.

II. LYMPHOMA

1. What is the diagnosis?

- Multiple lymph nodes which are discrete and not matted. Cut surface does not show caseation. It is homogenous. Hence, this is a specimen of Hodgkin's lymphoma.

2. How do you confirm the diagnosis?

- Lymph node biopsy

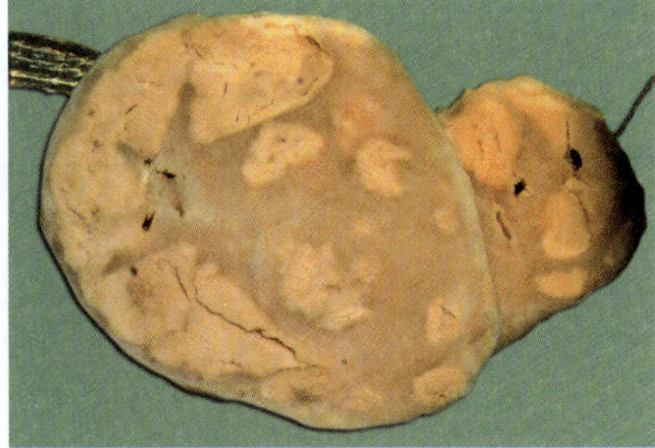

Fig. 69.1: Tuberculous (TB) lymphadenitis

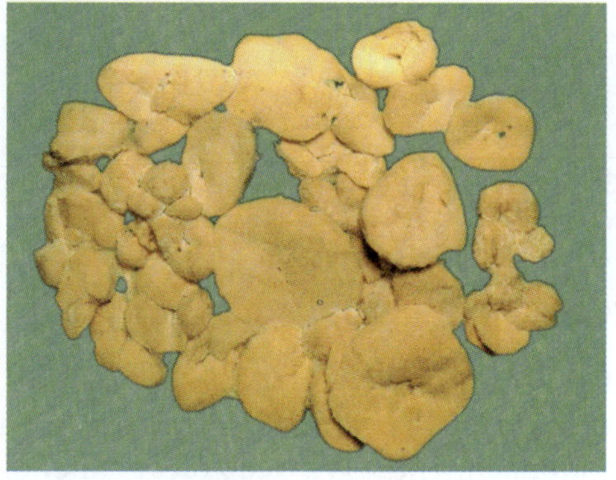

Fig. 69.2: Lymphoma

3. **What is the microscopic picture?**
   - Cellular pleomorphism: Lymphocytes, histiocytes, eosinophils, monocytes with giant cells containing mirror image nuclei—Reed-Sternberg cell.
4. **What are the common lymph nodes involved in Hodgkin's lymphoma?**
   - Cervical, axillary, para-aortic, iliac and inguinal lymph nodes.
5. **Is Waldeyer's ring involvement seen in Hodgkin's lymphoma?**
   - No, it is usually seen in non-Hodgkin's lymphoma.

III. SPECIMEN OF HEMIGLOSSECTOMY WITH HEMIMANDIBULECTOMY

1. **What is this specimen?**
   - Specimen showing growth arising from the tongue and infiltrating the mandible.
2. **What is the diagnosis?**
   - Advanced carcinoma tongue
3. **Is radiotherapy indicated in this situation?**
   - No, because chances of radionecrosis of the mandible are high.
4. **What type of X-ray is taken to look for involvement of the mandible?**
   - Orthopantomogram
5. **What is Commando's operation?**
   - Hemiglossectomy with excision of the floor of the mouth, hemimandibulectomy, with radical block dissection of the neck done in a single stage, with *en bloc* removal.

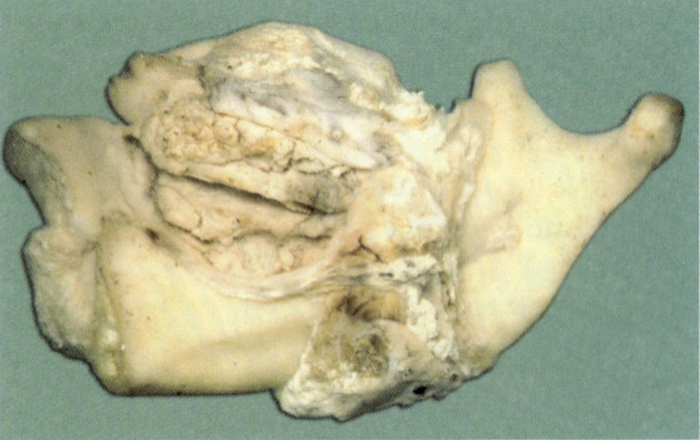

Fig. 69.3: Specimen of hemiglossectomy with hemimandibulectomy

IV. CHRONIC GASTRIC ULCER

1. **What is this specimen?**
   - Specimen of the stomach showing rugosity of the stomach. There is a deep ulcer crater along the lesser curvature.

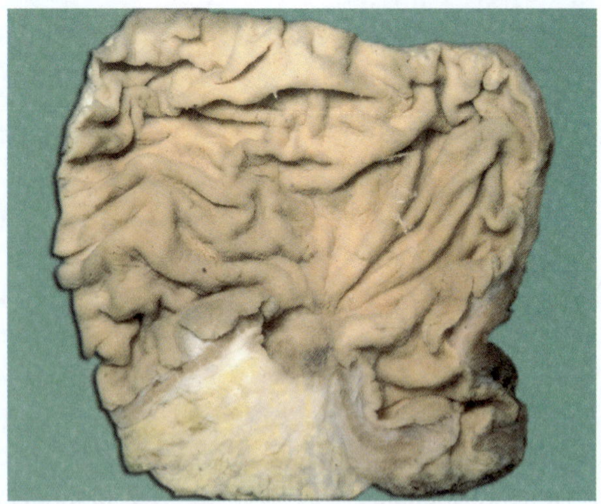

Fig. 69.4: Chronic gastric ulcer

2. **What is the diagnosis?**
   - Benign gastric ulcer
3. **Why is it a benign gastric ulcer?**
   - Since the rugae are of converging type, it is a benign gastric ulcer.
4. **How do you rule out malignancy in a gastric ulcer?**
   - Endoscopic biopsy
5. **What is the incidence of gastric ulcer turning into malignancy?**
   - 0.5 to 2%

V. LINITIS PLASTICA

1. **What is this specimen?**
   - Specimen of the stomach showing loss of normal rugosity. There is a nodular extensive infiltrating lesion along the entire length of the stomach.
2. **What is the diagnosis?**
   - Linitis plastica—leather bottle stomach.

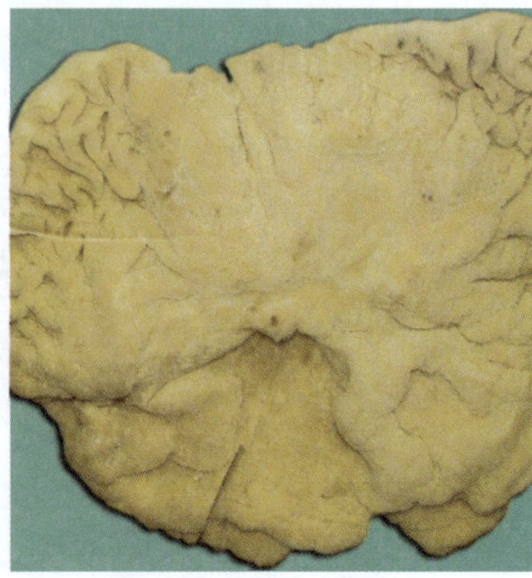

Fig. 69.5: Linitis plastica

3. **What is linitis plastica?**
   - It is an extensive fibrosis involving entire submucosa of the stomach initially and involves other layers also later.
4. **What is the treatment for linitis plastica?**
   - Radical total gastrectomy
5. **What is the D2 prognosis?**
   - Very poor

VI. INTUSSUSCEPTION

1. **What is this specimen?**
   - Specimen of intestine showing one portion of bowel invaginated within the other.
2. **What is the diagnosis?**
   - Intussusception
3. **What is the common type of intussusception?**
   - Ileocolic
4. **What are the parts of intussusception?**
   - Intussusceptum, intussuscipiens, neck and apex.
5. **What is the treatment in children?**
   - Hydrostatic reduction or operative reduction.
   - If there is gangrene—resection followed by end-to-end anastomosis.

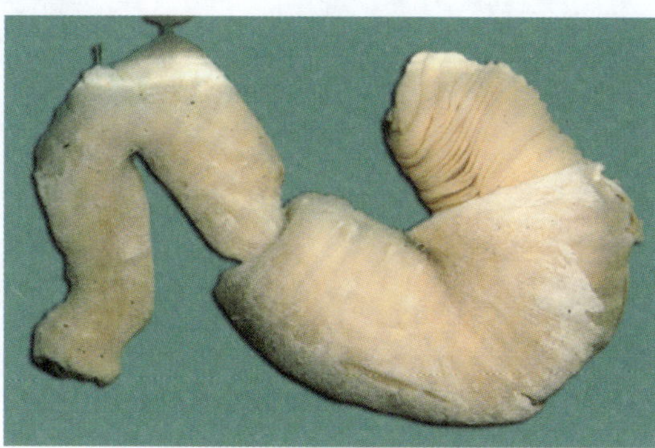

Fig. 69.6: Intussusception

VII. CARCINOMA RECTUM

1. **What is this specimen?**
   - Specimen of rectum showing ulceroproliferative growth in the middle of the rectum. Specimen also shows entire rectum and anal canal.
2. **What is the diagnosis?**
   - Carcinoma rectum
3. **What is this surgery?**
   - Abdominoperineal resection (excision) (APR). In this operation, entire rectum, anal canal, part of the sigmoid colon, fat, fascia, lymphatics and regional nodes are removed *en bloc* followed by permanent colostomy in the left iliac fossa.

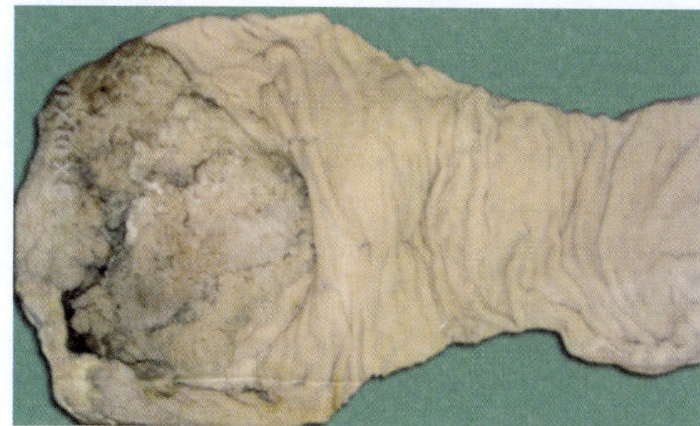

Fig. 69.7: Carcinoma rectum

4. **What are the indications for APR?**
   - Growth in lower rectum wherein sphincter cannot be saved.
5. **What is the position of the patient during APR?**
   - Supine with lithotomy called Lloyd Davis position.

VIII. GANGRENOUS APPENDICITIS

1. **What is this specimen?**
   - It is an appendicectomy specimen showing blackish discolouration of the appendix.
2. **What factors cause gangrene of the appendix?**
   - Gangrenous appendicitis occurs usually in elderly patients, where there is decreased vascularity due to atherosclerosis. It can also occur when the lumen is blocked due to faecolith, thereby causing ischaemia.
3. **What is the one simple investigation which is useful in diagnosing appendicitis?**
   - Total WBC count. Above 10,000 cells/cu mm of blood with increased neutrophil count.

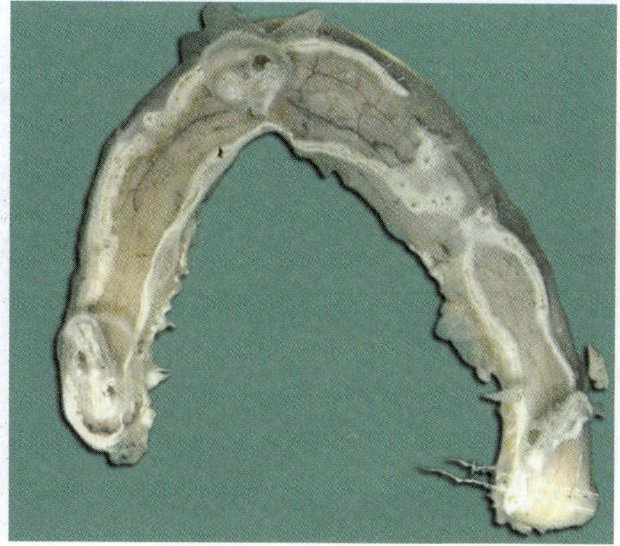

Fig. 69.8: Gangrenous appendicitis

4. What are the complications of acute appendicitis?

- Appendicular mass (in untreated cases)
- Perforation with an abscess
- Perforation with generalised peritonitis
- Pylephlebitis, portal pyaemia
- Septicaemia, gram-negative shock

5. How do you treat an appendicular mass?

- Conservative line, Oschner-Sherren regime—liquid and semisolid diet, antibiotics, intravenous fluids, etc.

IX. CARCINOMA ASCENDING COLON

1. What is this specimen?

- Specimen of terminal ileum, caecum and right colon with removal of involved lymph nodes and fat fascia. Nowadays, only 4–6 cm of ileum is removed.

2. What is the surgery?

- Right radical hemicolectomy done for growth in the ascending colon.

3. How do you identify colon?

- *Taenia coli* and appendix are seen. The colon has a larger diameter compared to small intestine.

4. What are the investigations?

- Barium enema will show persistent filling defect. However, colonoscopy is the investigation because the growth can be visualised and biopsy can be taken.

5. What do you mean by limited resection?

- It is done for ileocaecal tuberculosis wherein diseased segment is removed.

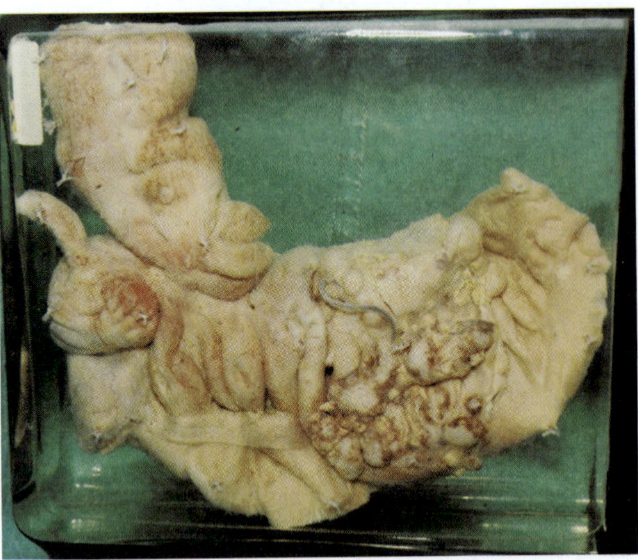

Fig. 69.9: Carcinoma ascending colon

X. MECKEL'S DIVERTICULUM

1. What is the specimen?

- Resected specimen of intestine showing a diverticulum. Hence, it is a Meckel's diverticulum.

2. Why is it a Meckel's diverticulum?

- Because it is a single diverticulum arising from antimesenteric border of the intestine.

3. What are common symptoms?

- Bleeding per rectum, abdominal pain due to inflammation, intestinal obstruction and peritonitis due to perforation.

4. What is the cause and what are the types of bleeding?

- Ulcer in the ectopic gastric mucosa. Bleeding can be occult, in small quantities or rarely can be massive.

5. How do you diagnose Meckel's diverticulum?

- Radio-nuclear (^{99m}Tc pertechnetate) scan is helpful when there is active bleeding.

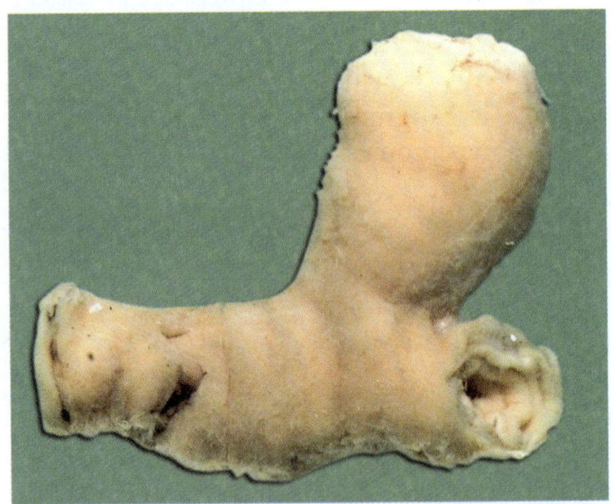

Fig. 69.10: Meckel's diverticulum

XI. POLYCYSTIC KIDNEY

1. What is this specimen?

- Specimen of kidney with multiple cystic lesions. Entire kidney is involved.

2. What is the diagnosis?

- Polycystic kidney

3. Why do you say it is polycystic kidney?

- Kidney is grossly enlarged
- Outer surface is bosselated
- Multiple cysts are present

4. What are clinical features of polycystic kidney?

- Women: 30–50 years
- Bilateral renal mass
- Hypertension

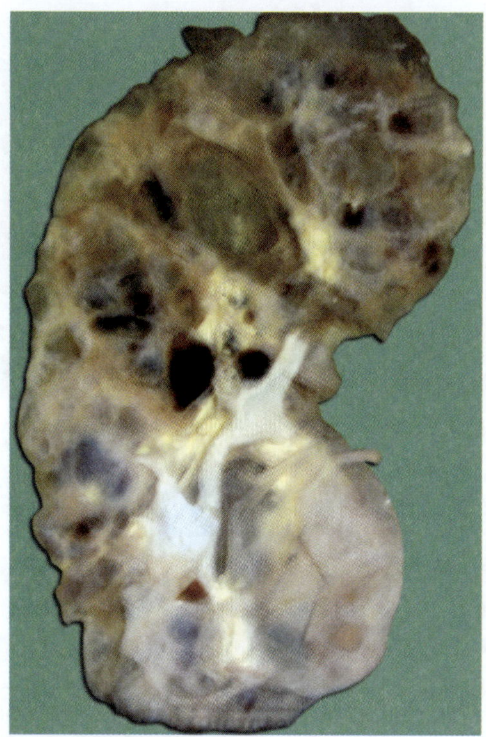

Fig. 69.11: Polycystic kidney

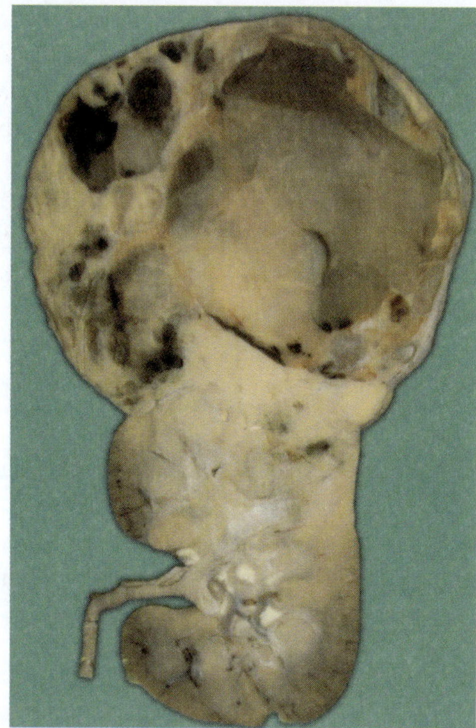

Fig. 69.12: Renal cell carcinoma

- Haematuria
- Renal failure

5. **What is the treatment?**
   - If there is no renal failure, control hypertension.
   - If there is renal failure—dialysis followed by renal transplantation.

XII. RENAL CELL CARCINOMA

1. **What is this specimen?**
   - Specimen of the kidney because it is reniform shaped, ureter and calyces are seen.
   - In the upper pole, there is destruction of the calyces with solid mass. Cut surface is smooth.
2. **What is the diagnosis?**
   - Renal cell carcinoma.
3. **What is the microscopic picture?**
   - Cuboidal or polyhedral clear cells with deeply stained rounded nuclei—clear cell carcinoma. Sometimes, dark cells can coexist. In some cases, walls of blood vessels are lined by tumour cells.
4. **How does it spread?**
   - Lymphatic and blood spread
5. **What are the primary malignant tumours which spread by blood?**
   - Renal cell carcinoma, follicular carcinoma thyroid, carcinoma prostate, carcinoma breast, bronchogenic carcinoma.

XIII. HYDRONEPHROSIS

1. **What is this specimen?**
   - Specimen of the kidney with ureter showing dilatation of pelvicalyceal system. Calyces are club-shaped.
2. **What is the diagnosis?**
   - Hydronephrosis—probably due to pelvi-ureteric junction (PUJ) obstruction.
3. **Why PUJ obstruction?**
   - Ureter is not dilated

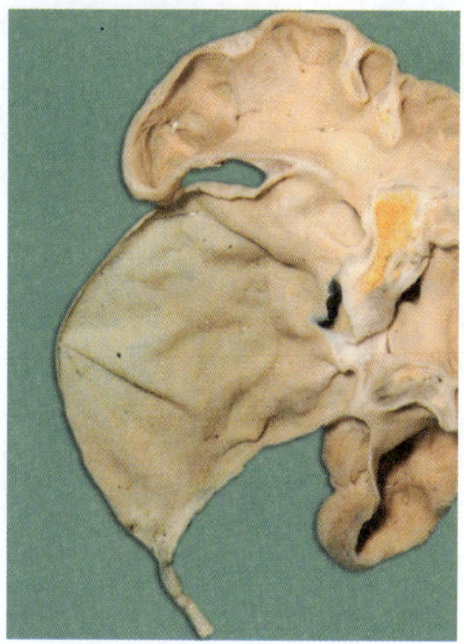

Fig. 69.13: Hydronephrosis

4. **What are the common causes of obstruction at PUJ?**
   - Stone in the pelvis
   - Aberrant vessels—a lower polar artery or vein arising from the main vessels in an aberrant position obstructs the upper ureter.
   - PUJ dyskinesia—occurs due to incoordination between neuromuscular impulses and pelvis.
5. **What is the treatment of PUJ dyskinesia?**
   - Anderson-Hynes pyeloplasty.

XIV. CARCINOMA PENIS

1. **What is this specimen?**
   - Specimen of penis, showing the glans. Prepuce is cut open showing the growth.
2. **What is the diagnosis?**
   - Partial amputation done for carcinoma penis
3. **What are the indications for partial amputation of the penis?**
   - Growth confined to the glans penis or to the prepuce.
4. **If shaft is involved, what is the treatment?**
   - Total amputation of penis followed by perineal urethrostomy.
5. **What are the complications of perineal urethrostomy?**
   - Bleeding, dermatitis and stenosis. The stenosis should be dilated by using Hegar's dilators.

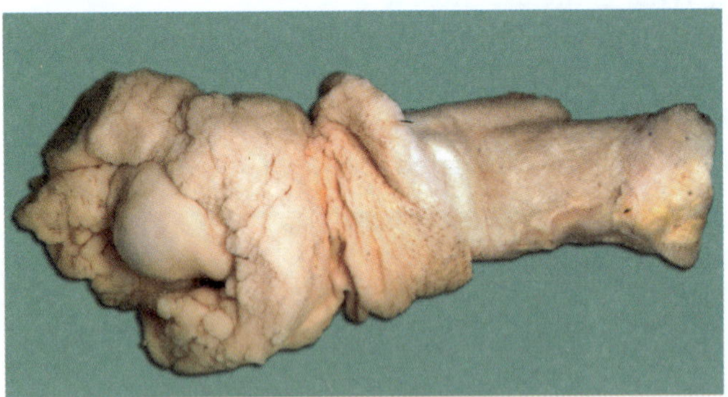

Fig. 69.14: Carcinoma penis

XV. SEMINOMA TESTIS

1. **What is this specimen?**
   - Specimen of testis showing spermatic cord. Cut surface of the testis is smooth and homogenous with a tumour in the upper part.
2. **What is the diagnosis?**
   - Seminoma
3. **Why not a teratoma?**
   - In a teratoma, the cut surface is not homogenous.

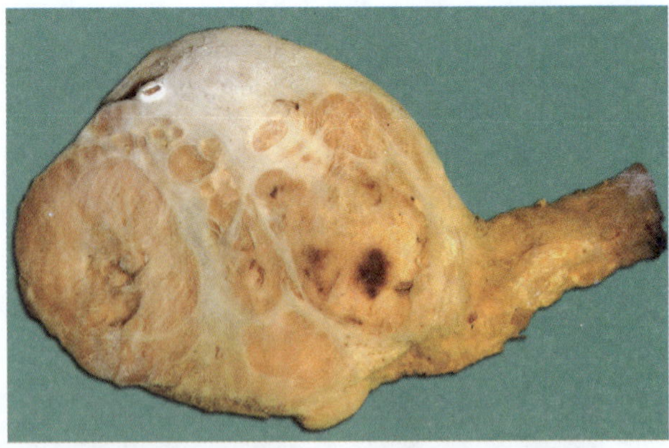

Fig. 69.15: Seminoma testis showing spermatic cord on the right side

4. **How does seminoma spread?**
   - Mainly by lymphatics.
5. **What type of orchidectomy is done for testicular tumours and why?**
   - High orchidectomy, through an inguinal incision. If scrotum is incised, chances of alternate pathway of lymphatics opening up are high. Hence, inguinal exploration is the choice.

XVI. CHOLECYSTECTOMY FOR GALLSTONES

1. **What is this specimen?**
   - Cholecystectomy specimen.
2. **What is the diagnosis?**
   - Multiple stones are present within lumen—diagnosis is probably chronic cholecystitis.
3. **Why do you say it is a gallbladder?**
   - It is pear-shaped with fundus, body and a narrow portion—cystic area.
4. **What is Hartmann's pouch?**
   - It is the distal angulated portion of gallbladder wherein a stone commonly lodges.

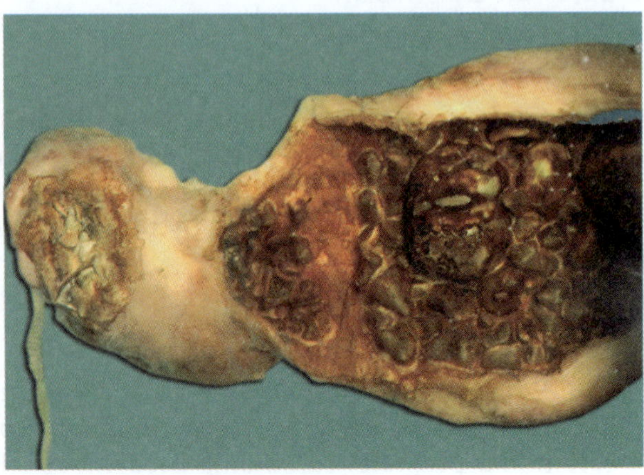

Fig. 69.16: Gallstones

5. **What are the common symptoms of gallstones?**
   - Flatulent dyspepsia, gallstone colic, acute and chronic cholecystitis are common symptoms of gallstones. Mucocoele, empyema, perforation and gallstone pancreatitis are other complications.

XVII. HYDATID CYST

1. **What is this specimen?**
   - Specimen of laminated membranes—this layer is also called ectocyst. It is thick and elastic resembling onion skin appearance.
2. **What is the diagnosis?**
   - Hydatid cyst—mostly liver
3. **What are the other layers of hydatid cyst?**
   - Outermost layer is called adventitial layer which blends firmly with liver tissue. The middle layer is ectocyst, also called laminated membrane. Inner layer is germinal epithelium, also called endocyst within which brood capsules and daughter cysts are present.
4. **What is the drug for hydatid disease?**
   - Albendazole 400 mg, a day for 15 days followed by no drug for 15 days. Then restart the cycle. Such treatment may have to continue for 6 months depending on the response rate.
5. **What are the common complications of hydatid cyst of the liver?**
   - Infection, rupture, calcification, cholangitis with jaundice are a few complications.

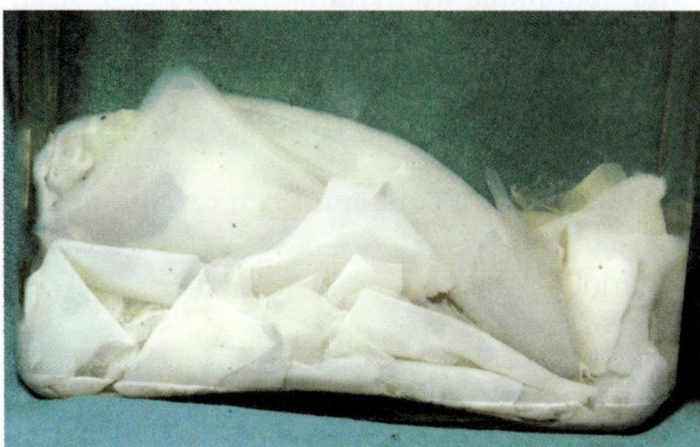

Fig. 69.17: Hydatid cyst

XVIII. RADICAL GASTRECTOMY INCLUDING REMOVAL OF THE COLON

1. **What is the specimen?**
   - Specimen of stomach with transverse colon.
2. **Why stomach and colon?**
   - It has lesser curvature and greater curvature—pylorus, body and proximal stomach. Colon is the immediate structure below the stomach.

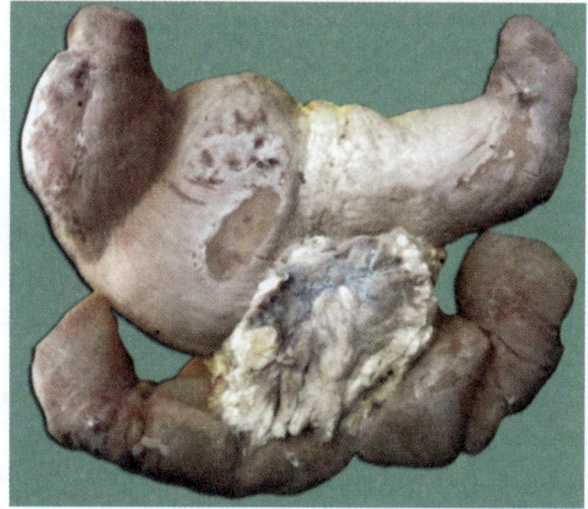

Fig. 69.18: Radical gastrectomy including removal of the colon

3. **What does it show?**
   - Exophytic growth infiltrating the colon
4. **What is the final diagnosis?**
   - Most probably it is carcinoma stomach infiltrating transverse colon.
5. **What is the best investigation in such cases to identify local infiltration?**
   - CT scan

XIX. LIPOMA

1. **What is this specimen?**
   - Specimen of lipoma
2. **Why do you say it is lipoma?**
   - It is lobular, yellow in colour
3. **What is the commonest site and type of lipoma?**
   - Flank is the commonest site. Single and subcutaneous variety is the commonest type.
4. **What are the common complications of lipoma?**
   - Liposarcoma and intussusception
5. **Which type of lipoma give rise to intussusception?**
   - Submucosal type

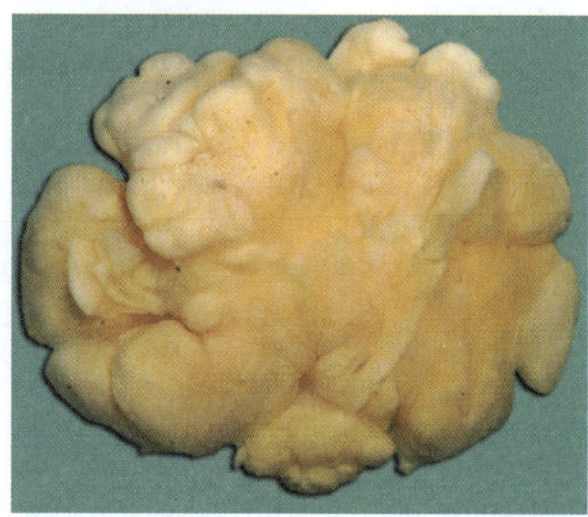

Fig. 69.19: Lipoma

XX. MALIGNANT MELANOMA

1. **What is this specimen?**
   - Specimen of foot showing a large ulcerated growth in the sole of the foot.
2. **What is the diagnosis and why do you say so?**
   - Malignant melanoma because the lesion is pigmented.
3. **What is the commonest type of malignant melanoma?**
   - Superficial spreading is the first followed by nodular variety.
4. **What are the staging systems available for this condition?**
   - Clark's level of invasion and Breslow's thickness are important staging systems in addition to TNM staging.
5. **What are the ABCDE of melanoma?**
   - Asymmetry
   - Border irregular
   - Colour variegation
   - Diameter >6 mm
   - Elevation

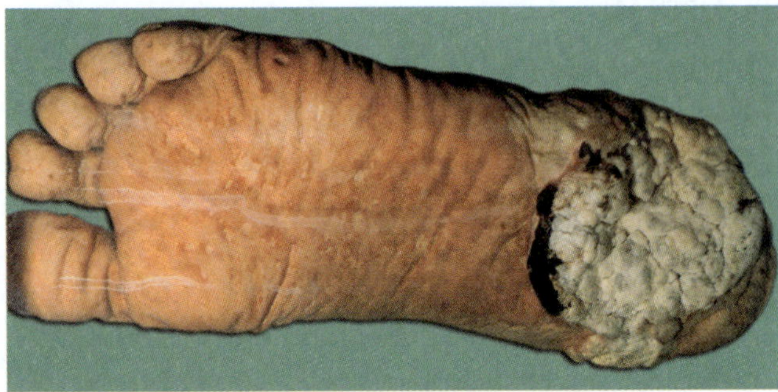

Fig. 69.20: Malignant melanoma

XXI. THYROIDECTOMY SPECIMEN

1. **What is this specimen?**
   - Specimen of thyroid gland showing both lobes and isthmus.
2. **What is the diagnosis and why do you say so?**
   - Probably it is a subtotal thyroidectomy specimen—surgery is done for multinodular goitre.
3. **What is the commonest type of malignancy of the thyroid gland?**
   - Papillary carcinoma—63%. 2nd common type is follicular carcinoma thyroid.
4. **What is the surgical treatment for well-differentiated carcinoma thyroid gland?**
   - Most centres follow total thyroidectomy. If the patient is in low-risk category, lobectomy can be done.

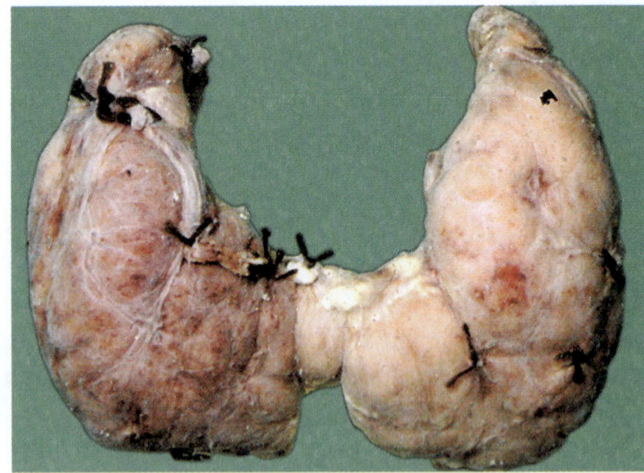

Fig. 69.21: Thyroidectomy specimen

5. **What blood investigation is useful in the follow-up period of papillary carcinoma thyroid gland?**
   - Thyroglobulin

XXII. WIDE EXCISION SPECIMEN OF SKIN

1. **What is this specimen?**
   - Specimen of skin which has been excised with normal skin. Hence, wide excision specimen.
2. **What is the diagnosis and why do you say so?**
   - Probably it is a squamous cell carcinoma because edges are everted.
3. **What are the common sites of squamous cell carcinoma skin?**
   - Areas with chronic irritation, e.g. Kangri cancer in the abdominal wall, chimney sweepers cancer, etc.
4. **What are the common precancerous lesions for squamous cell carcinoma?**
   - Leukoplakia, Bowen's disease, chronic irritation and scar tissues, etc.
5. **What do you call squamous cell carcinoma arising in a scar tissue?**
   - Marjolin's ulcer

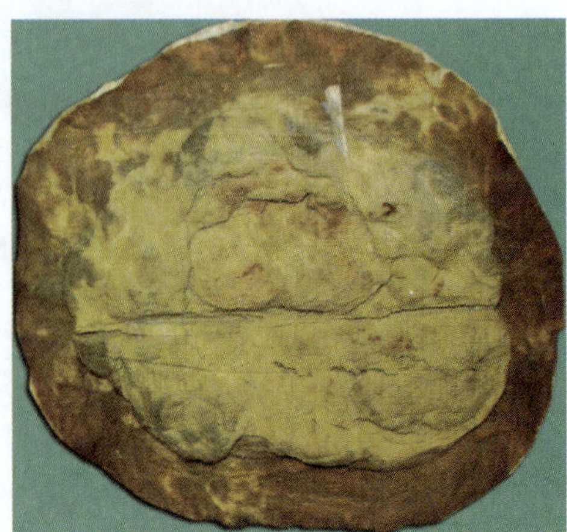

Fig. 69.22: Wide excision skin

XXIII. WHIPPLE'S PANCREATICODUODENECTOMY

1. **What is this specimen?**
   - Specimen showing distal stomach, duodenum, proximal jejunum and pancreatic head.
2. **What is the name of this operation?**
   - Whipple's pancreaticoduodenectomy
3. **Why is it done?**
   - Mostly due to periampullary carcinoma
4. **How can you get histopathological diagnosis?**
   - Endoscopic biopsy
5. **Is there any other indication for Whipple's surgery?**
   - Pancreatic head mass—doubt exists between chronic pancreatitis and carcinoma head pancreas. Provided experience of the surgeon is good.

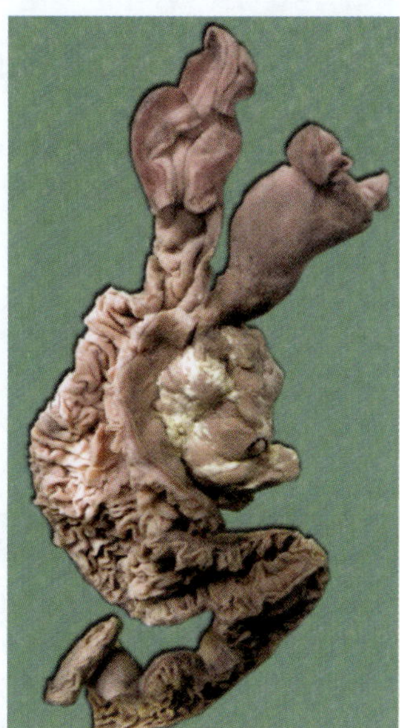

Fig. 69.23: Whipple's pancreaticoduodenectomy

XXIV. RIGHT HEMICOLECTOMY FOR CARCINOMA CAECUM

1. **What is this specimen?**
   - Specimen showing distal ileum, caecum, part of the ascending colon and a few lymph nodes
2. **What is the name of this operation?**
   - Limited colectomy
3. **Why is it done?**
   - Mostly due to ileo-caecal tuberculosis
4. **Why do you say so?**
   - Stricture is seen in the terminal ileum
5. **What was the indication for surgery?**
   - Acute intestinal obstruction

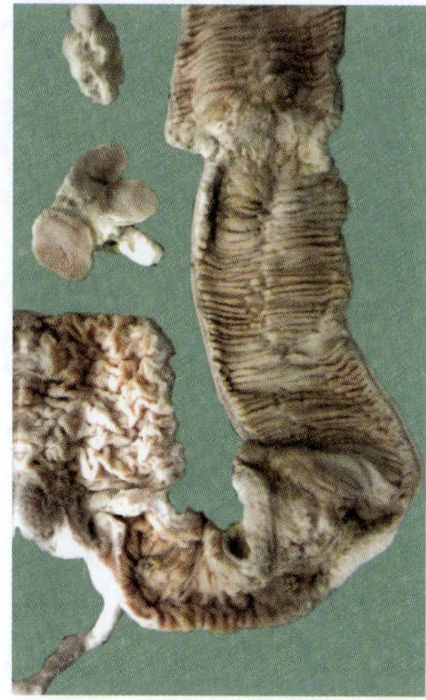

Fig. 69.24: Right hemicolectomy for carcinoma caecum

XXV. SPLENECTOMY SPECIMEN

1. **What is this specimen?**
   - Specimen showing spleen with laceration of the diaphragmatic surface.
2. **Why laceration?**
   - Blunt injury is the most common cause of rupture spleen.
3. **What will be clinical manifestation?**
   - Bleeding
4. **What other surgery can be done for bleeding?**
   - Partial splenectomy or splenorrhaphy
5. **What is the dangerous complication after splenectomy?**
   - Opportunistic post-splenectomy infections

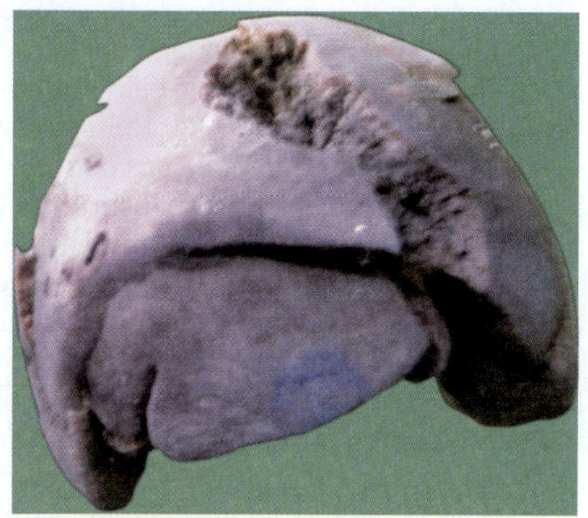

Fig. 69.25: Splenectomy specimen

Useful Tips
- Please look into the specimen carefully
- Please see both sides of the specimen
- Think which is the most likely organ involved
- Think what is the probable diagnosis.

CHAPTER

70

Operative Surgery, Laparoscopic Surgery and Accessories

- History of surgery
- Skin closure techniques
- Excision of swellings
- Surgery for hydrocoele
- Incision and drainage (I and D)
- Incision and drainage of breast abscess
- Circumcision
- Venesection or cut down
- Vasectomy
- Tracheostomy
- Thyroidectomy
- Amputations
- Amputations in leg
- Upper limb amputations
- Abdominal incisions
- Appendicectomy
- Bassini's herniorrhaphy
- Open cholecystectomy
- Vagotomy gastrojejunostomy (GJ)
- Intestinal resection and anastomosis
- Colectomy
- Staplers in surgery
- Laparoscopic surgery
- Hernia repair: TAPP (Transabdominal Preperitoneal Mesh Repair)
- SILS (LESS)
- Natural orifice transluminal endoscopic surgery (NOTES)
- VAAFT technique
- Robotic surgery
- Energy sources in surgery
- Harmonic scalpel
- Lasers in surgery

Introduction

Over a period of time, the number of operations an undergraduate is expected to know has become less and less. Today no MBBS doctor is supposed to do a surgical procedure because qualified surgeons are available even in a village. Hence, I have discussed only some common surgical procedures that an undergraduate student is expected to know. Every operation has been discussed along a certain basic pattern as given below and the key words used are given in Key Box 70.1. *Students should study surgical anatomy before reading this chapter.* Father of ancient surgery was an Indian, Sushrutha. Under history of surgery, I have listed a few eminent surgeons who have contributed to surgery in the past. It is followed by some basic aspects about skin closure techniques and knotting principles. Suture materials have been discussed under instruments section and surgical wound closure is discussed under appropriate surgeries. To give examples: the most common incision given is midline incision. The most common surgeries done are appendicectomy hernioplasty, etc. Students should study these surgeries in more detail. In this chapter common operations, laparoscopic surgeries and few other accessories related to surgery are discussed.

HISTORY OF SURGERY

- Surgery emerged as a specialty in the late 19th century.
- There are many eminent surgeons who have contributed significantly in the development of surgery. A few surgeons are uniquely associated with their work on a particular disease or specialty. There are numerous surgeons who have made distinct contribution in their respective specialty. Some of the commonly known works and the surgeons associated with them are listed below.

Surgeons	Associated work
Ambroise Pare	Haemorrhage control
Joseph Lister	Asepsis/antisepsis
Theodor Kocher	Thyroid surgery
Theodor Billroth	Gastric surgery
William Halsted	Breast surgery

Theodor Kocher (1841–1917): He was a student of Theodor Billroth and Bernhard von Langenbeck. He did extensive work on thyroid and excised the thyroid for goitre in 1876. Some of the contributions of Kocher are Kocher's transverse incision for thyroid surgery, Kocherization of duodenum, Kocher's sign for Graves' disease, Kocher's forceps, etc. He is known to be the father of thyroid surgery. He won the Nobel prize in 1909.

Theodor Billroth: He was the first surgeon to remove a part of the oesophagus in 1872. In 1873, he performed the first complete excision of a larynx. He was the first surgeon to excise a rectal cancer. He is credited with distinct eponymous work named after him that includes Billroth's 1 operation, Billroth's 2 operation, Billroth's cord, etc. He is considered to be the father of abdominal surgery.

Halsted (1852–1922): He is well known for radical operation for breast cancer. He introduced surgical gloves to protect the hands of his scrub nurse, Caroline Hampton. He developed surgery for inguinal hernia. He also developed topical anaesthesia.

Sushrutha: Ancient history showed Sushruta (600 BC) to be the pioneer in plastic surgery and his work is described in Sushruta Samhita. It describes various surgical procedures and instruments used. His famous surgery on ear lobe is believed to be a classical example of flap surgery used more than 2500 years ago in India. He is known to be "Father of Plastic Surgery".

Competency

SU14.3: Describe the materials and methods used for surgical wound closure and anastomosis (sutures, knots, and needles).

SKIN CLOSURE TECHNIQUES

- Good closure begins with a good incision
  - Incision should be made with scalpel at right angles to the skin.
  - It should be made along the relaxed skin tension lines, this also results in minimal scarring on healing.
- Skin should be handled gently to avoid devitalising the margins.
- The skin edges should be everted and approximated without tension.
- Circular incisions should be converted to elliptical incisions that are at least three times as long as wide, to allow the wound to heal without tension.
- Tension on the skin sutures can be minimised by using deep dermal and subdermal sutures.
  - It is better to leave the suture line lax than using too much tension, as postoperative oedema will often take up any slack in the suture material. Using too much tension can compromise the vascularity of the edges.

The commonly used suture techniques for skin closure are:

- Simple interrupted sutures.
- Mattress sutures: Can be either vertical or horizontal mattress sutures. These produce accurate approximation of wound edges.
- Subcuticular sutures: Good cosmetic outcomes.
- Other skin closure techniques include:
  - Tissue glue which are composed of cyanoacrylate
  - Skin adhesive strips, skin staples

Knotting Principles

Tying a knot is one of the most fundamental skills that a surgeon has to acquire and perfect.

The important principles of knotting are:

- The knot should be tied firmly, not too tight, without exerting too much tension on the tissues.
- The knot should not slip. A few suture materials, such as prolene, require additional throws to secure the knot.
- The knot should be compact and small to minimise the foreign material.
- The standard surgical knot is the reef knot, and additional throws are added for security. All knots should be squared.
- The suture should be cut appropriately after knotting leaving the thread at 1–2 mm length.
- In cases of continuous suture technique, an Aberdeen knot is used at the end.
- Abdominal incision closure has been given later.

Commonly used abbreviations are given in Key Box 70.1.

Key Box 70.1

Commonly Used Abbreviations

SA	Spinal anaesthesia
GA	General anaesthesia
LA	Local anaesthesia
OT	Operation theatre
NPO	Nil per oral
IV	Intravenous
RT	Ryle's tube

Steps of Operative Surgery

1. Indications
2. Contraindications
3. Position of the patient
4. Anaesthesia
5. Preparation of parts
6. Procedure
7. Closure
8. Postoperative management
9. Postoperative complications
10. Advice at discharge

Table 70.1 Sterilisation

Agents for sterilisation	Common of items
1. Autoclaving	Linen, operative instruments, glass syringes
2. Dettol or phenol	Sharp instruments (scissors, needles, blades)
3. Glutaraldehyde	Endoscopy and laparoscopy equipment
4. Ethylene oxide gamma radiation	Syringes
5. Formaldehyde	Disinfect rooms like OT
6. Skin	70% spirit, povidone iodine

Antiseptic Agents

- Povidone-iodine
- Spirit 70%
- Savlon

Autoclave and sterilisation: Table 70.1 and *see* Chapter 10 on sterilization.

EXCISION OF SWELLINGS

A. LIPOMA

1. Indications

- Large size (cosmesis/patient's wish)
- Recent rapid increase in size (sarcomatous change)
- Symptomatic naevo/neurolipomas
- Pressure symptoms based on site.

2. Contraindications

Strictly speaking, there are no contraindications. Excision of lipoma is a simple procedure. However, asymptomatic lipomas in a difficult location need not be excised. However, small the surgery may be, safety is an important principle to be kept in mind.

3. Position of the Patient

Supine/lateral/prone depending upon the location.

4. Anaesthesia

If small, under LA; if large, regional anaesthesia or GA.

5. Preparation of the Parts

Povidone-iodine and spirit

6. Surgical Procedure

- **Incision:** A linear incision over the summit of the swelling is placed and flaps raised on both sides of the incision.
- **Layers opened:** Skin and some part of the subcutaneous tissue till the capsule of the swelling is encountered.
- **Dissection:** Using an artery forceps or a mosquito forceps (if a small swelling), a plane is created between the raised flaps and the capsule of the swelling. Pressure is applied at the base of the swelling to deliver out the lipoma. A small vessel may be encountered as the base is being dissected that should be identified and cauterised or ligated. The specimen should be sent for histopathological evaluation.

7. Closure

If a large cavity is created due to excision of swelling, the excised skin flaps can be refreshed and excess skin can be removed. A few interrupted Vicryl sutures can be placed to close subcutaneous layer. The skin is closed with 2.0 ethilon vertical mattress suture. Sometimes, a drain may have to be kept in the cavity.

8. Postoperative Management

Nothing specific other than monitoring vitals and the operated area for bleeding. Majority of them can be done as day care surgery.

9. Postoperative Complications

- Infection, bleeding
- Injury to vital structures around
- Seroma formation, if large cavity remains

10. Advice at Discharge

Suture removal after 7–10 days, if non-absorbable sutures are used such as 3-0 silk. If absorbable sutures such as monocryl (3-0 Polyglactin) are used, there is no need to remove the sutures.

B. SEBACEOUS CYST

1. Indications

- Infection—results in abscess
- Complications such as **Cock's peculiar tumour**, horn and calcification.

2. Contraindication

No specific contraindication.

3. Position of the Patient

Supine/lateral/prone depending upon the location.

4. Anaesthesia

Mostly LA. Multiple cysts over scalp and scrotum may require GA or regional anaesthesia.

5. Preparation of the Parts

Povidone-iodine and spirit.

6. Surgical Procedure

- **Incision:** **Elliptical incision** around the summit of the swelling encircling the punctum.
- **Layers opened**
  - Incision should be superficial. Care should be taken not to cut open the cyst wall.
  - The principle is to **completely excise the cyst** with its wall and the overlying punctum and a bit of the surrounding skin around the punctum.
- **Dissection**
  - A plane is created between the skin and the cyst wall, carefully, preventing opening of the cyst wall.
  - An Allis forceps may be applied to the punctum and the elliptical skin to obtain traction. Flaps need to be raised gradually on either sides of the incision and then deliver the cyst *in toto.*
  - If the cyst wall opens up, the sebum is removed completely and an effort to remove all the cyst wall, in piecemeal, is made.

7. Closure

Single layer closure of the skin.

8. Postoperative Management

Nothing specific other than monitoring vitals and the operated area for bleeding. Majority of them can be done by day care surgery. In infected cases, antibiotics are given.

9. Postoperative Complications

- Infection
- Recurrence, if cyst wall is not completely removed.

10. Advice at Discharge

Suture removal after 7–10 days.

C. NEUROFIBROMA

1. Indications

- Cosmesis
- Symptoms of pain on pressure
- Pressure effects causing neurological deficits
- Sarcomatous changes

2. Contraindication

In von Recklinghausen's disease, only symptomatic neurofibromas should be removed.

3. Position of the Patient

Supine/lateral/prone depending upon the location.

4. Anaesthesia

Mostly LA, sometimes GA.

5. Preparation of the Parts

Povidone-iodine and spirit.

6. Surgical Procedure

- **Incision:** A linear incision over the summit of the swelling is placed and flaps raised on both sides of the incision.
- **Layers opened:** Skin and some part of the subcutaneous tissue till the capsule of the swelling is encountered.
- **Dissection:** Using an artery forceps or a mosquito forceps (if a small swelling), a plane is created between the raised flaps and the capsule of the swelling. Pressure is applied at the base of the swelling to deliver out the neurofibroma. Care should be taken not to injure the underlying nerve while dissecting.

7. Closure

It can be closed in two layers, subcutaneous—vicryl, interrupted and skin 2-0/3–0 sutures.

8. Postoperative Management

Nothing specific other than monitoring vitals and the operated area for bleeding. Majority of them can be done as day care surgery.

9. Postoperative Complications

- Infection
- Injury to the nerve causing weakness, loss of sensations of the affected part.
- If partially left behind, recurrence and chance of sarcomatous changes.

10. Advice at Discharge

Suture removal after 7–10 days.

SURGERY FOR HYDROCOELE

This is done as a day care surgery.

1. Indication

Vaginal hydrocoele. However, infantile and funicular hydrocoeles are also treated surgically in the same manner.

2. Contraindication

Secondary hydrocoele due to *testicular tumours*. They contain haemorrhagic fluid. It will be a big blunder to incise the scrotum mistaking it to be a vaginal hydrocoele. Suspect testicular tumours if the hydrocoele is recent and lax, if the testis is felt separately and is hard in consistency or transillumination is negative.

3. Position of the Patient

Supine

Pearls of Wisdom

Before incising scrotum for hydrocoele, palpate carefully testis and epididymis and rule out testicular tumour. When in doubt, get ultrasound examination of testis.

4. Anaesthesia

SA or LA

5. Preparation of the Parts

Savlon and spirit (iodine is better avoided because it can cause severe scrotal dermatitis and excoriation of skin, which can cause more discomfort to the patient than hydrocoele surgery).

6. Procedure (Key Box 70.2)

Incision

Hydrocoele is held tense by an assistant and 5–6 cm incision (depending upon size) is made over the most prominent part of the swelling parallel to the median raphe of the scrotum.

Layers Opened

- Skin
- Dartos
- External spermatic fascia

Key Box 70.2

Hydrocoele Surgery

- Aspiration: Not advised
- Lord's plication: Small hydrocoele
- Jaboulay's: Large hydrocoele

- Cremasteric fascia
- Internal spermatic fascia

At this stage, hydrocoele sac is visible and is delivered outside the incision (Fig. 70.1).

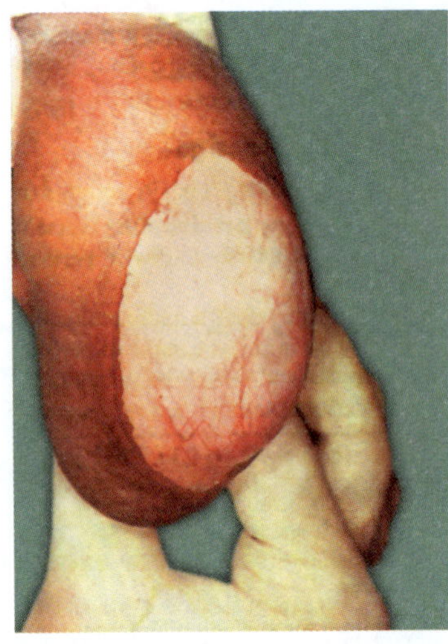

Fig. 70.1: Hydrocoele sac being delivered

Hydrocoele fluid is drained by using ***trocar and cannula.*** An opening is made in the tunica vaginalis sac and it is enlarged. All fluid is drained out. Testis and epididymis are inspected for any pathology, e.g. Craggy epididymis can be found in tuberculosis. Depending on the size of the hydrocoele and thickness of the wall of the sac, two types of surgery can be done.

a. **Small tunica vaginalis sac (TV sac):** The redundant tunica vaginalis is plicated by interrupted sutures. The sac gets crumpled up and surrounds the testis. This is called **Lord's plication** (Fig. 70.2). Advantage of this operation is minimal dissection, hence no complications.

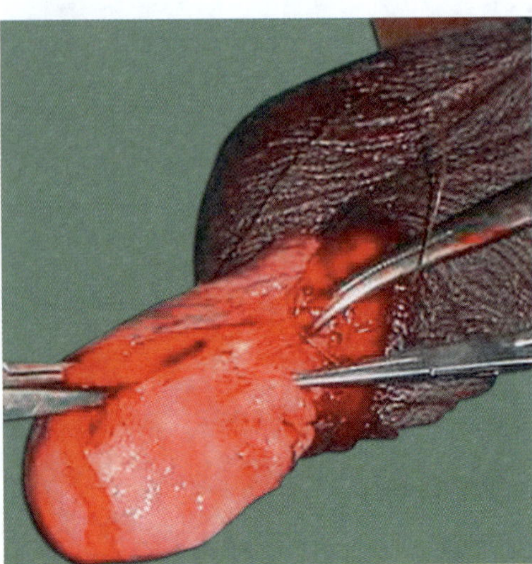

Fig. 70.2: The sac has been everted and edges of the sac sutured together

b. **Sac is large and thick or multilocular hydrocoele:** Partial excision of the hydrocoele sac is done leaving a margin of 1–2 cm. After obtaining hemostasis, eversion of sac is done. Here cut edge of the sac is everted and sutured behind the testis. This is called **Jaboulay's operation. By eversion of the sac, the secreting surface of the testis becomes anterior and secretions are absorbed by subcutaneous lymphatics** (Fig. 70.3A and B).

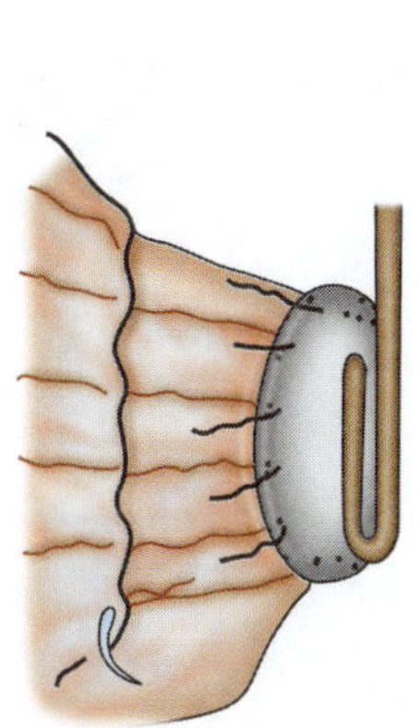

Fig. 70.3A: Lord's plication

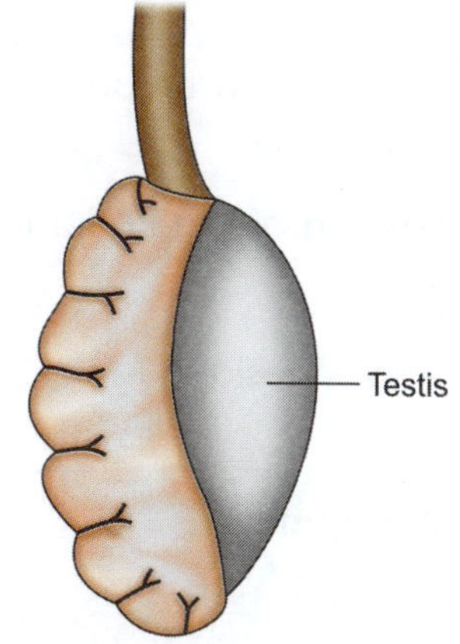

Fig. 70.3B: Jaboulay's operation

c. ***Sharma and Jhawer's technique:*** In this, minimum dissection of the sac is done to separate from surrounding region. This will avoid complications such as bleeding.

7. Closure

- In vast majority of the cases, if perfect hemostasis is obtained, draining the cavity is not required. A tube drain can be kept in the scrotum, if required. When kept brought out separately by making a stab incision and is anchored to the scrotal skin by white thread.
- Subcutaneous layer by using absorbable suture such as vicryl sutures.
- Skin—interrupted absorbable sutures (polyglactin—rapid vicryl). Silk is avoided for skin closure over the scrotum as black colour of the silk is not seen clearly over dark pigmented skin of the scrotum, making stitch removal difficult.
- Scrotal support is given to reduce oedema.

8. Postoperative Management

- NPO for 6 hours followed by soft diet.
- Prophylactic antibiotics are given. Postoperative antibiotics are not required.
- Use Monocryl which is a synthetic, absorbable suture—No need to remove sutures.

9. Postoperative Complications

- **Haematoma:** If it is large and increasing, wound should be reopened urgently and bleeders have to be ligated. It may be due to injury to the testicular artery, vein or pampiniform plexus of veins.

  Scrotal oedema can occur which resolves within 2–3 days.
- **Wound infection** can result in discharging pus.
- Testis can undergo necrosis. Such cases are treated with orchidectomy.
- **Injury to the spermatic cord**.

10. Advice at Discharge

Normal activity within 1 or 2 days.

Pearls of Wisdom

Even though surgery for hydrocoele is minor, it should not be taken lightly.

INCISION AND DRAINAGE (I AND D)

1. Indication

Pyogenic abscess, pyaemic abscesses.

2. Contraindication

Cold abscess.

3. Position of the Patient

Supine, prone or lateral depending upon site of abscess.

4. Anaesthesia

- Regional anaesthesia or GA is preferred because abscess is multiloculated and infiltration of lignocaine into the abscess cavity does not act because of the acidic pH of the pus.
- However, a superficial abscess which is pointing can be managed without GA.

5. Preparation of the Parts

Iodine and spirit.

6. Procedure

- **A stab incision** is made over the most prominent part of the swelling where skin is red, thinned out and is pointed.
- Pus that is drained is ***sent for culture and sensitivity.***
- A sinus forceps or finger is introduced within the abscess cavity and all the loculi are broken. When fresh blood oozes out, it indicates completion of the procedure.

- The cavity is irrigated with antiseptic agents such as iodine solution. It is followed by irrigation with normal saline.
- If the cavity is large, it is packed with roller gauze soaked in iodine and it is removed after 24–48 hours. Packing helps in controlling the bleeding, and keeps the abscess cavity open. By 7–10 days, the cavity collapses, granulation tissue fills up the cavity and healing takes place.

Hilton's method of drainage: When an abscess is located over a major vessel, as in axilla or neck, **do not make a stab incision**. An incision is made on the skin and subcutaneous tissue and sinus forceps is introduced. Later, it is treated like the treatment of an abscess. This method is followed to avoid injury to major vessels and nerves. It is also indicated in parotid abscess to avoid damage to facial nerve. Sinus forceps is selected because it is blunt tipped instrument without lock system so that opening and closing the blades are easy. It has a few serrations at the tip so that, if necessary, biopsy of the wall can be taken.

7. Closure

An abscess should not be closed, as it contains pus, bacteria (*see* also breast abscess drainage). However, in breast abscess, once all loculi are broken and after a thorough wash, the wound is closed with sutures, a drain is kept in the dependent position and brought out by a separate incision.

8. Postoperative Management

- Antibiotics
- Control of diabetes (if patient is diabetic)
- Regular dressings of the wound with antiseptic agents.

9. Postoperative Complications

- During the process of breaking the loculi, vessels underneath may be injured causing haematoma which requires drainage. Otherwise, there are no specific complications.
- Injury to vessels or nerves can occur, if basic principles of drainage of an abscess are not followed.

10. Advice at Discharge

Control of diabetes (if present).

INCISION AND DRAINAGE OF BREAST ABSCESS

1. Indication

Breast abscess (Key Box 70.3)

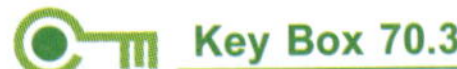 **Key Box 70.3**

Breast Abscess Drainage

- GA is preferred
- Do not wait for fluctuation
- Throbbing pain is an indication for surgery
- Small curved incision
- Keep in mind, mastitis carcinomatosa

2. Contraindication

None. However, ultrasound-guided aspiration of breast abscess should be done first especially in unilocular breast abscess.

3. Position of the Patient

Supine

4. Anaesthesia

GA

5. Preparation

Iodine and spirit

6. Procedure (Figs 70.4 and 70.5)

About 3 to 4 cm semicircular incision is made over the swelling where there is maximum tenderness. It is

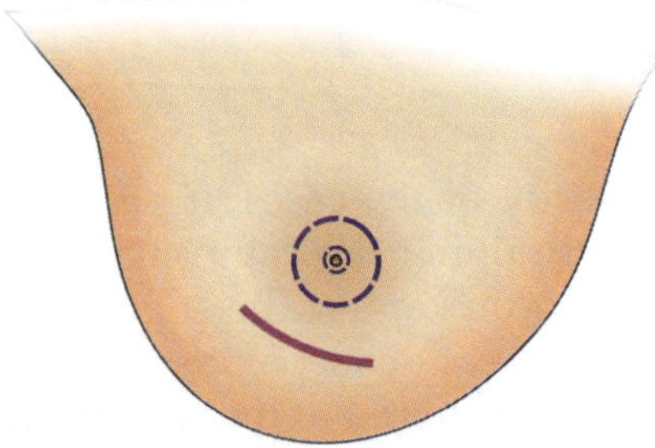

Fig. 70.4: Incision for breast abscess

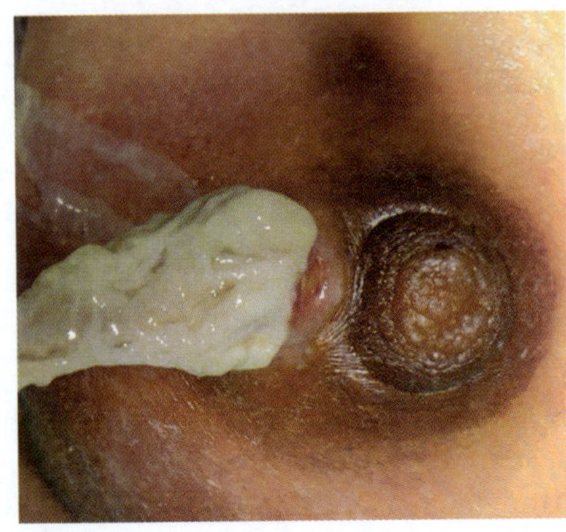

Fig. 70.5: Drainage and usage of corrugated rubber drain

drained just like pyogenic abscess. Another stab incision is made in the dependent position and tube drain is brought out through this incision. Corrugated drains are not used often now.

Pearls of Wisdom

Radial incision can be given, if abscess is in the peripheral part of the breast.

7. Closure

- If infection is very severe, **do not close the incision**.
- Otherwise, main wound is sutured and tube drain is brought down at the dependent position. Once the drainage is minimal, the drain is removed.

Pearls of Wisdom

Minor breast abscess need not be drained. Ultrasound-guided one or two aspirations may be curative in many cases.

8. Postoperative Management

- NPO for about 6 hours
- Antibiotic of choice is **cloxacillin** 500 mg 6th hourly because the common organism is *Staphylococcus aureus*. Please refer to MRSA and breast abscess on page 460.
- It may take 7–15 days for complete healing.
- One should not wait for fluctuation to develop in a breast abscess. If pain and tenderness does not subside by 48 hours, breast abscess is incised. Otherwise, breast tissue gets damaged.

9. Postoperative Complications

Haematoma needs evacuation.

10. Advice at Discharge

Lactating women should clean the nipple after every breastfeed and keep it clean.

CIRCUMCISION

Circumcision refers to removal of the preputial skin.

1. Indications

a. Ritual: Religious

b. Phimosis

2. Contraindication

Hypospadias

Pearls of Wisdom

Preputial skin is required for repair of hypospadias.

3. Position of the Patient

Supine

4. Anaesthesia

a. In children—GA

b. In adults—LA

5. Preparation of the Parts

Savlon and spirit

Pearls of Wisdom

Use plain lignocaine (without adrenaline) for LA during circumcision. Dose: 2% lignocaine 10–15 ml.

6. Procedure

In Adults (Fig. 70.6)

- Skin of the tip of the penis is held in two places by using artery forceps, prepuce is separated from the glans and is slit up in mid-dorsal line to a point a little beyond the middle of the glans.
- Preputial layers are trimmed away in a line parallel to the corona. ***On the ventral surface, frenular artery needs to be ligated by using figure of 8 stitch.*** Two layers of prepuce are united by interrupted fine chromic vicryl sutures/vicryl. Dressings are applied.

In Children (Fig. 70.7)

- Prepuce is held by two artery forceps and gentle traction is applied. A small artery clamp is applied distal to the glans and skin distal to the clamp is removed.
- Once clamp is removed, bleeding points are identified and ligated.
- Two layers of prepuce are approximated by using 5–0 vicryl.

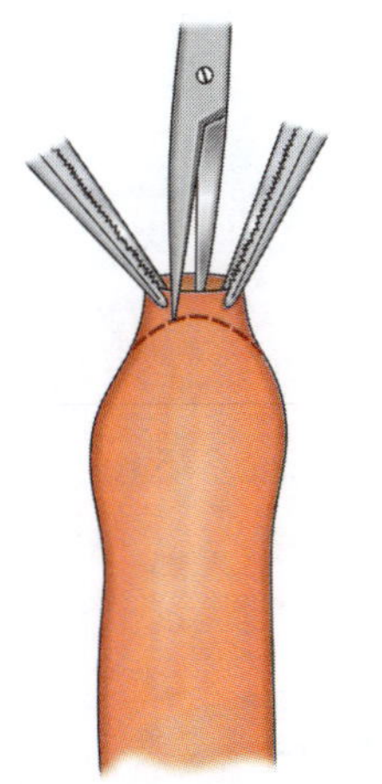

Fig. 70.6: Circumcision in adults

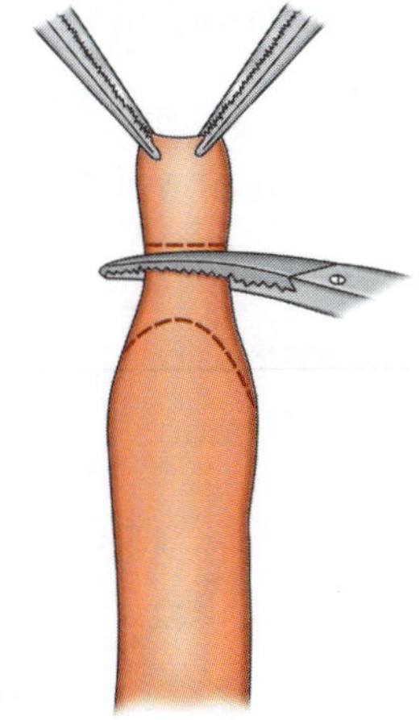

Fig. 70.7: Circumcision in children

7. Closure

Two layers of prepuce by using vicryl sutures.

8. Postoperative Management

- Sedatives and analgesics
- Antibiotics
- Removal of sutures is very painful. Hence, **do not use nonabsorbable sutures**.

9. Postoperative Complications

a. Injury to the glans penis can occur when there are extensive adhesions between prepuce and glans. It needs suturing.
b. **Haematoma:** Due to injury to the corpora cavernosa or due to the bleeding from cut edges.
c. **Tension at suture line,** if too much skin is removed. This may cause painful erection at a later date.

10. Advice at Discharge

This surgery in adults is done on an outpatient basis. Patients are discharged within a few hours. Hence, patients are advised to report, if there is bleeding and also not to wet the area for 2–3 days.

VENESECTION OR CUT DOWN

1. Indications

- Shock: Hypovolaemic, haemorrhagic, burns, etc.
- When peripheral veins are not visible due to shock, burns or massive haemorrhage, an incision is made in the anatomical sites of the vein. The vein is identified, isolated and cannulated for transfusion of fluids. This procedure is called *venesection* or *cut down* (Fig. 70.8).

2. Contraindication

None

3. Position of the Patient

Supine

4. Anaesthesia

Local infiltration by using 2% lignocaine 3–5 ml.

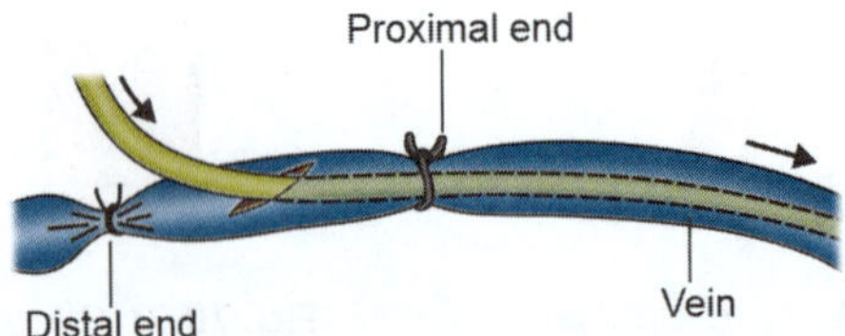

Fig. 70.8: Venesection

5. Preparation

Iodine and spirit

6. Procedure

Cephalic vein cut down is the most popular and an ideal procedure. A transverse incision about 5 cm is made in the deltopectoral groove. The cephalic vein is isolated and the distal end of the vein is ligated so that venous blood does not leak. A nick is made in the vein, through which a sufficient sized cannula (infant feeding tube can be used) is introduced. A silk ligature is applied above, just tight enough to hold cannula in place. Free flow of venous blood in the cannula indicates that it is inside the vein. The cannula is advanced further for about 10–15 cm. It is connected to IV line containing fluid (Fig. 70.8).

Precautions

- Take care not to inject air bubbles. Remove all air bubbles present in the drip set also to avoid air embolism.
- **Upper ligature should not be tight.** It may obstruct the flow of fluids.
- **Strict antiseptic principles** must be followed to avoid septicaemia.

Other Veins Selected for Cut Down

- Basilic vein in arm.
- Cubital vein at the elbow.
- Long saphenous vein in the leg. Veins in the leg, as far as possible, should be avoided to prevent deep vein thrombosis.

7. Closure

Skin—interrupted silk

8. Postoperative Management

- Care of wound by dressing
- To avoid air bubbles in the drip set

9. Postoperative Complications

- Infection, chills, rigors and septicaemia
- Air embolism

10. Advice at Discharge

Nil

Advantages of Cephalic Vein Cut Down

- Reliable vein and easy to do.
- If cannula is advanced into the right heart, CVP can be measured.

- Mobility of the patient is not restricted.
- Substances which cannot be given in a peripheral vein, such as 50% dextrose, etc. can be given without risk of thrombosis of the vein, for hyperalimentation purposes.

Pearls of Wisdom

Cannulate vein, not an artery for venesection. Thin-walled nonpulsatile bluish structure is vein.

VASECTOMY

Division and removal of a part of the vas deferens is vasectomy.

1. Indications

- Family planning
- To prevent epididymo-orchitis after prostatectomy. (Nowadays not routinely done.)

2. Contraindications

- **Relative:** Tuberculosis epididymo-orchitis. The incision may result in a nonhealing sinus. Hence, control of tuberculosis is done first followed by vasectomy.
- **Absolute:** Suspicion of testicular malignancy.

3. Position of the Patient

Supine

Cleaning and draping: Parts are cleaned and draped. Vas is palpated.

4. Anaesthesia

Local anaesthesia using 3–5 ml of 2% lignocaine.

5. Preparation of the Parts

- Savlon and spirit
- Iodine is better avoided.

6. Procedure

Feeling the Vas Deferens

After cleaning and draping, the vas is felt, at the root of scrotum between the index finger and thumb. It feels like a cord (Fig. 70.9). Lignocaine is infiltrated and wait for 1–2 minutes for lignocaine to act.

Incision

An incision of 2–4 cm is made in root of scrotum and it is deepened through layers of scrotum. An 'Allis forceps' is introduced within the incision and spermatic cord is held. During this step, fingers of the other hand help in guiding/locating/stabilising the cord. The coverings of the cord are incised.

Precautions

- Do not damage testicular vessels.
- Vas is separated. It is confirmed by its white colour, and it feels like a cord.
- Division of vas by three clamp method (Fig. 70.10).
- Vas is cut in two places A and B so that a piece of vas is removed, which can be sent for histopathology to confirm that it is vas.
- Since a piece of vas is removed, reunion of the cut ends will not occur.
- The two cut ends of vas are doubly ligated by using silk.

7. Closure

The skin is closed by absorbable one or two sutures so that removal not required.

8. Postoperative Management

- Rest for a few hours
- Antibiotics and analgesics

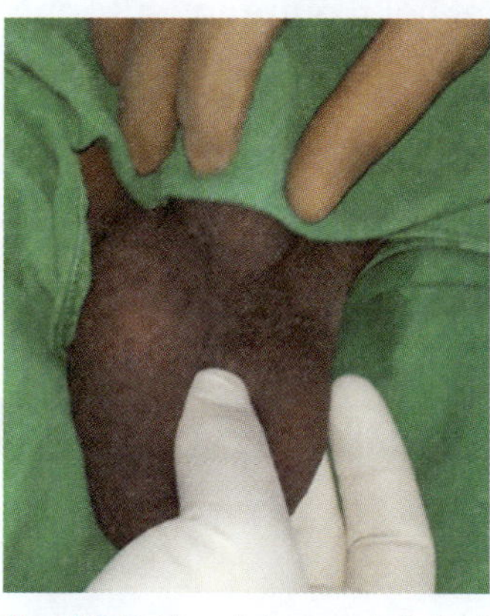

Fig. 70.9: Vas deferens is felt at the root of the scrotum

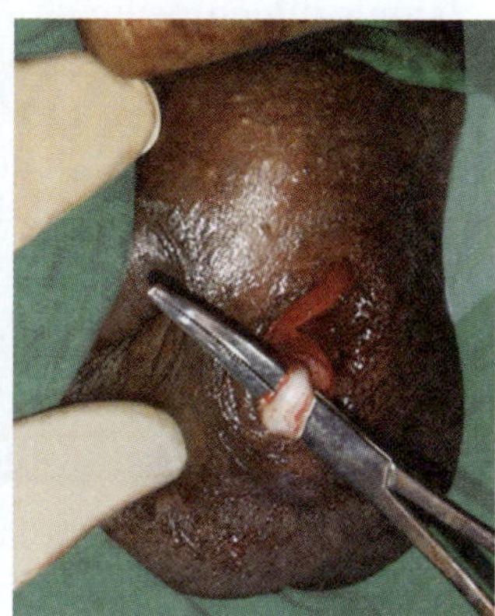

Fig. 70.10: Vas deferens is isolated from spermatic cord structures

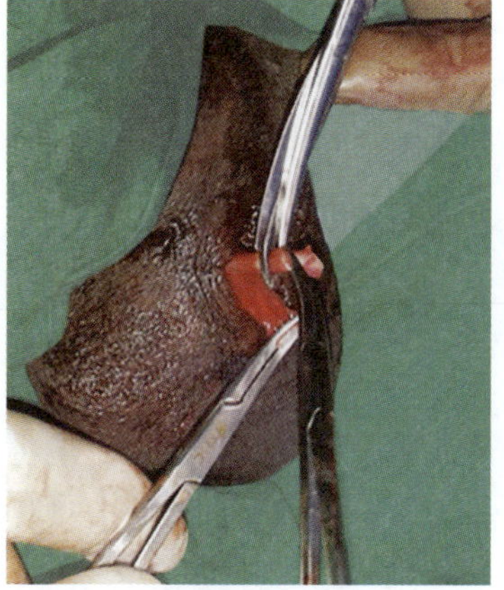

Fig. 70.11: Vas deferens is cut and a piece is sent for histopathology

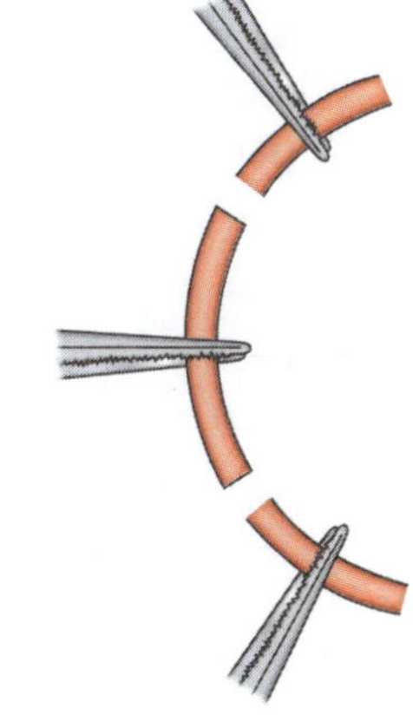

Fig. 70.12: Division of vas deferens by three clamp method

Pearls of Wisdom

The procedure is repeated on the other side.

9. Postoperative Complications

- Injury to the vessels, resulting in a large haematoma.
- Infection
- Testicular atrophy can occur a few years later. It is due to immunological reaction rather than disuse atrophy.

10. Advice at Discharge

To use other methods of family planning for two months while having sexual intercourse, as some sperms may be present in the distal end of the vas and seminal vesicle.

Pearls of Wisdom

Vasectomy being a part of family planning project, every student should be familar with this.

No Scalpel Vasectomy

- It is a novel technique to do vasectomy through one single puncture which does not require any suturing. It is less traumatic than conventional vasectomy and shortens recovery time.
- The procedure is done with LA.
- A special instrument is used to puncture the scrotum and grasp the vas deferens. Vas is then cut and through the same puncture, the other side is also operated.

TRACHEOSTOMY

An opening made in the trachea is tracheostomy.

1. Indications

a. Emergency

- Choking of the larynx due to dentures, foreign bodies, fish bones, etc.
- Stridor due to diphtheria, carcinoma larynx and bilateral recurrent laryngeal nerve paralysis after thyroidectomy.

b. Elective

- Coma
- Tetanus
- Barbiturate poisoning
- Head injuries
- Prolonged respiratory failure

2. Contraindications

- Absence of any specific indication. In patients with anaplastic carcinoma of thyroid presenting with stridor due to infiltration of growth into trachea, it may not be possible to do a tracheostomy or an attempt to do tracheostomy may result in the growth fungating through the incision (which is best avoided). In such patients, **endotracheal intubation** is done, if possible. If not possible, no other intervention is done.
- In very urgent cases, needle cricothyrotomy can be done.

3. Position of the Patient

Supine with extension of the neck and head by keeping a sandbag or a pillow under the shoulders.

4. Anaesthesia

Local infiltration anaesthesia

5. Preparation of the Parts

Iodine and spirit

6. Procedure

- **Incision:** Transverse curved incision for about 3–4 cm is made at the level of 2nd tracheal ring.
- **Dissection:** Skin, subcutaneous tissue and deep fascia are incised. Isthmus of thyroid is separated.
- **Procedure:** A transverse cut is made in the 2nd tracheal cartilage, its edge is held with Allis forceps and a small cuff of cartilage is removed. 'Cricoid hook' can be used to stabilise the trachea (found more useful in children).
- A suitable-sized tracheostomy tube is introduced within.
- The cuff of tracheostomy tube is inflated by using 2–5 ml of air and is held in place by passing a tape around the neck.
- Confirm that the **tube** is in the **trachea**, not in the subcutaneous plane.
- Confirm **air entry** on both sides of lung.

7. Closure

A few interrupted skin sutures by the side of the tracheostomy tube and dressing is applied.

8. Postoperative Management

- Suction of tracheostomy tube, regular dressing
- Humidification of air
- Check for air entry

9. Postoperative Complications

- Wound infection
- Air leakage
- Improper air entry
- Cricoid stenosis (high tracheostomy).

Closure of Tracheostomy

- Once patient improves and is able to take care of his own airway, the tracheostomy tube is blocked. Observe for 24–48 hours.
- If there is **no respiratory distress**, the cuff is deflated and the tube is removed. A few skin sutures can be put or dressing is applied. It closes automatically.

10. Advice at Discharge

- Tracheostomy done after laryngectomy is permanent. Patients should learn to use metal tracheostomy, cleaning the tubes, etc.
- Inner tube should be removed, cleaned and replaced in cases of respiratory distress.

THYROIDECTOMY

1. Indications

- All goitres with symptoms—MNG, toxic goitre, colloid goitre and malignant goitre.
- In all cases of toxic goitres, patients have to be optimised into normothyroid or euthyroid before surgery to avoid dangerous complications such as thyrotoxic storm or crisis.

2. Contraindications

Asymptomatic goitre, Hashimoto's thyroiditis, anaplastic carcinoma thyroid.

3. Position of the Patient

- Supine with extended neck by keeping a sandbag under the shoulders.
- Head end of the patient is elevated to about 30° to reduce venous congestion. This position is called **anti-Trendelenburg position**.

4. Anaesthesia

GA.

5. Preparation of the Parts

Iodine and spirit

6. Procedure

Incision (Figs 70.13A and B)

6–8 cm collar neck incision (Kocher's incision) or crease incision is given about 2 cm above the suprasternal notch along the natural crease of the neck or just above it.

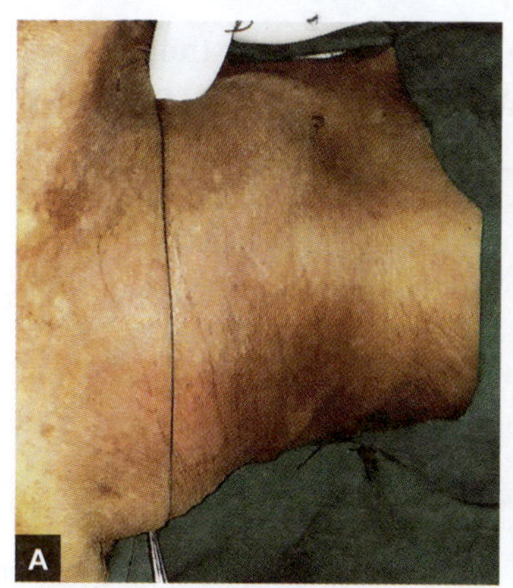

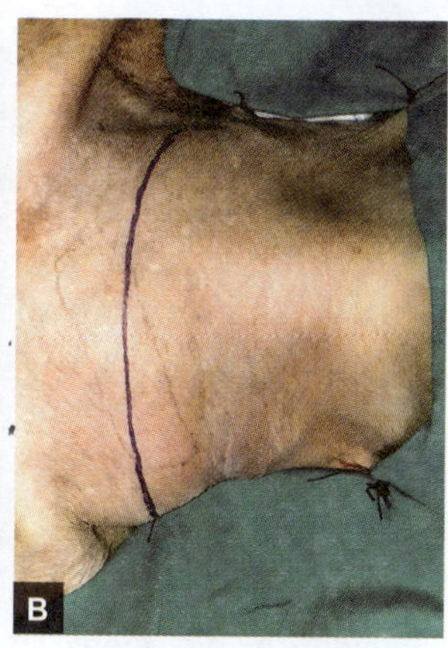

Fig. 70.13A and B: Neck incision is marked by using silk, and marker pen. This incision is also called Kocher's collar neck incision

Layers Opened

- Skin, platysma, subcutaneous tissue in the line of incision. Small bleeders are coagulated.
- Deep fascia is incised vertically (Fig. 70.14).
- Strap muscles are separated (can be cut in very large goitres). Sternothyroid, thyrohyoid and sternohyoid muscles. Most superficial muscles are sternohyoid.
- Pretracheal fascia is incised.
- Thyroid gland is mobilised by using blunt dissection.
- Assess the entire gland to know whether it is a solitary nodule or multinodular goitre.
- One of the lobes is mobilised by dividing middle thyroid vein (single, short, thin, vein).
- Then, upper pole is dissected. This pedicle contains superior thyroid artery and veins. They are ligated and divided in between. Please apply double ligature proximally. Let the dissection be close to the gland. Dissection and retraction of the upper pole of the right thyroid lobe laterally will open up a space called **cricothyroid space of Reeves**. Here we can find the external branch of the superior laryngeal nerve.

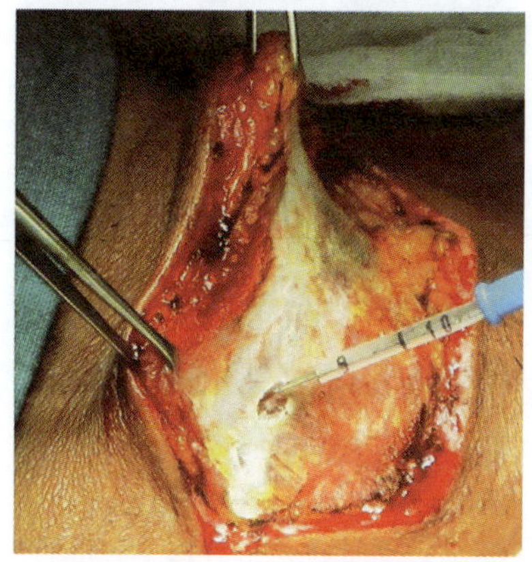

Fig. 70.14: Upper flap is raised. Plane of dissection is deep to platysma and superficial to pretracheal fascia

- Upper pole should be ligated as close to the gland as possible to avoid damage to external laryngeal nerve.
- Inferior thyroid artery used to be ligated[1] well away from the gland. It has a horizontal course. It is thick and pulsatile. Nowadays branches of inferior thyroid artery rather than the main artery are ligated. This will avoid injury to recurrent laryngeal nerve and it will prevent hypoparathyroidism also. Multiple veins, present in the lower pole, are ligated and divided.

Pearls of Wisdom

All major arteries should be ligated twice proximally. Example: Superior thyroid artery, facial artery, left gastric artery, cystic artery, renal artery.

- Isthmus is separated from trachea, both above and below.
- In subtotal thyroidectomy, the entire isthmus, parts of the right and left lobes are removed in flush with tracheal surface, leaving behind tissue in the tracheoesophageal groove to protect recurrent laryngeal nerve and parathyroid gland. Cut edges of thyroid gland are sutured by using vicryl sutures. In total thyroidectomy, almost entire gland is removed (Fig. 70.15).

Precautions

- Any structure directly entering the gland is unlikely to be RLN and hence, can safely be divided.
- Always identify the RLN. That is the best way to avoid injury to the nerve. Recurrent laryngeal nerve enters the thyrohyoid membrane, after running a vertical course, in the tracheoesophageal groove.

7. Closure

- A suction drain is kept in the thyroid bed.
- Deep fascia is sutured with 2-0 vicryl

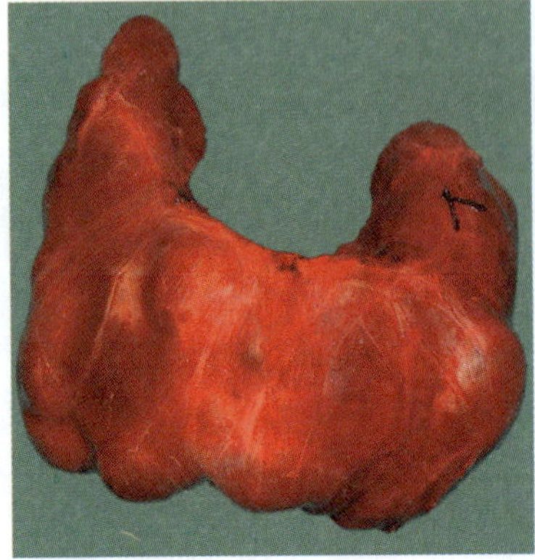

Fig. 70.15: Total thyroidectomy specimen for papillary carcinoma thyroid

- Subcutaneous fat—vicryl
- Skin—interrupted silk/subcuticular sutures or clips
- A bandage is applied.

8. Postoperative Management

- NPO for 6–8 hours followed by liquid diet.
- Antibiotics are not necessary.
- **Head end must be elevated** to reduce oedema of the wound.
- In toxic goitres, propranolol must be continued after surgery and slowly tapered over a week.
- Blood transfusion depending upon blood loss.
- Drain removal after 2–3 days (once it stops draining).
- Suture removal after 4–5 days.

9. Postoperative Complications

(for details see Chapter 37, page 431)

- **Haemorrhage: Tension haematoma.** Reactionary haemorrhage is due to slipping of ligature due to coughing, hypertension, etc. If it is alarming, deep fascial sutures have to be opened, haematoma drained and haemostasis has to be achieved.
- **Thyrotoxic crisis** in patients with toxic goitre
- **Tracheomalacia**—resulting in stridor
- Recurrent laryngeal nerve paralysis

TEN COMMANDMENTS: OF THYROIDECTOMY

1. All thyroidectomies should be done in euthyroid patients. If there is any toxicity, it should be very well controlled.
2. Collar neck incision should be given properly.
3. Haemostasis should be perfect at every stage of surgery.
4. Identify external laryngeal nerve at cricothyroid space of Reeves.
5. Identify recurrent laryngeal nerve in the tracheoesophageal groove—**Riddle's triangle**.
6. Identify and preserve all parathyroids by their location posterior to lobes and size of a small pea and yellow colour with a capsule. It has a separate blood supply from posterior branch of inferior thyroid artery.
7. Use bipolar cautery while coagulating a vessel near the RLN.
8. Upper pedicle is ligated—artery and vein are ligated separately.
9. Inferior thyroid artery branches are ligated.
10. When in doubt, keep a drain.

[1]Today, branches of inferior thyroid artery are ligated—not the main artery so as to preserve blood supply to parathyroid gland.

- Hypothyroidism
- Hypoparathyroidism
- Wound infection

10. Advice at Discharge

This depends on the type of indication for thyroid surgery, e.g. those who undergo subtotal thyroidectomy for thyrotoxicosis have to be closely followed for recurrent thyrotoxicosis or hypothyroidism. If calcium levels are low, it has to be supplemented.

Pearls of Wisdom

Thyroidectomy is an operation which provides a surgeon to demonstrate his skills and meticulousness.

Different Types of Thyroidectomy (Table 70.2)

Table 70.2 Different types of thyroidectomy

Diseases	Before surgery	After surgery	Name of the operation
1. Solitary nodule (benign)	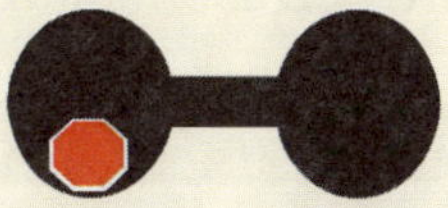	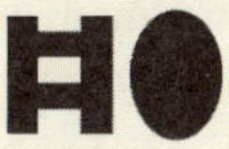	Hemithyroidectomy means removal of one lobe with isthmus (*see* page 426)
2. Multinodular goitre	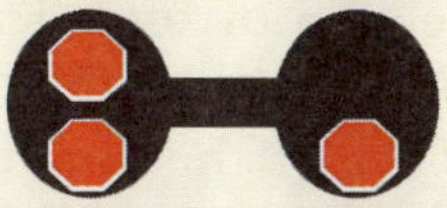	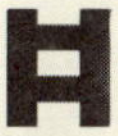	Total thyroidectomy (*see* page 405)
3. Toxic multinodular goitre	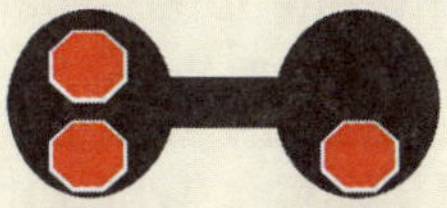	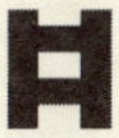	Total thyroidectomy (*see* page 412)
4. Primary thyrotoxicosis	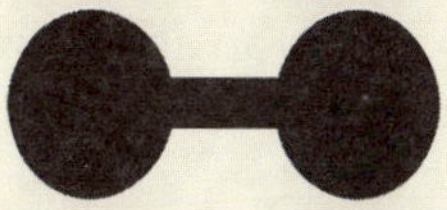	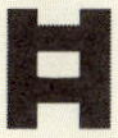	Total thyroidectomy (*see* page 407)
5. Malignant neoplasm	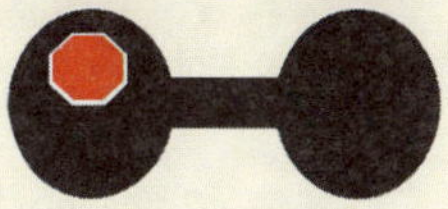	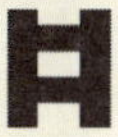	Total thyroidectomy (*see* page 414)

What is Zuckerkandl's tubercle?

- Zuckerkandl's tubercle is a pyramidal extension of the thyroid gland, located at the most posterior side of each lobe.
- The structure is important in thyroid surgery as it is closely related to the recurrent laryngeal nerve, the inferior thyroid artery, Berry's ligament and the parathyroid glands.
- It is also important to remove this in toto while doing thyroidectomy for malignancies.

AMPUTATIONS

Competency

SU27.4: Describe the type of gangrene and principles of amputation (refer page 207).

Definitions/Terminologies of Amputation

- End bearing: Weight is taken by the body.
- Non-end bearing: Here weight is taken by the joint.
- *Guillotine* amputation: Here no flaps are raised, all the tissues are divided at the same level and the stump is kept open.
- Formal amputation: In this case depending upon the indications and the decisions taken by the surgeon, amputation is done with closure of the stump.

Indications

1. Vitality of the part is destroyed by injury or disease—***dead limb.***
2. Life of patient is threatened by spread of a local condition—***deadly limb.*** *Examples:* Gas gangrene, extensive melanoma.
3. Patient may be better served by an artificial limb because of deformity or paralysis—***deformed limb. In such cases, better to amputate and fit in an artificial limb.***
4. Dying limb—acutely ischaemic limb, late presentation.

Optimum Levels of Amputation

Level of amputation depends not only upon the extent of disease but also function desired in the remaining stump. This differs markedly in the upper and lower limbs.

Ideal Stump

- Should have ideal length for proper fitting of prosthesis. Examples: Below knee: 8 to 12 cm from tibial tuberosity, above knee: 23 cm from greater trochanter and above and below elbow: 20 cm stump.
- Should be conical and rounded.
- Should not be tender.
- Should have adequate muscle padding so that its movements are adequate.
- Should have adequate blood supply so that it heals with primary intention in the postoperative period.
- Should have a thin scar which should not interfere with prosthetic function.
- Should not have any redundant soft tissue hanging.
- Skin and scar should not be adhered to the underlying tissue.

Incisions

Depending upon the site of the level of amputation and keeping in mind the blood supply of the part, different types of incision are given. They are as follows:

- *Racquet incision:* This is used in amputation for digits or toes.
- Elliptical or oval incision is given for metatarsal amputations.
- Circular incision is given especially in *Guillotine* amputation.
- U-shaped incisions: These are given to raise flaps—anterior and posterior flaps as in below knee or above knee. By convention equal flaps are used for above knee and a long posterior and short anterior flaps are used for below knee amputation. This is because, vascularity of the posterior flap is good below the knee due to bulky muscles with good blood supply when compared to the thin, muscle less anterior flap (*see* ten commandments).

AMPUTATIONS IN LEG

Skeleton of foot: To have a better understanding of amputations kindly study Figs 70.16 and 70.17 first.

- One of the common indications for lower limb amputations is diabetic ulcer/gangrene foot. Various types and various levels of amputations are done with the main aim is to conserve as much as possible. However, when the limb is a useless limb, a below knee or an above knee amputation is done depending upon the seriousness of the problem.

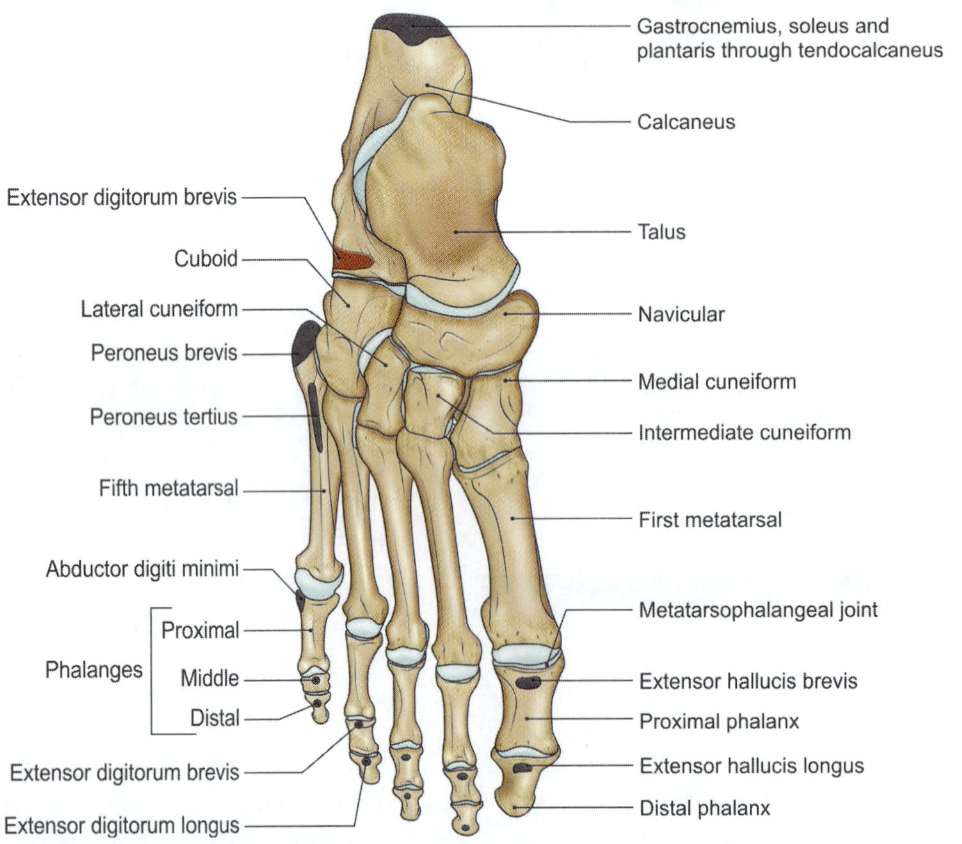

Fig. 70.16: Skeleton of the foot as seen from the dorsal aspect

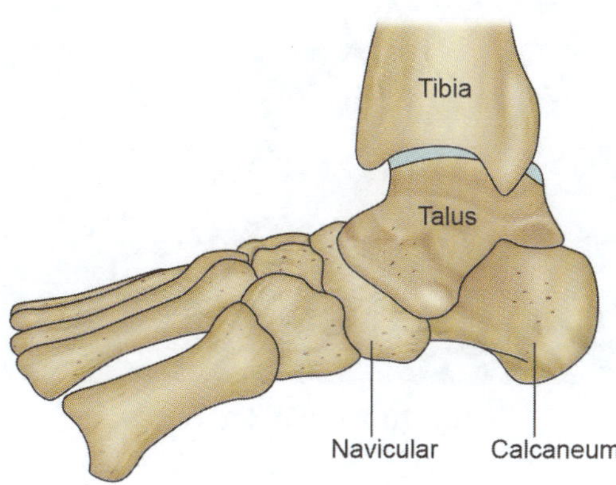

Fig. 70.17: Tarsal bones

1. **Ray amputation:** It is amputation of the toe with head of metatarsal or metacarpals.
2. **Transmetatarsal/metacarpal amputation:** It is called Gilles' amputation. When multiple toes are involved with gangrene as in vasculitis syndromes or in diabetic patients, amputation is done through metatarsal bones—proximal to the neck, distal to the base. Long volar flap is created and sutured to the dorsal skin.
3. **Lisfranc's amputation (tarsometatarsal amputation):** Tarsometatarsal articulations are called Lisfranc joint. The bones forming these are the first, second, and third cuneiforms, and the cuboid, which articulate with the bases of the metatarsal bones. The bones are connected by dorsal, plantar, and interosseous ligaments. These ligaments have to be divided. A long volar flap is used. Patient needs a surgical boot.
4. **Chopart's amputation:** Francis Chopart first described disarticulation through midtarsal joint. It is midtarsal amputation. Disarticulation of the foot is completed through talonavicular joint and through calcaneocuboid joint. Thus, Chopart amputation removes the forefoot and midfoot, saving talus and calcaneus. Tibialis anterior muscle is sutured to the drilled talus bone.
   - **Contraindication:** Ischaemic feet as in atherosclerosis.
   - **Disadvantages:** It is a very unstable amputation, because most of the tendons supporting the foot will be removed. Thus, it will go for equinus and must usually be fitted with a prosthesis that extends up to the patellar tendon level.
5. **Syme's amputation:**
   - The tibia and fibula are divided at or immediately above the level of ankle joint and their ends are covered with a single flap obtained from heel.
   - The end of the stump is at a height of about 6–8 cm from the ground.
   - 50% of people will be able to walk on the stump without prosthesis.
   - It is of value in patients who do not have access to modern artificial limbs.
   - **Pirgroff's modification of Syme's amputation** retains a small portion of calcaneum in the flap obtained from heel (Fig. 70.18).
   - Heel flap is supplied by medial and lateral calcaneal vessels, both are branches of posterior tibial artery.
   - Those who will not be able to walk after this amputation, can be fitted with elephant boot.

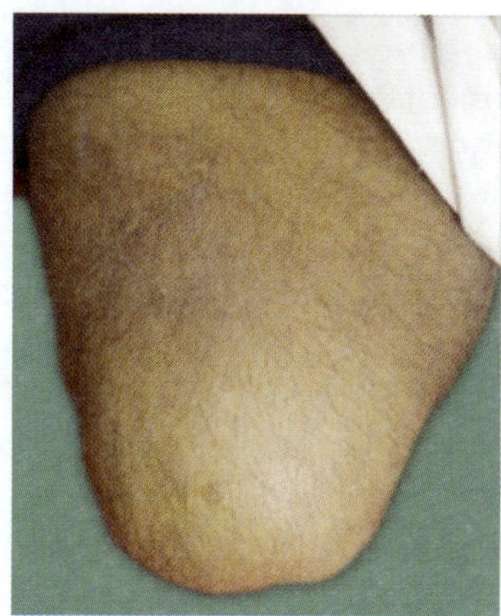

Fig. 70.18: Conical stump

TEN COMMANDMENTS: GENERAL PRINCIPLES IN AMPUTATIONS

1. Should mark the incision
2. Should give prophylactic antibiotics
3. Should avoid tourniquet in arterial occlusive diseases.
4. Should ensure adequate blood supply to the flaps—if raised as in below knee and above knee amputations.
5. Should ligate the blood vessels securely to avoid haematoma and then infection in the postoperative period.
6. Should not clamp the nerves but they are pulled down and transected as high as possible so that nerve ends are not caught in the suture line.
7. Should saw the anterior part of the bone obliquely to give a smooth anterior bevel which prevents pressure necrosis of the flap.
8. Should excise the bulky muscles so as to give a good conical stump (Fig. 70.18). Example: Excise soleus muscle in below knee amputations.
9. Should use absorbable sutures to unite the muscle ends.
10. Should drain the cavity with a suction drain which is brought out through the skin clear of the wound.

6. Below knee amputation:

- It is the operation of choice when it is not possible to preserve the foot or heel.
- The ideal length of the tibial stump is 14 cm.
- Minimum length required to fit an artificial leg is 8 cm. Stump shorter than this tends to slip out of the socket of an artificial limb.
- The stump is covered by creating long posterior flap.
- This is the amputation commonly done in patients who are in severe sepsis involving the leg with uncontrolled diabetes and life is in danger.
- All the rules mentioned above in ten commandments are followed here such as division of the nerve, flap vascularity, reduction of bulky muscles and the anterior scar, thus prosthesis will not cause discomfort while walking.
- Advantages of below knee amputation include greater range of movements without limp and without support.
- This amputation is also called Burgess amputation.
- POP cast should be put to prevent contractures (Fig. 70.19).

7. Amputations through thigh

- Ideal length is 25–30 cm as measured from tip of trochanter.
- It is done when it is not possible to save at least 8 cm of tibia as in some cases of diabetes or spreading infections of the leg and when muscles involved are not bleeding at surgery.
- When this amputation is done in children, as much length as possible should be preserved (growing epiphysis of femur is at lower end).
- Unlike, below knee amputation, equal flaps are raised—anterior and posterior.

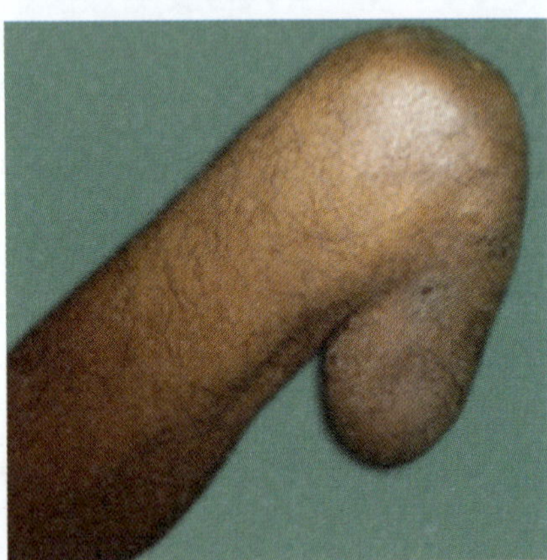

Fig. 70.19: Amputation contracture

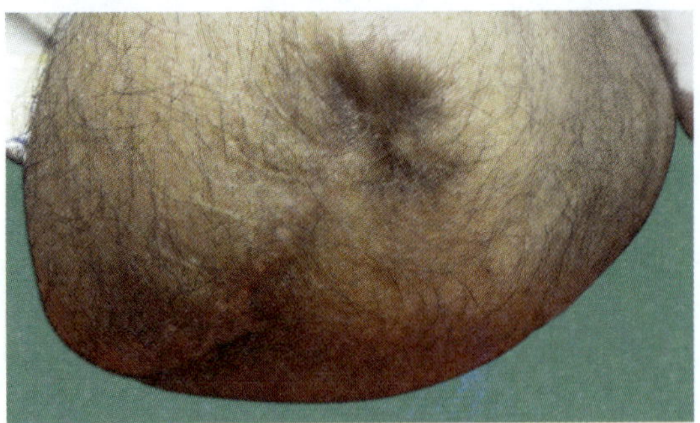

Fig. 70.20: Infected scar

- Any length less than 10 cm of femur will not help. In such cases, hip disarticulation is done.
- In peripheral arterial occlusive disease, an attempt is made first by raising below knee flaps. If edges of the skin flaps do not bleed, better to go ahead with above knee flaps because vascularity of above knee flaps are better. Above knee amputation stump healing is better than below knee.
- Disadvantages of this amputation are difficult rehabilitation (not easy), prosthesis fitting is not good, invariably patient needs one more support (Fig. 70.20).

8. Hip disarticulation

- When it is not possible to get minimum of 10 cm length of stump of the femur, hip disarticulation is done. This situation can occur in trauma or malignancies to get a wide clearance. Examples: Sarcomas or in cases of malignant melanomas.
- Usually a single posterior flap is raised—Solcum's approach.
- Anterior approach can also be used (2nd option)—Boyd's approach.

9. Hindquarter amputation

- In this amputation—one side of pelvis with innominate bone, pubis, muscles and vessels are removed. Hence, it is called hemipelvectomy today.
- Indications are trauma and tumour (malignancy).
- In the original description, common iliac artery used to be ligated. However, now the branches of external and internal iliac artery are ligated.
- A large posterior flap based on superior gluteal artery is used.
- Variations in this amputation are: Extended hemipelvectomy with removal of posterior part of the sacrum.
- Limb preserving hemipelvectomy: It is called internal hemipelvectomy.

UPPER LIMB AMPUTATIONS

GENERAL PRINCIPLES

- Conserve as much tissue as possible.
- Skin closure should not be under tension.
- Soft tissue cover over bony stump is desirable. Otherwise, painful adherent scar will result.
- Amputation through middle or terminal phalanx is preferred to disarticulation at interphalangeal joints since attachment of flexor tendons is thereby preserved.
- Every effort should be made to preserve as much of the thumb.

AMPUTATION THROUGH FOREARM AND UPPER ARM

- Ideal stump is 16–20 cm measured from olecranon.
- Stump less than 8 cm is useless for transmitting movement to an artificial elbow joint.
- A stump measuring 20 cm from acromion is ideal for fitting prosthesis.

Krukenberg's amputation: In this amputation, a gap is created between radius and ulna like a claw. It helps in holding objects.

Interscapulothoracic Amputation (Forequarter Amputation)

- Indications are for malignancy involving axial skeleton such as sarcoma. Sepsis involving the upper limb is another indication such as gas gangrene.
- It is a very radical mutilating operation, hence all possible limb saving attempts should be done first.
- Entire upper limb with scapula and lateral 2/3rds of the clavicle with all the muscles attached to it are removed.

Complications following Amputation

1. **Wound infection:** Especially it is common in amputations done for diabetic gangrene cases. Stitches may have to be opened to release pus followed by secondary suturing at a later date.
2. **Flap necrosis:** It is a common complication because of several reasons, important one being decreased blood supply to the limb either due to arterial occlusive disease or due to diabetes. Necrotic skin and subcutaneous tissues should be removed followed by secondary suturing at a later date. Hence, blood supply of the flap has to be kept in mind when raising the flaps.
3. **Stump ulcers** are common in the initial stages of wearing artificial limbs.
4. **Contracture:** If the artificial limb is not fitted, the stump will develop flexion contracture.
5. **Amputation neuroma:** This is an end neuroma. The cut end of the nerve is entrapped in the scar tissue and gives rise to pain. To avoid this, nerve end is pulled and cut so that after division of the nerve, the end gets retracted.
6. **Phantom limb:** A **phantom limb** is the sensation that a missing limb is attached to the body. Approximately 60 to 80% of individuals with an amputation experience phantom sensations in their amputated limb, and the majority of the sensations are painful. It is probably due to presence of a severe pain at the amputated site before surgery and the corresponding site in the brain has registered this sensation.

ABDOMINAL INCISIONS

Introduction

Incisions are given to approach an organ for removal or repair. The most important 3 criteria when incisions are given are: 1. Accessibility, 2. Extensibility, and 3. Safety. Many examples can be given for each one of these. However, one example for each one of the above 3 criteria has been given below.

1. Accessibility

When an incision is given, if a surgeon should be able to reach the organ without many difficulties. Classical example is: McBurney incision given at the site of maximum tenderness. As soon as peritoneum is opened, you can see appendix. (More details later). Subcostal incision on the left side gives direct access to the spleen for splenectomy.

2. Extensibility

Surprises are known inside abdomen and hence it is called as Pandora's box. When a upper midline incision is given for perforation peritonitis, if a lesion is identified in the lower abdomen, incision can be extended easily till midline incisions are popular and have this great advantage. If a surgeon has given McBurney incision for suspected appendicitis, after opening the abdomen he finds that the appendix is normal but it is a case of perforation of Meckel's diverticulitis, often the McBurney incision has to be closed and midline incision given to facilitate removal of Meckel's diverticulum.

3. Safety

Midline incisions are safe during laparotomy because no important nerve or artery is present in the midline. If precautions are not properly taken in paramedian incisions, traction on the nerves while retracting the muscles can result in nerve injuries. This may weaken the rectus abdominis muscle.

Various Incisions (Key Box 70.4)

Midline incisions, paramedian incisions (not done nowadays), McBurney grid iron incision, Kocher's subcostal incision, Pfannenstiel incision are commonly used incisions. Left abdominothoracic—an oblique incision above the umbilicus crossing along the 7th or 8th intercostal space for removing large spleens or exposure of lower oesophagus and right midline incision with right posterolateral thoracotomy through 5th intercostal space for oesophageal cancer are other incisions used. Details are not required for undergraduate students. Those of you are interested can refer to operative surgery books. Midline incision is given here, the rest have been covered along with respective operative surgery.

Key Box 70.4

Midline: Upper and lower
Paramedian: Upper, lower, right and left
Grid Iron: McBurney's
Kocher's: Subcostal
Pfannenstiel: Used by gynaecologists
Roof top-incision—Chevron incision
Left thoracoabdominal
Midline with right posterolateral thoracotomy through 5th intercostal space—Ivor Lewis operartion

MIDLINE INCISIONS

Upper and lower midline and mid-midline are commonly used incisions which give exposure to every viscus in the abdominal cavity. They are described here. Other incisions and approach have been given later with the procedure of surgery.

- To understand the formation of rectus sheath and linea alba which forms basis of midline incisions, refer page 955 in Chapter 52.
- **Upper midline incision:** Layers opened are—skin, subcutaneous fat, linea alba, preperitoneal fat and peritoneum. Closure is done mainly by taking good bites from the linea alba and skin. Peritoneum heals with proliferation of mesothelial cells. A few surgeons also take bites through peritoneum with absorbable sutures such as 2–0 polyglactin, linea alba with 2–0 prolene/PDS and skin with silk sutures.
- **Lower midline incision:** Layers opened are—skin, subcutaneous fat, linea alba. However, linea alba is not present in the lower part of lower abdomen below linea semilunaris line. Then preperitoneal fat and peritoneum are incised. Closure is done mainly by taking good bites from the linea alba and skin. Closure is similar to that of upper midline incision.

APPENDICECTOMY

This is the most commonly done emergency surgery by general surgeons all over the world. Today almost every appendicectomy is done by laparoscopic approach. Basic concepts of laparoscopy have been given in the later pages.

Pearls of Wisdom

Appendicectomy can be one of the easiest and sometimes one of the most complicated surgeries.

1. Indications

- Acute appendicitis—emergency appendicectomy
- Recurrent appendicitis—elective appendicectomy

2. Contraindications

Appendicular mass

3. Position of the Patient

Supine

4. Anaesthesia of the Parts

This surgery can be done either under GA or regional anaesthesia (spinal or epidural).

5. Preparation

Parts are cleaned with iodine and spirit, from the level of umbilicus above to the upper part of thigh below.

6. Procedure

Incision

1. McBurney's grid-iron incision is the most popular incision. It is at right angles to spino-umbilical line placed at McBurney's point. It is about 6–8 cm in length (Fig. 70.21).
2. **Lanz** incision is a curved transverse incision, placed at the McBurney's point. Cosmetically, it is a better incision (Fig. 70.22).

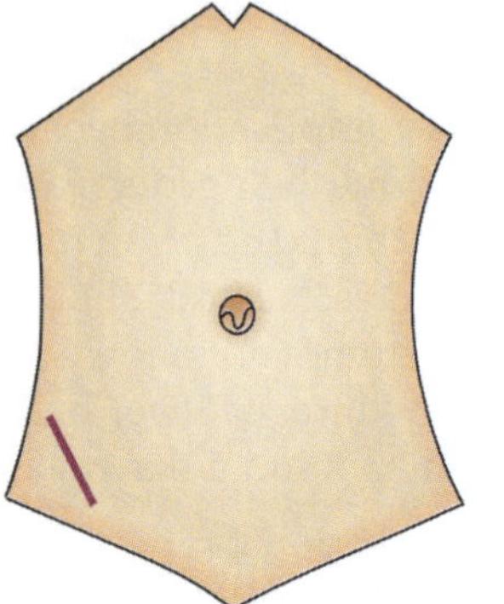

Fig. 70.21: Grid iron incision

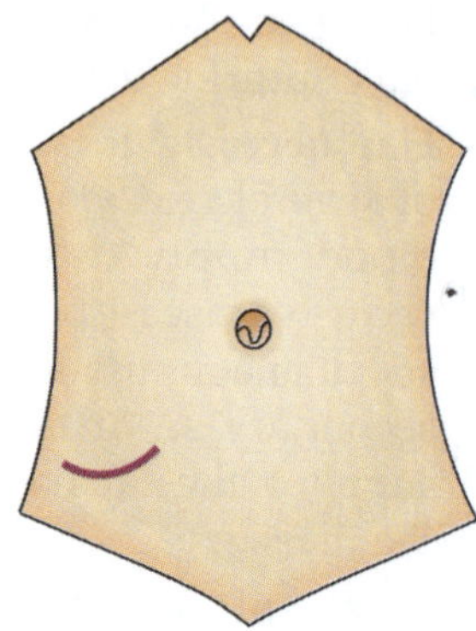

Fig. 70.22: Lanz incision

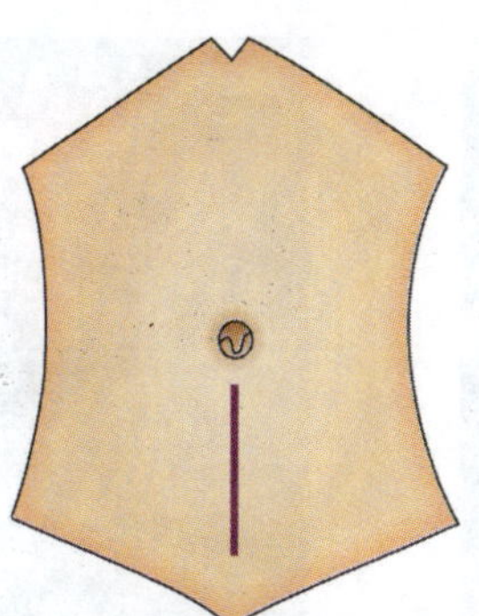

Fig. 70.23: Midline incision

3. Midline incision is made when diagnosis is in doubt as a part of **exploratory laparotomy**. This is also preferred in females where there is a gynaecological pathology such as ovarian cyst which may be the cause of right iliac fossa pain (Fig. 70.23).

Layers Opened

- Skin
- Two layers of subcutaneous tissue—superficial fatty (Camper's), deep membranous (Scarpa's). (C: comes first, S: later). There is no deep fascia in the abdomen.
- External oblique aponeurosis is seen running downwards and medially. It is incised in the direction of its fibres.
- Internal and transverse abdominal muscles are split (grid iron—right angle to each other).
- Peritoneum is incised.

Features of Acute Appendicitis at Operation

- Inflamed, turgid appendix—send pus/inflammatory exudate for culture/sensitivity
- Pus in the right iliac fossa
- Presence of omentum in the right iliac fossa
- Black or green appendix (gangrenous)
- Faecolith

Identification of the Appendix

- Trace taenia coli. They will lead to the base of appendix (**all roads lead to Rome**).
- Identify round structure—caecum and then look for appendix
- Often it is retrocaecal. In such cases, you need to mobilise right paracolic space by incising posterior peritoneal reflection.
- When you are tracing taenia coli, if you are not able to identify the appendix, it means most probably you are tracing taenia coli of the sigmoid colon.
- It may be subhepatic in cases of undescended caecum.

Surgical Procedure

- Appendix is gently held at mesoappendix by using Babcock's forceps and blood vessels in the mesoappendix are divided. These include appendicular artery, branch of ileocolic artery (accessory appendicular artery of Seshachalam, is a branch of posterior caecal artery). Once appendix is freed up to the base (caecum), a **purse string suture** is applied all round appendix, taking bites from caecum, using 2–0 atraumatic silk (Fig. 70.24).
- Appendix is crushed at base and is held 1 cm above the crush. A tight silk ligature is applied at the crushed site and appendix is cut in between. Stump is cleaned with spirit, invaginated and purse string is tightened. This is called burial of the stump. Perfect haemostasis is obtained (Fig. 70.25).
- Look for Meckel's diverticulum and if found make a note of this in the operative surgery notes.

Pearls of Wisdom

Look for Meckel's diverticulum, which may be the cause of right iliac fossa pain. You may find Meckel's diverticulum with narrow lumen, inflammation with band—remove it.

7. Closure

- Peritoneum—continuous 2–0 vicryl
- Split muscles—sutured together by a few interrupted sutures using 2–0 vicryl
- External oblique is sutured with silk
- Subcutaneous fat is sutured with vicryl
- Skin with interrupted silk.
- Peritoneal wash with saline is given and the area is dried with mop.
- Tube drain is not kept routinely unless there is gangrenous appendicitis or a lot of pus in the peritoneal cavity.

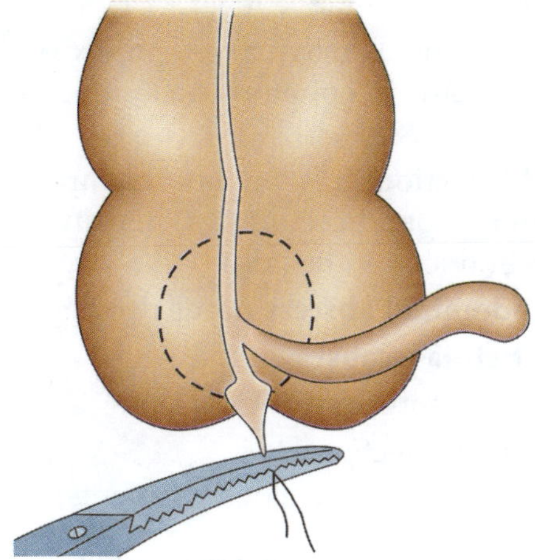

Fig. 70.24: Purse string suture

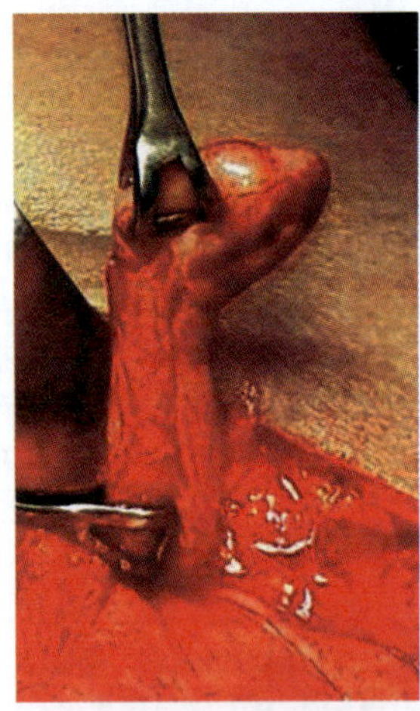

Fig. 70.25A: Acute appendicitis. Turgid swollen appendix. You can see Babcock's forceps used to hold the mesoappendix

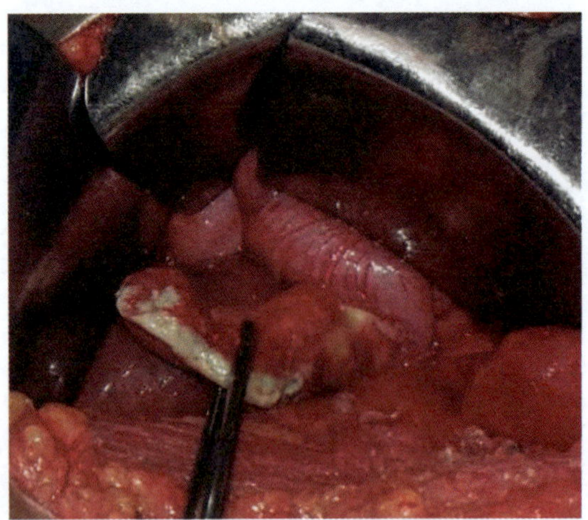

Fig. 70.25B: Perforated appendicitis at surgery due to a large faecolith

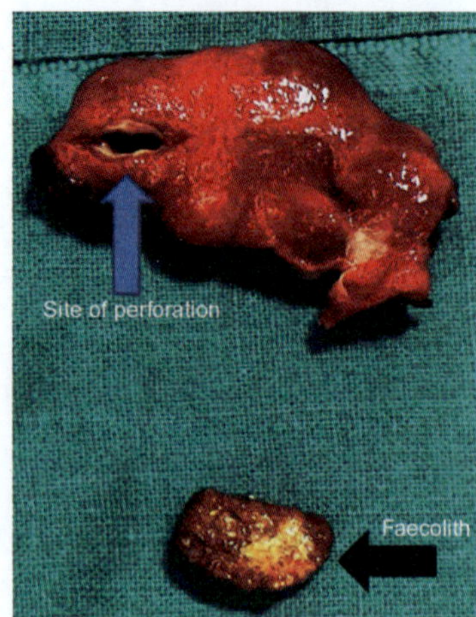

Fig. 70.25C: Specimen of appendix and a large faecolith

8. Postoperative Management

- RT aspiration is only in cases of peritonitis or persistent vomiting. Otherwise, nasogastric aspiration is not required.
- IV fluids 2.5 litres/day for one or two days.
- Oral fluids are allowed within 6–8 hours or very next day once abdomen is soft and bowel sounds are heard.
- Appropriate antibiotics to cover gram-positive, gram-negative and anaerobic organisms.
- Suture removal by 7–10 days.

9. Complications after Appendicectomy

A. **Postoperative fever** can be due to various factors. Thrombophlebitis, urinary tract infection and IV fluids are common causes. In the absence of these, wound infection, intraperitoneal abscess secondary to gangrenous appendicitis, may have to be considered.
  - Change of antibiotics according to culture and sensitivity reports of urine, pus and blood help in treating postoperative fever.
  - Elderly patients may have a pre-existing pulmonary disease. Respiratory tract infection also has to be considered.

B. **Wound infection:** It is the most common complication after appendicectomy. When in doubt open stitches and let out the pus.

C. **Intra-abdominal abscess** needs drainage

D. **Faecal fistula—causes**
  a. Gangrene spreading into caecum
  b. Persistent infection
  c. Carcinoma caecum (elderly patients)
  d. Ileocaecal tuberculosis
  e. Crohn's disease (uncommon in India)
  f. Actinomycosis (rare)[1].

Pearls of Wisdom

Most of the faecal fistulae will heal by themselves provided there is no distal obstruction.

E. **Septicaemia,** portal pyaemia, gram-negative shock in late cases of peritonitis due to perforated appendicitis are uncommon but dangerous complications.
  - Mortality of appendicular perforation and peritonitis is around 2%.

10. Advice at Discharge

To report, if any fever or discharge from the wound.

BASSINI'S HERNIORRHAPHY

- This means herniotomy and approximation of conjoined tendon to inguinal ligament to strengthen the posterior wall of the inguinal canal. With availability of the mesh, this surgery is not routinely done. **However, in strangulated hernias, after resection of the bowel, one cannot repair with mesh. Bassini's herniorrhaphy is still a good option.**
- In large, long-standing hernias and in sliding hernias, especially in elderly patients, it is better to catheterise their bladder before surgery for two reasons. Firstly, to avoid injury to the urinary bladder and secondly, they invariably develop retention of urine in the postoperative period.

[1]In *viva voce* examination, when a question is asked as to what is the common cause of faecal fistula following appendicectomy, the usual answer by students is actinomycosis. Remember it is the answer to be told last.

1. Indication

Inguinal hernias. Strangulated hernias.

2. Contraindication (Relative)

Severe cardiopulmonary insufficiency

3. Position of the Patient

Supine

4. Anaesthesia

Regional anaesthesia or GA. **Local anaesthesia** can be preferred in **high-risk patients**.

5. Preparation of the Parts

Like that for appendicectomy

6. Procedure

Incision

4–6 cm incision is made parallel to the inguinal ligament at the level of deep ring in the medial two-thirds of the inguinal ligament.

Layers Opened

- Skin
- Two layers of superficial fascia
- External oblique is incised in the line of direction of fibres, till external ring is slit open.
- Thin cremasteric box—thin covering is opened
- Identification of the sac—glistening white colour.
- Isolate the cord from the sac—by blunt and sharp dissection. The cord is held separately by using cord holding forceps.
- Mobilisation of the sac: The sac is mobilised up to the deep ring (Fig. 70.26). Mobilisation is complete when inferior epigastric artery pulsations and extraperitoneal pad of fat are seen.

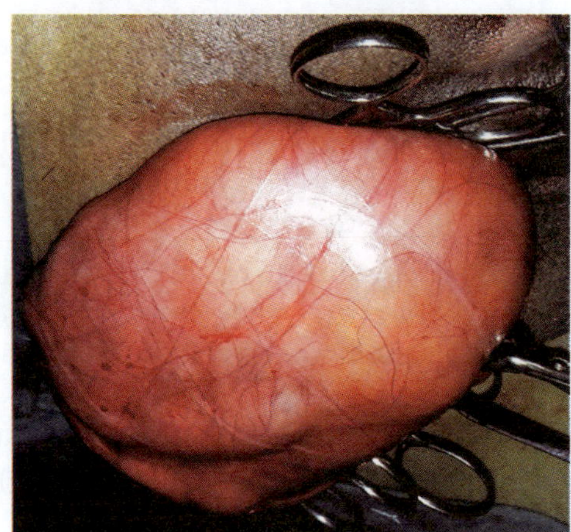

Fig. 70.26: Hernial sac is identified—glistening white in colour

- Opening of the sac: **The sac is opened and contents are examined.**
- Reduction of contents: **The contents are reduced into the peritoneal cavity carefully by using blunt forceps. Check carefully in bleeding from omental vessels** (Fig. 70.27).
- **Twist the sac** so that contents get reduced completely so as to avoid injury to the contents of the sac later while excising the sac (Fig. 70.28).
- **Transfixation ligature: It means suture ligature is passed through the sac:** It is applied as high as possible at the neck of sac and it is tightened.
- **Excision of the sac: As a rule, after excision, the ligated end of the sac should disappear from the operative field (means it will go into the peritoneal cavity).** After excision, see the excised sac and see whether omentum or intestine have been injured. Up to this stage, it is called **herniotomy**.

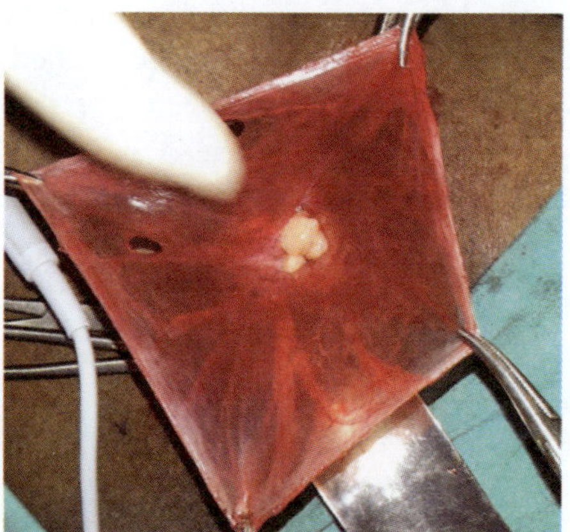

Fig. 70.27: Contents of the sac omentum—omentocele

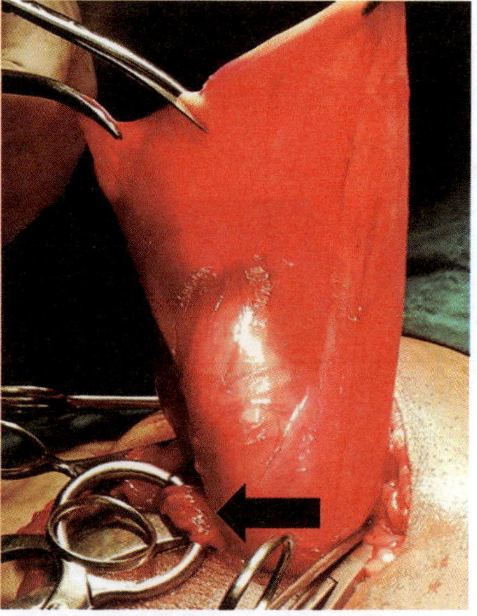

Fig. 70.28A: Sac is isolated and opened. You can see cord holding forceps with cord which is isolated and held separately

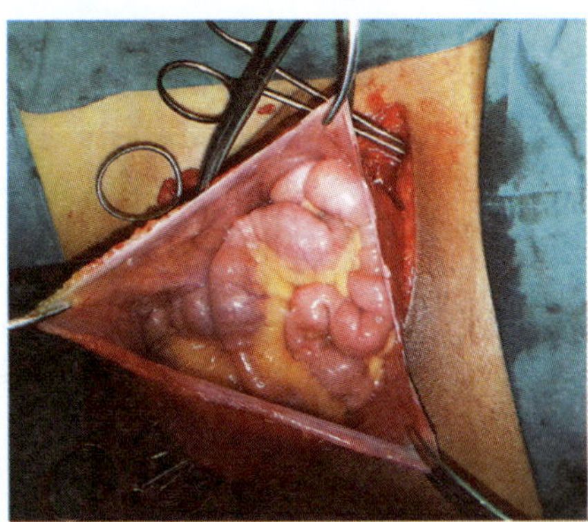

Fig. 70.28B: Contents of the sac—enterocele

- Conjoined tendon above is approximated to the inguinal ligament below by using nonabsorbable suture such as nylon or prolene. However, in strangulated hernias, PDS (polydioxanone)—a synthetic but absorbable sutures can be used. It gets absorbed between 130 and 180 days.
- Nonabsorbable suture is used so that its strength remains for a long time. This repair is called **Bassini's herniorrhaphy** (Key Box 70.5).

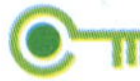 Key Box 70.5

Herniorrhaphy

- Identify the sac and identify the cord
- Isolate the sac and isolate the cord
- Mobilise the sac and open the sac
- Release adhesions, if any, and reduce the contents
- Twist the sac, transfix and ligate the sac

Excision of the sac and posterior wall repair

7. Closure

- External oblique is sutured with chromic catgut or silk (Fig. 70.29).
- Subcutaneous fat with absorbable catgut suture.
- Skin with silk.

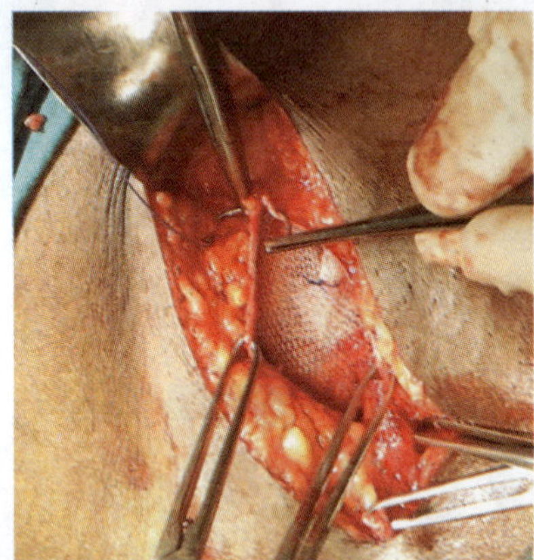

Fig. 70.29: External oblique aponeurosis is sutured

Pearls of Wisdom

Do not twist the sac in direct hernias and in sliding hernias.

Precautions (Key Box 70.6)

1. Ilioinguinal nerve should not be caught in ligature.
2. Conjoined muscles should not be strangulated.
3. There should not be any tension in the suture lines.

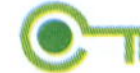 Key Box 70.6

Take Care of

- 1 nerve—ilioinguinal nerve. Entrapment causes inguinal neuralgia (*see* page 944)
- 1 bone—pubic bone do not take a stitch from the bone. It may cause periostitis pubis
- 1 cord—spermatic cord do not tighten the deep ring too tight
- 1 artery—inferior epigastric artery—see the pulsations near the deep ring and protect it
- 1 large artery—external iliac artery—while inguinal ligament being sutured to conjoined tendon on the lateral sides. Feel the pulse and protect
- 1 organ—urinary bladder—especially in elderly patients, large hernias and sliding hernias

8. Postoperative Management

- NPO for 6–8 hours, oral fluids and soft diet later.
- Analgesics.
- Prophylactic antibiotics, 1 dose is given 6 hours before surgery.
- Scrotal support, if the dissection is more (complete hernia).
- Suture removal after 7–10 days.

9. Postoperative Complications

1. **Immediate:** Haematoma due to injury to the pampiniform plexus of veins or improper haemostasis. It may need re-exploration.
2. **Wound infection** may result in discharging pus which is the cause of postoperative fever. Infection is the chief cause of recurrence.
3. **Severe periostitis pubis** (to avoid this nowadays, the repair is not done by taking bites through pubic bone). X-ray of the bone may have to be taken for diagnosis.
   - It is managed by analgesics and in intractable cases, injection of corticosteroids locally may reduce the pain.
4. **Nerve entrapment causing pain.**

10. Advice at Discharge

- Not to strain or lift heavyweights (e.g. bucketful of water) or to carry load on the shoulders for 3 months.
- If there is any precipitating cause such as chronic cough or difficulty in passing urine, etc. they have to be treated first. Otherwise, hernia will recur once again.

Pearls of Wisdom

Dissecting an inguinal canal and performing a good repair is a good exercise for a postgraduate because he has to dissect various anatomical layers, preserve nerves, vessels, vas deferens and do a good repair. Various steps of herniorrhaphy teach a postgraduate basic fundamental principle of surgery—Prof. CR Ballal, *former* Professor and Head, Kasturba Medical College and Hospital, Mangalore.

Please note: Today, the procedure of choice for inguinal hernia is mesh repair—Lichtenstein's repair. It is given in hernia Chapter 52, page 941). Please refer to hernia chapter on other repairs.

DESARDA REPAIR

Principle of Desarda repair: In normal individuals, the transversus abdominis aponeurosis (aponeurotic extensions) in the posterior wall is strong and elastic because of its aponeurotic nature and healthy muscles around keep it physiologically dynamic to give lifelong protection against hernia formation. This transversus abdominis aponeurosis is absent or deficient in hernia patients. **The Desarda repair technique uses an undetached strip of nearby external oblique aponeurosis to replace those absent aponeurotic extensions. This gives again a strong and elastic posterior wall.** Another fact noted in hernia patients is weakness of the muscle arch muscles that fail to keep the posterior wall physiologically dynamic. In Desarda repair, the strip is continuous with its original strong muscle and this nearby external oblique muscle gives additional strength to the muscle arch muscles to keep this posterior wall physiologically dynamic.

Anaesthesia: Surgery can be done under local or spinal anesthesia.

Surgery:

1. Skin and fascia are incised through a regular oblique inguinal incision to expose the external oblique aponeurosis.
2. The external oblique is cut in line with the upper crux of the superficial ring, which leaves the thinned-out portion in the lower leaf so a good strip can be taken from the upper leaf. The external oblique, which is thinned out as a result of aging or long-standing large hernias, can also be used for repair if it is able to hold the sutures.
3. Upper and lower leaves are cleared from surrounding tissue by proper undermining.
4. Sac is excised protecting ilio-inguinal nerve.
5. The upper leaf of the external oblique aponeurosis (EOA) is sutured to the inguinal ligament from the pubic tubercle to the internal ring using PDSII no. 1 or '0' (Monofilament Polydioxanone violet, Ethicon) continuous sutures (Fig. 70.30). The first suture is taken in the anterior rectus sheath part of the external oblique aponeurosis upper leaf above and the medial most part of the inguinal ligament below near the pubic tubercle. The last suture is taken so as to sufficiently narrow the new internal ring without constricting the spermatic cord by pushing the cord against the arching muscle fibers to its maximum extent (Fig. 70.30). ***Here, we are creating a new internal ring in the EOA with the help of the strip while suturing strip's lower border to the inguinal ligament. The original internal ring becomes defunct.*** Lateral pushing of spermatic cord against the arching muscle fibers to maximum extent is necessary while this suturing is done. Each suture is passed first through the inguinal ligament and then the external oblique upper leaf. Needle bites are taken as close to the border of the EOA as possible (about 1–2 mm). The index finger of the left hand is used to protect the iliac vessels and retract the cord structures laterally while taking lateral sutures.
6. A splitting incision is made in this sutured upper leaf, partially separating a strip of 1–2 cm width but never more than 2 cm. Normally 1.5 cm wide strip is

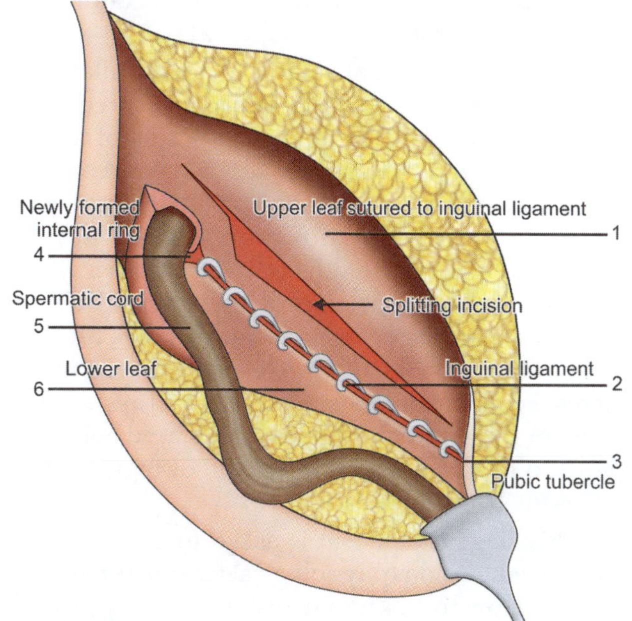

Fig. 70.30: The medial leaf of the external oblique aponeurosis is sutured to the inguinal ligament and a splitting incision is taken (*Courtesy:* Prof. Desarda Mohan Phulchand, (MB; MS; FICS; FICA) Professor of surgery and Chief of the hernia centre, Poona Hospital and Research Centre, Pune (INDIA)

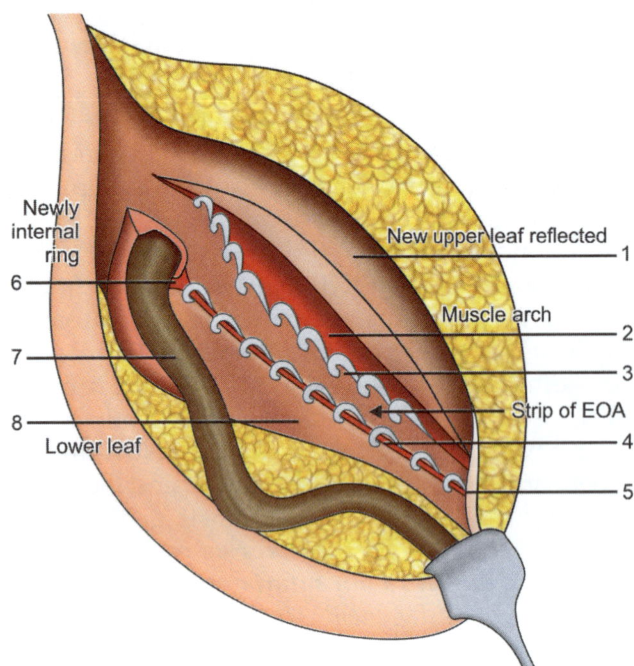

Fig. 70.31: Undetached strip of external oblique aponeurosis forming the posterior wall of inguinal canal. 1. New upper leaf; 2. Internal oblique muscle; 3. Sutures between the upper border of the strip and conjoined muscle; 4. Sutures between the lower border of the strip and the inguinal ligament; 5. Pubic tubercle; 6. Newly formed internal ring; 7. Spermatic cord; and 8. Lower leaf.

sufficient for most of the patients. This splitting incision is extended medially up to the pubic symphysis and laterally 2–3 cm beyond the internal ring. The medial insertion and lateral continuation of this strip is kept intact (Fig. 70.31).

7. A strip of the external oblique is now available, the lower border of which is already sutured to the inguinal ligament. The upper free border of the strip is now sutured to the internal oblique or conjoined muscle lying close to it with PDSII no. 1 or '0' (Monofilament Polydioxanone violet, Ethicon) continuous sutures throughout its length (Fig. 70.32). The aponeurotic portion of the internal oblique muscle is used for suturing to this strip wherever and whenever possible; otherwise, it is not essential for the success of the operation. This will result in the strip of the external oblique being placed behind the cord to form a new posterior wall of inguinal canal (Figs 70.32 to 70.34).
8. At this stage the patient is asked to cough and the increased tension (physiological tension) on the strip exerted by the external oblique to support the weakened internal oblique and transversus abdominis is clearly visible.
9. The spermatic cord is placed in the inguinal canal and the lower leaf of the external oblique is sutured

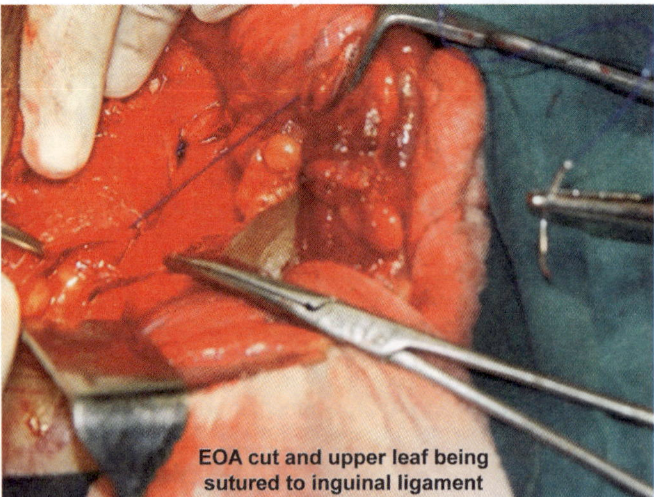

Fig. 70.32: Upper leaf of EOA being sutured to inguinal ligament

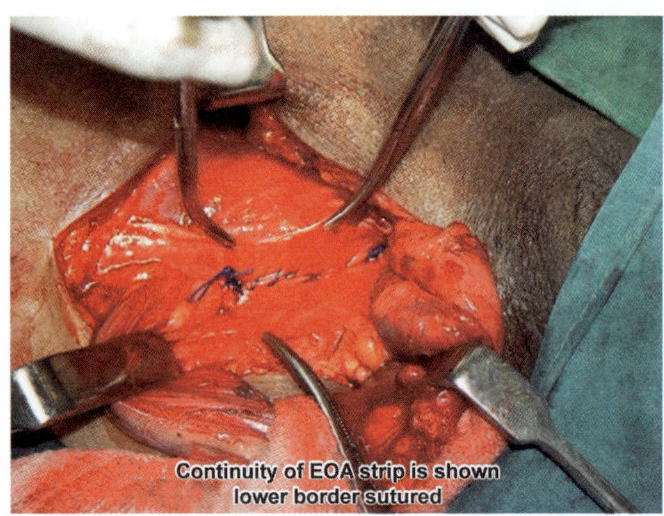

Fig. 70.33: Lower border of strip is sutured to inguinal ligament and upper border is lifted with two artery forceps. Continuity is kept intact

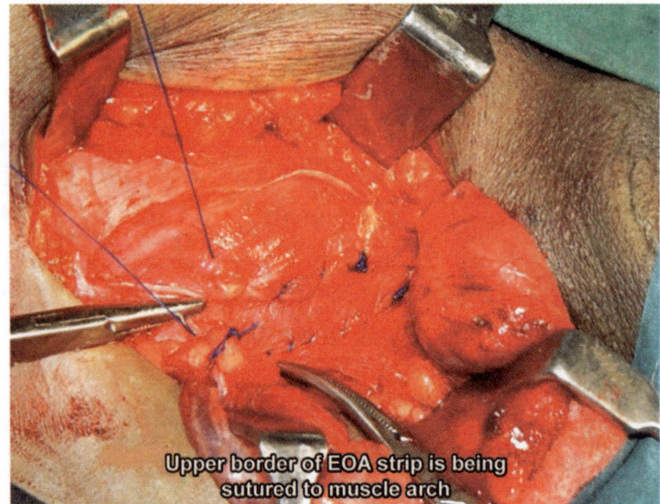

Fig. 70.34: Upper border of strip is sutured to the nearby internal oblique muscle with absorbable continuous sutures

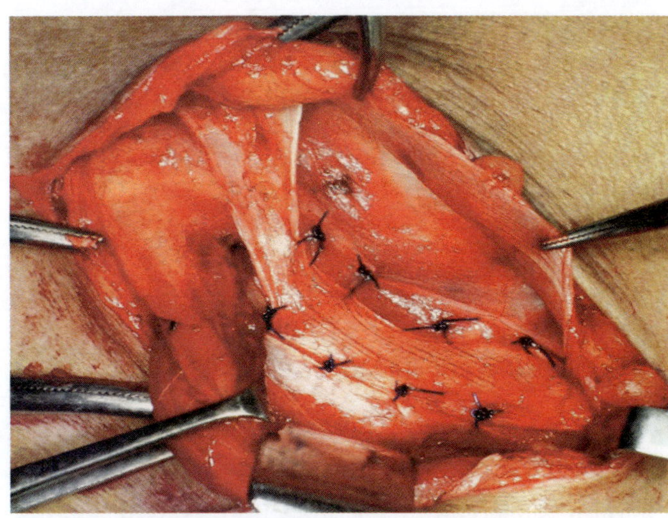

Fig. 70.35: Desarda repair completed

to the newly formed upper leaf of the external oblique in front of the cord, as usual, again using PDSII no.1 or '0' (Monofilament Polydioxanone violet, Ethicon) continuous sutures. Undermining of the newly formed upper leaf on both of its surfaces facilitate its approximation to the lower leaf. The first stitch is taken between the lateral corner of the splitting incision and lower leaf of the external oblique. This is followed by closure of the superficial fascia and the skin as usual (Fig. 70.35). This repair is written by Prof. Desarda and has been edited by authors.

Further Reading

A short handbook of Desarda Repair for inguinal hernia-published on electronic and print media—Author: Prof. (Dr) Desarda Mohan Phulchand (MB, MS, FICS, FICA), Professor, Department of Surgery and Chief of the hernia centre, Poona Hospital and Research Centre, Pune (India).

OPEN CHOLECYSTECTOMY

In the vast majority of the cases, gallbladder is removed by laparoscopic route. Details have been given in the gallbladder chapter. In this chapter, we will be studying gallbladder removed through open method—after doing a laparotomy.

DEFINITION

Removal of the diseased gallbladder by a laparotomy.

1. Indications

Laparoscopic cholecystectomy is now the gold standard for cholecystectomy. However, the role of open cholecystectomy is present when laparoscopic cholecystectomy fails due to extensive adhesions, **excessive bleeding**, CBD injury, impacted gallbladder, etc. (complications of laparoscopic cholecystectomy)

- Symptomatic gallstones
- Acute/chronic/acalculous cholecystitis
- Empyema gallbladder
- Mucocoele of gallbladder
- Asymptomatic gallstones—patients with high risk such as diabetes, haemolytic anaemias such as sickle cell anaemias and hereditary spherocytosis.

2. Contraindications

- Unfit for surgery
- Chronically debilitated patients

3. Position of the Patient

Supine: In laparoscopic cholecystectomy, the head end is elevated and a slight tilt is given to left side so that omentum and bowel fall away from the operating field.

4. Anaesthesia

GA

5. Preparation of the Parts

From level of nipple to lower abdomen, parts are cleaned with povidone-iodine and spirit.

6. Surgical Procedure

- **Incision:** Right subcostal incision (**Kocher's incision**) preferred/right paramedian.
- **Layers opened:** Skin, subcutaneous tissue, muscles (external oblique, internal oblique and transversus abdominis), preperitoneal fat and peritoneum.
- **Dissection**
  - After opening the abdomen, colon and stomach are retracted away.
  - Fundus of the gallbladder is held with a sponge holding forceps and retracted.
  - Assistant retracts the liver using a Deaver retractor.
  - **Calot's triangle is identified.** The cystic artery is identified, doubly ligated with 2.0 silk sutures and cut.
  - Cystic duct is now identified, skeletonised, doubly ligated with silk or vicryl sutures and cut.
  - The gallbladder is dissected off the gallbladder fossa using electrocautery and haemostasis is achieved.
  - Rarely, fundus first approach: When Calot's triangle anatomy is not clear due to inflammation and adhesions, the dissection is started from the fundus and proceeded towards the cystic duct which is ligated in the end.
  - Intra-abdominal drain is placed.

7. Closure

- Inner muscle layer—No. 1 prolene continuous interlocking.
- Outer muscle (2nd layer of muscles)—same suture.
- Subcutaneous layer—2.0 vicryl interrupted.
- Skin—2.0 ethilon/silk vertical mattress.

8. Postoperative Management

- Nil per oral till patient passes flatus
- To continue antibiotics in diabetic patients
- Watch for hypotension (bleeding), tachycardia, abdominal distension, pain (bile leak).
- If drain is kept, it is usually removed within 2–3 days.
- To avoid having oily foods

9. Postoperative Complications

- Infections and subphrenic abscess
- Bleeding from cystic artery
- Injury to CBD or hepatic duct—presents with jaundice in the postoperative period.
- Bile leak and fistulae
- Biliary stricture formations (late)
- Injuries to colon, duodenum and mesentery.

Pearls of Wisdom

If bile leak continues or CBD clipping is suspected, ask for ERCP and treat accordingly. Cystic duct stump leak is best treated by ERCP and stenting of CBD as early as possible.

10. Advice at Discharge

- Not to strain for 30 days—to prevent incisional hernia developing later.
- To avoid fatty food
- To report if jaundice develops (CBD injury or retained stone in CBD) or fever which may be due to subphrenic collection. (It can be treated with ultrasound-guided aspiration.)

Pearls of Wisdom

Identification of Y junction at open surgery and identification of cystic duct joining the infundibulum at laparoscopic surgery (dilated portion resembling elephant trunk) are the key points, which will help in avoiding bile duct injuries to a very large extent.

VAGOTOMY GASTROJEJUNOSTOMY (GJ)

Vagotomy GJ, as it was called, is a procedure that was commonly performed by surgeons until the invention of proton pump inhibitors increasing awareness and advent of upper GI endoscopies. Earlier, the incidence and complications of peptic ulcer were high and the commonly performed surgery for peptic ulcer was vagotomy GJ. It was also done for the complications of gastric ulcers such as gastric outlet obstruction due to strictures. However, nowadays this procedure is rarely done.

1. Indications

- Symptomatic peptic ulcer disease not responding to medical management.
- Complications of gastric ulcers such as stenosis and bleeding.

2. Contraindication

Vagotomy needs a bit of dissection near the hiatus. Hence, a risk of mediastinitis is present, if vagotomy is done in cases of perforation. Hence, a simple closure of perforation is done in emergency situations.

3. Position of the Patient

Supine

4. Anaesthesia

GA

5. Preparation of the Parts

From level of nipple to lower abdomen, parts are cleaned with povidone iodine and spirit.

6. Surgical Procedure

- **Incision**—upper midline
- **Layers opened**—skin, subcutaneous tissue, linea alba, preperitoneal fat, peritoneum.
- **Dissection**
  - After opening the abdomen, the pathology in the stomach or duodenum is noted and confirmed.
  - Gentle traction is given at the anterior stomach wall. The stomach is delivered out of the wound.
  - The oesophagus is palpated with the *in situ* nasogastric tube between the thumb and the fingers.
  - The peritoneum over the overlying distal oesophagus is incised and the oesophagus is gently mobilised. The oesophagus is encircled with a Penrose drain and lifted to visualise the anterior vagus. Once identified, it is cut after ligating or applying clips. A 2 cm portion of the nerve may be excised.
  - Similarly, the posterior nerve is found as a taut band between the right crus of diaphragm and the oesophagus which is identified and cut.
  - The duodenogastric junction is identified after lifting the transverse colon and its mesentery.

– The first loop of the jejunum (1 foot from the DJ) is taken and gastrojejunal anastomosis is performed in 2 layers—inner full thickness continuous suture with 3.0 vicryl and outer seromuscular interrupted sutures with 3–0 silk. The loop is usually taken posterior to the transverse colon through a surgically made rent in the transverse mesocolon (retrocolic) and is isoperistaltic.

7. Closure

- Peritoneum along with linea alba is sutured with no 1 prolene or loop ethilon continuous interlocking suture.
- Subcutaneous —2.0 vicryl interrupted sutures.
- Skin —2.0 ethilon vertical mattress sutures.

8. Postoperative Management

- NPO for 2 days till patient passes flatus—indication that there is no anastomotic leak. Ryle's tube is removed, then followed by clear fluids by mouth for 2–3 days followed by soft diet.
- Suture removal by 7–10 days
- Fluid and electrolytes have to be checked in the postoperative period.

9. Postoperative Complications

- Postvagotomy diarrhoea, due to denervation of the gut.
- Afferent loop obstruction/stomal oedema.
- Gallstone formation due to denervation of gall-bladder.
- Stomal ulcers due to bile reflux
- Bile reflux gastritis

10. Advice at Discharge

- To avoid large heavy meals
- Small frequent feeds better
- Avoid spicy and oily foods

All details about complications of vagotomy and GJ are given on page 586.

Competency

SU14.3: Describe the materials and methods used for surgical wound closure and anastomosis (sutures, knots, and needles).

INTESTINAL RESECTION AND ANASTOMOSIS

Introduction

Bowel anastomosis involves the surgical join between two intestinal segments. Bowel anastomosis is usually done to restore bowel continuity as part of surgery for diseased bowel or to bypass unresectable bowel. It may be accomplished either by handsewn technique or by the use of stapler devices. It has been stated that the key to a successful anastomosis is the accurate union of two viable bowel ends with complete avoidance of tension (Key Box 70.7). If anastomosis is not successful, complications can be very, very disastrous as shown in Fig. 70.36.

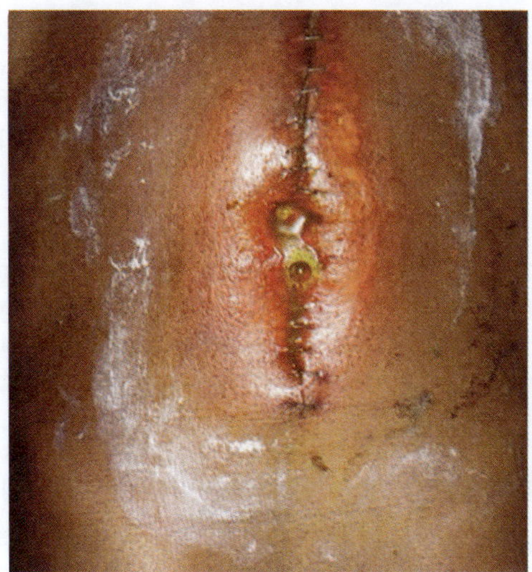

Fig. 70.36: Anastomotic leak

Physiology of Anastomosis Healing

The healing process at the anastomotic site is divided into three phases:

1. **Inflammatory phase:** The inflammatory phase lasts for the first 4 days during which the anastomosis is dependent on the mechanical strength provided by the sutures or staples. Hence, any AL occurring during the first two postoperative days is likely to be due to technical factors.
2. **Proliferative or fibroplasia phase:** The second phase of proliferation starts from the 5th postoperative day and lasts up to the 14th postoperative day. There is an increased collagen deposition during this phase to give tensile strength to the anastomosis.

Key Box 70.7

Key Factors for Successful Intestinal Anastomosis

- Good exposure in the operative field
- Gentle handling of the bowel
- Meticulous surgical technique
- Approximation of well vascularized bowel
- Avoid tension at anastomosis
- Minimize faecal contamination
- Good haemostasis

3. **Reparative or remodelling phase:** The last phase of remodelling occurs up to 1 year after the surgery. During this phase, rebuilding of the intestinal wall layers occurs at the anastomotic site.

Blood Flow and Anastomosis

The blood supply to the bowel is derived from the mesentery with vessels travelling on either side of the bowel wall to reach antimesenteric border. Hence, the anastomosis is centred on the antimesenteric border when possible (Fig. 70.37).

Instruments used for Intestinal Anastomosis (Fig. 70.38)

- Straight artery forceps for stay sutures, scissors to cut the intestines and forceps to hold the edge of the intestines to see carefully the layers taken while suturing.
- Curved small artery forceps for catching the bleeders followed by coagulation.
- Babcock's forceps for holding the intestines together, thus getting ready for anastomosis.

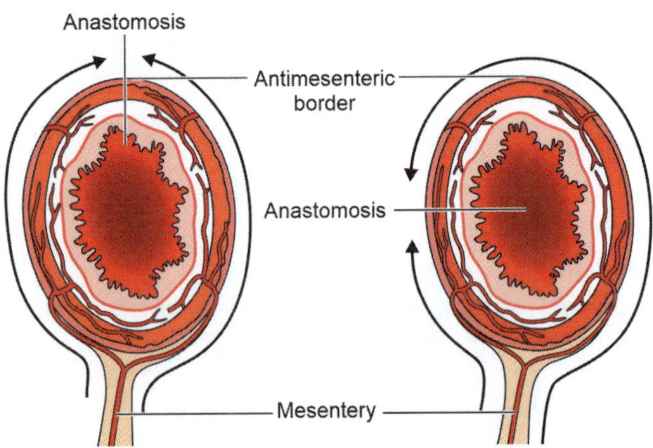

Fig. 70.37: Blood flow at anastomotic site

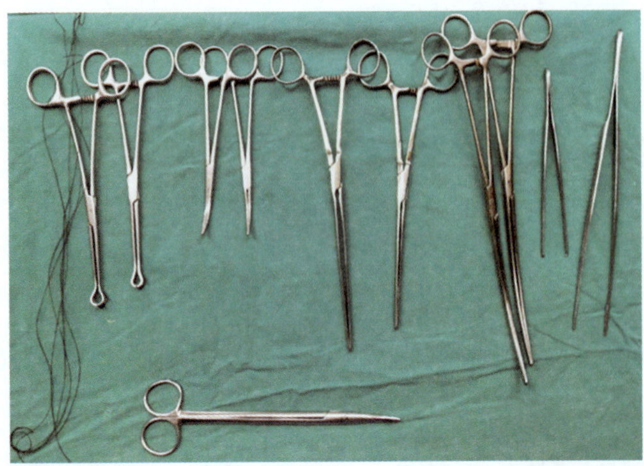

Fig. 70.38: Instruments used for intestinal anastomosis

- Moynihan's occlusion clamps—straight and curved—are applied to occlude the lumen so that contents of the intestine are not spilled over and also to control bleeding.

Suture Materials Used

Intestines: Inner absorbable such as 2–0 polyglactin (Vicryl) and outer 2–0 atraumatic silk.

Handsewn Anastomosis

It can be performed in a single layer or double layer fashion. Single layer anastomosis usually employs full thickness bites of the bowel wall (Fig. 70.39). In a double-layered anastomosis, the inner layer consists of full thickness bites whilst the outer layer consists of sero-muscular bites. There is no proven advantage regarding the type of suture material used. The ideal suture material should provide good tensile strength during the anastomotic site healing process with minimal local tissue reaction. Commonly used suture materials are 2–0 vicryl continuous for inner mucosal sutures and 2–0 interrupted for outer seromuscular layer.

Stapler Anastomosis

Stapler anastomosis drastically reduces the operating time, however, it requires the surgeon to be familiar with the stapling devices. They are usually not preferred, if the bowel is edematous due to high risk of anastomotic leak. There are different types of surgical staplers available for resection and anastomosis of bowel.

- **Transverse anastomosis (TA) staplers:** They are non-cutting staplers that require the specimen to be cut with scalpel or scissors after laying down the stapler rows.
- **Linear staplers:** They are popularly known as gastrointestinal anastomosis (GIA) staplers. They have a cutting mechanism for transection of bowel

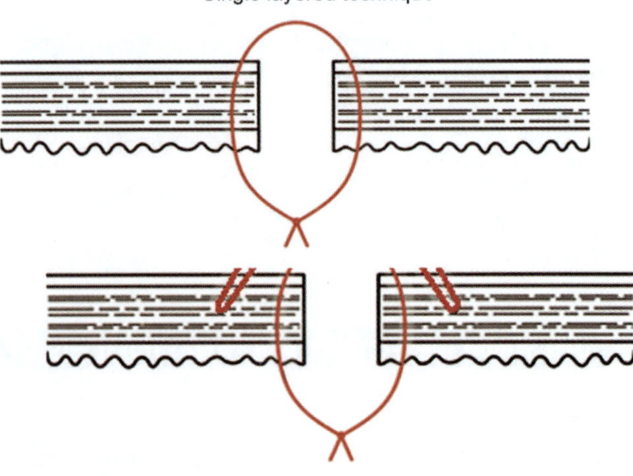

Fig. 70.39: Types of handsewn anastomosis

in addition to laying down stapler rows. These types are very commonly used for bowel resection and anastomosis in small and large bowel (Fig. 70.40).

- **End-to-end anastomosis (EEA) staplers:** These are circular cutting staplers that place several rows of staples. These are used in coloerectal and oesophago-gastric anastomosis.

Staplers are available in different staple line lengths and configurations. The cartridges are colour coded to indicate the height of the staples which are used based on the thickness of bowel being anastomosed (Fig. 70.41). One example of using blue cartridge is shown in Fig. 70.42.

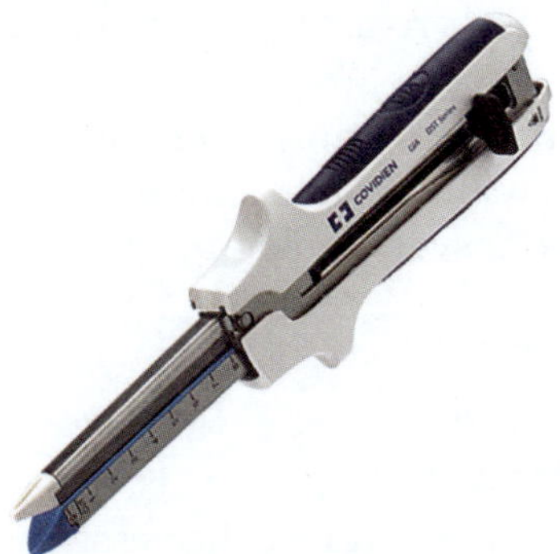

Fig. 70.40: GIA stapler device

Color	Tissue type	Open staple height	Closed staple height
Grey	Mesentery	2.0 mm	0.75 mm
White	Vascular	2.5 mm	1.0 mm
Blue	Standard	3.5 mm	1.5 mm
Gold	Standard/ thick	3.8 mm	1.8 mm
Green	Thick	4.1 mm	2.0 mm

Fig. 70.41: Colour coding of the cartridge

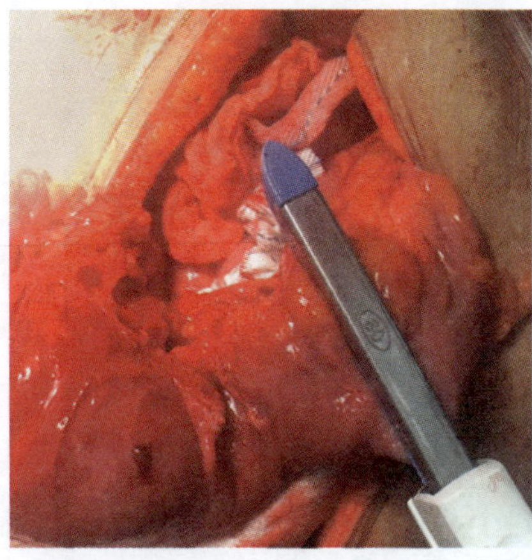

Fig. 70.42: Stapler resection of bowel

Type of Anastomosis (Fig. 70.43–70.45)

Anastomosis between two bowel segments can be created in various ways.

- **End-to-end:** This is performed when two bowel segments are of roughly equal caliber. In case of an unequal caliber, a Cheatle slit on the smaller caliber bowel will aid in anastomosis.
- **End-to-side:** This type is preferred when one bowel segment is wider than the other.

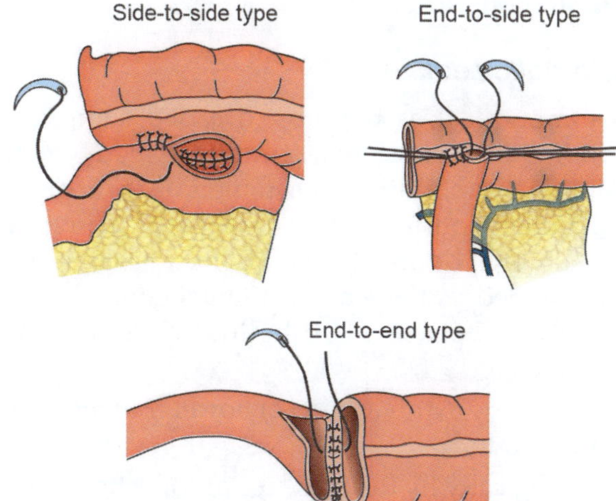

Fig. 70.43: Types of anastomosis

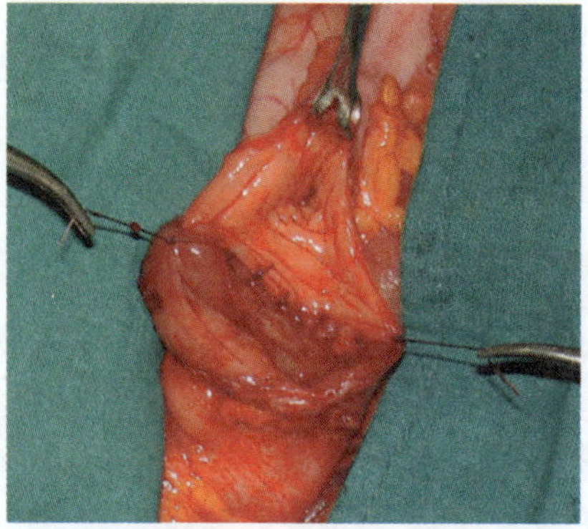

Fig. 70.44: End-to-end anastomosis

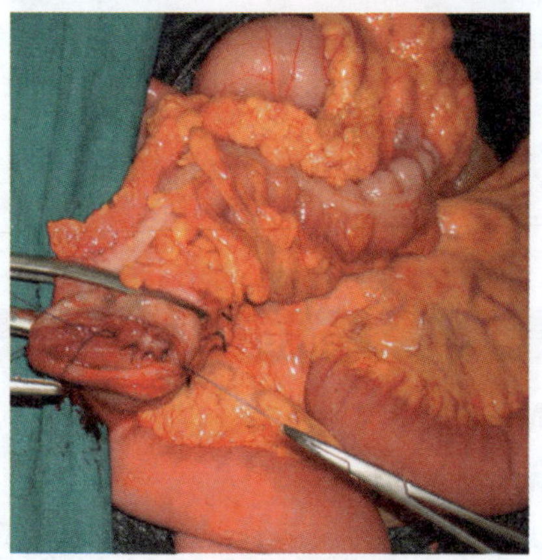

Fig. 70.45: Ileo-colic anastomosis

- **Side-to-side:** This type of anastomosis is carried out on the antimesenteric side of two bowel segments. It is the most commonly employed type of anastomosis.

Complications of Bowel Anastomosis

- Anastomotic leak
- Bleeding
- Wound infection
- Prolonged ileus
- Anastomotic stricture

Anastomotic Leak

Anastomotic leak is the most dreaded complication following intestinal resection and leads to high morbidity and mortality. Anastomotic leaks are usually identifiable by postoperative day 3–5. It occurs due to the breakdown or insufficiency at the anastomotic line and is defined as the leak of luminal contents from a surgical join between two hollow viscera which is identified.

- Clinically by extravasation of bowel content through drain/wound.
- Radiologically by the presence of collection adjacent to anastomosis.
- Intraoperatively during re-exploration.

Risk factors for anastomotic leak: They may be categorized into patient factors and technical factors. Some of the risk factors (Table 70.3) like smoking and consumption of alcohol may be modifiable.

Table 70.3: Risk factors for anastomotic leak

Patient factors	Technical factors
• Old age (>60 years)	• Emergency surgery
• Male gender	• Poor surgical technique
• High dose steroids	• Faecal contamination
• Smoking	• Haematoma formation
• Alcohol abuse	• Prolonged operating time
• Preoperative radiotherapy	• Intraoperative blood loss
• High-risk site of anastomosis	
• Diabetes mellitus	
• Anaemia	
• Uraemia	

COLECTOMY

RIGHT HEMICOLECTOMY

Indications

1. Carcinoma of the caecum or ascending colon
2. Tumours of appendix
3. Extended right hemicolectomy for carcinoma of hepatic flexure and proximal 1/3rd transverse colon and for closed loop obstruction in carcinoma of the transverse colon.
4. Modified right hemicolectomy for tuberculosis, Crohn's disease involving terminal ileum (Fig. 70.46).

Structures Removed

1. Terminal 5–10 cm of ileum
2. Caecum
3. Ascending colon
4. Proximal 1/3rd of transverse colon with hepatic flexure.
5. Extended right hemicolectomy—all the above structures with the proximal two-thirds of the transverse colon.
6. **Modified right hemicolectomy**—all the above structures with variable length of hepatic flexure or proximal transverse colon preserved.

Vessels Ligated

1. Ileocolic vessels
2. Right colic vessels
3. Right branch of middle colic vessels
4. Ileal vessels are ligated last

Surgical Techniques

1. **Laparotomy** through midline/right paramedian incision.
2. **Exploration** of the abdomen for liver deposits, peritoneal deposits, ascites and other synchronous lesions.
3. **Assessment** of the tumour for site, extent, mobility, serosal involvement and local extension.
4. **Mobilisation of the right colon** done by incising along the avascular lateral peritoneal fold or **white line of Toldt** and rotating the caecum and the ascending colon anteriorly and medially.

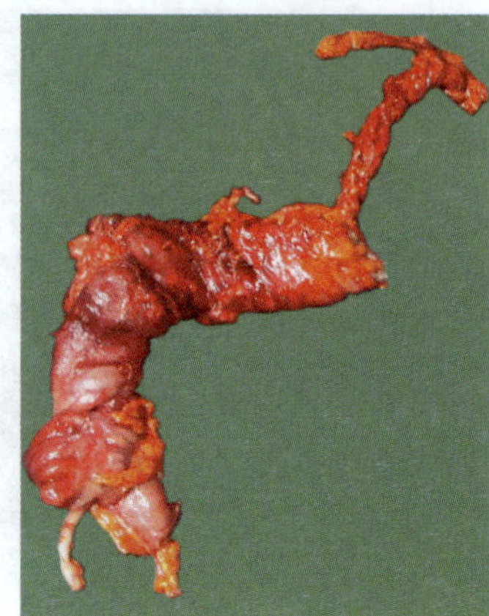

Fig. 70.46: Right hemicolectomy

5. **Retroperitoneum is entered** through the incision and dissection carried up towards the third and fourth part of duodenum.
6. Retroperitoneal structures encountered during dissection are the right kidney with **ureter, right gonadal vessels and duodenum**. Care must be taken to avoid injury to these structures.
7. **Turnbull's technique or no touch isolation technique**—early ligation of the vessels before manipulation of the tumour should be followed to prevent dissemination of the tumour cells during handling.
8. Ileocolic, right colic, right branch of middle colic and lastly ileal **vessels are isolated, ligated and divided.** Ileocolic and right colic vessels are ligated at the origin to include all the associated lymph nodes.
9. Ileum is transected at 5–10 cm from the ileocaecal junction and transverse colon at the junction of the proximal 1/3rd and distal 2/3rds. This is followed by an **ileotransverse colon anastomosis**.
10. Abdominal wall is closed in layers.

LEFT HEMICOLECTOMY

Indications

1. Carcinoma of the descending colon
2. Carcinoma of the splenic flexure
3. High-risk polyps

Structures Removed

Carcinoma of the Descending Colon

1. Distal 1/3rd of transverse colon
2. Splenic flexure
3. Descending colon
4. Sigmoid colon

Carcinoma of the Splenic Flexure

1. Distal 2/3rds of transverse colon
2. Splenic flexure and descending colon

Vessels Ligated

1. Left branch of middle colic vessels
2. Left colic vessels
3. Inferior mesenteric and sigmoidal vessels in case of carcinoma of descending colon.

Surgical Techniques

1. Laparotomy through midline/left paramedian incision.
2. Exploration of the abdomen for liver deposits, peritoneal deposits, ascites and other synchronous lesions.
3. Assessment of the tumour for site, extent, mobility, serosal involvement and local extension.
4. Mobilisation of the left colon done by incising along the avascular lateral peritoneal fold or white line of Toldt and rotating the descending colon and the sigmoid colon anteriorly and medially. Splenic flexure is mobilised by dividing the gastrocolic ligaments and phrenicocolic ligaments.
5. **Retroperitoneum is entered** through the incision and dissection carried medially towards the ligament of Treitz.
6. Retroperitoneal structures encountered during dissection are the **left kidney with ureter and left gonadal vessels.** Care must be taken to avoid injury to these structures.
7. **Turnbull's technique** or no touch isolation technique—early ligation of the vessels before manipulation of the tumour should be followed to prevent dissemination of the tumour cells during handling.
8. **Left colic and left branch of middle colic vessels** are isolated, ligated and divided in case of carcinoma of splenic flexure. Inferior mesenteric and sigmoidal vessels are also ligated in case of carcinoma of descending colon.
9. **Level of colonic transection and anastomosis:**
   - Carcinoma of the splenic flexure: Proximally at the junction of right 1/3rd and left 2/3rds of transverse colon and distally at the junction descending and sigmoid colon. Colocolic anastomosis is done.
   - Carcinoma of the descending colon: Proximally at the junction of right 2/3rds and left 1/3rd of transverse colon and distally at the rectosigmoid junction.
   - Colorectal anastomosis is done
10. **Abdominal wall is closed in layers**

TRANSVERSE COLECTOMY

Indication

Carcinoma of transverse colon

Structures Removed

Whole of the transverse colon including the hepatic and splenic flexures.

Vessels Ligated

1. Middle colic vessels
2. Left branch of right colic vessels
3. Right branch of left colic vessels

Surgical Techniques

1. Laparotomy through midline incision
2. Exploration of the abdomen for liver deposits, peritoneal deposits, ascites and other synchronous lesions.
3. Assessment of the tumour for site, extent, mobility, serosal involvement and local extension.
4. Mobilisation of the hepatic flexure is done by incising along the right avascular lateral peritoneal fold or white line of Toldt and rotating the hepatic flexure anteriorly and downwards. Splenic flexure is mobilised by dividing the gastrocolic ligaments and phrenicocolic ligaments.
5. **Turnbull's technique or no touch isolation technique**—early ligation of the vessels before manipulation of the tumour should be followed to prevent dissemination of the tumour cells during handling.
6. Isolation of middle colic, left branch of right colic and right branch of left colic vessels done and ligated.
7. Proximal transection is done just proximal to the hepatic flexure and the distal transection is done just distal to the splenic flexure.
   - Colocolic anastomosis is done
8. Abdominal wall is closed in layers

SIGMOID COLECTOMY

Indications

1. Carcinoma sigmoid colon
2. Diverticular disease
3. Sigmoid volvulus

Structures Removed

1. Sigmoid colon
2. Associated mesosigmoid
3. Lymph nodes in malignancy

Vessels Ligated

1. Inferior mesenteric vessels distal to the origin of left colic vessels.
2. Sigmoidal vessels
3. Left branch of left colic vessels

Surgical Techniques

1. **Laparotomy through midline**/left paramedian incision.
2. Exploration of the abdomen for **liver deposits**, peritoneal deposits, ascites and other synchronous lesions.
3. **Assessment of the tumour** for site, extent, mobility, serosal involvement and local extension.
4. **Mobilisation of the left colon** is done by incising along the avascular lateral peritoneal fold or white line of Toldt and rotating the descending colon and the sigmoid colon anteriorly and medially.
5. **Retroperitoneum is entered** through the incision and dissection carried medially towards the origin of inferior mesenteric artery.
6. Retroperitoneal structures encountered during dissection are the **left ureter and left gonadal vessels**. Care must be taken to avoid injury to these structures.
7. **Turnbull's technique or no touch isolation technique**—early ligation of the vessels before manipulation of the tumour should be followed to prevent dissemination of the tumour cells during handling.
8. **Inferior mesenteric vessels** distal to the origin of left colic vessels, sigmoidal vessels and left branch of left colic vessels done are isolated, ligated and divided.
9. **Colonic transection** done proximally at the junction of descending colon and sigmoid colon and distally at the rectosigmoid junction. Colorectal anastomosis is done.
10. Abdominal wall is **closed in layers.**

STAPLERS IN SURGERY

Principle

They are used for apposition of tissues.

Types

1. Cutaneous staplers
- Used after thyroidectomy. It is quick and gives clean apposition.
- Needs a special instrument for removal.

2. Linear staplers
- Used to close the bowel partially or completely.

3. Circular staplers
- Are also called EEA stapler: End-to-end anastomosis.
- Uses in surgery:
  a. After low or high anterior resection done for carcinoma rectum
  b. After oesophagogastrectomy
  c. Any other intestinal resection

4. GIA stapler (Fig. 70.47)
- Gastrointestinal anastomosis stapler: Used for side-to-side anastomosis.

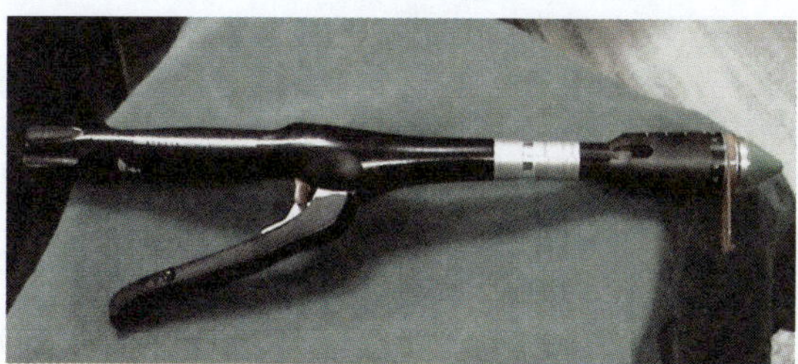

Fig. 70.47: GIA stapler

5. Endostapler

- With the increasing use of laparoscopy surgeries for facilitating a quick and safe anastomosis, endostaplers are used for intestinal anastomosis.
- Endovascular staplers are used to ligate vascular pedicles. Examples: **Renal pedicles** during laparoscopic nephrectomy, **adrenal veins** during laparoscopic adrenalectomy.

Advantages of Staplers

- Saves operating time
- The low rectal and oesophageal anastomosis have higher incidence of leakage rates. However, it can be decreased by using staplers.

Disadvantages

- Expensive
- Improper apposition results in leakage

Parts of the Stapler

1. Handle
2. Shaft
3. Head, detachable anvil + a staple cartridge.

The staples (approximately 15 in number) are present in the cartridge. The cartridge also has a circular knife.

Pearls of Wisdom

The doughnuts (rings of excised tissue) should be complete after the stapled anastomosis. Incomplete doughnut means incomplete wound closure (Fig. 70.48).

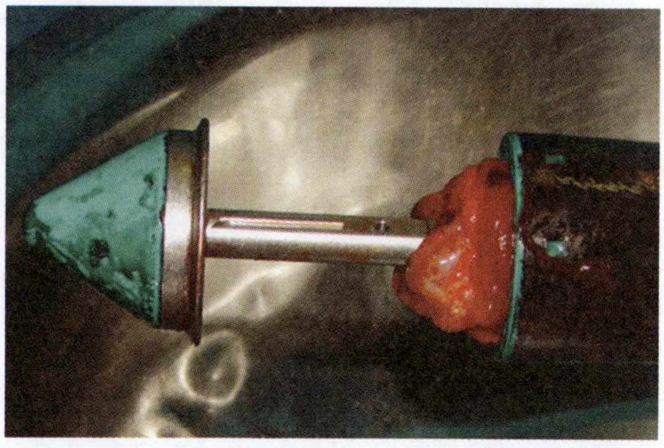

Fig. 70.48: Doughnut of stapler haemorrhoidopexy

Contraindications

1. If the tissues which have to be approximated are under tension, they should not be stapled.
2. Different lumen diameters should not be stapled end-to-end.
3. If the circular head is of greater diameter than the lumen, it should not be used.

LAPAROSCOPIC SURGERY

Introduction and History

- Laparoscopy made marked advances in the 1990s. Although the term minimally invasive surgery (MIS) is relatively recent, the history of its component parts is nearly 100 years old. What is considered the newest and most popular variety of MIS, laparoscopy, is in fact the oldest.
- Primitive laparoscopy, placing a cystoscope within an inflated abdomen, was first performed by Kelling in 1901.
- In the late 1950s, Hopkins described the rod lens, a method of transmitting light through a solid quartz rod with no heat and a little light loss.
- Muhe in Germany began performing laparoscopic-assisted cholecystectomies in 1985.
- In 1987, Mouret and Dubious performed the first video-laparoscopy in France.
- The explosion of **video-assisted surgery** in the past 20 years was a result of the development of compact, high-resolution, charge-coupled devices (CCDs) that could be mounted on the internal end of flexible endoscopes or on the external end of a Hopkins telescope.
- Coupled with bright light sources, fibreoptic cables, and **high-resolution video monitors**, the video endoscope has changed our understanding of surgical anatomy and reshaped surgical practice.

Basic Instrumentation

- **0° or 30° angled laparoscope** either 5 or 10 mm in diameter attached to camera connected to video source and monitor, ports for gas connection.
- **5 mm laparoscopic instruments** including Maryland dissector, blunt-tip dissecting forceps, cup-biopsy forceps, atraumatic grasping forceps, liver retractor, Babcocks forceps and scissors.
- **5 or 10 mm suction/irrigation device**
- **Laparoscopic ultrasound probe** (optional)

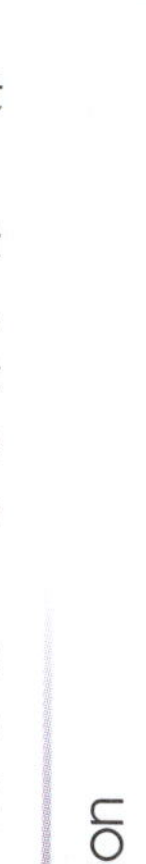

Equipment

1. **Telescope:** 30°, 0° or 45°
2. **Video camera:** A high-resolution video camera attached to the eyepiece of the telescope acquires the image for projection on the monitor. The video image is transmitted *via* a cable to a video unit, where it is processed into either an analog or a digital form (Fig. 70.49).
   - Analog is an electrical signal with a continuously varying wave or shift of intensity or frequency of voltage. Digital is a data signal with information represented by ones and zeros and is interpreted by a computer. These are the methods by which the picture is transmitted to the video monitor.
   - **The camera and cable are designed so that they can be sterilised in glutaraldehyde**.
3. **Light sources:** High-intensity light is created with bulbs of mercury, halogen vapour or xenon. Since light is absorbed by blood, any procedure in which bleeding is encountered may require more light. The light is carried to the fibreoptic bundles of the laparoscope *via* a fibreoptic cable. The current systems create even brightness across the field.
4. **Insufflators:** An insufflator delivers gas from a high pressure cylinder to the patient at a high rate with low and accurately controlled pressure (Fig. 70.50).

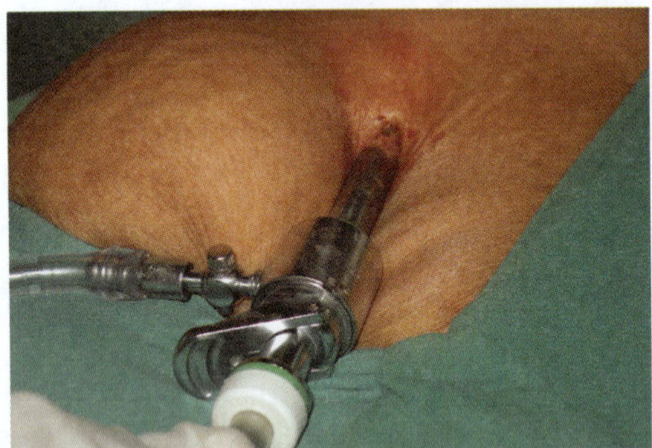

Fig. 70.49: Camera port (umbilical port)

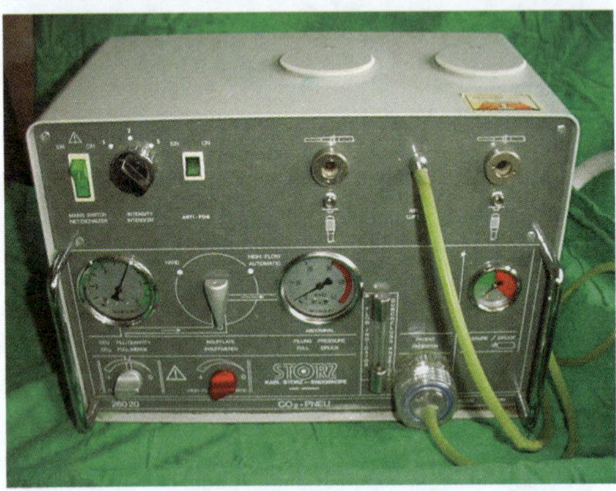

Fig. 70.50: Insufflator

5. **Video monitors:** High-resolution video monitors are used to display the image. These monitors may be positioned optimally.

Anaesthesia

- Usually done under general anaesthesia.
- Laparoscopic surgeon can influence cardiovascular performance by **reducing or removing the CO_2 pneumoperitoneum**.
- **Insensible fluid losses are negligible**, and therefore, IV fluid administration should not exceed that necessary to maintain circulating volume.
- Minimally invasive surgical procedures are often outpatient procedures. So, short-acting anaesthetic agents are preferable.
- Since, the factors that require hospitalisation after laparoscopic procedures include the management of nausea, pain and urinary retention, the anaesthesiologist should minimise the use of agents that provoke these conditions and maximise the use of medications that prevent such problems.
- Critical to the anaesthesia management of these patients is the **use of non-narcotic analgesics** (e.g. diclofenac) when haemostasis allows it, and the **liberal use of antiemetic** agents, such as **ondansetron and steroids.**

Procedure and Principles

The unique feature of laparoscopic surgery is the need to lift the abdominal wall from the abdominal organs by creating pneumoperitoneum.

Gases Used

Gases	Advantages	Disadvantages
Air	Historical importance	Poorly insoluble in blood so slower absorption More painful
CO_2	Inert	Rapidly absorbable Respiratory acidosis
N_2O	Inert Less painful Reduced intraoperative end tidal CO_2	Rapidly absorbable Danger of combustion Not safe in pregnancy

Laparoscopic Access (Fig. 70.51)

- The requirements for laparoscopy are more involved because the creation of a pneumoperitoneum requires that instruments of access (trocars) contain valves to maintain abdominal inflation (Key Box 70.8).
- Two methods are used for establishing abdominal access during laparoscopic procedures. The first, direct puncture laparoscopy, begins with the

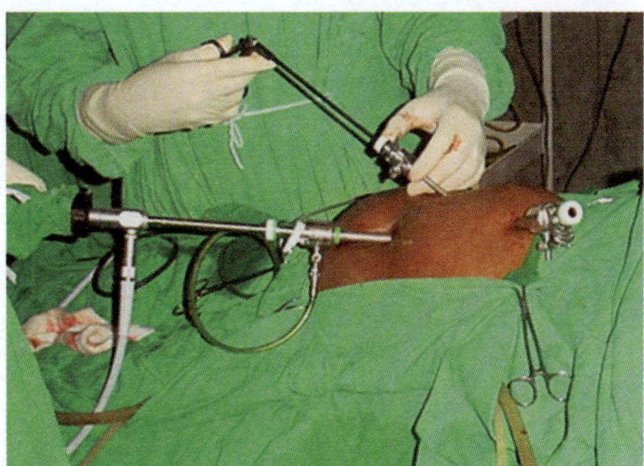

Fig. 70.51: 3 ports in place

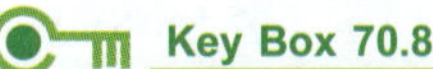

Key Box 70.8

Laparoscopic Access

1. Closed Veress needle technique
2. Open technique: Hasson's technique
3. Direct trocar insertion
4. Access using umbilical cicatrix tube
5. Disposable optical trocar

elevation of the relaxed abdominal wall with two towel clips or a well-placed hand. A small incision is made in the umbilicus, and a specialised springloaded (Veress) needle is placed in the abdominal cavity (Fig. 70.52). With the **Veress needle,** two distinct pops are felt as the surgeon passes the needle through the abdominal wall fascia and the peritoneum. The umbilicus usually is selected as the preferred point of access because, in this location, the abdominal wall is quite thin, even in obese patients. The abdomen is inflated with a pressure-limited insufflator. CO_2 gas is used usually with maximal pressures in the range of 14 to 15 mmHg. During the process of insufflation, it is essential that the surgeon observe the pressure and flow readings on the monitor to confirm an intraperitoneal location of the Veress needle tip (Key Box 70.9).

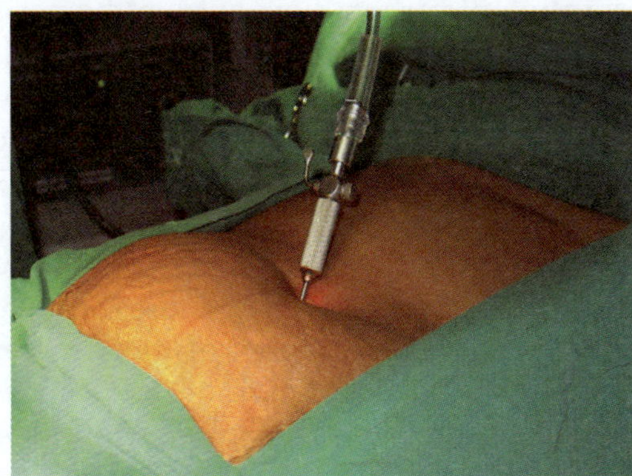

Fig. 70.52: Veress needle is used to create pneumoperitoneum

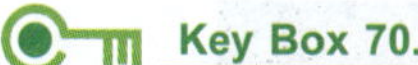

Key Box 70.9

Veress Needle

12–15 cm length with 2 mm external diameter. It has got outer and inner cannula. Outer cannula sharp cutting edge and inner cannula blunt edge with spring action.

Confirmation of Veress needle position

1. Hiss test
2. Aspiration test
3. Drop test
4. Percussion test
5. Reading of the insufflator

   Preferred position for Veress needle insertion is sub-umbilical or Palmer's point (3 cm below the middle of left subcostal margin).

- Occasionally, the direct peritoneal access (Hasson) technique is advisable. With this technique, the surgeon makes a small incision just below the umbilicus and under direct vision locates the abdominal fascia.

Utility and Scope

I. Basic

- Appendicectomy
- Cholecystectomy (Fig. 70.53)
- Hernia repair

II. Advanced

- Nissen fundoplication
- Heller's myotomy
- Gastrectomy
- Oesophagectomy
- Enteral access
- Bile duct exploration
- Colectomy (Fig. 70.54)
- Splenectomy
- Adrenalectomy

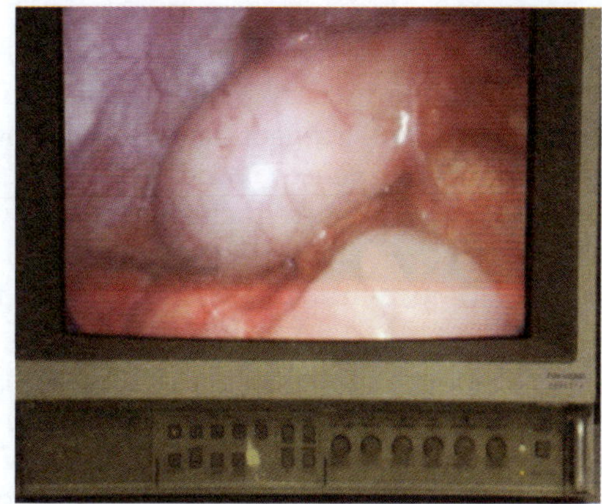

Fig. 70.53: Laparoscopic view of the gallbladder

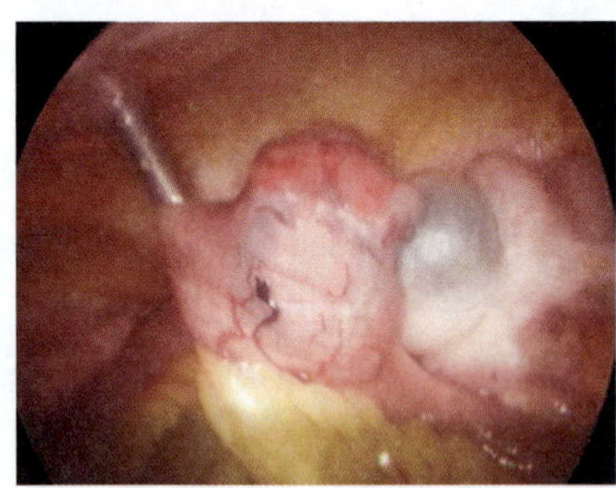

Fig. 70.54: Laparoscopic-assisted mobilisation of colon

- Lymph node dissection
- Nephrectomy
- Robotics
- Stereo imaging
- Telemedicine

III. Laparoscopy-assisted procedures

- Hepatectomy
- Pancreatectomy
- Prostatectomy
- Hysterectomy

The Physiologic Effects of Pneumoperitoneum

- The pneumoperitoneum has many effects that are only partially known despite years of study in humans and in animal models. There are effects resulting from the pressure within the abdomen and effects resulting from the composition of the gas used, generally carbon dioxide.
- The pressure within the abdomen from pneumoperitoneum decreases venous return by collapsing the intra-abdominal veins, especially in volume-depleted patients.
- This decrease in venous return may lead to decreased cardiac output.
- To compensate (Key Box 70.10), there is an elevation in the heart rate, which increases myocardial oxygen demand.
- High-risk cardiopulmonary patients cannot always meet the demand and may not tolerate a laparoscopic procedure. In volume-expanded healthy patients with full intra-abdominal capacitance vessels (veins), the increased intra-abdominal pressure actually may serve as a pump that increases right atrial filling pressure.
- Urine output often is diminished during laparoscopic procedures and usually is the result of diminished renal blood flow owing to the cardiovascular effects of pneumoperitoneum and direct pressure on the renal veins.

Key Box 70.10

Absolute Contraindications

- Advanced generalised peritonitis
- Massive abdominal distension secondary to obstruction
- Irreducible hernia
- Uncorrected coagulopathy, hypovolaemic shock
- Inability of the patient to tolerate a formal laparotomy
- Surgeon's lack of experience in performing laparoscopic procedures

Relative Contraindications

Previous surgery	Adhesions leading to visceral injury
Ongoing intra-abdominal sepsis	Friable bowel prone to injury
Bowel obstruction	Friable bowel prone to injury
Morbid obesity	Difficult access, requirement for longer instruments.
Pregnancy	Foetal distress, injury to gravid uterus
Aortic or iliac aneurysmal disease	Vascular injury
Cardiopulmonary compromise	Raised intra-abdominal pressure may significantly reduce cardiac preload. CO_2 insufflation may result in CO_2 retention

- In addition to direct effects, elevated intra-abdominal pressure results in release of antidiuretic hormone (ADH) by the pituitary, resulting in oliguria that may last up to 60 minutes after the pneumoperitoneum is released.

Complications of Laparoscopy

1. Injury to bowel/bladder
2. Injury to major vessels
3. CO_2 related complications
   a. **Hypercapnia:** Hypercapnia and acidosis are seen with pneumoperitoneum and are likely due to the absorption of carbon dioxide from the peritoneal cavity. Hypercapnia and acidosis that are difficult to control may follow, especially in elderly patients, those undergoing long operations and patients with pulmonary insufficiency.
   b. **Carbon dioxide embolus:** The incidence of clinically significant CO_2 embolism is very low, although recent reports using more sensitive tests suggest that tiny bubbles of gas are present commonly in the right side of the heart during laparoscopic procedures. Clinically important CO_2 embolism may be noted by unexplained hypotension and hypoxia during the operation.

c. **Capnothorax/pneumothorax:** Capnothorax can be caused by carbon dioxide escaping into the chest through a defect in the diaphragm or tracking through fascial planes during dissection of the oesophageal hiatus. It can also be due to opening of pleuroperitoneal ducts most commonly seen on the right side.

HERNIA REPAIR: TAPP
(Transabdominal Preperitoneal Mesh Repair)

KEY POINTS IN LAPAROSCOPIC INGUINAL ANATOMY

Space of Bogros

This 'preperitoneal space' is divided into two by the posterior lamina of the transversalis fascia. The posterior compartment of this space is called the 'Space of Bogros (proper)', described by French anatomist Bogros in 1923. The anterior space has been termed as the 'Vascular Space'. Medially it is continuous with the space of Retzius.

Prevesical Space of Retzius

The preperitoneal space that lies deep to the supravesical fossa and the medial umbilical fossa is the prevesical space of Retzius (described in 1858, by Swedish anatomist Retzius). Dissection of this space during a laparoscopic hernia repair is mandatory to enable proper mesh overlap of the hernial defect to aid in proper mesh placement/fixation.

Corona Mortis/Crown of Death/Circle of Death

- The pubic branch of the inferior epigastric artery courses in a vertical fashion inferiorly, crossing the Cooper's ligament and anastomosing with the obturator artery. In 25–30% of individuals (can be as high as 70–80%), the pubic branch is large and can replace the obturator artery.
- This large arterial branch is called aberrant obturator artery can partially encircle the neck of a hernia sac and be injured in a femoral hernia repair. It could also be injured while exposing the Cooper's ligament by freeing it of areolar adipose connective tissue.
- Because of this possibility an enlarged pubic branch of the inferior epigastric artery has in the past been known as the 'Corona Mortis'. The danger of injury in this area is more significant for obturator veins.

Triangle of Doom

- It is a misnomer. It is not a triangle. It indicates an area where it is dangerous to place staples or sutures during laparoscopic hernia surgery.

The "triangle of doom" is an inverted "V"-shaped area with its apex at the internal (deep) inguinal ring. The "triangle of doom" is bound laterally by the gonadal vessels, and medially by the vas deferens in the male, or the round ligament of the uterus in the female.

- Within the boundaries of this area you can find the external iliac artery and vein.
- Injury to these vessels can be catastrophic.

Triangle of Pain

Formed medially by gonadal vessels, laterally by iliopubic tract and inferiorly by peritoneal reflection. It contains lateral femoral cutaneous nerve, genital femoral nerve.

Introduction

Novel method used for hernias wherein transabdominally (intraperitoneal) dissection is done through a laparoscope, and a mesh placed in the preperitoneal space.

Indication

Large indirect hernias and irreducible hernias.

Procedure

- **10 mm infraumbilical port** is used for the laparoscopic camera.
- **5 mm ports** are placed one on each side on pararectal point at or above the level of umbilicus, so as to achieve adequate triangulation.
- Once ports are inserted, the hernial sac is recognized and the contents are reduced by pulling it transabdominally using a dissector (laparoscopic).
- Hernial sac is dissected in the preperitoneal plane after incising at the upper part of the hernial sac opening.
- Once the sac is dissected and excised, a prolene mesh is placed in the preperitoneal space. It is fixed to the pubic bone using tacks. Peritoneum is closed with prolene sutures.

Complications

- Mesh displacement
- Intestinal obstruction, if the mesh displaces into the peritoneum.
- Expensive
- Higher recurrence rates

HERNIA REPAIR: TEP (TOTALLY EXTRAPERITONEAL REPAIR)

Indications

1. Recurrent hernia
2. Bilateral inguinal hernias
3. Indirect/direct/femoral hernias

Contraindications

1. Obstructed/strangulated hernias
2. Ascites
3. Bleeding disorders

This surgery has surpassed the TAPP procedure and is turning out to be a promising procedure for management of hernias.

Procedure (Figs 70.55 to 70.57)

- Subumbilical incision (10 mm) placed
- **Extraperitoneal space** is created by passing the scope between the rectus muscle and the posterior rectus sheath medial to the muscle bundle edge.
- Initial dissection is carried out using laparoscope itself and **inflation of CO_2.**
- 2 more 5 mm ports are placed in the midline **4 cm and 8 cm below the 1st port respectively**.
- **Dissection** is carried out medially till the pubic tubercle, iliopectinate ligament and laterally till the iliac vessels and inferior epigastric vessels. Once adequate space is dissected, the sac is reduced by pulling it down from the inguinal canal (reduction of sac) and a 15 × 15 cm mesh is placed and spread.
- Mesh may be sutured, left as it is or fixed with tackers.
- Both sides can be done together through the same ports.

Complications

1. Cord/vas injuries
2. Inadvertent opening of the sac/peritoneum and creation of pneumoperitoneum
3. Seroma formation
4. Infection

Advantages of TEP

1. Approach is totally extraperitoneal
2. Smaller incisions
3. No need for fixing mesh
4. Peritoneum is intact

SILS (LESS)

Introduction

- Single port access (SPA) surgery, also known as laparoendoscopic single-site surgery (LESS), single incision laparoscopic surgery (SILS) or single port incision less conventional equipment-utilising surgery (SPICES) or embryonic natural orifice transluminal endoscopic surgery (E-NOTES) is an advanced minimally invasive surgical procedure in which the surgeon operates almost exclusively through a single entry point, typically the patient's navel.
- SPA surgical procedures are like many laparoscopic surgeries in that the patient is under general anaesthesia; insufflated and laparoscopic visualisation is utilised.
- In laparoendoscopic single-site surgery (LESS), a single small incision is used at the entry point rather than four to five small incisions.
- All surgical instruments are placed through this small incision and also the incision site is located in the left abdomen or umbilicus. In general, SILS techniques take the same amount of time to do as traditional laparoscopic surgeries.
- However, SILS is recognised as to be a more complicated procedure because it involves manipulating three articulating instruments through one access port.

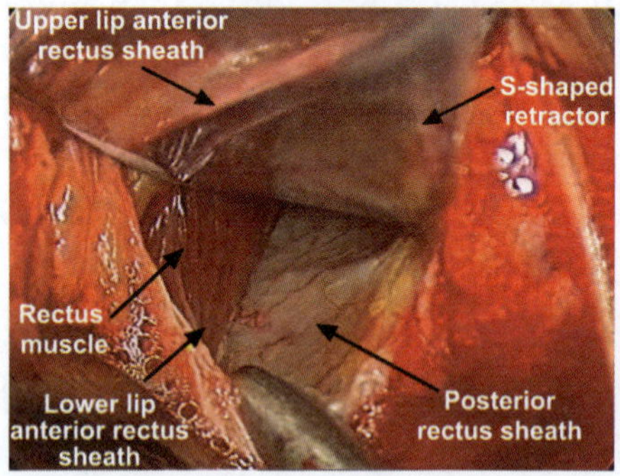

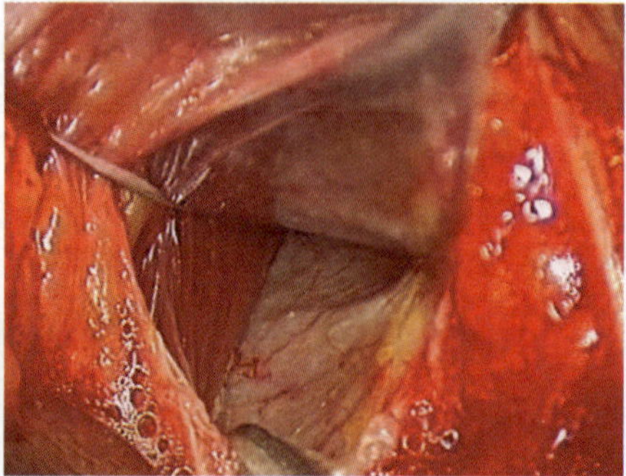

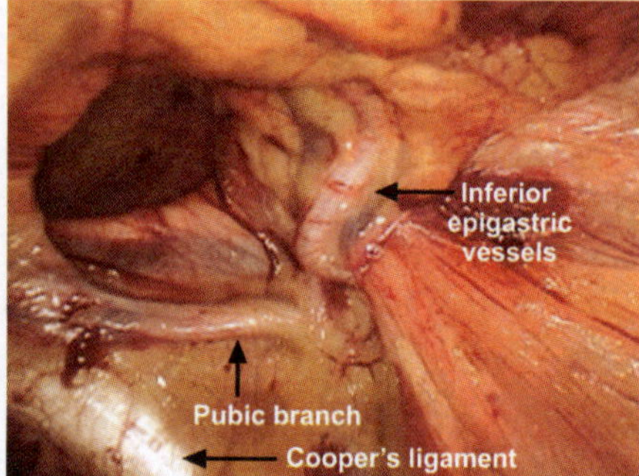

Figs 70.55 to 70.57: Totally extraperitoneal repair (TEP) (*Courtesy:* Dr Praveen Bhatia, Consultant Surgeon and Medical Director, Bhatia Global Hospital and Endosurgery Institute, New Delhi)

- Obesity, severe adhesions, or scarring from previous surgeries are a few cases, SILS may not be possible. Failure rates are high.

How SILS Differs from Traditional Laparoscopic Surgery?

- In single incision laparoscopic surgery, only one incision of around 1.5–2 cm is made just below the umbilicus to allow placement of three thin 5 mm port side by side parallel to each other.
- Port, a specially designed port is inserted into the abdomen; this port carries the telescope and laparoscopic instruments.
- Steps of surgical procedure are similar to the conventional laparoscopic surgery.
- As there is only one incision, pain is less as compared to traditional laparoscopic surgery and recovery is faster. The healed incision leaves practically no scar, thus making SILS cosmetically a superior option.
- In 5 to 10% patients, it may not be possible to complete the operation by SILS due to technical difficulties. One has to place one or two additional ports and completes the procedure in the traditional laparoscopic manner.

NATURAL ORIFICE TRANSLUMINAL ENDOSCOPIC SURGERY (NOTES)

Introduction

It means surgery performed endoscopically by initially passing the flexible endoscope through the body's natural orifices, like the mouth, anus, vagina, or urethra, to achieve access into areas that would not otherwise be accessible endoscopically, such as the abdomen and pelvis. Kalloo's did the first transgastric peritoneoscopy in 2004. In India, Dr GV Rao and Dr Nageshwar Reddy from Hyderabad, performed the first—NOTES in a patient who had appendicitis with extensive scars over the abdominal wall. The entry from abdomen was not possible. They performed transoral, transgastric appendicectomy.

Advantages

- Less invasive
- No abdominal incision
- Reduction in postoperative pain
- Wound infection, hernia formation and adhesions are very less.

Commonly Performed NOTES

- Transgastric appendectomy
- Transvaginal cholecystectomy

Future Upcoming Technologies

- Magnetically anchored and guidance systems (MAGS) are designed to manoeuvre intra-abdominal instruments. They use the external handheld magnet.
- The fundus of the gall bladder can be retracted above the costal margin by coupling the interior aspect of an external magnet. The graspers are situated on the gall bladder with the help of endoscopic biopsy forceps.
- Magnets may become valuable, within the operating room.

VAAFT TECHNIQUE

Introduction

It is performed for the surgical treatment of complex anal fistulas and their recurrences. Key points are the exact localisation of the internal fistula opening under vision, the fistula treatment from inside, and the hermetic closure of the internal opening. No risk of faecal incontinence as no sphincter damage—one of the great advantages over the conventional treatment.

Materials

- Fistuloscope, a unipolar electrode connected to a high frequency unit, a fistula brush and a forceps.
- A semicircular or linear stapler and 0.5 ml of synthetic cyanoacrylate with a tiny catheter are used as well.
- The fistuloscope is equipped with an optical channel, a working channel and an irrigation channel. The working length adds up to 18 cm; the use of a handle reduces it to an effective length of 14 cm.
- The optimal patient positioning is the lithotomy position. Spinal anaesthesia is required.
- The fistuloscope is connected to the Karl Storz equipment and to the washing solution bag (5000 cc glycine and mannitol 1% solution).

The Technique

It comprises a diagnostic phase and an operative phase.

The Diagnostic Phase

- The fistuloscope is inserted through the external fistula opening with the washing solution (glycine 1% and mannitol 1%) already running. Thus, it provides clear view of the fistula pathway which is seen on the screen.
- With right index finger in the rectum, fistuloscope is guided slowly into the fistula.
- Complete relaxation of the surrounding tissue induced by the spinal anaesthesia helps in gentle up and down movements to advance the fistuloscope.

- The continuous flow of the glycine-mannitol solution allows for an optimal view of the fistula's inside up to the internal opening.
- At this stage, insert an anal retractor in order to localise the internal fistula opening by looking for the light of the telescope in the rectum or anal canal.
- When the fistuloscope exits through the internal opening the rectal mucosa clearly appears on the screen. At this point, two or three stitches are put, in two opposite points of the internal opening margin in order to isolate those points and not to lose them.

The Operative Phase

- First locate the internal opening. From the internal opening to external opening, the fistula wall and all granulation tissues are coagulated. Procedure is done slowly so that fistula is destroyed under vision using a unipolar electrode. All the necrotic material is removed. Abscess cavity is irrigated.
- Fistuloscope is removed at this stage. The assistant stretches the threads towards the internal rectal space or rather the anal canal using a straight forceps in order to lift the internal fistula opening at least 2 cm into the shape of a volcano.
- Subsequently, stitch is inserted at the volcano's base and complete the mechanical cutting and suturing by using a linear stapler. The hermetic closure of the internal fistula opening can also be accomplished. This also depends on the internal opening position. Using a semicircular stapler, the suture will be horizontal. Using a linear stapler, the suture will be vertical.
- Last step is insertion of 0.5 ml of synthetic cyanoacrylate after the suture/staple line via the fistula pathway to further reinforce the suture. It helps in perfect closure of the fistula opening.
- This procedure assures a perfect excision and a hermetic closure of the internal fistula opening, excluding the risk of stool passage. Since the suture is situated tangential to the sphincter, the postoperative pain is low even if the suture falls both in the anal canal and the rectum.

Conclusion

- The advantages of the VAAFT technique are: No surgical wounds on the buttocks or in the perianal region, there is complete certainty in the localization of the internal fistula opening, and the fistula can be completely destroyed from the inside.
- Since operations are done from inside, no damage is caused to the anal sphincters. The risk of post-operative faecal incontinence is excluded.

ROBOTIC SURGERY

The term **robots** was introduced and coined in 1921, ***"robota"*** meaning forced labour. The first documented use of robotic-assisted surgery was in 1985. PUMA 560 robotic surgical arm was used successfully in a delicate neurosurgical biopsy, a non-laparoscopic surgery. The first laparoscopic procedure involving a robotic system was a cholecystectomy done in 1987. The following year the same PUMA system was used to perform a transurethral resection. da Vinci Surgical System is the first robotic system approved by the FDA for general laparoscopic surgery. The da Vinci system's 3D magnification screen allows the surgeon to view the operative area with the clarity of high resolution. The "Endo-wrist" features of the operating arms precisely replicate the skilled movements of the surgeon at the controls and filter out any shaking, greatly improving accuracy in small operating spaces. da Vinci system has been approved by the FDA for use in: Urological surgeries, general laparoscopic surgeries, general non-cardiovascular thoracoscopic surgeries and thoracoscopically-assisted cardiotomy procedures.

There are three different types of robotic surgery systems currently in use. The main difference between each system is how involved a human is in the process.

1. **Supervisory controlled systems:** The surgeon inputs data into the robot and the robot does all of the following surgery.
2. **Tele-surgical systems:** Cutting and sewing is performed by a surgeon at a console remote from the patient. The surgeon can be miles away at another site while performing this type of surgery.
3. **Shared control systems:** Doctors perform the work with the assistance of the robot technology, simultaneously.

Advantages

- Surgeons are able to perform more complex tasks (increases precision), physically easier, less awkward positioning for the surgeon. Procedures reduce the risk of death, complications, and hospital stay. It provides enhanced 3-D high-definition visualisation.
- For the patients: Reduced trauma to the body, less risk of infection along with faster recovery.

Disadvantages

- More expensive than traditional surgery.
- Removal of physical contact with surgery surface.
- The procedure can take nearly twice as long, depending on how well the surgeon knows the equipment.
- The size of the actual equipment can take up a lot of space inside the operating room.

- All operating instruments are NOT compatible with the technology required for robotic surgery.

Common procedures which can be done by da Vinci surgical system

Bladder cancer	Obesity
Colorectal cancer	Prostate cancer
Coronary artery disease	Throat cancer
Endometriosis	Uterine fibroids
Gynaecologic cancer	Uterine prolapse
Kidney cancer	Mitral valve prolapse

ENERGY SOURCES IN SURGERY

HIGH FREQUENCY (HF) ELECTROSURGERY

Principle involves passage of electric current through tissue by means of potential difference (voltage). The resultant flow of electrons excites the tissue molecules, notably water, creating heat energy which causes water evaporation and tissue coagulation. HF electrosurgery can be monopolar or bipolar. Here, the current escapes from electrode tip into the receptive tissue and exits through the grounding pad. Unmodulated continuous sine wave in voltage range 200–500 mV is used for **electrocutting** (Fig. 70.58).

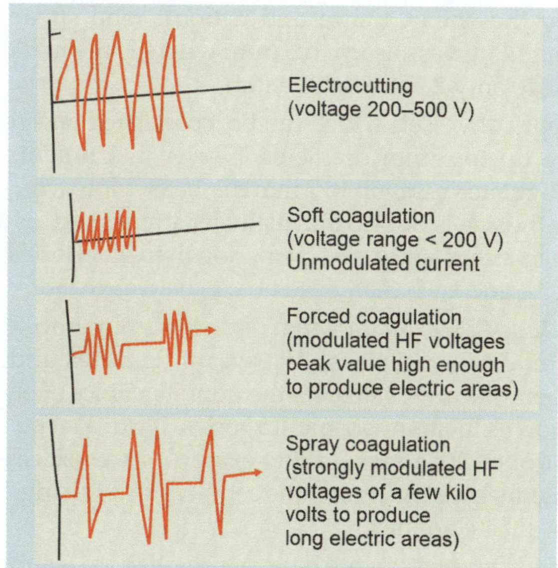

Fig. 70.58: Electrocautery

Uses of Electrocautery

1. To achieve haemostasis
2. Removal of skin tags
3. Treating very small, early basal cell carcinoma
4. Removal of erosions of cervix
5. Removal of condylomata, cutaneous acanthoma, warts, etc.

Bipolar Electrocautery

Heat energy is concentrated between two electrodes and does not dissipate throughout the tissue. Hence,

- Small volume of tissue is injured
- Less risk of burning injury
- Safe with pacemakers
- Excellent for obtaining haemostasis in areas that may be in close proximity to delicate structures, e.g. head and neck surgery.

Pearls of Wisdom

Effective in wet fields, uses coagulation current only.

Monopolar Electrocautery (Fig. 70.59)

Heat energy and thus tissue injury can extend for some distance away from the point of contact. Hence, great care should be taken to avoid:

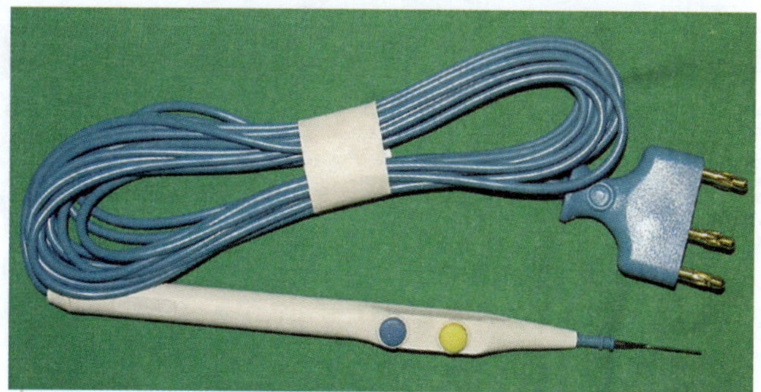

Fig. 70.59: Cautery cord: Yellow button is for cutting current and blue button is for coagulation

- Direct contact with a hollow viscus as this may lead to perforation.
- Close proximity to a major blood vessel as it may cause vessel wall injury.

Pearls of Wisdom

Not effective in wet fields, uses both cutting and coagulation current. Therefore, dissection is possible.

HARMONIC SCALPEL

- It is a high frequency mechanical energy device which uses ultrasound technology. This instrument has a hand held ultrasound transducer and scalpel. While using by hand or foot pedal, scalpel vibrates in the range of 20,000–55,500 Hz. During this process it cuts the tissues and seals the tissues. Process of sealing is by protein denaturation. No ligatures are required and perfect haemostasis is obtained. Scalpels have different sizes. It has three compatible probes that are the shear, blade and a hook. The shear can coagulate vessels up to 5 mm, whereas the hook and blade only 2 mm in diameter.

- Types of vessels which can be coagulated and sealed are up to 5 mm diameter. Newer instruments can coagulate vessel up to 7 mm diameter. However, to be on the safer side, 4–5 mm diameter arteries such as right colic artery and veins, superior thyroid arteries and veins and such many vessels can be sealed and cut.
- ***Advantages of harmonic scalpel:*** No smoke, no lateral thermal tissue injury, no ligatures and less operative time. Thus it is the popular choice of energy sources in laparoscopic surgeries. It can also be used for open surgeries—a few examples are excision of pile masses (haemorrhoidectomy) and raising flaps for mastectomies.
- ***Disadvantages:*** More time for coagulation. A spurting artery can be ligated by a haemostat or coagulated by cautery than harmonic scalpel. It is costly.

LASERS IN SURGERY

- **L**ight **A**mplification by **S**imulated **E**mission of **R**adiation
- Molecules which are placed in a compact area are activated when power is passed through. As a result of this, they move in different directions, they hit each other, releasing energy. This energy is used as laser to the area whenever required.

Types

1. Argon laser
2. Neodymium: Yttrium-aluminium-garnet laser (Nd:YAG laser)
3. CO_2 laser
4. Neon laser

Advantages and Disadvantages

- Most important advantage is a bloodless field—specially useful in head and neck surgeries and ENT surgeries.
- It is quick and there is less tissue trauma
- Expensive

Precaution

To avoid injuries to normal tissues, all reflecting instruments should be avoided so that the laser does not get reflected.

Pearls of Wisdom

All theatre personnel should wear special protective goggles.

Clinical Applications

1. Vascular malformation of the GIT
2. Endoscopic laser for advanced carcinoma oesophagus to relieve obstruction and dysphagia.
3. Obstructed colorectal cancer
4. **Liver resections:** Nd:YAG laser combined with CUSA can be used for liver resections.
5. CO_2 laser and Nd:YAG laser can be used for haemorrhoidectomy.

MISCELLANEOUS

WHEN TO DO PROPHYLACTIC SURGERY?

- Prophylactic bilateral mastectomy in BRCA 1 and BRCA 2 patients.
- Prophylactic total colectomy and ileoanal pouch in familial polyposis coli patients.
- Prophylactic total thyroidectomy in familial medullary carcinoma thyroid patients.
- Prophylactic cholecystectomy in Pima Indians.
- Prophylactic vagal sparing transhiatal oesophagectomy (THE) for severe dysplasia.
- Prophylactic gastrectomy-E-cadherin mutation.

PLEASE READ THESE INSTRUCTIONS

Students are requested to confirm the list of operations which will be asked in the examination with their teachers in their respective medical colleges and be prepared for exams. You should realise that what operation an undergraduate student is expected to know in more detail is not stated clearly in the syllabus. Nevertheless, you do not lose anything trying to understand more operations. Rather, it may help you in your postgraduate entrance examinations.

- The last four chapters are important for viva voce examination in general surgery. The questions given in these chapters are most commonly asked. This does not mean, however, that they are the only questions asked. As the subject is vast, the number of questions that can be asked can be unlimited. The purpose of viva voce section is to see how much the student knows as well as the depth and understanding of the subject.

Our best wishes to you once again. Enjoy reading Manipal Manual of Surgery, 6th edition—Authors

Index

This Index consists of two sections.

First section lists out important points for ease of reference during examination time grouped as:

- Classifications
- Criteria
- Disease
- Grading
- Method
- Operation
- Point
- Procedure
- Repair
- Rule
- Scoring system
- Signs
- Space
- Staging
- Syndromes
- Technique
- Tests
- Triads
- Triangles

Second section contains key-terms/keywords arranged alphabetically according to standard format.

Classifications

Abdominal tuberculosis 755
Amit Jain's classification 164, 170
ASA classification 48
Bismuth classification 628
Beahrs classification 880
Boyd's classification 177
Broder's classification 256
Bormann's classification 576
D'egidio classification 657
Enneking classification 299
European Hernia Society 935
Fontaine classification 179
Forrest classification 563
Gharbi classification 673
Gilbert 935
Gries Field modification of Martin's classification 850
Hinchey classification 813
Japanese 575
Johnson classification 556
Lauren's classification 575
Marseille's classification 646
Mathur's classification 691
Memorial Sloan-Kettering Cancer Centre: Lateral lymph node classification 339
Modified Atlanta classification 646
Modified Savary-Miller classification 515
Nyhus 935
Park's classification 891
Prague classification 520
REAL 221
Rutherford classification 179
Shamblin classification 330
Siewert classification 534
Standard classification of fistula *in ano* 890
Strasberg classification 628
Todani classification 631
WHO classification—testicular tumurs 1105
WHO classification—lymphoma 221
WHO classification of colorectal cancer 802
WHO-informal working group of echinococcosis (WHO-IWGE) (USG classification) 673
Woolner classification 415

Criteria

Amsterdam criteria II 796
Azzopardi and Salvadori criteria 472
Balthazar-Ranson criteria 651
Bathesda criteria 428
Epstein criteria 1088
Modified child's criteria 691
RECIST criteria 272

Disease

Caroli's disease 632
Cowden's disease 478
Menetrier's disease 574
Ormond's disease 745
Reeclin's disease 472
Schimmelbusch disease 463
Von-Recklinghausen's disease 293
Wilkie's disease 594

Grading

Crile's grading 404
Elston-Ellis modification of the SBR grading system (Nottingham grading system) 487
Roger Barnes' grading 1083
Splenic injury CT scan grading 703
Wagner grading system 167

Method

Bisgaard's method 241
Crile's method 401
Lahey method 401
Naffziger's method 409
Pizzillo's method 401
Zieman's method 938

Operation

Bishop-Koop operation 850
Charles excision operation 219
Cockett and Dodd 240
Commando's operation 345
Crile's operation 343
En bloc oesophagectomy—McKeown 533
Fowler's operation 146
Hartmann's operation 874
High operation of McEvedy 951
Ivanissevich operation 1104
Ivor Lewis operation 532
Kuntz operation 943
Low operation of Lockwood 950
May-Husni operation 241
Miles-Walker operation 871
Milnes-Walker operation 693
Palma operation 241
Palomo's operation 1104
Peustow's operation 636
Santulli operation 851
Sistrunk operation 324
Swiss-roll operation (Thompson's) 219
Transhiatal resection—Orringer 533
Trendelenburg's operation 239
Triple bypass 627
Whipple's resection 626
Zadik's operation 146

Point

Griffith's point 791
Murphy's point 617
Sudek point 791
McBurney's point 916
Sir Philip Manson-Bahr's amoebic point 775

Procedure

Altemeier's procedure 881
Bascom's technique 896
Bunnell's procedure 151
Chevasu's procedure 1108
Csendes procedure 559
Delorme's procedure 881
Devascularisation procedure 693
Duhamel's pull-through surgery 848
Frey procedure 636
Gastric transection of Tanner 694
Hans Beger procedure 636
Hartmann's procedure 829
Head coring procedure 636
Karydaki's procedure 896
Ladd procedure 858
Ober's and Barr's procedure 151
Ombredanne's procedure 1103
Paul Brand's procedure 151
Portosystemic shunt procedure 694
Silber's procedure 1103
Sugiura and Futagawa operation 694
Traverso-Longmire procedure 626
Wangensteen invertogram 851
Warren's shunt 697

Repair

Lichtenstein repair 941
Mayo repair 955

Nyhus repair 942
Shouldice repair 942
Stoppa repair 943

Rule

Goodsall's rule 891
Rule of 10 for cleft palate repair 373
Rule of 2 for Meckel's diverticulum 831
Rule of 6 for pseudocyst 658
Rule of 10 for cleft lip 373
Shenoy's Manipal rule of 2 381
Wallace rule of 9 278

Scoring system

Alvarado scoring system 920
APACHE II score 722
Child-Turcotte-Pugh (CTP) score 681
Courvoisier's law 617
Johnson-DeMeester's scoring system 515
Ranson's score 651
SOFA score 722
The Manheim peritonitis index (MPI) score 721

Signs

Angell's sign 1105
Ballance's sign 704
Berry sign 401
Blumberg's sign 725, 824, 918
Boas' sign 609
Branham's sign 336
Characterless loop of Wangensteen 825
Chilaiditi's sign 997
Chovstek's sign 438
Colon 'cut-off' sign 650
Cullen's sign 650
Curtain sign 383
Dalrymple's sign 408
Dance's sign—signe de dance 837
Deming's sign 1104
Dunphy sign 725, 918
Enroth sign 408
Fleischner's sign 757, 1232
Football sign 561
Froment's sign 203
Gaur sign 950
Gifford's sign 408
Grey Turner's sign 650
Hamman's sign 538
Homan's sign 163
Hook sign 143
Howship Romberg sign 964
Hutchinson's sign 263
Joffroy sign 408
Kanavel's sign 143
Kehr's sign 704
Kocher's sign 408
London sign 989
Lyre sign 330
Mercedez Benz sign 610
Milian's ear sign 120
Moebius sign 408
Moses' sign 163
Murphy's sign 608
Nicoladoni's sign 336
Pemberton's sign 406
Platysma sign 340
Prehn's sign 1105
Pseudokidney sign 837
Quincke's sign 181
Raccoon's eye sign 449
Rigler's sign 561
Rust sign 337
Rovsing sign 918, 1041
Sea Gull sign 610
Sentinel loop sign 650
Sign of groove 1098
Split pleura sign 1134
Stellwag sign 408
Stemmer's sign 216
Stierlin's sign 757, 1232
String sign of Kantor 772
Target sign 826
Torricelli-Bernoulli sign 586
Troisier's sign 754
Trousseau's sign 438, 641
Ugly duckling sign 260
Von Graefe's sign 408

Space

Cricothyroid space of Reeves 396
Prevesical space of Retzius 1305
Space of Bogros 1305
Space of Parona 142

Staging

Amit Jain's staging 165
Astler-Coller modification of Dukes' staging 802, 867
Cotswolds revision of the Ann Arbor staging system 222
Dukes' staging for colorectal cancer 802
Masaoka's clinical stage 1137
Modified Dukes' staging of carcinoma of rectum 867
TNM staging of cancers
  basal cell 252
  breast 487
  bronchogenic 1142
  colon 803
  epithelioma 252
  hepatocellular 681
  melanoma 264
  oesophagus 531
  oral cavity 352
  penis 1094
  prostate 1085
  rectum 867
  renal cell carcinoma 1057
  soft tissue sarcoma 299
  stomach 578
  testis 1107
  thyroid 417
  urinary bladder 1067

Syndromes

Abdominal Cocoon syndrome 856
AIDS anus syndrome 153
Bloom's syndrome 297
Boerhaave syndrome 538
Crest syndrome 199
Cronkhite-Canada syndrome 777
Carotid body syndrome 330
Cushing's syndrome 447
Digeorge syndrome 438
Eisenmenger's syndrome 1144
Fanconi syndrome 297
Felty syndrome 714
Fitz-Hugh-Curtis syndrome 720
Frey's syndrome 389
Gorlin syndrome 250
Horner's syndrome 347
Hovels-Evans syndrome 526
Kasabach-Merritt syndrome 677
Klinefelter's syndrome 470
Klippel-Trénaunay syndrome 229
Leriche's syndrome 179
Lesch-Nyhan syndrome 1043
Li-Fraumeni syndrome 473
Lynch's syndrome I and II 796
Mallory-Weiss syndrome 569
MEN syndromes 425
Mirizzi syndrome 613
Murphy's syndrome 918
Ogilvie's syndrome 829
Osler-Rendu-Weber syndrome 335
Pancoast's syndrome 347
Pendred's syndrome 398
Peutz-Jeghers syndrome 776, 906
Plummer-Vinson syndrome 523
Poland's syndrome 456
Postcibal syndromes 589
Prader-Willi syndrome 597
Sezary syndrome 226
Sipple syndrome 425
Sjögren's syndrome 390
SMA syndrome 595
Stewart-Treves syndrome 498
Sturge-Weber syndrome 335
TURP syndrome 1084
Valentino syndrome 723
Vasculitis syndromes 206
Von Hippel-Lindau syndrome 450
Wiskott-Aldrich syndrome 708
Zollinger-Ellison syndrome 552, 645

Technique

Fowler-Stephens technique 1102
Lilly's technique 632
Tessari technique 238

Tests

Adson's test 203
Allen's test 204
Card test 203
Copes test 918
Elevated arm stress test (EAST) 204
Fegan's method (test) 235
Gornall's test 939
Halsted test 203
Kocher's test 401
Mallampati test 1167
Military attitude test 23
Modified Perthes' test 235
Morrissey's test 234
Multiple tourniquet test 235
Pemberton's test 222
Traction test 1099
Trendelenburg test 234

Triads

Beck's triad 68
Borchardt's triad 592
Carney's triad 779
Charcot's triad 618
Cushing's triad 1155
Gilroy Benan triad 834
Hutchinson's triad 151
Mackler's triad 638
Murphy's triad 918
Reynold's pentad 619
Rigler's triad 836
Saint's triad 519
Tillaux's triad 744, 1017
Triad of Sandblom 697
Trotter's triad 340
Virchow's triad 243
Whipple's triad of insulinoma 644

Triangles

Beahrs triangle 396
Calot's triangle 602
Hesselbach's triangle 935
Passaro's triangle 645
Riddle's triangle 396
Sherren's triangle 918
Triangle of Doom 1305
Triangle of Grynfelt 963
Triangle of Petit 963
Triangle of pain 1305
Triangle of safety 1130

ABCDE
  acute abdomen 562
  mole 261
  perforation 562
Abdominal mass 1004
  clinical examination 1004
  mass in the epigastrium 1019
  mass in the right hypochondrium 1020
  mass in the right iliac fossa 1012
  mass in the right lumbar region 1022
  mass in the umbilical region 1015
  renal mass 1059
  the cystic mass 1016
Abdominal tap 727
Abdominal wall 971
  dehiscence 971
  divarication of recti 974
  rectus sheath hematoma 975
  wound closure 974
Abdominoperineal resection 871
ABG 82
ABPI 183
Abscess 111
  chronic 120
  cold 113, 329, 337
  pyaemic 112
  pyogenic 111
  ulnar nerve 151
Acid–base disorders 78
Acral lentiginous melanoma 262
Acrocyanosis 209
Actinomycosis 148
  abdominal 149
Acute adrenal insufficiency 67
Acute arterial occlusion 191
  embolic occlusion 191
Acute lower limb ischaemia
  signs 191
Adamantinoma 369
Adenoid cystic carcinoma 387
Adenolymphoma 386
Adenomatous polyp 574
Adoptive cell transfer 272
Adrenal glands 446
  adrenal insufficiency 448
  anatomy, physiology 446
  disorders of adrenal cortex 447
  neuroblastoma 448
  phaeochromocytoma 450
AIDS 152
Ainhum 195
Albumin 94
Amelanotic melanoma 262
Amelita Galli-Curci nerve 396
Amit Jain's
  triple assessment 172
Amoebic dysentery 778
Amoebic typhlitis 775
Amoeboma 776
AMPLE 988
Anaesthesiology 1165
  airway 1168
  caudal 1180
  complications of anaesthesia 1181
  endotracheal intubation 1169
  epidural 1178
  general anaesthetic agents 1166
  local anaesthetics 1174
  monitoring in anaesthesia 1173
  muscle relaxants
  preoperative assessment and
    premedication 1166
  regional anaesthesia 1173
  spinal anaesthesia 1177
Anal incontinence 898
Anal intraepithelial neoplasia 897
Analgesia 24
Anderson-Hynes pyeloplasty 1050
ANDI 461
Andy Gump deformity 356
Aneurysm
  carotid 329
  effects 310
  popliteal 194
Angiodysplasia 911
Angiogram
  CT 185
  magnetic resonance 186
Angiography 1232
  CT 1233
  retrograde 1233
Angioplasty 193
Anion gap 81
Anorectal abscess 889
Anterior resection 870
Antibiotics 44
  prophylaxis 44, 125
  therapeutic 45
Anticoagulation 245
Antisepsis 34 ,125
Antiseptics 36
Antithyroid drugs 412
Aorta
  aneurysm 1149
  coarctation 1145
  ruptured aneurysm 1150
Aortoiliac endarterectomy 189
Apathetic thyrotoxicosis 413
Appendix 914
  acute appendicitis 916
  appendicular abscess 924
  appendicular mass 923
  complications 923
  development and anomalies 914
  differential diagnosis 920
  faecal fistula 927
  mucocele 928
  neoplasm 928
  surgical anatomy 915
  Valentino appendix 929
Arc of Riolan 791
Aromatase inhibitors 494
Arterynof Drummond 791
Ascitic fluid analysis 757
Asepsis 34, 125
Aspergilloma 1139
Ataxia telangiectasia 472
Atherosclerosis 182
Audit 14
Auriculotemporal nerve 389
Autologous transfusion 75
AV fistula 335
AVPU system 983
Axillary tail hypertrophy 470
Axillary vein thrombosis 206

Balloon angioplasty 190
Balloon tamponade 693
Bariatric surgery 597
Barium studies 1226
  barium enema 1231
  barium meal 1227
  barium swallow 1226
Barron's band application 885
Batson's venous plexus 458
Batwing excision 505
Bazin's ulcer 163
Bile 603
Biliary ascariasis 640
Biliary hydatid 640
Biochemotherapy 271
Biological mesh 942
Biomedical waste (BMW) 27
BIRADS 484
Bisphosphonates 445, 497
Block dissections
  axillary 491
  catalona 1095
  ilioinguinal 267
  inguinal 270

radical neck 339
retroperitoneal 1108
selective neck 343
Blood transfusion 72
autologous 75
cryoprecipitate 73
complications 74
fresh frozen plasma 73
massive 63, 75
packed red blood cells 72
platelets 73
Blunt abdominal trauma 978
blast injuries 984
blunt abdominal trauma 987
chest injuries 1126
colonic injuries 996
duodenal injuries 996
gunshot wounds 985
liver injuries 992
mass casualities 986
missile wounds 985
pancreatic injuries 997
prehospital phase 978
primary survey 978
retroperitoneal haematoma 999
small bowel injuries 994
soft tissue injuries 1000
triage 979
vascular injuries 1001
warfare injuries 984
Bogota bag 732
Boil 118
Botulinum toxin 525, 960
Bowen's disease 249, 897, 1092
Brachial plexus block 1180
Brachytherapy 1206
Brainstem death 1162
Brain tumours 1160
Branchial cyst 328
BRCA 472
Breast 455
aberrations of normal development and involution 463
acute bacterial mastitis 458
angiosarcoma of the breast 499
antibioma 460
breast reconstruction 499
carcinoma breast 472
BCS 492
clinical 478
colloid 478
ductal carcinoma *in situ* (DCIS) 474
inflammatory 477
invasive 476
LABC 494, 505
lobular carcinoma *in situ* 475
medullary 477
mucinous 478
Paget's disease 477
radiotherapy 493
treatment 489
congenital anomalies 456
duct papilloma 469
fibroadenoma
galactocele 468
galactorrhoea 469
gynecomastia 470
idiopathic granulomatous mastitis 467
intracystic carcinoma of breast
macrocysts 468
male breast carcinoma 503
oncoplastic breast conservation surgery 504
phyllodes tumours 471
plasma cell mastitis 466
retromammary abscess
surgical anatomy 456
Breslow thickness 261
Bronchogenic carcinoma 1140
Bronchopleural fistula 1135
Buerger's
angle 181
disease 182
exercises 187
lymphoma 226
postural test 181
Burkitt's lymphoma 226
Burns 277
care 280
chemical 283
classification 278
electrical 282
management 278
shock 278
surgery 282
Bursa 315
Burst abdomen 972
Buschke-Lowenstein tumour 1092
Bypass grafts 188

CABG 1146, 1148
Café au lait spots 293
Calciphylaxis 445
Calcium 91, 438
Cancer 295
adrenocortical carcinoma 448
basal cell 249
breast 472
buccal mucosa 354
chimney sweep 255
colon 796
countryman's lip 255
early detection 1215
epithelioma 249
gastric 572
kang 255
kangri 255
lip 362
Marjolin's 249
maxillary antrum 365
melanoma 259
nasopharynx 366
oesophagus
oral cavity 349
salivary glands 383
screening 1217
thyroid 414
tongue 358
Cancer-en-cuirasse 498
Cancrum oris 209
Capsule endoscopy 907
Capsule obstruction 857
Carbuncle 30, 119
Carcinoembryonic antigen (CEA) 805
Cardiac tamponade 67
Carotid body tumour 330
CBNAAT 117
CEAP classification 232
Cellulitis 109
Cells of Cajal 779
Central venous pressure 69
Cervical rib 202
Chain of lakes appearance 622
Chassaignac tubercle 401
Chemodectoma 330
Chemotherapy 1212
breast 493
gastric cancer 585
lymphoma 223
melanoma 272
neoadjuvant 495
Chest trauma 1125
blunt trauma 1126
mediastinal emphysema 1133
myocardial contusion 1132
pulmonary injuries 1127
surgical emphysema 1132
tracheobronchial injuries 1131
Chiba needle 622
Chlonorchiasis 640
Choledochal cyst 630
Choledocholithiasis 618
Chordoma 295
Christmas disease 76
Chromoendoscopy 529
Chronic hyperplastic candidiasis 351
Chyluria 226
Circular anal dilator 887
Cleft lip 371
Cleft palate 372
Clinical examination
varicose veins 233
Clinical research 16
Cock's peculiar tumour 313
Cold abscess 113
Colectomy 806
Collar stud abscess 115
Collateral circulation 176
Colloids 93
Colon screening 811
Colonic pouch 890
Colonic stricture 816
Colonoscopy 810
virtual 1236
Colostomy 871, 875
Common bile duct stricture 628
Communication 6
Compartment syndrome 104
Computerised tomography 1036
Complications
MRM 490
thyroidectomy 431
Compound palmar ganglion 314
Congenital biliary atresia 639
Congenital megacolon 826
Conley's pointer 385
Consent 6
Constipation 792
Contractures 282
Core biopsy 484
Corn 274

Corona mortis 1305
Counselling 7
Courvoisier's law 617
Cowden's disease 478
Critical limb ischaemia 192
Crohn's disease 770
Crystalloids 93
CT scan 1235
CVP 69
CyberKnife 1211
Cystic pancreatic neoplasms 643
Cystic swellings 308
    epidermal cyst 312
Cystogastrostomy 658
Cystojejunostomy 658
Cystourethrography 1034
Cytokines 54

Damage control surgery 983
Deep vein thrombosis 243
Denonvilliers' fascia 862
Dentigerous cyst 368
Dermoid cyst 310, 321
Desmoid tumour 975
Devascularisation procedure 694
Dextran 94
Diabetic foot 164
    neuropathy 164
Diagnostic laparoscopy 728
Diagnostic peritoneal lavage 705, 990
Diaphragm
    hernia
    injuries 1131
DIC 75
Dietl's crisis 1049
Dieulafoy vascular malformation 570
Disappearing pulse 181
Diverticular disease of the colon 811
Doppler 236
Doppler-guided haemorrhoidal artery ligation 888
Duodenum
    blow out 591
    chronic duodenal ileus 594
    duodenal ulcer 553
    obstruction
Duplex scan 184, 236

ECOG 681
Ectopic salivary gland tumour 373
Electrolytes 42, 85
Elephantiasis neuromatosa 293
Eloesser drainage 1135
Embolism
    air 196
    atheroma 191
    fat 196
Empyema 1134
Empyema necessitans 460, 1136
Endometriosis 976
Endoscopic retrograde cholangiopancreaticography (ERCP) 621
Endotherapy 692
Endoscopy 556, 691, 1036
Endovenous laser ablation 238
Enhanced recovery program 808
Enteroclysis 1228
Enterocutaneous fistula 783, 927

Epididymal cyst 1101
Epididymis 1098
Epididymo-orchitis 1100
Epithelioma 254
Epulis 370
ERAS 808
ERCP 621
Erysipelas 120
Erythroplasia of Queyrat 1092
ESWL 1045
Ethics 10, 16

Fascial nerve 377
    repair 390
FAST 990
FASTHUG 1131
Feeding gastrostomy 41
Feeding jejunostomy 41
Felon 140
Femoropopliteal occlusion 189
Fibroma 289
Fibromatosis 975
    penis 1097
Filarial elephantiasis 215
Finney pyloroplasty 559
Fissurectomy 895
Fistula 127
    branchial 328
    colovesical fistula 803
    enterocutaneous 815
    fecal fistula 803, 815
    internal fistula 803, 813
    parotid 390
    salivary 386
    thyroglossal 324
    tracheo-oesophageal 543
Fistula *in ano* 890
Fistulectomy 891
Fistulotomy 891
Flail chest 1127
Flaps 254, 284
    Abbe 254, 363
    Boari 1053
    Estlander 254, 363
    Karapandzic 364
    PMMC 254, 286, 358
    Webster-Bernard 254
Fluids 85
FNAC 484
Focussed assessment with sonography for trauma 990
Fogarty catheter 193
Foley criteria 1051
Footballer's ulcer 161
Fournier's gangrene 1109
Frostbite 195

Gallbladder 601
    acute cholecystitis 607
    carcinoma 638
    Caroli's disease 632
    cholangiocarcinoma 636
    cholecystoses 611
    choledochal cyst 630
    chronic cholecystitis 611
    chronic pancreatitis 633
    congenital anomalies 603
    congenital biliary atresia 637
    empyema and perforation 612
    gallstones disease 603
    laparoscopic cholecystectomy 613
    mucocele 611
    obstructive jaundice 615
    physiology 602
    sclerosing cholangitis 630
    stricture of CBD 628
    surgical anatomy 601
Ganglion 314
Gangrene 208
    drug use and abuse 209
    dry 208
    embolic 191
    gas 133
    ICU 196
    synergistic 975
    thrombosis 191
    wet 208
Gastrectomy 559, 581
Gastric antral vascular ectasia (GAVE) 570
Gastric outlet obstruction 570
Gastrinoma 552, 646
Gastrojejunocolic fistula 587
GI tract bleeding
    lower 902
    upper 565
Giant cell arteritis 206
Giacomini vein 231
Gilmore's groin 949
Glasgow coma scale 1155
Glasgow—check list 260
Glomus tumor 314
Glossectomy 361
Glucagonoma 646
Goitre 402
    iodine deficiency 403
    multinodular 402
    puberty 403
Golf hole ureter 1053
Gossypiboma 738
Graves' disease 407
Griffith's point 791
Gumma 152

H. pylori 527
Haemangioma 332
Haematuria 1114
Haemetemesis 565
Haemophilia 76
Haemorrhage 60
    control 64
    peptic ulcer 563
Haemorrhoidectomy 886
Haemothorax 1130
Hamartoma 295
Hand-held Doppler 183, 236
Hand infections 138
    deep palmar 141
    suppurating tenosynovitis 143
    terminal pulp space 140
    web space infection 141
Hartmann's pouch 601
Hashimoto's thyroiditis 430
Head injuries 1152
    chronic subdural haematoma 1156
    CSF rhinorrhoea 1158
    extradural haematoma 1154
    fracture skull 1157
    raised intracranial pressure 1157

Heart 1143
- atrial septal defect 1146
- congenital 1143
- patent ductus arteriosus 1144

Heinecke-Mickulicz pyloroplasty 558
Heller's cardiomyotomy 524
Hemicolectomy 806
Henderson equation 79
Hepatic resection 682
Hepatitis B 126
Hepatitis C 126
Hepatoma 677
HER 2 receptor 485
Hernia 932
- aetiology 935
- Bochdalek 542
- classification 935
- clinical examination 937
- complications 944
- direct 936
- epigastric 960
- femoral 949
- giant 946
- hernioplasty 941
- incisional 955
- indirect 935
- inflamed 946
- inguinal defence mechanism 934
- interparietal 961
- Littre's 948
- lumbar 963
- Maydl's 948
- Morgagni 542
- Narath's 952
- obturator 964
- Ogilvie 937
- parastomal 65
- perineal 964
- prevesical 948
- recurrent 946
- sliding 948
- Spigelian 962
- sportsmana 949
- umbilical 952
- ventral 958

Herpetic whitlow 140
Hidradenitis suppurativa 899
Highly selective vagotomy 557
Hill Ferguson haemorrhoidectomy 887
- stapler haemorrhoidopexy 887

Hilton's line 791
Hilton's method 112
HIPEC 742
Hippocratic facies 725
History of surgery 1268
Hodgkin's lymphoma 220
Homan's sign 163
Homeostasis 52
Hour glass contracture 572
Human chorionic gonadotrophin 1107
Hunterian chancre 152, 1098
Hurthle cell carcinoma 423
Hutchinson's melanotic freckle 261
Hydrocephalus 1158
Hydrocoele 1099
- bilocular 1099
- canal of Nuck 1100
- congenital 1099
- encysted 1099
- infantile 1099

Hydroxyethyl starch 94
Hyperbaric oxygen 77, 103
Hypercalcaemia 92
Hyperhomocysteinaemia 177
Hyperkalaemia 90
Hypermagnesaemia 91
Hypernatraemia 89
Hyperparathyroidism 439
- primary 439
- secondary 439
- tertiary 439

Hypertrophic scar 106
Hypervolaemia 87
Hypocalcaemia 92
Hypokalaemia 90
Hypomagnesaemia 91
Hyponatraemia 87
Hypoparathyroidism 438
Hypospadias 1076
Hypovolaemia 86

Idiopathic retroperitoneal fibrosis 745
Ileosigmoid knotting 855
Ilioinguinal nerve 933
Immunohistochemistry 32, 485
Immunonutrition 40
IMRT 1210
Incidentaloma 452
Induration 158
Infertility 1111
Ingrown toenail 146
Inguinodynia 944
Injury 53
- immune response 54
- neuroendocrine response 54

Instruments 1245–1254
Insulinoma 644
Intercostal tube 1129
Interferon alfa 270
Interleukin 54
Intermittent claudication 177
Internal anal sphincter 882
Interstitial cell tumours 1108
Intestinal fistulae 783
Intestinal obstruction 819
- abdominal Cocoon 856
- adhesions and bands 833
- arrested rotation with bands 850
- atresia and stenosis 848
- basic principles in management 826
- caecal volvulus and bascule 830
- food bolus obstruction 856
- gallstone ileus 836
- Hirschsprung's disease 846
- imperforate anus 851
- intussusception 837
- malrotation and midgut volvulus 858
- Meckel's diverticulum 831
- meconium ileus 850
- mesenteric vascular occlusion 842
- paralytic ileus 852
- pathophysiology 821
- sigmoid volvulus 828
- strictures 845
- volvulus neonatorum 850

Intraosseous cannulation 62
Intravenous fluids 66
Intussusception
- retrograde 587

Investigations 30
IRIS 116
Ischaemia
- lower limb 176

Ischemic colitis 911
Ischiorectal abscess 889
IVC filters 246

Jack-knife position 895
Jackson's zones 278
Jehovah's witness 12
Jod Basedow's disease 398

Keloid 106
Kernonhan's notch 1155
Kidney 1038
- horseshoe 1040
- hydronephrosis 1047
- perinephric abscess 1060
- polycystic 1039
- pyonephrosis 1060
- renal cell carcinoma 1055
- renal stones 1042
- renal tuberculosis 1051
- surgical anatomy 1038
- ureteric stone 1046
- Wilms' tumour 1054

Klatskin's tumour 617
Krukenberg tumours 457, 577
Ksharasutra 892

Laparoscopic mesorectal excision 870
Laparostomy 730
Large intestine 789
- carcinoma colon 796
- colon screening 811
- colonic function 792
- colonic stricture 816
- diverticular disease of colon 811
- faecal fistula 815
- surgical anatomy 789
- tumours 793
  - familial polyposis coli 794
  - hereditary nonpolyposis
  - polyps 793

Laryngocele 331
Lasers
- CO_2 254

Lateral anal sphincterotomy of Notaras 890
LDH 265
Leprosy 150
Leptospirosis 113
Leptin 597
Leukoplakia 350, 351
Leydig cell tumour 1108
LIFT (ligation of internal fistula tract) 892
Ligaments
- inguinal 932
- lacunar 932
- Poupart's 932

Lindsay tumour 415
Lip reconstruction 364
Lip repair 373

Lipodermatosclerosis 240
Lipoma 289
Liver
- amoebic abscess 669
- ascites in portal hypertension 696
- benign tumours 676
- Budd-Chiari syndrome 697
- fibrolamellar carcinoma 679
- haemangioma 676
- haemobilia 698
- hepatoma 678
- hydatid cyst 672
- liver resection 684
- liver transplantation 697, 1192
- liver cystic diseases 676
- physiology 667
- polycystic liver 676
- portal biliopathy 697
- portal gastropathy 697
- portal hypertension 688
- pyogenic abscess 668
- secondaries 685
- segmental anatomy 678
- surgical anatomy 666

Lloyd-Davies position 871
Lord's dilatation 895
Ludwig's angina 110, 320
Lumbar sympathectomy 187
Lund and Browder chart 278
Lymph nodes
- cloquet 950
- epitrochlear 225
- Irish 296, 577
- Lund 602
- Rotter's 457
- Virchow 1011

Lymphadenopathy 319
- cervical 320
- metastasis 338

Lymphangioma 317
Lymphangitis 111
- hand 139

Lymphoedema 210
Lymphoma
- anaplastic large cell 226
- gastric MALT 225
- HIV related 154

Madura foot 145
Maduramycosis 145
Maggot therapy 174
Malignant exophthalmos 410
Malignant lymphoma 781
Malignant melanoma 259
- clinical 263
- treatment 266
- types 262

Mammography 482
Mandibulectomy 357
Marjolin's ulcer 249
Martorell's ulcers 156, 163
Masaoka's clinical stage 1137
Mastalgia 463
Means-Lerman scratch 412
Mediastinum 1136
- anatomy 1136
- masses 1137

Medicolegal aspects
- burns injuries 286
- gunshot 985
- organ transplantation 1201

MELD score 1193
Meleney's gangrene 121, 975
Menetrier's disease 574
Meningioma 1161
Meningocele 319
Merkel cell carcinoma 274
Mesenteric cyst 744
Mesenteric venous thrombosis 843
Mesentery 743
Mesh rectopexy 881
Metabolic acidosis 80
Metabolic alkalosis 81
Metabolic response 52
MIBG scan 441
Mickey Mouse' sign 236
Micturating cystourethrography 1033
Mikulicz disease 390
Milker's nodes 144
Milligan-Morgan ligature and excision 886
Misty mesentery 743
Mithramycin 445
Moh's surgery 253
Mondor's disease 503
Morrant-Baker's cyst 316
Moynihan's hump 603
MRI 1238
MRSA infections 560
MR urography 1037
Mucoepidermoid tumours 386
Mucous cysts 374
Mycosis fungoides 222
Myonecrosis 135
Myopectineal orifice of Fruchaud 933

Naevus 259
Neck
- surgical anatomy 338
- lymphadenopathy 338
- dissections 341
- secondaries 338

Necrotising fasciitis 121
Needle thoracocentesis 68
Needles 1256–1258
Nerve repair 391
Neurilemmoma 293
Neuroblastoma 448
Neurofibroma 292
Neuroma 292
Non-Hodgkin's lymphoma (NHL) 224
NOTES 1303
Nosocomial infection 122
Null hypothesis 17
Numerical rating scale 23
Nutrition 38, 19
- BMR 39
- enteral 41
- malnutrition 38
- parenteral 42
- perioperative 40

Obstipation 823
Obstructive jaundice 615
Octreotide 697
Odontomes 367
Oesophagus 511
- achalasia cardia 523
- anatomy of the diaphragm 541
- Barrett's oesophagus 520
- carcinoma of 526
- corrosive oesophageal stricture 537
- diaphragmatic hernia 542
- differential diagnosis dysphagia 539
- diverticulum of 539
- fundoplication 517
- gastro-oesophageal reflux disease (GORD) 514
- hiatus hernia 518
- manometry 516
- nutcracker 526
- oesophageal perforations 538
- oesophagectomy 533
- physiology 513
- Plummer-Vinson syndrome 522
- rolling hernia 519
- sliding hernia 518
- surgical anatomy 511
- tracheo-oesophageal fistula 543

Operative surgery 1268
- abdominal incisions 1286
- amputations in leg 1282
- appendicectomy 1286
- Bassini's herniorrhaphy 1288
- circumcision 1275
- colectomy 1298
- Desarda repair 1292
- energy sources in surgery 1309
- excision of swellings 1270
- harmonic scalpel 1309
- incision and drainage (I and D) 1273
- incision and drainage of breast abscess 1274
- intestinal resection and anastomosis 1295
- laparoscopic surgery 1301
- lasers in surgery 1310
- natural orifice transluminal endoscopic surgery (NOTES) 1307
- open cholecystectomy 1293
- robotic surgery 1308
- SILS 1307
- skin closure techniques 1269
- staplers in surgery 1300
- surgery for hydrocele 1272
- TAPP 1305
- TEP 1306
- thyroidectomy 1279
- tracheostomy 1278
- upper limb amputations 1285
- VAAFT technique 1307
- vagotomy gastrojejunostomy (GJ) 1294
- vasectomy 1277
- venesection or cut down 1276

Organ transplantation 1191
- immunosuppression 1194
- islet cell 1198
- kidney 1194
- liver 1193
- small intestines 1196

Orphan Annie-eyed nuclei 415
Osmolality 86
Osmolarity 86
Osteomyelitis 128
OTC—On-table cholaniography 625

Pachydermatocoele 294
Paget's disease
- penis 1092

bone 1086
nipple 477
Pain 22
chronic pain 25
neuropathic pain 25
nociceptive pain 25
psychogenic pain 25
PAIR 675
Pancoast's tumour 347
Pancreas
acute pancreatitis 646
annular 660
carcinoma of 640
chronic pancreatitis 633
cystic fibrosis 661
distal pancreatectomy 659
ectopic 660
endocrine tumours 644
islet cell transplantation 663
pancreatic abscess 656
pancreatic ascites 663
pancreatic divisum 661
pancreatic fistula 662
pancreatic necrosectomy 654
pseudocyst 657
surgical anatomy 615
Papilloma 288
Paradoxical aciduria 571
Paraneoplastic syndromes 297
Parathyroid glands
acute hypercalcaemic crisis 445
autotransplantation 443
cryopreservation 444
endoscopic parathyroidectomy 444
hyperparathyroidism 440
physiology 438
surgical anatomy 437
tetany 438
minimally invasive endoscopic parathyroidectomy (MIP) 445
Paronychia 138
Parotid gland 377
acute parotitis 378
parotidectomy 385
surgical anatomy 377
tumours 382
Patey's modified radical mastectomy 490
PCNL 1045
Pelvic congestion syndrome 246
Penis 1091
fracture 1110
carcinoma 1092
paraphimosis 1092
Peyronie's disease
phimosis 1092
surgical anatomy of 1091
ulcer 1097
Percutaneous endoscopic gastrostomy 41
Perianal abscess 889
Pericardiocentesis 68
Pericolic abscess 803
Periodic peritonitis 741
Perioperative care 19, 92
Peritoneum 719
abdominal compartment syndrome 730
acute peritonitis—scoring system 720
complications of peritonitis 732
pelvic abscess 732
subphrenic abscess 733
intra-abdominal sepsis 720
peritoneal lavage 729
special types of peritonitis 736
tumours 741
carcinoma peritonei 742
pseudomyxoma peritonei 741
PET scan 1241
Peterson's hernia 965
Peyronie's disease 1097
Phaeochromocytoma 450
Pharyngeal pouch 332
Phrygian cap 603
Pigtail catheter drainage 672
Piles 884
Pleomorphic adenoma 382
Plethysmography 237
Plexiform neurofibromatosis 293
Preoperative care 19
Plummer disease 412
Pneumothorax 990, 1127
POEM 525
Portal hypertension 688
Portocaval shunt 695
mesentericocaval shunt 695
Portosystemic shunts 694
Portwine stain 333
Postcibal syndromes 589
Postoperative care 20
Pott's puffy tumour 313, 1158
Pressure sore 153
Pretibial myxoedema 410
Priapism 1110
Primary hyperaldosteronism 447
Proctalgia fugax 899
Proctocolectomy 768
Proctoscopy 863
Prostate 1081
carcinoma 1084
Gleason score 1087
prostatitis 1088
surgical anatomy 1081
benign prostatic hyperplasia (BPH) 1082
Prostate specific antigen 1087
Pruritus ani 899
Psammoma bodies 415
Pseudohyponatraemia 89
Pseudointestinal obstruction 854
Pseudomesenteric cyst 760
Pseudosclerosing cholangitis 697
Psoas abscess 746
PUJ dysfunction 1049
Pulmonary thromboembolism 246
Push enteroscopy 907
Pyloric stenosis 570
Pyogenic granuloma 146, 363
Pyomyositis 122
Splenorenal shunt 695

QUART therapy by Veronesi 492

Radiation 1203
electronic beam therapy 1206
exposure 36
reactions 1209
sources 1205
Radiofrequency ablation 239
Radioisotope scanning 1036
Ram's horn penis 210
Ramstead pyloromyotomy 594
Ranula 318
Raynaud's disease 199
Reeclin's disease 472
Rectum and anal canal 861
anal incontinence 898
anorectal abscess 889
anorectal physiology 883
carcinoma rectum 864
fissure *in ano* 893
fistula *in ano* 890
haemorrhoids 884
malignant tumours 897
pilonidal sinus 895
prolapse rectum 877
rectal ulcer 866
rectovesical pouch 862
sacrococcygeal teratoma 896
surgical anatomy 861
surgical anatomy of anal canal 882
VAAFT 893
Recurrent laryngeal nerve 396
paralysis 431
Renal arteriography 1033
Reperfusion injuries 194
Research studies 17
Respiratory acidosis 80
Respiratory alkalosis 81
Retrograde pyelography 1030
Retroperitoneal cyst 746, 1018
Retroperitoneal abscess 746
Retroperitoneal sarcoma 747
Retroperitonel tumour 746
Retroperitoneum 745
Retrosternal goiter 406
Riedel's thyroiditis 430
Risus sardonicus 131

Saegesser's splenic point of tenderness 704
Safe surgery 50, 51
Salivary gland 380
anatomy 380
calculi 380
tumours 382
sialoadenitis 380
Salmon patch 333
Saphenous eye sign 236
Schatzki ring 536
Schimmelbusch disease 463
Schwannoma 295
Schwartz test 235
Sclerosing cholangitis 630
Sebaceous cyst 312
Seldinger's technique 69, 185
Self-expandable metal stents 874
Semimembranosus bursitis 316
Seminoma 1105
SEMS 535
Sengstaken's tube 693
Sentinel node
breast 491
melanoma 267
penis 1095
SEPS 240

Sertoli cell tumours 1109
Sestamibi scan 442
Seton 892
Sezary syndrome 226
Shock 59
- anaphylactic 67
- cardiogenic 65
- distributive 65
- haemorrhagic 61
- hypovolaemic 64
- neurogenic 67
- obstructive 67
- septic 65

Shock lung 1130
Short saphenous varicosity 243
Sigmoidopexy 829
SILS 1303
Sinus 126
- congenital sinus 126
- median mental sinus 295, 370
- pilonidal sinus
- tuberculous 115

Sister Mary Joseph's nodule 577
Skin 248
- premalignant lesions 249
- tumours 248

Skin grafting 283
Skin substitutes 286
Small intestine 752
- abdominal tuberculosis 755
- adenocarcinoma 777
- anatomy 752
- Crohn's disease 770
- embryology and development 752
- GIST 778
- ileostomy 769
- inflammatory bowel diseases 763
- intestinal amoebiasis 775
- intestinal fistulae 783
- intestinal tuberculosis 760
- neuroendocrine tumours 779
- Peutz-Jeghers syndrome 776
- physiological functions 754
- radiation enteropathy 776
- short gut syndrome 781
- small intestinal diverticula 786
- surgical complications of enteric fever 774
- tuberculous mesenteric lymphadenitis 760
- tuberculous peritonitis 758

Soft tissue sarcoma 298
- angiosarcoma 305
- dermatofibrosarcoma protuberans 273, 305
- Kaposi's 273, 305
- liposarcoma 291, 302
- lymphangiosarcoma
- malignant fibrous histiocytoma 302
- neurofibrosarcoma 292
- retroperitoneal 302
- rhabdomyosarcoma 305
- synovial 305

Solar keratosis 249
Somatic cells 56
Specimens 1259–1267
SPECT 443
Spermatocoele 1101
Sphincter of Lutkens 602
Spina bifida occulta 319
Spitz naevus 259
Spleen 701
- acquired autoimmune haemolytic anaemia 711
- complications of splenic injuries 704
- congenital abnormalities 703
- functions of 702
- hairy cell leukaemia 715
- hereditary spherocytosis 709
- idiopathic thrombocytopaenic purpura 708
- overwhelming postsplenectomy infection 716
- partial splenectomy 706
- rupture of the spleen 703
- sickle cell anaemia 712
- splenectomy 705
- splenectomy for other conditions 713
- splenic artery aneurysm 714
- splenorrhaphy 706
- surgical anatomy 701
- thalassaemia 711

Squamous cell carcinoma 255
Stag horn calculi 1043
Stem cells 56
Stephen's line 851
Sterilization 34
Sternomastoid tumour 331
Stomach 545
- acute dilatation of stomach 591
- bezoars 593
- carcinoma 572
- chronic complications of peptic ulcer 570
- chronic duodenal ileus 594
- complications of gastrectomy 587
- duodenal anatomy and obstruction 595
- gastric lymphoma 586
- gastric physiology 548
- gastritis 551
- gastrointestinal stromal tumours (GIST) 585
- *H. pylori* infection 549
- haemetemesis 563
- idiopathic hypertrophic pyloric stenosis 593
- non-ulcer dyspepsis 551
- peptic ulcer disease 553, 568
- perforated peptic ulcer 560
- surgical anatomy 545
- volvulus of the stomach 593

Stove in chest 1127
Strawberry angiomas 334
Stricturoplasty 762
Stump carcinoma 588
Subclavian steal syndrome 210
Subfascial ligation of Cockett and Dodd 240
Subhyoid bursitis 322
Submandibular salivary gland
- anatomy 380
- lymph node 326
- stones 380
- tumours 382

Submucous fibrosis 351
Superior laryngeal nerve 432
Surgical care bundle 124
Surgical emphysema 1132
Surgical site infections 123
Sutures 1257
Swellings 308, 326
Synchronous carcinoma 797
Syphilis 151
T tube cholangiogram 1238
Takayasu's arteritis 206
TASC guidelines 194
TATA 112
Tea pot deformity 572
TEM (transanal endoscopic microsurgery) 874
Temporal arteritis 206
Tendon transfer 146
Tension gastrothorax 1129
Tension pneumothorax 68, 1128
Teratoma 1106
Testis 1098
- anatomy 1098
- ectopic 1103
- retractile 1102
- torsion 1104
- tumours 1105
- undescended 1102

Tetanus 130
Tetany 438
Tetralogy of Fallot 1143
Thiersch wiring 881
Thimble bladder 1053
Third space losss 92
Thoracic outlet syndrome 201
Thrombolysis 193, 245
Thrombophebitis 182
Thymoma 1136
Thyroglobulin 423
Thyroglossal cyst 323
Thyroid gland
- adenoma 414
- anaplastic carcinoma 424
- clinical examination 399
- ectopic thyroid 434
- follicular carcinoma 420
- goitre 403
- Graves' disease 407
- incidentaloma 430
- lingual thyroid 433
- lymphoma 426
- malignant tumours 414
- medullary carcinoma 425
- multinodular goiter 405
- papillary carcinoma 414
- physiology 395
- radioisotope scan 128
- retrosternal goiter 406
- solitary nodule 426
- surgical anatomy 394
- thyroid function tests 395
- thyroiditis 430
- toxic goiter 407

Thyrotoxic storm/crisis 432
TIPSS 693
TIRADS 417
Tissue engineering 56
Tongue
- carcinoma 358
- glossectomy 362
- hemangioma 367
- macroglossia 367
- syphilitic lesions 367
- ulcers 366

Total mesorectal excision (TME) 869
Tourniquet 64
Toxic megacolon 765

Toxic shock syndrome 121
TRALI 74
TRAM flap 499
Transposition of great vessels 1143
Trastuzumab 494
Traube's space 1010
Traumatic fat necrosis 470
Triage 979
Trigeminal neuralgia 1162
Triple assessment 481
Trismus 131, 355
TRUS (transrectal ultrasonography) 868
Tubercle of Zuckerkandl 394
Tuberculous
 intestines 760
 investigations 117
 kidney 1050
 lymphadenitis 113
 mastitis 461
 peritoneum 758
 spine 337
 treatment 118
 urinary bladder 1053
Tubes 1254–1256
Tunnel of love 627
Turban tumour 274
TURP 1084
Tylosis 526
Tyndallisation 35

Ulcerative colitis 763
Ulcers
 arterial 162
 dressings 160
 leg ulcers 153, 158
 neuropathic 163
 penis 1098
 phagedenic 163
 post-thrombotic 163
 rodent ulcer 250
 traumatic 157
 trophic 158, 162
 tropical 163
 tubercular 158
 venous 162, 240
Ultrasound 1234
Umbilicus 968
 umbilical fistulae 969
 umbilical hernia 970
 umbilical inflammation 969
 umbilical neoplasms 970
 umbolith 970
Upper GI tract bleeding 565
Upper limb gangrene 199
Ureteric colic 1046
Urethra 1072
 anatomy 1072
 posterior urethral valve 1078
 rupture 1072
 stricture 1075
Urethrography 1035
Urethroscopy 1036
Urinary bladder 1063
 acute cystitis 1069
 carcinoma of 1065
 diverticula 1069
 ectopia vesicae 1069
 interstitial cystitis 1070
 rupture bladder 1071
 schistosoma haematobium 1070
 surgical anatomy 1063
 urinary diversion 1071
 urinary fistulae 1069
 vesical calculus 1064
Urinary retention 1077
Urinary tract infections 1118
Urine examination 1029

VAAFT 1307
VAC therapy 171
VACTER anomalies 543
Vale of Kerckring 625
Valve of Gerlach 915
Valve of Heister 602
Varicose veins 229
 anatomy 230
 complications 240
 deep veins 231
 foam sclerotherapy 238
 perforators 230
 RFA 239
 saphena varix 232
 short saphenous vein 242
 tests 234
 treatment 237
 venography 236
 venous ulcer 240
VATS 1135
Veress needle 1303
VGP 571
Vincent's angina 371
Vitellointestinal duct 831
VSD 1143

Wart 274
Water regulation 86
White bile 663
Wilkie's disease
Wolfe graft 284
Wolff-Chaikoff effect 433
Wound 99
 healing 100, 103
 negative pressure assisted closure 103
 surgical 107
 suturing 102

Xeroderma pigmentosum 249
X-ray KUB 1030

Zenker's diverticulum 539
Zollinger-Ellison syndrome 552, 645